Encyclopedia of Women's Health

Edited by

Sana Loue, JD, PhD, MPH
Case Western Reserve University School of Medicine
Cleveland, Ohio

and

Martha Sajatovic, MD
University Hospitals of Cleveland
Case Western Reserve University School of Medicine
Cleveland, Ohio

Core Editors

Keith B. Armitage, MD
University Hospitals of Cleveland
Case Western Reserve University School of Medicine
Cleveland, Ohio

Deanna Dahl-Grove, MD
Department of Pediatric Emergency Medicine
Rainbow Babies and Childrens Hospital
Cleveland, Ohio

Siran M. Koroukian, PhD
Case Western Reserve University School of Medicine
Cleveland, Ohio

Merrill S. Lewen, MD
Huntington Memorial Hospital
Pasadena, California

Linda S. Lloyd, DrPH
Alliance Healthcare Foundation
San Diego, California

Margaret L. MacKenzie, MD
Cleveland Clinic Foundation
Willoughby Hills, Ohio

Angela Pattatucci Aragon, PhD
Graduate School of Public Health
University of Puerto Rico
San Juan, Puerto Rico

Alicia M. Weissman, MD
Crystal Run Healthcare
Middletown, New York

Kluwer Academic/Plenum Publishers
New York   Boston   Dordrecht   London   Moscow

Library of Congress Cataloging-in-Publication Data

Encyclopedia of women's health / edited by Sana Loue and Martha Sajatovic.
  p. cm.
 Includes bibliographical references and index.
 ISBN 0-306-48073-5
  1. Women—Health and hygiene—Encyclopedias. 2. Women—Diseases—Encyclopedias.
I. Loue, Sana. II. Sajatovic, Martha.

RA778.E5825 2004
613'.04244—dc22
                           2003064026

ISBN 0-306-48073-5

© 2004 Kluwer Academic/Plenum Publishers
233 Spring Street, New York, New York 10013

http://www.wkap.nl/

10 9 8 7 6 5 4 3 2 1

A C.I.P. record for this book is available from the Library of Congress

Preface

The field of "women's health" is not a solitary discipline. Women's health consists, instead, of knowledge and expertise of professionals in many disciplines who work together to improve women's health status. Accordingly, the *Encyclopedia of Women's Health* brings together the knowledge and experience of professionals from a wide range of fields including medicine, law, psychology, social work, demography, education, epidemiology, dentistry, cosmetology, massage, nutrition, physical fitness, history, and many others. This broad foundation allows us to explore women's health from a biopsychosocial perspective, and to consider the many facets of women's health and the many factors that impact women's health status. This text is intended as a reference both for nonhealth professionals who wish to have a more in-depth understanding of various topics, and for health professionals searching for an introduction to fields outside of their own.

The first portion of the *Encyclopedia* serves as an introduction to the study of women's health. It includes an in-depth examination of various foundational aspects of women's health, including the history of women's health, women in the health professions, the impact of work on women's health, and women's role in providing health care to others. The second portion of the *Encyclopedia* is organized alphabetically by entry. These entries focus on all aspects of women's health, from medicine, to legal issues, to history, to beauty, to complementary and alternative approaches to health. The information that is presented is meant to be practical and informative. Each entry is followed by a list of suggested readings, as well as a listing of resources available on the Internet and elsewhere. We trust that you will find these pages both exciting and informative in their depth and coverage.

Sana Loue
Martha Sajatovic

Contents

I. Foundation Topics in Women's Health

History of Women's Health in the United States

Siran M. Koroukian

This chapter provides a brief overview of the history of women's health and the array of factors that have played a central role in shaping it. First, it presents a background describing gender-based disparities in health care. It then discusses the cultural context in which women have been perceived by society, their representation in the health care workforce, and the development of the medical specialty of obstetrics and gynecology (OB/GYN), as well as social, economic, and political forces that have shaped the medical care provided to women. It concludes with thoughts on future directions in women's health, while considering the many advances made toward gaining equality with men in education, employment, societal role, and political empowerment.

BACKGROUND

As discussed by Ruzek et al. (1997), the World Heath Organization (WHO) recognizes several elements as prerequisites for health: freedom from the fear of war; equal opportunity for all; satisfaction of basic needs for food, water, and sanitation; education; decent housing; secure work; useful role in society; and political will and public support. These elements provide a framework to study women's health in the United States in a temporal context, and to draw a trajectory of it through history. Inequalities in these elements between men and women have greatly contributed to health disparities observed in today's societies throughout the world, particularly in regard to education and to social, economic, and political empowerment. These inequalities have existed in the past and persist through contemporary times.

The dramatic improvements in women's health during the 20th century should be noted at the onset. These changes are described in detail in a document compiled by the U.S. Department of Health and Human Services (DHHS), Office of Women's Health. From 1900 to 1990, women's life expectancy increased by more than 30 years—from 48.3 years to about 80 years. Even in the first 40 years of the 20th century, a significant reduction was observed in maternal mortality (from 600–900 to 11 deaths per 100,000 live births), infant mortality (from 146 to 34 per 1,000 live births), and in the number of deaths from tuberculosis (fourfold). These dramatic changes occurred even before the introduction of antibiotics; further improvements followed the development and availability of antibiotics, the improvement of hygiene, and numerous advances in medical practices. Unfortunately, however, increases in longevity were accompanied by an increased likelihood of developing chronic diseases, as shown by the shift in the causes of death in women from infectious diseases in the early 1900s (tuberculosis, syphilis, pneumonia, and influenza) to chronic illnesses at the end of the 20th century (cardiovascular disease [CVD], cancer, stroke, chronic obstructive pulmonary disease, and diabetes). Also, due to advances in medicine and technology, many women with disabling conditions are now able to survive and participate in various activities at a rate higher than ever. By the end of the 1990s, 24% of adult women were living with disabilities; 70% of those with nonsevere disabilities and 25% of those with severe disabilities were part of the U.S. workforce.

Despite the improvements highlighted above, gender disparities in health persist today, with significant gaps observed in the prevention and treatment of a number of clinical conditions. This is in part a result of the failure to integrate women's health in general medical practice due to (1) a view of women's health as encompassing only the reproductive system, consisting of pregnancy and childbirth, abortion, contraception, menstruation, and menopause, and (2) the assumption that women's health care needs are identical to those of men, except for the differences in reproductive health.

In recent years, medical research has been redirected to determine whether, and in what aspects, disease prevention, presentation, and treatment may differ between men and women. Because until recently medical research has almost exclusively included men, the symptoms, progression, and management of nonreproductive diseases have been, and still are, based on what has been observed in men and not in women. In turn, these observations have been incorporated in didactic courses taught in medical schools. Health care professionals who have received teaching from this perspective have been trained to associate certain symptoms with a given diagnosis. Consequently, they may miss an opportunity for early diagnosis and disease management if the disease is presented and/or described by women differently than by men or if the disease presentation is not consistent with what is described in the mainstream medical literature. For example, the presentation of coronary artery disease (CAD), the leading cause of death in women in contemporary times, may be very different in men than in women. In a study by Philpott, Boynton, Feder, and Hemingway (2001), gender-based differences were reported in pain location when describing chest pain, with women referring to pain in such locations as the throat, neck, jaw, or even central and lower abdomen, more often than men. As noted by Philpott et al. (2001), Such locations are described as "atypical" in cardiology textbooks, a term used to mean "not like men." Similarly, women complained of shortness of breath, palpitations, lack of energy, back pain, nausea, and dizziness more

often than men—symptoms that are not viewed as specific to CAD. Such patterns of "atypical" and/or nonspecific symptomatology greatly contribute to an underestimation of the extent of the problem by the physician, and consequently to inadequate disease management. In fact, it has been found that women are referred for coronary artery bypass graft at a more advanced stage of the disease than men. As a result, they are more likely to experience, in addition, a higher rate of perioperative mortality. Another study by Ayanian et al. (1993) examining the rates of diagnostic and therapeutic procedures among patients hospitalized for CVD has documented higher rates of such procedures in men than in women. However, investigators have been unable to determine whether these findings indicated that these procedures were overused by men or underused in women.

Attention to differences in how diseases should be treated in men compared with women has also been neglected, reflecting the longstanding belief in the medical community that treatment for nonreproductive diseases should be identical in men and in women. Findings from research in more recent years have highlighted the important roles played by female hormones in maintaining not only reproductive health, but general health as well. One example is the role played by estrogen in protecting women against CVD. Such a finding has led us to better understand changes in the likelihood of developing CVD in the peri- or postmenopausal periods. Similar observations about disease presentation and treatment may be made about other clinical conditions as well.

A committee of the American College of Physicians (1997) recently recommended that women's health care refer to the "prevention, screening, diagnosis, and management of conditions that are unique to women, more prevalent in women, more serious among women, have different risk factors for women, and/or require different interventions in women." The committee places a special emphasis on expanding "women's health from the narrower concept of reproductive health care." This change in paradigm, along with the very important gains that women have made in mustering political forces in the last century, particularly in the last few decades, is highly promising for vast improvements in women's health in the decades to come. To understand gender-based disparities, however, it is important to consider women and their health in a cultural context through time. How women were viewed by the society, and how the medical profession perceived their health care needs—and changes thereof over time—are paramount in understanding women's health in contemporary times.

CULTURAL CONTEXT

For centuries, women have been perceived as weak, sickly creatures. Assumptions have been made about the smaller size of their brains and their inferior intelligence, as well as their frailty. This position has shaped the beliefs and attitudes of the medical community, leading to an almost a priori assumption that most health complaints presented by women may be psychosomatic in nature or have a psychological underpinning. For example, nausea in pregnancy was believed to have resulted from the ambivalence or the resentment of women who were not well prepared for motherhood.

Women were believed to have been "dominated by their uterus and ovaries." To illustrate the extent to which such stereotypes are embedded in our culture, it is worth noting that the term "hysteria" that originates from the Latin root of "hyster," meaning *uterus*, is a term used in common language today to refer to "wild uncontrollable emotion or excitement," as defined in the *Oxford American Dictionary* (1980). To date, the term "hysteria" is used in the medical lexicon to refer to a nervous affection occurring mostly in women. According to the Merriam-Webster Online Medical Dictionary, hysteria is "1. a psychoneurosis marked by emotional excitability and disturbances of the psychic, sensory, vasomotor, and visceral functions without an organic basis, and 2. behavior exhibiting overwhelming or unmanageable fear or emotional excess." Given such attitudes, it comes as no surprise, for example, that removal of ovaries, or female castration, was performed to treat psychological ailments.

There are several elements—or events—in female reproductive health that have shaped society's perceptions of women and their health over time. From a biological perspective, the fact that menstruation and childbirth are unique to women and that they are often accompanied by a level of pain and discomfort (such as bleeding and cramps in menstruation and labor pains in childbirth) are likely to have helped develop the notion of women being sicker and weaker than men. Menopause has led a clear understanding of the presence of a biological clock in women's reproductive functions; in cultures in which women are valued almost exclusively for their reproductive abilities, reaching menopause implied a sense of finality and worthlessness, and even an end to sexuality as well. Conversely, the sustained sexual functions in men and their (apparently) sustained reproductive function in older age may have contributed to their feeling of superiority in that regard. From a socioeconomic perspective, the traditional role of women in attending to their families has been greatly responsible for the reduced devotion of their mental and physical energy to the personal development of their mind and body; this focus has contributed to gender inequalities in education, secure work, and income observed throughout history and persisting until today. It is through the consideration of the complex and strongly linked set of biological, social, legal, political, and economic factors that women's health and their quality of life should be studied. The following sections provide a brief overview of some of these factors.

Menstruation

Menstruation, in some cultures, has been perceived as mystical, while in others, menstruating or postmenstrual women have been viewed as "unclean." This perception varied widely across various cultures. For example, Chinese sages considered menstrual blood the essence of Mother Earth. At the other extreme, between the 8th and 11th centuries, the Christian Church refused communion to menstruating women.

It is believed that the concept of calendar developed first in women, as they followed their body rhythm in relation to their observations of the moon. Some refer to Chinese women's establishment of the lunar calendar 3000 years ago. It has also been claimed that the origin of mathematics may have derived from the concept of counting that is so deeply embedded in the menstrual cycle.

It is worth noting the issues of quality of life that are associated with menstruation. From sponges to menstrual cups that had to be inserted in the vagina to collect blood, to reusable pads, women have had to use a wide array of menstrual products. According to the DHHS document (2002), disposable pads were developed following World War I and marketed in the 1920s; they were manufactured using materials and techniques similar to those used in manufacturing war bandages. This technology was later used to develop adult diapers and special pads for adults with urinary incontinence. Tampons were developed during the same time period, and widely used in the 1940s. However, there were several concerns with the use of tampons. One concern was that tampons would compromise a girl's virginity. Fears about their safety were intensified in 1980, when toxic shock syndrome in young women (813 cases and

38 deaths) was linked to a type of superabsorbent tampons. More recently, false rumors spread through the Internet also raised concerns that tampons may contain asbestos and dioxin.

Female Sexuality

Historically an interest in and enjoyment of sexual relations were considered unhealthy for women. As an example, masturbation and sexual arousal were thought to lead to insanity. The suppression of sexual feelings could be achieved by removing the clitoris; clitoridectomies were performed in America until the late 1930s and continue to be performed to date in many regions of Africa.

Female sexuality remains severely underresearched. In 1953, a report published by Michael Kinsey caused a major controversy, as it showed that many of the 5,500 women interviewed for the study actually enjoyed sexual life. These findings challenged the widely held belief that women's role in lovemaking was to satisfy the husband. The biological framework in which sexuality is studied, and the medicalization of it, explain why the evaluation of sexuality has been restricted to that of physical performance during intercourse, without consideration of factors such as love, passion, freedom from fear, emotional involvement, and cooperative contraception. In the medical context, erectile function is considered paramount in the study of male sexuality, with numerous studies on impotence. It had been hypothesized that the clitoris may suffer from similar vascular anomalies as the penis. However, the number of studies on female sexual dysfunction and its association with chronic diseases, medications, or lifestyle, is dwarfed in comparison to that of studies on male sexual dysfunction (see Tiefer, 1994).

Pregnancy and Childbirth

Pregnancy and childbirth historically have been considered to be focal events in reproductive life. However, the male-centered understanding of these events and their management have shaped women's health and its research in very important ways. For example, as discussed by Duffin (1999), it was believed in the late 1600s that a sperm included a fetus that a woman would carry for nine months and later deliver. The human egg was not discovered until early 1800s, although it is much larger in size than the sperm.

Female midwives, many of whom were educated and trained like surgeons, were primarily in charge of childbirth. They were often respected as prominent members of their communities. Male midwives started appearing in the 17th century in birthing rooms, mostly in affluent homes.

Obstetrics was slow to be incorporated in the medical profession; it was rejected by the American College of Physicians as an "ungentlemanly profession." By the early 19th century, however, obstetrics became part of the medical curriculum. The study of the gravid uterus, its pathology, and details in measuring the pelvis to predict difficulties in childbirth became important components of obstetrics. Ergotamine was introduced in the early 1800s to control postpartum hemorrhage. A significantly higher rate of infections was observed among women attended by physicians, compared to those who were attended by midwives. It was hypothesized that the high rate of infections may have been associated with inadequate hand-washing techniques by physicians performing autopsies on women who had died as a result of postpartum fever, and who later attended to women during delivery, resulting in the transmission of infectious agents. Infection control was later introduced with a hand-washing program of chlorine solution.

The concept of pain control during delivery encountered stiff resistance, however, due to a strong belief that women were meant to suffer in childbirth, pursuant to the Biblical imposition of labor pain as a punishment for the "original sin." It is unclear why physicians increasingly came to rely on the use of anesthetics, despite the higher cost, although some historians believe women advocated for it. Pain control evolved from general anesthesia to regional anesthesia, which was shown to be safer for the infant; later, pain was managed using Lamaze education and psychoprophylaxis.

Use of instrumentation during childbirth, such as forceps, electronic monitoring of fetal heartbeats and uterine contractions, and cesarean delivery, increased steadily as well. The use of diagnostic and interventional technology in pregnancy followed; this included diagnostic ultrasounds, amniocentesis, and in utero surgery on the fetus. The treatment of infertility, which led to a dramatic increase in multiple births, also advanced rapidly in the 20th century, through hormonal treatments, in vitro fertilization, and more recently, cloning.

The movement favoring natural childbirth and breast-feeding, which recognizes pregnancy and childbirth as natural events, and mother's milk as the best source of nutrition for the infant, originated in the 1970s. The profession of midwifery experienced a rebound during this time. Later, birthing centers were developed and were designed to simulate a homelike environment in a hospital setting. There was also heightened interest in home deliveries and doulas, or laypersons providing physical, emotional, and informational support to the birthing mother and her partner during childbirth and postpartum care.

Abortion

Abortions were not considered illegal until the 19th century when Britain and the United States passed their first antiabortion laws. During this antiabortion period, abortions continued to be performed, but they were done in highly septic environments, using any means that a woman could find: knitting needles, coat hangers, vaginal douches with toxic solutions, or ingestion of strong chemicals. Resorting to such measures reflected women's resolve to find any means to abort when facing an unwanted pregnancy. Such practices resulted in high rates of mortality, mostly from infections; when not fatal, severe complications such as sepsis and perforation of the uterus often resulted. Sepsis often led to secondary infertility, due to the obstruction of the Fallopian tubes, as well as other chronic conditions. The psychological stress was also significant. And, because the tradition of early abortion had been well rooted in these societies, abortions continued to be performed openly, and juries refused to convict abortionists.

In 1973, the U.S. Supreme Court held that limiting a woman's right to terminate her pregnancy violated the Due Process Clause of the 14th Amendment of the Constitution (*Roe v. Wade*). In 1976, the Hyde Amendment banned the use of Medicaid funds for abortion, except when the woman's life was endangered. Nearly 20 years later, the law was broadened to allow Medicaid coverage for abortion services in the cases of rape or incest. To date, many faiths and institutions, such as the Roman Catholic Church, consider abortion unacceptable, except when performed in the cases of rape or incest.

During the antiabortion era of the late 1800s, an estimated 2 million abortions were performed. One hundred years later, approximately 1.5 million abortions are now performed every year. These, statistics as noted in *Our Bodies, Ourselves,* speak to the inability of laws to control *the extent, to which* women utilize abortions. However, the laws affect the *practice* of abortions, as antiabortion laws encourage illegal and clandestine practice of abortions, most often performed in nonoptimal conditions, leading to adverse outcomes, and even maternal death. The legalization of abortions has contributed to dramatic reductions in maternal mortality.

Contraception

Efforts to prevent pregnancy can be traced to as far back as ancient Greece. Until a few decades ago, however, women relied on breast-feeding that serves as a fairly effective means of contraception, through the suppression of ovulation. Throughout the centuries, women's diaries described their lives in a perpetual transition from pregnancy to breast-feeding and then back to pregnancy. Freeing themselves from the constant function of reproduction was perceived as the key to emancipation.

The first birth control clinic was opened in 1916, in Brooklyn, New York, by Margaret Sanger who became a major catalyst for changing laws pertaining to the use and dissemination of contraception. The clinic remained open for 10 days and served 500 women during that time. It was forced to shut down, however, as it was challenged by the Comstock Law of 1873, which considered information on birth control as obscene, and outlawed its distribution. In 1936, in *U.S. v. One Package*, Margaret Sanger and the Federal Legislation on Birth Control were successful in arguing that physicians were exempted from the provisions of the Comstock Law that prohibited the dissemination of information on contraceptives. In *Griswold v. Connecticut* (1965), the Supreme Court overturned one of the last state laws prohibiting the use of contraceptives by married couples. Numerous initiatives aimed at funding family planning services were introduced, first in 1965 through the War on Poverty, by the Office of Economic Opportunity; and later in 1970 (Title X), a federally funded program to serve low-income women.

In the early 20th century, coitus interruptus, the rhythm method, early versions of condoms and diaphragms, abortion, and surgical sterilization were common methods of birth control. Toward the end of the century, the birth control pill, which was first approved as a treatment for irregular periods and menstrual cramps, became the most commonly used form of reversible contraception. The Food and Drug Administration (FDA) approved the use of birth control pills in 1960. Early versions of the birth control pill contained high levels of estrogen; their use was associated with elevated risks of blood clots, heart disease, and stroke. As a result, increasing use was made of contraceptives that carried lesser systemic effects, such as the diaphragm and the condom.

The intrauterine device (IUD), first introduced in the 1960s, was later discontinued in the 1980s, following the FDA's 1974 ban on the use of one type, the Dalkon Shield, due to its association with uterine infections. In the 1990s, long-lasting and reversible forms of contraceptives were introduced, such as Norplant (implant) and Depo-Provera (injectable). The latter product, which was often prescribed to young, sexually active women, was viewed as a product that may have contributed to the decline in teen births in the United States during the last decade. The use of condoms increased later as a result of the HIV/AIDS epidemic, as it also presented an effective method to prevent sexually transmitted diseases (STDs).

Despite these advances in the development of effective methods of contraception, the topic of birth control remains taboo, and many pregnancies occur without planning, and/or are terminated deliberately. The use of contraceptives requires careful planning; unfortunately, access to contraceptives may be limited in some circumstances. The use of some of the most effective forms of family planning methods requires consultation with a physician and a willingness to undergo a gynecologic exam. This poses a significant impediment to young women who may find the physical exam and the disclosure of their sexual history to health care providers too embarrassing and/or frightening. To others, this process is difficult or impossible because of financial barriers, including lack of adequate insurance, or logistical difficulties, such as travel and childcare. While the responsibility of ensuring family planning is ideally shared by sexual partners, the burden engendered by unprotected sexual activity is typically borne by women.

Lesbian Health

Lesbian health has been part of public debate only in recent years, and the Healthy People 2010 (the federal government's guidelines for health care in the next century) has specifically called for the elimination of disparities in the health of gay and lesbian communities. It is estimated that 6.5 million women (or 4% of the adult female population) in the United States are lesbian. Consequently, a given provider attending to the adult

female population is likely to serve lesbian women as well as women of other sexual orientations (heterosexual and bisexual) and the physician must be prepared to provide an adequate environment for optimal care.

It is of note that lesbians are significantly less likely than their heterosexual counterparts to seek gynecologic care for prenatal care or family planning. It follows then that they are less likely to also undergo screening exams for breast and cervical cancer, or for STD, a pattern that has contributed to increased risk of cancer and STD in this population.

Numerous other barriers to care for lesbians are identified. Health care providers rarely receive adequate training on gay, lesbian, bisexual, and transgender (GLBT) health care issues. For instance, it has been reported that only a few hours are devoted to the study of such issues in the course of several years of training in medical schools. Providers' attitudes range from homophobia to "heterosexism" (a term that mirrors sexism or racism), making the environment unwelcoming to the GLBT population. Finally, the effects of financial barriers are not to be underestimated, as lesbians are less likely than heterosexual women to have health care insurance, because they may not be eligible to receive coverage under their partners' policies. It has been reported that in 2000, only 99 (or 20%) of Fortune 500 companies, and 8 state governments offered benefits to domestic partners. Even when those benefits were available, many employees were reluctant to disclose their sexual orientation in the workplace for fear of compromising their employment position.

Menopause

Negative attitudes toward menopause have persisted throughout the centuries. Some have attempted to explain cessation of menstrual blood flow through the presence of "insufficient pumping force through blood vessels." Vaginal atrophy, bladder symptoms, cancer, gout, and arthritis were believed to occur during menopause. The boundaries between normal physiology and pathology with regard to menopause were not delineated until recently. That menopause was a natural process and that symptoms were not fatal was first explained in a 1904 publication by Pancoast and others, entitled *Beautiful Womanhood: Guide to Mental and Physical Development*.

With menopause, an array of changes occurs gradually over a period of several years, involving changes in bleeding patterns, hot flashes, sleep disturbances, weight changes, vaginal discomforts, changes in sexuality, osteoporosis (or loss of bone mass), as well as changes in mood and cognition. In the 1960s, estrogen therapy was proposed as a remedy to menopausal symptoms and aging. A number of studies were initiated in later years as part of the Women's Health Initiative to investigate the risks and benefits of hormone replacement therapy (HRT). HRT is believed to provide relief from menopausal symptoms, and offer protective effect against osteoporosis and CVD. However, HRT also entails additional risks, such as an increased likelihood of some cancers. Results from studies currently under way are expected to further elucidate the effects of HRT.

Body Image

Throughout history, women have been expected to meet a certain body image to conform to a contemporary standard of appearance and beauty, which is usually set by male views. Preoccupation with body image at the turn of the century was enhanced with the greater availability of mirrors in private and public places and the development of photography. Interest was accelerated through the 20th century with the enhancement of photography, and with the advent of television, motion pictures, and, more recently, the Internet. The idealized female body shape has transitioned from corsets and the narrow waist in the 19th century, to the natural shape early in the 20th century, the svelte look in the 1920s, and the fuller bust and rounded hourglass figures in the 1930s to 1950s. During the era of short hemlines of the 1960s and 1970s, increased attention was focused on the size and shape of women's thighs and buttocks.

The link between changes in body look and fashion is evident through several examples. For instance, the desired image of a fuller bust gave way to breast augmentation surgery, which was achieved through the insertion of silicone breast implants. These procedures have been associated with a number of complications, including infection, bleeding, and leakage of the silicone, and even a systemic disease. The concern about thigh size fueled efforts to develop cellulite-fighting creams, and liposuction to remove fatty tissue.

Other items that were perceived to enhance body image but actually had potentially harmful effects include "beauty products" for makeup, hair coloring, and footwear. The use of hair and facial products may be associated with inflammation of the eyelid, chemical burns, and hair loss. Nail salons have been identified as a possible venue for the transmission of various infectious agents, including hepatitis B and C, and HIV; transmission can be avoided through the use of proper techniques for sterilizing instruments. A large proportion of women wear shoes smaller than their feet, and many develop arthritic changes over the years as a result of the damage caused by footwear. Narrow toe-boxes in shoes can exacerbate joint problems such as bunions and hammertoes; 90% of surgeries to correct bunions are performed in women. High heels may be responsible for a number of health problems resulting from an alteration in the normal function of the ankle and the ability to maintain balance. These include an increased risk of injury due to falls, low back pain due to compensatory reliance on different parts of the musculoskeletal system to achieve balance, and osteoarthritis of the knee.

Body image has also been incriminated in the steadily increasing rates of eating disorders throughout the 20th century, from self-starvation, to binge eating. The creation of Barbie doll in 1959, setting an unrealistic standard of beauty, has been blamed for encouraging girls to adopt unhealthy habits in an attempt to attain that body image. An estimated 5–10 million women were identified with such disorders in the 1990s, with prevalence believed to have been higher among white, middle-class, educated young women, presumably because of differences in standards of beauty and body image. Some argue, however, that eating disorders may be underdiagnosed among women of color.

Since the late 1970s, the preference for body image has shifted to a more athletic look, with increasing numbers of women participating in sports and regular exercise, while emphasizing a healthy lifestyle. The female population is growing older and significantly heavier in body weight, with increasingly higher rates of obesity in the United States and elsewhere in the world, and women are in search of an image that is both healthy and realistic. Obesity and lack of exercise have been identified as some of the most important *modifiable* risk factors for CVD and cancer, the two leading causes of mortality in women.

On a more positive side, considerations for body image became a catalyst to reconsider radical mastectomy for the treatment of breast cancer. This procedure, developed by William Halstead in 1915, remained the standard of care until 1985, when lumpectomy (removal of lump), combined with radiation therapy, was shown to be as effective as radical mastectomy.

REPRESENTATION OF WOMEN IN THE HEALTH CARE WORKFORCE

White men have dominated the medical profession, and until the 1990s, most clinical studies that have led to important guidelines in disease prevention and management have enrolled white male subjects only. Findings from these studies have been assumed to apply to women or to minority men in a comparable way.

There are accounts of female physicians having practiced obstetrics in ancient Greece and Rome. However, with the advent of male midwives in later times, women's presence faded from obstetrics and medical practice, and their practice remained limited to rural areas, where physicians were scarce. In modern history, one of the first women to have practiced medicine did so by hiding her sex. For example, the sex of Canada's first known woman physician, Dr. James Miranda Barry, a British military officer and surgeon in the mid-1800s, was not known until after her death. Simultaneously, however, history witnessed the founding of the first medical college of women by Elizabeth Blackwell (1868).

In the Western Hemisphere, men had no presence in birthing rooms until the 17th century and there was a general discomfort with the physician–patient (male–female) relationship. It is recounted that in Victorian society, a doctor performing a pelvic exam had to gaze into the patient's eyes, or off into space, rather than looking on the patient's naked body. In Chinese society, women used dolls to indicate the location of symptoms, so the physician would not have to see or touch her body. Such levels of discomfort persist to date, especially in certain cultures, and many women in the United States choose female physicians and report greater satisfaction with them.

In the 19th century, women joined the health care workforce by entering the profession of nursing, which initially included both men and women. Florence Nightingale, considered one of the founders of nursing, developed the profession on "womanly virtues" including cleanliness, patience, order, and service. Feminists have claimed that this approach was responsible for the subservience that nurses (mostly female) were expected to display toward physicians (mostly male) and for the development of sexism in the nursing profession. Over the course of the 20th century, nursing had become a primarily female field, and this is believed to have contributed to the lower status and pay for the profession, relative to other medical professions.

The role and status of midwives also declined despite the fact that the training and practice of midwifery was becoming more professionalized and regulated. This was due in part to a dramatic decline in the number of home births (from 90% in 1900 to 10% in 1950). This shift from home births to hospital deliveries occurred simultaneously with the steady reduction in the proportion of births attended by midwives (from 40% in 1915 to 11% in 1935), and the increase in male predominance in the specialty of OB/GYN. With the movement of natural childbirth, the profession experienced a rebound in the 1970s. More recently, the role of certified nurse midwives has been expanding into the primary care arena.

Women began enrolling in medical schools in the mid 19th century. In 1900, 6% of physicians were women. This proportion remained unchanged through 1960, due to quotas that restricted women's admission to medical schools. A lawsuit by Women's Equity Action League against certain medical schools in 1970 changed this course, and by the year 2000, nearly half of the students enrolled in medical schools were women. Not surprisingly, women's health issues began to be included in medical school curricula. In 1990, Dr. Antonia Novello became the first woman—and the first minority person—to be appointed and serve in the position of Surgeon General.

Despite this progress, only eight U.S. medical schools had women deans in the late 1990s. Although the ratio of female to male medical students has been increasing steadily, there are numerous indications that medical schools remain ill-suited to educate women. Even in the most renowned medical schools, women students report sexist attitudes and insensitive comments from their male educators, such as women being in medical schools because of "unresolved penis envy." To date, women experience difficulty in being accepted as true professionals both by their peers and their patients.

The dominance of men in the OB/GYN specialty has undoubtedly shaped women's health, as they theorized about birth, conception, and the woman's body. First came the overmedicalization of pregnancy and childbirth that in turn has been responsible for the dramatic increase in the use of procedures in the practice of obstetrics. This is best evidenced by the high rates of cesarean deliveries (up to one in four deliveries in the 1980s in the United States); the gynecologic surgery also developed. Several strategies were developed to remedy psychological ailments in women. The practice of "preventive" oophorectomy originated, with the belief that it prevented ovarian cancer, especially, but not exclusively, among women with a strong family history of breast or ovarian cancer. Unfortunately, the effectiveness of this procedure in cancer prevention, and the costs and benefits of surgical menopause have not been studied with rigor, even though a considerable proportion of hysterectomy procedures also entailed oophorectomy. This procedure can be likened to castration, and the decision to undergo such drastic therapy should be evaluated in light of the potential physical and emotional consequences and the availability of other treatment options.

POLITICAL FORCES

The dominance of men in politics has also been a key factor in shaping policies on women's health. As outlined in *Our Bodies Ourselves* (OBOS) and the *Boston Women's Health Book Collective*, a premier book that introduced key ideas, women are often catalysts for social change. Women are often well-informed health care consumers and they are overrepresented in the health care workforce and among health care consumers. However, they remain underrepresented in positions of policymaking.

Following the numerous political successes outlined above, ranging from the legalization of contraception and abortion to the increased representation of women in academic medicine, women found themselves in an increasingly stronger position to participate in policy debates and bring about important changes in the health care system. In the 1990s, in an effort to address longstanding inequalities in women's participation in medical research, and the significant lack of clinically relevant biomedical and health services research for women, the 1993 National Institutes of Health (NIH) Revitalization Act established the Office of Women's Health at the NIH. This Act requires that women and minorities be adequately represented in all government-supported research projects. As part of this Act, the NIH sponsored the Women's Health Initiative, a 15-year, $625 million, multisite project, consisting of prevention studies to examine heart disease, osteoporosis, and breast and colon cancer. These studies are aimed primarily at ensuring that the 30-year gain in longevity during the 20th century be translated into a true improvement in quality of life. In 1996, the Office on Women's Health established National Centers of Excellence in Women's Health, with the goal of integrating women's health research, medical training, public health education, community outreach, and clinical services. These centers are to strive to recruit, retain, and promote women in academic medicine.

As outlined in the U.S. Department of Health and Human Services Office of Women's Health (2002) *A Century of Women's Health: 1900–2000*, women have accomplished other significant political achievements including the passage of:

- Title IX of the Education Amendments (1976) prohibiting sex discrimination in all educational programs receiving federal funding
- the Pregnancy Discrimination Act (1978), prohibiting sex discrimination in employment based on pregnancy, childbirth, or related medical conditions
- the Breast and Cervical Cancer Mortality Prevention Act (1990) requiring the provision of mammograms and pap smears to underserved women
- the Mammography Quality Standards Act (1992), establishing national standards and a uniform system of quality control of mammography clinics across the country
- the Infertility Prevention Act (1992), providing screening, treatment, counseling, and follow-up treatment to women diagnosed with STDs
- the Family and Medical Leave Act (1993), enabling women and men to take up to three months of leave in a 12-month period to care for family, without losing their jobs
- the Violence Against Women Act (1994), defining new federal crimes of violence against women and establishing enhanced penalties to fight against sexual assault and domestic violence

Other accomplishments include:

- the appointment of Patricia Harris, an African American, as the first female Secretary of Health, Education, and Welfare (1979)
- the consolidation of maternal, infant, child, and adolescent health at the state level through Maternal and Child Health Services Block Grant (1981)
- the establishment of the Women Race for the Cure (1983) to raise funds for breast cancer research, education, screening, and treatment programs

- the appointment of Margaret Mary Heckler as the first Secretary of the Department of Health and Human Services (1983), best known for the initiation of set rates for Medicare payments to hospitals

With each president and administration, the political climate engendered by the ideology of elected officials is likely to facilitate or hinder efforts to gain grounds on issues of health and social justice. Issues of reproductive health are highly affected by such changes, although the state of public health dictates a public policy agenda that may appear to be paradoxical with a contemporary political outlook. For example, despite a conservative government during the Reagan and Senior Bush administrations, the high prevalence of HIV/AIDS prompted the then-U.S. Surgeon General Dr. C. Everett Koop to discuss in public messages the use of condoms, with the intention of curbing HIV/AIDS transmission.

FUTURE DIRECTIONS

Women in the United States constitute an immensely diverse group of individuals. Their emancipation, achievements in higher education, and representation at the highest level of business, government, and public policy, will enable women to capitalize on the successes accomplished over the last century and to shape the health care system to adequately meet the needs of the contemporary female health care consumer.

At the one end of the spectrum, we see women who seek a balance between family responsibilities and achievement in professional life, and between beauty and health; women who are highly educated, with a level of sophistication that demands information and knowledge about health conditions and illnesses; a collaborative dynamic of decision-making between health care provider and patient; a far better integration of women's physical and mental health in general medical practice; a holistic approach to healing; a recognition of spirituality as a new and integral dimension of health; a network of support for women throughout the health spectrum; and a health care system that can accommodate the diversity in ethnicity, creed, origin, languages, and sexual orientation in the female population.

At the other end of the spectrum, the female population includes the younger women with unwanted pregnancies; those who never seek prenatal care; those struggling to provide a living for their family; those who

transition from welfare to work and encounter multiple barriers to adequate childcare; those who did not have the knowledge and/or the means to seek preventive/ routine health and cancer screening services because they were uninsured or underinsured, and presented with metastatic cancer upon diagnosis; those whose STD went undiagnosed and/or untreated and have secondary infertility; those who are sexually assaulted and abused; and those who are victims of domestic violence.

The challenges are numerous and diverse, and there are multiple areas that require immediate attention. Meeting these challenges will require a fundamental change in the way health care is financed and delivered, and the extent to which academic medicine and allied health professions are able to integrate these changes in their curricula and produce a cadre of health professionals who are adequately trained to serve this population. Women must continue to build and expand on the successes made in the past century and prepare the social, political, and health care environments for future generations.

Suggested Reading

American College of Physicians. (1997). Comprehensive women's health care: The role and commitment of internal medicine. *American Journal of Medicine, 103,* 451–457.

Ayanian, J. Z., & Epstein, A. M. (1993). Differences in the use of procedures between women and men hospitalized for coronary heart disease. *New England Journal of Medicine, 325*(4), 221–225.

Ayanian, J. Z., Guadagnoli, E., & Cleary, P. D. (1995). Physical and psychosocial functioning of women and men after bypass surgery. *Journal of the American Medical Association, 274*(22), 1767–1770.

Clancy, C. M., & Massion, C. T. (1992). American women's health care. A patchwork quilt of gaps. *Journal of the American Medical Association, 268*(14), 1918–1920.

Duffin, J. (1999). *History of medicine. A scandalously short introduction.* Toronto, Canada: University of Toronto Press.

Kerrigan, D. C., Todd, M. K., & O'Reiley, P. (1998). Knee osteoarthritis and high-heeled shoes. *Lancet, 351,* 1399–1401.

Moss, N. E. (2002). Gender equity and socioeconomic inequality: A framework for the patterning of women's health. *Social Science and Medicine, 54,* 849–861.

Oberle, K., & Allen, M. (1994). Breast augmentation surgery: A women's health issue. *Journal of Advanced Nursing, 20,* 844–852.

Philpott, S., Boynton, P. M., Feder, G., & Hemingway, H. (2001). Gender differences in descriptions of angina symptoms and health problems immediately prior to angiography: The ACRE study. *Social Science and Medicine, 52,* 1565–1575.

Rousseau, M. E. (1998). Women's midlife health. Reframing menopause. *Journal of Nurse-Midwifery, 43*(3), 208–223.

Rousseau, M. E. (1998). Hormone replacement therapy: Short-term versus long-term use. *Journal of Nurse-Midwifery, 47*(6), 461–470.

Ruzek, S. B., Olesen, V. L., & Clarke, A. E. (Eds.). (1997). *Women's health: Complexities and differences.* Columbus: Ohio State University Press.

Stotland, N. (1994). Conception and abortion: Challenges for now and the next century. In A. J. Dan (Ed.), *Reframing women's health: Multidisciplinary research and practice* (pp. 142–150). Thousand Oaks, CA: Sage.

Tiefer, L. (1994). Sexuality: Not a matter of health. In A. J. Dan (Ed.). *Reframing women's health: Multidisciplinary research and practice* (pp. 151–161). Thousand Oaks, CA: Sage.

United States Department of Health and Human Services Office of Women's Health. (2002). *A century of women's health: 1900–2000.*

Utian, W. H. (1997). Menopause—a modern perspective from a controversial history. *Maturitas, 26,* 73–82.

Suggested Resources

American Academy of Dermatology. www.aad.org

Association of Reproductive Health Professionals. www.arhp.org

Boston Women's Health Book Collective. Our Bodies, Ourselves. www.ourbodiesourselves.org

Doulas of North America. www.dona.org

Feminist Women Health Center. www.fwhc.org

History World. www.historyworld.net

Kellermeier J. *How menstruation created mathematics.* http://faculty.plattsburgh.edu/john.kellermeier/Menses/Menses.htm

Medline Plus Health Information Merriam-Webster Medical Dictionary. http://www2.merriam-webster.com/cgi-bin/mwmednlm

On-line Medical Dictionary. http://www.nlm.nih.gov/medlineplus

The Society of Chiropodists and Podiatrists. www.feetforlife.org

The Women's Health Information Center. www.4women.gov

The World Health Organization. www.who.org

Disparities in Women's Health and Health Care

Sana Loue and Nancy Mendez

The United States is a large, multicultural society. The total U.S. population in the year 2000 was 281.4 million; women comprised 50.9% of this total. Focused attention on women's health is critical for numerous reasons, in addition to the fact that women constitute slightly more than half of our population. First, various health concerns exist that are unique to women, such as ovarian and cervical cancer, while still other health concerns exist that impact women to a far greater degree than

men, such as eating disorders and specific autoimmune disorders. Women are also major consumers of health care services and prescription drugs and often play a critical role in deciding matters related to the health care of family members. Finally, women and men differ biologically and with respect to health indicators. For instance, women tend to have higher rates of illness and disability than men, but also tend to live longer than men (Centers for Disease Control and Prevention, 1995).

Significant diversity exists even among women. Almost one third of women in the United States self-identify as other than white. The number of adult women in the various subgroups in the United States varies widely ranging, for instance, from 24,500 Alaskan Native women to 15.3 million African American women. However, health, health care, and health access are not equivalent across subgroups of women.

These differences are known as health disparities. Health disparities have been defined as "differences in the incidence, prevalence, mortality, and burden of disease and other adverse health conditions that exist among specific population groups in the United States" (National Institutes of Health, 2003). This chapter begins with an overview of the role of biological sex in the determination of gender role and the impact of that relationship on women's health care. The chapter continues with a discussion of historical and cultural issues that are relevant to the existence of health and health care disparities across subgroups of women.

CULTURAL AND HISTORICAL CONTEXT: SEX AND GENDER

Consider the following health disparities between men and women:

1. Although women have both a lower threshold and a lower tolerance for pain than men do, they are more likely to be inadequately treated for pain (Hoffman & Tarzian, 2001).

2. Manifestations of HIV/AIDS are different in women than in men. However, until 1993, the definition of AIDS formulated by the Centers for Disease Control and Prevention did not include the symptoms that are common to women. As a result, many women with AIDS were unable to provide documentation to qualify for benefits, such as Medicare and Social Security Disability, even though they were as sick as many of the men who were able to qualify.

3. Research has found that among patients with presumed coronary heart disease, women with positive radionuclide exercise tests were referred for coronary angiography less frequently than men (Tobin et al., 1987).

4. Women are often referred for coronary artery bypass surgery at a more advanced stage of the disease than men, resulting in higher perioperative mortality (Khan et al., 1990).

5. Researchers studying hospital discharges in Massachusetts and Maryland found that women who were hospitalized for coronary heart disease underwent fewer diagnostic and therapeutic procedures than men. It was not clear whether these differences represented overuse by the men or underuse by the women (Ayanian & Epstein, 1991).

6. Until relatively recently, women were often excluded from clinical trials to test medications, even though they would be consumers of the medication if it were to later be approved for marketing. This was problematic because women may respond differently than men to pharmacologic agents.

Sex differences have often been attributed to one or more of the following factors: (a) biological factors, such as hormones; (b) acquired risks through work and leisure activities; (c) psychosocial aspects of symptoms and care; (d) health reporting behavior; and (5) the effect of previous health care on future health (Verbrugge, 1990). However, the historical and cultural context in which illness and health seeking occur is also relevant to understanding why these disparities may exist.

Prior to the late 18th century, women in the United States were viewed as fundamentally similar to men, but inferior, due to the underdevelopment of their reproductive organs. Beginning with the late 18th century, women were seen as biologically different from men, but still inferior, as evidenced by their smaller skulls and resulting smaller brain capacity (Fee, 1979). A division of labor by sex, it was argued, was justified and necessary because women's lives were tyrannized and controlled by their reproductive systems, from menstruation, through childbearing and menopause. Consequently, women were not only debilitated, but also disabled and unsuited for larger societal roles (Smith-Rosenberg, 1973).

Unlike men who, it was believed in the 19th century, had the power to indulge or repress their sexual impulses (Skene, 1889, cited in Smith-Rosenberg, 1973), women were subject to cyclical periods of pain, weakness, irritability, and insanity (Wiltbank, 1854, cited in Smith-Rosenberg, 1985). Puberty represented a precipitous crossing into womanhood, fraught with danger of diseases should there be either an "excess or a deficiency of the proper influence of these organs [ovaries] over the other parts of the system" (Kellogg, 1895, p. 371, cited in Smith-Rosenberg, 1985). The preservation of health, then, demanded full attention to the development of healthy reproductive organs, which could be accomplished by adherence to a regimen of rest, a simple diet, and an unchallenging routine of domestic tasks (Smith-Rosenberg, 1973).

Menopause was similarly ominous, resulting in numerous diseases including diarrhea, vaginal inflammation, paralysis, tuberculosis, diabetes, depression, hysteria, and insanity, due to the cessation of menstruation and the "violation of the physiological and social laws dictated by [a woman's] ovarian system" (Smith-Rosenberg, 1973, p. 192). Such violations included education, attempts at birth control or abortion, a failure to adequately attend to the needs of one's husband or children, an overly indulgent lifestyle, and engaging in sexual intercourse during or after menopause (Smith-Rosenberg, 1973).

The late 19th century medical view of women and their role rested, then, on four assumptions. First, women had a closed energy system, whereby the use of the brain would result in the theft of energy from the ovaries. Second, bodily functions were organized in a hierarchical fashion with the ovaries maintaining a position superior to that of the brain. Third, females were physiologically fragile. Finally, male and female functions operated in a polarized fashion with men embodying the brain and mind, and women, the body and ovaries (Smith-Rosenberg, 1985). Women who rejected these premises and engaged in violative behaviors were characterized by physicians as an "intermediate sex," fusing the female and male to become the "Mannish lesbian" (Smith-Rosenberg, 1985). In other words, women who rejected the traditional female gender norms were considered abnormal.

The emergence in the late 1800s and through the mid-1900s of the "New Woman" violated existing taboos. "New Women" abandoned the domestic setting, seeking an education not equal, but identical, to that received by men (Smith-Rosenberg, 1973). It was predicted that such women would disrupt a delicate psychological balance through the emphasis on the mind rather than the ovaries. Within men, however, the brain and heart were dominant permitting them to pursue such intellectual activities.

The women's health movement was to have a lasting impact on women's health and health care and, not surprisingly, their social roles as well. The beginning of the movement has been traced to 1970, when women protested over their exclusion from congressional hearings on the use of the birth control pill (Eagan, 1994). The first printing of *Our Bodies, Ourselves* was released in 1971, providing women with a basic source of information. Abortion was legalized in 1973, with the decision in *Roe v. Wade*. The publication of *Why Me?* challenged medicine's reliance on the Halsted radical mastectomy, requiring the removal of the entire breast, the axillary lymph nodes, and the underlying chest wall, to treat breast cancer (Kushner, 1975).

These advances notwithstanding, women were often excluded from research and the benefits it produced until relatively recently. The exclusion of women was defended based on the need for homogeneity among research participants in order to facilitate the analysis, the potential liability of a woman and/or her offspring were injured as a result of participation, and the belief that it is morally wrong to include women in studies because they may be, or may become, pregnant (Merton, 1996). The exclusion of women may have contributed to our lack of understanding about differences in such things as disease presentation and drug metabolism between men and women.

DISPARITIES AMONG WOMEN

Health disparities also exist across subgroups of women. Consider the following examples.

1. The cancer incidence per 100,000 women for the years 1992–1998 ranged from 140.1 per 100,000 among American Indian women to 400.1 per 100,000 among Alaskan Native women. American Indian women experienced the lowest rate of cervical cancer (6.2 per 100,000), while Hispanic women experienced the highest rate (14.4 per 100,000) (Glanz, Croyle, Chollette, & Pinn, 2003).

2. Minority women have been disproportionately impacted by HIV/AIDS. By the end of 1998, more than 77% of women infected with HIV were from minority groups; 57% were African American and 20% were Hispanic.

3. Systemic lupus erythematosus affects approximately 239,000 individuals in the United States. Women are disproportionately affected. The disease can affect many parts of the body, including the skin, kidneys, lungs, heart, and brain. Out of every 10 cases of this disease, 9 are in women. As many as 1 in every 250 African American women will develop lupus in their lifetimes, compared to 1 in 400 Hispanic women and 1 in 600 white women. The increased incidence among African Americans has been attributed to both genetic factors (Hochberg, Petri, Machan, & Bias, 1991) and environmental factors (Kardestuncer & Frumkin, 1997). The mortality rate among African American women with the disease is triple that in white women with this illness.

4. Scleroderma is an autoimmune disease that results in the hardening of the skin. This can potentially affect tissues in the lungs, heart, kidneys, intestinal tract, muscles, and joints. This illness is especially prevalent among Native American women.

5. Homicide accounts for 40% of work-related injury among women (Bell, 1991). The highest work-related homicide rates are among African Americans and women over the age of 65 (Bell, 1991).

6. In 1998, 68.1% of white women reported having had a mammogram within the previous 2 years, in comparison with 44.6% of Alaskan Native women. Eighty percent of white women reported having had a Pap smear within the previous 3 years, as compared with 46% of American Samoan women.

7. African American women are more likely to have had inadequate prenatal care than non-Hispanic white women.

8. Compared to other Hispanic subgroups, Cuban women appear to utilize preventive services, such as mammograms and Pap smears, at a higher rate than women in other Hispanic subgroups.

9. Among Hispanics, Puerto Rican women are most likely to have health insurance. African Americans are less likely than whites to have a usual source of care.

10. Among older women enrolled in Medicare managed care, non-Hispanic black and African American women are more likely to report fair or poor health (Bierman, Haffer, & Hwang, 2001).

11. Among men and women who are infected with HIV, women are less likely than men to receive highly active antiretroviral therapy (HAART) to treat their infection, even when they had equally likely come to their medical appointment in the previous 6 months and their illness was similar in severity.

12. Twenty-two percent of white women reported smoking in 1998, compared to 7% among some Asian American groups and almost 40% among some American Indian tribes.

Disparities in Women's Health and Health Care

An understanding of how these disparities may have come to exist requires an examination of relevant historical and cultural factors.

African American Women

It is critical to remember that the African ancestors of persons now known as African Americans were brought to the New World forcibly, as slaves. As of the 2000 census, approximately 34.7 million individuals, representing 12.3% of the U.S. population, self-identified as African American, while another 36.4 million individuals, or an additional 12.9% of the population, indicated that black or African American is one of their racial affiliations. Women constitute slightly more than half of all African Americans.

Despite the general tendency to view African American women as constituting a homogeneous group, there is, in fact, great diversity. Approximately 5% of black Americans were born outside of the United States. This includes, for instance, French-speaking individuals from Haiti, Portuguese-speaking individuals from Brazil, Dutch-speaking individuals from Aruba, and English-speaking individuals from Belize.

More than three quarters of the black population live in urban areas and more than half live in 13 southern states. Almost one quarter of all black Americans lived below the poverty level as of 1999 and almost one third of all black women lived in poverty as of 1995. One sixth of employed black women earn incomes below the federal poverty level. Blacks continue to experience racism and discrimination in access to adequate housing, improved education, employment, and health care. These circumstances are associated with

- increased levels of violence associated with internalized rage due to frustration and anger
- increased levels of hypertension associated with stress
- higher rates of specific respiratory diseases due to increased exposure to hazards in the living and work environments
- decreased access to health care insurance and health care
- inadequate treatment when health care is sought
- a lack of neighborhood facilities for the treatment of illness and consequent reliance on emergency departments as the usual source of care

American Indian Women

It is believed that between 12 and 15 million American Indians lived in North America prior to the arrival of the Europeans. However, as of the 2000 census, only 2.5 million individuals self-identified as American Indian or Alaskan Native and an additional 4 million indicated that they were part American Indian or Alaskan Native. The category "American Indian or Alaskan Native" includes individuals who trace their origins to the indigenous peoples of North and South America and who continue to maintain a tribal affiliation or community attachment.

American Indians and Alaskan Natives comprise 556 federally recognized tribes; each tribe belongs to one of seven nations. There are 300 reservations in the mainland United States and 500 government units in Alaska that are home to the tribes. These tribes are diverse in terms of culture, language, and habitat. However, they share numerous common characteristics and experiences, including:

- loss of their land and forced migration, often to reservations or urban areas
- the outlawing of their language and spiritual practices, many of which were critical in addressing health and illness
- the deaths of generations to war and infectious diseases
- a coerced dismantling of a clan-based society and reorganization to a nuclear family-based system
- racism and discrimination, often resulting in a lack of employment and poverty
- lack of adequate health care, despite a treaty obliging the U.S. government to provide a reasonable level of health care to American Indians and Alaskan Natives

These circumstances, in turn, are associated with

- reliance on unhealthy diets due to poverty and unemployment, and reliance instead on government commodity foods that are high in fat and calories
- an increase in obesity and associated diseases, such as cardiovascular disease, due to decreases in hunting and gathering following the loss of lands and the assumption of a sedentary lifestyle
- an increase in family violence, associated with frustrations arising from the extinction of traditional gender roles

- a decrease in self-esteem and resulting increases in rates of substance use, due to discrimination and poverty
- an inability to utilize preventive care due to large distances between providers and women's residences

Asian and Pacific Islander Women

Almost 14% of women in the United States self-identified as Asian or Pacific Islander in the 2000 census. This designation includes individuals who have their origins in original peoples of the Far East, the Indian subcontinent, or Southeast Asia, such as Cambodia, China, and India, as well as individuals who trace their origins to the indigenous peoples of Hawaii, Guam, Samoa, or other Pacific Islands. Asians represent more than 60 different ethnic groups and speak more than 100 different languages.

The majority of Asian Americans now live in urbanized areas. In 1998, the five cities with the largest Asian and Pacific Islander populations were Los Angeles, New York, San Francisco, Honolulu, and Washington, DC. Among the states, California, New York, and Hawaii have the largest Asian and Pacific Islander populations.

Like American Indians and Alaskan Natives, Asian and Pacific Islanders are distinct in many ways, including language, religion, customs, education, and health beliefs. As communities they also share common experiences and characteristics that may impact their health status and their health care from Western medicine, including:

- the experience of prejudice and discrimination
- difficulties related to migration to the U.S. mainland, including immigration bans against specific groups for discrete periods of time
- a high proportion of members born outside of the United States
- alternative systems of health care
- an increased emphasis on the role of the family in decision-making

These circumstances are associated with

- decreased access to health care providers due to the scarcity of health care providers who speak the languages of the consumers
- decreased willingness to seek health care due to fear of difficulties in communicating
- decreased access to health care information due to linguistic differences

- decreased access to health care due to lack of employment-based health care insurance and publicly funded health care insurance associated with immigration status
- increased substance use related to attempts to cure certain illnesses without relying on Western medicine

Hispanic/Latino Women

Hispanics now account for 35.3 million individuals in the United States and an additional 3.8 million individuals in the Commonwealth of Puerto Rico; this constitutes 12.5% of the U.S. population. Women account for 17 million individuals, or slightly less than half of all Hispanics.

The major subgroups of Hispanics in the United States are Mexican Americans, Puerto Ricans, and Cuban Americans. Sizable portions of the Hispanic population also are from countries in Central America, South America, and the Dominican Republic. Almost 40% of all Hispanics were born outside of the United States, more than 90% of the population live in urban areas, and slightly more than three quarters of the population reside in seven states (Arizona, California, Florida, Illinois, New Jersey, New York, and Texas).

As of 1998, slightly more than one quarter of Hispanics were living in poverty. In 1999, more than one quarter of Puerto Rican women and more than one quarter of Mexican women were living in poverty. This poverty level is attributable in part to relatively high levels of unemployment, as well as to a greater number of female-headed households, which are more likely than others to have incomes below the federal poverty level.

Many Hispanic women are employed in relatively low wage jobs. Hispanics are three times as likely as non-Hispanic whites to be employed on a full-time basis and to still lack health care insurance. Almost one third of all Hispanics did not have health insurance for the entire year during 1999; even those who were employed were less likely to be provided with health insurance by their employers.

Acculturation appears to play a major factor in both health and health care access. For instance, greater acculturation to U.S. culture has been found to be associated with increased rates of substance use, while lower levels of acculturation have been found to be associated with a reduced risk of diabetes and heart disease, as well as a lower incidence of low-birthweight babies. It has been suggested that individuals who are highly acculturated to

17

Disparities in Women's Health and Health Care

U.S. culture may experience increased levels of frustration due to an inability to access educational and other resources due to prejudice and discrimination.

As a result of these circumstances, many Hispanics may experience

- decreased access to health care due to a lack of health insurance and additional economic barriers
- difficulties in accessing care due to language and/or immigration-related issues
- increased difficulty in seeking care for certain types of issues, such as domestic violence, due to fears associated with immigration status or language barriers
- increased risk of disease associated with sedentary lifestyles due to environmental and economic barriers to accessing fitness facilities and safe recreational areas

Elderly Women

"Elderly" has been defined as persons who are 65 years of age or older. However, distinctions have been made between those who are between the ages of 65 and 74, who are referred to as the young-old; those between the ages of 75 and 84, who are considered to be the old; and those who are over the age of 85, who are referred to as the older-old. Some subpopulations within the United States, however, may view old age as beginning as early as 40.

Approximately 12% of the U.S. population is now considered to be elderly; that proportion is expected to increase. The geographic distribution of elderly persons is not uniform, however, across the states. In addition, there are more female than male elderly. For instance, in the age group from 65 to 74 years old, there are 82 men for every 100 women, while among those 85 years old or older, the sex ratio is 49 males for every 100 females. Women are also more likely to be widowed than are men and, because they are living longer, are also more likely to suffer from chronic disease, disability, and dependency.

As many elderly women age and their partners die, an increased number of women may be living in poverty. And, even though those over the age of 65 are eligible for the receipt of Medicare, access to care may be impaired nevertheless, because Medicare does not cover all health care costs that may be incurred. As a result, Medicare must be supplemented by private insurance, Medicaid, and/or private resources. However, many elderly women may not have such supplemental coverage due to either eligibility restriction or financial resources.

Many elderly may have immigrated from other countries. Depending upon their age at the time of immigration, they may not have acquired skills in English and sufficient knowledge of the U.S. health care system that would enable them to access care more easily. For instance, in 1990, almost 40% of older Hispanics reported that they did not speak any English.

Many elderly women may not have had a formal education. It has been reported that 31% of all women aged 65 and older, who are enrolled in Medicare managed care, have not had a high school education (Bierman et al., 2001).

These circumstances may be associated with

- inadequate access to health care due to financial, immigration, and/or language barriers
- low health literacy
- increased difficulty in making complex health care decisions
- increased incidence of psychosocial problems associated with isolation

Rural Women

Even within subgroups of women, disparities may exist in health status and health care access between those women living in urban areas and those who reside in rural locales. For instance, a recent study of perinatal and infant health among rural and urban American Indian and Alaskan Native women found that rural women were much more likely to have received inadequate prenatal care (Baldwin et al., 2002). In addition, both rural and urban American Indian and Alaskan Native women were more likely to receive inadequate prenatal care compared with white women.

Compared to their urban counterparts, rural women

- are more likely to be migrants, thereby decreasing the likelihood that they will have time off for sick leave or to seek care
- are less likely to have access to mental health services, to pharmaceuticals, and to specialized care due to a shortage of professionals and other health care services in rural areas
- are less able to access care due to a lack of insurance and transportation difficulties (Gaston, 2001)

Lesbian and Bisexual Women

Nonheterosexuality has been variously seen as a reflection of degeneracy, a criminal tendency, and/or a matter for medical concern. The apparent medical consensus that homosexuality was a form of pathology resulted in its inclusion as a sociopathic personality disturbance in the 1952 edition of the American Psychiatric Association's *Diagnostic and Statistical Manual of Mental Disorders* (DSM-I). It was not until 1973 that homosexuality was declassified as a mental disorder.

Nevertheless, a number of states continue to criminalize same-sex sexual behavior. Relatively few jurisdictions in the United States prohibit discrimination on the basis of sexual orientation. Homophobic attitudes have been noted among diverse groups of health care providers, including physicians (Matthews, Booth, Turner, & Kessler, 1986) and social workers (Berkman & Zinberg, 1997). In addition, relatively few employers provide health insurance coverage to nonspouse partners, although same-sex marriage and legally recognized partnerships are still relatively rare.

These circumstances have been found to be associated with

- decreased access to health insurance coverage and, consequently, to care (Mays, Yancey, Cochran, Weber, & Fielding, 2002)
- decreased quality of care
- increased risk of substance use
- an increased risk of suicide

CONCLUSION

Such disparities can and should be eliminated. First, such inequalities are fundamentally unfair when poor health results from "an unjust distribution of the underlying social determinants of health" (Woodward & Kawachi, 2000, p. 923). Our brief review of the historical and cultural contexts that have given rise to these disparities evidences an unjust distribution of the underlying social determinants of health as the source of such health disparities.

Second, it has been argued that health inequalities ultimately affect everyone. For instance, infectious diseases, such as tuberculosis and HIV/AIDS, do not limit their impact based on classifications that we may have established based on socioeconomic status, sex, or ethnicity. Mental illness and substance use affect not only the individual, but also those around him or her.

Third, inequalities are avoidable to the extent that they can be modified through policy interventions. As an example, the transmission of HIV/AIDS can be reduced among populations at higher risk through increased government action and funding.

Finally, public health interventions that reduce health inequalities may also produce financial savings. As an example, improving access to cervical cancer screening among groups with low access may in the long term result in lesser spending due to earlier intervention (Woodward & Kawachi, 2000). Similarly, the cost of preventing a case of HIV/AIDS far surpasses the lifetime cost of treating an infected individual (Gorsky, Macgowan, Swanson, & Delgado, 1995).

References

Ayanian, J. Z., & Epstein, A. M. (1991). Differences in the use of procedures between women and men hospitalized for coronary heart disease. *New England Journal of Medicine, 325*, 221–225.

Baldwin, L. M., Grossman, D. C., Casey, S., Hollow, W., Sugarman, J. R., Freeman, W. L., et al. (2002). Perinatal and infant health among rural and urban American Indians/Alaska Natives. *American Journal of Public Health, 92*, 1491–1497.

Bell, C. A. (1991). Female homicides in United States workplaces, 1980–1985. *American Journal of Public Health, 81*, 729–732.

Berkman, C. S., & Zinberg, G. (1997). Homophobia and heterosexism in social workers. *Social Work, 42*, 319–332.

Bierman, A. S., Haffer, S. C., & Hwang, Y. T. (2001). Health disparities among older women enrolled in Medicare managed care. *Health Care Financing Review, 22*, 187–198.

Centers for Disease Control and Prevention (1995). *Health United States, 1996–97*. Hyattsville, MD: Department of Health and Human Services (DHHS Publ. [PHS] 95-1232).

Eagan, A. B. (1994). The women's health movement and its lasting impact. In E. Friedman (Ed.), *An unfinished revolution: Women and health care in America* (pp. 15–27). New York: United Hospital Fund of New York.

Fee, E. (1979). Nineteenth century craniology: The study of the female skull. *Bulletin of the History of Medicine, 53*, 425–433.

Gaston, M. H. (2001). 100% access and 0 health disparities: Changing the health paradigm for rural women in the 21st century. *Women's Health Issues, 11*, 7–16.

Glanz, K., Croyle, R. T., Chollette, V. Y., & Pinn, V. W. (2003). Cancer-related health disparities in women. *American Journal of Public Health, 93*, 292–298.

Gorsky, R. D., Macgowan, R. J., Swanson, N. M., & Delgado, B. P. (1995). Prevention of HIV-infection in drug abusers: A cost analysis. *Preventive Medicine, 24*, 3–8.

Hochberg, M. C., Petri, M., Machan, C., & Bias, W. B. (1991). HLA class II alleles DrB1*1501/15.3 and DqB1*0602 are associated with systemic lupus erythematosus (SLE) in African-Americans [abstract]. *Arthritis and Rheumatism, 34*, S140.

Hoffman, D. E., & Tarzian, A. J. (2001). The girl who cried pain: A bias against women in the treatment of pain. *Journal of Law, Medicine, and Ethics, 29*, 13–27.

Kardestuncer, T., & Frumkin, H. (1997). Systemic lupus erythematosus in relation to environmental pollution: An investigation in an African-American community in north Georgia. *Archives of Environmental Health, 52*, 85–90.

Khan, S. S., Nessim, S., Gray, R., Czer, L. S., Chaux, A., & Matloff, J. (1990). Increased mortality of women in coronary artery bypass surgery: Evidence for referral bias. *Annals of Internal Medicine, 112*, 561–567.

Kushner, R. (1975). *Why me?* New York: W. B. Saunders.

Matthews, W. C., Booth, M. W., Turner, J. D., & Kessler, L. (1986). Physicians' attitudes towards homosexuality—A survey of a California medical society. *Western Journal of Medicine, 144*, 106–110.

Mays, V. M., Yancey, A. K., Cochran, S. D., Weber, M., & Fielding, J. E. (2002). Heterogeneity of health disparities among African American, Hispanic, and Asian American women: Unrecognized influences of sexual orientation. *American Journal of Public Health, 92*, 632–639.

Merton, V. (1996). Ethical obstacles to the participation of women in biomedical research. In S. M. Wolf (Ed.), *Feminism and bioethics: Beyond reproduction* (pp. 216–251). New York: Oxford University Press.

Skene, A. J. C. (1889). *Education and culture as related to the health and diseases of women.* Detroit: George S. Davis. (Cited in C. Smith-Rosenberg (1973). The cycle of femininity: Puberty to menopause in nineteenth century America. *Feminist Studies, 1*, 58–72. [Reprinted in *Disorderly conduct: Visions of gender in Victorian America*, by C. Smith-Rosenberg, 1985, New York: Alfred A. Knopf.])

Smith-Rosenberg, C. (1973). The cycle of femininity: Puberty to menopause in nineteenth century America. *Feminist Studies, 1*, 58–72. (Reprinted in *Disorderly conduct: Visions of gender in Victorian America*, by C. Smith-Rosenberg, 1985, New York: Alfred A. Knopf.)

Smith-Rosenberg, C. (1985). *Disorderly conduct: Visions of gender in Victorian America.* New York: Alfred A. Knopf.

Tobin, J. N., Wassertheil-Smoller, S., Wexler, J. P., Steingart, R. M., Budner, N., Lense, L., et al. (1987). Sex bias in considering coronary bypass surgery. *Annals of Internal Medicine, 107*, 19–25.

Verbrugge, L. M. (1990). Pathways of health and death. In R. D. Apple (Ed.), *Women, health, and medicine in America: A historical handbook* (pp. 11–79). New York: Garland.

Wiltbank, J. (1854). Introductory lecture for the Session, 1853–54. Philadelphia, PA: Edward Gratton. Cited in C. Smith-Rosenberg (1985). *Disorderly conduct: Visions of gender in Victorian America,* New York: Alfred A. Knopf.

Woodward, A., & Kawachi, I. (2000). Why reduce health inequalities? *Journal of Epidemiology and Community Health, 54*, 923–929.

Suggested Reading

Department of Health and Human Services, National Cancer Institute. (2003). *Cancer in women of color monograph.* Bethesda, MD: Author. Available at http://www.cancercontrol.cancer.gov/womenofcolor/.

Department of Health and Human Services, National Institutes of Health. (2000). *Strategic research plan to reduce and ultimately eliminate health disparities: Fiscal years 2002–2006.* Bethesda, MD: Author.

Loue, S. (1999). *Gender, ethnicity, and health research.* New York: Plenum.

Women in the Health Professions

Martha Sajatovic, Susan Hatters-Friedman, and Isabel Schuermeyer

INTRODUCTION

Women make up 50% of the global population and 51% of the U.S. population, representing a large and diverse group of individuals (United Nations, 1995; U.S. Bureau of the Census, 1999). In the United States, employment patterns for women have changed tremendously over the last several decades. For example, in 1950, women represented 34% of the workforce compared to 60% in 1997 (Wagener et al., 1997). The occupational roles and working conditions of women also vary dramatically and have changed over the last decades, profoundly influenced by economics and sociopolitical culture.

Currently, women in the health care professions deliver a vast array of diverse services, including preventative care, primary care, acute and specialized services, and care in a variety of settings. In 1996, registered nurse was the fourth and nurse's aide/orderly was the sixth leading occupation for women (U.S. Department of Labor, 1997). The growing trend for higher education among women has helped spur growth in the number of women in the health care workforce. Among occupations expected to grow the fastest between 1996 and 2006, those where the majority of employees are women include dental assistant (99.1% women), physical therapists (61.9% women), and respiratory therapists (58.4% women) (Welstedt, 2000).

The types of roles that women play in the delivery of health care services have changed substantially as well. This is well demonstrated by changes over the last three decades in the medical profession. In 1970, 7.7% of actively practicing allopathic physicians were women. By 1996 this had increased to 22.0% and is expected to increase to 29.7% by 2010 (American Medical Association, 1997/1998; Council on Graduate Medical Education, 1995). This trend is likely to continue as women currently make up approximately half of medical student classes compared to only 11% in 1970.

Over 60% of women physicians are clustered in the specialties of internal medicine, family practice, obstetrics–gynecology, pediatrics, and psychiatry (Clancy, 2000). The fact that a majority of women physicians are younger and are primary care providers has important implications in the delivery of preventative care services as well as on patient satisfaction and communication issues. Age and gender of physician significantly impact likelihood of adherence with evidence-based guidelines for medical care, and independent of physician age, women physicians are more likely to provide Pap tests, breast examinations, and recommend regular mammography screening to women patients (Franks & Clancy, 1993; Lurie et al., 1993). It has also been suggested that women health care providers have communication styles that enhance patient satisfaction and the provider–patient relationship (Clancy, 2000). Women physicians spend more time in interactive communication and listen more closely to patient concerns (Clancy, 2000), and in situations where personal violence or sexual abuse has occurred, patients are more likely to reveal this information to their women physicians (Roter, Lipkin, & Korgnard, 1991).

It must be noted that while women overall have made substantial gains in representation in the health professions, this is not the case for all women. The numbers of minority women in medicine have increased only slightly, and remain far behind Caucasian women (Clancy, 2000). Additionally, women still rarely occupy positions of leadership in professional medical organizations.

OPPORTUNITIES AND BARRIERS FOR WOMEN IN THE HEALTH CARE PROFESSIONS

Throughout their life span women use health services more than men (Verbrugge & Steiner, 1981). This, along with a developing focus on women's health issues, a more informed consumer base, and a frequent preference by women patients for women health care providers, all create growing opportunities for women in the health care professions. Job satisfaction, financial remuneration, and personal empowerment are all potential benefits for successful women health care providers. A report from the U.S. Department of Health and Human Services (1989) found that women in professional specialty occupations were the group with the highest self-assessment of general health status in the total labor force. Additionally, the growing numbers of women in most health-related occupations offer greater potential for social support, mentoring, and relative freedom from sexual harassment and discrimination.

However, as described by Stellman and Lucas (2000), there are a variety of basic socioeconomic factors that affect all women workers. These factors are relevant to women health care professionals as well, and represent potential barriers to successful employment by women in health care fields. Factors described by Stellman and Lucas (2000) as affecting working women in general, are discussed below in relation to women in the health care professions.

1. *Occupational segregation.* As is the case for women workers in general, women health professionals tend to be overrepresented in a relatively small number of health occupations, particularly nursing and health support/health aid capacities (U.S. Department of Labor, 1997). These traditionally "female" occupations have tended in the past to be less well paid than many traditionally "male" occupations (Stellman & Lucas, 2000). When barriers that tend to keep women within narrow occupational boundaries are lessened, some professions may experience staffing losses such as the current nursing "shortage."

2. *Barriers to advancement/attainment.* For women in medicine, the "glass ceiling" may be an invisible, yet powerful force preventing advancement in job status. Women in academic medicine are most likely to hold lower level ranking such as instructor or assistant professor while there are relatively few women department heads or deans (McMurray et al., 2002; Nora, 2002).

3. *Underemployment.* Many women work part time, with the proportion of all working women who work full time remaining at approximately 73% over the last two decades (U.S. Department of Labor, 1988; U.S. Department of Labor, 1997). Twenty to fifty percent of women physicians in primary care practice work part time (McMurray et al., 2002). This is often in response to other personal commitments such as parenting/child care. A growing issue in the United States is "elder care" where women, usually employed daughters, care for aging parents (Messing, 1997). In general women consistently perform significantly more "unpaid" hours of home/family-related work compared to men with fewer "paid" hours of work outside the home (Stellman & Lucas, 2000).

4. *Lower remuneration.* Women in medicine continue to earn less than their male counterparts. Some of this is due to working fewer hours (McMurray et al., 2002) as well as working in lower paying specialties. The absolute numbers of women entering more highly paid surgical fields remain low, and women are rare in the higher paying medical specialties such as cardiology, where only 5% of practicing cardiologists and 10% of trainees are women (American College of Cardiology, 1998).

5. *Lack of seniority.* Employees who are younger or with less seniority may be more likely to suffer layoffs or employment termination in times of economic hardship or corporate downsizing. This is most likely to affect women who are entering a health occupation only recently. Managed care and reduction in hospital-based services have eliminated many health care positions and reduced job satisfaction (Davis, Scott Collins, & Schoen, 2000) for women, such as women physicians in health maintenance organizations (HMOs).

6. *Multiple burdens.* While opportunities to experience multiple social and occupational roles offer women more choices and potential for overall better physical and mental health (Barnett & Baruch, 1987), the presence of multiple, conflicting obligations may lead to stress, exhaustion, and "burnout." Many women have substantial domestic and childcare responsibilities (Messing, 2000) in addition to their occupations as health care providers. For example, nurses who work full time and have young children report more fatigue than those without children, particularly in circumstances where domestic tasks are not shared (Tierney, Romito, & Messing, 1990). Lee, Duxbury, and Higgen (1994) have noted that working women utilize organizational, planning, and negotiating skills to balance work and family life. However, a continued lack of mentors, role models, and women in leadership positions may make these skills difficult to acquire for young women just entering the health care professions.

7. *Sexual harassment and discrimination.* Sexual harassment and discrimination against women may occur in all the health professions, most particularly in areas that have been traditionally male dominated. Palepu and Herbert (2002) recently reported that three-quarters of U.S. women medical faculty experience sexual discrimination or harassment during their careers. Devaluation of the nursing profession, a traditionally "female" occupation, may represent a form of systematized and pervasive discrimination against women, which has resulted in lack of empowerment

(Gary, 2002), lower pay (Scott, 2002), and nurses leaving the profession (Rosenstein, Russell, & Lauve, 2002).

Variability among the Health Professions

While there are a number of factors that may be substantial obstacles to career choice, development, and advancement, the number of women in the health professions continues to increase. Women are successfully overcoming barriers and entering nontraditional fields in record numbers. However, variability exists in opportunities and growth among the health care specialties. Some areas, such as nursing, are currently experiencing staff shortages of crisis proportions (Ross, 2002). It remains to be seen how trends such as these will affect health care practice and service delivery.

Nursing

History and Early Experience. Nursing is the practice of caring or nurturing for others. The history of nursing goes back many centuries, with the earliest groups having minimal training and typically associated with religious orders. Later, during the Crusades, knights took part in nursing care of the wounded. At the end of the 18th century, hospitals were considered improper for young women. Modern nursing began in earnest during the mid-19th century. Florence Nightingale, a British nurse, is credited with making nursing a desirable and respected profession. She was a major force in securing a critical and valued role for nurses in health care.

Nursing Today: Career Satisfaction and Career Stress. Nurses are the largest group of professional health care workers and have one of the largest percentages of women in an occupation. The nurses of today have a degree in nursing ranging from a diploma to a doctoral degree. Most commonly they become licensed practical or registered nurses. Work locations cover a broad spectrum from hospitals to nursing homes and private practice offices. Furthermore, nurses have a wide range of specialties to choose from, including surgery, medical units, critical care, psychiatry, and home health care.

In recent times, nurses have suffered from the common angst of the working woman—specifically, the challenges in combining professional ambition with motherhood and family life. Some feel that nurses endure more than other female professionals because their occupation is more stressful. Examples of current stressors in the nursing profession include a severe nursing shortage, corporate health care downsizing, health resource restrictions inherent in managed care, daily crisis, and long, irregular hours.

Many descriptions of nurses indicate that they must be submissive, subordinate, and passive. These descriptions have long been applied to traditional housewife and mother roles as well. In contrast to the commonly perceived central role of physicians for curing, nurses may receive little credit for their important role in illness treatment and recovery. There are many stereotypes of nurses including "angels of mercy," servants to physicians, as well as "old maids" and "battleaxes." Some feel that the female domination of nursing has been one of the reasons this field's development has been hampered; specifically, that nursing has been socialized to be a female career and in a way is considered an extension of work at home. Throughout the time of the feminist movement, society in general has been quick to criticize women who have a family and work for not putting their family first. Others point out that the ideal nursing traits of compassion, sensitivity, and compliance are not useful in career success—where autonomy and competitiveness are valued (Castledine, 1983).

In spite of the fact that most nurses are women, the feminist movement has not always actively benefited the nursing profession. This is true in general of female-dominated professions, such as nursing and social work, which have traditionally been identified with a housewife role. The feminist movement has at times ignored women nurses, as the strongest emphasis has been on improving access for women into traditionally male dominated fields. Because of this, some nursing groups feel that their field is devalued by the feminist movement (Letvak, 2001).

Job satisfaction and commitment to the profession has been studied among nurses, as it has been noted that there is a high turnover rate in nursing. Multiple explanations have been proposed including that women will never be satisfied in careers as they value relationships above all else. Some have observed that men and women have different approaches toward morality. For example, it has been suggested that women value caring and connections with others, while men value justice, autonomy, and independence (Letvak, 2001). A study by Magnussen (1998) evaluated career perceptions of nurses who entered the field between 1910 through 1980. Each woman represented a different decade and it was hoped that this would shed some light on the perceptions of the field. This report found that women in nursing had a desire to serve others, and found the field to be financially accessible with regard to education. Women who entered nursing in the latter decades also noted that the work was satisfying, flexible, respected, and always in demand (Magnussen, 1998). Letvak (2001) recently suggested that women nurses may be able to improve their job satisfaction through united effort and by obtaining flexible work schedules, thus leading to better attendance at work and fewer nurses leaving the field.

Sexual harassment is an issue in the nursing field that has been closely examined in recent times. This is an important issue on many fronts—with regard to nurse employees, nursing management, and health care administrators. In addition to the destructive effects on the victim, sexual harassment can lower staff morale, efficiency, and productivity. Sexual harassment is illegal and the employer can be held liable if it happens while a nurse is at work. A 1994 study (Libbus & Bowman, 1994) found that 72% of women nurses experienced sexual harassment while at work. Twenty-five percent of the perpetrators were physicians, approximately 54% were patients, and the remainder were colleagues or family members of the patients. Many of the women reported confronting patients for this behavior, although fewer nurses did this if the perpetrator was a physician or a coworker. It is felt that this may be secondary to the power differential at play in a hospital setting where physicians and male nurses traditionally have had more power than female nurses. Interestingly, most female nurses do not report feelings of self-blame as is common for many female victims of sexual harassment. It is possible that the ego strength developed through nursing education and experience allows many nurses to avoid the self-blame typically seen in victims of sexual harassment. While it has been suggested that women nurses directly confront the perpetrator of sexual harassment, it is essential for nurse managers and executives to take responsibility for providing a safe work environment and ensure that sexual harassment does not occur (Libbus & Bowman, 1994).

Verbal abuse has also been examined in the nursing profession (Bruder, 2001). Although this type of abuse appears to be fairly common, it is not often openly addressed. Almost all nurses have experienced verbal abuse at some time from peers, physicians, or patients (Bruder, 2001). This type of abuse can lead to decreased self-esteem and job dissatisfaction. Of note, male nurses are at much lower risk of verbal abuse than are female nurses. A recent report emphasized the importance of open communication regarding this issue, role-play to come up with ways to confront a person who is verbally abusive, and to refer to those in power by their first name, if that is how they refer to the nurse in question (Bruder, 2001).

Nurses are considered to be at relatively high risk of substance use, possibly because of the high stress nature of their work combined with access to controlled substances. A survey of 1,951 female nurses (Collins, Gollnisch, & Morsheimer, 1998) assessed lifetime illegal drug use. This report noted that 37% of nurses had used marijuana, 16% had used opiates, and almost 3% had used hallucinogens. In the past month, approximately 1% had used marijuana and almost 2% had used opiates. Prescribed drugs were also included in this study; lifetime use of tranquilizers was 20% and amphetamines, 12%. It was noted that the rate of prescription drug use was comparable to that of male and female physicians and this may relate to the fact that both nurses and physicians have easy access to controlled substances. Collins et al. (1998) suggested that neuroticism, which is how stress is perceived, may be a risk factor for substance use, and that female nurses with higher neuroticism have higher perceptions of stress and therefore are more likely to use alcohol to cope with this stress (Collins et al., 1998).

Gender Differences in the Nursing Profession. Men have always been a minority in nursing. In 1940, only 1% of nurses were men and in 1984, only 4%. Compared to women nurses, men are typically older upon entering the field, more likely to be married, and have a history of being in the military. One study comparing job satisfaction between male and female nurses found that men appear to be more satisfied with their supervisors and felt more motivated by their job compared to women (Zawacki, Shahan, & Carey, 1995). As is true in the other health professions, patients may have gender preferences for nurses. A recent study from Australia surveyed patient gender preferences for nurse providers in 1984 and in 2000 (Chur-Hansen, 2002). This study demonstrated that as the intimacy of a situation increases the more likely it is that patients would prefer a nurse of their own gender. Furthermore, this was found to be particularly true for female patients compared to male patients (Chur-Hansen, 2002).

It has been noted that male nurses gravitate to critical care, psychiatry, and general medicine. On the other hand, female nurses tend to work in pediatrics, midwifery, and geriatrics, which are specialty areas considered more traditionally "female." In a study conducted in Ireland (Muldoon & Kremer, 1995), questionnaires were given to 123 student nurses to examine their career aspirations, gender role, and job commitment. The study found that career aspirations are influenced by perceived gender role and motivation, but not by job commitment (Muldoon & Kremer, 1995).

Physicians

History and Early Experience. Early women doctors learned through apprenticeships and cared primarily for women and children. In the 1770s, Frances Coomes may have been the first American woman physician. She practiced in Kentucky and, although she was known as Mrs. Coomes, she apprenticed along with a man who was thereafter known as a practicing physician. During the Civil War, Mary Walker served as a doctor, while disguised as a man (Dickstein, 1996).

Elizabeth Blackwell, the first woman formally academically trained as a physician in the United States, was a governess in a physician's home and studied his books (Levin, 1988). In 1847, Blackwell was accepted to the Geneva College of Medicine in New York, and graduated at the top of her class in 1849 (Chin, 2002; Friedman, 1994; Levin, 1988). In 1850, the Women's Medical College of Pennsylvania opened (Chin, 2002), and in 1864, Rebecca Lee Wright was the first African American female physician trained in the United States (Hart-Brothers, 1994).

This progress was not without controversy. In 1874, Harvard professor Edward Clarke reported that women who attended medical school would develop "monstrous brains and puny bodies; abnormally active cerebration and abnormally weak digestion; flowing thought and constipated bowels" (Chin, 2002). In spite of these dire predictions, by 1900 there were 19 women's medical schools in the United States (Chin, 2002), and by 1900, 5% of U.S. physicians were women. This number remained below 10% until the 1970s (Chin, 2002).

By 1893, the *Women's Medical Journal* had been launched, and in 1915, the Medical Women's National Association was founded (Chin, 2002). In 1915, women were also finally admitted into the American Medical Association (Chin, 2002). Some specialties within medicine were less accessible to women as the decades progressed, and the first woman was not certified by the American Board of Surgery until 1940 (Jonasson, 2002). Federal legislation facilitated the increased numbers of women in medicine into the 1970s and beyond. Within two years of the 1972 passing of Title IX of the Higher Education Act, which prevented universities receiving federal funding from discrimination based on gender, over 20% of medical school entrants were women (Chin, 2002).

Education and Training. A typical medical school curriculum lasts 4 years after completion of an undergraduate degree. Medical school mixes classroom learning and clinically based "rotations" in health care settings. More than 40% of medical students in the United States, Canada, England, and Australia are now women, consistent with increases in female applicants (McMurray et al., 2002), and 44.6% of U.S. medical students in 2000–2001 were women (Jonasson, 2002).

Residency is the training after medical school, in the new doctor's choice of generalist or specialty field. Residencies range in length based on specialty, with most being 3–5 years long. In residency, women physicians are often confused for nurses or aides. Residency often falls during a woman's childbearing years, and is quite physically as well as mentally challenging due to long and often unpredictable work hours.

Despite the increase in women completing medical school in the last quarter century, differences persist in choice of specialty and patterns of practice compared with their male colleagues (McMurray et al., 2002). The highest percentages of women residents can be found in obstetrics–gynecology (67%) and pediatrics (65%), caring for other women and children (Fye, 2002). Less than 5% of women residents choose surgery (McMurray et al., 2002). One former obstetrical resident who left her program due to her desire to be a mother wrote "residency is a barbaric training process during which new physicians can have the humanity literally worked out of them ... the dogma maintained is that residents must work as many hours as are humanly possible because of the vast amount of knowledge to be learned ... " (Becker, 2002).

Specialty Choice, Career Advancement, and Job Satisfaction. In 1980, there were 37,189 female physicians in the United States. In 2000, this rose to 148,768, an increase of over 300% (Salsberg & Forte, 2002). The influence of women in medicine is suggested by an increased emphasis on the importance of the doctor–patient relationship and the growth of preventive medicine (Chin, 2002). The majority of women physicians practice in primary care settings such as pediatrics or internal medicine. Female pediatricians increased from 28% in 1980 to 48% in 1998, and women are soon expected to represent the majority of pediatricians. Women pediatricians are more likely than men to work part time (26% vs. 4%), primarily due to childcare responsibilities. This may lead to a need for more total pediatricians to treat patients (Cull et al., 2002).

From 1988 to 1998, the income of women physicians was "gaining on" the income of men at a rate of about 1% per year (Wallace & Weeks, 2002). However, women in internal medicine still earn less than 80% of what their male counterparts make (Wallace & Weeks, 2002), and female physicians have been consistently noted to receive less pay than male physicians (McMurray et al., 2002). This difference persists even after adjustment for age and hours worked (Wallace & Weeks, 2002). Wallace and Weeks (2002) reported that if the trend of increase in women physicians' pay continues, women and men primary care physicians should receive the same hourly pay by the year 2014.

In academic settings, women medical school faculty earn less, and receive promotions more slowly than their male counterparts (McMurray et al., 2002). A Harvard study showed that women with children received professorship less frequently than men or women without children, and women with children were less satisfied with their careers (Epstein, 2002). Women are promoted less often than men with similar qualifications, and only 8% of medical school chairs are women (Nora, 2002).

Women physicians often must balance family demands with the demands of work, suffering "fatigue, stress, guilt, and role strain" (Palepu & Herbert, 2002). Physician "burnout" occurs when doctors under pressure are "overloaded with the demands of caring for sick patients within constraints of fewer organizational resources." Physicians with burnout may experience exhaustion, headaches, sleep problems, relationship disturbances, anxiety, depression, heart attack, as well as being more vulnerable to addictions and errors in judgment (Spickard, Gabbe, & Christensen, 2002). This has been explained as "the silent anguish of the healers" (Spickard et al., 2002). Unfortunately, women physicians are much more likely to report "burnout" than male physicians (Spickard et al., 2002). Women physicians in the United States experience more "burnout" than their male U.S. counterparts and more than physicians in the Netherlands (Linzer et al., 2002).

Women in the Health Professions

Manson et al. (2002) reported that women physicians with children had the lowest level of career satisfaction and that women in general reported less satisfaction with career goals and work compared to men. Some of these career satisfaction differences may be due to the demands of multiple role obligations. For example, in a survey of surgeons (Sonnad & Colletti, 2002), women surgeons' spouses were more likely to work outside the home than were male surgeons' spouses, and women surgeons spent twice the number of hours parenting compared to men. Women surgeons were somewhat more likely to miss work for family obligations, while male surgeons were more likely to miss family obligations for work (Sonnad & Colletti, 2002).

Midwives

History and Training. The word "midwife" is derived from "mid" or "with" and "wife" or "woman" (Rooks, 1997), and it has been said that midwives truly epitomize the commitment of women to be with women during childbirth (Reed & Roberts, 2000). In early times, midwives were also known as "wise women" or "witches." They discovered herbal remedies, such as ergot for labor pain, and belladona to inhibit uterine contractions in threatened miscarriages. This was unpopular with the church, because of the belief that only God could heal (Garratt, 2001) and the view that labor pain was a punishment for Eve's original sin (Ehrenreich & English, 1973).

Midwives, as women healers, were felt to have special knowledge about the "female mystery" of birth. During the Middle Ages, midwives were persecuted for using pagan birth rituals, and witch hunts of the 1400s and 1500s killed many midwives. Midwives were accused of offering babies to the devil if the baby died (Rooks, 1997). Men were often excluded from childbirth, and male "barber-surgeons" were called in only when forceps (invented in the 1600s) were needed (Rooks, 1997). Women were not permitted to practice surgery (Ehrenreich & English, 1973).

The history of midwives in the United States began with dependence on them in the Colonies, a near disappearance in the early 1900s, and reemergence of midwifery later in the 20th century (Reed & Roberts, 2000). Bridget Lee Fuller was a British midwife brought over on the Mayflower and salaried as the town midwife in Plymouth (Rooks, 1997). Many early American midwives were minority women or immigrants who had trained in other countries (Reed & Roberts, 2000).

For example, Southern plantation owners often had slaves serve as midwives, and skills were passed along during apprenticeships (Rooks, 1997).

The first publicly funded midwife training program began in 1911 (Rooks, 1997). A decade later, the Sheppard Towner Act of 1921 allowed nurses to supervise midwives, and this was an impetus to begin educating nurses as midwives (Reed & Roberts, 2000). After the development of midwifery schools, midwives practiced in underserved areas, especially in New York, New Mexico, and Kentucky (Reed & Roberts, 2000). The first nurse-midwifery service in the United States, the Frontier Nursing Service in Kentucky, was founded in 1925 (Reed & Roberts, 2000). In the White House Conference on Child Health and Protection that same year, it was noted that "trained midwives surpass the record of physicians in normal deliveries" (Rooks, 1997). However, by the 1930s, midwives attended only one eighth of U.S. births (Rooks, 1997).

Midwifery Outside the United States. Midwifery is seen as a standard model of care in other developed countries (Rooks, 1997). Australian and Canadian studies have demonstrated that continuity of midwifery care can lead to a significant reduction in cesarian section rates, and in the United Kingdom there is a growing use of midwifery-led, freestanding birth centers (Brodie, 2002).

A recent study of Australian midwives showed that they were underrecognized and underutilized (Brodie, 2002). In this same report, Australian midwives reported feeling "dominated by medicine" as the amount of medical intervention in pregnancy was on the rise. There was also concern raised about difficulties in keeping up skills in rural areas, due to lack of continuing education (Brodie, 2002).

In many Latin countries, there are no schools for professional midwifery, and in the poorer areas, 70–95% of births are attended by traditional midwives. Notable exceptions are Costa Rica and Chile, in which almost all births occur in hospitals, due to national campaigns (Romero, 2002). Possibly as a consequence, Chile also has the highest cesarian section rate in the world, at 40–80% (Romero, 2002). In many parts of the world, the willingness of midwives to practice in underserved areas, and to focus on prevention, education, and breast-feeding are important advantages.

Midwives in the United States. In the United States, approximately 99% of midwives are women (Rooks, 1997). A midwife provides independent care of normal pregnancies, delivery, postpartum period care, new-born care, and family planning (Schuiling & Slager, 2000). Although midwifery and medicine differ, there are some similarities as well (Rooks, 1997). Midwifery has been described as "a celebration of life" rather than a medical procedure (Romero, 2002) and the midwife tends to focus on the woman and the experience of pregnancy. Examples of midwife interventions during pregnancy include efforts for smoking cessation and domestic violence prevention. Additionally, midwives collaborate with obstetricians and try to avoid obstetric interventions when possible (Rooks, 1999).

Ideally, a pregnant woman is followed by the same midwife throughout a pregnancy, with an obstetrician providing medical review periodically during the pregnancy (Waldenstrom, 1997). A prevailing strategy is that of the "midwife as a present but nondominant force" in childbirth who has the ability to take more authority if needed (Kennedy, 2002). Hospital births attended by midwives may vary greatly in technique from those managed by obstetricians; for example, there may be fewer procedures and pain medications, more changes in position, and the woman may often drink during labor (Rooks, 1997).

In 1971, the American College of Obstetricians and Gynecologists (ACOG) endorsed the role of the nurse-midwife in maternity care, and in the past several decades, nurse-midwifery has expanded significantly (Reed & Roberts, 2000). Training, scope of practice, and licensing standards for midwives vary from state to state (Reed & Roberts, 2000; Rooks, 1997). However, national certification is necessary for the practice of nurse-midwifery in almost all states. Sixty-eight percent of nurse-midwives have a master's degree while 5% have a doctorate. In 2000, there were 45 programs accredited for training nurse-midwives (Reed & Roberts, 2000). Direct entry midwives (midwives not previously trained as nurses) are legally prohibited in nine states (Reed & Roberts, 2000), while in the majority of states, nurse-midwives may prescribe medications to patients (Reed & Roberts, 2000).

As of 1997, midwives attended 6% of U.S. births (Rooks, 1997). Native Americans have the highest percentage of midwife births, followed by African Americans and Hispanics, at much higher rates than Caucasian and Asian women (Rooks, 1997). Often, mid-wives continue to practice in underserved areas such as Appalachia, and minority and immigrant communities (Rooks, 1997). Finally, nurse-midwives' salaries are much lower than that of obstetricians (Achterberg, 1990).

Pharmacists

History and Employment Patterns. Among the health professions, pharmacy has one of the highest percentages of women in the field. With current growth trends, the proportion of women in pharmacy may eventually exceed the proportion of women in the nursing field (Francke, 1987). However, this pattern is a change from the past. Women in pharmacy practice are rather novel in the United States and the first women graduated from a college of pharmacy in 1883. This is not true in other countries. For example, in Russia and the Philippines almost all pharmacists are women (Slining, 2000). However, pharmacy schools were open to women before they were allowed into medical, dental, or law schools (Henderson, 2000). During World War II, women made up 10% of pharmacy students; this number dropped after the war ended (Henderson, 2000). In 1950, 95% of practicing pharmacists were men. This dropped to 91% in 1970 (West, 2000), and by 1983, 25% of pharmacists were women (Henderson, 2000).

Enrollment in pharmacy schools has also seen an upward trend for women. In 1950, 9.4% of enrollees were women and this increased in 1972 to 24% (West, 2000). Projected data suggest that pharmacy is currently a female-dominated profession (Francke, 1987; Henderson, 2000). There are concerns that this will lead to a shortage in the field, as women tend to work fewer years compared to men (West, 2000). This concern is partially fueled by the recruitment pitch that a career in pharmacy can allow a woman to combine work with having a family, and pharmacy can be practiced part time while still earning a good salary (West, 2000).

It has been suggested that there are many reasons why women are interested in the field of pharmacy. These include the ability to use scientific knowledge while being able to serve people. This field may be attractive to women because there is the ability to move to other fields and to specialize (Slining, 2000). It has been suggested that women pharmacists are superior in dealing with women's health issues such as gynecological, sexual, and contraceptive problems (Slining, 2000).

Academic institutions have been slow to hire female pharmacists and 50 years ago faculty were almost exclusively male. In 1973 women made up 4.8% of faculty. It is thought that women are not hired as frequently because women had not pursued Pharm.D. degrees in the past. As the female enrollment in doctorate degrees increases, the prevalence of male-dominated faculty is likely to decline (West, 2000). The first female dean of a pharmacy school was appointed in 1987, and in 2000 approximately 36% of full-time professors were women (Henderson, 2000).

Pay and Job Satisfaction. In 1981, the American Pharmaceutical Association's Task Force on Women in Pharmacy Final Report recommended that women insist on equal pay and should seek out management positions. Women earned $32.30 per hour compared to $33.50 per hour that men earned in the year 2000. The difference in pay was attributed to women working part-time, as the part-time hourly wage was lower than the full-time hourly wage (Henderson, 2000).

A 1978 study compared male and female pharmacists' salary and benefits (Shoaf & Gagnon, 1980). This study found that 29% of women worked part-time, compared to only 5% of men. There was no difference in disability insurance, sick days, or paid vacation. It was found that men had higher salaries, because they had higher level positions, such as management. Women were also less satisfied with their work compared to men—again, this was attributed to men having higher level positions (Shoaf & Gagnon, 1980).

Another study examined the perceptions of work between men and women pharmacists (Quandt & McKercher, 1982). This study found no difference in the perceived amount of time spent performing clinical activities. However, women felt that they spent more time in dispensing activities such as screening drug orders. As had been seen in previous studies, men reported a greater job satisfaction and women had a greater likelihood of leaving the profession (Quandt & McKercher, 1982).

In a study looking at career commitment (Wolfgand, 1995), no difference was found between the genders. It was found that for both men and women, there was a negative relationship between career commitment and professional recognition stress.

Other Health Professions

There are a multitude of other health professions in which women find employment. As noted in the fields already discussed, women have historically dominated some professions, while women are relative newcomers to other health professions. Health professions in which women are well represented include dentist/dental assistant, physical therapist, respiratory therapist, occupational therapist, and music therapist. These fields

are briefly discussed, although it must be noted that this is by no means a complete list of health professions that women practice.

Dentistry. Dentistry is the field that is centered on the treatment and prevention of tooth, mouth, and gum diseases. There are many different health care professionals in this field including dental hygienist, dental assistant, and dentist.

The education for dental hygienists varies from a 2-year degree to master's level work. Dental hygienists typically are responsible for performing tooth cleaning, assistance with x-rays, and initially obtaining patient histories. While dentistry is a fast-growing occupational area for women, barriers to job advancement and career satisfaction may continue to occur for women entering these professions. Garvin and Sledge (1992) found that almost 27% of dental hygienists reported sexual harassment, with the majority reporting their employer/dentist as the perpetrator. Patients were responsible for 37% of the incidents reported in this study.

Dental assistants are, in general, responsible for managing the office, recordkeeping, and sterilizing equipment. They usually would have participated in a dental assistant program at a community college level.

To become a dentist, one must complete undergraduate level coursework and then graduate from a dental school. Dentists can then choose to specialize in one of eight fields including orthodontics and periodontics. It has been noted that as recently as the 1960s women in dentistry were expected to enter certain areas of the profession, such as maternity and child welfare services (Stewart & Drummond, 2000). Initially, women were more common only in the supporting dental fields such as dental hygienist. Recent data show that women make up 38% of dental school students and approximately 14% of active practitioners. Scarbecz and Ross (2002) recently studied gender differences in the motivation of dental school students. This study found that female students ranked people-oriented motives higher than their male counterparts. Male students felt that self-employment and business-related reasons were more important. Both male and female students rated financial gains and flexibility of career as being equally important.

Solomon and Hayes (1995) evaluated gender differences and type of practice of pediatric dentists. This study specifically evaluated stage of career as well, by classifying participants into groups of early career (1–5 years in practice) versus established career (>10 years). In the early career group, more men were in private practice whereas more women were faculty at dental schools. In the established career group, more men were group practice owners and women were more likely to be in a solo practice.

In a study of job satisfaction of women dentists, 80% of respondents reported that they were satisfied with their career (Price, 1990), and that they had a good working relationship with male and female colleagues and their staff.

In studies looking at career patterns of female dentists, it has been found that women are more likely than men to take breaks during their career (Newton, Buck, & Gibbons, 2001; Newton, Thorogood, & Gibbons, 2000). The median length of career break taken by a woman dentist has been reported to be 9 months, that of hygienists 11 months, and that of dental assistants 11.5 months (Newton et al., 2000, 2001). Almost 61% of women dentists take a career break whereas only 27% of men do. Most of the career breaks taken by women dentists are for childcare reasons. It has also been noted that female dentists who take a break are expected to have a 25% shorter career life than those who do not (Newton et al., 2000, 2001).

Physical Therapists. Physical therapy is the discipline where scientific physical procedures are used to treat people with disabilities or diseases with the goal of functional recovery. Physical therapists work in a variety of locations including hospitals, rehabilitation centers, nursing homes, clinics, and in private practice. This type of treatment started in ancient times, and there are records of this being used by ancient Greeks and Romans. Modern physical therapy started in the 19th century in Britain, and became popular in the United States shortly after its start in Britain. The field was female dominated and most graduates from physical therapy school during that time were young women. The numbers of indiduals in the field dramatically increased after World War II secondary to the increased demand. Physical therapy had shown impressive results in the treatment of those injured in battle.

Rozier, Raymond, Goldstein, and Hamilton (1998) evaluated career success of 1,906 men and women physical therapists. It was found that family issues are the primary factor responsible for success or lack of success in the career of physical therapy. Specifically, success for female physical therapists appears to depend largely on their family responsibilities (Rozier et al., 1998).

Respiratory Therapists. Respiratory therapists are often critical in the care of patients suffering from breathing disorders. The majority of respiratory therapists are women. They treat all ages, from premature infants, who have immature lung function, to adults with chronic lung diseases. Approximately 80% of respiratory therapists work in hospitals, while others work in doctor's offices and in home care settings. Respiratory therapists play a role in evaluation of respiratory disorders including testing as well as treating the disorders with oxygen, aerosols, and chest physiotherapy (which is used to loosen mucus from the lungs).

Respiratory therapists, on average, work 35–40 hours per week. Their training is varied and qualifications may include specific degrees, or certificate programs. Most states have licensure requirements for respiratory therapists. There is an expected future increase in employment opportunities for respiratory therapists, due to an increase of middle-aged and elderly Americans, many of whom may develop chronic obstructive pulmonary disease (COPD), pneumonia, or cardiac conditions with pulmonary complications (U.S. Department of Labor, 2003).

Occupational Therapists. Women have traditionally been the primary caregivers of children and those with disabilities; and they dominate the field of occupational therapy (Froehlich, 1992). In fact, 93–95% of occupational therapists are women (Froehlich, 1992; Miller, 1992). However, male occupational therapists have traditionally been better paid and have held proportionally more roles of administration than their female counterparts (Miller, 1992).

Occupational therapists believe in the importance of meaningful work to the overall well-being of patients, and work with patients to empower them (Froehlich, 1992). They must work against prevailing negative attitudes of the population against persons with disabilities.

Music Therapists. The great majority of music therapists are women (Lathom, 1982). While they are found in many health care sectors, a large percentage of music therapists work in psychiatric facilities (Lathom, 1982).

Music therapists treat patients using "the marriage of science and art for the purpose of healing" (White, 2001). Musical healing has been used in the United States since the late 1700s (White, 2001). In the late 1800s, music recordings were used to help with sleep and surgery-related anxiety and anesthesia (White, 2001). In 1926, Isa Maud Ilsen, a nurse, established the National Association for Music in Hospitals (White, 2001). In the 1940s, music was used to treat wounded and "shell-shocked" veterans, as well as patients undergoing dental procedures (White, 2001).

Music therapists use music to "bring about changes from undesirable, unhealthful, and uncomfortable conditions to more acceptable states" (White, 2001). Music is selected for specific elements including rhythm, harmony, and melody (White, 2001). For example, lower pitched music can decrease tension, and some music can bring up memories (White, 2001). Studies have established that music therapy can cause changes in respiration, heart rate, blood pressure, pain, nausea, and anxiety (White, 2001).

CONCLUSIONS

Women in the health professions today are a powerful force, delivering a vast array of services in a variety of settings. The entry of women into formerly male-dominated professions is changing the face of medicine for both patients and health care providers. In traditionally female-dominated professions such as nursing and midwifery, issues of empowerment and autonomy are increasingly emphasized. In many instances, women patients prefer to be cared for by women providers, and women patients are more likely to share information with their women health care providers regarding such sensitive and stigmatized issues as domestic violence and addictions. Over time, this is likely to lead to improved health care for women and their families.

A number of challenges exist for women in the health professions including barriers to career access (e.g., there are still few women physicians in surgical specialties) and multiple job stressors. Some career stressors for women in the health professions are similar to those experienced by male colleagues such as long and unpredictable hours and corporate downsizing. Other stressors are particularly profound for women, such as balancing the multiple demands of parenting and career. Finally, the gains made by women in the health professions have not been equally distributed, with women of color still grossly underrepresented in the greatest areas of growth.

References

Achterberg, J. (1990). Women as health-care provider: Realities of the marketplace. In J. Achterberg (Ed.), *Woman as healer* (pp. 171–187). Boston, MA: Shambhala.

American College of Cardiology. (1998). The ACC professional life survey: Career decisions of women and men in cardiology. A report of the committee on women in cardiology. *Journal of the American College of Cardiology, 32*, 827–835.

American Medical Association. (1997/1998). *Physician characteristics and distribution in the U.S.* Chicago: Author.

Barnett, R. C., & Baruch, G. K. (1987). Social roles, gender and psychological distress. In R. C. Barnett, L. Biener, & G. K. Baruch (Eds.), *Gender and stress* (pp. 122–143). New York: Free Press.

Becker, J. E. (2002). What's a smart woman like you doing at home? *Obstetrics and Gynecology, 99*(5), 832–834.

Brodie, P. (2002). Addressing the barriers to midwifery—Australian midwives speaking out. *Australian Journal of Midwifery, 15*(3), 5–14.

Bruder, P. (2001). Verbal abuse of female nurses: An American medical form of gender apartheid? *Hospital Topics, 79*(4), 30–34.

Castledine, G. (1983). Opening the gates on gender traits. *Nursing Mirror, 156*(15), 16.

Chin, E. L. (2002). Historical perspective. In E. L. Chin (Ed.), *This side of doctoring*. Thousand Oaks, CA: Sage.

Chur-Hansen, A. (2002). Preferences for female and male nurses: The role of age, gender and previous experience—year 2000 compared with 1984. *Journal of Advanced Nursing, 37*(2), 192–198.

Clancy, C. M. (2000). Gender issues in women's health. In M. D. Goldman & M. C. Hatch (Eds.), *Women and health* (p. 52). San Diego, CA: Academic Press.

Collins, R. L., Gollnisch, G., & Morsheimer, E. T. (1998). Work stress, coping, and substance use among female nurses. In D. L. Wetherington & A. B. Roman (Eds.), *Drug addiction research and the health of women: Executive summary* (pp. 319–337). Washington, DC: National Institutes of Health, National Institute on Drug Abuse.

Council on Graduate Medical Education. (1995). *Women in medicine*. Rockville, MD: U.S. Department of Health and Human Services.

Cull, W. L., Mulvey, H. J., O'Connor, K. G., Sowell, D. R., Berkowitz, C. D., & Britton, C. V. (2002). Pediatricians working part-time: Past, present, and future. *Pediatrics, 109*(6), 1015–1020.

Davis, K., Scott Collins, K., & Schoen, C. (2000). Women's health and managed care. In M. D. Goldman & M. C. Hatch (Eds.), *Women and health* (pp. 55–63). San Diego, CA: Academic Press.

Dickstein, L. J. (1996). Overview of women physicians in the United States. In D. Ware (Ed.), *Women in medical education: An anthology of experience*. NY: State University of New York Press.

Ehrenreich, B., & English, D. (1973). *Witches, midwives, and nurses*. Old Westbury, NY: Feminist Press.

Epstein, L. C. (2002). Sex differences in career progression and satisfaction in an academic medical center. *Journal of the American Medical Women's Association, 57*, 195–207.

Flores, G. (2002). Mad scientists, compassionate healers, and greedy egotists: The portrayal of physicians in the movies. *Journal of the National Medical Association, 94*(7), 635–658.

Francke, G. N. (1987). Women in a changing profession. *American Journal of Hospital Pharmacy, 44*(12), 2708.

Franks, P., & Clancy, C. M. (1993). Physician gender bias in clinical decision making: Screening for cancer in primary care. *Medical Care, 31*, 213–218.

Friedman, E. (1994). *An unfinished revolution: Women and health care in America* (p. 285). United Hospital Fund of New York.

Froehlich, J. (1992). Proud and visible as occupational therapists. *American Journal of Occupational Therapy, 46*(11), 1042–1044.

Fye, W. B. (2002). President's page: Women cardiologists: Why so few? *Journal of the American College of Cardiology, 40*(2), 384–386.

Garratt, R. A. (2001). The midwife as healer. *Complementary Therapies in Nursing and Midwifery, 7*(4), 197–201.

Garvin, C., & Sledge, S. (1992). Sexual harassment within dental offices in Washington State. *Journal of Dental Hygiene, 66*(4), 178–184.

Gary, D. L. (2002). The why and wherefore of empowerment: The key to job satisfaction and professional advancement. *Nursing Forum, 32*(3), 33–36.

Grumbach, K. (2002). Women in medicine: A four-nation comparison. *Journal of the American Medical Women's Association, 57,* 185–190.

Hart-Brothers, E. (1994). Contributions of women of color to the health care of America. In E. Friedman (Ed.), *An unfinished revolution: Women and health care in America* (p. 285). United Hospital Fund of New York.

Henderson, M. L. (2000). Women in pharmacy: Twenty-five years of growth. *The Annals of Pharmacotherapy, 34,* 943–946.

Jonasson, O. (2002). Leaders in American surgery: Where are the women? *Surgery, 131,* 672–675.

Kennedy, H. P. (2002). The midwife as an "instrument" of care. *American Journal of Public Health, 92*(11), 1759–1760.

Lathom, W. B. (1982). Survey of current functions of a music therapist. *Journal of Music Therapy, 19*(1), 2–27.

Lee, C., Duxbury, L., & Higgen, C. (1994). *Employed mothers: Balancing work and family life.* Ottawa: Canadian Center for Management Development.

Letvak, S. (2001). Nurses as working women. *Association of Operating Room Nurses Journal, 73*(3), 675–682.

Levin, B. (1988). *Women and medicine: Pioneers meeting the challenge* (2nd ed.). Lincoln, NE: Media.

Libbus, M. K., & Bowman, K. G. (1994). Sexual harassment of female registered nurses in hospitals. *Journal of Nursing Administration, 24*(6), 26–31.

Linzer, M., McMurray, J. E., Visser, M. R. M., Oort, F. J., Smets, E. M. A., & DeHaes, H. C. J. M. (2002). Sex differences in physician burnout in the United States and the Netherlands. *Journal of the American Medical Women's Association, 57*(4), 191–193.

Lurie, N., Slater, J., McGovern, P., Ekstrum, J., Quam, I., & Margolis, K. (1993). Preventative care for women. Does the sex of the physician matter? *New England Journal of Medicine, 329,* 478–482.

Magnussen, L. (1998). Women's choices: An historical perspective of nursing as a career choice. *Journal of Professional Nursing, 14*(3), 175–183.

Manson, J. A., Rockhill, B., Resnick, M., Shore, E., Nadelson, C., Horner, M., et al. (2002). Sex differences in career progress and satisfaction in an academic medical center. *Journal of the American Medical Women's Association, 57*(4), 194.

McMurray, J. E., Cohen, M., Angus, G., Harding, J., Gavel, P., Horvath, J., et al. (2002). Women in medicine: A four-nation comparison. *Journal of the American Medical Women's Asociation, 57*(4), 185–190.

Messing, K. (1997). Women's occupational health: a critical review and discussion of current issues. *Women Health, 25*(4), 39–68.

Messing K. (2000). Multiple roles and complex exposures: Hard to pin down risks for working women. In M. D. Goldman & M. C. Hatch (Eds.), *Women & health* (pp. 455–461). San Diego, CA: Academic Press.

Miller, R. J. (1992). Interwoven threads: Occupational therapy, feminism, and holistic health. *American Journal of Occupational Therapy, 46*(11), 1013–1019.

Muldoon, O. T., & Kremer, J. M. (1995). Career aspirations, job satisfaction, and gender identity in female student nurses. *Journal of Advanced Nursing, 21*(3), 544–550.

Newton, J., Buck, D., & Gibbons, D. (2001). Workforce planning in dentistry: The impact of shorter and more varied career patterns. *Community Dental Health, 18*(4), 236–241.

Newton, J., Thorogood, N., & Gibbons, D. (2000). The work patterns of male and female dental practitioners in the United Kingdom. *International Dental Journal, 50*(2), 61–68.

Nora, L. M. (2002). Academic medicine gets a poor report card—what are we going to do? *Academic Medicine, 77*(10), 1062–1066.

Palepu, A., & Herbert, C. P. (2002). Medical women in academia: The silences we keep. *Canadian Medical Association Journal, 167,* 877–879.

Price, S. (1990). A profile of women dentists. *Journal of the American Dental Association, 120*(4), 403–408.

Quandt, W. G., & McKercher, P. L. (1982). Perceptions of work among men and women pharmacists in nonadministrative positions. *American Journal of Hospital Pharmacy, 32*(11), 1948–1951.

Reed, A., & Roberts, J. E. (2000). State regulation of midwives: Issues and options. *Journal of Midwifery and Women's Health, 45*(2), 130–149.

Romero, L. C. (2002). Midwifery in Mexico. *Midwifery Today International Midwife, 63,* 47–50.

Rooks, J. P. (1997). *Midwifery and childbirth in America.* Philadelphia: Temple University Press.

Rooks, J. P. (1999). The midwifery model of care. *Journal of Nurse-Midwifery, 44*(4), 370–374.

Rosenstein, A. H., Russell, H., & Lauve, R. (2002). Disruptive physician behavior contributes to nursing shortage. *Physician Executive, 28*(6), 8–11.

Ross, J. A. (2002). Looming public health crisis: The nursing shortage of today. *Journal of Perianesthesia Nursing, 17*(5), 337–340.

Roter, D., Lipkin, M., & Korgnard, A. (1991). Sex differences in patients and physicians communication during primary care medical visits. *Medical Care, 29,* 1083–1093.

Rozier, C. K., Raymond, M. J., Goldstein, M. S., & Hamilton, B. L., (1998). Gender and physical therapy career success factors. *Physical Therapy, 78*(7), 690–704.

Salsberg, E. S., & Forte, G. J. (2002). Trends in the physician workforce, 1980–2000. *Health Affairs, 21*(5), 165–173.

Scarbecz, M., & Ross, J. (2002). Gender differences in first-year dental students' motivation to attend dental school. *Journal of Dental Education, 66*(8), 952–961.

Schuiling, K. D., & Slager, J. (2000). Scope of practice: Freedom within limits. *Journal of Midwifery and Women's Health, 45*(6), 465–471.

Scott, H. (2002). The nursing profession must be more assertive over pay. *British Journal of Nursing, 11*(19), 1228.

Shoaf, P. R., & Gagnon, J. P. (1980). A comparison of female and male pharmacists' employment benefits, salary, and job satisfaction. *Contemporary Pharmacy Practice, 3*(1), 47–51.

Slining, J. (2000). Women's role in pharmacy practice in the year 2000. *The Annals of Pharmacotherapy, 34,* 950–954.

Solomon, E., & Hayes, M. (1995). Gender and the transition into practice. *Journal of Dental Education, 59*(8), 836–840.

Sonnad, S. S., & Colletti, L. M. (2002). Issues in the recruitment and success of women in academic surgery. *Surgery, 132*(2), 415–419.

Spickard, A., Gabbe, S. G., & Christensen, J. F. (2002). Mid-career burnout in generalist and specialist practices. *Journal of the American Medical Association, 288*(12), 1447–1450.

Stellman, J. M., & Lucas, A. (2000). Women's occupational health: International perspectives. In M. D. Goldman & M. C. Hatch (Eds.), *Women & health* (pp. 514–522). San Diego, CA: Academic Press.

Stewart, F., & Drummond, J. (2000). Women and the world of dentistry. *British Dental Journal, 188*(1), 7–8.

Tierney, D., Romito, P., & Messing, K. (1990). She ate not the bread of idleness: Exhaustion is related to domestic and salaried work of hospital workers in Quebec. *Women Health, 16*, 21–42.

United States Department of Health and Human Services, Public Health Service, Centers for Disease Control, National Center for Health Statistics. (1989). *Health characteristics of workers by occupation and sex: United States, 1983–85* (Adv. Data, No. 168). Washington, DC: Author.

United States Department of Labor, Bureau of Labor Statistics. (1988). *Labor force statistics derived from the current population survey, 1948–87* (Bulletin 2307, pp. 195–300). Washington, DC: U.S. Government Printing Office.

United States Department of Labor, Bureau of Labor Statistics. (1997). *Employment and earnings.* Washington, DC: U.S. Government Printing Office.

United States Department of Labor, *Occupational outlook handbook.* Bureau of Labor Statistics. (2003). Respiratory therapists. Retrieved April 7, 2003, from www.bls.gov/oco/ocos084.htm

Verbrugge, L. M., & Steiner, R. P. (1981). Physician treatment of men and women patients: Sex bias or appropriate care? *Medical Care, 19*, 609–632.

Wagener, D. K., Walstedt, J., Jenkins, L., Burnett, C., Lalich, N., & Fingerhut, M. (1997). *Women: Work and health* (DHHS Publication No. PHS 97-1415). *Vital Health Statistics, 3*(31), 1–91.

Waldenstrom, U. (1997). Challenges and issues for midwifery. *Australian College of Midwives Incorporated Journal, 10*(3), 11–17.

Wallace, A. E., & Weeks, W. B. (2002). Differences in income between male and female primary care physicians. *Journal of the American Medical Women's Association, 57*(4), 180–184.

Welstedt, J. (2000). Employment patterns and health among U.S. working women. In M. D. Goldman & M. C. Hatch (Eds.), *Women & health* (pp. 447–454). San Diego, CA: Academic Press.

West, S. (2000). Women in pharmacy: Some predictions for women students and faculty. *The Annals of Pharmacotherapy, 34*, 947–949.

White, J. M. (2001). Music as intervention. *Nursing Clinics of North America, 36*(1), 83–92.

Wolfgand, A. P. (1995). Job stress, coworker social support, and career commitment: A comparison of female and male pharmacists. *Journal of Social Behavior and Personality, 10*(6), 149–160.

Zawacki, R. A., Shahan, R., & Carey, M. (1995). Who has higher job satisfaction: Male or female nurses? *Nursing Management, 26*(1), 54–55.

Suggested Resources

United Nations. (1995). 1992 statistics projected to 1995. Sex and age distribution of the world's population. www.un.org

United States Bureau of Census, Population Division. (1999). United States population estimates by age, sex, race, and Hispanic origin, 1990–1997. Retrieved July 1999, from www.census.gov/population/estimates/nation

Women in the Workforce

Lorann Stallones

Historically, women have been found working in six key tasks in a majority of societies: provision of food; care of the home; child care; nursing the sick; teaching; and manufacture of clothing. As women have moved into wage labor, they often have been found to perform these same activities in a commercial form, that is, tasks that are centered around care of and service to others. Vast numbers of women are found working as teachers, nurses, cleaners, and garment makers. Women also are likely to work indoors at work considered to be lighter than men's work. Often the jobs involved are considered clean and safe and are physically undemanding, repetitive in nature, and boring. Some jobs require dexterity, but not skill; and often jobs lack mobility, with women working in one particular workstation for long hours. As a result of the perception that women are working in safe environments, studies have not focused on the hazards encountered in those work sites. The work of women has traditionally been viewed as marginal and temporary, with the expectation that they would leave paid employment once they married and began child-rearing. This perception has had a marked impact on the inclusion of women in studies of occupational hazards. There is limited information about the occupational hazards related to those occupations where women have been the majority of workers.

Division of labor within factories, offices, schools, and hospitals has evolved into sexual division of tasks with distinct patterns of segregation that are somewhat masked by the manner in which information is reported in labor statistics. Although there has been a marked decline in the number of occupations that completely excluded one sex or the other, there is an increased likelihood that men will work in occupations where coworkers will be predominately men. While women are gradually making inroads into occupations that have previously been male dominated, a similar trend of males entering female-dominated occupations has not been as evident. This results in a persistent pattern of gendered work segregation. Men may work in environments where there are few women, but women rarely work in environments where there are more women than men. Traditional jobs that women have held have often become mechanized, and have moved from a domestic activity to a marketplace activity. Often, as a result the jobs then become men's work rather than women's work. An example of this would be the transformation of sewing done by women as seamstresses in their homes to factories devoted to sewing where men operate the large equipment. Work of higher status and higher pay has traditionally been men's work and as certain jobs are upgraded, that work becomes men's work. Women's entry into work that has been traditionally held by men has the opposite effect, salaries decline, and the status of the occupation similarly declines. Gender differences in the workplace are of two types, employment conditions (salaries, work hours, length of contracts, and benefits) and job content. These differences influence women's occupational health and safety.

In the United States in 2001, there were 43.6 million women aged 16 years and older working full time. This represents about 60% of women in those age groups. These women comprised 44% of the total workforce of full-time workers. An additional 14 million women were employed part time. Women represented 68% of the part-time workforce. One of the most notable issues to consider in the health and safety of women working in the United States is the continued discrepancy between salaries of men and of women. Table 1 contains data on the number of women employed in specific occupations, the percentage of the total workforce they represent, and their weekly median income, contrasted to that of the men in the same occupational categories. Traditional women's jobs have been defined as those that include 75% or more of the workers. Using that definition, there are not any major occupational categories except administrative support services that would be considered traditionally women's work. There are occupations within the major groupings where the work would be considered women's work, notably registered nurses and health technicians, including licensed practical nurses. In those occupational groups, women's median weekly incomes are below men's median weekly incomes. In occupations where women comprise more than 50% of the group, professional specialties, administrative support including clerical workers, and service occupations, median weekly incomes for women are below incomes of their male counterparts. However, there does not appear to be a correlation between the percentage of women in any occupational category and the magnitude of salary differential

between women and men. For example, among equipment operators women comprise only 5% of the workforce, but their salary is 90% of men's salaries, while among nurses women comprise 91% of the workforce and their salaries are 88% of men's. The greatest differential in salaries is seen in the sales occupations, where women comprise 45% of the total workforce and their salaries are 62% of their male counterparts. Although studies of the distribution of diseases in populations have consistently associated lower income with poorer health status, the extent to which income differentials contribute to occupational illness and disease outcomes among women has not been assessed in a comprehensive manner. Access to high-quality medical care services is influenced by the ability to pay. For example, if women's salaries are lower than men's a larger portion of their income goes to paying medical insurance. Conversely, if women are employed part time they may not receive medical insurance as a benefit of their employment and will have to pay out of pocket for medical care. This coupled with the perception that women's work environments are safe and healthy results in little exchange about workplace between a woman and a physician when a woman does seek medical attention. As women move into more nontraditional work settings, the absence of occupational medicine training among primary care physicians will only serve to exacerbate the problem of correctly attributing diseases to working conditions.

Within major occupational groupings there are a large number of specific occupational titles. Several of the categories will be described. Managerial and professional specialties include financial managers, personnel and labor relations, purchasing managers, educational administrators, medicine and health managers, real estate managers, funeral directors, accountants, auditors, financial officers, buyers, purchasing agents, and construction inspectors. Professional specialties include architects, engineers, surveyors, computer system analysts, mathematical scientists, chemists, atmospheric scientists, geologists, physicians, dentists, veterinarians, registered nurses, pharmacists, dieticians, respiratory therapists, occupational therapists, physical therapists, teachers, librarians, economists, psychologists, social workers, recreation workers, clergy, lawyers, musicians, actors, photographers, dancers, public relations specialists, and athletes. Technicians and related support include clinical laboratory technicians, dental hygienists, radiological technicians, licensed practical nurses, electrical technicians, engineering technicians,

Women in the Workforce

Table 1. Median weekly earnings among full-time employed women aged 16 years and older by occupation, percentage of workforce, and percentage of median male weekly income, United States, 2001[a]

Occupation[b]	Total number of women	Women as percentage of total workforce	Women's weekly median income ($)	Women's income percentage of men's median income
Total	43,671,000	44	511	76
Managerial	15,956,000	49	732	70
Professional	8,510,000	52	749	73
Chemists	54,000	36	800	74
Physicians	161,000	32	958	70
Registered nurses	1,459,000	91	820	88
Therapists	246,000	71	782	96
Teachers—college	244,000	37	844	75
Teachers—except college	3,232,000	73	707	91
Technicians and related support	1,883,000	50	580	74
Health technicians	1,099,000	79	534	76
Engineering technicians	187,000	20	608	82
Science technicians	98,000	41	558	81
Technicians, other[c]	499,000	41	705	74
Sales occupations	4,574,000	45	429	62
Administrative support including clerical	10,954,000	77	469	81
Service	5,812,000	52	335	76
Farming, forestry, fishing	222,000	15	308	84
Precision production, craft and repair	1,012,000	8	479	74
Mechanics/repairers	201,000	5	594	89
Construction trades	94,000	2	437	72
Operators, fabricators, and laborers	3,258,000	22	368	73
Machine operators	2,119,000	35	369	72
Production inspectors	329,000	50	400	67
Transportation and material moving occupations	356,000	8	439	75
Motor vehicle operators	299,000	9	422	71
Equipment operators	51,000	5	486	90
Handlers, equipment cleaners	783,000	20	342	85

[a] Data from the United States Bureau of Labor Statistics.
[b] Occupations listed under the major headings are representative of the types of occupations included but do not include all possible occupations under the major grouping, therefore the numbers will not sum.
[c] Includes airplane pilots, navigators, legal assistants, and computer programmers.

biological technicians, chemical technicians, airplane pilots and navigators, broadcast equipment operators, computer programmers, tool programmers, and legal assistants. Sales includes insurance, real estate, securities and financial services, advertising, mining, manufacturing, wholesale, motor vehicle and boat sales, apparel, furniture, appliances, parts, news vendors, and models. Clearly the broad occupational categories reflect a wide array of hazards, some unrelated to others within the broader occupational group, others closely related to categories found within other occupational groupings. For example, dentists and dental technicians, and chemists and chemical technicians are more likely to have similar exposures to hazards than to other categories within the broad heading of professional or technical specialties. For this reason, within Table 1, some of the specific occupational groups are presented under the major occupational category.

Table 2. Number and median weekly earnings of part-time employed workers aged 16 years and over by selected characteristics, United States, 2001[a]

Characteristic	Number of men	Men's median weekly income ($)	Number of women	Women's median weekly income ($)	Women's income percentage of men's median income
Age					
16–24	3,590,000	140	4,538,000	136	97
25+	3,077,000	219	9,721,000	218	99
Race/ethnicity					
White	5,575,000	168	12,452,000	187	111
Black	722,000	160	1,240,000	175	109
Hispanic	712,000	185	1,266,000	179	97

[a] Data from the United States Bureau of Labor Statistics.

Table 2 contains information about the part-time employed workforce. Among part-time workers, women comprise 68% of the total workforce. Benefits are not usually available for part-time workers, therefore women are less likely than men to be employed in circumstances that would provide full access to medical care and disability insurance as part of their employment. Among part-time workers, women who are Caucasian and African American receive higher salaries than their male counterparts, but women who are Hispanic receive lower salaries. This may be due to the length of time women are employed as part-time workers. Women may leave the workforce to raise their children and then return to part-time work as their children get older.

OCCUPATIONAL INJURIES AND ILLNESSES

Annually, the United States Bureau of Labor Statistics publishes data on the number of nonfatal occupational illnesses and injuries that occurred, which required the person to miss days of work. For women the common injuries by frequency are sprains and strains (47%), bruises and contusions (10%), soreness and pain (8%), fractures (6%), cuts, lacerations, and punctures (4%), multiple injuries (3%), carpal tunnel syndrome (3%), back pain and tendonitis (3%), heat burns (1%), chemical burns (<1%), and amputations (<1%). Table 3 contains the numbers of injuries and illnesses and rates per 1,000 by occupation and a comparison between women and men. While women have long been described as safer workers than men, in 16 of the

28 occupational categories presented, their rates are higher than the rates for their male counterparts. In five of the occupational groupings women's rates were more than two times greater than men's rates of injury and illness. These occupations were physicians, registered nurses, therapists, college teachers, and sales occupations.

The majority of information available from the Bureau of Labor Statistics is related to occupational injuries, not occupational illnesses. Acute episodes of trauma, back pain, and chemical burns are far easier to link with the workplace than are illnesses that develop over long periods. Other types of data collection systems are necessary to access information about occupational illnesses.

Although the majority of information available about occupational illnesses and injuries relates to the occupation of the individuals, there are also data on the industry in which someone is employed. The industry influences hazardous exposures in a significant manner. For example, a clerical worker may work in a manufacturing plant, in a library, or at home. Conversely, a nurse working in home health care or in a public health department may experience very different exposures than a nurse working in a hospital. Similarly, within the hospital a surgical nurse will be exposed to different hazards than a nurse working as a supervisor on the pediatric floor. Therefore, data are sometimes presented related to industry in combination with occupation or industry alone. The major industries are agriculture, mining, construction, manufacturing, transportation/public utilities, wholesale trade, retail trade and finance, insurance, and real estate. Whether information is presented by industry or by occupation,

Women in the Workforce

Table 3. Nonfatal occupational injury and illness rates per 1,000 full-time workers involving days away from work among women and men, 2000[a]

Occupation	Women—Number of illnesses/ injuries	Women's illness/injury rate per 1,000	Men—Number of illnesses/ injuries	Men's illness/injury rate per 1,000	Rate ratio (female:male)
Total	555,722	12.72	1,097,104	19.62	0.64
Managerial	64,346	4.03	34,552	2.12	1.90
Professional	43,403	5.10	16,103	2.03	2.51
Chemists	48	0.89	62	0.64	1.39
Physicians	170	1.06	131	0.39	2.72
Registered nurses	22,047	15.11	2,408	16.61	0.91
Therapists	3,066	12.46	564	5.64	2.21
Teachers—college	68	0.28	48	0.11	2.54
Teachers—except college	4,936	1.53	1,192	1.00	1.53
Technicians and related support	154,620	13.66	98,036	11.03	1.23
Health technicians	21,256	19.34	5,895	20.33	0.95
Engineering technicians	916	4.90	5,057	6.87	0.71
Science technicians	1,439	14.68	1,297	9.33	1.57
Technicians, other	2,097	4.20	8,383	11.91	0.35
Sales	62,380	13.64	36,082	6.44	2.11
Administrative support including clerical	66,515	6.07	41,322	12.66	0.48
Service	180,091	30.99	96,167	18.04	1.72
Farming, forestry, fishing	6,984	31.46	34,540	27.17	1.16
Precision production, craft, and repair	18,933	18.71	278,522	25.28	0.74
Mechanics/repairers	3,716	18.49	102,768	9.33	1.98
Construction trades	2,531	26.92	127,629	28.96	0.93
Operators, fabricators, and laborers	128,937	39.58	550,096	48.64	0.81
Machine operators	46,846	22.11	111,039	28.08	0.79
Production inspectors	5,604	17.03	5,813	18.00	0.95
Transportation and material moving occupations	17,273	48.52	171,832	41.41	1.17
Motor vehicle operators	14,990	50.13	144,992	48.27	1.04
Equipment operators	2,087	40.92	25,050	25.02	1.63
Handlers, equipment cleaners	42,310	54.04	214,158	66.78	0.81

[a] Data from the United States Bureau of Labor Statistics.

the assumption that specific exposures have occurred or have not occurred to individuals must be viewed with caution. Table 4 contains the occupational injury and illness rates among women and men based on industry codes rather than occupational codes. From this comparison, women would be viewed as far less likely to report occupational injuries when contrasted with their male counterparts. However, those comparisons include such a wide difference in actual job tasks that the conclusion would be suspect, especially when compared with the results presented in Table 3.

TOXICOLOGY

Acute toxicity testing of xenobiotics has usually been conducted in test animals of a single sex in order to conserve animals. Differences in metabolism, transformation, and toxicity by sex have been documented in rats, mice, and humans. Sensitivity to the lethality of xenobiotics has also been described with female rats being more sensitive than males in some cases, but for others, male rats were more sensitive. Little evidence has accumulated in human research to provide

Table 4. Rates of nonfatal occupational injuries and illnesses involving days away from work per 1,000 workers by sex and industry, 1996[a]

Industry	Rate among women	Rate among men	Ratio female:male
Agriculture	9.7	11.0	0.88
Mining	4.3	29.9	0.14
Construction	5.5	24.9	0.22
Manufacturing	17.5	24.8	0.71
Transportation	15.6	29.3	0.53
Wholesale trade and retail trade	12.6	22.1	0.57
Finance, insurance, real estate	4.6	6.3	0.73
Services	9.9	10.1	0.98

[a] Data from the United States Bureau of Labor Statistics.

evidence of specific examples in which these differences have ultimately been linked with different disease outcomes, with the exception of effects that are gender specific, such as menstrual dysfunction.

OCCUPATIONAL CANCERS

Almost every type of cancer has been linked with occupational exposures, but certain cancers such as leukemia and cancers of the lung, bladder, and brain appear to be more strongly related to occupational exposures. These associations appear to be similar for women as for men. Breast cancer and tumors of the female reproductive system have been less well studied and cannot be evaluated in studies where women have been excluded. Long-term follow-up studies are required to determine the association between occupational cancers and chemical exposures; however, these studies have typically included only men.

Leukemia among women has been associated with exposure to benzene, solvents, vinyl chloride, antineoplastic drugs, and x-ray machines. Lung cancer in women has been associated with exposure to asbestos, mercury, environmental tobacco smoke, solvents, arsenic, chromium, nickel, and polycyclic aromatic hydrocarbons. Bladder cancer among women has been associated with dyes, metals, and other chemicals. Brain cancer has been found to be elevated among women employed in electronics industries, textile industries, candy manufacturing, construction industries, the telephone industry, and grain farming. Working women at

high risk of breast cancer include teachers, nurses, other health care workers, chemists, airline attendants, and physicians. Increased risk of ovarian cancer has been found among women employed as chemists, engineers, in laboratories, cosmetologists, teachers, carpenters and woodworkers, and those in textile manufacturing, stone, clay, and glasswork, dry cleaning, telephone operation, and nursing. Women exposed to herbicides have been reported to have an increased risk of ovarian cancer.

Table 5 contains an abbreviated list of industries and occupations where specific exposures have been associated with cancers in women. Due to the overlap of exposures associated with adverse reproductive outcomes, both are included in the same table.

OCCUPATIONAL REPRODUCTIVE HAZARDS

Normal reproductive function in women requires integration and proper functioning of the hypothalamic–pituitary–ovarian axis (HPOA). Disruption of the HPOA can result in lack of menses, menstrual irregularity, or reduced fertility. A number of toxics in the workplace may act on the HPOA, including lead, mercury, carbon disulfide, formaldehyde, tetrachloroethylene, toluene, estrogens, anesthetic gases, nitrous oxide, antineoplastic drugs, ethylene oxide, cadmium, pesticides, and solvents. Physical agents that have been associated with adverse reproductive health include ionizing radiation, nonionizing radiation, noise, and vibration. Biological agents that women workers may be exposed to that are associated with adverse reproductive outcomes include infectious agents such as toxoplasmosis, listeriosis, German measles, herpes, chickenpox, hepatitis B and C, cytomegalovirus infection, parvovirus infection, and HIV infection. Women may also be exposed to mycotoxins from fungi. Adverse reproductive outcomes may also result from exposure to shift work, long work hours, physical exertion, and psychosocial job stress.

Adverse reproductive outcomes that have been associated with occupational exposures among women include pregnancy-induced hypertension, spontaneous abortion, low-birthweight babies, preterm deliveries, and birth defects. Pregnancy-induced hypertension has been associated with shift work, noise, physical work, psychosocial job stress, lead, and cadmium. Spontaneous abortion has been associated with ionizing radiation, nonionizing radiation, low-frequency electromagnetic fields (EMF), contagious diseases, and all the chemicals

Women in the Workforce

Table 5. Industries and occupations and exposures to reproductive and cancer hazards

Industry/occupations	Hazardous exposure
Agriculture	Pesticides[a,b], solvents[a,b], petroleum, mycotoxins[a]
Service industries	
Cosmetology	Formaldehyde[a,b], hair dyes[a,b], standing[a]
Dry cleaning	Solvents[a,b], standing[a]
Food service	Tobacco smoke[a,b], cooking fumes[a,b], standing[a]
Health care	Antineoplastic drugs[a,b], anesthetic gases[a,b], standing[a], shift work[a,b], viruses[a,b], antibiotics[a], lifting[a], ionizing radiation[b], microwave exposure[a]
Clerical workers	Video-display terminals[a]
Flight attendants	Standing[a], viruses[a]
Manufacturing	
Computers, electronics	Lead[a], metal fumes[a,b], solvents[a,b]
Furniture	Wood dust[b], solvents[a,b], glues[b], formaldehyde[a,b]
Motor vehicle manufacturing	Paints[b], fumes[b], lead[a], solvents[a,b], machining fluids[b]
Chemical/plastics/rubber	Vinyl chloride[b], benzene[b], solvents[a,b], nitrosamines[b], fluoride[a], toluene[a,b], metals[a,b], mercury[a,b], arsenic[a,b]
Textile, apparel	Asbestos[b], dyes[b], lubricating oils[b]
Ceramics	Lead[a], chromium[a,b], cadmium[a], copper[a], cobalt[a], manganese[a]
Paint	Metal[a,b], formaldehyde[a,b], antimicrobial agents[a,b]
Slaughterhouses, canneries	Cold[a], irregular work schedules[a]

[a] Associated with adverse reproductive outcomes.
[b] Associated with cancers.
Sources: Goldman & Hatch (2001); Paul (1993).

listed in the previous paragraph. Low birthweight has been associated with microwaves, short waves, high-frequency EMF, noise, shift work, long working hours, physical exertion, and pesticides. Preterm delivery has been associated with lead, pesticides, mycotoxins, noise, shift work, physical exertion, and psychosocial job stress. Birth defects have been associated with anesthetic gases, antineoplastic drugs, solvents, pesticides, contagious diseases, and physical exertion.

Table 5 contains reproductive exposures that have been found associated with specific industries and occupations among working women.

WORK ENVIRONMENT AND TASKS

In terms of size, strength, visual acuity, and color recognition, women differ from men. These differences influence hazards in the workplace in a subtle fashion. Materials, tools, workstations, chairs, and other equipment designed for the average-sized man will not fit the ergonomic needs of the average-sized woman and may create strain that leads to injuries and cumulative trauma disorders. Biological makeup certainly influences the ability to do certain tasks; however, the structure of the workplace can influence the ability of someone to perform the work. Adaptation of workstations

by individuals may provide a better and more cost-effective mechanism for promoting health and safety than by selection of individuals with specific characteristics, especially in jobs where turnover rates are high.

Statistics are used to summarize information. In the case of occupational studies, one job title combines information that is inferred about income, training, job content (tasks and activities), and hazardous exposures. In order to define occupational health and safety hazards for women, the actual job content associated with a specific occupation or job title needs to be understood. As more work is conducted, it has been increasingly recognized that men and women with the same job title do not perform the same tasks. Therefore, the risks associated with the job title may not equally reflect the hazardous exposures for both groups.

Conditions that affect women to a greater extent than men in the workplace are closely linked to the types of work environments where women predominate. Fibromyalgia, repetitive strain injuries, "sick building syndrome," and multiple chemical sensitivity are found twice as often among women as among men. These conditions are among the most hotly contested as real illnesses, being often attributed to "hysteria" or neurosis. Mass hysteria, that is, physical symptoms suggesting an organic illness but arising from a psychological cause, has been used to explain periodic episodes of sick building syndrome when a specific exposure cannot be identified as the "cause." Females have been shown to be more exposed to factors that may increase the risk of reporting symptoms associated with sick building syndrome including tobacco smoke, working in open plan offices or reception areas, holding a lower position in the office, handling more paper, and perceiving psychosocial and physical work as being worse compared with men. In addition, women were often found living in apartment buildings, increasing the complexity of indoor air exposures from multiple sources. In most occupational health and safety research, factors outside the workplace are not considered in the exposure assessment.

PSYCHOSOCIAL JOB STRESS

Stressors that have been studied in the workplace include job insecurity, lack of control, role ambiguity, role conflict, scheduling, interpersonal conflict, work–family conflict, sexual harassment, long work hours, monotony, and boredom. Job insecurity is a concern of losing one's job due to layoffs and to downsizing. Lack of control is having no say in the tasks one performs, how they are performed, and when they must be completed. Job control is measured by a worker's ability to develop skills, to learn new things, to use creativity, to perform varied work, and to make decisions about the task and the pace of work. Role ambiguity is the uncertainty of a worker about what expectations are resulting from a lack of feedback on performance or job tasks. Role conflict is when there are expectations that are not compatible, for example, when one supervisor assumes a worker is responsible for one set of tasks and another assumes the worker is responsible for a different set of tasks and one person cannot accomplish both sets of tasks. Scheduling issues can include shift work, rotating shifts, night shifts, or inflexible schedules. Interpersonal conflict is not getting along with coworkers. Work–family conflict is complex but relates to the need to respond to family issues and to work issues where the demands cannot both be met.

The effects of stress include depression, anxiety, aggression, low self-esteem, substance abuse, physiological effects (elevated blood pressure and elevated cholesterol), and diseases (cardiovascular disease, pregnancy-induced hypertension, and preterm delivery). Studies of the relationships between job stress and health have only begun to integrate the notion that women have different types of work experiences than men and that the stressors they experience may differ or may be responded to in different ways. For women, the highest level of job control is found in gender-integrated occupations. The top stressor reported among women is interpersonal conflict, while men in the same occupation report the top stressor to be wasted work or time.

Evidence continues to accumulate that the psychosocial aspects of work differ for women and for men. However, how these differences relate to risk of distress, mental disorders, and cardiovascular diseases have not been well described among women. Social support appears to buffer the adverse effects of some occupational exposures among women. Pregnancy outcomes in relation to job stress have been shown to be better for working women in the presence of support from others. Other illnesses may benefit as well, but less work has been done assessing potential protective effects.

One area where the interaction between work and home can be demonstrated is that of workplace violence. Homicide is the leading cause of occupational traumatic death among women, comprising 42% of all traumatic injury deaths. While robbery was the primary motive of job-related homicides, domestic disputes accounted for one sixth of the workplace homicides among women workers. Almost half of the homicide victims work in retail, including grocery stores and eating and drinking establishments, common workplaces for women. The fact that domestic disputes do enter the workplace for women but not for men is an important issue when developing workplace violence prevention programs. If programs address only coworkers and clients, family violence will not be addressed.

One area that has not received a great deal of attention is the experience of women related to sexual harassment. The most extreme example would be rape and there is little written about rape in the workplace. The stress of working in an environment where harassment is accepted has not been extensively addressed in medical literature. Perhaps these issues have been viewed as legal issues, not medical ones, but clearly they are likely to have profound long-term medical consequences that are worthy of attention by occupational health professionals.

SUMMARY

While women are moving into new jobs and experiencing new exposures, information about how the hazards will affect the health and safety of the women has not been developed. The most significant difference between women's and men's work is the persistence of a salary differential. Income does influence health, through access to medical care, quality food, and safe housing. The roles women play at home also will influence their capacity to work safely. Fatigue, lack of affordable day care for children and aging parents, low salaries, inadequate design of tools and work tasks, and lack of control over work hours contribute to other hazards that are present in work environments. A more integrated approach, including social, biological, and physical exposures external to the workplace, is needed to benefit women and men who work. Care must be taken when comparing illness and injury experience between women and men or any two groups of workers, to account for actual exposures at a particular job. Use of broad industry categories may lead to erroneous conclusions about the safety risks for specific groups of workers.

SEE ALSO: Agricultural work, Cancer, Carpal tunnel syndrome, Sexual harassment, Socioeconomic status.

Suggested Resources

Bradley, H. (1989). *Men's work, women's work.* Minneapolis: University of Minnesota Press.

Drudi, D. (1997). A century-long quest for meaningful and accurate occupational injury and illness statistics. *Compensation & Working Conditions,* Winter, 19–27.

Gold, E. B., & Tomich, E. (1994). Occupational hazards to fertility and pregnancy outcome. *Occupational Medicine: State of the Art Reviews, 9,* 435–469.

Goldman, M., & Hatch, M. (Eds.). (2001). *Women & health* (pp. 441–527). San Diego, CA: Academic Press.

Hubbard, R. (1990). *The politics of women's biology.* New Brunswick, NJ: Rutgers University Press.

Infante, P. F., & Pesak, J. (1994). A historical perspective of some occupationally related diseases of women. *Journal of Occupational Medicine, 38,* 826–831.

Islam, S. S., Angela, A. M., Doyle, E. J., & Ducatman, A. M. (2001). Gender differences in work-related injury/illness: Analysis of workers compensation claims. *American Journal of Industrial Medicine, 39,* 84–91.

Messing, K. (1998). *One-eyed science: Occupational health and women workers.* Philadelphia: Temple University Press.

Paul, M. (1993). *Occupational and environmental reproductive hazards: A guide for clinicians.* Baltimore: Williams & Wilkins.

Reid, J., Ewan, C., & Lowy, E. (1991). Pilgrimage of pain: The illness experience of women with repetition strain injury and the search for credibility. *Social Science & Medicine, 32,* 601–612.

Stellman, J. M. (1994). Where women work and the hazards they may face on the job. *Journal of Occupational Medicine, 36,* 814–825.

Stenberg, B., & Wall, S. (1995). Why do women report "sick building symptoms" more often than men? *Social Science & Medicine, 40,* 491–502.

Zahm, S. H., Pottern, L. M., Lewis, D. R., Ward, M. H., & White, D. W. (1994). Inclusion of women and minorities in occupational cancer epidemiologic research. *Journal of Occupational Medicine, 36,* 842–847.

Women in Health: Advocates, Reformers, and Pioneers

Sana Loue

Throughout our history, women have played a critical role in advocating for improvements in the health and health care of not only women, but also the population as a whole. Advocacy has been defined as "taking a position on an issue, and initiating actions in a deliberate attempt to influence private and public choices" (Labonte, 1994, p. 263). Advocacy can assume multiple forms, including community organizing, coalition building, advocacy through politics, the courts, legislatures, or regulatory agencies, and advocacy through the press. These mechanisms are not mutually exclusive, and many are used simultaneously to effectuate important goals.

Other women have made significant contributions to health through their professional achievements in science and medicine. Some women have asserted the right of women to practice in a health care profession, such as Elizabeth Blackwell, who became the first female physician in the United States. Others, like Helen Brooke Taussig, were pioneers in their fields and made outstanding discoveries that led to improved health and/or health care for others.

Still other women have created significant change by acting as reformers, creating change by establishing organizations, shelters, and other institutions designed to promote health and cure disease. Although many of these reform efforts, such as those of Matilda Evans, were accomplished almost single-handedly, they brought numerous benefits to the communities and populations who were their focus.

This chapter reviews many health advocacy efforts and pioneering achievements of women. The women who are highlighted in this chapter are only a fraction of those who have worked for or advocated for improvements in health; it would be impossible to describe the efforts of so many in only one chapter. Instead, this chapter illustrates the breadth of contributions that women have made to improve health and health care and provides examples of their inspirational efforts.

WOMEN AS ORGANIZERS

Many women have been able to effectuate significant change in health and health care as a result of efforts to organize. Some of these efforts have involved efforts to organize communities. This type of organizing has been described as "the process of organizing people around problems or issues that are larger than group members' own immediate concerns" (Labonte, 1994, p. 261). Many times, community organizing utilizes a "bottom-up" approach that allows community members to direct the effort themselves. Power and empowerment are key to this process. Power allows people to predict, control and participate in their environment," while empowerment is the "process by which individuals and communities are enabled to take such power and act effectively in changing their lives and their environment" (Minkler, 1992, p. 3). Activities often associated with community organizing include small group meetings, town hall meetings, and marches and rallies.

Community organizing may sometimes evolve into the development of coalitions in order to accomplish stated goals. Oftentimes, organizing efforts evolve, as well, into the formation of new organizations, such as Mothers Against Drunk Driving (MADD), described below. Those involved in such efforts may work or volunteer in diverse fields including politics, health, and social work, to name a few.

Occupational Health

Lucy Gonzalez Parsons (1852–1942) is best known as a leftist writer and a labor organizer. Parsons had a long history, though, of political involvement. In 1872, she and her husband Albert were forced to leave Texas due to their political involvement in opposing the Jim Crow segregation laws that were being instituted at the

time. The legality of their marriage was questioned because the then-existing nonmiscegenation laws prohibited cohabitation and marriage between members of different races; Lucy was of African American and Mexican heritage and her husband was African American. When they arrived in Chicago in 1873, the country was in the midst of a depression due to high rates of unemployment. Chicago workers, in particular, were impacted by mill closings and low wages at the railroad companies. As a labor activist, Parsons supported the International Ladies' Garment Workers Union, and advocated for fair wages, equal pay for women, and an 8-hour workday. She argued vociferously against the system of involuntary servitude that was imposed on African Americans under the laws of southern states following the conclusion of the Civil War. She attributed women's enslavement by men to their lack of economic independence.

Public Health Nursing

The establishment of public health nursing as a profession has been credited to Lillian D. Wald (1867–1940). In 1893, with financial assistance from philanthropists, Wald opened the Nurses Settlement in New York. She expanded its services to include nurses' training, educational programs for the community, and youth clubs and, eventually, the center became known as the Henry Street Settlement. The number of nurses associated with the center grew from 2 in 1893 to more than 250 by 1929. Wald was key in the decision to extend nursing service to a local public school on a trial basis in 1902. Ultimately, this experiment resulted in the establishment of a citywide public school nursing program, the first such program in the world.

Relief Work

Annie Turner Wittenmyer (1827–1900) was known for her work establishing special diet kitchens at army hospitals during the Civil War. She was instrumental in training other women, who also followed her example by opening other similar kitchens. By the end of the war, the army's medical department had adopted Wittenmyer's ideas. Later, Wittenmyer led a campaign to establish a home for Civil War nurses and for the mothers and widows of veterans. Wittenmyer is also known for her support of the temperance movement and women's suffrage.

Substance Use and Public Health

MADD came into being as a nonprofit organization in August 1980, largely through the single-minded efforts of Candy Lightner, who had lost her 13-year-old daughter as the result of a car accident caused by a drunk driver. At the time of the accident, the driver was on probation for previous DUI (driving under the influence) convictions and had been released on bail, posted by his wife, for another hit-and-run DUI offense that had occurred several days prior to the accident involving Cari Lightner (Reinarman, 1988). The organization was funded with the proceeds from Cari's insurance settlement, Candy Lightner's own savings, and various small grants from the American Council on Alcohol Problems, the National Highway Traffic Safety Administration, and the Levy Foundation (Reinarman, 1988).

From its inception, MADD portrayed itself as the voice of the victim: the individually harmed victim, who survived an accident caused by a drunken driver; the bereaved victim, who has lost a loved one due to the actions of a drunken driver; and the general community activist, who is convinced that community involvement is a key to the resolution of social problems and the restoration of justice (see Weed, 1990).

The organization focused its attention on three primary areas of activity: public awareness, legal advocacy, and victim assistance. Chapters were urged to educate communities about the seriousness of DUI and to recognize individual responsibility for a decision to drive while intoxicated. Community awareness and education also included working with the media and developing Speaker's Bureau programs, poster contests, and annual candlelight vigil and educational programs designed for school-age children and youth. MADD chapters also provided supportive services to families who had lost loved ones, such as the provision of appropriate referrals to community resources, the Victim Information Packet, grief brochures, and sufficient information to enable victims to assert their rights through the court case.

WOMEN AND THE COURTS

Health and Civil Rights

Urvashi Vaid (1958–), born in India, worked on the National Prison Project for the American Civil Liberties Union in Washington, DC. She was instrumental in focusing national attention on injustices within the prison system through the numerous class-action lawsuits that she filed. In 1984, her focus shifted to address the rights of HIV-infected prisoners. Vaid became the executive director of the National Gay and Lesbian Task Force in 1989. She remained active in advocating for health care for HIV-infected persons and for recognition of gays and lesbians.

Mental Health and Civil Rights

During the late 1800s, it was not unusual for lax commitment laws to be used against family members as a means of resolving family conflict. Illinois law provided one such example. Under the then-existing law, married women and invalids could be committed to a mental hospital in the absence of any legal safeguards. Elizabeth Packard (1816–1897) dared to disagree publicly with her clergyman-husband regarding his religious admonitions. In 1860, he had her involuntarily confined to a mental hospital, claiming that she was a threat to her family. Elizabeth claimed that this commitment was retribution for her then-unorthodox religious beliefs. She was not released from the asylum for 3 years. Following her release, she sued her husband for wrongful confinement and worked to reform the commitment laws. Her efforts resulted in the passage of "Packard laws," which provided mentally ill persons with greater legal safeguards against wrongful commitment. Packard was also the founder of the now-defunct Anti-Insane Asylum Society.

Reproductive Health

Sara Ragle Weddington (1945–) successfully argued the case of *Roe v. Wade* before the United States Supreme Court in 1973; that decision resulted in the legalization of abortion. Weddington had had personal experience with difficulties associated with obtaining an abortion; she had an unplanned pregnancy during law school and, in order to obtain an abortion, traveled across the border to Mexico.

Abortion had actually been legal in the United States until the mid-1880s. At that time, a male-dominated medical profession lobbied to make abortions not performed by physicians illegal, in order to restrict the ability of women to practice midwifery, which included abortions, and to prevent "race suicide" among middle- and upperclass white women who were obtaining abortions. By 1900, abortion had become an underground activity.

These "backstreet abortions" not infrequently resulted in serious complications or death. The decision in *Roe v. Wade* increased women's access to safe procedures.

Sex Discrimination

Catherine MacKinnon (1947–) focused her attention as a lawyer on issues related to pornography, which she views as a form of sex discrimination that encourages and legitimizes the exploitation and abuse of women. MacKinnon is credited with successfully arguing before the United States Supreme Court that sexual harassment in the workplace is sex discrimination and should be considered, therefore, a violation of federal law. She is the author of numerous books including *In Harm's Way: The Pornography of Civil Rights Hearings* (1999) and *Sexual Harassment of Working Women* (1978).

WOMEN, LEGISLATION, AND POLITICS

Health and Civil Rights

Although she is best known for her efforts to abolish slavery, Sojourner Truth (1797–1883) played a key role in securing the right of African Americans to use public transportation. Originally named Isabella Baumfree at her birth, Truth escaped from slavery 1 year before the state of New York granted emancipation. Her narratives about her experiences as a slave helped to dispel the widely held belief that slaves were cared for by their masters and were content to remain in that condition. In 1865, after suffering a dislocated shoulder when a conductor tried to evict her from a streetcar, Truth filed a lawsuit in Washington, DC. That verdict affirmed the right of African Americans to utilize public transportation.

Health and Human Rights

The Universal Declaration of Human Rights, passed by the General Assembly of the United Nations in 1948, came about largely through the efforts of Eleanor Roosevelt (1884–1962). In 1946, Roosevelt was appointed as the Head of the United Nations Human Rights Commission and served as the only female member of the United States delegation to the United Nations. Upon the passage of the Declaration, the members of the General Assembly arose and gave her a standing ovation. The Universal Declaration of Human

Rights recognizes significant health interests in that it specifically prohibits slavery and the slave trade (Article 4), torture, or cruel, inhuman, or degrading treatment or punishment (Article 5), provides for marriage by consent only and the protection of the family as a unit (Article 16), assures reasonable limitation of working hours and periodic holidays (Article 24), and specifies the right to a standard of living that is adequate for the health and well-being of individuals and their family members, including medical care and the right to security when sick or disabled (Article 25). Prior to this effort, Roosevelt had been active in speaking out against the then-Senator Joseph McCarthy and his persecution of suspected communists and in support of equal pay laws and civil rights.

Health Care Reform

Like Eleanor Roosevelt, Hillary Rodham Clinton (1947–) was deeply involved in politics. During her husband Bill Clinton's tenure as President of the United States, she headed the Task Force on National Health Care Reform. The task force included six Cabinet secretaries in addition to other White House officials. More than 50 congressional meetings were held in order to develop proposals that would fundamentally reshape the health care system in the United States. Ultimately, the recommendations of the task force were not adopted. However, the effort to reform the health care system may have served to galvanize organizations and legislatures to reconsider various mechanisms for the provision of health care. In 2000, Clinton was elected as New York State's first female senator. In the Senate, she serves on the Health, Education, Labor, and Pensions Committee.

Mental Health

Improved treatment of mentally ill patients and prisoners came about during the 1800s largely through the efforts of Dorothea Dix (1802–1887). In 1841, Dix began a Sunday school class for women in an East Cambridge, Massachusetts, jail. She argued vociferously with prison officials to remedy the harsh conditions of the mentally ill individuals who were housed in the jails, only to be told that "lunatics" were unable to feel cold and would burn themselves if given a source of heat. Her exposé to the Massachusetts legislature of the conditions of almost 1,000 mentally ill inmates resulted in the renovation of the asylum in Worcester, Massachusetts. Dix eventually expanded her efforts to improve the conditions of the mentally ill to Rhode Island, Connecticut, New York, New Jersey, and Tennessee. Additional reforms came about as a result of Dix' lobbying and organizational efforts including the founding in 1844 of Medical Superintendents of American Institutions for the Insane, the establishment of 32 mental hospitals in the United States, and the removal of many mentally ill individuals from jails. Unfortunately, although Congress passed her proposed legislation permitting the use of income from the sale of western lands to fund mental health programs, the bill was ultimately vetoed by the then-President Franklin Pierce, who feared that the government would become responsible for indigent persons as a result. During the Civil War, Dix served as the Union's Superintendent of Female Nurses and, in this position, sought to improve the conditions of the soldiers and the nurses who cared for them.

Sex Discrimination

Many times, major changes are effectuated by proposing legislation to interested legislators and championing its passage. These efforts can occur at the local, state, or national level. Bella Savitsky Abzug (1920–1998) worked to effectuate change at the national level. She was elected to the United States House of Representatives in 1971, after having worked as a labor law attorney for 23 years. Although its ratification by the states ultimately failed, she worked diligently for the passage of the Equal Rights Amendment to the U.S. Constitution. Abzug also supported abortion rights and a women's credit rights bill and was the first person to introduce gay rights legislation into Congress. She authored several bills while in Congress, which were designed to improve the status of women and to prevent discrimination on the basis of sex. Abzug returned to her law practice following her tenure in the House of Representatives.

WOMEN IN THE MEDIA

Environmental Health

The modern environmental movement essentially came into being through the efforts of Rachel Carson (1907–1964). Carson is perhaps best known for her publication entitled *Silent Spring*, which has been called one of the most influential books ever written on conservation. *Silent Spring* was initially published in the *New Yorker*, a short month after publications linking the use of thalidomide to birth defects. At the time of *Silent Spring*'s publication, the public was particularly concerned about the potentially adverse health effects of radioactive fallout from atomic testing. *Silent Spring* detailed the damage that was being caused to the environment by DDT and various other pesticides that were then in use. Carson's book influenced the then-President John F. Kennedy to call for the testing of chemicals that were highlighted in the book and, in addition, prompted the drafting by state legislatures of 40 bills to regulate the use of pesticides. Five years after Carson's death, the federal government phased out the use of DDT.

Health, Violence, and Civil Rights

Ida Bell Wells-Barnett (1862–1931), an African American journalist, challenged in the courts her forcible removal from a first-class railroad car because of her race. Sixteen years old at the time of the incident, Wells hired a white attorney to press her claim in court. Although she prevailed in the circuit court, the Tennessee Supreme Court later reversed the verdict and found in favor of the railroad. Wells was required to pay court costs and return the $500 award. Her article describing this experience marked the beginning of her career as a journalist.

Wells' writing focused on the loss of rights that African Americans had experienced under Reconstruction. In 1889, she acquired a one-third ownership in the *Memphis Free Speech and Headlight* and became its editor. Following the lynching of three of her friends on manufactured charges of inciting a riot, Wells prevailed upon African Americans to leave Memphis, since it failed to protect the lives or property of African Americans. In response, 6,000 African Americans left Memphis for the newly admitted state of Oklahoma, resulting in an economic crisis for white Memphis businessmen. Her investigation of lynching and the publication of her findings as *Southern Horrors* (1892) and *Red Record* (1895) contributed to the development of public awareness of lynching and its condemnation.

Immigrant Health

Grace Abbott (1878–1939) played a key role in raising public awareness about the plight of immigrants to the United States with her book entitled *The Immigrant and the Community* (1917). Her efforts stemmed from her work with poverty-stricken immigrants living in the slums of Chicago and her study of the conditions on Ellis Island, where intending immigrants were processed by immigration officials for entry into the United States. She testified before Congress against immigration restrictions and, in a series of weekly articles in the *Chicago Evening Post*, attacked the exploitation of immigrants. In addition to her work on behalf of immigrants, Abbott is known for her work in support of child labor laws and her role in planning the social security system as a member of the then-President Franklin Delano Roosevelt's Council on Economic Security.

Mental Health

Elizabeth Cochrane Seaman (1864–1922), writing under the name of Nellie Bly, was largely responsible for exposing the inhumane conditions that beset the mentally ill women housed at the Blackwell Island (now Roosevelt Island) women's asylum. Seaman pretended to be mentally ill in order to observe and record the conditions at that hospital. She published her exposé in *New York World*; these articles were later collected and published as *Ten Days in a Mad House* (1887). Her work precipitated a grand jury investigation of the conditions in that asylum. Seaman was also known for her effort to beat Phileas Fogg's 80-day tour around the world in Jules Verne's fictional account, *Around the World in Eighty Days*. Seaman set the record, with a journey that required 72 days, 6 hours, 11 minutes, and 14 seconds. She has been called the best known journalist of her day.

Reproductive Health

Margaret Sanger (1879–1966) is known as the founder of the United States birth control movement. In 1912, Sanger began writing a column entitled "What Every Girl Should Know" for the Socialist daily, *The Call*. She discussed the reproductive process in the column, but avoided any direct mention of contraception because the 1873 Comstock law, which was then in effect, criminalized the publication, distribution, or possession of information about devices or medications for abortion or contraception.

Sanger viewed birth control as both a social issue and a reproductive issue. Family planning, she believed, would liberate poor women from the economic oppression that they suffered as a result of unwanted pregnancies. Sanger argued that "no woman can call herself free who does not own and control her own body." Following her publication of a pamphlet entitled "Family Limitation," Sanger moved to Europe. Her experiences there impressed upon her the need for birth control as a mechanism of women's sexual liberation.

Sanger opened the first birth control clinic in Brooklyn, New York, in 1916. After distributing contraceptives to approximately 400 women, she was arrested and ultimately served time in prison for distributing contraceptives. The following year, she began publication of the *Birth Control Review* and, in 1921, she established the American Birth Control League that eventually evolved into the Planned Parenthood Federation of America in 1942. In 1923, she opened the Birth Control Clinical Research Bureau in New York City, which was to become the first permanent birth control clinic in the United States.

Sanger's efforts were opposed by the medical establishment and the church. Physicians warned that diaphragms would cause cancer and madness and that interference with "God's will" would lead to mental and physical illness. Finally, in 1937 the American Medical Association recognized the provision of contraception as a legitimate medical service. And, although the federal Comstock Law was overturned in 1938, many states retained similar laws. It was not until 1965, with the Supreme Court decision in *Griswold v. Connecticut*, that women were assured of their right to privacy that included the decision to use contraceptives.

WOMEN AS HEALTH PIONEERS

Cardiology

Helen Brooke Taussig (1898–1986) is known as the pioneer of the surgical technique that is used to save "blue babies." Taussig had originally studied medicine at Harvard Medical School, but left there because of sex discrimination (see entry on Discrimination). She earned her medical degree, instead, from Johns Hopkins University. In 1930, she became the Head of the Johns Hopkins pediatric heart clinic. She became interested in studying the condition popularly known as "blue baby" syndrome, which was actually an infantile heart malformation, pulmonary stenosis, that would prevent the baby's heart from pumping oxygen into the blood. Taussig, together with the surgeon Alfred

Blalock, developed an artificial duct that could be implanted surgically to carry blood past the constricted part of the artery. This mechanism is known as the Blalock–Taussig shunt. This discovery is credited with paving the way for open-heart surgery with the heart–lung machine. In 1962, Taussig worked to alert physicians about the dangers associated with the use of thalidomide, prescribed as a sedative during pregnancy. (See entry on Thalidomide.)

Occupational Health

Alice Hamilton (1869–1970) has become known as "the matriarch of industrial medicine." Hamilton was a professor of pathology at Northwestern University, located near Chicago. Her 1910 study of the poisoning of approximately 600 workers implicated seven different industrial processes as the cause. Her research ultimately resulted in the development and implementation of new testing and safety regulations in the state of Illinois.

Dr. Harriet Hardy was largely responsible for the identification of beryllium as the cause of an outbreak of sarcoidosis of the lung among predominantly female employees at a fluorescent light plant in Massachusetts. Although scientists at the state's Division of Occupational Medicine suspected that occupational exposures were responsible for the outbreak, their findings were suppressed as a result of industry pressure. Hardy, then an employee of the Division, proceeded with an investigation. As a result of her findings, women were able to sue successfully for injuries resulting from exposure to beryllium while washing their husbands' work clothes or from exposure while living near the beryllium plants.

Pediatrics

Ethel Collins Dunham (1883–1969) set the standard of care for the treatment of premature infants. At the turn of the 20th century, some cities were experiencing a 30% mortality rate among infants under the age of 1 year. Dunham was the first researcher to recognize the association between prematurity and infant death. Her text, entitled *Premature Infants: A Manual for Physicians*, became a standard text in this field.

Psychiatry

Karen Danielson Horney (1885–1952) is best known as a feminist psychiatrist who rejected Freud's theory that women suffered from "penis envy," asserting instead that men might be suffering from "womb envy," which led them to claim their superiority in other areas of life. Horney argued that environmental and social conditions, rather than instinctual or biological drives, as maintained by Freud, determined individual personality. She objected to Freud's concept of libido, a death instinct, and the Oedipus complex. Horney argued that the primary condition for the later development of neurosis was the infant's experience of basic anxiety arising from the infant's feeling of helplessness in a potentially hostile world. She further asserted that the source of much of women's psychological distress was due to a male-dominated culture that had produced Freudian theory. Horney authored multiple texts, taught at the New York Psychoanalytic Institute, and, together with Erich Fromm, founded the *American Journal of Psychoanalysis*.

Reproductive Health

Bertha Van Hoosen (1863–1952), while on staff of Illinois University's Medical School, invented what has become known as "twilight sleep" anesthetic, a combination of scopolamine and morphine, to ease the pain of childbirth while still retaining consciousness. Van Hoosen delivered over 2,000 babies using this technique, although many of her male colleagues refused to use it.

WOMEN AS REFORMERS

Health and Spirituality

Mary Baker Eddy (1821–1910) is best known as a founder of Christian Science. Although this represents a religious or spiritual orientation, its tenets are intimately tied to efforts to improve health. Eddy's first edition of *Science and Health*, which addressed the concept of mind healing, was published in 1875.

Ellen G. White (1827–1915) cofounded the Seventh Day Adventist Church, together with her husband James White, in 1863. That year, following a severe illness, White received a vision telling her that Adventists should refrain from meat, alcohol, tobacco, tea, and coffee, and should rely on natural remedies in lieu of physicians. Through her efforts, the Western Health Reform Institute was established in Battle Creek in 1866 and, shortly thereafter, the College of Medical

Evangelists, now known as Loma Linda University, was established in southern California. Although many had conceived of White as a prophet, foreshadowing changes in health care, critics have suggested that her ideas derive from those of others who preceded her.

Health Care

During the early to mid-1900s, South Carolina was known for its lack of attention to the health problems plaguing its African American residents. Even when attention was paid to diseases that disproportionately affected the African American populace, it was often to prevent the transmission of disease to whites. Matilda Evans, an African American physician in Columbia, South Carolina, sought to address the unmet health care needs of African American families. In 1930, she began a clinic for expectant mothers, infants, and children. The Evans Clinic was supported by African American businessmen and, eventually, state and local governments.

Immigrant Health

Jane Addams (1860–1935) devoted her life to three causes: social reform on behalf of the poor, woman's suffrage, and pacifism. Her social reform efforts included the founding of the settlement house, Hull House, to serve Chicago's poor immigrant population. Unlike many of her predecessors, Addams believed that poverty resulted from social dynamics rather than from personal defects. Hull House offered numerous services including day care, vocational training, citizenship and literacy classes, child and medical care, music and art classes, and leisure activities. Volunteers of Hull House were instrumental in the passage of state child labor laws, compulsory education laws, and the establishment of the first juvenile court in the United States.

During her lifetime, Addams authored more than 450 articles and 12 books; she had her books printed in only union shops. Her advocacy of labor unions and her stance as a pacifist during World War I led to her loss of support and her identification on a "traitor list" of the Senate Judiciary Committee. However, in 1931, Addams became the first woman to receive the Nobel Peace Prize and, to this day, remains the only social worker to have ever been awarded that honor.

Public Health

Sara Josephine Baker (1873–1945), a physician in New York, was perhaps best known for her role in locating and apprehending "Typhoid Mary" Mallon, a cook who infected seven families with typhoid. However, her impact extended far beyond this one incident. During the early 1900s, the United States had one of the highest infant and maternal death rates in the Western world. In 1908, Baker was appointed to head the Bureau of Child Hygiene within New York's Department of Health; this was the first tax-supported child health agency in the United States. As a public health administrator, Baker worked ceaselessly to decrease the rate of infant mortality. Her policies emphasized the need for preventive medicine and good hygiene; during her tenure, the agency distributed pamphlets on hygiene, trained midwives, and taught mothers to care for their infants. Ultimately, Baker's efforts led to a reduction in the rate of child mortality from 1 in 7 births to 1 in 14.

Evangeline Cory Booth (1865–1950) was the daughter of William Booth, who had left the ministry to found an independent evangelical organization that became known as the Salvation Army. In 1904, Evangeline Booth assumed the leadership of the Salvation Army in the United States. During her tenure, the Salvation Army established soup kitchens, shelters, hospitals for unwed mothers, and disaster relief efforts.

Substance Use and Pediatrics

Clara Hale (1905–1992), a social worker, was the founder of Hale House, the first official home for babies who were born addicted to drugs. Hale began babysitting in her home during the 1930s and first became a foster parent in 1940. She is credited with having raised 40 foster children. Hale first took care of a drug-addicted baby in 1969. In 1975, Hale House became the Center for the Promotion of Human Potential, which was the first black childcare volunteer agency in the United States. In the 1980s, Hale began to devote her attention to the care of HIV-infected infants.

Women in the Health Professions

Florence Nightingale (1820–1910) is known as the founder of modern nursing. Nightingale supervised a unit of field nurses in British army hospitals during the Crimean War, with an emphasis on hygiene and the need for prompt attention. In 1860, she founded a training school for nurses, which became the model for other training programs.

Elizabeth Blackwell (1821–1910), the first female physician in the United States, lived during the same period of time as Nightingale and considered Nightingale a friend. Blackwell was denied admission to every medical school in New York and Philadelphia because of her sex. Geneva College in upstate New York voted to admit Blackwell, believing that the completion of the application by a woman was a prank. Her sister Emily Blackwell (1826–1910) experienced similar difficulties securing admission to a medical school, but was finally able to complete her medical education at Western Reserve University in Cleveland. Blackwell, Emily, and Marie Zackrzewska founded the New York Infirmary for Women and Children in 1857. The infirmary established a training course for nurses in 1858 and began the first charitable in-home medical service in the United States in 1866. By 1860, this institution was providing services to more than 3,600 patients each year. The institution was later expanded in 1868 to include the first college for the training of female physicians. The college remained operational until 1898, when Cornell University Medical College began accepting female medical students. At that time, the Women's Medical College closed and transferred its students to Cornell. While settled in London, Blackwell helped to establish the London School of Medicine for Women, where she served as a professor. Her book, *Pioneer Work in Opening the Medical Profession to Women*, details these efforts.

CONCLUSION

As indicated, women have contributed to the improvement of health across time and across disciplines. Ultimately, one must ask why these women embarked on these paths. Few received any financial remuneration for their efforts. Many would never have anticipated that they would later receive recognition and awards for their work. Still others, such as Jane Addams and Lucy Parsons, were condemned for their work when it became politically undesirable.

Carol Gilligan has maintained that the process of moral development in women differs from that among men. Her research findings indicate that, while men may emphasize fairness and rules in the resolution of moral dilemmas, women are more likely to focus on the preservation of relationships. It is possible that this process is reflected in the life choices that these and other women have made and continue to make.

Many times, these contributions are not recognized or remembered. However, they serve as an inspiration to future generations of women to contribute to society.

References

Labonte, R. (1994). Health promotion and empowerment: Reflections on professional practice. *Health Education Quarterly, 21*(1), 253–268.

Minkler, M. (1992). Community organizing around the elderly poor in the United States: A case study. *International Journal of Health Services, 22*, 303–316.

Reinarman, C. (1988). The social construction of an alcohol problem: The case of Mothers Against Drunk Drivers and social control in the 1980s. *Theory and Society, 17*, 91–120.

Suggested Resources

Apple, R. D. (Ed.). (1990). *Women in health & medicine in America: An historical handbook*. New Brunswick, NJ: Rutgers University Press.

Cullen-DuPont, K. (2000). *Encyclopedia of women's history in America*. New York: Facts On File.

Edmondson, C. M. (1999). *Extraordinary women: Women who changed history*. Holbrook, MA: Adams Media.

Goodwin, J. L. (Ed.). (2002). *Encyclopedia of women in American history*. Armonk, NY: M.E. Sharpe.

Langston, D. (2002). *A to Z of American women leaders and activists*. New York: Facts On File.

II. Topics in Women's Health

Abdominal Pain

Abdominal pain is the most common gastrointestinal symptom for which medical evaluation is sought. It is a nonspecific, unpleasant sensation that can be associated with a multitude of conditions originating both within and outside the abdomen. Causes may range from common normal physiologic processes to life-threatening emergencies. There are many factors that contribute to the sensation and perception of pain, including underlying pathology, psychosocial disorders, and an individual's pain tolerance. Thus, abdominal pain is one of the most complex complaints that clinicians encounter.

The sensation of pain is produced by mechanical stimuli, chemical stimuli, or a combination of both. The most common mechanical stimulus is stretch. There are stretch receptors located in the muscular layer of the hollow organs (gastrointestinal, urinary, and biliary tracts), mesentery (membranous attachment of intra-abdominal organs to the posterior abdominal wall), and in the capsule (membranous outer covering) of solid organs (e.g., liver, spleen, kidneys). Thus, any process which leads to distention, stretching, and traction may generate abdominal pain. Chemical stimuli can increase the sensitivity of these pain receptors. Pain receptors located in the mucosa (lining of the esophagus, stomach, bladder, and intestines) are stimulated primarily by chemical stimuli released in response to local injury due to inflammation, infection, ischemia (decreased or absent blood flow), necrosis (cell death), or radiation.

Broadly speaking, abdominal pain may be produced by obstruction, inflammation, perforation, or ischemia of any hollow organ. Infection, obstruction of drainage or blood flow, and infiltration (e.g., by tumor cells) may cause capsular distention in solid organs leading to pain. Normal physiologic processes like menstruation and ovulation may also cause abdominal pain. Abdominal pain may be a feature of a number of extra-abdominal conditions including heart attack, pneumonia, testicular torsion, and a variety of metabolic disorders (e.g., lead poisoning, kidney failure). A herpes zoster flare ("shingles") affecting a nerve that innervates the skin over the abdomen may be a misleading cause of pain before the characteristic rash appears.

Although most episodes of abdominal pain are due to mild self-limited conditions, it is essential to be able to discern the signs and symptoms that represent potential emergencies and require immediate intervention. Medical attention should be sought immediately when abdominal pain is accompanied with any of the following "alarm" signs or symptoms: red blood in the stool; maroon stool; black tarry stool; fever; sudden onset of constipation or bloating; persistent vomiting; vomiting red blood or "coffee grounds"; history of recent abdominal trauma; known or suspected pregnancy; or progressively increasing pain severity.

The clinician must interpret the complaints and physical findings in the particular context of the patient in order to first assess the level of urgency and then implement an efficient diagnostic and treatment strategy. A thorough history and physical examination is the first crucial step in the assessment of abdominal pain. Important information to be obtained are the onset of pain, location, temporal qualities (e.g., intermittent vs.

constant), radiation (e.g., to the back, shoulder, groin), relationship with gastrointestinal functions (e.g., eating, defecation), associated symptoms (e.g., fever, vomiting, jaundice, diarrhea), and any exacerbating or alleviating factors. Other characteristics include the quality of the pain (e.g., sharp, dull, cramping, or gnawing) and its severity. A detailed menstrual history in female patients should also be obtained.

The description of the onset of pain distinguishes acute abdominal pain, lasting hours to days, from chronic pain, occurring over a period of weeks to months. A perforated ulcer, dissecting aortic aneurysm, ruptured ectopic pregnancy, or kidney stones may cause pain that is sudden in onset and reaches peak severity within minutes. Acute abdominal pain that progresses to severe pain within a few hours should alert the clinician to consider acute appendicitis, cholecystitis, diverticulitis, intestinal ischemia, or intestinal obstruction. Acute abdominal pain associated with passing blood either from the upper or lower gastrointestinal tract can be a sign of ulcer disease, intestinal ischemia, or inflammatory bowel disease.

Chronic abdominal pain occurring over a period of weeks to months in the absence of any alarm signs or symptoms may be less urgent, allowing for a more systematic evaluation. Chronic intermittent pain may, at times, be particularly difficult to diagnose whereas chronic persistent pain usually has an identifiable cause, such as chronic pancreatitis, disseminated malignancy, or severe inflammatory bowel disease. Examples of conditions causing intermittent abdominal pain, often associated with meals, include gastroesophageal reflux disease, peptic ulcer disease, biliary tract disease, and chronic pancreatitis. Pain that is temporally associated with a woman's menstrual cycle may be due to endometriosis or ovulation. Chronic pain associated with anorexia and weight loss may indicate an underlying malignancy. The symptoms of irritable bowel syndrome, a functional disorder characterized by abdominal discomfort or pain associated with an alteration in bowel habit, are often precipitated or worsened by stress or anxiety. Chronic intractable abdominal pain (CIAP) is another functional disorder seen predominantly in women, often with a history of sexual or physical abuse, in which pain is longer than 6 months in duration and organic causes have been excluded.

Although abdominal pain may not be as precisely localized as it is elsewhere (e.g., the skin), the location of pain may provide some useful clues. Traditionally, the abdomen is divided into four parts, referred to as the patient's right upper, left upper, right lower, and left lower quadrants. Other locations of clinical importance are the epigastrium (in the central upper abdomen), periumbilical area (around the umbilicus or navel), and suprapubic area (below the umbilicus and above the pubic bone). Pain arising in the right upper quadrant may represent acute cholecystitis (inflammation of the gallbladder) or hepatitis. Pain in the left upper quadrant may be due to impaired blood flow to the spleen or left colon. Pain caused by appendicitis often begins in the periumbilical area and then settles in the right lower quadrant. Pain due to disorders involving the kidneys, ovaries, or fallopian tubes is usually perceived on the same side of the abdomen as the affected organ. Because diverticulosis most often involves the sigmoid colon, which is located in the left lower quadrant, the pain of diverticulitis (acute diverticular inflammation) is usually perceived in this region. Suprapubic pain may be seen in urinary tract infections, pelvic inflammatory disease, and endometriosis. Central abdominal pain may be due to gastroenteritis, peptic ulcer disease, or acute pancreatitis. Diffuse abdominal pain may represent infectious peritonitis, appendicitis, inflammatory bowel disease, or a perforated duodenal ulcer.

An important feature of abdominal pain is the tendency for pain to be located at a site remote from the affected organ. The term for this is referred pain. For instance, pain from an inflamed gallbladder may sometimes be perceived in the right shoulder. Abdominal pain may also radiate, for example, the epigastric pain from pancreatitis may radiate to the back; and flank pain from a kidney stone may radiate to the groin.

A careful, gentle physical examination plays a vital role in the physician's evaluation of abdominal pain and is often more informative than laboratory studies. The clinician assesses the general appearance of the patient along with the vital signs. Alarm signs including confusion, restlessness, sweating, rapid heart rate, drop in blood pressure, or high fever usually dictate urgency in the evaluation. A history of abdominal pain associated with unresponsiveness, shock, or cardiac arrest suggests that a catastrophic abdominal event has occurred that requires emergent treatment. The presence of abdominal distention, scars, rashes, bruising, or hernias may aid in the diagnosis. Absence of bowel sounds (after listening for at least 1 min) may indicate the presence of an ileus (the failure of intestinal contents to pass through the gastrointestinal tract in the absence of an anatomical obstruction), whereas hyperactive or high-pitched tinkling sounds suggest intestinal obstruction. Guarding (involuntary abdominal muscular wall contraction) on palpation suggests the presence of peritonitis. The abdomen is also examined for the presence of masses as well as liver and spleen findings such as enlargement, nodularity, or tenderness. In women with lower abdominal pain, a pelvic examination should be performed to assess potential uro-gynecological causes. Tenderness, blood, or a mass lesion found on rectal examination provides other important diagnostic information.

Laboratory and radiologic studies can provide additional information in making the diagnosis. Specific tests ordered should reflect the clinical suspicion. In general, a complete blood count, serum chemistries, and urine studies are performed. A pregnancy test should be considered in all women of reproductive age with lower abdominal pain. Other laboratory tests, including stool studies, liver function tests, amylase, and lipase, are ordered when clinically appropriate.

A variety of diagnostic imaging tests are available which may aid in the evaluation of abdominal pain. Plain x-rays of the abdomen, in upright and supine (lying down) positions, is obtained when perforation or bowel obstruction are suspected. Ultrasonography is useful in the evaluation of the liver, biliary tract, spleen, kidneys, and tubo-ovarian system. Doppler technology allows evaluation of the large vessels. Computed tomography (CT), the most versatile imaging tool, is highly sensitive for the detection of inflammatory, neoplastic, and vascular lesions, as well as for identifying obstruction, perforation, and fluid collections. Other potential radiologic examinations available, depending on the clinical circumstances, include angiography, contrast imaging, nuclear medicine scans, or magnetic resonance imaging (MRI). Clearly the specific management of abdominal pain will vary greatly depending on the acuity and cause. The evaluation and treatment of both acute and chronic abdominal pain often require input from a number of medical/surgical specialists including surgeons, obstetrician/gynecologists, and gastroenterologists. The decision of which specialist(s) to involve and when is dictated by the clinical circumstances. Surgeons perform not only a great number of curative operative procedures, but also both invasive (e.g., exploratory abdominal surgery) and minimally invasive diagnostic (e.g., laparoscopy) procedures.

Obstetrician/gynecologists are skilled in the evaluation of women with a suspected gynecologic cause of pain and perform a wide variety of diagnostic and curative procedures such as transvaginal ultrasound, diagnostic and therapeutic laparoscopy, and a number

of other pelvic surgical procedures. Gastroenterologists offer a variety of procedures for the diagnosis and treatment of abdominal pain including upper and lower endoscopy (insertion of a flexible tube containing a camera into the mouth or rectum) of the digestive and pancreas–biliary tracts, motility studies, and pH (acid) monitoring.

Chronic abdominal pain is often difficult to diagnose and treat. At times, the involvement of an anesthesiologist or other pain management professional is helpful. They are skilled in the management of pain with medications, therapeutic nerve blocks (injection of an anesthetic agent near a specific nerve or group of nerves), and counseling. If there appears to be a psychiatric component to abdominal pain, referral to a mental health professional is appropriate. Chronic functional abdominal pain syndromes require a combined approach of education, reassurance, dietary changes, medications, and, at times, behavioral therapies (e.g., relaxation and biofeedback techniques).

SEE ALSO: Chest pain, Chronic pain, Nausea, Pelvic pain, Peptic ulcer disease

Suggested Reading

Pasricha P. J., et al. (1999). Abdominal pain. In T. Yamada, D. H. Alpers, L. Laine, C. Owyang, & D. W. Powell (Eds.), *Textbook of gastroenterology* (3rd ed., pp. 795–815). Philadelphia: Lippincott, Williams & Wilkins.

Suggested Resources

U.S. National Library of Medicine: http://www.nlm.nih.gov/medline/ency/article/003120.htm

SAPNA THOMAS
MARGARET F. KINNARD

Abortion   According to the U.S. Centers for Disease Control and Prevention, 1.18 million legal abortions were performed in the United States in 1997.

The risk of death from legal abortion is 0.4 per 100,000 induced abortions. Most abortions are performed surgically by vacuum curettage. Medical abortion (abortion induced by the use of medications) has recently become an option in this country. In most medical abortions, expulsion of the pregnancy occurs at home. About 1% of women require surgical evacuation to complete the process.

TECHNIQUE FOR SURGICAL ABORTION

Surgical abortion can be performed in an office or hospital setting. The success rate of surgical termination is 99%. It is usually a single-step process that requires one visit to the practitioner. In early pregnancy (less than 7 weeks), a small flexible plastic cannula (5–6 mm) is inserted into the uterus under sterile conditions. Plastic syringes (50 ml) are used as the vacuum source and the uterine contents are suctioned out. Adequate pain relief is provided by injecting local anesthetic into the cervix and administering intravenous sedation and analgesics.

After 7 weeks, a larger rigid plastic cannula (8–10 mm) is used with an electric pump as the vacuum source. After 18 weeks, a dilation and evacuation (using larger bore cannulae) usually must be performed under general anesthesia.

Typically, seaweed (laminaria) or a synthetic version is inserted into the cervix to prepare it for the procedure. The seaweed absorbs water, swells, and gently dilates the cervix over a 24-hour period. This facilitates the use of a cannula to extract the fetus and placenta at the time of the procedure.

The risks associated with pregnancy termination increase with gestational age and the use of general anesthesia. Risks include hemorrhage, infection, and perforation of the uterus if a surgical instrument slips through the uterine wall. Uterine perforation can cause bladder, bowel, or vascular injury necessitating further surgery for repair. The most common complication is uterine infection (0.1–4.7%).

MEDICAL ABORTIONS

Medical termination requires the close observation of a practitioner. It usually requires two or more visits, and there is a potential need for emergency intervention during the process. Finally, it requires close follow-up to ensure that the process of abortion is complete.

The earlier the gestational age is, the higher the complete abortion rate. The complete abortion rate ranges from 92 to 96% if medication is begun before 56 days. The pregnancy age should be confirmed by clinical evaluation and/or ultrasonography. Most medication regimens require patients to be no more than 50 days pregnant (as calculated from the first day of the last menstrual period).

The bleeding resulting from a medical abortion is heavier than that experienced during a normal menses and is accompanied by severe cramping. Most patients require pain medication. In rare instances, women who are having a medical abortion require an emergency dilation and curettage because of heavy bleeding (1%). Postabortion follow-up with a practitioner is extremely important because not all women are able to determine whether they have completely aborted based on their symptoms. In some studies, only half of the women who thought they had aborted actually had done so. Medical abortion is contraindicated in women on long-term systemic corticosteroid therapy or anticoagulant therapy and in those with chronic kidney, liver, or respiratory disease, severe anemia, a known coagulopathy, uncontrolled hypertension, angina, valvular disease, cardiac arrhythmias, or cardiac failure.

Three medications are currently used in medical abortion: misoprostol, mifepristone (RU 486), and methotrexate.

Misoprostol is the most common medication used in medical abortion. It was originally approved to prevent gastric ulcers in persons taking anti-inflammatory drugs. It causes softening of the cervix and uterine contractions, resulting in the termination of a pregnancy. Because misoprostol is potentially teratogenic (it can cause physical malformations of the fetus), a surgical abortion must be performed in the event of a continuing pregnancy.

Mifepristone is a progestin-like structure that occupies the progesterone receptor and prevents its activation (antiprogesterone effect). This may cause an alteration in the lining of the uterus (decidua) resulting in termination of the pregnancy. It also softens the cervix so the pregnancy can be expelled.

Methotrexate blocks DNA synthesis by blocking enzymes. This halts the process of implantation (attachment of the embryo to the uterine wall). All three medications can cause side effects including pain, nausea, bleeding, vomiting, diarrhea, warmth or chills, dizziness, headache, and fatigue.

Repeated use of medical termination has not been well studied in the medical lecture. However, there is no medical basis to believe that repeated medical abortion has an untoward effect on fertility.

SEE ALSO: Birth control, Ultrasound

http://www.acog.org

Habibeh Gitiforooz

Access to Health Care

Access to health care
has dominated the health policy scene for several
decades. In the early 1990s, national legislation, "universal access" to health care, was introduced by
President Clinton and the Congress as a way to provide
health security for all Americans. Lively debates were
generated and the topic commanded national attention.
The effort, although unsuccessful, has kept the problem
of health care access on the public agenda. Access to
care generally refers to the timely use of personal health
services to achieve the best possible outcomes. Initially,
the premise was access to physicians and hospitals.
More recently, health care access has included a variety
of providers, services, and facilities. In addition, access
describes the actual use of health services and factors
that facilitate or impede health care.

Aday (2001) and Anderson (see Anderson et al.,
1996) describe six types of access: *Potential access*
refers to health care system characteristics that influence
the use of services. *Realized access* is the actual use of
health services. *Equitable access* is the use of health services determined by demographic characteristics and
need. *Inequitable access* refers to the use of health
services that is determined by social characters and
available resources. *Effective access* is the use of health
services that improves health status or satisfaction.
Efficient access minimizes the cost of health care services and maximizes health status or satisfaction. Thus,
each type of access to care is influenced by a number
of characteristics and events. In an effort to understand
the influences on access to health care, numerous
studies have examined the barriers to care in specific
populations.

PERSONAL/FAMILY BARRIERS

Acceptability

Services must be desirable and viewed as acceptable to the patient/client and family. Physical setting,
demeanor, and scope of services all must be acceptable.

Language/Literacy

Patients/clients experience significant barriers
when important information is complex and not in their
native language. Complicated systems such as application for Medicaid present perceived and real barriers in
literacy and native language. Further, workforce studies
underscore the lack of providers who speak the language and are from the same culture as the populations
they serve. Thus, barriers are influenced by provider
and patient factors.

Culture

Health care providers and facilities that do not
understand the cultural expectations and norms of the
service populations present obstacles to accessing care.
Lack of knowledge about the culture further creates difficulty in achieving compliance with necessary medical
treatments.

Attitudes, Beliefs

The relationship between the provider of services
and the patient/client involves mutual respect and
understanding. Barriers occur when patients/clients perceive attitudes and beliefs about the nature of their
health as negative and not consistent with their own
beliefs about their health. This results in delays and lack
of compliance that undermines successful treatment outcomes. Provider negative attitudes (fear, homophobia,
discomfort of dying patients) in caring for HIV/AIDS
patients is one example.

Human Behaviors

Individual characteristics may serve as barriers to
treatment. Patients with physical or emotional disabilities may find it difficult to find services to meet their
needs. Health care providers, on the other hand, behaving in a courteous and respectful manner are likely to
facilitate the engagement of at-risk patients/clients.

Education/Income

Multiple studies have documented that lower
income and less educated populations do not access the
health care system to the same extent that more educated affluent populations do. Utilization and quality
are notably less for some groups and higher utilization

(such as emergency rooms) occurs in other populations. With increasing health care costs, more of the population is experiencing "out-of-pocket expenses" as a barrier to obtaining services.

FINANCIAL BARRIERS

Insurance Coverage

Insurance coverage, tied to employment, is the admission ticket to health services. While there are several government programs to provide services, substantial numbers fall into the "near poor" and uninsured or underinsured groups. Patients/clients are reluctant to seek care without insurance and providers/facilities are reluctant to provide care since services may not be reimbursed. Insurance reform is a health policy issue currently under discussion at the federal and state levels to stimulate investment in health care for all Americans.

Reimbursement Levels

Reimbursement levels for health services have been a major disincentive for providers and health care facilities. While government programs and private insurance companies have attempted to implement cost containment and reasonable reimbursement, significant gaps exist and exacerbate the barriers that populations at risk may experience.

STRUCTURAL BARRIERS

Availability

Access to health service, in particular, a regular source of medical care, is contingent upon services being available where and when needed by the service population. Barriers based on availability, for example, occur when services are located only in more urban areas creating barriers for remote rural populations or during hours when those working are unable to come for services. Lack of access to the appropriate health service and extended waiting times are also examples of access limited by availability.

Transportation

Lack of transportation is frequently cited as a barrier to access to care. Innovative approaches to support bus fare and transportation vans have been developed to complement basic medical services. These efforts may not be sustained since they are not a reimbursable service. Women frequently encounter this barrier when they are dependent on others for transportation.

It is clear that groups and individuals at risk may experience multiple barriers in trying to access health care. These are often individuals and groups who are vulnerable and need multiple services. Aday (2001) notes that the principal health needs of vulnerable populations are *physical* (high-risk mothers and infants, chronically ill and disabled, persons living with HIV/AIDS); *psychological* (mentally ill and disabled, alcohol or substance abusers, suicide or homicide prone); *social* (abusing families, homeless persons, immigrants and refugees). Many of these vulnerable groups have crosscutting health needs such as battered pregnant women, pregnant, homeless, substance-abusing women. These women are all at increased risk, requiring specialized services and experiencing multiple barriers to accessing care. A single-parent Hispanic woman with three children and no insurance, living in a rural area, likely experiences the following barriers:

- Fewer providers in rural areas
- Providers may not take uninsured
- Providers may not understand language and culture
- Transportation and childcare may not be available
- Fearful of her immigrant status being questioned

Concern over access to health care services is generated by the observations that some population groups may experience differences in access to health and subsequently experience poorer outcomes. Testing the equity of access involves measuring utilization of services as well as outcomes and determining barriers to care. In a landmark report, Access to Health Care in America (1993), the Institute of Medicine proposed five indicators for assessing access:

- Promoting successful birth outcomes
- Reducing the incidence of vaccine-preventable diseases
- Early detection and diagnosis of treatable diseases
- Reducing the effects of chronic disease and prolonging life
- Reducing morbidity and pain through timely and appropriate treatment

Acculturation

Access to timely prenatal care, immunizations, Pap tests, chronic disease management, and dental visits, for example, are all personal health services that contribute to favorable health outcomes. Thus, measurement of these indicators provides useful clues to how Americans access health care. In these selected examples, notable differences in access to care and health disparities can be determined. For example:

- There is a striking difference between Caucasians and African Americans receiving prenatal care (73.5% and 50.7% respectively) and a notable gap in black/white infant mortality rates (black rates twice as high as Caucasians).
- Childhood immunization rates reveal differences based on race, ethnicity, and geography.
- Elderly white women were more than twice as likely as younger white women to never have had a Pap test in 1987.
- Persons from poor areas are two thirds as likely as those from high-income areas to have access to hospital admission and referral services.
- Those with dental insurance made an average of about one more visit to the dentist than those without insurance. Differences by race persist after insurance.

Insurance, as a key to accessing health services in this country, deserves special note. Studies support that Americans without health insurance are generally sicker, die sooner, and when they receive care, it is likely to be of poorer quality than those with insurance. The 43 million uninsured Americans and 30 million underinsured reveal further racial, ethnicity, and income disparities. Hispanics, Asian Americans, American Indians, Alaskan Natives, and African Americans are all less likely to have insurance, have more difficulty getting care, and have fewer choices than Caucasians. Those in the population who are low-income can expect to have only limited access to preventive and primary, specialty care and subsequently suffer from poor health/outcomes. While many strides have been made in improving access for women to prenatal care, many services essential to low-income women are government-supported programs (food stamps, WIC, etc.). These programs are subject to the availability of resources and women are often left vulnerable by changing eligibility requirements, work program time limits, lack of culturally and linguistically sensitive services, and cross-cutting health issues.

While numerous federal and state initiatives have attempted to provide universal access to specific groups, to date a fragmented system with large numbers of uninsured is the current reality. The implications for women are significant. As high users of health services, access to appropriate care has a significant impact. Women are likely to have lower wages when they work and are more likely to be uninsured or underinsured. Women also need preventive services to maintain their health, Pap tests, family planning services for example. Women are frequently heads of household and experience barriers such as childcare and transportation. Minority women, low-income women, and immigrant women are at particular risk for experiencing barriers to care resulting in negative health outcomes. Access to health care will be a major area of concern for women and will require policy actions to remediate this gap.

SEE ALSO: Health insurance, Medicaid, Medicare

Suggested Reading

Aday, L. A. (2001). *At risk in America: The health of vulnerable population in the United States.* San Francisco: Jossey-Bass.

Anderson, R. M., Rice, T. M., & Kominski, G. F. (Eds.). (1996). *Changing the U.S. health care system.* San Francisco: Jossey-Bass.

Institute of Medicine. (2002). *Unequal treatment: Confronting racial and ethnic disparities in health.* Washington, DC: National Academy Press.

Millman, M. (Ed.). (1993). *Access to health care in America.* Washington, DC: National Academy Press.

BETH E. QUILL

Acculturation Acculturation has been defined as the process of cultural change that immigrants undergo when they enter in contact with a new, host culture. Immigrants bring their own cultural identity, language, values, beliefs, and behaviors, which might differ from those of the host culture. Although it is less common to acknowledge that the host culture can also change through contact with immigrants, acculturation is a dynamic, reciprocal process that generates change in both groups, because culture is a dynamic and evolving configuration of cognitions, identities, behaviors, values, and norms.

There are two types of acculturation: group level and individual. Group-level change involves change at the societal level, such as a change in economic or political regime to which the entire population must adapt. For instance, due to colonization, revolution, or modernization, great economic and political changes take place that impact the society at large. Simultaneously, changes can occur at the individual level, and as individuals shift from an agricultural economy to an industrial economy, changes in values, behaviors, and competences take place. Individual-level acculturation can be a consequence of group-level acculturation, but not exclusively, as it also occurs when a single individual migrates to a different culture. It is possible that individuals are suddenly confronted with the need to survive and therefore have to adapt and change former behaviors, learn a new language, and live by different rules.

Acculturation may take place at a variable pace. At the group level it is possible that some changes happen very slowly. For instance, the evolution of attitudes toward vaccination or toward boiling water may require a long time in some societies, particularly if the indigenous medical beliefs differ from those of the host or colonial society.

In the early years of acculturation research, it was believed that immigrants would lose their culture while gaining the culture of the host society. Research has found that, rather than acculturation being a linear process, it is a dual process in which individuals can acquire the skills necessary to live in the host country, while retaining their own cultural skills. Such is the case of language. Immigrants do not lose their native language unless they migrate at an early age and are unable to practice their native language. Learning a new language does not have to happen at the expense of the native language. Many immigrants are bilingual; one does not have to forget one's own language in order to learn English. European countries exemplify bilingual or multilingual societies in which bilingualism is not perceived as interfering with cognitive processes.

While language acquisition may be relatively fast, particularly if immigrants are exposed to education and training in the new language, cultural identity may change more slowly. Most immigrants continue to identify as Dominican, Brazilian, Vietnamese and, even after naturalizing and becoming citizens of the host country, they continue to identify with their original culture or their ethnicity. In fact, the history of the world reveals multiple examples in which ethnic identity is more powerful than national unity. The Basque people have retained their own ethnic identity and language despite having been assimilated by Spain. A Basque identifies first as Basque, and may even refuse to identify as Spanish. In Cyprus, a Greek Cypriot will not identify with a Turk Cypriot, even if both have been born on the island.

The tendency in the United States is to encourage "melting" into the pot rather than preserving a diversified, multicultural society. This is particularly true for European-descent Americans, who may say "I am American" rather than "I am Irish American." However, assimilation has not been easy for people of color because they have been less welcome in the United States than white European groups. Descendants of enslaved African immigrants, of indigenous Latinos, or of the East Asians who migrated in the 19th century are often seen as strangers and foreigners in what has been their own land for a number of centuries. Thus, it makes more sense for them to identify as African American, Latino/Hispanic American, and Asian American rather than as American.

Immigration can be stressful because there are many losses and challenges that individuals face throughout this process. The resulting stress has been labeled acculturative stress. These pressures may come from the host society and involve the requirement of learning the language, customs, and mores, or they may come from the culture of origin and involve the retention of traditions, contacts with family, and potential disapproval from loved ones. The latter type of acculturative stress is common among second- or third-generation immigrants whose communities expect them to retain the behaviors and traditions of their parents. This type of acculturative stress has been less studied and it has often been disregarded in the literature.

Acculturative stress can result in poorer mental or physical health outcomes. For instance, women who had to leave children behind and cannot send for them until much later often experience depression due to separation from their loved ones. Immigrants who have fled war situations often suffer from posttraumatic stress disorder in addition to acculturative stress. In order to alleviate their pain, some immigrants may resort to alcohol or substance use, which, in turn, is related to greater risk for accidents, HIV/AIDS, and social isolation.

In sum, acculturation is a process that is multidimensional and complex, and that deserves careful study. It requires interventions not only to help immigrants adapt to the new society but also to help the host culture to successfully integrate the contribution of new immigrants.

Acne

SEE ALSO: Asian and Pacific Islander, Immigrant health, Latinos

Suggested Reading

Balls Organista, P., Organista, K. C., & Kurasaki, K. (2003). The relationship between acculturation and ethnic minority mental health. In K. Chun, P. Balls Organista, & G. Marín (Eds.), *Acculturation: Advances in theory, measurement, and applied research* (pp. 139–161). Washington, DC: American Psychological Association.

Berry, J. W., & Sam, D. (1997). Acculturation and adaptation. In J. W. Berry, M. H. Segall, & C. Kagitcibasi (Eds.), *Handbook of cross-cultural psychology: Social behavior and applications* (2nd ed., pp. 291–326). Boston: Allyn & Bacon.

Chun, K., Balls Organista, P., & Marín, G. (2003). *Acculturation: Advances in theory, measurement, and applied research.* Washington, DC: American Psychological Association.

Rodriguez, N., Myers, H. F., Flores, T., & Garcia-Hernandez, L. (2002). Development of the multidimensional acculturative stress inventory for adults of Mexican origin. *Psychological Assessment, 14,* 451–461.

Stonequist, E. V. (1937). *The marginal man: A study in personality and culture conflict.* New York: Russell & Russell.

Zea, M. C., Asner-Self, K., Birman, D., & Buki, L. (2003). The abbreviated multidimensional acculturation scale: Empirical validation with two Latino/a samples. *Cultural Diversity and Ethnic Minority Psychology, 9,* 107–126.

MARIA CECILIA ZEA

Acne

Acne Acne vulgaris is a common disorder affecting the skin. It specifically involves the pilosebaceous unit, consisting of the hair follicle and sebaceous gland. The cause is multifactorial and the four major causal components are proliferation of the bacteria *Propionibacterium acnes*, abnormal shedding of the cells lining the pores, androgen-induced sebum production, and inflammation. It primarily affects teenagers but is not confined to this age group. The lesion types in acne are divided into two major groups, inflammatory and noninflammatory. Noninflammatory lesions include open and closed comedones, also known as whiteheads and blackheads, respectively. Inflammatory lesions are more prominent, appearing as red papules, pustules, or, the most severe, cysts. Acne predominates in areas rich in sebaceous glands such as the face, chest, and upper back. Although acne does not constitute a life-threatening condition, multiple studies have demonstrated that the psychosocial ramifications of this highly visible condition occurring during the formative teenage years can seriously impact self-esteem and quality of life.

Multiple categories of drugs have proven efficacy in the treatment of acne. Awareness of the multifactorial pathogenesis of acne has facilitated the rational application of combination therapies with different mechanisms of action. Milder cases of acne are generally treated with topical products including benzoyl peroxide, antibiotics, and vitamin A derivatives. The side effects of topical products are generally limited to local irritation or drying of the skin. In more severe cases, systemic antibiotics are used in combination with the topical agents. The most commonly prescribed systemic antibiotics are in the tetracycline class including tetracycline, doxycycline, or minocycline. An increasing prevalence of *Propionibacterium acnes* resistance to the usual antibiotics used to treat acne is being seen, and the treatment period should be kept as brief as possible for this reason. For the most severe cases of acne, a systemic retinoid, isotretinoin, may be prescribed. All of the systemic drugs are associated with various side effects necessitating proper patient selection and counseling before starting the medication and careful monitoring during the treatment course.

Adult female acne is significantly influenced by the effect of androgens on the pilosebaceous unit. An index of suspicion for overproduction of androgens from the adrenal glands or ovaries must be considered, but in the majority of patients hormone levels are normal and there appears to be a peripheral alteration whereby the sebaceous gland is more sensitive to normal circulating androgen levels. Acne in this population is particularly challenging to treat because it tends not to respond to the traditional therapies employed in teenage patients. Efficacious treatments such as oral contraceptives, some of which are now approved by the Food and Drug Administration for the treatment of acne, and antiandrogens, none of which are approved for this indication, alter the hormonal milieu of the pilosebaceous unit.

The most important aspect of acne treatment is patient compliance with medications. Contrary to popular belief, particular foods are not implicated in the development of acne. However, the Western diet, high in sugar and refined carbohydrates, may have an adverse effect on acne. Poor hygiene is also not a significant factor in acne and, in fact, overzealous cleansing can worsen the irritation. In most cases, the acne is self-limited peaking in severity during the teenage years and eventually remitting. The presence or absence of acne in teenage girls is not predictive of who will go on to develop the adult female variety. Early and appropriate treatment will reduce the likelihood of long-term scarring as will avoidance of manipulating the lesions.

See Also: Adolescence, Oral contraception, Skin disorders

Suggested Reading

Baldwin, H. E. (2002). The interaction between acne vulgaris and the psyche. *Cutis, 70,* 133–139.

Goulden, V., Stables, G. I., & Cunliffe, W. J. (1999). Prevalence of facial acne in adults. *Journal of the American Academy of Dermatology, 41,* 577–580.

Shaw, J. C. (1996). Antiandrogen and hormonal treatment of acne. *Current Therapy, 14,* 803–811.

White, G. M. (1998). Recent findings in the epidemiologic evidence, classification, and sub-types of acne vulgaris. *Journal of the American Academy of Dermatology, 39,* S34–S37.

MARY GAIL MERCURIO

Acquired Immunodeficiency Syndrome

(AIDS) AIDS is a medical diagnosis by a physician of a set of symptoms or conditions based on specific criteria established by the Centers for Disease Control and Prevention (CDC). These criteria include infection with human immunodeficiency virus (HIV) *and* either the presence of one or more defined AIDS indicator diseases or other indicators of a suppressed immune system based on certain blood tests (CD4+ counts). The "opportunistic" diseases associated with AIDS occur following the depression of an individual's immune system, allowing susceptibility to unusual infections or malignancies.

AIDS, the end stage of HIV disease, is caused by the infection and spread of HIV within the body. A positive HIV test result alone does not mean that a person has AIDS, only that HIV infection has occurred. HIV destroys CD4+ T blood cells that are crucial to the normal function of the human immune system. Most HIV-infected people carry the virus for years before the immune system is damaged enough for AIDS to develop. There is a direct correlation between the amount of HIV in the blood, the decline in CD4+ T cell numbers, and the onset of AIDS. Progression from initial HIV infection to AIDS may take 10 years or more, but varies greatly depending on many factors, including a person's health status and their health-related behaviors. Reducing the amount of virus in the body with anti-HIV drugs can slow down the rate at which HIV weakens and destroys the immune system.

The natural history of HIV infection in adults is well documented in the medical literature. The impact of gender on the outcome of HIV infection is still being investigated. HIV appears to progress more rapidly in women than men and to present with a different array of opportunistic conditions. These factors may also be compounded by the tendency of women to receive less care and to present with more advanced disease.

HIV TRANSMISSION

HIV can be transmitted through blood, semen (including pre-seminal fluid or "pre-cum"), vaginal fluid, or breast milk. The most common modes are: sexual intercourse (anal, vaginal, or oral sex) with an HIV-infected person; sharing needles, syringes, or injection equipment with an injecting drug user (IDU) infected with HIV; and from HIV-infected women to babies before or during birth, or through breast-feeding after birth. HIV can also be transmitted through transfusions of infected blood or blood clotting factors, but routine screening of all donated blood since 1985 has made this risk extremely low. Some health care workers have become infected after being stuck with needles containing HIV-infected blood.

Transmission of HIV can be influenced by several factors, including characteristics of the HIV-infected host, the recipient, and the quantity and infectivity of the virus. Having a sexually transmitted disease (STD) can increase a person's risk of becoming infected with HIV. In addition, if an HIV-infected person is also infected with another STD, that person is 3–5 times more likely to transmit HIV through sexual contact. HIV cannot be transmitted from casual (i.e., hugging or shaking hands) or surface (i.e., toilet seats) contact or from insect bites. Intact, healthy skin is an excellent barrier against HIV and other viruses and bacteria.

In the United States in 2001, CDC estimated that 66% of adult/adolescent women reported with AIDS were infected through heterosexual exposure to HIV; of these, 24% were infected through sex with an IDU. Direct risks associated with drug injection (sharing needles) accounted for 32% of all cases among women. Additionally, women who use noninjection drugs (e.g., "crack" cocaine, methamphetamines) are at greater risk of acquiring HIV sexually, especially if they trade sex for drugs or money.

HIV TESTING

The only way to determine for sure whether some-one is infected is to be tested for HIV infection. Many people who are infected with HIV do not have any symptoms for many years. The tests commonly used detect antibodies produced by the body to fight HIV. Most people will develop detectable antibodies within 3 months after infection, with the average being 25 days; in rare cases, it can take up to 6 months.

Many women in care are not routinely screened for HIV. Since women of color are less likely to receive regular health care, they are also even less likely to be tested for HIV.

HIV testing and counseling provides an opportunity for women to find out whether they are infected and gain access to medical treatment that may help to delay disease progression. For infected pregnant women, it may provide a viable opportunity to access treatment to prevent transmission of HIV to their child. For women who are not infected, HIV counseling offers an opportunity to learn important prevention information.

STATE OF THE HIV/AIDS EPIDEMIC

Worldwide, the World Health Organization estimates that the number of people living with HIV/AIDS is rapidly approaching 50 million, of whom almost 50% are women. In several regions of the world, the proportion of women exceeds 50%. The United Nations AIDS (UNAIDS) program estimates that 5 million new HIV infections occurred in 2001, or approximately 14,000 new cases per day. An estimated 3 million adults and children died of HIV/AIDS in 2001.

In the United States, the CDC estimates that approximately 800,000–900,000 people are living with HIV or AIDS, of whom 30% are women. Approximately 40,000 new HIV infections occur in the United States every year. Of the 240,000–270,000 women living with HIV disease in the United States, more than one half do not know their serostatus, meaning whether they are HIV-positive or HIV-negative, or that of their partner. Many will not be tested for HIV until they seek prenatal care, give birth, develop an AIDS-related illness, or until their partner develops an AIDS-related illness.

Through December 2001, 816,149 U.S. cases of AIDS had been reported to the CDC. Since 1985, the proportion of all AIDS cases reported each year among adult and adolescent women has more than tripled, from 7% in 1985 to 26% in 2001. The epidemic has continued to increase most dramatically among women of color. African American and Hispanic women together represent less than one fourth of all U.S. women, yet account for more than three fourths (78%) of AIDS cases reported to date among women. In 2001 alone, African American and Hispanic women represented an even greater proportion (80%) of cases reported in women.

During the mid-to-late 1990s, advances in HIV treatment led to dramatic declines in AIDS deaths and slowed the progression from HIV to AIDS in the United States. As a result, more people are now living with AIDS in the United States than ever before. This growing population represents an increasing need for continued HIV prevention, care, and treatment services. Even as HIV/AIDS-related deaths among women continued to decrease in 1999, largely as a result of recent advances in HIV treatment, HIV/AIDS was the fifth leading cause of death among U.S. women aged 25–44, and the third leading cause of death among African American women in this same age group. HIV/AIDS-related deaths among women of color also have declined less rapidly than their white/Caucasian counterparts.

Despite the dramatic advances made in understanding the natural history of HIV disease and the development of effective antiretroviral therapies, the AIDS epidemic continues to grow with some disturbing trends. HIV/AIDS morbidity and mortality increasingly impact the poor, the disenfranchised, and the young, groups in which women are traditionally overrepresented.

PREVENTING HIV TRANSMISSION

Abstaining from engagement in any behavior that carries risk of acquiring HIV (e.g., sexual intercourse or using and injecting drugs) is the most effective way to avoid HIV, but not always the most realistic. To minimize risk for those who choose to be sexually active, the CDC recommends the following: engage in sex that does not involve vaginal, anal, or oral sex; have intercourse with only one uninfected partner; and/or use latex condoms every time you have sex. For IDUs who cannot or will not stop injecting drugs, the following steps are recommended to reduce risk: never reuse or "share" syringes, water, or drug preparation equipment; only use syringes obtained from a reliable source (such as pharmacies or needle exchange programs);

use a new, sterile syringe to prepare and inject drugs; if possible, use sterile water to prepare drugs; otherwise, use clean water from a reliable source (such as fresh tap water); use a new or disinfected container ("cooker") and a new filter ("cotton") to prepare drugs; clean the injection site prior to injection with a new alcohol swab; safely dispose of syringes after one use. If new, sterile syringes and other drug preparation and injection equipment are not available, then previously used equipment should be boiled in water or disinfected with bleach before reuse.

Medical therapy (ZDV—zidovudine, also known as AZT or Retrovir) is available to effectively reduce the chance of an HIV-infected pregnant woman passing HIV to her infant before, during, or after birth. In 1998, the U.S. Public Health Services released updated recommendations for offering antiretroviral therapy to HIV- positive pregnant women.

Programs focusing on reducing the transmission of HIV among women should include an increased emphasis on prevention and treatment services for young women and women of color; address the intersection of drug use and sexual HIV transmission; develop and widely disseminate effective female-controlled prevention methods; and better integrate prevention and treatment services for women across the board, including the prevention and treatment of other STDs and substance abuse and access to antiretroviral therapy. More options are urgently needed for women who are unwilling or unable to negotiate condom use with a male partner.

CARE AND TREATMENT

The field of HIV/AIDS care is advancing at a breathtaking speed. New developments are rapidly superseded by even newer data. Recommendations for antiretroviral treatment and alternative regimens continue to evolve as new medications are developed and additional data from clinical trials is presented. As a consequence, treatment protocols will not be described here in deference to a recommendation to review the most current HIV/AIDS treatment guidelines available through AIDS Treatment Information Service (ATIS) (*United States & Canada:* 1-800-HIV-0440; *TTY:* 1-888-480-3739; *International:* 1-301-519-0459; *Mailing Address:* HIV/AIDS Treatment Information Service, P.O. Box 6303; Rockville, MD 20849-6303; *Web site:* http://hivatis.org; *E-mail:* atis@hivatis.org).

Early medical treatment and a healthy lifestyle can help an individual with HIV stay well. Prompt medical care may delay the onset of AIDS and prevent some life-threatening conditions. A person who has learned that he/she is HIV-positive should see a doctor, even if he/she does not feel sick. Drugs are now available to treat HIV infection and to assist in maintaining health.

Because they are often diagnosed later and generally have poorer access to care and medications, women tend to have higher viral loads and lower CD4 counts upon entering care. Even in care, the health status of HIV-positive women continues to compare poorly to that of their male counterparts. Despite increased attention in recent years, HIV-positive women in care are less likely than men to receive the current standard of care, including regular visits with an experienced clinician, antiretroviral therapy, combination therapy, and/or a protease inhibitor(s). Receipt of care from a less experienced provider is a critical problem, since provider expertise and experience directly affect quality of care and disease progression. Women are less likely to know their viral load or CD4 count, and their medical charts are less likely to contain this information. All of these factors are further exacerbated for poor women and women of color.

Research and experience indicate the following set of conditions to facilitate HIV care for women. (a) The risk for HIV must be perceived. (b) HIV status must be known and the need for and promise of medical care understood. (c) Caregiving responsibilities to children and family members must be met. (d) Basic life needs for food, shelter, and community must be met. (e) Treatment for other problems including substance abuse and mental health disorders must be ongoing. (f) Transportation to appointments must be available. (g) Childcare must be available. (h) Financial means to pay for health care and medications must be available. (i) The patient must encounter medical personnel qualified to treat HIV infection in women. (j) HIV-positive mothers must encounter care that is "family-centered" and coordinated—care that addresses the impact of HIV and barriers to care for the family. (k) All prescribed medications must be available. (l) Informational, psychological, and emotional support from peers and care providers must be ongoing.

At present, the approach to management of HIV disease is the same for both women and men. The clinical course of HIV infection in women does not seem to differ significantly from that in men, with the exception of the associated gynecologic and obstetric conditions and issues. Women may have lower HIV viral loads than men with an equivalent degree of immunosuppression, but do not tend to differ in overall survival or complication-free survival. As both women and men live longer with HIV disease and AIDS, general preventive strategies and health maintenance have become part of routine care. These include smoking cessation, control of hypertension, minimizing cardiovascular risk factors, and routine screening for malignancy (cervical, breast, colon).

SOCIAL/PSYCHOSOCIAL CHALLENGES AND NEEDS

Many social/psychosocial issues, including homosexuality, drug use, mental illness, racism, homelessness, and poverty, are linked inextricably to the context of HIV/AIDS by association with the communities that it has heavily impacted, in addition to the clinical challenges of the disease itself and its toll on the health and well-being of those infected. For many women with HIV/AIDS, specific challenges and needs impact their ability to protect themselves from HIV and/or access care. These are: (a) parenthood and caregiving, with approximately 62% of all HIV-positive women taking care of at least one child under age 20, with their first priority to their children; (b) lack of awareness of risk and serostatus; (c) discrimination due to HIV status, and racial discrimination for women of color; (d) poverty, with most HIV-positive women already poor before becoming infected and becoming poorer as their disease progresses; (e) psychological distress, including fear, depression, and anxiety about their serostatus, compounded by high incidences of poverty, discrimination, caregiving responsibilities, addiction, sexual abuse, and domestic violence; (f) substance abuse of both injected and noninjected substances, a prominent problem among women at risk and with HIV disease, impacting health care utilization and outcomes; (g) comorbidities, with women of color in particular having less exposure to health information, preventive health services, and primary care than men, and subsequently suffering higher rates of certain cancers, cardiovascular disease, hypertension, obesity, tuberculosis, and diabetes, further complicating HIV care; (h) STDs, with women of color, particularly African American women, having higher rates of chlamydia, syphilis, and gonorrhea than white women.

SEE ALSO: African American, Condoms, Discrimination, Heroin, Homosexuality, Latinos, Lubricants, Preventive care, Safer sex, Sexually transmitted diseases, Substance use

Suggested Reading

Anderson, J. (Ed.). (2001). *A guide to the clinical care of women with HIV.* Rockville, MD: U.S. Department of Health and Human Services, Health Resources and Services Administration, HIV/AIDS Bureau.

The Body: Resources for HIV Positive Women. (2003). New York (February 4, 2003); http://thebody.com/women/women.html.

Centers for Disease Control and Prevention. (2002). CDC's answers to frequently asked questions about HIV/AIDS. Atlanta, GA (May 16, 2002); http://www.cdcnpin.org/hiv/faq.htm.

Centers for Disease Control and Prevention. (2002). HIV/AIDS among US women: Minority and young women at continuing risk. Atlanta, GA (March 11, 2002); http://www.cdc.gov/hiv/pubs/facts/women.html.

Centers for Disease Control and Prevention. (2002). *HIV/AIDS Surveillance Report, 13*(2), 1–44

The Henry J. Kaiser Family Foundation. (2001). *Key facts: Women and HIV/AIDS.* Menlo Park, CA: Author.

HIV Disease in Women of Color. (1999, May). *HRSA care action.* Rockville, MD: U.S. Department of Health and Human Services, Health Resources and Services Administration, HIV/AIDS Bureau.

Mann, D. (1998, December). Four perspectives from women serving women. *HRSA care action.* Rockville, MD: U.S. Department of Health and Human Services, Health Resources and Services Administration, HIV/AIDS Bureau.

Project Inform—Project Wise; HIV/AIDS Treatment Info and Advocacy for Women (2003). New York (February 24, 2003); http://www.projinf.org/pub/ww_index.html.

Women and HIV/AIDS. (1998, December). *HRSA care action.* Rockville, MD: U.S. Department of Health and Human Services, Health Resources and Services Administration, HIV/AIDS Bureau.

DANIEL P. O'SHEA

Activities of Daily Living The ability of an individual to provide self-care or function independently is often referred to by the phrase "activities of daily living." This phrase is often used to describe physical functioning, or those functions an individual performs daily for his or her own safety and health maintenance. In the early 1960s, Katz et al. described the six areas that are considered the functions essential to physically care for oneself. They are typically listed in the order in which functions are lost due to physical illness or dementia: bathing, dressing, toileting, transferring, continence, and feeding.

Instrumental activities of daily living (IADL) are functions that are essential for independent living. IADL involve the ability to plan, organize, maintain a dwelling, and manage the condition of oneself or others. Several activities may be considered, including meal preparation, doing laundry, providing for a clean living space, paying bills and managing business affairs, taking medications as recommended, telephoning, scheduling appointments, arranging transportation or driving, traveling to both familiar and unfamiliar locations, shopping for groceries, remembering to refill prescriptions, and remembering holidays and scheduled events. Some of these activities may be culturally bound, or gender specific. For example, if the husband always handled the finances, a woman who finds herself suddenly widowed may be unable to carry out these activities simply because she never learned how. In evaluating both activities of daily living and IADL, the focus is the ability to care for oneself. When this is not possible, some assistance may be required.

See Also: Assisted living, Long-term care, Nursing home

Suggested Reading

Functional Activities Questionnaire. (1982). *Journal of Gerontology, 37*, 323–329.

Katz, S., Ford, A. B., Moskowitz, R. W., Jackson, B. A., & Jaffe, M. W. (1963). Studies of illness in the aged: The index of ADL: A standardized measure of biological and psychosocial function. *Journal of the American Medical Association, 185*, 914–919.

EVANNE JURATOVAC

Acupuncture Acupuncture is a medical treatment that has emerged from the naturalist school of thought in China over 2,000 years ago. It has been modified and perfected over the course of its existence and has been adapted by other cultures. Acupuncture is one part of a Chinese medical system based on the production and flow of Qi (pronounced "chi"), which may be described loosely as vital energy. Qi circulates through meridians and organs in an orderly fashion and it is the disruption in the production and flow of Qi that results in disease and pain. As a system of medicine quite different than the Western system, acupuncture has its own language and references to organs may be thought of as metaphorical when compared to the Western definition of organ function. Traditional acupuncture treatments consist of insertion of thin sterile needles at specific locations along the meridians. The exact locations used are determined by a careful assessment by the acupuncturist or the patient and the problem being treated. This assessment involves questioning, observation of the patient, assessment of the pulses and tongue, and locating areas of tenderness on examination through palpation. In essence, a history and physical exam similar to that done in Western medicine is performed, but with a different emphasis. Treatments are thus individualized, such that the same Western diagnosis may well be treated quite differently in different patients.

In Western countries, acupuncture has been primarily used to treat pain, but is increasingly receiving attention for treatment of other conditions. Due to the nature of the individualized treatments, acupuncture does not lend itself well to the constraints of controlled clinical studies, leading many Western trained physicians to doubt or underestimate its effectiveness. Despite these limitations, efforts to clarify the role of acupuncture are receiving more attention. A National Institutes of Health consensus panel has recently concluded that acupuncture is probably effective for postoperative and chemotherapy-induced nausea as well as postoperative dental pain. Further it was stated that acupuncture may be an acceptable alternative treatment for a number of other conditions including headache, menstrual cramps, low back pain, osteoarthritis, carpal tunnel syndrome, addiction, stroke rehabilitation, tennis elbow, fibromyalgia, myofascial pain, and asthma.

During an acupuncture treatment, needles are inserted at various points along a meridian. This usually involves the use of both local and distal points. A local point is a point at the location where the discomfort or pain is present. Distal points are chosen for their traditional effects and are distant from the location of pain. These acupuncture needles are extremely thin and solid—unlike the hollow needles used to draw blood.

Although treatments involve minimal discomfort, an aching or radiating sensation may be noted. This phenomenon of "De Qi" is often sought by the practitioner and is thought by many to be important for a treatment to be effective. Needles may then be manipulated manually or stimulated by low-level electricity. A smoldering herb may also be used to warm the needles in the technique known as moxibustion. As acupuncture has evolved, multiple different styles and approaches have emerged. One such approach involves the use of "reflex microsystems." Reflex microsystems are localized areas of the body that have representations of the entire body within them. The most commonly used microsystem is the ear. Thus, for example, treatment of the ear can have effects on the entire body. Other microsystems commonly used include the scalp and the hand. These are frequently stimulated in conjunction with other acupuncture treatments. In addition to the use of needles, stimulation of acupuncture points with lasers, magnets, and pressure show considerable promise.

A treatment may last up to 45 min and the patient not uncommonly experiences a sense of relaxed well-being following a treatment. Transient fatigue or euphoria is a less common effect. Other side effects that may be seen include bruising and pain at the needle insertion site, and a transient aggravation of the underlying problem. Of note, a mild increase in symptoms is often seen followed by improvement. Fainting may uncommonly occur, especially during a first treatment, but future treatments can usually be continued with caution. Serious complications are exceedingly rare, but could include bleeding, infection, and puncture of an organ. While one treatment may on occasion produce dramatic results, acupuncture is not magic, and usually 8–12 treatments are required. Periodic treatments may be necessary to maintain a response.

Acupuncture is used in conjunction with Western medicine and a recommendation to discontinue other treatments should be regarded with suspicion and discussed with your physician. Acupuncture practitioners may be medical doctors who have received further training in acupuncture, or licensed acupuncturists who also undergo extensive training. Further study should help further elucidate the role of acupuncture. For now it can be stated that acupuncture has been shown to be safe and effective for a number of conditions.

SEE ALSO: Back pain, Chronic pain, Headache, Pain

Suggested Reading

Acupuncture. NIH Consensus Statement Online 1997 Nov 3–5; *15*, 1–34.

Helms, J. (1995). *Acupuncture energetics: A clinical approach for physicians.* Berkeley, CA: Medical Acupuncture Publishers.

Kaptchuk, T. J. (2000). *The web that has no weaver: Understanding Chinese medicine* (2nd ed.). Chicago: Contemporary Books.

DOUGLAS FLAGG

Acute Myocardial Infarction
Cardiovascular disease is the leading cause of death among women in the United States. In fact, according to the 2003 statistical update from the American Heart Association, cardiovascular disease kills over 7 million women annually in the United States, more than the next seven causes of death combined. Of these cardiovascular deaths, the most common cause is acute myocardial infarction (MI). An MI occurs when blood supply to the heart is suddenly interrupted for some period of time. This process may occur because of the development of a thrombus on the surface of a previously existing cholesterol plaque in the coronary arteries. If this blockage is complete and persists for some time—often greater than 30–60 min—the result may be death to the myocardium supplied by this vessel, a so-called transmural infarction. In other situations, the blockage may not completely obstruct all myocardial blood flow, yet it persists and leads to damage. The resulting infarction is termed nontransmural, indicating that the damage has not been as extensive. On occasion, MIs may also be caused by spasm of the coronary artery or very transient obstruction that cannot be identified on later angiographic evaluation.

The pathophysiology that leads to an MI is the same in women and men; however, there are important gender differences that are apparent on presentation with MI. Women are less likely than men to present with an acute transmural infarction (also called an "ST-elevation MI" because of the typical EKG pattern). Instead, women more often experience nontransmural ("non-ST-elevation") infarctions or acute coronary symptoms not resulting in an MI. This more subtle presentation may be one reason why physicians and laypersons tended to consider coronary heart disease less as a disease of women than of men. In fact, multiple studies have shown that, compared with men, women present later to the hospital with an MI, are less likely to receive important thrombolytic drugs when appropriate, and are less likely to be referred for coronary angiography. Furthermore, because MI is often not correctly diagnosed, women are less likely to receive appropriate medications and cardiac rehabilitation.

Recent findings have effectively destroyed the myth that MI is a less important disease in women than in men. On the one hand, women have important differences from men who present with MI—on average, the women are 10–20 years older, with more elevated cholesterol levels and possibly more hypertension, but a lower prevalence of cigarette smoking. Women also are more likely to have diabetes, which is a major risk factor for poor outcome with MI and, when present, negates any gender benefit for women. In addition, women who sustain an MI are also as much as 50% more likely to die in the short term as are men. Finally, perhaps because of their older age and greater extent of other illness, women are more likely to suffer so-called mechanical complications of MI, such as cardiac rupture.

In addition to the different characteristics of women and men with MI, there are important differences in the symptoms that each gender tends to report upon presentation. The classic symptoms, such as the sudden onset of pressure centered in the chest, radiating down one or both arms, and associated with a "cold sweat" (or diaphoresis), should be considered more as the typical middle-aged male symptoms associated with MI. While both genders certainly experience a full range of symptoms, women are much less likely to have these so-called "classic" symptoms and are more likely to have a wider range of complaints, including shortness of breath (dyspnea), nausea or vomiting, and pains in the jaw, back, or even abdomen, with or without chest pain. Women are also more likely to sustain an MI without any characteristic symptoms—the so-called "silent MI." It is now recognized that any individual—either physician or layperson—who relies on more stereotypical chest pain symptoms for diagnosis will fail to appreciate early symptoms of an MI more often in women than in men.

Good news is that the therapies for MI have, almost uniformly, provided strong benefit to both genders. Unfortunately, there is mounting evidence that women do not receive these therapies as often as men. For patients with an ST-elevation MI, the accepted beneficial therapies include thrombolytic therapy and "primary angioplasty," which involve emergent coronary angiography to identify the occlusion and then angioplasty to open the artery. Both of these therapies work in women and men, and in the multitude of medical studies to evaluate these treatments, it appears that the benefit for women is similar to the benefit extended to men. However, because women with MI tend to be older, with greater comorbidity, and because they are on average smaller in body size than men, they may have more problems with bleeding with all therapies and may sometimes not be eligible for thrombolytic therapy. Furthermore, among older patients, there is a concern that women may have more complications with thrombolytics, and some investigators have proposed that primary angioplasty is a better treatment for women. However, it is also true that women may arrive at the hospital too late for thrombolysis, emphasizing that women, their families, and their physicians need to recognize possible signs of MI and present to emergency departments promptly so that appropriate therapy may be pursued.

Just as important as rapid treatment for ST-elevation MI, is appropriate therapy for non-ST-elevation MI, the more common presentation for women. While thrombolytic therapy is not an effective treatment for this condition, a wide range of medical therapies significantly reduce the risk associated with this type of infarction. Relative to management of this condition, debates within the cardiology community have recently focused on the routine use of certain medications, most notably the glycoprotein IIb/IIIa inhibitors, and the routine use of an "early aggressive strategy," which involves early catheterization and intervention as needed for patients with non-ST-elevation MI. While there has been some evidence that women do not receive as great a benefit with IIb/IIIa inhibitors as do men, a recent study that used these agents in the evaluation of early catheterization demonstrated that the benefit of an "aggressive strategy" was just as strong in women as in men, but of particular benefit in high-risk women.

Medications that should be considered for all patients with MI provide benefits to both genders, in the setting of ST-elevation or non-ST-elevation infarction. The most important of these drugs remains aspirin, which in the early studies of ST-elevation MI provided benefit equal and in addition to that of thrombolytic therapy. Other drugs that must be considered include beta-blockers (which may provide even stronger benefits to women than to men), ACE inhibitors, and statin medications. The statins, which lower blood cholesterol levels, have demonstrated on average a 20% reduction in mortality in all patients with coronary disease, and there is no evidence of preferential effect by gender. One note specific to women is that the majority of evidence now indicates that hormone replacement therapy does not provide any special level of protection before or after MI.

After recognition of an appropriate therapy for MI, other procedures and treatments may be appropriate for women. Some of these, such as nuclear cardiac scans or echocardiograms, can give a better indication of individual levels of risk and guide intensity of treatment. Other treatments, such as cardiac rehabilitation, including exercise training and secondary prevention, are powerful tools that, again, physicians have been less likely to offer to women than to men.

Scientific knowledge has increased the understanding of the burden of cardiovascular disease in women. With a better appreciation of the clinical characteristics and symptoms that mark acute MI in women, we are now much more able to provide therapies of proven benefit to all patients.

Addiction Ethics

SEE ALSO: Cardiovascular disease, Chest pain, Cholesterol, Diabetes, Hormone replacement therapy, Smoking

Suggested Reading

American Heart Association. (2002). *2003 heart and stroke statistical update* (pp. 1–29). Dallas, TX: Author.

Douglas, P. (2001). Heart disease in women. In E. Braunwald (Ed.), *Heart disease: A textbook of cardiovascular medicine* (6th ed., pp. 2038–2051). Philadelphia: W. B. Saunders.

Glaser, R., Hermann, H., Murphy, S., et al. (2002). Benefits of an early invasive management strategy in women with acute coronary syndromes. *Journal of the American Medical Association, 288,* 3124–3129.

Miller, C. L. (1997). A review of symptoms of coronary artery disease in women. *Journal of Advanced Nursing, 39,* 17–23.

Tsang, T. S., Barnes, M. E., Gersh, B. K., & Hayes, S. N. (2000). Risk of coronary heart disease in women: Current understanding and evolving concepts. *Mayo Clinic Proceedings, 75,* 1289–1303.

Welty, F. K. (2001). Cardiovascular disease and dyslipidemia in women. *Archives of Internal Medicine, 161,* 514–522.

Suggested Resources

www.americanheart.org: Website of the American Heart Association. Fact sheets on women and heart disease can be referenced by searching for "Women and cardiovascular disease."

JASON H. COLE
NANETTE K. WENGER

Addiction Addiction is a common language term for the clinical entity known as Chemical Dependence. For decades Americans have known the term addiction to indicate an individual who is out of control in their use of mood-altering drugs. The term addiction has taken on a connotation that is highly stigmatized (like the term "alcoholic" is much more stigmatized than the term "drinking problem"). In reality, addiction is a primarily genetic, chronic progressive disease of the brain that is characterized by the intermittent inconsistent loss of control over the use of mood-altering drugs, resulting in repetitive adverse consequences to the user. The basic brain problem of addiction appears to be an inability to consistently control the use of drugs that produce an acute or quick surge of dopamine in the brain. This surge of dopamine leads to a feeling of euphoria or "high." Addiction to mood-altering drugs other than nicotine affects 10–13% of Americans at some time in their lives. A more complete description of addiction is in the entry entitled Substance use.

SEE ALSO: Chemical dependency, Substance use

Suggested Resources

www.jointogether.org: A national service for addiction treatment and prevention education funded by the Robert Wood Johnson Foundation.

TED PARRAN JR.

Addiction Ethics Although women today make up nearly a third of those persons who abuse substances in the U.S. population, they have often been neglected in research and clinical care. Since the 1970s, increasing academic and governmental attention has been focused on the needs of addicted women. However, significant ethical challenges remain in the effort to provide compassionate, competent, and equitable treatment for women suffering from addictions.

EPIDEMIOLOGICAL BACKGROUND

In 1994, the United States Department of Health and Human Services estimated that 200,000 women died of illnesses related to drug abuse. The figure was more than quadruple the number of women predicted to die of breast cancer. Large epidemiological studies estimate that 4.4 million women had used an illicit drug in the month prior to being surveyed, and that half of all women 15–44 years of age have used an illicit drug at least once in their lives.

The media have offered often highly stigmatizing accounts of an epidemic of substance abuse among contemporary women. Although the scientific evidence does not support such a dramatic rise in alcohol and drug abuse among women, there are disturbing trends. Heavy drinking is increasing in younger women and students on college campuses, with women in the prime reproductive years of 21–34 having the highest rates of problem substance use. Seventy percent of AIDS cases in women are related to illicit drug use, and at least half are the result of sexual contact with a partner who is an intravenous drug user.

ETHICAL PRINCIPLES

There is a consensus among Western ethicists that respect for persons, autonomy, veracity, beneficence, nonmaleficence, and justice are cardinal principles of modern medical ethics. These principles have received wide acceptance and are especially relevant to the ethical issues involved in the treatment and research of women with addictive disorders. Respect for persons requires that health professionals and researchers honor the fundamental dignity of each human being. Autonomy is self-determination, the ability of an individual to make her own medical decisions. Veracity is the obligation of the physician to tell the truth about medical conditions and treatment. Beneficence mandates that health professionals place promoting the good and avoiding harm of a patient or research participant above all other considerations. Nonmaleficence literally means to "do no harm" to the patient through medical care. Justice means that the burdens and benefits of prevention research and treatment must be distributed fairly and impartially.

STIGMA

Stigma in the context of addictions has been defined as "a mark that sets a person apart linked to an undesirable characteristic leading to rejection." Although men in nearly every society are heavier and more destructive users of substances, women have consistently been more highly stigmatized. Historically, women in many cultures have been acculturated to view the use of drugs and alcohol as behavior contrary to their role in society. These cultural expectations play a protective role in discouraging substance use. On the other hand, women who do use substances are disparaged and may be blamed for domestic violence or sexual trauma that befalls them in the context of substance use. In ethical terms, stigmatization fails to respect the intrinsic worth of women suffering from addictive disorders as persons. Stigmatization has contributed to the failure of the medical profession to fulfill the duties of nonmaleficence through adequate attention to issues of domestic victimization and social inequities that contribute to addictions in women.

ETHICAL DIMENSIONS OF CRIMINAL JUSTICE SYSTEM INVOLVEMENT

Women with addictions are frequently involved with the criminal justice system. Although in many cases this involvement is due to serious criminal behavior, in other cases it is due to the criminalization of addictive behavior. There is a growing trend toward diverting individuals with petty drug-related offenses from incarceration to treatment. However, this progress is opposed by punitive attitudes toward substance abusers, rooted in stigma as described above.

Beyond the stigma attached to substance abuse irrespective of gender, women have been punished for abusing substances under a double standard that treats them differently from men who abuse substances. During the last decade, state legislatures have taken punitive action against women abusing drugs during pregnancy, creating a climate of fear for those seeking help. A 1992 survey found that 150 women in 24 states had been prosecuted for drug use during pregnancy. Ethnic minorities were 10 times as likely to face charges. At least 10 states currently have laws that require mandatory reporting to child protective services of any newborn who tests positive for drugs. It is estimated that thousands of children have been removed from their mothers who were incarcerated rather than sent to drug rehabilitation.

Health professionals often experience ethical dilemmas when treating women who are involved with the criminal justice system. Reporting requirements (e.g., to a probation officer) may create a conflict between veracity (truthfulness) and nonmaleficence (the obligation to do no harm). Mandated treatment compromises autonomy and may seem disrespectful. For clinicians, the ethical mandate is to honestly negotiate with the patient a treatment agreement which acknowledges the constraints imposed by the legal system and professional ethics, and which is on the whole beneficial to the patient. Court-ordered treatment in fact tends to have significant positive consequences for the patient. Since documentation of treatment compliance is often a condition of release, such reporting can literally keep the patient out of jail. Such requirements moreover serve as a strong, albeit coercive, incentive to participate in treatment.

SPECIAL FEATURES OF ADDICTION IN WOMEN

Fair (just) and effective (beneficent) treatment of substance use disorders in women requires adequate knowledge. In particular, it is crucial to understand how addicted women tend to differ from addicted men, rather than blindly to apply models that were developed for men. Social and environmental influences are strong determinants of addictive behavior in women. Many addicted women are involved with partners who abuse substances and frequently are also perpetrators of domestic violence. Without family system treatment, these women have a poor chance of recovering. Women are often without the job skills, income, or insurance that would enable them to access and afford health care. Many women with addictions are single mothers, yet few programs have childcare available. The highly successful 12-step approach, originally developed by and for white men, emphasizes the surrender of power. This model may be less appropriate and effective for women, and minority women in particular, who have been lifelong victims of exploitation.

Medical and psychiatric comorbidity in women with addictions is different from that found in men. Women become dependent upon substances more rapidly than men even though they tend to consume smaller quantities per body weight. Women also more quickly develop the medical sequelae of alcohol and other drug use for physiological reasons such as lower levels of the enzyme that metabolizes alcohol, and a higher percentage of body fat, which influences how long a drug remains active in the body. Liver disease, hypertension, cardiomyopathy, peptic ulcer, and anemia all have a more severe course in women. Women who abuse substances also have a higher rate of comorbid psychiatric disorders than men. Depression is particularly common and frequently precedes the substance abuse, suggesting that depression may play a causal role. A number of barriers to care have prevented addicted women from receiving appropriate and high-quality care for both addictive and psychiatric disorders.

SEE ALSO: Depression, Domestic violence, Informed consent, Mental illness, Pregnancy, Substance use

Suggested Reading

Beauchaump, T., & Childress, J. F. (2001). *Principles of biomedical ethics* (5th ed.). New York: Oxford University Press.

Blume, S. B. (1998). *Understanding addictive disorders in women.* Annapolis Junction, MD: American Society of Addiction Medicine.

Galanter, M., & Kleber, H. D. (1999). *Textbook of substance abuse treatment* (2nd ed.). Washington, DC: American Psychiatric Press.

Link, B. G., Struening, E. L., Rahav, M., Phelan, J. C., & Nuttbrock, L. (1997). On stigma and its consequences: evidence from a longitudinal study of men with dual diagnoses of mental illness and substance abuse. *Journal of Health and Social Behavior, 38,* 177–190.

Wetherington, C. L., & Roman, A. B. (Eds.). (1998). *Drug addiction research and the health of women.* Rockville, MD: U.S. Department of Health and Human Services, National Institute on Drug Abuse.

CYNTHIA M. A. GEPPERT
MICHAEL BOGENSCHUTZ

Adolescence

Adolescence Adolescence, by many accounts, is a period rooted in culture and society. Prior to the industrial revolution, children were treated like adults and worked side by side with their parents in the factories. Industrialization during the 19th century led to new patterns of work that excluded children, lengthened the amount of formal schooling, and brought increased economic dependence of youth on their families. These events ushered in the period of the life cycle we now call adolescence, defined as a transitional stage whose chief purpose is to prepare children for adulthood. Broadly speaking, this developmental period spans the second decade of life and ends with the assumption of adult work and family roles.

Adolescence is characterized by a series of dynamic and interactive changes across several spheres, including biology, psychology, cognitive functioning, social interactions, and emotions. While these changes proceed in relatively the same sequence for most teens, they occur at varying rates and times for youth and are shaped by the environments in which they take place. Thus, it is typical for teens to mature in some respects before others. A more complete understanding of these changes is achieved by using a multidisciplinary contextual perspective that incorporates the impact of culture, families, peers, schools, communities, neighborhoods, and society. Indeed, youth face unprecedented challenges in society today compared to 20 years ago, and these challenges shape their long-term functioning in fundamental ways. Today, more than ever, teens are confronted with an array of confusing messages about their responsibilities, sexual behavior, health risks, life choices, job opportunities, interpersonal relationships, and future potential. Yet, despite these added challenges, most young people traverse the teen years with relative ease and success. Research indicates that youth have the capacity to cope with these challenges, and in fact, it is through the successful resolution of these experiences that most youth achieve significant personal growth.

STATUS OF ADOLESCENTS

In 1999, there were approximately 39.5 million youth between 10 and 19 years of age in America. Recent census data show that the majority of these youth lived in Western states and metropolitan areas. Based on current projections, the racial and ethnic makeup of the adolescent population in the United States will become increasingly heterogeneous, including a decrease in whites, an increase in other racial/ethnic groups, and growing numbers of Hispanics. One in six youth less than 18 years of age live at or below the poverty line, and ethnic minorities constitute a large percentage of poor youth; nearly one third of black and Hispanic youth live in poverty. Poverty is related to a host of conditions that negatively affect youth's development, including increased exposure to crime and unemployment, poor health status, low-quality schools, and limited access to health care and adequate housing. Moreover, economic hardship on the family influences adolescents' functioning and well-being through increased parental distress and less effective parenting behavior. The percentage of adolescents living in two-parent households has fallen sharply over the past 20 years particularly for minority youth, and nearly 42% of teens living in single-parent female-headed households are poor.

TRENDS IN ADOLESCENT PHYSICAL AND MENTAL HEALTH

The majority of adolescents appear to be in good-to-excellent physical health. They show low rates of cancer, hypertension, and other physical disorders, and mortality rates have dropped dramatically for all adolescents over the past two decades. Nonetheless, trends in mortality rates underscore the health disparities for males and females and different ethnic groups. Mortality increases with age, and males are three times more likely to die than females. The rate of death among black males continues to be much higher than for any other group. The leading causes of death for teens are no longer a natural phenomenon but instead constitute injury and violence resulting from motor vehicle accidents, homicide, suicide, and other unintentional injuries. Thus, a large majority of the deaths are preventable, and understanding these behaviors is critical to public health prevention efforts.

The Surgeon General recently released a report on mental health indicating that nearly 21% of youth aged 9–17 meet criteria for a diagnosable mental or addictive disorder, and 11% report significant impairment as a result of their mental health problems. There is additional evidence that mental health disorders are under-diagnosed among youth, and that more than 30% may have some mental health symptoms. Obesity has emerged as a major health and mental health concern because evidence points to serious risks associated with poor nutrition and excess weight. Indeed, the percentage of overweight youth rose from 5% in 1980 to 20% in 2002 with black adolescents at greatest risk.

TRENDS IN ADOLESCENT RISK BEHAVIOR

Experimentation and risk taking are hallmarks of adolescence, yet the negative health consequences today are more serious than ever before. Unprotected sex will not only result in unwanted pregnancy, but it may also lead to HIV transmission. Illegal substances are more potent and more addictive, and cars and guns are easily accessible. Specific risk behaviors show divergent patterns among adolescents. Tobacco use peaked in 1997 but appears to have stabilized, while alcohol use remains high. Almost half of all high school seniors report using marijuana at some point in their lifetime, although recent use (in the past 30 days) has fallen in the past 5 years. The trends for sexual behavior are more mixed. For the first time in two decades, fewer adolescents are having sexual intercourse and more teens are using condoms. However, only 30% report using condoms consistently, and almost 75% of high school seniors have had sexual intercourse. Furthermore, teens account for approximately 25% of new sexually transmitted diseases reported annually, and adolescents are one of the only groups for which rates of HIV infection are increasing. The primary mode of HIV transmission for adolescents is through unprotected sexual activity, and adolescent females are now almost as likely to become infected with HIV as males, comprising 59.7% of new HIV cases in 2001. These trends underscore the new predominance of heterosexual HIV transmission among youth.

ADOLESCENT DEVELOPMENT IN CONTEXT

Biological Changes

Adolescence marks the most rapid and significant biological changes throughout the life span with the exception of infancy. Puberty and menarche (see entries in this encyclopedia) end with the ability to reproduce and the appearance of a physical adult form. The main physical manifestations of these changes are a dramatic growth in height and weight, further development of the gonads or sex glands (i.e., ovaries in females), growth of secondary sex characteristics (e.g., breasts, pubic hair, sex organs), changes in the distribution of fat and muscle in the body, and increased tolerance for exercise resulting from improved circulation and respiration. The changes in appearance evoke mixed reactions from the teenager about herself and mark critical shifts in family relationships, peer relationships, and societal expectations (see below).

Cognitive Changes

There are important changes in cognitive functioning during adolescence that have far-reaching implications for achievement and interpersonal relationships. Advanced reasoning abilities emerge and teens become increasingly capable of abstract and logical thought. They are able to consider multiple hypothetical outcomes and view events from perspectives other than their own, although shifts in emotions may impair their judgment at times. Teens acquire a greater capacity to think in a multidimensional way rather than being limited to a single issue, and they begin to think more about the process of thinking or metacognition. However, adolescence also brings a heightened focus on the self, or egocentrism, and the belief that one's own experiences are unique. These cognitive changes may lead to increased conflict in the family as youth become increasingly aware of their parents' limitations. Youth typically assume they are immortal and invulnerable, and these beliefs have been implicated in elevated risk-taking behavior, such as unprotected sexual activity and substance use.

Social Changes

Social relationships change in distinct ways during adolescence. It is common for teenagers to evoke complex reactions from parents, peers, and society, especially with the development of secondary sex characteristics and need for increased autonomy. There is a shift in focus from parental relationships to greater intimacy with peers. Peer groups become larger and more complex during adolescence, and they form around similar interests (e.g., hobbies, sports teams). Adolescents may adopt the values of their peers, but

there is extensive evidence to suggest that teens assume transient peer values such as music, fashion, clothes, and makeup, but not more rooted beliefs such as antisocial behavior or political views. Romantic relationships increase in significance with age with early romantic feelings characterized by distant crushes developing into intimate adult-like relationships in later adolescence. Developing sexual interests and impulses are linked to increases in hormones (estrogen and testosterone) and other elements in the adolescents' social context. The emergence of close social ties is an important developmental milestone during adolescence and failure to achieve close interpersonal relationships is associated with distress.

Families play a central role in helping youth traverse the second decade of life. Family relationships shift with the transformation of the parent–child relationship. Parental control over adolescent behavior is more limited, and there is a redefinition of the boundaries between autonomy and connectedness among family members. A key challenge for the family during this transition is to permit individuation and identity exploration and at the same time stay connected to one another. Autonomy and connectedness in the family may be viewed along a continuum with either end leading to impaired adolescent development. When there is too much autonomy or chaos, reliable parental figures are absent, and teens seek a secure environment outside the home, for example, among peers by joining a gang. At the other extreme are families who maintain rigid roles and relationships, adhere unbendingly to rules, and show little tolerance for deviance. Adolescent identity formation is compromised because there is minimal acceptance of self-expression, differing opinions, and independence.

Optimal adolescent development occurs in the context of supportive and nurturing family relationships, parental flexibility and adaptability to the individuation process, tolerance for role experimentation and confusion, and the transformation of the parent–child relationship to a more equal give-and-take. Parents must continue to set firm and consistent limits and follow through on consequences, but discipline is most effective in the context of a warm and loving parent–adolescent relationship. There is a popular belief that adolescence is a time of "storm and stress," when family relationships become highly argumentative and hostile. Some conflicts can positively facilitate the process of redefining rules, roles, and relationships, but most families do not experience significant disagreement. Indeed, most adolescents and parents successfully modify and renegotiate their relationship to accommodate the adolescent's increasing maturity. Of note, adolescents report that parents remain the most important confidants during this transitional period.

Psychological Changes

There are unique psychological changes that take place during the second decade of life. Youth begin to question and formulate new identities and definitions of the self. They seek out novel experiences in order to explore different options, experiment with diverse roles and values, identify potential role models, and test the limits of their newfound autonomy. Adolescents look for ways to separate and individuate while at the same time feel pulled to remain a child. As a result, youth will often vacillate between rebelliousness and dependence. The desire for individuation increases with age, but all youth continue to yearn for closeness with others including their families.

Changes in emotional development have important implications for future functioning. Teens experience mood swings from happiness to sadness and may be unfamiliar with how to adapt to these shifts. During adolescence, the first gender disparity in rates of depression emerges, with teenage girls reporting significantly more depression than boys. Explanations for this increase include hormonal changes, increased cognitive processing and the tendency to compare one's self to others, greater sensitivity to life events and stressors, and negative perceptions of body image. Some girls have difficulty adapting to their altered appearance as they mature, specifically around normal weight gain during puberty. Girls gain on average 40 lb over the course of adolescence, and this increase sometimes leads to eating disorders, such as anorexia nervosa and bulimia.

Cultural Issues

Many cultures do not have an "adolescence" or a transition period between childhood and adulthood. In agrarian societies, for example, girls begin to work in the home at a very young age observing their mothers and performing the adult roles they will eventually assume. On the other hand, some cultures mark the transition to adulthood using unique rituals or rites of passage. For example, in Jewish tradition, a girl performs a series of rituals as part of her Bat Mitzvah that culminate in her becoming a "woman." As another example, in many

Latino communities, girls are initiated into adulthood through a coming-out ceremony called the Quinceañera. These examples illustrate the importance of cultural influences on adolescent development. Some theorists suggest that youth need an event to demarcate the transition to adulthood, and they hypothesize that the absence of socially sanctioned "rites of passage" in America explains the growing involvement of youth in gang activity where initiation rituals are enacted.

Legal Issues

The second decade of life is fraught with confusing messages about the transition to adulthood. Consider, for example, the laws that allow youth to consent for health care at age 12, but drive at age 16. They are permitted to watch R-rated movies at age 17, but they must be 18 years old to vote. Moreover, they are not allowed to drink alcohol until age 21. These inconsistent messages about youth's decision-making ability, maturity, and adult status are confusing and unsettling.

Conclusions and Recommendations

Today's youth are tomorrow's leaders. They will shape the future of our society, and they will determine our role and status in the world. Investing in our nation's youth will yield significant benefits, while not investing in them will have far-reaching consequences. Indeed, America has devoted few resources to nurture our young people, and it shows. The United States has the highest death rate among youth than any other developed nation. Access to drugs, alcohol, guns, and cars have produced high morbidity and mortality rates among adolescents. Our mass media bombards youth with positive images of risk behavior, violence, and unbridled pleasures without corresponding messages about the need for responsibility to others and productive roles in society. Institutional opportunities to learn how to function in adult roles are limited in scope and restricted to certain populations, and there are few chances to achieve outside the mainstream (e.g., those without a college degree, poor). In sum, we have a significant challenge ahead of us to help youth achieve their full potential, but it can be done. Our future depends on it.

SEE ALSO: Child abuse, Environment, Menarche, Puberty, Sexual abuse, Socioeconomic status, Substance use

Adoption

Suggested Reading

DiClemente, R. J., Hansen, W. B., & Ponton, L. E. (1996). *Handbook of adolescent health risk behavior.* New York: Plenum Press.

Robin, A., & Foster, S. (1989). *Negotiating parent–adolescent conflict.* New York: Guilford Press.

Schulenberg, J., Maggs, J. L., & Hurrelmann, K. (1997). *Health risks and developmental transitions during adolescence.* Cambridge, England: Cambridge University Press.

Journal of Adolescent Health (December 2002) (Vol. 31, No. 6, Supplement health future of youth II: Pathways to adolescent health. Guest editors: Charles E. Irwin & Paul Duncan.

GERI R. DONENBERG

Adoption   Adoption is both a legal event and a life-long experience that affects birth parents, adoptees, and adoptive parents. The birth family, the adoptee, and the adoptive family are known as the adoption triad. It is estimated that 2–5% of American households include adopted children. This translates into over 100,000 adoptions occurring in the United States each year. Based on a national survey of adoption attitudes reported by the Evan Donaldson Institute for Adoption, in 2002, most Americans (64%) knew a birth parent, someone who is adopted, or an adoptive parent. Adoption is a part of the national fabric of family life in the United States.

Adoption philosophy has changed since the 1970s. The paradigm has changed from finding infants for infertile couples (i.e., parent-centered adoption practice) to finding adoptive families who can meet the needs of children (i.e., child-centered adoption practice)—be they infants, older children, children with special health, developmental, or behavior needs; or children adopted from other countries.

The pool of adoptees has changed over the last few decades. Stepparent adoptions, usually an unrelated man adopting the minor children of a women he marries, represents about half of all adoptions in the United States. Children adopted from the public child welfare system comprise the second largest group of adoptees. These children often have a history of abuse, neglect, and trauma prior to their adoptions. The children from the public system represent about 20% of adoptions. International adoptees represent the next group and have grown over time, reaching to almost 20,000 children adopted from other countries into the United States in 2001. This is about 15% of all adoptions. Infants placed for adoption comprise the last group of children. Many of these children are placed through private attorneys and private agencies. They represent the last 15% of the pool of adoptees.

Adoption practices are undergoing radical changes. Until recently in our culture, adoption has been marked by secrecy and denial. The usual practice in adoption was to seal birth records, amend the birth certificate to reflect as if the child was born to the adoptive parent, and sever all contact with any member of the immediate or extended biological family. Now, adoptions have an option of being more open, including having ongoing contact between adoptees and biological family members.

Adoption is a women's health issue in several ways. Women are triad members in that they are birth mothers, adoptees, and adoptive mothers. Unique issues emerge for all of the members of the adoption triad, each revolving from loss.

Birth mothers, while an intrinsic member of the adoption triad, are often the least acknowledged and understood member for a variety of reasons. While we have a better understanding of some of the issues encountered by birth mothers who relinquished infants, we have very little knowledge about birth mothers who had parental rights involuntarily terminated or whose children were placed for adoption internationally. The next few paragraphs discuss the issue only from the perspective of the first group of birth mothers.

In the past, there was a greater societal stigma against unmarried women being pregnant. The shame and secrecy that was part of adoption was due, in part, because the pregnancy was a clear indication of women's sexuality. Social mores attempted to regulate women's sexuality and having sex outside of marriage resulted in ostracism for many birth mothers. They were often hidden from the community in maternity homes or at family members not living in the same community. These women were often pressured to place their child for adoption.

Birth mothers were encouraged to put the relinquishment of the child behind them emotionally and go on with their life. For many birth mothers, the act of surrendering the baby for adoption was a traumatic experience—a physical, emotional, and psychological loss that had implications for the rest of the mothers' lives. This loss, complicated by the isolation, shame, and secrecy surrounding the relinquishment of the child, affected self-esteem, sexuality, marital relationships, subsequent childrearing, relationships with the family of origin, and the birth mother's capacity for trust and intimacy in all relationships. The loss was compounded by the institution of closed adoptions that put legal, social, and emotional barriers on contact between birth mothers and the adoptee or adoptive parents. Today, women who have lost children to adoption have many more avenues to speak openly about and deal with this loss. Some search for their now adult children and others hope to be found. With changing societal attitudes, many birth mothers now reach out for support from family, friends, and organizations that were not available to them in past generations.

One of the biggest issues facing adoptees is the resolution of identity issues. Adoptees experience a variety of issues around identity, varying in intensity and frequency, throughout the life span.

Identity issues are compounded by the lack of information, in closed adoption, about basic physical and mental health information from their biological family members. In closed adoption, unless this information was gathered at the time of adoption and given to the adoptive family, this information is generally inaccessible to the adoptee. The building blocks of identity are basic information. Because they lack information about their biological origins, some adoptees experience identity difficulties in the form of "genealogical bewilderment"—a sense that one's genetic history is hidden by legal barriers that result in difficulty forming a complete self-identity.

To fill gaps in knowledge, some adoptees make the decision to search for the birth family. Although the decision to search is a multidimensional issue for adoptees, one reason for searching is to resolve identity issues related to developing a healthier and more self-aware sense of self, including seeking answers to questions regarding physical resemblance, genetic health issues, and emotional resolution about relinquishment. In domestic cases of adoption, adoptees have been largely successful at gaining access to previously confidential identifying information. In contrast, the majority of international adoptees often have no identifying information about birth parents due to cultural attitudes about relinquishment and adoption. For example, in China, no formal mechanism exists for parents to relinquish a child for adoption. Birth parents are forced to abandon their children, who are primarily female, in a safe place such as a market, residential area, or factory, where they know their children will be found and placed in a social welfare institution. In turn, adoptive families are encouraged to give their children a cultural and ethnic history since a biological history may never be available to them.

Therefore, the issue of search and identity is more complicated for international adoptees.

Adoptive families, in particular, adoptive mothers, often have gone through a lengthy process of trying to get pregnant before they pursue the option of adoption. One of the most salient health issues for adoptive mothers is dealing with infertility. About 19% of all U.S. couples have a fertility problem. Many adoptive mothers build or add to their families through adoption after multiple unsuccessful attempts at reproductive technologies. These technologies are stressful on the mental and physical health of women and often involve increased physician visits, out-of-pocket costs to families, and time lost from employment; women may experience an emotional rollercoaster each month, especially if pregnancy is not achieved.

Some adoptive parents have been reluctant to have an open adoption. Some fear contact or feel threatened by the presence of the birth mother. With the advent of openness in adoption, a new era in adoptions has begun where both birth parents and adoptive parents can reach an agreement upon the type of disclosure and contact they will share as the adoption continues. Openness is seen to be in the best interest of the child, and is now embraced as a positive trend by the adoption community.

The adoption of a child impacts all members of the adoption triad throughout their lives and for generations to come. The unifying point for all adoptive families is that adoptive parenting has special issues related to adoption and these issues need to be addressed throughout the family life cycle. In each case, differences between adoptive parenting and biologic parenting must be acknowledged, addressed, and celebrated as a unique element specific to each individual family.

In conclusion, while the more difficult issues of adoption are discussed above, it is important to have a balanced view. There are many strengths to be acknowledged about adoption. First, all adoptions are planned and the parents want children. Second, adoptive parents have demonstrated basic competence in motivation, problem-solving skills, and mental health in order to adopt by successfully completing a home study. Third, a broader definition of family through adoption raises awareness that relationships build families, not necessarily biology.

A significant part of the child population is affected by adoption. Adoption is a social arrangement that has more positives than it does negatives and remains the best solution for children who cannot be raised with their biological parents.

Suggested Reading

Brodzinsky, D., & Schecter, M. (1990). *The psychology of adoption.* New York: Oxford University Press.

Groza, V., & Rosenberg, K. (Eds.). (2001). *Clinical and practice issues in adoption: Bridging the gap between adoptees placed as infants and as older children, revised and expanded.* Westport, CT: Bergen & Garvey.

Sachdev, P. (1989). *Unlocking the adoption files.* Lexington, MA: Lexington Books.

Winkler, R., Brown, D., van Keppel, M., & Blanchard, A. (1988). *Clinical practice in adoption.* New York: Pergamon Press.

Suggested Resources

Adoption.org http://www.adoption.org/bparents/html/body_birthpar. htm Retrieved February 2, 2003. A site that addresses all aspects surrounding birth parent's concerns, such as coping with grief, romantic relationships, parenting issues, birth and placement, searching, support groups, how to cope, and counseling resources.

Joint Council on International Children's Services http://www.jcics. org/miss.on.html Retrieved February 2, 2003. The Joint Council on International Children's Services is an organization that advocates for ethical practices within international adoption agencies.

National Adoption Information Clearinghouse http://www.calib. com/naic Retrieved February 2, 2003. The National Adoption Information Clearinghouse (NAIC) is a service of the Children's Bureau; Administration on Children, Youth, and Families; the Administration for Children and Families; and the Department of Health and Human Services. The NAIC provides information for professionals, adoptees, birth relatives, and adoptive parents.

North American Council on Adoptable Children http://www.nacac. org/postadoptionservices.l Retrieved February 2, 2003. North American Council on Adoptable Children offers useful information regarding postadoption services that include articles that relate to issues regarding adoption and post-adoption.

VICTOR GROZA
LINDSEY HOULIHAN

Adultery

Adultery   Adultery is consensual sexual intercourse between a married person and someone other than that person's spouse. Adultery is rarely charged as a crime. It is more often a concern as a part of a divorce case.

Adultery is one of many possible grounds for divorce in the majority of states in the United States. Historically, adultery was one of the few grounds, and in one state the only reason, on which divorce would be allowed. Adultery was also historically important in states that linked child custody or property decisions to the grounds for divorce. Now that most states have "no fault" grounds for divorce, adultery is much less legally significant. Some states even have a requirement that the grounds for divorce not be taken into account when the judge decides issues of child custody and property distribution.

Proving adultery can be very difficult because sexual acts rarely take place in front of witnesses. Some courts have considered adultery proven when the parties had motivation and opportunity, such as checking in to a motel together, to engage in sexual conduct. A few courts have even been called upon to determine whether graphic sexual communication over the Internet constitutes adultery, but there is no clear law yet established.

SEE ALSO: Divorce

Suggested Reading

The American Bar Association guide to family law: The complete and easy guide to the laws of marriage, parenthood, separation and divorce. (1996). New York: Times Books/Random House.

SHEILA SIMON

Advance Directives   Since the mid-1970s, a great deal of attention has been focused on advance or prospective health care planning as a way for individuals to maintain some control over their future medical treatment even if they eventually become physically and/or mentally unable to make and express important decisions about their own care. Proponents of advance care planning also claim that it may help individuals and their families avoid court involvement in medical treatment decisions, conserve limited health care resources in a way that is consistent with patient autonomy or self-determination, and reduce the emotional or psychological stress on family or friends in difficult crisis situations.

There are two main legal mechanisms available for use in prospective (i.e., before-the-fact) health care planning. One is the proxy directive, ordinarily in the form of a durable power of attorney (DPOA), while the second is the instruction directive, usually referred to as a living will, health care declaration, or natural death declaration. In the United States, these legal mechanisms have their basis in various statutes enacted by state legislatures. In some countries (e.g., Great Britain), advance directives have been recognized by the courts even though they have not been codified in the form of statutes.

In their advance directive statutes, many state legislatures have attempted to draw distinctions between artificial means of feeding and hydration, on one hand, and other forms of life-sustaining medical treatment (such as ventilators and antibiotics), on the other. Specifically, many statutes try to make it more difficult procedurally for families or other decision-makers for incompetent patients to refuse or withdraw artificial feeding or hydration than to refuse or withdraw other forms of life-sustaining medical treatment. Some persons argue that these legal provisions are necessary to protect very vulnerable patients from unfair undertreatment and medical neglect; however, advance directive statutes that discriminate on the basis of the type of medical treatment being refused by the patient or surrogate probably are unconstitutional.

The courts and legislatures consistently have made it clear that state advance directive statutes are not intended to be the only means by which patients may exercise the right to make future decisions about medical treatment. For instance, a patient might convey wishes regarding future medical treatment orally to the physician during an office visit, with the physician documenting the patient's words in the medical chart. When that patient later becomes unable to make medical decisions, the patient's oral instructions are just as valid legally as would be a written document executed in compliance with all the statutory formalities found in the state's advance directive statute.

There is a substantial body of evidence indicating that very often patients' stated wishes regarding life-sustaining medical treatment are not respected and implemented. In actuality, critically ill patients frequently receive more aggressive medical treatment than they earlier had said they would want.

State advance directive statutes all excuse a health care provider who chooses, for reasons of personal conscience, not to implement the expressly stated treatment preferences of a patient or surrogate, as long as that provider does not impede that patient being transferred to the care of a different provider if that is what the patient or surrogate wishes. Similarly, courts have declined to hold health care providers legally liable for failing to follow a patient's or surrogate's instructions to withdraw or withhold particular forms of treatment, on the grounds that providing life-prolonging intervention cannot cause the sort of injury or harm for which the legal system is designed to supply financial compensation.

See Also: Durable power of attorney for health care, Living wills

Suggested Reading

American Medical Association Council on Ethical and Judicial Affairs. (1998). Optimal use of orders not to intervene and advance directives. *Psychology, Public Policy, and Law, 4*, 668–675.

King, N. M. P. (1996). *Making sense of advance directives* (rev. ed.). Washington, DC: Georgetown University Press.

Ulrich, L. P. (1999). *The patient self-determination act: Meeting the challenges in patient care.* Washington, DC: Georgetown University Press.

Marshall B. Kapp

Affirmative Action

Even with the passage of the Civil Rights Act of 1964, the fight for equality and against discriminatory practice has continued. Although the Act is the nation's strongest civil rights law, minority groups still lack basic equal opportunities. Affirmative action is a proactive policy used to provide equal opportunities for groups such as women, blacks, and other disadvantaged social and ethnic groups. Before the adoption of affirmative action, women and minorities were not being hired for jobs and were being denied admission into higher educational programs because of their race or gender. Affirmative action is an essential tool in correcting the widespread and wrongful discriminatory practices of this past century, which have kept minorities and women from pursuing higher education and employment opportunities. Specifically, affirmative action requires organizations to establish programs that ensure equal access be given to disadvantaged social and ethnic groups.

The term affirmative action was first used by President John F. Kennedy in an executive order to the Equal Employment Opportunity Commission (EEOC). Executive Order 10925 charged the EEOC to use "affirmative action" to ensure that employment practices did not discriminate. This was followed by Executive Order 11246, which was issued by President Lyndon B. Johnson in 1965, requiring government contractors to use "affirmative action" in their employment practices in order to increase equality for minorities. Two years later, the executive order was expanded to include women.

Not only was the support of President Johnson essential in ensuring the passage of the Civil Rights Act of 1964, he was also the key figure in the advancement of affirmative action. The strong support from President Johnson eventually led to the adoption of a governmental requirement that all federal programs provide equal opportunity and treatment for minorities. In one speech, President Johnson championed affirmative action by stating, "We seek not just freedom but opportunity—not just legal equity but human ability—not just equality as a right and a theory, *but equality as a fact and as a result*" (*Timeline of Affirmative Action Milestones*, Brunner).

Although affirmative action had never been embraced with open arms, it was not until 1978 that it was first challenged in federal court. Alan Bakke, a white student, claimed that the University of California Davis Medical School's affirmative action program discriminated against him because it used a quota system reserving 16 seats for minority students. Consequently, minority students with lower grade and standardized test scores than Bakke were admitted, while his application was denied for two consecutive years. Even though the Supreme Court ruled that the use of quotas was unlawful, it did rule that it was lawful for the school to use race as a factor in the admission process.

The three branches of government have all taken differing views as to the future of affirmative action. For instance, in 1989, the Reagan administration pushed for the Supreme Court to declare affirmative action unlawful. While the Court did not abolish affirmative action outright, it did substantially limit the scope and use of the policy. Most of these rulings were handed down within a 3-month period shortly after Justice Rehnquist became the Chief Justice. The Democrats who were then in control of the Congress responded by attempting to pass legislation in 1990 that would overturn the Court's decisions, but were unsuccessful in overriding President Bush's veto. In 1991, a compromise between the Democrats and the Bush administration was reached which prohibited the use of quotas, and allowed legislation to pass that would overturn the Court's decisions which limited affirmative action. However, during the Clinton administration, a 3-year moratorium on new affirmative action programs was imposed, coupled with a promise not to end affirmative action.

While the federal government grappled with the future of affirmative action, more than a few state governments have pressed hard to eliminate it altogether. In 1997, California passed Proposition 209, which abolished the use of affirmative action throughout the state. Washington and Florida soon followed suit; Washington abolished affirmative action in 1998 with Initiative 200, and in 2000, Florida abolished the use of affirmative action in education. More recently, two cases arising out of the admission policy of the University of Michigan may determine the future of affirmative action. In *Grutter*

v. Bollinger and *Gratz v. Bollinger*, the plaintiffs challenged before the U.S. Supreme Court the use of race as a factor in the school's admission process. In *Grutter v. Bollinger*, the United States Supreme Court held that the University of Michigan's consideration of race as a factor in law school admission was not unconstitutional. However, the awarding of points based on minority status alone in the consideration of undergraduate admissions was found unconstitutional in *Gratz v. Bollinger*.

These two cases reflect very different schools of thought on affirmative action. Proponents of its continued use argue that affirmative action is responsible for providing minorities with equal opportunity and access. Equal opportunity and access are critical because of the underrepresentation of minorities and women in higher education, in higher paying employment, and in professional positions. Furthermore, proponents argue that if factors such as athletics, legacies, and other relationships to benefactors are all given special consideration in admission, then a student's diverse background should be taken into account as well. Opponents of affirmative action argue that if it is wrong to discriminate based on race and gender, then it is equally wrong to use such factors to help an applicant in the selection process because it leads to reverse discrimination against whites. This is because affirmative action programs use preferential treatment and quota systems to give undeserving applicants a free ride at the expense of a better qualified white student. Opponents emphasize that this goes against the grain of the American value of self-reliance.

For women, affirmative action has meant that they now enjoy nearly the same opportunities as men in employment, education, and business opportunities. In 1987, the Supreme Court held that it was lawful for an employer to use affirmative action to increase the ratio of female employees. Although affirmative action has helped women make progress, women still have not realized the promise of "equality as a result" in President Johnson's speech. Women do not receive equal treatment and parity in the workforce. When compared to men, women earn only 74 cents per dollar; African American and Hispanic women earn even less at 63 and 57 cents, respectively. Furthermore, there is still a gap in professional education programs because only 25% of doctors and lawyers in the country are women, and only 8.4% of engineers are women. Affirmative action programs for women are still widely supported abroad. In 1997, the European Court of Justice held that affirmative action for women is lawful in the private sector and has become the legal precedent for all European Union members.

Affirmative action has been instrumental in providing equal access and opportunities for minorities and women. Although several states have abolished affirmative action, the Supreme Court has been reluctant to immediately follow suit. Now, the future of affirmative action is uncertain. The July ruling expected by the Court will either support its continued existence or abolish it altogether. Whether or not affirmative action has a future in the United States, history has shown the demonstrably positive impact it has had on minorities and women. Today, both groups enjoy opportunities in employment and education that would not have been possible otherwise.

SEE ALSO: Discrimination

Suggested Reading

Bacchi, C. L. (1996). *The politics of affirmative action.* London: Sage.

Brunner, B. *Timeline of affirmative action milestones,* Family Education Network, Inc. http://www.infoplease.com/spot/affirmativetimeline1.html (Last accessed January 12, 2004)

Clayton, S. D., & Crosby, F. J. (1995). *Justice, gender, and affirmative action.* Ann Arbor: University of Michigan Press.

Ooiman Robinson, J. A. (2001). *Affirmative action: A documentary history.* Westport, CT: Greenwood Press.

ELIZABETH M. VALENCIA

African American

quilting*

somewhere in the unknown world
a yellow eyed woman
sits with her daughter
quilting.

some other where
alchemists mumble over pots.
their chemistry stirs
into science. their science
freezes into stone.

in the unknown world
the woman
threading together her need
and her needle
nods toward the smiling girl
remember
this will keep us warm

how does this poem end?
do the daughters' daughters quilt?
do the alchemists practice their tables?

*From Lucille Clifton, *Blessing the Boats: Poems New and Selected, 1988–2000.* Copyright © 2002, 1991 by Lucille Clifton. Reprinted with permission of BOA Editions, Ltd.

do the worlds continue spinning
away from each other forever?

Lucille Clifton

African American (AA) women's health care has been and continues to be unacceptably poor. Some AA women are numbered in the lowest socioeconomic status for both wealth and education. Many of them live and raise their families under conditions of poverty with a primary concern for the basic needs of food, clothing, and shelter. Health care for some of these women is a luxury and is attended to in an emergency situation only. Many women who live in poverty were born into an environment of poverty and have had limited exposure to formal education. There are other AA women who are well educated and affluent—some are categorized as middle class and others as wealthy. However, research studies have shown that across the spectrum of class and socioeconomic status, AA women's health care remains unacceptably poor. The reasons for this seem to be multifaceted and reflect several barriers to health care for AA women.

The U.S. Department of Health and Human Services Office of Women's Health describes some of the barriers as being related to: "the current state of medical practice, medical education, medical research and medical leadership in the United States creates its own obstacles for minority women. These four areas of medicine have traditionally ignored the health of women and minorities." These obstacles take into account the physical location of medical practice facilities, many of which tend to be inaccessible to a sizeable portion of the AA female population who live under conditions of impoverishment. The lack of access to health care resources results in a decrease in the receipt of preventive care and continuity of care. This can result in an increase in hospitalizations and higher health care costs.

According to the census report for year 2000, while most women across racial and ethnic groups had an office-based usual source of care, white woman were more likely to have office-based care than nonwhite women. AA women were more likely to use a hospital outpatient department or emergency room for their usual care. Hospital outpatient departments often have high-volume practices and as a result physicians in these settings have less time to spend with patients. And sometimes these physicians provide less preventive care counseling than do physicians in other medical practices.

The lack of access to health care providers in minority communities does not address the full scope of the problem. In April 2000, *The New England Journal of*

Medicine published an article based on a survey by Dr. Sean R. Morrison et al. The authors reported that they had observed that many AA and Hispanic patients who were receiving palliative care at a major urban teaching hospital were unable to obtain prescribed opioids from their neighborhood pharmacies. Dr. Morrison and colleagues surveyed a randomly selected sample of 30% of New York City pharmacies to obtain information about their stock of opioids.

> Our data demonstrated that many New York City pharmacies do not stock sufficient medication to treat patients with severe pain. Furthermore, pharmacies in predominantly nonwhite neighborhoods are significantly less likely to stock adequate supplies of opioids than are pharmacies in predominantly white neighborhoods. These results suggest that nonwhite patients maybe at even greater risk for the under treatment of pain than previously reported...

This practice impacts the heath care of AA women who live in neighborhoods that consist of a predominantly minority population.

There are many other health care system barriers related to medical practice; it would require a separate volume to address them all. Two additional issues that will be addressed here are AA women and mammography, and AA women and the practice of cardiac catheterization.

Many studies have focused attention on AA women and the use of mammography: the results have shown that AA women are less likely to undergo mammography and are more often diagnosed with advanced-stage breast cancer than are white women. The question that remains unanswered is why are AA women more often diagnosed with advanced-stage breast cancer? Is the access to providers for primary prevention the issue or are the providers not referring AA women for mammography? According to Ellen P. McCarthy et al., in their study "Mammography Use Helps to Explain Differences in Breast Cancer Stage at Diagnosis between Older Black and White Women":

> We previously found that greater mammography use was associated with an increasing number of visits to a primary care provider among Black and White women but receipt of primary care was not enough to correct the disparity in mammography use between Black and White women. Furthermore, many studies show that a physician's recommendation is the most important determinant of mammography use.

In the case of cardiac catheterization, it has been well publicized that there is a clear racial difference in the referral pattern practice of physicians when presented with patients who have a complaint of chest pain. AA women are less likely than white women and men, AA and white, to undergo a cardiac catheterization or coronary artery bypass graph surgery, when they are hospitalized with a diagnosis of chest pain or myocardial infarction.

The Department of Health and Human Services has also listed medical education, medical research, and medical leadership as barriers limiting access to health care. Medical education was targeted because of limited training in the area of cultural competence in health care training programs. In addition, the enrollment of AA students into traditionally white medical school matriculation has declined as expressed by Jack H. Geiger in an article titled "Comment: Ethnic Cleansing in the Groves of Academe." The article was published in *The American Journal of Public Health* in September 1998. As a consequence of the decrease in minority enrolment in health care training programs, there is, as well, a disparity in the number of minorities who serve in all areas of health care. This is especially evident in the lack of diversity among the medical school faculty members, researchers, and administrators. Disparity in the racial/ethnic mix of the providers can add to the stress and uncertainty of care that is experienced by the patient.

To accurately assess the issues of health care in AA women, we need researchers and participants. Lessons learned from the Tuskegee Syphilis Study have stressed the importance of informed consent and health care ethics in every research situation. It is imperative that AA women become more actively involved in research projects and fulfill the roles of both the researcher and the educated consenting participant.

HEALTH STATISTICS

The average life expectancy between 1950 and 2000 increased by an average of 8 years for males and females of all races. But, the most significant increase in life expectancy was among AA females whose average life expectancy increased by 12.3 years. This improvement has raised the average life expectancy to 75 years for AA women, but it remains below the 79.5 years average life expectancy for all race females.

The Health Resources and Services Administration Office of Women's Health also looks at the years of potential life lost as a measure of population health. This measure calculates the years of life lost by people who died before their full life expectancy. In 1998, AA women had more than 10,000 years of potential life lost due to all causes. That number is double that of white women and more than three times the number for Asian women.

What are the leading causes of death for AA women? Heart disease, cancer, and stroke rank as the top three with diabetes listed as fourth. Obesity and hypertension, although not listed as major causes of death in AA women, contribute to the disease process for both heart disease and stroke. According to the year 2000 census report, 35.8% of AA women self-reported that they were obese. Obesity can lead to heart disease, stroke, and diabetes. It has also been implicated in some forms of cancer. Obesity is a treatable condition that requires full participation by the patient along with medical advice and support.

Not all threats to the health and well-being of the AA women are as treatable as obesity. AIDS has a high incidence and prevalence in AA women. According to the U.S. Health Status Morbidity Report, the age and prevalence are as listed:

Age in years	AIDS cases
13–19	1,112
20–24	4,443
25–34	27,885
35–44	28,863
45–64	11,717
65 and older	967

These figures are staggering and will continue to grow if we allow it; therefore, as AA women we must move forward as advocates for an improved health care system that will meet the needs of a diverse population of consumers.

See Also: Access to health care, Discrimination, Education, Racism, Socioeconomic status

Suggested Reading

Fiscella, K., et al. (2000). Inequality in quality: Addressing socioeconomic, racial, and ethnic disparities in health care. *Journal of the American Medical Association, 283*(19), 2579–2584.

Fremgen, B. F. (2002). *Medical law and ethics.* Upper Saddle River, NJ: Prentice–Hall.

Gamble, V. N. (1997). Under the shadow of Tuskegee: African Americans and health care. *American Journal of Public Health, 87*, 1773–1778.

Geiger, J. H. (1998). Comment: Ethnic cleansing in the groves of academie. *American Journal of Public Health, 88*(9), 1299–1300.

McCarthy. E. P., et al. (1998). Mammography use helps to explain differences in breast cancer stage at diagnosis between older black and white women. *Annals of Internal Medicine, 128*(9), 729–736.

Morrison, S. R., et al. (2000). "We don't carry that"—failure of pharmacies in predominantly nonwhite neighborhoods to stock opioid analgesics. *New England Journal of Medicine, 342*(14), 1023–1026.

Schulman, K. A., et al. (1999). The effect of race and sex on physicians' recommendations for cardiac catheterization. *New England Journal of Medicine, 340*(8), 618–626.

Suggested Resources

Office of Women's Health. Health Resources and Services Administration (HRSA) Department of Health and Human Services, http://www.hrsa.gov/womenshealth/ (accessed May, 2003)

The health of minority women. Office of Women's Health, www.4woman.gov. (accessed May, 2003)

Anne Simpson

Age Spots *see* Liver Spots

Ageism

The term "ageism," a set of beliefs about age, was coined in the late 20th century. It is a form of stereotyping that refers to prejudgment or discrimination against *any* particular age group, although it is typically viewed today as a negative perspective about the aged. Categorizing by chronological development, ageism can be framed either in positive or negative terms: babies are dependent/uninteresting, toddlers are explorers/oppositional, teenagers are defining their values/unreliable and self-centered, young adults are energetic/unfocused, middle-aged workers are successful/entrenched, retirees are carefree/useless, the elderly are to be honored/forgetful and frail. One's chronologic age or stage of development may influence the nature of the stereotypes held. Whether in the context of ageism, sexism, or racism, attributes which are viewed as positive in one group may be negative for another (such as labeling the same behavior as "forcefulness" in males and "aggressiveness" in females, or "forgetfulness" in the young as "senility" in the old).

References to ageism obtained through an Internet search and a review of the medical literature predominately refer to prejudice against the elderly—such as inequities in work opportunity, portrayal of the elderly in the media, and inappropriate medical care. In 2002, the American Psychological Association specified that "ageism is defined as a prejudice toward, stereotyping of, and/or discrimination against any person or persons directly and solely as a function of their having attained a chronological age which the social group defines as 'old'." The U.S. Department of Health and Human Service's Administration on Aging defines ageism as "a term expressing prejudice against older adults through attitudes and behavior."

Government financial support for elderly individuals with little to no resources was initiated in the 1930s and 1940s as Social Security in the United States, and as Old Age Pensions in Britain, coupled with mandatory retirement ages. In the 1970s, political activists such as Maggie Kuhn in the United States pursued the notion that mandatory retirement was ageism, and by 1978, mandatory retirement was effectively abolished. Recent changes have raised the lower limit of "retirement age" (eligibility for full Social Security pension benefits) from 65 to 67, because of concerns regarding the solvency of the Social Security system.

Contemporary definitions of "old" or "elderly" are variable: old enough for membership in the American Association of Retired Persons (AARP) at 50; retired from the workforce (which may be, depending on one's occupation, as early as age 40 in the military/police/firefighter sphere, or 55, 60, or 75 as negotiated with employers); eligible for Social Security and Medicare benefits; gray-haired or wrinkled; unable to appreciate the current generation's popular music/fashion/aspirations.

Ageism in its limited meaning (regarding discrimination against the elderly) tends to assume that the elderly are no longer able to contribute to society in a meaningful way, and drain the broader society's resources because of a continuous decline in health and well-being. Census Bureau statistics challenge this concept, noting that a relatively small number of the elderly are in fact in nursing homes, and that these individuals tend to be the very oldest. Some research and anecdotes indicate that being segregated with other aged people and having limited opportunities for decision-making leads to declining function. Chronological age does not solely define function, though health and social policy might suggest otherwise.

While it is understood that discrimination against the *elderly* is prohibited, it is less well known that the Age Discrimination Act of 1975, which affects programs or activities receiving U.S. federal financial assistance, "applies to persons of all ages." In both industrialized and nonindustrialized societies, there are generally accepted ages or stages for the definition of childhood (dependent status) or adulthood (the age of consent or majority), with variation by societal norm or law. For example, adulthood may be defined as the onset of puberty, becoming a parent, entering a career, completing education, living independently, or solely by age (e.g., 13 or 18 or 21 years). In medical care, the context of the visit may determine the age of consent: minors may not be treated for injury without permission from a parent or guardian, but may receive care for sexually transmitted diseases or family planning without such permission.

Even though chronological age or distinguishing between "childhood" and "adulthood" are convenient ways to categorize people, this can overlook the possibility of continuing growth and development throughout the human life cycle. Just as children can be seen as progressing through recognizable stages or streams, so can adults. There are, not surprisingly, different models of child development rooted in various theories such as those of Piaget, Freud, Gesell, and Bandura. The work of Eric Erickson extended the notion of childhood developmental stages into adulthood, pairing ranges of chronological age (early adulthood, middle age, and later years) with psychosocial conflicts and their resolutions. Subsequently, the scholarly and popular literature has addressed various formulations of such phases or stages of adulthood and now includes the elderly.

Overall, we expect that age and experience will yield maturity; we expect a 3-year-old to handle adversity differently than a 30-year-old. But a 16-year-old may be wise and a 60-year-old foolish; a 30-year-old well settled into a career or still unfocused. Stages of development may overlap or be revisited. In contemporary society, we are likely to have multiple roles in family, work, friendship, and community. We may achieve maturity in one role but find it elusive in another, or devote energies to one sphere of life (work vs. family) or stream of development (intellect vs. social relationships) at the expense of another. Further, we may interrupt career or postpone family for a period of time, then reassess and refocus, no matter what our chronological age. In the late 20th century, individuals as unlike as Julia Child and Jimmy and Roslyn Carter publicly embarked on new directions in their lifework at a time that many would be simply "retired."

Age, like gender or race, may have less importance in defining one's place in modern society than in previous generations. A new and positive "ageism" may take the forefront in the 21st century, expecting and encouraging persons to develop their strengths and skills without respect to chronological age.

SEE ALSO: Activities of daily living, Affirmative action, Dementia, Discrimination, Social support, United States Civil Rights Act of 1964, Youth

Suggested Reading

Carter, J. (1998). *The virtues of aging*. New York: The Library of Contemporary Thought, The Ballantine Publishing Group.

Department for Work and Pensions. (2003). "Age positive—tackling age discrimination and promoting age diversity in employment," Department for Work and Pensions, Sheffield, England, http://www.agepositive.gov.uk. (Accessed May 2003).

Erikson, E. H. with new chapters by Erikson, J. M. (1997). *The life cycle completed–extended version*. New York: W.W. Norton.

Friedan, B. (1993). *The fountain of age*. New York: Simon & Schuster.

Gleitman, H. J., Fridlund, A. J., & Reisberg, D. (1999). *Psychology* (5th ed.). New York: W.W. Norton.

Levinson, D. J., Darrow, C. N., Klein, E. B., Levinson, M. H., & McKee, B. (1988). *The seasons of a man's life*. New York: Alfred A. Knopf. (See also Levinson, D. J. in collaboration with Levinson, J. D. (1996). *The seasons of a woman's life*. New York: Ballantine Books.

TERESA TROGDON ANDERSON

Agoraphobia

Agoraphobia Agoraphobia is a psychiatric illness in which individuals are anxious about being in situations where escape may be difficult or embarrassing. Nervousness may also occur if someone is not available to help in case a panic attack or panic-like symptoms occur. Due to these apprehensions, individuals with agoraphobia begin to avoid situations, or experience intense anxiety or fear having a panic attack or panic-like symptom attack while in them, or require a companion to accompany them. Individuals with agoraphobia typically avoid being alone either at home or otherwise. Other typical situations that are avoided are places that are difficult to leave abruptly like public transportation, tunnels, theaters, restaurants, and the like.

To understand agoraphobia, the notion of panic must first be elucidated since it is a key component in diagnosis. Panic attacks are episodes of intense anxiety in which at least four of the following thirteen symptoms peak very quickly: increased heart rate, sweating, shakiness, shortness of breath, choking feelings, chest pain, abdominal distress, dizziness, feelings of unreality or detachment from self, fear of losing control or dying, tingling, chills, or hot flushes.

Panic-like symptoms are fewer in number than is required for a full-fledged panic attack, but can also include other incapacitating symptoms (e.g., severe headache). Panic attacks or panic-like symptoms can be either unexpected or situationally predisposed. The former occur unpredictably whereas the latter can be in response to some stimulus, but at other times attacks do not occur with that stimulus at all (e.g., an attack may occur after entering a mall but at other times this may not happen).

A diagnosis of panic disorder with agoraphobia is given when agoraphobia occurs along with unexpected full-fledged panic attacks with a month of concern about one of the following: fears of another attack, or the implications of the attack, or a marked change in behavior associated with the attacks. On the other hand, a diagnosis of agoraphobia without history of panic disorder is made when agoraphobia symptoms are related to fears of developing the panic-like symptoms without a history of full-fledged panic attacks.

There is considerable controversy about the incidence of agoraphobia without a history of panic attack. The unitary model postulates that panic and agoraphobia are variations of the same underlying disorder whereas the dualistic model postulates that they are discrete disorders. Although an epidemiologic study reported a 68% rate of agoraphobia without panic attacks or disorder, it is rarely seen in clinical settings. Another study found that agoraphobia without panic occurred in 7.8% of study participants as opposed to agoraphobia with panic in 0.8% of a young sample (ages 14–24). Others report that the occurrence of agoraphobia without panic disorder is rare as most individuals (95%) have past or present panic disorder. Differences in the results obtained are blamed on flawed study methodology.

Agoraphobia generally develops between the ages of 18 and 35. The exact cause is unknown; however, it is thought to be a combination of biology, gender, and environment. Panic disorder with agoraphobia is three times as likely to occur in women than men. Community samples of individuals with panic disorder indicate that from one half to one third also have agoraphobia. It is estimated that clinical samples (individuals being treated for psychiatric disorders) have even higher rates of agoraphobia. Agoraphobia usually occurs within the first year of frequent panic attacks and can continue even though panic attacks may remit. Most individuals with limited symptom attacks have experienced full-fledged panic attacks at some point. Panic attacks, as opposed to limited symptom attacks, are associated with greater impairment. In some cases a decrease in agoraphobia follows a decrease in panic symptoms. Cases of agoraphobia without a history of panic seem to have a more difficult course and outcome. Individuals who experience more severe agoraphobia tend to experience other anxiety disorders as well. The course of agoraphobia varies. Some individuals experience a waxing and waning course, while others will have periods of brief improvement or remission.

Treatment of agoraphobia targets the panic symptoms with antipanic medications such as tricyclics, benzodiazepines, serotonin reuptake inhibitors, and monoamine oxidase inhibitors. Psychotherapy using cognitive-behavioral therapy (CBT) focuses on changing the dysfunctional beliefs and behaviors associated with the interpretation of panic symptoms and the agoraphobic avoidance. Exposure-based therapies seem to be most effective for agoraphobic avoidance. A 70% improvement in agoraphobia symptoms has been documented when the treatment used was in vivo exposure. Depending on the assessment of symptoms and their severity, either medication or psychotherapy is used, or a combination of both.

SEE ALSO: Anxiety disorders, Depression, Panic attack, Phobia, Posttraumatic stress disorder

Suggested Reading

American Psychiatric Association. (1994). *Diagnostic and statistical manual of mental disorders* (4th ed.). Washington, DC: American Psychiatric Association.

Eaton, W. W., & Keyl, P. M. (1990). Risk factors for the onset of Diagnostic Interview Schedule/DSM-III agoraphobia in a prospective, population-based study. *Archives of General Psychiatry, 47*, 819–824.

Hedley, L. M., & Hoffart, A. (2001). Agoraphobia without history of panic disorder. *Clinical Psychology and Psychotherapy, 8*, 436–443.

Hollander, E., Simeon, D., & Gorman, J. M. (1999). Anxiety disorders. In R. E. Hales, S. C. Yudofsky, & J. A. Talbott (Eds.), *Textbook of psychiatry* (3rd ed., pp. 567–634). Washington, DC: American Psychiatric Press.

McLean, P. D., & Woody, S. R. (2001). *Anxiety disorders in adults: An evidence-based approach to psychological treatment.* New York: Oxford University Press.

Wittchen, H.-U., Reed, V., & Kessler, R. C. (1998). The relationship of agoraphobia and panic in a community sample of adolescents and young adults. *Archives of General Psychiatry, 55*, 1017–1024.

VIRGINIA E. AYRES

Agricultural Work

Approximately 22,200 women in the United States are employed in agriculture as farm owners, managers, workers, and in other related occupations. Although women employed in agriculture represent a small portion of the total agricultural workforce—less than 15%—this number underestimates the contribution of women to agricultural productivity. Women contribute untold hours of unpaid work on farms.

As informal and formal workers on farms, women are exposed to a multitude of biological, chemical, physical, and mechanical hazards. Occupational diseases in women working on farms will go undiagnosed if a physician assumes she does not work or if a physician is unfamiliar with occupational diseases. Hazards encountered on farms include heavy equipment; enclosed spaces such as silos, grain bins, and manure storage structures; toxic and irritant gases and dusts including carbon dioxide, nitrogen dioxide, anhydrous ammonia, pesticides, endotoxins, fungi, and molds; weather extremes; and animals. Respiratory diseases, traumatic injuries, musculoskeletal disorders, noise-induced hearing loss, skin disorders, chemical poisoning, infectious diseases, cancer, infertility, low birthweight, birth defects, and Parkinson's disease are associated with hazards encountered in agriculture.

Due to the fact that women are often employed off the farm, their contribution to farm work may put them at higher risk of injuries due to fatigue. In addition, since the work changes seasonally and is often done under time pressure, women are likely to be at a high risk of injury comparable to new workers in other occupational settings. Inexperience and lack of familiarity with equipment often leads to work-related injuries. Equipment designed for an average male may increase ergonomic strain for women and result in increased risk of musculoskeletal injuries.

Women who have been exposed to agricultural chemicals have been found to have excesses of non-Hodgkin's lymphoma, leukemia, multiple myeloma, soft tissue sarcoma, and cancers of the breast, ovary, lung, bladder, cervix, and sinonasal cavities. Exposure assessments to toxic substances have largely been derived from male animal models. Genetic and other biological differences may contribute to differing susceptibility to agricultural chemicals between men and women. Susceptibility may be increased or it may be reduced due to gender. Therefore, patterns of cancer among women exposed to agricultural chemicals may well differ from patterns observed among men.

Emotional and psychological gender differences related to the isolation of rural farm life have not been assessed. Mental health in rural areas has been a neglected issue in medical care service access. The absence of services may have a detrimental effect on the health and well-being of farm women.

Women who are migrant farm workers are exposed to the same hazards as men who are migrant workers. However, they are likely to experience greater ergonomic problems than their male counterparts. In addition, migrant women who work during their pregnancy are likely to experience problems due to bending and lifting. Exposure to pesticides in the fields has been a persistent problem for all migrant workers and should also be of concern for the children exposed in utero. Women who migrate from other countries may also experience high levels of exposure to farm chemicals that are no longer in use in the United States, increasing their risk of medical problems. Cultural differences, differences in perception of risk, differences in prevention strategies, and language barriers create unique problems for addressing the medical problems of migrant women.

Women who work on the farm are often excluded from consideration of agricultural safety and health programs. Role definition as homemakers or employed workers in settings other than agriculture may influence women's perception of risk, involvement in safety programs, and identification of diseases related to agricultural exposures.

In general, safety measures to reduce problems among women working in agriculture are the same as those proposed for men. However, women who work infrequently with equipment may need to be retrained when they have been away from it for a while. Women need to be aware that they are exposed to dusts and chemicals that should be mentioned to their physicians when they are having health problems.

SEE ALSO: Cancer, Immigrant health, Rural health, Women in the Workforce (pp. 37–40)

Suggested Reading

McDuffie, H. H., Dosman, J. A., Semchuk, K. M., Olenchock, S. A., & Sentihilselvan, A. (1995). *Agricultural health and safety: Workplace, environment and sustainability.* Boca Raton, FL: Lewis.

Messing, K. (1998). *One-eyed science: Occupational health and women workers.* Philadelphia: Temple University Press.

Murphy, D. (1992). *Safety and health for production agriculture.* St. Joseph, MO: American Society of Agricultural Engineers.

LORANN STALLONES

AIDS *see* Acquired Immunodeficiency Syndrome

Alcohol Use Although patterns of drinking and behavior when inebriated vary cross-culturally, alcohol consumption affects men and women differently in all cultures for biological as well as social reasons. Women's bodies metabolize alcohol differently from men's because of their generally smaller body size, greater fat-to-muscle ratio, and fluctuating hormonal levels. Although the capacity to drink alcohol without showing strong effects of inebriation varies individually and can be modified by experience, in general, women get drunker faster on less alcohol than men. In addition, negative effects of chronic overconsumption of alcohol such as liver disease, anemia, peptic ulcers, high blood pressure, and hepatitis develop more quickly in women. Not only has breast cancer been linked to alcohol consumption in women, but also the well-cited protective factors of moderate consumption against heart disease only apply to women after menopause, and then only if women consume half the quantities permitted in men. Women have been found to suffer psychological harm from alcohol addiction more strongly than men, and addiction among women in most societies is so heavily stigmatized that female problem drinkers are at higher risk than men for depression, low self-esteem, and suicidal impulses. However, because most research on problem drinking has focused on men, health providers know less about female addiction and how best to treat it.

Alcohol use during early pregnancy can cause birth defects. Even a single instance of consuming 5–7 drinks in the first trimester can lead to fetal alcohol syndrome, which causes characteristic facial deformities, developmental disabilities, and seizure disorders. Heavy drinking can also trigger miscarriages. The effects of alcohol consumption in the second and third trimesters are poorly understood, but preliminary evidence suggests a link between moderate drinking (4 drinks or less per session) in later pregnancy and dyslexia, learning disabilities, and other forms of brain damage. Rates of fetal damage may vary by ethnic group, possibly because of differences in drinking behavior and access to prenatal care. Concern over the effect of maternal drinking on fetal health has led to attempts to impose sometimes oppressive restrictions on drinking by women of reproductive age.

Heavy drinking has social as well as biological costs for women. Socially it makes women vulnerable to violence and sexual abuse. Although the exact nature of the link between alcohol use and violence, especially sexual violence, remains an object of debate, researchers have discovered some patterns. A double standard of women's drinking can lead men to see inebriated women as legitimate targets for sexual aggression. Alcohol outlets such as bars vary in terms of the respectability of women who enter. In outlets at the lower end of the scale, men may regard any woman who enters as, by definition, sexually available, putting them at risk for harassment or rape.

Drinking impairs decision-making, makes people clumsy, and can lead to unconsciousness. This decreases women's awareness of possible impending danger, and lowers their ability to respond to a hazardous situation. Because alcohol use can also increase a person's risk of perpetuating a violent act (whether male or female), as well as intensify the degree of violence, women can be at risk of violence not only because of their own drunkenness but also because of that of their male partners. Even at moderate levels, alcohol encourages aggressiveness; at higher levels it can inhibit cognitive capacity. Drinking heavily forms part of male status-building in groups: men often encourage one another in capacity competitions. The combination of male status-building through heavy drink and impairment of reasoning capacity in both men and women can lead to violent escalation of sexual conflicts. Even moderate drinking can impair women's ability to negotiate sexual behavior, increasing their risk for pregnancy and sexually transmitted diseases as well.

Culturally based excusing of inebriate behavior means that drunkenness can absolve personal responsibility in what anthropologists call a "time-out" phase, in which inebriates are not held to the same standards of behavior as sober people. For example, a rapist who demonstrates inebriation at the time of the assault may face a lesser legal penalty. Ironically, double standards often mean that juries see inebriated female rape victims as having invited assault, or confusing the rapist

as to her intent, lessening his attributed guilt. Alcohol use also increases risk of conjugal violence. Women with a drinking problem are more likely to be slapped, beaten, kicked, hit, or have their lives threatened by their husbands. Conflicts related to finances, jealousy, and gender role transgressions can be heightened through regular alcohol abuse by both partners. Alcohol addiction can increase risk for codependency and economic dependence on men, constraining women from leaving abusive relationships, creating a vicious circle that is difficult to escape.

Concern over alcohol's effects on women's sexual continence and the health of their children has led to restrictive laws against female drinking and even against women entering bars. Feminist-led changes in sexual mores and the entrance of large numbers of middle-class women into the workplace have opened more opportunities to drink for women desiring social connotations surrounding drinking, such as glamour, independence, free choice, and masculine privilege, as women increasingly try to fit into a male-dominated world, to compete with men on equal footing in all levels, and see the double standard which governs drinking as oppressive. While employed men generally drink more heavily than employed women, women's drinking rates increase with some types of employment. Women are generally more likely to drink if they earn enough to buy alcohol, have completed higher education, live in an urban area, and have professional employment, but researchers cannot make any strong connection between employment in itself and drinking problems among women. Greater access to alcohol and greater social freedom to drink among women can be seen as positive; increased moderate drinking among employed women does not necessarily imply a greater rate of problem drinking.

Since the 20th century, U.S. feminists have seen women's drinking in terms of greater freedom. Historically, though, in the United States, Mexico, and Great Britain, women led the 19th century temperance movement against drinking by both men and women. In the contemporary world, female-led antidrinking movements have arisen in many developing countries in which women agitate politically against male drinking and also take steps to smash breweries and boycott alcohol products. In the United States and Great Britain, women have led political movements to criminalize driving under the influence, citing maternal grief at the loss of children to drunk driving crashes. Ironically, both women who seek to expand female access to alcohol, and women who seek to restrict alcohol use by both sexes see their efforts as improving women's lives.

SEE ALSO: Addiction, Pregnancy, Rape, Violence

Suggested Reading

Ames, G., & Rebhun, L. A. (1996). Women, alcohol and work: Interactions of gender, ethnicity, and occupational culture. *Social Science and Medicine, 43*, 1649–1663.

Eber, C. (1995). *Women and alcohol in a highland Maya town: Water of hope, water of sorrow.* Austin: University of Texas Press.

Fallaw, B. (2002). Dry law, wet politics: Drinking and prohibition in post-revolutionary Yucatán, 1915–1935. *Latin American Research Review, 37*, 37–65.

Morgan, P. (1987). Women and alcohol: The disinhibition rhetoric in an analysis of domination. *Journal of Psychoactive Drugs, 19*, 129–133.

Randall, C. L. (2001). Alcohol and pregnancy: Highlights from three decades of research. *Journal of Studies on Alcohol, 62*, 554–562.

Van der Walde, H., Urgenson, F. T., Weltz, S. H., & Hanna, F. J. (2002). Women and alcoholism: A biopsychosocial perspective and treatment approaches. *Journal of Counseling and Development, 80*, 145–154.

L. A. REBHUN
YASMINA KATSULIS

Alpha-Fetoprotein Screening

The value of alpha-fetoprotein (AFP) in detecting neural tube defects was recognized over 30 years ago. AFP is a glycoprotein synthesized by the fetal yolk sac, gastrointestinal tract, and liver. When the fetal integument is not intact, markedly elevated levels of AFP occur in the amniotic fluid and maternal serum. Hence, elevated AFP levels are associated with neural tube defects, such as anencephaly and spina bifida, and abdominal wall defects. Other causes of high AFP levels include renal anomalies, decreased maternal weight, and multiple gestation. Conversely, low AFP levels are associated with chromosomal trisomy, fetal demise, and increased maternal weight. Inaccurate estimation of gestational age is the most common reason for an abnormal AFP value.

AFP screening is recommended for all pregnant women in order to help detect those among the general population who may require further diagnostic evaluation. In most regions of the United States, AFP is combined with two additional analytes produced by the placenta, human chorionic gonadotropin (hCG) and unconjugated estriol (uE3). These markers, commonly referred to as the triple screen, can be done from 15 to 22 weeks gestation, but are most accurate between 16 and 18 weeks gestation. The triple screen is designed to identify pregnancies complicated by neural tube defects, trisomy 18, and trisomy 21. An increased hCG value is the most sensitive marker for detecting trisomy 21, while low hCG levels are associated with trisomy 18. Levels of uE3 are decreased in pregnancies affected by trisomy 21 and trisomy 18. Of the markers, only AFP has value in screening for neural tube defects. Absolute values of the three serum analytes are converted to multiples of the median (MoM) and used to calculate a woman's age-related risk of fetal anomaly. Gestational age, maternal race, and maternal weight are also factors used to adjust the level of risk.

Maternal serum AFP screening can detect about 90% of anencephaly cases and 80% of all open spina bifida cases. The three serum analytes combined detect 60–70% of trisomy 21-affected fetuses with a false positive rate of 5%. Ongoing research aims to improve detection rates using better combinations of maternal serum markers. Inhibin A, free βhCG, and plasma protein A (PAPP-A) are among the serum analytes proposed either to increase screening sensitivity or to allow detection earlier in gestation.

Appropriate diagnostic testing after positive screen result depends on the analyte levels. For AFP, a MoM value greater than 2.0–2.5 is considered abnormal. Next an ultrasound examination is done to rule out inaccurate estimation of gestational age as a source of error. Because elevated AFP levels persist with neural tube defects, a repeat maternal serum measurement is sometimes obtained. If the AFP remains elevated and gestational age is confirmed, the patient should be referred for a high-resolution ultrasound. When performed by an expert, ultrasound can detect nearly all cases of anencephaly and spina bifida. Amniocentesis may also be utilized to assess karyotype, amniotic fluid AFP, and acetylcholinesterase.

Trisomy 21 screening uses a series of age-specific risk cutoff levels for each triple screen analyte. Many labs select a risk cutoff of 1 in 270, the risk of a 35-year-old woman for carrying a fetus with trisomy 21. Amniocentesis and detailed ultrasound are offered to women whose triple screen values place them in an at-risk group.

Although triple screening is noninvasive and does not physically harm the mother or fetus, receiving abnormal results can cause great emotional stress. Awareness of congenital anomalies in the fetus leads to ethically complex decisions like whether to terminate the pregnancy or not. Before prenatal serum marker screening is done, women should understand how the test may affect them. Counseling should include explanations of the accuracy of the test, the conditions detectable by screening, and the follow-up diagnostic testing recommended for a high-risk screen.

See Also: Neural tube defects, Pregnancy, Prenatal care

Suggested Reading

Cunningham, F. C., & MacDonald (Ed.). (1997). Prenatal diagnosis and invasive techniques to monitor the fetus. *Williams obstetrics* (pp. 919–941). Stamford, CT: Appleton & Lange.

Evans, M. I., Krivchenia, E. L., & Yaron, Y. (2002). Screening. *Best Practice and Research Clinical Obstetrics and Gynecology, 16,* 645–657.

Graves, J. C., Miller, K. E., & Sellers, A. D. (2002). Maternal serum triple analyte screening in pregnancy. *American Family Physician, 65,* 915–920.

N. K. Yeaney

Alternative Medicine   *see* Complementary and Alternative Health Practices; *see also* specific treatment, for example, Acupuncture

---

Alternative Treatment   *see* Complementary and Alternative Health Practices; *see also* specific treatment, for example, Acupuncture

---

Alzheimer's Disease   The syndrome of dementia is an irreversible decline in cognitive abilities that causes significant dysfunction. Like most syndromes, dementia can be caused by a number of diseases. In the 19th century, for example, a main cause of dementia was syphilis. Currently, as a result of dramatic increases in average human life expectancy, dementia is caused primarily by a number of neurological diseases associated with old age. Dementia is distinguished from "pseudodementia" because the latter is reversible—for example, depression, extreme stress, and infection can cause dementia, but with treatment, a return to a former cognitive state is likely. Dementia is also distinguished from "normal age-related memory loss," which affects most people by about age 70 in the form of some slowing of cognitive skills and a deterioration in various aspects of memory. But "senior moments" of forgetfulness do not constitute dementia, which is a precipitous and disease-related decline resulting in remarkable disability. Since 1997, a degree of cognitive impairment that is greater than normal age-related decline but not yet diagnosable as dementia has been labeled "mild cognitive impairment," or MCI, with about a third of those in this category "converting" to dementia each year. These cognitive conditions from normal age-related forgetfulness to dementia form a continuum. Specialized clinics that were once called Alzheimer's Centers are increasingly changing their name to Memory Disorders Centers in order to begin to treat patients at various points along the continuum prior to the onset of dementia.

Although dementia can have many causes, the primary cause of dementia in our aging societies is Alzheimer's disease (AD). Approximately 60% of dementia in the American elderly and worldwide in industrialized nations is secondary to AD. About two thirds of those with AD are women. This is because women in industrialized countries tend to outlive men, and age is the most significant risk factor for AD. It is also the case that women's brains may be adversely affected by diminished estrogen levels. One epidemiological study in the United States estimated that 47% of persons 85 years and older (the "old-old") had probable AD, although this is considered somewhat inflated. Epidemiologists differ in their estimates of late-life AD prevalence, but most studies agree roughly on the following: about 1–2% of older adults at age 60 have probable AD, and this percentage doubles every 5 years so that 3% are affected at age 65, 6% at age 70, 12% at age 75, and 24% by age 80. While some argue that those who live into their 90s without being affected by AD will usually never be affected by it, this is still speculative. According to a Swiss study, 10% of nondemented persons between the ages of 85 and 88 become demented each year. There are very few people in their late 40s and early 50s who are diagnosed with AD. Without delaying or preventive interventions, the number of people with AD, in the United States alone, will increase to 14.3 million by 2050. These numbers represent a new problem of major proportions and immense financial consequences for medicine, families, and society.

AD family caregivers are predominantly women across the world. In many countries, like Japan, it is even assumed that the daughter-in-law married to the oldest son will take on caregiving duties for her mother- or father-in-law. In other societies, the youngest daughter in a family has often had to sacrifice marriage and other plans to stay home and care for aging parents. About 80% of family caregivers in the United States are women.

Men tend to focus on indirect forms of care, such as managing finances and other needs that do not involve direct caring. This is especially significant for women's health because AD caregivers are typically under stress, and studies show high susceptibility to stress-induced caregiver illnesses such as depression. Financially, women who care for their husbands will be impacted by Medicaid "spend down" policies, which require an expenditure of the couple's assets before qualification for assisted living or nursing home benefits. This contributes to the feminization of poverty.

Filial duties between an adult child and a parent raise complex ethical questions. That women are assumed to have these duties in the sense of demanding everyday care, and must therefore bear the brunt of caregiver stress, suggests that men must learn to accept a more engaged caregiving role.

Women have especially high stakes in many aspects of AD care and policy. They are deeply impacted by policies that preclude federal support of respite care for family caregivers. Women will be especially affected by successful research into treatments for AD, as well as in the ethical policies surrounding treatment decisions and end of life. Because there are more women than men in nursing homes, they are impacted more significantly by nursing home policies. Women do most of the direct caring, and they are at greater risk of AD. Thus, this is a disease with clear feminist implications.

SEE ALSO: Activities of daily living, Assisted living, Disability, Medicaid, Medicare, Nursing home, Quality of life

Suggested Reading

Aevarsson, O., & Skoog, I. (1996). A population-based study on the incidence of dementia disorders between 85 and 88 years of age. *Journal of the American Geriatrics Society, 44*, 1455–1460.

Firlik, A. D. (1991). "Margo's logo." *Journal of the American Medical Association, 265*, 201.

Gauderer, M. (1999). Twenty years of percutaneous endoscopic gastrostomy: Origin and evolution of a concept and its expanded applications. *Gastrointestinal Endoscopy, 50*, 879–882.

Gillick, M. R. (2000). Rethinking the role of tube feeding in patients with advanced dementia. *New England Journal of Medicine, 342*, 206–210.

Ikels, C. (1998). The experience of dementia in China. *Culture, Medicine and Psychiatry, 3*, 257–283.

Kitwood, T. (1997). *Dementia reconsidered: The person comes first.* Buckingham, UK: Open University Press.

Post, S. G. (2000). *The moral challenge of Alzheimer disease: Ethical issues from diagnosis to dying* (2nd ed.). Baltimore: The Johns Hopkins University Press (1st ed. 1995).

STEPHEN G. POST

Amenorrhea   *see* Menstrual Cycle Disorders

Americans with Disabilities Act

Signed in July 1990, the Americans with Disabilities Act (ADA) provides the disabled with protections similar to those already covering discrimination on the basis of sex, national origin, race, religion, and veteran status. An individual is protected under the ADA if his/her ability to perform one or more major life activities (such as hearing, sight, self-care, walking, breathing, speaking, or learning) is hampered by a physical or mental condition, if they have a record of having such a condition, is thought of as such, or associates with such a person. The law is designed to open up employment opportunities, government services, public accommodations, transportation services, and telecommunications to the disabled on an equal-opportunity basis. Unfortunately, successive Supreme Court rulings have steadily weakened the ADA.

The ADA prohibits discrimination against qualified disabled people in all employment-related activities, including: hiring, promotion, training, and compensation. Except in cases where a person's disability poses a direct threat to their own and/or others' health and safety in the performance of the job, disability cannot be used as a basis for discrimination. Except where it would be infeasible, or impose a significant expense or effort (an "undue hardship") on the part of the employer, organizations employing 15 or more must provide reasonable accommodations to disabled employees and job applicants as they request or indicate. Such reasonable accommodations can include, for example, accessibility modifications to existing facilities, changing work schedules, providing adaptive or modified equipment (such as speech-recognition computer software for someone with cerebral palsy), or adjusting training.

In covering the provision of government services, the ADA obligates states and localities to ensure that the disabled enjoy equal access to government employment, programs, and services. Besides being subject to similar employment and access rules to those governing private employers, state and local entities also must remove discriminatory barriers to the disabled for participation in and eligibility for programs, activities, and services. Additionally, these organizations must provide for "public accessibility," that is, they need to ensure that the disabled can access all of their programs, activities, and services, by providing them in accessible locations, whether in their own facilities, or at an offsite location.

Some of the most visible changes brought by the ADA stem from the law's "public accommodations" provisions, which apply to a private company or other organization which owns or operates a facility open for public access, such as a theater, restaurant, shopping mall, park, museum, or any other of a wide range of facilities. These provisions, which include both major renovations of existing buildings and new construction, are intended to ensure the accessibility of new and newly renovated public facilities. Such places include a variety of access-minded features, providing, for example, parking lots with curb cuts and a number of designated accessible spaces, elevators, barrier-free design and layout, accessible bathrooms, tables of wheelchair-appropriate clearance and height, and sufficiently wide doorways. Under the ADA, reasonable accommodations for such public establishments go beyond just physical access; they can include, for example, reading a price tag to a blind customer, retrieving a book from an unreachable shelf for a wheelchair user, and providing straws and cutting up food for a patron with limited arm function at a restaurant.

Public and private transportation services are similarly enjoined by the ADA against discriminatory behavior to the disabled; they must provide an equal or at least equally effective level of service as that provided to the nondisabled. Airlines, taxi lines, train and bus lines, and other transportation providers must make reasonable accommodations, including, for example, ensuring the accessibility of: new and refurbished buses and depots, commuter and light rail train cars, stations, and providing access-enabling services to physically or mentally disabled riders.

Another major area covered by the ADA is that of telecommunications services for those with hearing and/or speech impairments. Telecommunications providers (phone companies), for example, must allow telecommunications device for the deaf (TDD) and teletype usage and communication with operators. In addition, in states lacking their own telecommunications relay service (TRS) programs (TRS allows, through an intermediary, a person using a TDD to communicate with an unimpaired person without one), providers must provide impaired customers with these services continuously 24 hours a day, 7 days a week, at no extra cost or limitation (such as call length).

SEE ALSO: Disability, Discrimination

Suggested Reading

A Guide to Disability Rights Laws, DOJ; Civil Rights Div., Disability Rights Section (August 2001).

Americans with Disabilities Act: Questions and Answers, DOJ; Civil Rights Div., Equal Employment Opportunities Commission (August 23, 2002).

The Americans with Disabilities Act: A Primer for Small Business, DOJ; Civil Rights Div., Equal Employment Opportunities Commission (September 10, 2002).

JANET L. LOWDER
CHARLES GROVER

Anorexia Nervosa The *Diagnostic and Statistical Manual of Mental Disorders* (DSM-IV) categorizes eating disorders as anorexia nervosa (AN), bulimia nervosa (BN), and eating disorder not otherwise specified (ED-NOS). AN is characterized by an intense fear of gaining weight, refusal to maintain a normal body weight, disturbed perception of one's own shape or size, and, if female, amenorrhea of at least three consecutive cycles. Individuals lacking insight are frequently brought to professional attention by a family member after marked weight loss. AN is subcategorized as either restrictive eating or binge-eating/purging type with self-induced vomiting, misuse of laxatives, diuretics, or enemas. Up to 50% of patients with AN develop bulimic symptoms, and some patients who are initially bulimic develop anorexic symptoms. Psychiatric comorbidities include depressive symptoms like sadness, social withdrawal, irritability, insomnia, or decreased sexual interest. These may be secondary to physiological sequelae of semistarvation and resolve only after partial or complete weight restoration. Obsessive-compulsive features like frequent thoughts of food, hoarding food, picking/pulling apart small portions of food, or collecting recipes, along with anxiety and concerns of eating in public, are common. Other comorbid conditions include substance abuse, sexual abuse, and bipolar disorder.

Although AN frequently begins in the midteens, the onset is in the early 20s for 5% of patients. Estimates of male-to-female ratio range from 1:6 to 1:10. The reported lifetime prevalence of AN among women has ranged from 0.5% when narrowly defined to 3.7% for more broadly defined AN. Eating disorders are more frequent in industrialized societies, where there is an abundance of food and being thin, especially for females, is considered attractive. In the United States, eating disorders are common in young Hispanic, Native American, and African American women, but the rates are still lower than in Caucasian women. Female athletes involved in running, gymnastics, or ballet dancers, male body builders and wrestlers are also at increased risk. Biological and psychosocial factors are implicated in the cause of anorexia, but the etiology and underlying mechanisms of eating disorders remain unknown. Antidepressants often benefit patients with AN and implicate a role for serotonin and norepinephrine. Starvation results in many biochemical changes such as hypercortisolemia, nonsuppression of dexamethasone, suppression of thyroid function, and amenorrhea. Monozygotic twins, other first-degree female relatives, and children of patients as well as low levels of nurturance and empathy are reported in families of children presenting with eating disorders. In addition to the clinical interview, rating scales such as the Eating Attitudes Test, Eating Disorders Inventory, or Body Shape Questionnaire can be used for assessment of eating disorders.

Medical comorbidity and complications of AN are related to weight loss, starvation, purging, and laxative abuse. Generalized weakness, dehydration, electrolyte and cardiac rhythm abnormalities, and amenorrhea are common. AN should be differentiated from malignancy, seizures, AIDS, depressive disorders, somatization disorder, schizophrenia, and BN.

A comprehensive treatment plan includes a combination of good nutritional rehabilitation, psychotherapy, and medications. Weight, cardiac, and metabolic status of the individual with AN determine the acuity of the illness and the need for hospitalization. Aims of treatment are to restore the patient's nutritional status by establishing healthy eating patterns, treat medical complications, correct core dysfunctional ideations related to eating disorders, enlisting family support, and providing for family counseling. Medications for treatment of AN can be initiated before or after weight gain. Medications can maintain normal eating behaviors as well as treat associated depressive or obsessive-compulsive symptoms. Antidepressants like the serotonin-specific reuptake inhibitors, for example, fluoxetine (Prozac), are commonly considered. Low doses of antipsychotics for marked agitation with psychotic thinking and benzodiazepene anxiolytics for extreme anticipatory anxiety are helpful. Long-term follow-up shows recovery rates ranging from 44% to 76% with mortality of up to 20% primarily from cardiac arrest or suicide. Treatment guidelines are readily available with an abridged, up-to-date version at www.guidelines.gov/index.asp.

See Also: Body image, Bulimia nervosa, Depression, Eating disorders, Weight control

Suggested Reading

American Psychiatric Association. (1994). *Diagnostic and statistical manual of mental disorders* (4th ed.). Washington, DC: American Psychiatric Association.

American Psychiatric Association. (2000). Eating disorders measures. In *Handbook of psychiatric measures* (pp. 647–673). Washington, DC: Author.

American Psychiatric Association Work Group on Eating Disorders. (2000). Practice guideline for the treatment of patients with eating disorders (revision). *American Journal of Psychiatry, 157,* 1–39.

Fairburn, C., & Brownell, K. (2002). *Eating disorders and obesity* (2nd ed., pp. 233–237). New York: Guilford Press.

Kaplan, H. I., & Sadock, B. J. Eating disorders. In *Synopsis of psychiatry* (8th ed., pp. 720–736). Philadelphia: Lippincott, Williams and Wilkins.

KATHLEEN N. FRANCO
RASHMI DESHMUKH

Anovulatory Uterine Bleeding   *see* Vaginal Bleeding

Anxiety Disorders

The term Anxiety Disorders refers to a category of psychiatric illnesses that are generally more chronic than substance use or affective (mood) disorders. It is estimated that 25% of the population have had some type of anxiety disorder in their lifetime. The fourth edition of the *Diagnostic and Statistical Manual of Mental Disorders* (DSM-IV) classifies 12 anxiety disorders: panic disorder without agoraphobia, panic disorder with agoraphobia, agoraphobia without history of panic disorder, specific phobia, social phobia, obsessive-compulsive disorder, posttraumatic stress disorder (PTSD), generalized anxiety disorder (GAD), acute stress disorder, anxiety disorder due to a general medical condition, substance-induced anxiety disorder, and anxiety disorder not otherwise specified.

The two most common anxiety disorders are social phobia (13% lifetime prevalence) and simple phobia (11% lifetime prevalence). Risk factors for anxiety disorders include lower socioeconomic status, female gender, and living in the Northeast region of the United States. Women are twice as likely to have any anxiety diagnosis, except social phobia, where the women-to-men ratio is 3:2. Adults between the ages of 25 and 34 have the highest prevalence rates. There are no differences among races. Individuals with anxiety disorders are highly likely to have another coexisting mental disorder, but only a small number actually seek treatment.

Anxiety is a universal feeling that is normal and adaptive in the right circumstances; however, when the level of anxiety begins to interfere with functioning or cause considerable emotional distress, it is important to evaluate for the presence of an anxiety disorder. In most of the disorders outlined here, the level of anxiety experienced causes the suffering person to seek refuge by avoiding the source of anxiety, or by performing some neutralizing behavior until the lifestyle is drastically hampered, or to experience intense anxiety in the face of the source. Panic attacks are a central feature of several of the anxiety disorders. These are episodes of intense anxiety in which at least four of the following thirteen symptoms peak very quickly: increased heart rate, sweating, shakiness, short of breath, choking feelings, chest pain, abdominal distress, dizziness, feelings of unreality or detachment from self, fear of losing control or dying, tingling, chills, or hot flushes. Panic-like symptoms are fewer in number than is required for a full-fledged panic attack, but can also include other incapacitating symptoms (e.g., severe headache).

Panic attacks or panic-like symptoms can be either unexpected, situationally bound, or situationally predisposed. The first type occurs unpredictably whereas the situationally bound type occurs in the presence of a trigger. Situationally predisposed can be in response to some stimulus but at other times attacks do not occur with that stimulus at all (e.g., an attack may occur after entering a mall but at other times this may not happen).

A diagnosis of *panic disorder with agoraphobia* is given when agoraphobia occurs along with unexpected full-fledged panic attacks with a month of concern about one of the following: fears of another attack, the implications of the attack, or a marked change in behavior associated with the attacks. *Panic disorder without agoraphobia* has the same criteria for diagnosis except that it occurs in the absence of agoraphobia symptoms. On the other hand, a diagnosis of *agoraphobia without history of panic disorder* is made when agoraphobia symptoms are related to fears of developing the panic-like symptoms without a history of full-fledged panic attacks.

Specific phobia and *social phobia* are similar in that the increased anxiety is situationally bound to a specific trigger(s). In specific phobia, this can be anything from animals, to storms, to public transportation. When these triggers can be easily avoided, functioning is rarely impaired (e.g., fear of buses, but no need to travel by bus). However, when the specific phobia is something occurring in everyday life, the impairment can be considerable (e.g., fear of tunnels when living in New York City). In social phobia, the anxiety arousal is linked to social interactions and feared negative evaluations by others. Since anyone can speak to you at any time, individuals may experience more of a general anxiety arousal than those with other anxiety disorders. Individuals with this disorder will adopt a range of avoidance behaviors to manage their anxiety, at times with significant consequences (e.g., turning down a promotion that requires more social interaction).

Individuals with *obsessive–compulsive disorder* (OCD) experience recurrent intrusive thoughts or behaviors that are time consuming enough to impair functioning or cause significant distress. Obsessions are not worries about everyday problems, but instead can be about contamination (touching a public door handle), order (distress when objects are asymmetrical), or aggressive imagery (hurting a child). Attempts are made to ignore these thoughts or to neutralize them with some repeated action (e.g., hand washing). These repeated actions (compulsions) serve to lower the

90

anxiety associated with the unwanted thoughts or impulses. At times this may also take the form of mental acts (e.g., repeating words to oneself or counting). Compulsions can be related to the obsession (e.g., checking that the iron is unplugged in response to fear that the iron was left on and may start a fire), but in other cases, may have nothing to do with them (e.g., counting backwards from 100 to neutralize fear of hitting someone while driving). Attempts to avoid provoking situations or objects can lead to even greater decrease in functioning.

PTSD develops after exposure to some extreme traumatic stressor that was either experienced directly, was witnessed, or learned about that involved either actual or threatened death or injury or threat to physical integrity of others or self. The person's reaction to the event is one of intense horror. Triggers can be anything reminiscent of the original event including similar sounds, smells, dreams, or internal body sensations. Symptoms include a feeling that one is reexperiencing the event, avoidance of any cues that are related to the original trauma, and increased arousal (e.g., sleep difficulties, irritability) that persist for more than a month. Those who develop PTSD continue to experience a myriad of symptoms long after a typical recovery period. *Acute stress disorder* is similar to PTSD but it involves significant dissociative symptoms (e.g., dazed, numb) and the duration is shorter, a minimum of 2 days and a maximum of 4 weeks after the traumatic event occurs.

Individuals who worry excessively and are unable to control it may be experiencing GAD. Associated body symptoms include feeling restless, irritable, and easily fatigued. Sore muscles and sleep disturbance may also accompany the anxiety. The focus of worry is usually everyday things like work, school, or family finances but it is severe enough to cause impairment in functioning or cause significant distress.

Anxiety disorder due to a general medical condition and *substance-induced anxiety disorder* are diagnosed when anxiety symptoms from panic, GAD, or OCD occur in direct relation to a medical condition in the former or, in the latter, as a response to a medication or drug. A diagnosis of *anxiety disorder not otherwise specified* is given when anxiety symptoms are predominant but do not meet criteria for any of the specific disorders listed above.

Hypotheses regarding individual differences in vulnerability to anxiety include genetic, cultural, and personality factors, early childhood experiences, and other learned factors. Various interventions have been used to target specific anxiety symptoms. More common treatments include exposure-based therapies, behavioral therapy, cognitive restructuring, and relaxation training. Numerous medications are available to treat specific anxiety disorders, most notably the selective serotonin reuptake inhibitors, monoamine oxidase inhibitors, buspirone, tricyclics, beta-blockers, carbamazepine, venlafaxine, and benzodiazepines.

SEE ALSO: Depression, Panic attack, Phobia, Posttraumatic stress disorder

Suggested Reading

American Psychiatric Association. (1994). *Diagnostic and statistical manual of mental disorders* (4th ed.). Washington, DC: American Psychiatric Association.

Beck, A. T., Emery, G., & Greenberg, R. I. (1985). *Anxiety disorders and phobias: A cognitive perspective.* New York: Basic Books.

Brown, T. A., & Barlow, D. H. (1992). Comorbidity among anxiety disorders: Implications for treatment and DSM-IV. *Journal of Consulting and Clinical Psychology, 60,* 835–844.

Foa, E. B., & Wilson, R. (1991). *Stop obsessing!* New York: Bantam Books.

Hollander, E., Simeon, D., & Gorman, J. M. (1999). Anxiety disorders. In R. E. Hales, S. C. Yudofsky, & J. A. Talbott (Eds.), *Textbook of psychiatry* (3rd ed., pp. 567–634). Washington, DC: American Psychiatric Press.

Kessler, R. C., McGonagle, K. A., Zhao, S., Nelson, C. B., Hughes, M., Eshleman, S., et al. (1994). Lifetime and 12-month prevalence of DSM-III-R psychiatric disorders in the United States: Results from the National Comorbidity Survey. *Archives of General Psychiatry, 51,* 8–19.

McLean, P. D., & Woody, S. R. (2001). *Anxiety disorders in adults: An evidence-based approach to psychological treatment.* New York: Oxford University Press.

VIRGINIA E. AYRES

Arthritis Osteoarthritis and rheumatoid arthritis are the two most common types of generalized arthritis. Unfortunately, many think that the two terms are interchangeable but in fact, they are two very different diseases with different treatments. As treatments differ, it is vital that the correct diagnosis is made.

OSTEOARTHRITIS

Osteoarthritis is the most common form of arthritis. It is primarily a disease of the cartilage that cushions the joints, leading to progressive thinning of that cushion.

More than just "wear and tear" leads to osteoarthritis. Cartilage undergoes constant recycling of removing old cartilage and replacing it with new. With aging, the recycling process breaks down and osteoarthritis then begins to form.

The most common joints affected are the fingers, base of the thumb, hip, knee, spine, and the great toe (a bunion). Risk factors for developing osteoarthritis include: obesity, aging, and situations that put one at risk at certain joints. For example, occupations that involve repetitive knee bending, kneeling, squatting, or stair climbing are associated with an increased frequency of knee osteoarthritis.

The symptoms of osteoarthritis include pain, stiffness, and disability. Initially, the pain is only intermittent, typically associated with the use of the joint. With time, the pain can be more constant as the disease advances. With inactivity, the joint stiffens and can give the sensation of locking up when trying to move it again. Morning stiffness, after a full night of inactivity, usually lasts about 15–30 minutes. This is in contrast to rheumatoid arthritis where morning stiffness can last for hours. The mainstay of treatment for osteoarthritis is nonsteroidal anti-inflammatory drugs. Osteoarthritis is discussed in greater detail elsewhere.

RHEUMATOID ARTHRITIS

Rheumatoid arthritis is a disease of a disordered immune system in which inflammatory cells attack the joints. Because of the aggressive joint inflammation, the pain is much more severe and disabling than that of osteoarthritis. Like most autoimmune diseases, rheumatoid arthritis is more common in women. Other risk factors for rheumatoid arthritis include age greater than 50, smoking, and relatives with rheumatoid arthritis. Because this is an immune system process, multiple joints are involved at the same time. The most common joints include the hands, wrists, knees, and feet, but any joint can be involved. The disease is usually symmetrical, in that the same joint is affected on both sides of the body. Because of the inflammation, morning stiffness can last for hours. Some patients develop rheumatoid nodules, which are bumps on their elbows. This is a sign of severe progressive rheumatoid arthritis.

Abnormal blood tests in rheumatoid arthritis patients include an elevated erythrocyte sedimentation rate (ESR) and C-reactive protein, which are both signs of inflammation. A positive rheumatoid factor can be suggestive of rheumatoid arthritis but it is not absolutely necessary to make the diagnosis. The presence of a positive rheumatoid factor means that a more aggressive form of rheumatoid arthritis is present which requires more aggressive therapy. Treatment of rheumatoid arthritis has two goals: to control pain and to stop the joint destruction. To control pain, nonsteroidal anti-inflammatory medications or sometimes prednisone can be used to control the inflammation. With decreased inflammation in the joints, the pain and stiffness will decrease. However, these medications cannot stop the abnormal immune system from attacking the joints: other medications are needed for this.

The mainstay of rheumatoid arthritis treatment has been methotrexate, which was originally a cancer drug. A low dose of methotrexate given once a week has been shown to significantly improve the symptoms of rheumatoid arthritis in most patients. Other immune system altering medications are used if methotrexate is ineffective.

Recently, technology has allowed medical researchers to create medications that specifically target immune molecules that are known to be the cause of the inflammatory process in the joint. One such molecule is tumor necrosis factor (TNF), which is a highly destructive molecule in rheumatoid arthritis, causing lots of inflammatory debris in the joints. One medication that targets TNF is etanercept (Enbrel), given by subcutaneous injection twice a week. Etanercept is a TNF receptor that binds up the circulating TNF and prevents it from affecting the joint. Imfliximab (Remicade) is an antibody to TNF that binds it so that the TNF cannot affect the joint. Imfliximab is given by intravenous infusion every 4–8 weeks. Both of these medications have revolutionized how rheumatoid arthritis is treated. These medications, as with all immune system altering medications, can increase the risk of infections. All patients who use these drugs should be closely monitored by their physicians.

We now approach rheumatoid arthritis much like we treat cancer, by attempting to put the disease into remission. Aggressive therapy can prevent future joint damage and avoid disability. Of course, aggressive therapy is associated with more potentially harmful side effects. Anyone who uses these medications must consider the potential risks and benefits of therapy.

SEE ALSO: Autoimmune disorders, Osteoarthritis

Suggested Reading

Klippel, J. H. (Ed.). (2001). *Primer of rheumatic diseases* (12th ed.). Atlanta, GA: Arthritis Foundation.

Koopman, W. J. (Ed.). (1997). *Arthritis and allied conditions* (13th ed.). Philadelphia: Williams & Wilkins.

MARIE KUCHYNSKI

Asian and Pacific Islander

The women of Asia and the Pacific Islands are the world's largest demographic group, comprising over one quarter of humankind. They inhabit regions as diverse as cosmopolitan Taipei and Tokyo, snowy Himalayan peaks, and the tropical isles of the Philippines. Over 10,000 years ago, Asians journeyed across land bridges and the ocean to become the first inhabitants of what is now known as the Americas. After the founding of the United States, Asian immigration was severely limited by more than two centuries of laws such as the 1790 Immigration and Naturalization Act that only allowed naturalized citizenship for "white" persons, and the Chinese Exclusion Act in effect from 1882 to 1943. In 1965, immigration quotas favoring those of European national origins were replaced by those favoring skilled professionals. Whereas 19th century Asian immigrants were mostly Chinese and Japanese male agricultural and railroad laborers, the post-1965 Asian immigration wave largely consisted of highly educated Chinese and Asian Indians. With the fall of Saigon to communist forces in 1975, Southeast Asians sought refuge in the United States. Initially comprised of the Vietnamese upper class fleeing political persecution, later waves consisted of rural populations from Laos, Cambodia, Vietnam, and other parts of Asia. Although now largely abandoned, anti-Asian laws continue to exist, such as those prohibiting Asians from owning land in Florida and New Mexico. However, because of civil rights legislation, these laws are unenforced.

According to the 2000 U.S. census, over 5.6 million Asian and Pacific Islander American women live in the United States, totaling approximately 2% of the U.S. population. They are remarkably diverse in terms of ethnic origin, educational status, socioeconomic status, and degrees of acclimatization to the Western world. The very concept of "Asia" originates from Europe and many who we consider "Asian" may not feel that they share a common ethnic identity. For example, Chinese and Japanese, who have a long history of war and genocidal conflict, see themselves as distinct as Germans and Jews. With the passing of the Civil Rights Act of 1964, legal bans on interracial marriage, existent in many states, were lifted. Today, many Asian and Pacific Islander Americans are of mixed race, further defying categorization.

Asian and Pacific Islander American women have made notable achievements. During much of the 1990s, Maxine Hong Kingston was the most widely taught living American author. Elaine Chao currently serves as the U.S. Secretary of Labor. Nevertheless, Asian and Pacific Islander women often endure negative stereotypes of submissiveness and of being accepting of sexual exploitation, as put forth by media images such as Suzy Wong and Miss Saigon. In 1988, playwright David Henry Hwang won a Tony Award for "M. Butterfly," a play that critiques these stereotypes.

HEALTH BELIEFS

Many Asian and Pacific Islander cultures have highly evolved health practices. Examples include acupuncture, Chinese herbal remedies, yoga, meditation, and Ayurvedic medicine, all of which are gaining increasing acceptance into mainstream America and being incorporated into Western medical practices. Whereas many Asian and Pacific Islander women are well informed about the offerings of Western medicine, many elderly and recent immigrants may not understand Western medical concepts, or find them confusing. For example, a study of Southeast Asians in Ohio found that 94% did not know what blood pressure is. A survey of Vietnamese women in San Francisco revealed that 52% believed "there is little one can do to prevent cancer." In fact, traditional Chinese medical texts have no concept of cancer. Beliefs such as these can interfere with preventive mammograms and Pap smears that screen for cancer. Chinese medical doctors, prevalent throughout Asia, largely rely on examinations of the pulse and the tongue, and Asian and Pacific Islanders accustomed to seeing these physicians may find the extensive questioning and physical examinations of Western doctors intrusive. Western and Asian cultures have many dissimilar concepts and interpreters must therefore not only translate language, but culture as well, a difficult task during today's time-limited medical visits.

Asian and Pacific Islander

Many surveys have shown that Asian Americans are likely to use traditional Asian remedies even when they seek help from Western doctors. A 1992 study found that 69% of Asian American women and 39% of Asian American men used traditional Asian remedies. Often, this concomitant usage remains unknown to their Western physicians.

Many Asians believe that they are more sensitive to drugs than Caucasians and may therefore intentionally take lower doses of medicines than prescribed. A growing number of studies now support the validity of what has been considered to be an "old wives' tale." In a 1989 study, Zhou found that Asians respond more profoundly to propranolol, experiencing lower blood pressures and heart rates than Caucasians. The liver enzyme cytochrome P450-2D6, responsible for degrading numerous psychiatric medicines, exists in at least nine variations, with a less active form found in 33–50% of Asians and Africans. Several studies show that Asians experience higher plasma levels and more severe side effects than Caucasians in response to Haldol, an antipsychotic medication metabolized by P450-2D6. Similarly, studies confirm that Asians have higher plasma levels of the antidepressant desipramine (P450-2D6 metabolized) than Caucasians.

PHYSICAL HEALTH

Asian American women have the highest life expectancy of any ethnic group in the United States, at 85.8 years. Issues of major concern with Asian and Pacific Islander American women include: higher rates of osteoporosis, hepatitis B infection, and tuberculosis (TB). Lower incidences of screening for breast and cervical cancers are also of concern.

Osteoporosis

Osteoporosis is more common among women of Asian race than any other. Asian women tend to have small skeletal frames along with low dietary calcium intake, as many traditional Asian diets lack dairy products, given the high prevalence of lactose intolerance among the population. Despite a higher rate of osteoporosis, Asian women have a lower incidence of hip fractures than Caucasian women, but an equal prevalence of vertebral fractures.

Infectious Diseases

Worldwide, the vast majority of those infected with hepatitis B are in Asia. In the United States, many Asian immigrants have hepatitis B and women may transmit the virus to their children during birth. A study found that although Asian and Pacific Islander women accounted for only 3% of births in the United States, they accounted for 48% of births to hepatitis B carriers. TB is the number one infectious killer in the United States, and it is four times more common among Asian Americans than the general population. The risk of TB declines as time spent in the United States increases. HIV infection is rare among Asian and Pacific Islander Americans and accounted for less than 1% of AIDS cases in the United States in 1999.

Breast Cancer and Cervical Cancer

Asian and Pacific Islander American women have the lowest breast cancer death rate of any U.S. group at 13.1 per 100,000. However, an example of the heterogeneity of the population is that Native Hawaiians have the highest breast cancer death rate of any U.S. ethnic group at 37.2 per 100,000. The example of breast cancer in Asian women is often used as evidence of environmental rather than genetic causes of cancer. Breast cancer for Chinese and Japanese women living in Asia is lower than for American women, but with immigration to the United States, breast cancer rates rise. Ethnic Chinese, Japanese, and Pilipina women born in the United States have a breast cancer risk that is 60% higher than their counterparts born in Asia. Preventive screening for breast cancer and cervical cancer among Asian and Pacific Islander American women is a major public health concern as these women tend to have low rates of obtaining mammograms and Pap tests. Interfering with screening may be cultural biases against genital examinations by male physicians and beliefs that these exams might affect virginity. Subsequently, Asian and Pacific Islander American women tend to have more severe cases of cervical cancer due to late diagnosis.

MENTAL HEALTH

Suicide

Whereas Western cultures view suicide as a religious sin, such a taboo does not exist in most Asian cultures. For traditional Chinese and Japanese, suicide can be seen as an honorable way to save face and to remove shame from one's family. The Japanese language has over 20 words for suicide, mostly describing different means of accomplishing it. For women aged 15–24, and over age 65, Asian Americans have the highest rates of suicide.

Stigma

Mental illness holds great stigma for many Asian and Pacific Islanders, so that when they finally seek psychiatric help, they are severely ill. Mental illness is often underreported because of interdependence and duty between family members. For example, if mental illness in the family is revealed, relatives may become stigmatized, unemployable, or unmarriageable.

Trauma

Posttraumatic stress disorder and the psychological impacts of trauma are rampant within Asian and Pacific Islander American families. Many have endured torture, rape, starvation, and the witnessing of family members being murdered as a result of political persecution or difficult journeys of exile. This is especially true for recent Southeast Asian immigrants from Vietnam and Cambodia. Although most U.S.-born Asian Americans have not personally suffered these traumas, parents who have shaped their emotional and intellectual world-view may be heavily influenced by trauma inflicted by the Chinese Communist Revolution, the Korean War, or the internment of Japanese Americans in U.S. concentration camps during World War II.

Somatization

Many Asian and Pacific Islanders tend to express emotional distress through physical symptoms such as headaches, stomach upset, or various other symptoms with no discernible physical cause. For example, among a group of Cambodian American women who suffer psychosomatic blindness, 90% had witnessed the killing of a relative.

Alcoholism

About 80% of Asians and 10% of Caucasians metabolize alcoholic beverages in a manner that causes flushing and gastrointestinal upset, a reaction that can be protective against alcoholism. Many studies confirm ethnic differences in enzymes that metabolize alcohol.

SEE ALSO: Immigrant health, Posttraumatic stress disorder, Suicide

Suggested Reading

Adams, D. L. (Ed.). (1995). *Health issues for women of color, a cultural diversity perspective.* Thousand Oaks, CA: Sage.

Asian Women United of California (Ed.). (1989). *Making waves: An anthology of writings by and about Asian American women.* Boston: Beacon Press.

Gaw, A. C. (Ed.). (1993). *Culture, ethnicity and mental illness.* Washington, DC: American Psychiatric Press.

Kingston, M. H. (1976). *The woman warrior: Memoirs of a girlhood among ghosts.* New York: Alfred A. Knopf.

Leigh, W. A., & Lindquist, M. A. (1998). *Women of color health data book: Adolescents to seniors.* Baltimore: National Institutes of Health.

Loue, S. (1999). *Gender, ethnicity, and health research.* New York: Kluwer Academic/Plenum.

Pi, E., & Gray, G. (2000). Ethnopsychopharmacology for Asians. In: P. Ruiz (Ed.), *Ethnicity and psychopharmacology.* Washington, DC: American Psychiatric Press.

Takaki, R. (1989). *Strangers from a different shore: A history of Asian Americans.* Boston: Little, Brown.

Zane, N. W. S., Takeuchi, D. T., & Young, K. N. J. (Eds.). (1994). *Confronting critical health issues of Asian and Pacific Islander Americans.* Thousand Oaks, CA: Sage.

DORA L. WANG

Assisted Living
Individuals who need help with one or a few of the activities of daily living (such as meal preparation, dressing, bathing, and the like) can often continue to reside in the most independent setting possible if this help is provided. This is described as assisted living.

Assisted living can be provided in the home or in specially designed housing. Services typically provided in assisted living facilities include three meals per day (usually served in a restaurant-style common dining room), help with taking medications on schedule, transportation to local stores or medical appointments, housekeeping and laundry service, and social activities. Assistance with eating, bathing, dressing, toileting, and walking is usually restricted to *minimal* assistance with dressing and grooming, or supervision transferring into and out of the tub for safety. In general, residents of assisted living facilities must be able to feed and toilet themselves.

Asthma

Most facilities have staff available 24 hours per day to monitor, remind, or supervise. However, the staff members are there to assist only and are not medical professionals. If a resident requires close supervision, assistance with several of the activities of daily living, or 24-hour availability of a licensed nurse, then transfer to a nursing home is usually recommended.

Increasingly, individuals and their caregivers prefer to not have to move when their needs change. Because of consumer demand, some assisted living providers have responded with increased staffing levels of licensed nurses to help with medication administration, continuous oxygen treatment, and even hospice care. Assisted living apartments sometimes exist as part of a larger facility that includes a nursing home and perhaps transitional housing for those residents who need help with multiple activities of daily living but do not yet qualify for the nursing home. This arrangement is called a continuing care retirement community. These communities allow residents to maintain continuity with familiar staff members and a familiar environment, and allow spouses to remain close even when one enters the nursing home while the other remains in assisted living.

SEE ALSO: Activities of daily living, Long-term care, Nursing home

Suggested Reading

Anon. (2001). More reasons to stay. *Provider, 27,* 18–20, 23, 26–28.

Suggested Resources

AARP information on assisted living: www.aarp.org/contacts/housing/assistliv.html

EVANNE JURATOVAC

Asthma   Asthma is a chronic inflammatory disease characterized by periodic obstruction of the bronchioles. Two key features of asthma are *reversible* airflow obstruction and bronchial hyperresponsiveness to stimuli. Triggers of airway hyperresponsiveness include respiratory infections, exercise, cold or dry air, atmospheric pollutants, occupational irritants, or specific environmental allergens. Other risk factors for asthma include heredity, history of allergies, cigarette smoking, and socioeconomic status.

The overall prevalence of asthma is increasing. In the United States, asthma has a prevalence of approximately 6% and mortality is 1 in 10,000. In the last decade, the death rate from asthma in the United States has increased significantly, with the increase in women being more than twice that observed in men (54% compared to 23%).

In addition to having a higher mortality in females, asthma displays several other differences between genders. The gender differences in asthma begin in childhood in which the prevalence of asthma is higher in boys. This has been attributed to boys having smaller airways in proportion to lung volumes than girls, although it has also been suggested that there is an underdiagnosis of asthma in girls. The difference in asthma prevalence between genders reverses sometime during adolescence, when the asthma rate in females actually increases. Lung growth is dysynaptic in girls and their lungs stop growing in the late teens. The lungs of boys, on the other hand, demonstrate isotropic growth and their lungs continue to grow until the age of 20. These differences may be the result of pubertal changes in sex hormones.

In adulthood, asthma is more common in women than in men, and it appears to have a greater impact on quality of life in women. Recent studies have also found that obesity is associated with the development of asthma in women but not in men. This difference is believed to be due to the influence of obesity on levels of female sex hormones. Studies of patients reporting to the emergency department for asthma have found that although men typically have worse lung function as measured by flow spirometry, women are hospitalized more frequently than men and have longer hospital stays. In a longitudinal study of 914 patients with asthma in Kaiser Permanente, researchers found that women reported more symptoms, used more medication, and had greater health care use than men. In general, women tend to experience greater discomfort than men for the same level of airflow obstruction. Reasons for these gender differences are not entirely known but are thought to be multifactorial, including biological, social, and psychological factors.

Two aspects of asthma unique to women are premenstrual asthma and asthma during pregnancy. Premenstrual asthma has been reported in up to 30–40% of women and is associated with a worsening of asthma symptoms prior to and during menstruation. Several mechanisms for premenstrual asthma have been proposed, but the most widely studied is the influence of sex hormones on asthma. Studies demonstrating the relaxant effect of estrogen and progesterone on bronchial smooth muscle, as well as studies showing an improvement in asthma symptoms after estrogen administration, have led researchers to speculate that the premenstrual drop in estrogen levels may be responsible for the worsening of asthma symptoms.

Hormonal influences are also among the proposed mechanisms for the course of asthma in pregnancy. Asthma is a common problem during pregnancy and can have a potentially serious impact on pregnancy outcomes. Recent studies have found that, on average, asthma symptoms during pregnancy worsen in a third of women, improve in another third, and remain the same in the remaining third. Women with severe asthma prior to pregnancy are at greater risk for exacerbations during pregnancy. Furthermore, while symptoms tend to improve during the third trimester, they may worsen postpartum. However, the majority of women return to their prepregnancy asthma state in a few months. Proper management of asthma is essential during pregnancy, as poor control has been associated with increased maternal morbidity and adverse perinatal outcomes. Treatment of asthma during pregnancy is similar to treatment in nonpregnant women and includes the use of inhaled beta agonists, corticosteroids, theophyllines, and anti-allergy medications.

SEE ALSO: Adolescence, Lung disease, Menstruation, Pregnancy, Smoking

Suggested Reading

Chen, Y., Dales, R., Tang, M., & Krewski, D. (2002). Obesity may increase the incidence of asthma in women but not in men: Longitudinal observations from the Canadian National Population Health Surveys. *American Journal of Epidemiology, 155,* 191–196.

de Marco, R., Locatelli, F., Sunyer, J., & Burney, P. (2000). Differences in incidence of reported asthma related to age in men and women. *American Journal of Respiratory and Critical Care Medicine, 162,* 68–74.

Ensom, M. (2000). Gender-based differences and menstrual cycle-related changes in specific diseases: Implications for pharmacotherapy. *Pharmacotherapy, 20,* 523–539.

Singh, A., Cydulka, R., Stahmer, S., Woodruff, P., & Camargo, C. (1999). Sex differences among adults presenting to the emergency department with acute asthma. *Archives of Internal Medicine, 159,* 1237–1243.

Tan, K., & Thomson, N. (2000). Asthma in pregnancy. *American Journal of Medicine, 109,* 727–733.

RACHEL LANGE
MARILYN GLASSBERG

Augmentation Mammoplasty *see* Breast Augmentation

Autoimmune Disorders

The immune system is a highly complex system of cells and chemical reactions that fights off infection and protects the body from germs. When germs invade the body, the immune system detects proteins on the surface of the germs and then gears up to remove the foreign invasion. In general the system works very well. However, at times the immune system malfunctions and begins to see normal body proteins as foreign. The immune system then gears up to fight against this "foreign" protein that really is part of normal cells. This is called autoimmunity and causes autoimmune disease, including connective tissue diseases and inflammatory conditions such as arthritis and vasculitis. These are all diseases where the body fights against itself and its normal tissues.

The true reason for the reaction against normal body proteins is not well understood, but some autoimmune diseases are inherited. Some people may have the gene for an autoimmune disease but the gene must be turned on for the disease to occur. The exact triggers are not known and that is why some members of a family may develop disease whereas others do not. The most common belief is that exposure to an infection may be the trigger but the specific infection is unknown. Sometimes the apparent infection is not even noticed or the autoimmune disease develops long after the episode of infection.

Sometimes, an infection can trigger an autoimmune response even after the infection is cleared. This may happen if the protein of the infecting germ is almost identical to the person's normal cells. This is termed molecular mimicry. Aside from this, infectious particles can alter the immune system directly and alter the cell's ability to function properly or just interfere with some of the immune system functions. Another way to cause autoimmunity is by a change in the way cells die in the body. Cells in the body die and are cleared through specific pathways. If dying cells are not removed appropriately and linger about, they may start to seem foreign to the body. Another potential cause for autoimmunity may be a change in the way a body normally produces inflammation. Some cells in the body are assigned to police the inflammatory cells and

Autoimmune Disorders

chemicals so they do not get out of hand. The policing mechanism may not work and the system runs out of control. Other theories about autoimmunity exist. It is unlikely that there is a sole culprit, and more likely that small alterations at various levels cause the body to fight against itself.

Autoimmune disease can affect any body part. Because it is a disease that can affect lots of parts of the body at once, many organs can be affected at the start or only a few may be affected initially and then other symptoms occur over time. The diagnosis of an autoimmune disease is not easy and may require repeated history and physical examination sessions along with blood testing. Most of the signs and symptoms of the various autoimmune diseases are categorized into groupings that make up certain disease syndromes. Criteria for each have been established but the criteria are primarily for research purposes to ensure that patients in a study really have the same disease. Patients may be diagnosed with a specific disease without meeting full criteria and their symptoms can and should be treated as they arise. Autoimmune diseases must be diagnosed with extreme care and caution because many other diseases may mimic or appear to be autoimmune when they are not. The danger herein lies with the treatment. Since autoimmunity is a disease of almost a "hyperactive" immune system, the treatment is aimed at suppressing the immune system. Many of the diseases that look like they could be autoimmune disease are infections or cancer, and blocking the immune system in these instances could be fatal. Infections must be ruled out through vigorous testing before treating and diagnosing an autoimmune disease. Even if an autoimmune disease is diagnosed with certainty, the patient must be entirely free of infection before treatment begins.

Although any infection can rev up the immune system and cause changes that look like an autoimmune disease, there are certain classic mimics that will be discussed here. Subacute bacterial endocarditis, which is a bacterial infection of the heart valves, is frequently confused with rheumatoid arthritis and systemic lupus erythematosus (SLE) because all of these cause joint swelling, rashes, and positive laboratory tests. It is important to note that infections themselves cause a surge in inflammatory chemicals and cells and can cause unreliable laboratory tests. The infectious growth on the heart valves may become dislodged and land in the joints, skin, and kidney, causing symptoms that we also see with autoimmune disease. Blood cultures and careful evaluation should always be done to rule out bacterial endocarditis as a cause of the "autoimmune" symptoms.

Another disease that should not be missed is tuberculosis (TB). TB can cause disease all over the body including the lungs, kidneys, and skin. Syphilis and HIV diseases are also commonly misdiagnosed as autoimmune diseases. It is important to realize that the above diseases as well as others may give false-positive laboratory tests that may be confused with autoimmune diseases, but the diagnosis should be based primarily on history and physical examination. In some cases biopsy specimens are critical to confirm the diagnosis.

SLE is the classic autoimmune disease and is discussed in detail elsewhere. In SLE, the primary problem is the production of autoantibodies to several normal proteins found in the core of normal cells. The antibodies form clumps of proteins and cause injury when they deposit on various tissues. In SLE, first-degree relatives of patients with SLE will have a much higher chance of developing the disease: SLE occurs in approximately 25–50% of identical twins versus 5% of fraternal twins. This disease can affect virtually any organ system. The classic symptoms are the butterfly rash on the face, mouth sores, inflammation of the lining of the heart and lungs, and arthritis.

Rheumatoid arthritis is also a classic autoimmune disease and can affect organs other than joints. The nonjoint manifestations can involve the heart, lungs, skin, and eyes. The trigger for rheumatoid disease is not known.

The inflammatory muscle diseases are another group of diseases that have an autoimmune basis. These diseases cause breakdown of muscle and weakness. The hallmark of these diseases is muscle weakness of the shoulder and hip areas, with or without associated muscle pain. Patients have difficulty raising their arms to or above their heads, and difficulty getting out a chair or walking up stairs or inclines. In severe cases, the disease may affect the neck muscles and the head may feel heavy. Respiratory muscle weakness and breathing problems can also occur, as well as swallowing difficulties. As implied by the name, these diseases affect mainly the muscles, but the lungs themselves may also be affected, causing an inflammatory lung disease and resulting in heart failure. The skin may also display a classic rash. In children, the rash is called a heliotrope rash and it is a purple or violaceous discoloration of the upper and lower eyelids. In adults, the rash may appear as shiny plaque-like lesions over the knuckles of the hands. There may also be joint pain without joint swelling.

Laboratory tests in the inflammatory muscle diseases show breakdown of muscles but also signs of autoimmunity on special testing. Specific tests can predict lung involvement or worse prognosis. Muscle testing via electrical analysis of the muscles and nerves, and also muscle biopsy are critical since other muscle diseases that are not autoimmune related can only be diagnosed with a biopsy. In one of these diseases, adults with both skin and muscle disease (dermatomyositis) have a 25% increased chance of having cancer before, during, or after the disease develops.

Scleroderma is another interesting manifestation of autoimmune disease. Again, the exact cause is not clear, but cases have been noted to cluster within families that have other autoimmune diseases. Scleroderma causes skin tightening and hardening. Certain cells that are responsible for scarring and scar tissue formation appear hyperactive in this disease. The more scar tissue they deposit, the less able the tissues are to breathe and this loss of breathability or oxygenation causes even more scar tissue to be deposited. Autoantibodies are associated with scleroderma but it is not clear if they are a cause or a result of the process.

Patients with scleroderma may develop a wide variety of symptoms, ranging from Reynaud's phenomenon (sensitivity and skin color changes in response to cold) or calcium deposits, and some small amount of skin tightening, to kidney failure, lung damage, and severe thickening of the skin that encases the whole body. The gastrointestinal tract and heart may also be involved. Treatment of scleroderma is very difficult and can only slow the disease. However, it is important to be aware of the diagnosis and work toward treatment.

Another family of classic autoimmune diseases is a group of diseases causing inflammation of the blood vessels (vasculitis). Inflammation of the blood vessels in these diseases may be due to an allergic response, or cell changes within the vessel wall, or dying off of vessels. Each of these diseases tends to involve only the small, medium, or large arteries. Vasculitis is associated with fever, general illness, and can involve multiple organs. In situations where a diagnosis of vasculitis is considered, infection must be ruled out or treated, and the degree of organ involvement must be determined. Examination of the skin, hands, oral or vaginal lining, urine, stool, and complete blood work must be done to look for any abnormality. Often a biopsy will allow the disease to be categorized.

Small vessel vasculitis usually involves the skin, joints, and gastrointestinal tract. An example is hypersensitivity vasculitis, which is a response to something outside the body. Behcet's syndrome causes eye ulcerations and gastrointestinal problems in people of Mediterranean or Far East background. Small vessel diseases may also involve the brain, causing very subtle behavioral changes or obvious neurological symptoms. Medium vessel vasculitis commonly involves the lungs and kidneys. Some classic syndromes are polyarteritis nodosa, allergic granulomatosis and angiitis, Churg–Strauss vasculitis, and Wegener's vasculitis. The large vessel diseases include Takayasu's arteritis, temporal arteritis, and polyarteritis nodosa. A good and detailed history usually reveals classic symptoms of these disorders.

Autoimmunity does not only cause rheumatologic disorders. Diabetes, thyroid diseases, and other endocrine diseases may also be autoimmune, as well as some neurologic diseases and blood diseases. Many gastrointestinal illnesses are associated with abnormalities of the immune system. More than one autoimmune disease may be found in the same patient, or members of a patient's family may have different autoimmune diseases. It is important to look for those patterns to help diagnose some of these conditions, because diagnosis is often difficult. These diseases can get better or worse in cycles and more symptoms can occur over time. Often, the symptoms are treated while the entire process of disease is unfolding. Patience, thoroughness, and keeping an open mind will help to diagnose patients who have these relatively rare diseases.

SEE ALSO: Arthritis, Raynaud's phenomenon, Scleroderma, Systemic lupus erythematosus

Suggested Reading

Arthritis Foundation. (2001). *Primer on the rheumatic diseases* (12th ed.). Atlanta, GA: Author.

Klippel, J. H., & Dieppe, P. A. (1998). *Rheumatology* (2nd ed.). St. Louis, MO: C. V. Mosby.

Klippel, J. H., Dieppe, P. A., & Ferri, F. F. (1999). *Primary care rheumatology*. St. Louis, MO: C. V. Mosby.

LORI B. SIEGEL

B

Back Pain Back pain is the second most common reason for medical office visits. About 60–90% of people will have at least one significant episode of low back pain during their lifetime. Low back pain is the most common and the most expensive cause of work-related disability in the United States. Workers' compensation costs as well as medical expenses run as high as $100 billion per year. At any given time, at least 1% of the workforce is either permanently or temporarily disabled by back pain.

There are many risk factors for low back pain including increasing age, heavy physical work, obesity, smoking, drug abuse, and history of headache, job dissatisfaction, and monotonous work. Rarely, severe scoliosis (sideways curvature of the spine) can place a person at risk for low back pain. Minor postural problems including mild spinal curvatures, leg length differences, and physical fitness do seem to affect the development of low back pain. Most important, abnormalities on x-rays including lumbar spine films that are commonly taken by chiropractors as well as abnormalities seen with computerized tomography (CT) scans and magnetic resonance imaging (MRI) scans, do *not* match up with the existence of low back pain. In fact, abnormalities on spine films are found in the majority of adults, most of whom have no back pain at the time.

There are many causes for low back pain, and the more serious causes need to be excluded by an accurate history and physical examination. However, in acute low back pain, a definite source of pain cannot be found in about 85% of people.

Low back pain that does not send pain into a leg is rarely if ever caused by a ruptured disk in the low back. Usually, this kind of low back pain is related to muscle strain, spasm, or trigger points. Trigger points are areas in the muscle that are tender, feel like a taut band, and reproduce a patient's pain when pressed on. A lot of pressure on these trigger points can sometimes cause shooting pain, which may mimic a herniated disk. Another cause for acute low back pain is inflammation in the sacroiliac joint, where the base of the spine rests on the pelvis. This can cause pain that increases with walking, sitting, or standing, and improves with position change. Other symptoms include pain that travels to the groin, and pain that travels down the back of the leg or the side of the thigh. This can also mimic a herniated disk in the spine. However, pain from a trigger point or the sacroiliac joint usually stops near the knee, while the pain of a herniated disk more often travels all the way to the foot.

There are many causes of low back pain, including abnormalities of the spinal column, the joints between vertebrae, the disks between the vertebrae, and the ligaments and muscles that support the lower back. All of these problems can cause low back pain with or without pain going into a leg. In addition, acute and chronic low back pain may be caused by infections, either infection elsewhere in the body or localized to the spine and its surrounding structures. Other causes include autoimmune and inflammatory diseases such as ankylosing spondylitis, psoriatic arthritis, and reactive arthritis. Endocrine abnormalities and certain toxins can produce low back pain. Cancers beginning in the spine or metastasizing from other parts of the body, especially from the lung, bone, kidney, prostate, or thyroid gland, are also important causes of acute low back pain. Blood vessel problems such as strokes in the spinal cord and abdominal aortic aneurysms can produce pain localized to a particular region of the lumbar spine.

If the history and physical examination raise the suspicion of a serious cause for the pain, then more testing needs to be done. However, it is important to remember that even when abnormalities are seen on imaging studies such as CT scans and MRI scans, the abnormality often has nothing to do with the pain. Eight-five percent of patients with acute low back pain and approximately 65% of patients with chronic low back pain cannot be given a specific diagnosis.

The treatment of low back pain is usually nonsurgical. Ninety percent of patients with an initial acute episode of low back pain will recover with simple treatments. In large studies, elaborate treatments for acute, nonspecific, nonradiating low back pain have not been proven to be particularly effective. Bed rest in particular should be avoided after 1–2 days. During the first week or so of low back pain, physical therapy should be avoided, but after about 7–10 days gradual stretching and strengthening exercises of the spine and abdomen can help relieve the pain. Careful use of narcotic pain relievers and muscle relaxants can be helpful in severe, acute pain. However, over the long term, nonsteroidal anti-inflammatory drugs such as ibuprofen, naproxen, and similar prescription drugs are more effective. Surgery should only be considered if there is progressive weakness, bowel or bladder incontinence, or a significant structural deformity.

Back braces, except in rare instances, are not helpful, especially in someone who has chronic low back pain, since braces can lead to weakening of the muscles. Heat and cold can provide comfort. Epidural steroid injections have not been proven to be an effective therapy for back pain or radiating symptoms, according to researchers who reviewed lots of studies of back pain. In fact, some of the additives in steroid preparations, when injected in and around the spinal canal, can be toxic to the nerves. This can cause increased pain due to scarring and infection. Other treatments, such as spinal manipulations, acupuncture, and transcutaneous electrical nerve stimulation, are not very useful in acute back pain but may be helpful in chronic back pain.

Chronic low back pain should be treated with an aggressive regular exercise program and nonsteroidal anti-inflammatory drugs. A variety of other medications that are used for all kinds of chronic pain are also helpful in chronic low back pain. These medications include antidepressant medications and antiseizure and antispasticity drugs. Special programs that teach about pain and stress management and include physical reconditioning and an ergonomic evaluation can also be extremely helpful for people with chronic low back pain.

SEE ALSO: Arthritis, Autoimmune disorders, Chronic pain, Exercise, Physical examination

Suggested Reading

American Academy of Orthopedic Surgeons informational website: orthoinfo.aaos.org

Cherkin, D., Deyo, R., Battie, M., et al. (1998). A comparison of physical therapy, chiropractic manipulation, and provision of an educational booklet for the treatment of patients with low back pain. *New England Journal of Medicine, 339*, 1021–1029.

Deyo, R. A., & Weinstein, J. A. (2001). Low back pain. *New England Journal of Medicine, 334*, 363–370.

Kriegler, J. S. (1993). Medical management of chronic low back pain. In R. W. Hardy (Ed.), *Lumbar disc disease* (2nd ed., pp. 293–297). New York: Raven Press.

JENNIFER S. KRIEGLER

Behavior Therapy   *see* Cognitive-Behavioral Therapy, Psychotherapy

---

Bereavement

The death of a loved one, especially a child, spouse, or someone of similar closeness, is one of the most significant and traumatic events a person is likely to experience. Despite this, the majority of people handle the loss with minimum morbidity. For a small minority, the loss may lead to increased doctor visits for new or worsening medical conditions, increased use of substances (such as alcohol, benzodiazepines, and hypnotics), the development of chronic depression or a posttraumatic stress disorder (PTSD)-like syndrome termed "complicated grief," and even increased mortality. In order to understand the more pathologic outcomes, one must be familiar with the more expected reaction in the immediate post-bereavement period and in the year following.

Bereavement

Before proceeding with the normal reaction, it is necessary to clarify terms. *Bereavement* is the reaction to a loss by death. *Grief* is the emotional and/or psychological reaction to any loss, but not limited to death. *Mourning* is the social expression of bereavement or grief, sometimes defined by culture, custom, and religion. *Complicated or traumatic grief* is the disordered psyche and behavioral state present beyond 6 months following a loss; the term implies unresolved loss and impaired performance. With these definitions in mind, we will discuss bereavement and complicated or traumatic grief.

Most studies of the recently bereaved have delineated three stages. The first stage is termed *numbness*, since this is the term that the recently widowed used to describe themselves. It lasts from a few hours to a few days, perhaps a few weeks. Things that need to be done get done, but most of what is said and done is poorly remembered. Anxiety symptoms may appear. The second stage is *depression*. While symptoms of irritability and restlessness are prominent, all depressive symptoms are common. Many people are on their way to recovery by 6 months, although others continue to have symptoms through the first year and even into the second year. The survivor's mood is almost always disturbed on holidays, anniversaries, the birthday of the deceased, the anniversary of the death, and other personal or meaningful events and may partially be the cause of the much-discussed "Christmas depression."

In the recently bereaved, prominent symptoms of the second stage are crying, sleep disturbance, sadness, depression, loneliness, restlessness, poor appetite, feeling tired, poor memory, loss of interest in some things (but not necessarily neighbors and friends), difficulty concentrating, and weight loss. The weight loss can be profound. The sleep disturbance often remains entrenched, whereas the weight loss usually ends after the second month. From the third month on there is more likely to be weight gain. By one year, the most prominent symptoms are sleep disturbance and loneliness. The third stage, *recovery*, is acceptance of the death and a return to some level of functioning that was established before the death.

Since depressive symptoms are common, the question is how many of the recently bereaved experience the full depressive syndrome that we know as major depressive disorder. In studies of widowed persons, about 50% meet criteria for major depression at some time during the first year. About 10% of the recently widowed experience a chronic depression. There are very few predictors of this chronic depression. Those that have been verified across several studies include poor physical health prior to the loss, poor mental health prior to the loss (particularly a previous depressive episode or prior substance abuse), and depression at 1–2 months postloss. An unknown percentage of those with chronic depression develop complicated grief. These people experience preoccupation with the deceased, crying, searching, and yearning for the deceased, feeling stunned, disbelief, nonacceptance, anger, distress, detachment, avoidance, some replication of symptoms that the deceased experienced, loneliness, bitterness, and guilt. This syndrome demands an intervention.

There is still a good deal of controversy over the physical morbidity and mortality of bereavement. The bereaved do not have more physical symptoms than matched controls; and there is no increase in hospitalization, either psychiatric or general, after a loss. The most important outcome in the immediate bereavement period is that those who use substances, use more; those who drink, drink more; those who smoke, smoke more. This may explain some of the morbidity and mortality associated with bereavement. There have been numerous studies on mortality following the death of someone close. Men under the age of 75 (the "young-old") have an increased mortality in the first 6 months after a loss. Women do not clearly have this increased mortality.

The vast majority of people who experience a loss will recover gradually without any interventions. Those who become chronically depressed or develop complicated grief need psychiatric intervention. Although the treatment could be simple, such as education and self-help groups, a more logical treatment is psychotherapy (such as interpersonal therapy, IPT) or pharmacotherapy (such as antidepressant therapy). It is unclear how best to treat complicated bereavement. For postbereavement depression, open-label studies of antidepressants have demonstrated remission rates at or above 50% in the first 2–3 months of treatment; low relapse rates occurred following medication discontinuation. The field awaits a definitive study involving placebo controls.

See Also: Depression, Mood disorders, Posttraumatic stress disorder

Suggested Reading

Clayton, P. J. (2000). Bereavement. In G. Fink (Ed.), *Encyclopedia of stress*. London: Academic Press.

Clayton, P. J., & Darvish, H. S. (1979). Course of depressive symptoms following the stress of bereavement. In J. E. Barrett (Ed.), *Stress and mental disorder*. New York: Raven Press.

Clayton, P., Demariais, L., & Winokur, G. (1968). A study of normal bereavement. *American Journal of Psychiatry, 125,* 64–74.

Prigerson, H. G., Shear, M. K., Frank, E., Beery, L. C., Silberman. R., Prigerson, J., et al. (1997). Traumatic grief: A case of loss-induced trauma. *American Journal of Psychiatry, 154,* 1003–1009.

Zisook, S., & Shuchter, S. R. (1991). Depression through the first year after the death of a spouse. *American Journal of Psychiatry, 148,* 1346–1352.

PAULA A. HENSLEY
PAULA J. CLAYTON

Binge Eating Disorder Binge eating disorder (BED) is characterized by recurrent episodes of binge eating in the absence of inappropriate compensatory behaviors such as vomiting or excessive use of diuretics and laxatives. Currently, it falls under the category of Eating Disorder Not Otherwise Specified in the *Diagnostic and Statistical Manual of Mental Disorders,* fourth edition (*DSM-IV*). An individual with BED lacks control over his or her eating, rapidly consuming large quantities of food over an extremely short period of time. Commonly, they eat when not hungry and will continue to eat until they are uncomfortably full. They may eat alone out of embarrassment and disgust, experiencing depression and guilt over their eating patterns. The frequency of binge eating is at least twice a week, for 6 months or more.

BED affects 2% of the general population or 30% of obese patients in medical treatment. All eating disorders affect females more than males and perhaps 60% of BED patients are females. All socioeconomic classes and ethnic groups are affected. BED is distinct from anorexia nervosa (AN) and bulimia nervosa (BN) and rarely do patients with BED develop AN or BN. BED patients do not fixate on body shape or weight, are often overweight, and do not generally use vomiting, diuretics, or laxatives to control weight. Most patients with BED have physical complications of obesity such as hypertension, non-insulin-dependent diabetes mellitus, and menstrual disturbances. Patients with obesity and BED often become trapped in a cycle of desperately attempting to diet followed by losing control, binge eating, and gaining more weight.

Adopting a treatment approach with long-term focus on improved physical and psychological health could lead to behavioral changes and improved self-acceptance. The goals of treatment include cessation of binge eating, improved physical health mediated in part by weight loss, and reduction in psychological distress. Behavioral weight control, cognitive behavioral therapy, and interpersonal therapy are all advantageous. Behavioral weight control techniques include positive reinforcement of healthy eating, stimulus control by limiting exposure to unhealthy foods, and development of pleasurable alternatives to binge eating. These therapies reduce binge frequency and promote short-term weight loss in obese patients with BED. A variation to this approach is following a very low calorie diet with liquid nutritional supplements, but partial relapse during refeeding frequently occurs. Cognitive behavioral therapy (CBT) in group or individual therapy seeks to identify the thoughts, feelings, and circumstances leading to binge eating and to modify these by restructuring dysfunctional cognition. The specific focus is on examination of thoughts and feelings related to body image and in promotion of self-acceptance. Studies of CBT for BED have reported excellent short-term binge reduction but variable deterioration over the long term and no significant weight loss. Interpersonal therapy seeks to identify the problems between individuals that contribute to maintenance of this maladaptive pattern. A substantial reduction in binge eating may initially occur but by 1 year, some symptoms often return. An alternative is a sequential treatment model consisting of 12 weeks of CBT followed by 24 weeks of group behavioral weight loss treatment and subsequent follow-up for 1 year. This model, advocated by the Stanford group, was successful in reducing binge eating and maintaining the response at 1 year. The New York State Psychiatric Institute also promoted a combination of group behavioral weight control program and close follow-up.

Pharmacological interventions include use of serotonin reuptake inhibitors like sertraline (Zoloft) and fluoxetine (Prozac), venlafaxine (Effexor), and tricyclic antidepressants. However, weight loss is usually a short-term effect and none of these medications have been Food and Drug Administration (FDA) approved for treatment of BED. A retrospective review of venlafaxine (75–300 mg/day) used in obese BED patients showed a decrease in binge eating severity and frequency with 5% weight loss in 43% of the patients. Fluoxetine is approved by the FDA for treatment of BN and has been noted to decrease binge eating. A 6-week placebo-controlled trial of fluoxetine (20–80 mg/day) in 60 outpatients reported a significant reduction in frequency of binge eating, body mass index, and severity of illness. A recent 14-week placebo-controlled study of topiramate (Topamax) (50–600 mg/day) in obese BED patients reported a reduction in binge frequency, body mass index, body weight, and scores on the Yale Brown Obsessive Compulsive Scale (modified for binge eating). One small study suggests that the opiate antagonist naltrexone may also reduce binge eating and block the urge to eat.

Patients with obesity and BED face multiple challenges. A therapeutic plan tailored to the individual patient's needs is advisable. More information is available for the public at www.nationaleating disorders.org, the website for the National Eating Disorders Association.

SEE ALSO: Anorexia nervosa, Body image, Bulimia nervosa, Eating disorders

Suggested Reading

Arnold, L. M., McElroy, S. L., et al. (2002). A placebo controlled, randomized trial of fluoxetine in the treatment of binge-eating disorder. *Journal of Clinical Psychiatry, 63*(11), 1028–1033.

Devlin, M. J. (2001). Binge eating disorder and obesity. *Psychiatric Clinics of North America, 24*(2), 354–357.

Kaplan, H. I., & Sadock, B. J. (1998). Eating disorders. In *Synopsis of psychiatry* (8th ed., pp. 730–731). Philadelphia: Lippincott, Williams & Wilkins.

Malhotra, S., King, K. H., et al. (2002). Venlafaxine treatment of binge-eating disorder associated with obesity. *Journal of Clinical Psychiatry, 63*(9), 802–806.

McElroy, S. L., Arnold, L. M., et al. (2003). Topiramate in the treatment of binge eating disorder associated with obesity. *American Journal of Psychiatry, 160*(2), 255–262.

Powers, P. S., & Santana, C. A. (2002). Eating disorders. A guide for the primary care physician. *Primary Care: Clinics in Office Practice, 29*(1), 81–98.

KATHLEEN N. FRANCO
RASHMI S. DESHMUKH

Biofeedback *see* Psychotherapy

Bipolar Disorder

Bipolar disorder, also known as manic-depressive disorder, is a type of mood disorder, which occurs in approximately 1% of the population. This rate of occurrence is consistent across groups of diverse ethnicity and culture. In general, bipolar disorder is a long-term illness with an episodic and variable course. Unlike major depressive disorder that is significantly more common in women, the occurrence of bipolar disorder is equally common in men and women. Bipolar disorder is characterized by the presence of mania, or a manic episode, defined as a period of abnormal, persistently elevated, expansive, or irritable mood. An individual need only have one manic episode to fit lifetime diagnostic criteria for bipolar disorder. Additional symptoms that may occur in the context of mania include grandiosity or inappropriately elevated self-esteem, excessive or "pressured" speed, diminished need for sleep, racing thoughts, agitation, distractibility, and involvement in activities that potentially lead to negative consequences such as substance abuse, excessive spending, sexual promiscuity, or other high-risk behaviors. Although individuals with a manic episode frequently lack insight into illness (understanding and awareness of their illness), and will deny acknowledgment of their condition if confronted by it, manic symptoms are associated with severe impairments in functioning. Risk of harm to self or others may occur in the context of impulsive decision-making. Some individuals with mania become psychotic or paranoid, and may require hospitalization for protection of themselves and others.

Individuals with bipolar disorder may also experience depressive episodes characterized by depressed mood, diminished interest in everyday activities, difficulty sleeping, significant weight change, decreased energy, feelings of worthlessness or inappropriate guilt, diminished concentration, and thoughts of death or suicide.

Gender appears to be related to the order and frequency of manic and depressive episodes. In men, the first episode is more likely to be manic, and men may be more likely to experience subsequent manic episodes. Women are more likely to have the first mood episode in the form of depression, and may be more likely to experience depressive episodes compared to men. Additionally, women with bipolar disorder are particularly vulnerable to episode recurrence after childbirth, in the postpartum period. Postpartum psychosis may occur, with some women experiencing their first episode shortly after childbirth.

Mean age of onset of bipolar disorder is 21 years; however, there is frequently a 5- to 10-year interval between age of onset of illness and age at first treatment or first hospitalization. Bipolar disorder may occur in children and adolescents as well as may occur for the first time in adults over the age of 60. Bipolar disorder is generally a chronic illness, with multiple occurrences of mood episodes. More than 90% of individuals who have a single manic episode go on to have future episodes. Studies on the course of bipolar illness prior to the common use of treatment for the disorder suggest that an average of 4 episodes will occur over a 10-year period, and individuals with untreated bipolar disorder may have more than 10 episodes of abnormal mood states (highs or lows) during their lifetime. The duration of episodes and duration of between-episode periods frequently stabilize after the fourth or fifth episode.

In many cases, an individual will experience several bouts of depression before the occurrence of a first manic episode. For this reason, a diagnosis of bipolar disorder may be overlooked, particularly in the early phases of illness. It is not uncommon to see individuals who eventually are proven to have bipolar disorder being mistakenly diagnosed with depressive disorder, schizophrenia, or even some types of personality disorders.

Clarifying diagnoses can be sometimes difficult, especially in cases where patients may not be knowledgeable about bipolar disorder and its symptoms. This may lead to a nonreporting/underreporting of manic symptoms. It is critical that the diagnosing clinician be aware of such issues as individual history of mania or hypomania, family history of mood disorder or family history of manic episodes, substance abuse history, and any history of previous treatment. Consultation with family members or significant others is often extremely important. Bipolar disorder may be differentiated from major depressive disorder by the occurrence of mania/hypomania in bipolar illness. Individuals with schizophrenia primarily experience psychotic symptoms such as hallucinations or delusions in contrast to the primary disorder of mood seen in bipolar illness. Individuals with personality disorder, particularly borderline personality, may exhibit labile (rapidly fluctuating) mood state, impulsivity, and risk-taking behavior, which may mimic a manic state. Close observation of symptoms over a longer time period will assist in differentiating these disorders from bipolar illness.

Approximately 5–15% of individuals with bipolar disorder experience four or more episodes within a 12-month period. This variant of bipolar disorder is classified as rapid-cycling type and is more common in women. Other factors that favor the occurrence of the rapid-cycling variant of bipolar disorder, and which are particularly relevant to women, are borderline hypothyroidism (underactive thyroid functioning) and menopause.

Bipolar disorder has both genetic and biological underpinnings. Bipolar illness tends to run in families, and it is known that the concordance for bipolar illness is higher among monozygotic (identical) compared to dizygotic (fraternal) twin pairs. The specific biological factors that cause bipolar illness have not been clearly identified; however, most theories regarding possible biological origins of bipolar disorder involve dysregulation/dysfunction in neurotransmitter systems including the serotonergic, noradrenergic, dopaminergic, cholinergic, GABAergic, and glutamatergic systems.

In addition to the often-serious effects of acute symptoms of bipolar illness, individuals with bipolar disorder frequently have substantial psychosocial difficulties as a result of the disorder. Multiple aspects of life are frequently affected including marriage relationships, child-rearing, and occupational status. Divorce rates are generally higher among individuals with bipolar illness, approaching two to three times the rates of individuals who do not have bipolar illness. The occupational status of individuals with bipolar illness is twice as likely to be impaired as compared to individuals without bipolar illness.

Suicide is also a significant risk in bipolar disorder, with up to 19% of individuals with bipolar illness eventually committing suicide. The risk of suicide appears to be greatest when individuals have depressive symptoms and during the first few years after the onset of bipolar illness. Individuals with comorbid alcohol abuse are more likely to make suicide attempts compared to individuals with bipolar disorder who do not abuse alcohol. Additionally, stressful life events may precede suicide or suicide attempts among individuals with bipolar illness. On the positive side, treatment for bipolar illness, specifically the use of lithium carbonate, has been associated with a sixfold reduction in the rate of suicide attempts among individuals with bipolar illness.

Psychiatric comorbidity is defined as the presence of other psychiatric syndromes in addition to the principal psychiatric diagnosis. In the case of bipolar disorder, psychiatric comorbidity is relatively common, with estimates in the order of 35–65%. The rate of comorbidity between bipolar disorder and substance-related disorder is particularly high, and among all Axis I psychiatric conditions, bipolar disorder appears to have the highest prevalence of comorbid substance abuse. Prevalence rates of substance abuse in bipolar populations have been reported to range from 21 to 58%. Among individuals with bipolar illness, early age of onset is a risk factor for comorbid substance abuse. Although substance abuse is generally seen more often among men than among women, some researchers have reported that among individuals with newly treated bipolar illness, women are more likely to have a history of comorbid substance abuse or dependence compared to men with bipolar illness. However, the issue of substance abuse as it relates to gender in bipolar illness needs further study before definitive conclusions can be drawn regarding gender differences on this specific aspect of bipolar disorder.

GENERAL TREATMENT RECOMMENDATIONS

The goal of treatment in bipolar disorder is complete remission of symptoms with a return to baseline level of health and functioning. Unfortunately, at this time, there is no "cure" for bipolar disorder, but it is entirely possible for individuals with bipolar illness to experience long periods of freedom from symptoms or with minimal recurrence of mood episodes. Predictors of good outcome include good response to medications, older age at illness onset, good psychosocial supports, absence of comorbid psychiatric and medical conditions, and adherence with treatment.

It is known that psychotherapies may make biological treatments more effective in the management of bipolar illness. Thus, a general recommendation is the use of combined psychotherapy and medication management in optimizing treatment for bipolar disorder. Most studies of psychosocial treatments for bipolar disorder utilize contemporary psychotherapies such as cognitive behavioral therapy, tend to be fairly focused, and are delivered in the context of standard medication treatments. These therapies offer practical techniques for coping with stress, educate patients and families about bipolar illness, and encourage adherence with medication treatment. Types of psychotherapies that have been reported to be particularly beneficial in bipolar illness include family-focused treatment and interpersonal and social rhythm therapy. Psychosocial treatment of bipolar disorder may be delivered in individual, family/couples, or group formats.

The cornerstone of medication treatments in bipolar disorder is mood-stabilizing medication. As bipolar disorder tends to be a chronic, potentially relapsing condition, long-term treatment or prophylaxis treatment with mood-stabilizing medication is generally recommended. The two most commonly used mood-stabilizing medications are lithium carbonate and the anticonvulsant medication valproate (Depakote and others). Other medications that may be utilized in the management of mood episodes in bipolar illness include carbamazepine (Tegretol and others), lamotrigine (Lamictal), and other anticonvulsant compounds. Relatively recently, the atypical antipsychotic medication olanzapine (Zyprexa) received the Food and Drug Administration (FDA) approval for use in bipolar disorder, and use of newer antipsychotic mediations has become increasingly common in the management of bipolar illness.

Regular follow-up with medical care during the prophylaxis (maintenance) phase is extremely important. Choice of mood-stabilizing medication should generally be based upon an individual's history and clinical status. Both lithium and valproate have proven efficacy as first-line agents. Individuals having a good history of medication response to a particular compound are very likely to have a repeat good response with treatment with this same compound. During maintenance treatment visits, the treating clinician will generally review any occurrence of medication adverse events as well as monitoring of medication levels. Medication blood levels are routinely monitored with lithium, valproate, and carbamazepine. Psychoeducational interventions are typically most effective during the maintenance period, once individuals have achieved some degree of clinical stability. Best results are generally obtained when families or important individuals in the patient's social support network are engaged in treatment as well.

Individuals with bipolar disorder may develop severe depressive episodes in which substantial functional impairment is seen, and suicide vulnerability becomes an important issue. When this occurs, common treatment strategies involve optimizing mood-stabilizer treatment, addition of additional mood-stabilizing medication, and possible use of antidepressant medications. Families and support individuals should be alerted to possible suicide risks and psychosocial measures implemented as needed. Individuals with suicidal ideation may require hospitalization. Most newer, standard antidepressant drugs appear to be equally efficacious in bipolar depression and choice of agent should be based upon past history and current clinical status.

Less commonly, alternative, nonmedication biological therapies are used for the treatment of bipolar disorder. These include treatments such as electroconvulsive therapy (ECT), rapid transcranial magnetic stimulation (rTMS), and phototherapy/bright light therapy. ECT is a generally safe and effective treatment for depression and mania, which is done under general anesthesia. A brief electrical stimulus is administered via electrodes attached to the scalp, which results in a brief seizure (40–60 s). ECT is often done when individuals are unable to tolerate medication, or when medications have been ineffective. rTMS is a less established, noninvasive procedure in which a brief, nonconvulsive (nonseizure causing) stimulus is used for the treatment of depression. Light therapy involves use of high-intensity light exposure to treat depressive symptoms.

SEE ALSO: Depression, Mood disorders, Schizophrenia

Suggested Reading

American Psychiatric Association. (1994). *Diagnostic and statistical manual of mental disorders* (4th ed.). Washington, DC: Author.

American Psychiatric Association. (2002). *Practice guideline for the treatment of patients with bipolar disorder* (*revision*). Washington, DC: Author.

Brady, K. T., & Lydiard, R. B. (1992). Bipolar affective disorder and substance abuse. *Journal of Clinical Psychopharmacology*, Suppl. 12, 17S–22S.

Fuller, M. A., & Sajatovic, M. (2001). *Drug information for mental health*. Cleveland, OH: Lexi-Comp.

Goldberg, J. F., & Harrow, M. (Eds.). (1999). *Bipolar disorders: Clinical course and outcome*. Washington, DC: American Psychiatric Press.

Goodwin, F. K., & Jamison, K. R. (1990). *Manic-depressive illness*. New York: Oxford University Press.

Parry, B. L. (2000). Hormonal basis of mood disorders in women. In E. Frank (Ed.), *Gender and its effects on psychopathology* (pp. 3–21). Washington, DC: American Psychiatric Press.

Strakowski, S. M., Tohen, M., Stoll, A. L., et al. (1992). Comorbidity in mania at first hospitalization. *American Journal of Psychiatry*, *149*, 554–556.

Tondo, L., Baldessarini, R. J., Hennen, et al. (1998). Lithium treatment and risk of suicidal behavior in bipolar disorder patients. *Journal of Clinical Psychiatry, 59*, 405–414.

MARTHA SAJATOVIC

Birth Control Contraception is defined as the use of medications, devices, surgery, or sexual timing or practices to voluntarily avoid unintended pregnancy and to space childbirth. Birth control, family planning, fertility control, pregnancy prevention, and planned parenthood are other terms used for contraception. A general medical or gynecological health exam for girls and women of reproductive age is not complete unless the health caregiver has addressed the need for contraception. Appropriate counseling for the selection and use of a contraceptive method should include information regarding the benefits, risks, alternatives, and instructions for use presented in a noncoercive and nonjudgmental manner, as well as the opportunity for questions. The choice to use a contraceptive method is a decision made by the woman and her partner based on personal, social, religious, and financial considerations. In addition, other health factors including the possibility of exposure to sexually transmitted infections and personal health history should be considered. Noncoercive, collaborative, and thorough counseling increases the likelihood that the user will be comfortable and competent to use the selected method.

People have attempted to control their fertility since antiquity. As long as 4,000 years ago, the *Cahun Papyrus*, the oldest written document on fertility control, describes the use of pessaries made from crocodile dung and fermented dough. Condoms made from linen and the skins of sheep, goats, and even snakes were widely used. In the ruins of Pompeii, curettes and dilators similar to instruments used in modern-day abortion were discovered (*New Internationalist*, 1998).

Until the mid-19th century, few effective methods of fertility control existed. In the early 20th century, Margaret Sanger (1883–1966), a nurse and feminist, introduced the diaphragm into the United States. She founded the organization that would later become Planned Parenthood Federation of America. In 1965, the U.S. Supreme Court declared birth control to be a basic right in the *Estelle T. Griswold and C. Lee Buxton v. State of Connecticut* decision. Abortion, a subject that continues to divide the country today, was legalized in 1973 in the *Roe v. Wade* decision. This action by the Supreme Court limited the circumstances under which states could restrict the "right to privacy" under local law (Youngkin & Davis, 1998). In 1987, in the *Webster v. Reproductive Health Services* decision, the Supreme Court weakened the right to abortion on demand. This 5-4 decision allowed the states to restrict abortion in public facilities, to forbid the use of public employees in the performance of abortion, and to require viability testing for fetuses thought to be greater than 20 weeks gestation. This divisive national controversy continues to be far from resolved.

Socioeconomic and medical implications of unintended pregnancy are far-reaching and expensive in both economic and human terms. A 1995 report by the Institute of Medicine on the implications of unintended pregnancy on the well-being of women and families reports:

1. A woman with an unintended pregnancy is less likely to seek early prenatal care and more likely

to expose the fetus to harmful substances such as alcohol and tobacco.

2. Births from unintended pregnancies are more likely to occur to mothers who are adolescent, unmarried, or over age 40—characteristics that carry special medical risks and socioeconomic burdens.

3. Children born from an unwanted conception are at greater risk of being born at low birthweight, of dying in the first year of life, of being abused, and of having developmental disabilities.

4. Mothers who experience unintended pregnancy are at greater risk for depression and both parents may suffer economic hardship or failure to reach educational or career goals.

Teen pregnancy creates especially challenging social problems. According to the Alan Guttmacher Institute (1999), 78% of teen pregnancies are unplanned, accounting for one fourth of all accidental pregnancies annually. Seven in ten teen mothers finish high school but are less likely to go on to college. Partly because most teen mothers come from disadvantaged backgrounds, 28% are poor between the ages of 20 and 30 while only 7% who give birth after adolescence are poor at those ages.

There is ample evidence demonstrating the cost-effectiveness of contraceptive use. In a 1995 study, Trussel et al. measured the cost of contraceptive methods compared to the cost of unintended pregnancies when no contraception was used. They found the total savings to the health care system to fall between $9,000 and $14,000 per woman over 5 years of contraceptive use. These figures do not include the costs to women and families for the needs of children and the loss in earnings potential due to educational and employment discrepancies between those with planned and unplanned childbearing. It is estimated that for every $1.00 spent on publicly funded reproductive health care, $3.00 of Medicaid funding for prenatal and pediatric medical care is saved (Planned Parenthood Federation of America, 2001).

There are many types of contraception. They are categorized as abstinence, coitus interruptus, lactational amenorrhea method, barrier methods, hormonal methods, fertility awareness methods, intrauterine device, and surgical sterilization. Each of these methods has risks, benefits, and individual effectiveness rates. When deciding to use a method of contraception, safety, efficacy, and personal factors should be taken into consideration (Hatcher et al., 1998).

Virtually all methods of contraception are safer than pregnancy-related complications. Safety issues that should be taken into account are personal health risks, future fertility, side effects, and specific precautions that can make using the method safer. For instance, when using an IUD, minimizing the number of sexual partners decreases the risk of pelvic infection and subsequent decreased future fertility.

Efficacy of a method is determined by both the chosen method and user characteristics. Some sources document efficacy statistics as perfect use versus typical use. Typical use is affected by the frequency of use (taking a pill everyday vs. an injection every 3 months), whether the method interferes with spontaneity by requiring the partner(s) to use it at the time of intercourse, whether it requires cooperation of both partners, and whether it can be used consistently due to issues of availability and cost of supplies. Methods that require a prescription must be ordered by a medical provider thus incurring the additional cost of a medical visit. Over-the-counter methods are more easily available and less expensive but often less effective.

Personal factors that should be taken into consideration when selecting a contraceptive method include:

- personal preference and comfort with a method
- frequency of intercourse
- personal health factors that might be complicated or improved by a method (i.e., irregular periods improve with oral contraceptives)
- religious prohibitions to a given method
- previous positive or negative experience using a method

Barrier methods such as condoms, vaginal pouch, contraceptive sponge, and spermicidal foams, jellies, and inserts are widely available over the counter in most pharmacies. They do not require a prescription, are inexpensive, simple to obtain, and uncomplicated to use. The only barrier methods requiring a prescription and medical exam for fitting are diaphragms and cervical caps.

Hormonal contraception is the most common reversible method used in the United States. These methods include oral contraceptives (the pill), emergency contraception (morning-after pill), injectable medications (Depo-Provera), transdermal hormones (the patch), and vaginal hormones (the ring). All these methods require medical visits for prescriptions and/or injection or surgical placement. Some insurance carriers pay for the medical visits, medication, devices, and procedures for placement. Many cover only the cost of the medical visit. Checking insurance coverage and cost of the medical services and method prior to making a decision about use avoids unexpected expense. Many methods are available at reduced cost at Planned Parenthood, local family planning clinics, health departments, or free clinics for those who qualify for services.

The use of fertility awareness and lactational amenorrhea methods requires education by a knowledgeable professional. Fertility awareness is a complex method requiring motivated couples and a willingness to abstain from intercourse cyclically during fertile times. This method necessitates several hours of instruction and follow-up to assure accurate measurements and observations of signs of fertility. It is the only method currently authorized by the Catholic Church.

Intrauterine devices (IUDs) and sterilization (tubal ligation and vasectomy) require medical intervention and costs for medical evaluation and visits. Sterilization, particularly tubal ligation, may incur hospital costs as well. Insurance coverage for these procedures varies greatly. Some family planning clinics insert IUDs at reduced cost but do not perform surgical sterilization. Again, the key is to ascertain information about cost and insurance coverage prior to making decisions to use either of these methods.

The decision to use contraception is complex and multifactorial. It is essential to consider personal health and financial factors, safety, efficacy, and the impact that an unintended pregnancy may have. Unplanned pregnancy will have lifelong consequences whether it ends in termination, adoption, or personally raising a child. Trusting one's reproductive fate to chance may cause unforeseen and unwelcome consequences. With the widespread availability and increased numbers of options, the need for contraception can be met for everyone who desires to prevent unintended pregnancy.

SEE ALSO: Abortion, Condoms, Diaphragm, Dilation and curettage, Intrauterine device, Lubricants, Natural family planning, Oral contraception, Safer sex, Tubal ligation

Suggested Reading

Hatcher, R., Trussel, J., Stewart, F., Cates, W., Stewart, G., Guest, F., et al. (1999). *Contraceptive technology.* New York: Ardent Medica.

Institute of Medicine, National Academy of Sciences. (1995). *The best intentions: Unintended pregnancy and the well-being of children and families.* Washington, DC: National Academy Press.

Trussel, J., et al. (1995). The economic value of contraception: A comparison of 15 methods. *American Journal of Public Health, 85,* 494–503.

Youngkin, E. Q., & Davis, M. S. (1998). *Women's health: A primary care clinical guide* (p. 162). Stamford, CT: Appleton & Lange.

Suggested Resources

Alan Guttmacher Institute. (1999). Facts in brief: Teen sex and pregnancy. Retrieved September 1999, from http://www.agi-usa.org/pubs/fb_teen_sex.html

New Internationalist. (1998). A history of reproduction, contraception and control. Retrieved July 1998, from http://www.newint.org/issue303/history.htm

Planned Parenthood Federation of America. (2001). America's family planning program: Title X. Retrieved March 2001, from http://www.plannedparenthood.org/library/familyplanningissues/TitleX_fact.html

NANCY MYERS-BRADLEY

Blackwell, Elizabeth

Elizabeth Blackwell, the first woman awarded a medical degree in the United States, was born February 3, 1821, in Bristol, Gloucestershire, England. Hannah and Samuel Blackwell had nine children, of which Elizabeth was the third. Elizabeth's father was a highly prosperous sugar refiner and the Blackwell children, even the girls, were privately tutored. In 1831 the family moved to New York City, where Samuel Blackwell established another successful sugar refinery. However, in 1835 a fire destroyed it. The Blackwell family became involved in social reform and the antislavery movement. These beliefs led Samuel Blackwell to start a sugar refinery in Cincinnati, Ohio, using sugar beets. This method did not require the use of slave labor.

Elizabeth's father died shortly after moving to Cincinnati; the family was left in an impoverished state, and so the older children were forced to find work. Elizabeth and two of her sisters began teaching at a private school that their mother, Hannah, established in their home. Elizabeth then moved to Kentucky to find work, also as a teacher. Life in Kentucky did not suit her. Elizabeth's strong antislavery beliefs would not allow her to remain living in a slave state, so she moved back to Cincinnati. It was in Cincinnati that Elizabeth made her decision to become a doctor, in spite of inadequate preparation in the sciences and classical languages, and prior medical experience, which many medical schools required.

In 1845 Elizabeth went to South Carolina to teach and arranged to live in a physician's household, where she received some medical training and the opportunity to study Greek and Latin. During that time, she applied to many colleges, but none accepted her. Finally in 1847 the Geneva College in New York accepted her as a medical student. This really was an accident. The administration allowed the students, at this time all men, to vote as to whether to admit her or not. Thinking that the request was a joke, the students unanimously voted to allow her admittance. Elizabeth was a dedicated student, and graduated first in her class in January 1849.

During her medical studies at Geneva College, Elizabeth worked on a women's ward at Blockley Almshouse, a charitable hospital in Philadelphia. After graduating, Elizabeth went to Paris to intern at La Maternité, the only hospital that would accept her. It was there that her dreams of becoming a surgeon died. Elizabeth contracted an eye ailment that resulted in the loss of her left eye. However, this did not stop Elizabeth Blackwell from becoming a great doctor.

In 1850, Elizabeth went to England for an internship at St. Bartholomew's Hospital. It was here that she met the famous Florence Nightingale, with whom she became a close and lasting friend. One year later, Elizabeth returned to New York, but found those doors were closed to her; no one wanted to hire a woman doctor. So Elizabeth opened her own clinic. This was not an easy task, as no one wanted to rent to a woman doctor either. In 1853, she finally purchased a small home in Manhattan and opened her own clinic, the New York Dispensary for Poor Women and Children, now the New York Infirmary—Beekman Downtown Hospital. Two other women, her younger sister Emily and a Polish immigrant named Marie Zackrzewska, joined Elizabeth. Both women had attended Western Reserve College in Cincinnati, now known as Case Western Reserve University. This clinic was so successful that in 1857, the three women opened another clinic in Greenwich Village.

Even though Elizabeth was determined not to marry, this did not mean that she could not have a family. In 1854, she adopted a young orphaned girl named Katharine Barry, known as Kitty.

Showing her antislavery sentiments, during the 1860s Blackwell formed an organization called the Women's Central Association of Relief, a Civil War nursing program. In 1868, Elizabeth, with help from her friend Florence Nightingale, opened the Women's Medical College of the New York Infirmary with fifteen students and a faculty of nine, including Elizabeth as Professor of Hygiene and her sister Emily as Professor of Obstetrics and Diseases of Women. One year later, in 1869, Elizabeth moved to England and her sister Emily continued to run the College and the clinics. In 1875, Elizabeth became a professor of gynecology at the London School of Medicine for Children. She continued to teach there until she retired in 1907. In 1910, Elizabeth Blackwell died of a stroke in Sussex, England.

Not only was Elizabeth Blackwell a successful physician, but she also wrote several books. They include *The Laws of Life* (1858), *The Religion of Health* (1871), *Counsel to Parents on the Moral Education of Their Children* (1878), *The Human Element in Sex* (1884), *Essays in Medical Sociology* (1902), and her autobiography, *Pioneer Work in Opening the Medical Profession to Women* (1895).

See Also: Discrimination; Jacobi, Mary Putnam; Nightingale, Florence; Nurse, Physician, Women in the Health Professions, (pp. 20–32); Women in Health: Advocates, Reformers and Pioneers (pp. 40–48)

Suggested Reading

Blackwell, E. (1970). *Pioneer work in opening the medical profession to women.* New York: Source Book Press.

Edwards, J. (2002). *Women in American education, 1820–1955: The female force and educational reform.* Westport, CT: Greenwood Press.

Felder, D. G. (1996). *The 100 most influential women of all time.* New York: Carol.

Kline, N. (1997). *Elizabeth Blackwell: A doctor's triumph.* Berkeley: Conari Press.

Peck, I. (2000). *Elizabeth Blackwell: The first woman doctor.* Brookfield, CT: Millbrook Press.

Truman, M. (1976). *Women of courage.* New York: Morrow.

Suggested Resources

U.S. National Library of Medicine. (2002). National Institutes of Health, Department of Health and Human Services. Retrieved July 2003, from http://www.nlm.nih.gov/hmd/blackwell/ (accessed July, 2003)

TAMBRA K. CAIN

Blood Pressure   *see* Hypertension

Body Image   Cultural perception of the perfect female shape has varied over time from a full-figured fertility goddess and rounded Rubenesque figure to the pencil thin Twiggy and Ally McBeal. In Third World countries, women who are heavier are associated with high social status and having money to buy food, while the Western world worships thinness. Many women attribute to their bodies the power to define their lives. Physical and emotional health suffers when extreme obesity or anorexia occurs driven by a dictatorial body image. A negative body image can lower one's mood, self-esteem, and confidence. Social influences on body image begin early. Children and adolescents who are teased about being fat begin to "hate" the way they look and fear ostracism and isolation from peers. Even elementary aged girls now talk of diet, but severe pressure occurs at puberty when the natural process of rounding is counter to the desired image. In fact, girls who have a negative body image are more likely to have eating disorders and depression and are likely to consider suicide. Lower socioeconomic status, less education, and lower paying jobs are known associates of obesity and feeling ashamed of appearance.

A mother's body image has a significant impact on her daughter even without words. Is the mother happy with her body image; are diets continual; is she always worried she looks fat; or does the daughter perceive poor treatment of her mother and vows never to look the same? A feminist approach would urge each woman to formulate a cognitive image of physical and mental health. Rather than being "tyrannized" by society or caught in the male/mind, female/body dichotomy, women can begin to celebrate their unique bodies. Self-caring, not self-contempt, can encourage true improvement both inside and outside. Healthy nutrition and exercise habits can allow flexibility of what is seen as good. Each woman must decide what is most beneficial for her health. As a group older women are less concerned about weight and body image than middle-aged women, but the very old also tend to be thinner. Likewise ethnic minorities may be more accepting of their weight and body image than whites in this country. Peers and colleagues at school or work, income level, education, occupation, household size, marital status, activity level, parenthood, residential density, and region impact on weight and therefore indirectly on body image.

For centuries men's opinions about features that visually attracted them to females molded how women perceived themselves. Women have believed that if men found them attractive, they would be protected from violence. This offers little satisfaction to several million women each year who are victims of violent crime, most often at the hands of someone with whom they are intimate. Nonetheless, to appear more beautiful than others, women listen to weight loss and cosmetic industries and are forever seeking to appear youthful and thin. Many will select an "easy" quick and more dramatic attempt to achieve the perfect body with surgery.

In the recent past the media has made it impossible to escape reminders of how the attractive, healthy woman should look. Although humans performed nasal reconstruction for other reasons in ancient times, not until the 1950s did beauty surgery grow in popularity. Nose, ear, eye area, and lid surgeries increased as well as removal of blemishes. Many women feel they must aspire shapes displayed on television, magazines, or billboards. Albeit some women have breast reductions for health or athletic reasons, others request this procedure to appear thinner. The frequency of liposuction of thighs and tummy tucks (abdominoplasty) dramatically escalated in the 1990s as well as breast implants for those wishing to be more attractive to men. Rhinoplasty (nose), rhytidectomy (facelift), cheek and chin augmentation, brow lifts, ear and eye area surgery, and chemical peels are all designed to improve the facial image.

Society judges women by their appearance more often than men, particularly with respect to weight and body shape. "Stigmatization" and feelings of inadequacy encourage women to utilize technology available to make the body more attractive, which may vary from culture to culture. For example, in the Philippines reshaping skin lateral to the eyes to appear more European is the most popular plastic surgery procedure. There is little available data using standardized testing to discern how much body image may improve from procedures such as liposuction, laser eye surgery, or Botox injections, but it is likely there is some. Between 1992 and 2001, the incidence of breast augmentation in healthy patients increased by 533% according to the American Society of Plastic Surgeons. A recent study by Banbury reports 96% of women who have breast augmentation felt that surgery had a positive impact on their body image and 80% said they would have the surgery again.

Other body image concerns follow malignant illness and surgical procedures. Losing one's hair after chemotherapy is particularly common in women who face cancer treatment. Vulvectomy, mastectomy, and ileostomy (surgical procedures that remove portions of external genitalia, breasts, or bowel) are devastating blows, leaving some to describe they no longer feel like a woman. A woman may have been praised for her beautiful hair or told by her husband how he loved her breasts and now may find it harder to trust that she will still be valued as much as she was prior to the physical loss. Certainly many women with cancer have benefited greatly from multiple "image-boosters." Support groups and counselors recommend women consider possibilities from makeup classes and wigs to breast and vaginal reconstruction.

Although weight loss and exercise can improve body image for many, "phantom fat," the continued self-perception of being overweight and recollection of adverse consequences of being fat can limit improvement for others. Cognitive-behavioral therapy that reshapes body image and provides alternative interpretations can be quite helpful. With this therapy, individuals describe their ideals, learn relaxation techniques, participate in psychoeducational sessions, attack old distortions, develop positive activities, and explore interpersonal relationships. Feedback from other participants and practicing strategies to change negative mental schema and unhealthy behaviors support new efforts of an individual working to improve body image. There is no single correct treatment any more than a single correct body. Each woman must objectively reflect on her own health physically, mentally, and spiritually to guide her decisions.

SEE ALSO: Anorexia nervosa, Bulimia nervosa, Depression, Eating disorders

Suggested Reading

Baguet, C. (1995). Cancer and women. In R. P. Epps & S. C. Stewart (Eds.), *Women's complete healthbook* (pp. 639–648). New York: Delaconte Press.

Banbury, J. (in press). Prospective analysis of the outcome of subpectoral breast augmentation: Sensory changes, muscle function, and body image. *Plastic and Reconstructive Surgery*.

Cash, T. F. (2002). The management of body image problems. In K. D. Brownell & C. G. Fairburn (Eds.), *Eating disorders and obesity* (2nd ed., pp. 599–603). New York: Guilford Press.

Hutchinson, M. G. (1994). Imaging ourselves whole: A feminist approach to treating body image disorders. In P. Fallon, M. A. Katzman, & S. C. Wooley (Eds.), *Feminist perspectives on eating disorders* (pp. 152–168). New York: Guilford Press.

Petro, J. A., & Phillips, L. G. (1995). Reconstructive and plastic surgery. In R. P. Epps & S. C. Stewart (Eds.), *Women's complete healthbook* (pp. 627–638). New York: Delaconte Press.

Rosen, J. C. (2002). Obesity and body image. In K. D. Brownell & C. G. Fairburn (Eds.), *Eating disorders and obesity* (2nd ed., pp. 399–402). New York: Guilford Press.

Sobal, J. (2001). Social and cultural influences on obesity. In P. Björntorp (Ed.), *International textbook of obesity* (pp. 305–322). New York: John Wiley & Sons.

Tolman, D. L., & Debold, E. (1994). Conflicts of body and image; female adolescents, desire, and the no-body body. In P. Fallon,

M. A. Katzman, & S. C. Wooley (Eds.), *Feminist perspectives on eating disorders*. New York: Guilford Press.

KATHLEEN N. FRANCO
MOHAMMED ALISHAHIE
DAVID L. BRONSON

Body Mass Index Obesity is an important risk factor for many illnesses, especially heart disease and diabetes. However, body weight alone is not the best way to determine whether an individual is overweight. Whether the number of pounds a person carries is healthy or not depends on one's height and the amount of fat compared to the amount of muscle. The relationship between the amount of fat and muscle, weight and height is referred to as body composition. Extremely precise measures of body composition involve elaborate procedures such as underwater weighing or taking multiple measurements of the width of skin that can be "pinched" off the person's frame in numerous locations on the body.

The body mass index (BMI) is a much simpler way to estimate body composition and obesity by relating body weight to height. Indirectly, BMI measures body composition because a strong relationship has been found between the amount of body fat and BMI. BMI is often used to assess the level of health risk for obesity-related diseases. The equation used to calculate BMI is

$$BMI = \frac{\text{body weight in kilograms}}{(\text{height in meters})^2}$$

A BMI that is lower than 18.5 is considered underweight. Healthy, fit persons have BMI values from 18.5 to 24.9. When the BMI is between 25.0 and less than 30.0, a person is considered to be overweight. An individual with a BMI between 35 and 40 is considered obese. Extreme or "morbid" obesity is defined as a BMI of 40 or greater. People with BMIs above 30 have an increased risk for heart disease and adult-onset diabetes.

To reduce BMI, and therefore reduce the risk of illness, the best solution is to follow healthy eating and exercise guidelines, provided by your physician or a certified dietician/nutritionist. Particularly important is increasing the amount of low-fat protein, vegetables, and fruits in the diet, eating less high-fat or high-sugar foods, and engaging in aerobic exercise such as vigorous walking, jogging, bicycling, aerobic dance, or swimming.

See Also: Cardiovascular disease, Diabetes, Diet, Obesity, Weight control

Deborah Rosch Eifert

Suggested Resources

BMI calculator: http://nhlbisupport.com/bmi/bmicalc.htm
BMI tables: http://www.nhlbi.nih.gov/guidelines/obesity/bmi_tbl.htm

---

Breast Augmentation Over the last few decades, there has been a great deal of emphasis placed on the shape and size of women's breasts. Many women sometimes wish that their breasts were larger and for that reason seek breast enlargement or augmentation mammoplasty.

Women have diverse reasons for wanting to augment their breasts. Breast augmentation involves using implants to enlarge and shape the breasts, and permits a woman to wear clothes that, at one time, were not an option, such as swimsuits and dresses that fit in the hips and not the breast. Sometimes, women wish to go back to the size they were prior to pregnancy or after weight loss. Breast augmentation may also improve self-esteem and, indirectly, how a woman relates to others.

Approximately a decade ago, there was a great deal of negative publicity directed toward breast implants, particularly silicone implants. As a result, silicone implants were taken off the market. Since that time, studies have not found any association between silicone breast implants or breast cancer or autoimmune disorders. Still, the silicone implants are now used only in trial studies and have been replaced with saline (salt) implants. Salt is a natural constituent of our bodies and, therefore, allergic reactions are virtually nonexistent. Other substances such as peanut and soybean oil have been utilized, but have since been taken off the market.

One of the first important steps for seeking breast augmentation is an in-depth consultation with a board-certified plastic surgeon. There are always risks associated with any procedure and these should be provided in the consultation. Many women also obtain a wealth of information from the Internet. There are many websites dedicated to this subject as well as information through the American Board of Plastic Surgery.

Once a woman has decided to have the procedure performed, there are various options for how and where it is performed. This procedure is performed in an accredited outpatient facility, surgery center, or hospital and is almost always done on an outpatient basis. It is usually performed under general anesthesia, but conscious sedation can also be used. An incision can be made in the following places: around the edge of the areola (pigmented area around the nipple), just above the crease underneath the breast, within the armpit, or just at the edge of the navel. Once the incision is made, a space or pocket is developed and the implant is placed. The implant can be placed either underneath the breast tissue itself or underneath the muscle of the chest wall.

The technique that is used for the surgery depends not only on the surgeon's preference but also on the result that the patient desires. The surgeon may also suggest a procedure to enhance the desired result; for instance, if the breasts are saggy, a breast lift may be needed.

After surgery, there is a recovery period of 2–3 days and sometimes a week, depending upon the patient's threshold. Pain medication is given to help with the discomfort. Within a week following the surgery, the stitches are usually removed if they are not dissolvable. Generally, the woman will be able to shower and to return to nonstrenuous work. A period of time will elapse before the swelling resolves; during this time, a support bra must be used. Strenuous activity is usually permitted after a month.

There are many common questions women have regarding breast augmentation. How does a woman decide how large she wants to be? Many women look at pictures in a magazine. Although this can be of some assistance, the shape and size of the picture may not have any correlation to hers. There are some surgeons who have women put trial sizes in their bra. Others suggest buying an inexpensive bra of the desired size and placing water in a sandwich bag. It is a difficult decision to make, but the woman should really make a conscientious effort to be a part of that. Many women think when they have their breasts enlarged, they will go, for example, from a 32A to a 36C. This is a misconception because only the volume will become larger and not the circumference of the chest. For instance, a woman who wears a 32 bra, will continue to wear a 32 bra.

Another common question relates to the implant's durability over time. No one really can predict that figure. This is a manufactured device and can have defects. The manufacturing companies offer a lifetime warranty and will replace the implant at no charge. Sometimes, there is also a stipend offered to help pay for surgery that is necessary within the first 2 years. Some women wonder what may happen to them if there is a defect. If there is a defect in the implant, the only thing it can do is deflate. There is an obvious difference between the two sides and the implant will have to be replaced. However, the procedure to replace implants is relatively simple and does not require a lot of "downtime."

Some women wonder what will happen if they are unhappy about the size. If this occurs, the size can be changed with further surgery. If there is any uncertainty, there are implants which have a port through which more volume may be added. However, a small secondary operation is necessary to remove the port.

There are thousands of breast augmentations performed every year with successful and pleasing results on the patient's part. This is an important decision. Accordingly, it is critical that the surgeon chosen be qualified to perform the procedure and that he or she have good rapport with the patient.

SEE ALSO: Body image, Breast cancer, Breast reconstruction

Suggested Resources

www.implantinfo.com
www.plasticsurgery.org

JANET BLANCHARD

Breast Cancer   Over 200,000 women are diagnosed with breast cancer each year, and this number is expected to increase significantly over the next decade as more women will be living in the age-at-risk group. One out of eight women will be diagnosed in their lifetime, and at least 40,000 will die of the disease each year. Most women who get breast cancer will survive the disease, and the number of women dying per year is expected to decrease. For many reasons, this encouraging trend is expected to continue.

As advances in imaging techniques, treatment, and prevention continue to be made, women can expect their chances of surviving breast cancer to improve. The actual cause of most breast cancers is not known. However, many risk factors have been identified that include female gender, family history, early menarche, late menopause, increasing age, some forms of benign breast disease, prolonged exposure to exogenous estrogen, and recently identified mutations in the genes *BRCA 1* and *2*. The majority of women being diagnosed with breast cancer, however, do not have these risk factors, with the exception of increasing age and female gender.

Detecting breast cancer ("screening") involves self-examination, evaluation by a physician, and imaging. The relative importance and ability of each of these mechanisms to detect breast cancer (sensitivity) continues to be debated; a combination of the three will always be important in early detection of breast cancer. Early detection remains the best way to survive breast cancer.

Screening for breast cancer should be applied based on a woman's individual risk of getting breast cancer. A woman is considered at increased risk if she has a strong family history or genetic predisposition, has previously received therapeutic radiation to the chest for another condition, has a 5-year calculated risk (by special computer techniques) of 1.7%, or has had a breast biopsy showing atypical hyperplasia or lobular carcinoma in situ. These women should also have an annual physical examination. This group of women should have annual mammography (perhaps at an earlier age), and more frequent exams by a health care professional. Some women in this group may be candidates for chemoprevention, a newer treatment that involves taking a medication (tamoxifen) prophylactically, which is ordinarily given to women who have diagnosed breast cancers. Women at normal risk between the ages of 20 and 39 should be encouraged to do breast self-examination, and have an examination by a physician every 1–3 years. Women aged 40 and above should have an annual mammography and continue with breast self-exam.

Exciting new imaging techniques are being developed to diagnose early breast cancers, at smaller sizes than were previously detectable. Modalities for the treatment of breast cancers continue to evolve at a rapid rate. In the future, early breast cancer treatment may not actually involve surgery as we know it. Even the standard techniques of surgery are now dramatically less invasive, so that most women with breast cancer today are treated in the outpatient setting.

When a diagnosis of breast cancer is made, it is imperative that a thorough, nonhurried discussion occur with a surgeon who will present all treatment options. Most women will be deciding between two equally safe options. Breast cancers are typically slower growing tumors, which implies that a decision regarding the type of surgery need not be reached immediately, but rather after a woman understands fully the choices available to her. After sufficient consultation, which may involve seeking a second opinion, a woman can make an informed choice.

The two options that are available today are breast-conserving surgery (lumpectomy or wide excision/radiation) or mastectomy with or without reconstruction. Both offer equally good survival rates. A minimally invasive technique that accurately evaluates the axillary lymph nodes (sentinel node dissection) is part of either of the primary surgical procedures.

Once the surgical treatment is completed and the stage (size of tumor and status of the nodes) is determined, then a decision can be made regarding the need for chemotherapy. This involves a discussion with a medical oncologist, understanding that the recommendation for chemotherapy is not based on the surgery chosen, but the stage of the tumor. Most women with breast cancer today are treated by a multidisciplinary team comprised of several specialties.

As mentioned above, advances are being made daily in the diagnosis and treatment of breast cancer. Women should be encouraged that management of early-detected breast cancer involves increasingly less invasive approaches and will be addressed through the interaction of a team of dedicated specialists. New techniques in the fields of genetics, radiologic imaging, medical oncology, pathology, and surgery empower a woman to be actively involved in the management of her disease. Most women with breast cancer are surviving the disease, and can look forward to a future where prevention may actually be a reality.

See Also: Breast augmentation, Breast lumps, Cancer, Mammography, Mastectomy

Suggested Resources

CancerSource.com

DAVID FADDIS

Breast Enlargement   *see* Breast Augmentation

Breast Examination   A breast examination is a simple means of detecting changes in breast tissue. There are two kinds of examinations, self-exam and clinical exam. The goal of these procedures is early detection of breast cancer because early treatment can increase survival rates.

Breast cancer is not only the most common non-skin cancer in women, but is also the second deadliest as well. If a woman lives to age 90, she has a 1 in 8 chance of developing breast cancer. Breast cancer is mostly a disease of older women. Statistically, the 1-year incidence for breast cancer in a 40-year-old woman is 1 in 800, for a 50-year-old woman it is 1 in 400, and for women age 60 the incidence is 1 in 200. In younger age groups, breast cancer is uncommon and screening tests may be less effective. Therefore, we have different recommendations for different age groups. Screening recommendations are also different for patients with a strong family history of breast cancer or a personal history of breast cancer. This discussion is for women who are at average risk for development of breast cancer.

Much research in the last 40 years has been done on screening for breast cancer, but guidelines do not always agree on what type of screening method to use and frequency with which to screen. The screening methods currently in use include mammography, clinical breast exam (CBE), and breast self-exam. Mammography will be discussed elsewhere. This section will discuss the evidence and recommendations for CBE as well as breast self-examination.

The CBE is a breast exam performed by a health care professional on a patient without symptoms. Some women are more willing to accept CBE instead of mammography for breast cancer screening, which makes it an especially important clinical skill. To perform a CBE, one must know the distribution of breast tissue. Breast tissue extends from the breastbone medially to the underarm laterally and from the collarbone superiorly to the "bra line" inferiorly. Normal breast tissue can be lumpy due to the mammary ducts and lobules.

No randomized controlled trial has looked at CBE alone versus not screening at all for breast cancer. However, mammography has been evaluated with and without CBE for breast cancer detection. Mammography has been shown to be effective in decreasing breast cancer mortality. Since mammography is known to be an effective screening tool, a clinical trial that excludes it would be unethical. Therefore, we must look at indirect evidence to decide if CBE is effective in detecting breast cancer and decreasing mortality. Some of the indirect evidence comes from studies including the meta-analyses by Barton, Harris, and Fletcher (1999). Many of these patients had CBE and screening mammography for

Breast Examination

breast cancer detection. From these trials we see that breast cancer mortality decreased by about 25% in women aged 50–69 years and by 18% in women in their 40s. One of the studies reviewed by Barton 1999 was the Canadian National Breast Screening Study. This study looked at women from 50 to 59 years old and offered them CBE alone or CBE plus mammography each year for 5 years. The 7-year mortality rates were similar, suggesting that mammography may not decrease mortality in women in their 50s, and that careful CBE alone may be as good as CBE plus mammography. Another study reviewed by Barton et al. (1999) was the Edinburgh randomized trial of breast cancer screening, which found mammography detected 26% of breast cancers while CBE detected only 3%. However, another randomized trial done with the Health Insurance Plan of New York (HIP) found breast cancer detection rates of 33% with mammography and 45% with CBE. The HIP study was conducted with early mammography techniques, but still suggests that CBE does have a role in detection of breast cancer. Other studies report that CBE can find from 3% to 45% of breast cancers. The exact percentage of cancers found on CBE is not known.

One reason that cancer detection may vary is the difference in technique used. Rates of CBE sensitivity (finding disease in those who really have it) range from 53% to 68% in women between 40 and 49 years and 48% and 63% in women between 50 and 59 years. Different studies use different methods for performance of the CBE. Some studies did not report their method of CBE. The Mammacare method has been advocated for universal use since its components have been validated in independent investigations of CBE technique. The components include palpation, examination pattern, and duration and inspection. Palpation (physical examination) of the breast is most accurately done while the patient is lying down with her arm extended above her head (Figure 1). This flattens out the breast tissue. The entire breast is palpated using the boundaries previously outlined in a vertical strip pattern or lawnmower pattern. The pads of the index, middle, and fourth fingers palpate each row (Figure 2). In each row, the clinician should stop and make small circular motions as if tracing the outer edge of a dime at a superficial, intermediate, and deep pressure. Each CBE can take up to 3 minutes for each side in an average-sized breast (B cup). Checking the armpit and area above the collarbone for enlarged lymph nodes is usually performed, but has not been clinically tested. Palpation of the nipple area is usually performed as well. Expression of fluid from a nipple is not

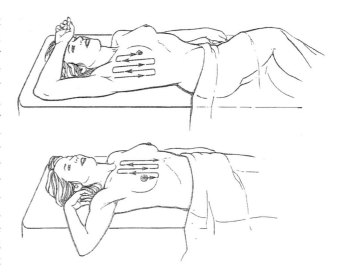

Figure 1. Position of patient and direction of palpation for clinical breast examination. Top figure shows the lateral portion of the breast and bottom the medial portion of the breast. Arrows indicate strip pattern of examination.

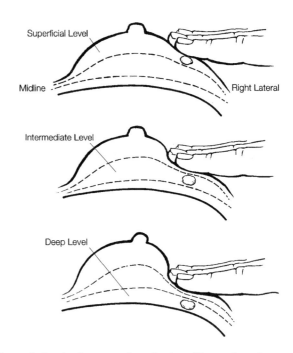

Figure 2. Levels of pressure for palpation of breast tissue in a cross-sectional view of the right breast. The examiner should make three circles with the finger pads, increasing the level of pressure (superficial, intermediate, and deep) with each circle.

a useful prognostic sign for cancer. However, spontaneous nipple discharge may need further evaluation.

Several guidelines recommend that CBE be performed every 1–2 years for all women over age 40.

However, women at higher than average risk need to discuss individual screening recommendations with their health care provider. Evidence shows that clinicians taught the Mammacare method of CBE were better at finding breast cancers. Barton et al. (1999) found in their review that a well-conducted CBE can detect breast cancers about 50% of the time in patients without symptoms. There is some overlap with mammography and CBE; 10% of breast cancers detected are invisible on mammography. Similarly, 40% of breast cancers detected are not found on CBE. Patients have a better long-term survival if their breast cancer is detected by mammography, probably because mammography can detect smaller cancers.

The second type of examination method is breast self-examination. This is a simple means for women to detect changes in their own breast tissue. It is performed each month, usually within a week after menstruation, when the breast is least bumpy. Technique is important in breast self-examination. Patients should ask their health care providers for help in learning the proper technique. The proper technique includes looking at the breast and systematically examining the breast using the middle three fingers. Breast self-examination is not a substitute for screening mammography or CBE.

Few studies have shown that the chance of dying of breast cancer is reduced by breast self-examination. However, there may be some small evidence to support this method of screening. Patients need to be aware that the evidence for self-breast examination is unproven and that it may increase their chances of having a benign breast biopsy. The American Academy of Family Physicians, the American College of Obstetricians and Gynecologists, and the American Cancer Society all recommend routine teaching of breast self-examination.

SEE ALSO: Breast cancer, Breast lumps, Fibrocystic breast disease, Mammography

Suggested Reading

Barton, M. B., Harris, R., & Fletcher, S. W. (1999). Does this patient have breast cancer? The screening clinical breast examination: Should it be done? How? *Journal of the American Medical Association, 282,* 1270.

Bobo, J. K., Lee, N. C., & Thames, S. F. (2000). Findings from 752 081 clinical breast examinations reported to a national screening program from 1995 through 1998. *Journal of the National Cancer Institute, 92,* 971.

Harvey, B. J., Miller, A. B., Baines, C. H., & Corey, P. N. (1997). Effect of breast self-examination techniques on the risk of death from breast cancer. *Canadian Medical Association Journal, 157,* 1205.

Miller, A. B., To, T., Baines, C. J., & Wall, C. (2000). Canadian National Breast Screening Study-2: 13-year results of a randomized trial in women aged 50–59 years. *Journal of the National Cancer Institute, 92,* 1490.

Suggested Resources

Mammacare, Inc. www.mammacare.com

National Alliance of Breast Cancer Organizations. www.nabco.org

National Women's Health Information Center information on breast self-examination. www.4woman.gov/faq/bsefaq.htm

SUSAN KIRSH

Breast-Feeding Human breast milk is now widely acknowledged to be the most complete form of nutrition for infants, with a range of physiological and psychological benefits for both the infant and mother. Through the ages, humans have been dependent on it for its sustenance and even contraceptive attributes. Research supports the observation of benefits for infants' growth, immunity, and development, as well as reduced financial cost to the family. Prevention of diarrheal diseases and even dental cavities are just some of its protective powers. Likewise, breast-feeding has been shown to improve maternal health, including reduction in postpartum bleeding, earlier return to prepregnancy weight, reduced risk of premenopausal breast cancer, and reduced risk of osteoporosis. Yet, in spite of these advantages, ambivalence surrounds the practice because of the myriad of factors that influence a woman's ability and decision to commit to breast-feeding.

PREGNANCY AND PREPARATION

This is an ideal time to assess attitudes and readiness for breast-feeding. A breast health assessment, including a review of breast self-examination and nipple evaluation, is prudent. Also, an understanding of the anatomy and physiology of lactation (milk production) is an essential complement to successful breast-feeding. Human breast tissue begins to develop in the sixth week of fetal life; thus, when you are born, you already have breast tissue (as does your newborn). These mammary glands or secretory glands undergo most of their maturation postnatally, during adolescence and adulthood. They are considered mature once capable of producing milk, and fully functional once lactation actually begins. Each portion of the breast has a function. The external dome is comprised of the *nipple* that is the exit point for all the milk ducts (aka lactiferous ducts) and the pigmented *areola* that houses the nipple, nerve endings, Montgomery's glands (small, pimple-like openings that secrete a substance that lubricates and protects the nipple and areola during pregnancy and lactation), lymph drainage ports, and hair follicles. Internally, there are four main types of tissues: *glandular* (alveolar) tissue that produces milk; *ducts* that transport the milk; *connective* tissue that supports the breasts' upright position; and *adipose* (fat) tissue that protects the breast from injury (note that adipose tissue determines the size of the breast, but size has absolutely no effect on milk production or quality). Arterial blood supplies nourishment to the actual breast tissue as well as essential nutrients and hormones to make milk. The lymphatic system removes cellular waste, and the nervous system is essential for, among other things, transferring the stimulus of suckling to trigger a hormonal pathway responsible for milk production and letdown.

In the early days of pregnancy, when the hormone estrogen (E) begins to increase, it directly stimulates the ductules to grow, while the surge in the hormone progesterone (P) stimulates the alveoli and lobular tissue (grape-like collection of alveoli) to grow; hence the feeling of breast fullness in the early phases of pregnancy. This glandular growth is also influenced by insulin and cortisol. In spite of the structural changes that occur in the breast because of E and P, these hormones inhibit actual milk production. The two main hormones responsible for milk production are prolactin and oxytocin. Prolactin, which has peak production at night, stimulates the production of specific milk proteins as well as attracts immunoglobulin A from gut-associated lymphoid tissue. Oxytocin, a trigger for uterine contractions, also contracts the myoepithelial cells surrounding the alveoli, causing them to squeeze the newly formed milk into the duct system. This process is also referred to as "milk ejection reflex" or "milk letdown." Both of these hormones are released from the pituitary gland, into the blood, in response to the ovarian hormones (E and P), as well as the stimuli from the senses (visual, tactile, auditory, and olfactory). A number of factors, typical to the nursing mother, can also affect prolactin levels, including psychogenic stress, anesthesia, surgery, exercise, nipple stimulation, and sexual intercourse, to name a few. The most specific and effective stimulus for prolactin secretion, however, is suckling or nursing.

The early stage of pregnancy is an opportune time to *acknowledge and assess your personal feelings and biases* toward breast-feeding. Whether a health professional, a first-time mother, father, or friend, understanding our health beliefs is an integral component of making healthy behavior choices. Many times these beliefs are rooted in cultural practices, past personal experiences of others or ourselves, and even the teachings of those we respect as authorities on the subject. For example, many people believe breast-feeding is "intuitive" because it is a "natural" phenomenon. The art of breast-feeding is a learned skill, irrespective of a woman's education level. Also, in some cultures, mothers who wish to breast-feed may be reluctant to give colostrum (premilk) to their newborn because they consider it unclean or harmful. Use this time to expand and *alter your knowledge, skills, and attitude based on fact*, not fiction or anecdotes (see resource list at the end of the chapter). Speak with a lactation consultant or attend a breast-feeding support class or group.

As delivery and childbirth become more of a reality, the opportunity to nurse or breast-feed should again be entertained, with focused choices to ensure a successful and positive experience. *Anticipating what will be needed, what to expect, and arming yourself with information and practical skills* are shared sentiments from lactation consultants and mothers who have had positive and negative experiences. Feeding all newborns (whether breast or bottle) will have challenging moments. Likewise, it seems that the support system you align yourself with during breast-feeding is one of the most important decisions a woman can make in this endeavor. Support can be defined as anything or anyone who provides healthy guidance or solutions to perceived stressors. This may be someone to burp a baby after a feeding or someone with words of encouragement. Choosing a health provider who supports the practice and is knowledgeable about breast-feeding, as well as surrounding oneself with experienced women, have been shown to dramatically increase the duration and success of nursing. Even the hospital or birthing center selected will impact on the decision to start or continue breast-feeding. The "Ten Steps to Successful Breastfeeding" as defined by the World Health Organization, the United Nations Children's Fund, and adopted by the Department of Health and Human Services, outlines key practices for health care institutions. It recommends:

- a written breast-feeding policy that is communicated to all health care staff
- staff training in the skills needed to implement the policy
- education of pregnant women about the benefits and management of breast-feeding

- early initiation of breast-feeding
- education of mothers on how to breast-feed and maintain lactation
- limited use of any food or drink other than human breast milk
- rooming-in
- breast-feeding on demand
- limited use of pacifiers and artificial nipples
- fostering of breast-feeding support groups and services

Selecting a "breast-feeding friendly hospital" or institution with the above policies and philosophy provides a good environment for a healthy start.

CAUTIONS ABOUT BREAST-FEEDING

Human milk provides the most complete form of nutrition for infants, including premature and sick newborns, with rare exception. When direct breast-feeding is not possible, expressed milk should be provided. In cases of maternal infection, the basic tenet is that breast-feeding is rarely contraindicated. The few exceptions are situations where infectious agents may be associated with significant morbidity and mortality. Advice against breast-feeding should be based on careful consideration of the general benefits for mother and baby, the risks of not receiving human milk, and the most current information about the condition.

REPRODUCTIVE FUNCTION DURING LACTATION

It is helpful to know that the elevation of prolactin, and the abrupt withdrawal of ovarian and gonadotrophin hormones after childbirth and during lactation may lead to decreased breast sensitivity during lovemaking, vaginal epithelium atrophy, dryness, and decreased cervical mucus as well. These changes may, in turn, lead to discomfort during sexual intercourse and increase dyspareunia. Locally applied lubricants are helpful, and these changes usually improve over time. These hormonal changes also produce a lactational amenorrhea, or a cessation of ovulation and menses. The length of this hiatus from the ovulatory cycle varies, lasting longer with exclusive breast-feeding. Consequently, a measure of conception protection occurs for the first few months; however, ovulation, menstruation, and regaining fertility become a reality with decreased lactation. Family planning, birth

intervals, and a reliable method of contraception should be addressed in advance of starting to breast-feed.

POSTPARTUM AND BEYOND

In the first few days of breast-feeding, immediately after delivery and before the mature milk comes in, a thick, yellowish liquid known as colostrum is produced in small quantities and secreted from the nipples. Yet this "premilk" is sufficient to nourish the baby, satisfy the baby, and protect the baby from jaundice and many infectious diseases during the first few days of life. Colostrum that can even be present early in the second trimester of pregnancy contains complex immunological proteins, white blood cells, and factors that activate bowel function, a necessary stimulus to excrete the yellow pigment bilirubin (a by-product of red blood cell damage) into the stool. "Foremilk," which is the first portion of expressed milk, is similar to skim milk in both appearance and fat content. It is also larger in volume than "hindmilk," the creamier milk with a higher fat content that comes toward the end of the feeding. The volume of milk production will only diminish if the hormonal pathway regulated by frequent suckling is inhibited, if there is severe malnutrition, or if the mother is more than 10% dehydrated.

Nursing frequency and its influence on both infant and maternal nutrition can be categorized into one of three breast-feeding patterns. *Exclusive breast-feeding* (also known as unrestricted breast-feeding) is the term applied when infants are fed *only* by this method, on demand, and for unrestricted periods. Typically this entails an average of 10–12 feedings per day and occurs during the first 6 months of life. *Partial breast-feeding* is the term coined when breast-feeding is *supplemented* with limited amounts of formula, juice, water, or solid foods. *Minimal breast-feeding*, sometimes referred to as "token" feeding, usually means that the infant receives nearly all sustenance from formula and other foods. Research has found that the benefits of breast milk increase with increased exclusiveness of breast-feeding, and in fact, "token" breast-feeding has little or no nutritional value.

The chemical makeup of breast milk changes with every feed, making it tailored for the infants' needs. Its nutritional content is primarily fat, protein, lactose, water, vitamins, and minerals, including calcium and iron. Nutritional requirements of the lactating mother should begin with a balanced diet and supplements based on maternal dietary deficiencies. Health care providers should give particular attention to vegetarians and malnourished women, as calcium and B vitamins, among other things, may need to be supplemented. Also, living in an industrialized, developed country is not a guarantee against malnourishment and thus every woman should have a nutritional assessment. Other supplements like vitamin D, iron, and fluoride may be recommended for the infant beyond 6 months of age depending on other environmental and lifestyle factors. Assessment of the infant's nutritional status begins with monitoring the number of wet and soiled diapers, weight gain, and signs of jaundice. A health provider should observe suckling techniques and evaluate feeding frequency if any concerns arise.

TRENDS AND PRACTICES

From the dawn of civilization women have entertained the use of special feeding flasks, wet nurses, and mixed concoctions of animal milk as alternate methods to nurture infants. Uninformed concerns about maternal beauty, nobility, and the etiquette of the wealthy fueled many of these practices. In the mid-1900s, when most advances in science were perceived as beneficial, the "scientifically" prepared formulas were marketed as medical and commercial solutions to the problems of infant feeding. "Scientific motherhood" coupled with the impact of urbanization and industrialization led to a worldwide downward trend in breast-feeding. This impact was especially harmful to the breast-feeding practices of mothers in developing countries. Modified "formulas" that were closer to human milk in nutrient quantity were still very different in quality and lacked immune factors. In developed countries, there were negligible differences in mortality between breast-fed and artificially fed infants; however, the evidence became increasingly clear regarding the prevention of infant and later illness among those breast-fed. In developing countries, artificially fed infants had an associated higher morbidity and mortality than breast-fed infants, primarily caused by infection and malnutrition. Poor access to clean water along with inadequate preparation, dilution, and storage of "formulas" are large contributors to these outcomes.

Global trends toward increasing breast-feeding have been noted since the late 20th century. Data from the International Breastfeeding Compendium suggest that in the unindustrialized countries, most children are breast-fed for a few months. This is due in great part to the strong work of mother support groups, more educated women, and available evidence as to the benefits of breast milk, along with control of the marketing of artificial formula preparations.

In the United States, a national health initiative, *Healthy People 2000*, was outlined in 1978. It defined clear targets for improved maternal and child health measures and included improving breast-feeding rates as a priority.

	Target (%)		
	1978	1998	2010
In early postpartum	30	64	75
At 6 months	<5	29	50
At 1 year	<5	16	25

The international community has similar objectives; however, the baseline rates are lower in many developing countries, with slow but steady advances toward the target rates. Studies confirm that the rate of breast-feeding is higher for married, well educated, higher socioeconomic status women. Maternal employment outside the home and non-Anglo American ethnicity were related to higher rates of bottle-feeding. Many of these women, well informed about the benefits of mother's milk, chose not to breast-feed because it was "too difficult" and "there were too many rules." The most frequent reasons cited for stopping breast-feeding by women who started at hospital discharge were (1) not enough milk, (2) felt tired, and (3) infant's pediatrician told mother to stop. Asking for help from lactation consultants, mother and father support networks, and trained health professionals allows access to practical guidance and accurate information and should be sought before making any decision to stop nursing. Nursing is a flexible practice that should be tailored to fit the lifestyle needs of you and your baby. Most problems, typically experienced in the first 2–3 weeks of breast-feeding, have simple solutions. *Proper positioning* and *feeding on demand* can lead to avoidance of many of the common problems that affect milk supply and breast health such as engorgement, sore nipples, and blocked ducts. Positioning is the single most important factor for getting breast-feeding started well. This refers to (1) the physical alignment of mother and infant, (2) the way the mother holds the infant, (3) the position of the mother's hand as it supports her breast, and (4) the position of the baby's mouth, lips, and tongue—often called the "latch-on"—around the areola and nipple. Addressing problems early is also important to prevent outcomes such as infant failure to thrive, mastitis, yeast infections, and maternal discouragement, all of which require professional attention. Recommendations for routine breast care involve washing the breast following each nursing session with only lukewarm water, if at all; and massaging a small amount of expressed milk onto the nipple and areola following every feed.

Milk *banking* and *pumping* are notable options in expressing breast milk that provide optimal infant nutrition while the mother is not physically able to nurse due to health problems, employment demands, physical absence, or simple fatigue. Special instructions are available in the cited references regarding these practices and the storage of expressed milk.

SUMMARY

The evidence for the short- and long-term benefits of breast-feeding on the health of the infant, women, and their families continues to grow. This has led a renewed commitment from the health care community to encourage and support this practice. The forces that improve success, however, lie not only in the guidance of health professionals, but seem grounded in the stories and support of mothers who have had positive or negative experiences. Understanding that breast-feeding is natural but is a learned skill is at the foundation of successful nursing. Consequently, the approach to breast-feeding requires a humble respect for the emotional, physical, and time commitment involved, as well as skill grounded in the experience of our ancestors. There are numerous books, videos, websites, support groups, and health professionals available to guide a woman and her family through this lifestyle practice. A referral listing with some of these resources is available at the end of this chapter.

SEE ALSO: Lactation, Pregnancy

Suggested Reading

American Academy of Family Physicians. (2001, Fall). *Position paper: Breastfeeding.* Leawood, KS: Author.

American Academy of Pediatrics. (1997). Policy statement: Breastfeeding and the use of human milk (RE9729). *Pediatrics, 100*(6), 1035–1039.

Association of Women's Health, Obstetric and Neonatal Nurses (AWHONN), & Johnson & Johnson Consumer Products, Inc. (1996). *Compendium of postpartum care* (1st ed., pp. 1.24–1.27). Skillman, NJ: Johnson & Johnson Consumer Products.

Bronner, Y. L., Bentley, M., Caulfield, L., et al. (1996). *Influence of work or school on breastfeeding among urban WIC participants.* Abstracts of the 124th Annual Meeting of the American Public Health Association, New York.

Kleinman, R. E. (Ed.). (1998). *Pediatric nutrition handbook* (4th ed.). Elk Grove Village, IL: American Academy of Pediatrics, Committee on Nutrition.

La Leche League International. (1987). *The womanly art of breastfeeding* (4th rev. ed.). Markham, Ontario, Canada: Penguin Books.

Lawrence, R. A., & Robert, M. (1999). *Breastfeeding: A guide for the medical profession* (5th ed.). St. Louis, MO: C. V. Mosby.

Mohrbacher, N., & Stock, J. (1997). *The breastfeeding answer book* (rev. ed.). La Leche League International.

Renfrew, M., Fisher, C., & Arms, S. (2000). *The new bestfeeding. Getting breastfeeding right for you.* Berkeley, CA: Celestial Arts.

Riordan, J., & Auerbach, K. G. (1999). *Breastfeeding & human lactation* (2nd ed.). Sudbury, MA: Jones & Bartlett.

Robin, P. (1998). *When breastfeeding is not an option. A reassuring guide for loving parents.* Rocklin, CA: Prima.

UNICEF & WHO. (1990). *Innocenti Declaration on the Protection, Promotion and Support of Breastfeeding.* Florence, Italy: Author.

U.S. Department of Health and Human Services, Office of Women's Health. (2000). *HHS blueprint for action on breastfeeding.*

Suggested Resources

www.breastfeeding.com
www.lalecheleague.com
www.nursingmothers.com
www.waba.org.br/

KARIN SMALL WURAPA

Breast Implant *see* Breast Augmentation

Breast Lumps
A woman's breast is composed internally of multiple glandular lobules and ducts surrounded by fatty tissue, and therefore by the nature of its design is often of lobular texture. Most women notice irregularities or lumps in their breast from time to time. Fortunately, the overwhelming majority of these breast lumps (80–90%) are benign. Despite this, almost all women will, at some point in their lifetime, be confronted with breast cancer either personally or in a friend or relative. In the United States, the current statistics are that 1 in 8 women will develop breast cancer in her lifetime and that 1 in 30 women will die of breast cancer. This may become a more sobering statistic the next time you are in a room with 30 or more women. Though

breast cancer survival is now actually improving as earlier breast cancer detection and improved cure rates take effect, for women, breast cancer remains the second leading cause of cancer-related deaths in the United States. It is important for each woman to have a good understanding of the changes in her breast and when and why it is important to see a medical professional early if a suspicious breast lump occurs.

Although normal changes and breast lumps can occur at any time, there are certain patterns that occur at specific times or ages in a woman's life. Before puberty, breast bud development in a young girl may occur one side at a time or one side larger than the other. This lump asymmetry is generally normal development. After breast development and with menstruation, many women experience cyclical changes in their breasts as hormone levels fluctuate monthly. Young women may develop smooth, rubbery, mobile, oval lumps in their breast known as fibroadenomas. Fibroadenomas are the most common breast tumor in young women, found especially from age 15 to 30, though they may occur later in life as well. Fibroadenomas are benign and do not carry an increased risk of cancer but may increase rapidly in size. Pregnancy and lactation may also result in irregular breast changes as milk-producing glands become engorged. Occasionally a duct may become plugged or infected resulting in a painful, tender, red mass. Breast infection or abscess may also rarely occur when a woman is not breast-feeding and may require antibiotics or surgical drainage. Trauma to the breast can cause bruising and internal bleeding resulting in a hematoma, or later a residual lump effect known as fat necrosis. The most extreme examples of cyclical hormonal breast changes are often labeled as "fibrocystic changes." These fibrocystic breast changes are worse 7–10 days before menses, may be painful, swollen, and tender, and often produce irregular ropey or granular lumps, which improve following menses. These lumps may be multiple and involve both breasts. Fibrocystic changes are more prominent from ages 30 to 50 and may become worse as menopause approaches. Treatment of severe, painful fibrocystic changes usually involves the use of salt restriction, avoiding caffeine, tea, and chocolate, and in some cases the use of hormone manipulation. These changes generally resolve after menopause if hormone replacement is not being used. Breast cysts, as a component of fibrocystic changes, are fluid-filled sacs that may become quite tense, firm, and painful and may mimic solid lumps. Breast cysts are most common from age 40 to menopause. After menopause, a breast lump may be any of the above benign conditions; however, the likelihood that it is cancer becomes much higher. Though breast cancer is more common as a woman grows older, it can occur even at a young age.

Any breast lump that persists through one menstrual cycle or any new lump in a postmenopausal woman should be brought to the attention of a medical professional. Workup usually consists of a thorough history, a clinical breast exam, and mammograms. This may be supplemented by ultrasound of the breast and/or fine-needle aspiration (withdrawal of fluid or solid cell material). Core biopsy (large-needle tissue sampling) or excisional biopsy (complete removal of the lump) is often indicated to rule out malignancy. Cysts often respond to simple needle aspiration. Recurrent or bloody cysts are generally an indication for excision. Only rarely are such imaging studies as magnetic resonance imaging (MRI) or positron emission tomography (PET) scanning indicated. Breast cancer can present as a lump (often painless) or as a suspicious finding on a mammogram. Other changes such as skin dimpling, bloody nipple discharge, new nipple retraction, or lumps under the armpit can occur with breast cancer. Some breast cancers are not detectable on physical examination and others are not seen on mammogram, thus both methods must be used to evaluate for the possibility of cancer.

Although some breast cancers (5–10%) are inherited (mutations in the *BRCA1* and *BRCA2* genes are identified examples), most breast cancers appear to occur sporadically. Certain conditions are associated with a higher incidence of cancer. These include risks related to family history such as breast cancer in more than one first-degree relative (sister or mother), breast cancer in a first-degree relative before age 50, bilateral breast cancer in a first-degree relative, or known *BRCA1* or *BRCA2* gene mutations in the family. Other risks are related to long-term unopposed estrogen exposure such as early onset of menses, lack of breast-feeding, no pregnancies or late pregnancies, obesity, or late menopause. The majority of benign fibrocystic lumps are not associated with any increased risk of breast cancer. However, certain benign diagnoses such as the hyperplasia seen with intraductal papilloma and sclerosing adenosis, and atypical hyperplasia are associated with an increased risk of breast cancer.

Breast cancer usually arises from two normal cell types in the breast, ductal cells that form the tubes that carry milk out to the nipple, and lobular cells that form the actual milk-producing glands of the breast. Breast cancer can either be noninvasive, so-called ductal carcinoma in situ (DCIS) or lobular carcinoma in situ (LCIS), or it can be invasive, so-called ductal carcinoma or lobular carcinoma. All of these are classified in the broad category of glandular cancers or so-called adenocarcinomas. DCIS is felt to be precancerous with a high likelihood of becoming invasive cancer with time. It thus requires aggressive treatment. LCIS behaves differently and while its presence is associated with a higher risk of cancer in either breast, it does not appear to become invasive cancer itself. Close monitoring or very rarely more aggressive prophylactic bilateral mastectomy is used. Ductal invasive carcinoma and lobular invasive carcinoma are malignant cancers that can potentially metastasize (spread to other parts of the body) and are treated similarly with aggressive therapy.

Breast cancer treatment occurs at two very different levels. The first is local treatment that involves treatment to the affected breast and its draining lymph nodes in the adjacent armpit (axilla). The second is systemic treatment that involves treatment to the rest of the body away from the breast, where cancer cells may spread in advanced cases. Surgery and radiation are both local treatments to treat only the breast and axilla. Chemotherapy and hormonal therapy are systemic treatments and are used to treat the rest of the body, if the risk of metastasis outside the breast is high enough.

Local breast cancer treatment generally involves two options. The first option is breast conservation treatment that consists of surgical lumpectomy and axillary node excision combined with radiation to the breast and axilla. This conserves most of the breast. The second option is mastectomy that involves removal of the entire breast and axillary node excision. Mastectomy may be accompanied by immediate or delayed reconstruction of the breast with plastic surgery. Radiation is often not required with mastectomy. In either option an important principle is the treatment of the entire affected breast, including the breast tissue that is away from the cancer itself, by either removing it (mastectomy) or irradiating it (radiation). The axillary node excision with either of the two above options can be accomplished in several ways depending on the clinical situation. One option is sentinel node biopsy where one or two axillary lymph nodes identified in a special technique as the first (or sentinel) node(s) to drain the breast are removed and inspected. If no cancer is found in the sentinel node the procedure is over. If the sentinel node is found to contain cancer, more axillary nodes are then removed. Axillary node excision may also be accomplished by axillary node sampling, in which at least 10 nodes are removed, or by formal axillary node dissection, in which most of the axillary nodes are removed. In many situations breast conservation treatment with axillary node excision and mastectomy with axillary node excision may be equivalent treatment in terms of both overall survival and local recurrence rates.

The prognosis and severity of breast cancer depends on whether the tumor has spread to the axillary lymph nodes or other areas of the body and on the original size of the tumor. The term grade refers to the microscopic appearance and aggressiveness of the cancer cells themselves and ranges from grade 1 (best) to grade 3 (worst). The term stage refers to the extent of the spread of the cancer and ranges from stage I (small tumor with no spread to the lymph nodes or elsewhere: excellent prognosis with proper local treatment) to stage IV (distant metastases: very poor prognosis even with aggressive local and systemic treatment). Other factors such as the patient's age and menopausal status, total number of lymph nodes involved with cancer, vascular or lymphatic invasion, estrogen and progesterone receptor status, DNA ploidy, S phase fraction, and HER-2/*neu* and p53 status also affect prognosis and the need for possible systemic treatment.

Systemic treatment, if indicated, is either chemotherapy or hormonal therapy or both. Chemotherapy is usually given primarily intravenously using a combination of different drugs in cycles often as an outpatient usually for 4–6 cycles lasting from 3 to 6 months. Recently, newer medications used to treat the side effects of chemotherapy have dramatically improved the tolerance for this type of treatment. Hormonal therapy in oral pill form (tamoxifen or aromatase inhibitors) is often indicated as systemic treatment for certain tumors or age groups.

The key to better breast cancer cure rates is early detection and treatment. For early breast cancer detection and as part of a healthy lifestyle, all women should practice a triple approach: monthly breast self-examination (beginning at age 20 and taught by a medical professional), yearly breast clinical examinations (beginning at age 25–30 and performed by a qualified medical professional), and routine screening mammography (beginning at age 35–40). Women at higher risk for breast cancer should seek and follow the advice of a breast care specialist for lifetime surveillance.

SEE ALSO: Body image, Breast cancer, Breast examination, Hormone replacement therapy, Mammary glands, Mammography, Mastectomy, Menopause

Suggested Reading

Love, S. M. (2000). *Dr. Susan Love's breast book.* Cambridge, MA: Perseus.

Winchester, D. P., & Cox, J. D. (1998). Standards for diagnosis and management of invasive breast carcinoma. *CA: A Cancer Journal for Clinicians, 48,* 83–107.

Suggested Resources

American Cancer Society. www.cancer.org
www.breastcancer.about.com
National Cancer Institute. www.cancer.gov

DAVID JOSEPH LOURIÉ

Breast Reconstruction

Breast cancer can be an extremely devastating disease. One in every seven women will develop breast cancer in her lifetime. There are many options that are available for treating breast cancer. The emphasis over the last decade has leaned toward breast conservation. However, there are times when a mastectomy is the only option. This leaves the woman with an asymmetry or deformity that she may find intolerable. The more conservative treatments may also leave a significant deformity.

Women now have options after mastectomy and/or lumpectomy. In the past decade, these options have been offered before the procedure is performed. Breast reconstruction is not for everyone. A diagnosis of breast cancer may be so overwhelming that a woman does not wish to think about this particular aspect prior to surgery or even ever. A thorough discussion between the patient and her doctor will help her decide what the best option is for her. She may also consider other options, such as radiation and/or chemotherapy.

The decision to have breast reconstruction may not stem from the fact that a woman is missing a breast. It is often more convenience-oriented than aesthetic. Women do not want to put a prosthesis into their bra everyday. They want to be able to wear a bathing suit, a low-cut dress, or an open blouse without having to worry about the prosthesis being seen. In addition, putting a prosthesis on everyday reminds them daily about their breast cancer.

The goal of breast reconstruction is to create a breast that looks and feels as natural as possible. However, it should be remembered that the reconstructed breast will never be the same as the natural one.

There is no evidence that reconstruction will increase the chance for recurrence nor hide recurrence.

Breast reconstruction requires a minimum of two procedures and may be performed either immediately at the time of mastectomy or at a later time. If delayed, it is often because the woman does not want to think about reconstruction. Other health issues may also preclude her from undergoing breast reconstruction immediately. In the majority of cases, women elect to have immediate reconstruction.

Surgery for reconstruction can be accomplished using one's own tissue (known as autologous) or using skin expansion. When a mastectomy is performed, there is a shortage of skin/tissue. If tissue expansion is used, a balloon expander is placed underneath the muscle of the chest wall. After healing, the tissue is gradually expanded in the office. When desired expansion is obtained, the second phase of the reconstruction is performed. The expander is removed, a permanent implant is placed, and a nipple is created (if desired). In addition, the opposite side may have to be adjusted for symmetry; for instance, if the opposite side is very large.

If autologous tissue is used, a skin flap from the back, abdomen, or buttocks is taken. This flap consists of skin, fat, and muscle with its own blood supply. In short, the tissue is elevated and transferred to the mastectomy site and a breast mound created. This is a more complicated procedure. It requires much more time, increases the possibility that blood transfusions will be needed, and necessitates a much longer hospital stay. However, the advantage is that there is no foreign body associated and there is usually less need for adjustment of the opposite side. The second stage entails nipple reconstruction and possible adjustment of the opposite side. One of the most popular flaps is called the "tummy tuck" or TRAM flap. This procedure entails taking skin, fat, and muscle from the bottom of the abdomen and transferring them up into the mastectomy site and creating a breast mound. The end result is the creation of a breast and the provision of a tummy tuck as the skin and so forth were removed from that site.

There are always risks and complications that can occur. These should be discussed in detail with the reconstructive surgeon. Any woman undergoing mastectomy should be told of all available options so that she and the team that is caring for her can make the best individual decision.

SEE ALSO: Body image, Breast cancer, Breast lumps, Mammography, Mastectomy

Suggested Reading

De Castro, C. C. (2002). Mastopexy and breast reduction. *Aesthetic Surgery Journal, 22*, 569–572.

Suggested Resources

www.plasticsurgery.org/public_education procedure/reductionmammaplasty.com

JANET BLANCHARD

Breast Reduction   There is a lot of emphasis placed on the size of women's breasts. Most of the time, the emphasis is focused on enlarging the size of the breasts. However, large breasts can be equally difficult for women. Usually the problem begins in early adolescence when puberty begins or after pregnancy, particularly when a woman has gained a great deal of weight. When a young teenager has large breasts, peers often make fun of them or make rude comments. This can create psychological problems that may persist into adulthood. In addition, a significant weight gain can cause the breasts to enlarge. The medical term for this is breast hypertrophy or macromastia. The increased weight from macromastia can cause a lot of stress on the shoulder, eventually creating poor posture which may lead to shoulder, neck, and back pain. In addition, women find it difficult to exercise due to "bouncing" and increased weight on their shoulders. Other symptoms may include skin irritation under the breasts, indentations in the shoulders from the bra, and a feeling of self-consciousness about the size of the breasts.

What are the options for correcting macromastia? First, height and weight criteria should be examined. If a woman is grossly overweight, a weight reduction program should be initiated. This may help to bring the size of the breasts into the correct proportion. If the breasts are still large, a surgical procedure can then be planned. There are literally thousands of such breast reduction surgeries performed every year.

Breast reduction surgery, also known as reduction mammoplasty, is a procedure designed to remove the excess breast tissue. When the breasts enlarge, the nipple and pigmented area around the nipple (the areola) descend down below a "normal" plane. In addition to removing the excess breast tissue, this procedure also raises this complex into a normal position. This involves a great deal of incisions and suturing. It is performed in an operating room under a general anesthetic, usually on a same-day surgical basis.

There are a variety of procedures available for reduction mammoplasty, which often results in a fair amount of scarring; this scarring is permanent, but may fade in 1–2 years. This is probably the drawback to this operation. However, women are often thankful to have the increased weight off their chest, back, and so forth, so that they consider this a fair trade off. It is very helpful to see pictures prior to surgery and these are usually shared with the woman at the initial consultation with the plastic surgeon. Additionally, in the last few years, a great deal of emphasis has been placed on reducing the scarring and preserving nipple sensation and increasing the ability to breast-feed if a woman is still within the childbearing age.

The type of procedure used will be discussed and determined during the initial consultation with the plastic surgeon. Although many incisions are necessary, there is usually not enough blood loss to necessitate a blood transfusion.

The timing for breast reduction surgery is individualized. However, if women are of the childbearing age and feel strongly about breast-feeding, the procedure should be postponed until after this period.

Some commonly asked questions include: How does a woman determine what size she wants to be after the operation? This is a decision that is made with the plastic surgeon. Factors that enter into this decision include body habitus and height and weight. Pictures are also extremely helpful and additional helpful information can be found on the Internet. Women who gain weight after breast reduction surgery will experience an enlargement of their breasts; the reverse is true as well.

Most insurance companies do not consider this a cosmetic procedure. However, they do set guidelines in order for this procedure to be covered. They will usually allow payment if more than 500 g or 1 lb is removed from each side. Preauthorization for medical necessity is required. This involves taking pictures, including height, weight, bra size, and symptomatology prior to the surgery. The insurance companies make the decision, not the doctor, as to whether this meets the criteria. Breast reduction surgery can be an extremely rewarding operation. However, a thorough consultation, examination, and understanding of the details of surgery should take place prior to making this commitment.

SEE ALSO: Body image, Mammary glands, Mammography, Mastectomy

Bulimia Nervosa

Suggested Resources

www.plasticsurgery.org/publiceducation

JANET BLANCHARD

Bulimia Nervosa According to the *Diagnostic and Statistical Manual of Mental Disorders*, fourth edition (DSM-IV), eating disorders can be classified as anorexia nervosa (AN), bulimia nervosa (BN), and eating disorder not otherwise specified (ED-NOS). BN is characterized by recurrent episodes of "out of control" or binge eating, occurring on average at least twice a week for 3 months with self-evaluation that is unduly influenced by body shape and weight. Unlike AN, BN patients are typically within the normal weight range or mildly overweight. Although not during a binge, they do restrict their total caloric consumption between binges.

The onset of BN is usually in adolescence but may be as late as early adulthood. Estimates of lifetime prevalence among women range from 1.1% to 4.2%, with the male-to-female ratio ranging from 1:6 to 1:10. Eating disorders are more frequent in industrialized societies. In the United States, among non-Caucasian races, African American women are more likely to develop BN as compared to AN and more likely to purge. Biological and psychosocial factors are implicated in the pathophysiology but only partially understood. Increased endorphin levels are found in patients with BN after purging and may be likely to induce feelings of wellbeing. Antidepressants often benefit patients with BN and suggest a role for serotonin and norepinephrine. First-degree female relatives and monozygotic twins of patients with AN have higher rates of AN and BN. Families of patients with BN have higher rates of substance abuse, particularly alcoholism, affective disorders, and obesity. High levels of hostility, chaos, and isolation and low levels of nurturance and empathy are reported in families of children presenting with eating disorders.

The essential features of BN are binge eating and inappropriate compensatory behaviors including fasting, vomiting, laxative use, or exercising to prevent weight gain. Binge eating is typically triggered by dysphoric mood states, interpersonal stressors, intense hunger following dietary restraints, or negative feelings related to body weight, shape, and food. Individuals are typically ashamed of their eating problems and binge eating usually occurs in secrecy. In addition to DSM-IV criteria, the Eating Attitudes Test, Eating Disorders Inventory, or Body Shape Questionnaire may be helpful in diagnosis and assessment of eating disorders. Comorbid conditions include major depressive disorder or dysthymia, bipolar disorder, obsessive–compulsive disorder, sexual abuse, and substance abuse. Patients with BN have been described as having difficulties with impulse regulation. Medical complications are related to obesity, vomiting, and laxative abuse. Differential diagnoses include medical conditions like abdominal epilepsy, brain tumors, Kluver–Bucy syndrome and Klein–Levin syndrome.

The recommended treatment plan combines both psychotherapy and medications. Antidepressants are used to reduce the frequency of disturbed eating behaviors and to treat any comorbid depression, anxiety, obsessive–compulsive features, and symptoms of impulse disorders. The only medication approved by the Food and Drug Administration (FDA) for BN is the serotonin-reuptake inhibitor fluoxetine (Prozac). Several studies have demonstrated efficacy of other serotonin-reuptake inhibitors like fluoxetine, sertraline, paroxetine, and citalopram; tricyclic antidepressants (TCA) like imipramine, nortriptyline, and desipramine; and monoamine oxidase inhibitors (MAOI). Doses of TCA and MAOI antidepressants parallel those used to treat depression, but higher doses of fluoxetine (60–80 mg/day) may be needed to treat BN. Bupropion has been associated with seizures in purging bulimic patients and its use is not recommended. Lithium continues to be used occasionally as an adjunct for comorbid disorders.

Little long-term follow-up data on BN exist. Short-term success is 50–70%, with relapse rates between 30% and 50% after 6 months but the overall prognosis is better than that for patients with AN. Poor prognostic factors are hospitalization, higher frequency of vomiting, poor social and occupational functioning, poor motivation for recovery, severity of purging and presence of medical complications, high levels of impulsivity, longer duration of illness, delayed treatment, and a premorbid history of obesity and substance abuse.

The clinical practice guideline for the diagnosis and treatment of eating disorders is found on the American Psychiatric Association (APA) website. An abridged, up-to-date version is available at www.guidelines.gov/index.asp.

SEE ALSO: Anorexia nervosa, Body image, Eating disorders, Weight control

Suggested Reading

American Psychiatric Association. (1994). *Diagnostic and statistical manual of mental disorders* (4th ed.). Washington, DC: American Psychiatric Association.

American Psychiatric Association. (2000). Eating disorders measures. In *Handbook of psychiatric measures* (pp. 647–673). Washington, DC: American Psychiatric Association.

American Psychiatric Association Work Group on Eating Disorders. (2000). Practice guideline for the treatment of patients with eating disorders (revision). *American Journal of Psychiatry, 157*(Suppl. 1), 1–39.

Kaplan, H. I., & Sadock, B. J. (1998). Eating disorders. In *Synopsis of psychiatry* (8th ed., pp. 720–736). Philadelphia: Lippincott, Williams & Wilkins.

Kay, J., Sansone, R. A., et al. (2001). Eating disorders. *Hospital Physician Psychiatry Board Review Manual, 5*(2), 1–12.

KATHLEEN N. FRANCO
RASHMI S. DESHMUKH

Byrne, Ethel

Ethel Byrne, along with her sister Margaret Sanger, founded the first birth control clinic in the United States in 1916. Ethel and Margaret grew up in Corning, New York. Their mother, Anne, suffered from tuberculosis. Contraception, in addition to being illegal, was unheard of in the girls' devout Catholic neighborhood. Anne became pregnant eighteen times and had seven miscarriages. She ultimately delivered eleven children and was further incapacitated with tuberculosis after each pregnancy.

Ethel and Margaret's father, Michael Higgins, was a tombstone engraver by trade, but spent much of his time studying politics and social issues. The family lived in increasing poverty with each additional child. Their economic situation worsened when Higgins invited one of his heroes to speak in town. His hero happened to be an agnostic as well as a socialist. The local priest was horrified, and advised his parish to shun Higgins like the devil himself and to purchase their tombstones elsewhere. When Ethel was in her early teens her mother died of tuberculosis. She and Margaret spent the next few years caring for their father.

Ethel became a nurse and helped her sister (also a nurse) distribute information about contraception through a weekly magazine called *The Woman Rebel* and through a pamphlet titled "What Every Girl Should Know." Until 1965, states could pass laws (known as Comstock Laws) that made distributing this type of information as well as the use of birth control methods in some states a crime. While Margaret had been arrested for obscenity stemming from the magazine, the charges had been dismissed. But when the sisters opened their clinic in Brooklyn in 1916, they were treated far more harshly.

After they had treated 500 patients, police raided the clinic on the tenth day of its operation and arrested Ethel, Margaret, and a third founder, Fania Mindell. Ethel was the first of the three to go to trial in 1917 and she was sentenced to 30 days in the women's workhouse on Blackwell's Island. Ethel decided to go on a work and hunger strike during her sentence to garner publicity for the birth control movement. When she got to prison, the warden's wife assigned her a job waiting tables and cleaning the warden's quarters. Ethel refused and began her hunger strike. She issued statements to the papers every day. The publicity increased when the warden issued an order that she be force-fed. After 185 hours of the hunger strike, Ethel became the first woman in U.S. history to be force-fed in prison. The governor of New York, Charles Whitman, offered Ethel leniency if she would promise not to violate the Comstock Laws again. Ethel refused. Margaret, however, told the governor that she would ensure that Ethel did not work in the birth control movement again. Ethel was released from prison and, as her sister promised, did no more work for the movement. Ethel lived into her 70s while Margaret continued to fight for contraceptive provision and information. In 1965, the Supreme Court ruled that laws like the one that sent Ethel to prison are unconstitutional.

SEE ALSO: Access to health care; Birth control; Comstock Laws; Pregnancy; Sanger, Margaret

Suggested Reading

Gray, M. (1979). *Margaret Sanger: A biography of the champion of birth control.* New York: Richard Marek.

Werner, V. (1970). *Margaret Sanger: Woman rebel.* New York: Hawthorne Books.

Suggested Resources

Planned Parenthood Federation of America. (1998). Retrieved March 2003, from http:\\www.plannedparenthood.org

POLLY HAMPTON

Calcium

Calcium Calcium is an important component of bones and teeth. The calcium in bone is constantly removed and replaced, so getting enough calcium is important to maintain strong bones. Calcium is absorbed in the stomach and small bowel, but only about 25% of ingested calcium is absorbed. About half of all adults do not get the recommended daily allowance (RDA) of calcium in their diet, and calcium supplements are needed (see Table 1).

Calcium is available as carbonate, citrate, phosphate, gluconate, lactate, oyster shell, bone meal, and dolomite. *Consumer Reports* has done extensive testing of calcium absorption from hundreds of supplements and found that almost all dissolve well. According to these experts, there is no scientific reason to buy more expensive supplements that make special health claims. They recommended choosing a calcium supplement based on cost. Calcium carbonate, which is found in many antacids, is often the least expensive.

Patients often overestimate the amount of calcium they consume in their supplements. The most important information on the supplement's label is the amount of elemental calcium. The amount of elemental calcium by weight varies from 9% in calcium gluconate to 40% in calcium carbonate. When reading the label, also check the serving size: the amount of calcium provided is often based on a serving size of two or more pills.

Calcium is most efficiently absorbed when taken in doses of no more than 500–600 mg at one time. Calcium carbonate is absorbed best in an acid environment, and some patients with low stomach acid (e.g., patients who take acid-blocking medication) may not absorb calcium

Table 1. Recommended daily calcium intake (from NIH consensus statement)

Group	Optimal daily intake (in mg of calcium)
Infant	
Birth–6 months	400
6 months–1 year	600
Children	
1–5 years	800
6–10 years	800–1,200
Adolescents/young adults	
11–24 years	1,200–1,500
Women	
25–50 years	1,000
Pregnant and nursing	1,200–1,500
51–65 years (postmenopausal)	
Not on estrogen	1,500
On estrogen	1,000
Over 65 years	1,500
Men	
25–65 years	1,000
Over 65 years	1,500

carbonate well. In this circumstance, calcium citrate is preferred since it does not depend on acid for absorption. Calcium carbonate should be taken with meals since food stimulates acid output. For those who cannot take a pill, chewable calcium supplements are available (Tums, Viactiv) as well as liquid preparations (Citracal effervescent tablets). Calcium can cause gastrointestinal (GI) adverse events such as bloating, gas, and constipation. Switching calcium brands or changing from carbonate to citrate can often alleviate this side effect. There has been some concern that calcium supplements may contain trace amounts of lead. However, calcium itself blocks lead absorption into the bloodstream. Also, the amount of lead found in supplements is less than the amount found in many foods. In general, lead levels in calcium tablets are well below levels that are considered unsafe.

Vitamin D is essential for adequate absorption of calcium. The major sources of vitamin D are fortified dairy products (mainly milk) and sunlight. Vitamin D deficiency is common and occurs in up to 20% of people as reported in some studies. Those living in northern latitudes are at higher risk, as are lactose-intolerant people and the elderly. Vitamin D supplementation is often needed. The RDA for vitamin D is 400 IU which is the amount in an adult multivitamin, although many experts believe that 600 IU or, in the elderly, 800 IU is the appropriate dose. Calcium supplements are available with and without vitamin D. People in higher risk groups, especially the elderly, should take vitamin D in a multivitamin or with their calcium supplement.

Several medical conditions affect calcium absorption and excretion. As mentioned above, low stomach acid decreases calcium carbonate absorption, and patients with GI disorders (celiac disease or surgery with removal of portions of the stomach or small bowel) may not absorb enough of the calcium and vitamin D that they take in. Patients taking glucocorticoids like prednisone also have reduced calcium absorption. Parathyroid hormone regulates calcium absorption and excretion, and abnormalities of the parathyroid glands can lead to dangerously high or low levels of calcium in the blood. Some patients lose too much calcium in the urine. This can occur in patients with renal tubular abnormalities and in patients who are on high-sodium diets. Hydrochlorothiazide, a diuretic used for high blood pressure, decreases the excretion of calcium into the urine.

The most obvious and probably the most important benefit of calcium is the prevention and treatment of osteoporosis. There have been many studies of calcium and its effect on bone mass and risk of fracture. Almost all show a beneficial effect on bone mass and several have demonstrated significant reduction in fractures of the spine and hip. It is important to note that calcium alone cannot prevent the accelerated bone loss that occurs in the first 5–6 years of menopause. The relatively sudden loss of estrogen at menopause overwhelms any beneficial effect of calcium. Similarly, calcium and

vitamin D are not adequate treatments for patients with established osteoporosis, especially those with fractures. In these patients, other drugs are required in addition to calcium and vitamin D. Some drugs used for osteoporosis block the removal of calcium from the bones, like estrogen, alendronate (Fosamax), risedronate (Actonel), or raloxifene (Evista), while others stimulate new bone formation, like teriparatide (Forteo).

In addition to preventing and treating osteoporosis, calcium supplements appear to lower blood pressure, protect against kidney stones, and may reduce colon cancer. The reduction in kidney stone formation occurs because most stones are made of oxalate. Calcium binds oxalate in the intestines and reduces the amount of oxalate in the urine. People with calcium-containing kidney stones should talk to their doctor before taking calcium supplements.

SEE ALSO: Osteoporosis and osteopenia, Vitamins

Suggested Reading

Chapuy, M. C., Arlot, M. E., Duboeuf, F., et al. (1992). Vitamin D3 and calcium to prevent hip fractures in elderly women. *New England Journal of Medicine, 327*(23), 1637–1642.

Dawson-Hughes, B., Harris, S. S., Krall, E. A., et al. (1997). Effect of calcium and vitamin D supplementation on bone density in men and women 65 years of age or older. *New England Journal of Medicine, 337*(10), 670–676.

Heaney, R. P. (1996). Nutrition and the risk for osteoporosis. In R. Marcus, D. Feldman, & J. Kelsey (Eds.), *Osteoporosis* (p. 483). San Diego, CA: Academic Press.

Heaney, R. P. (2000). Lead in calcium supplements. Cause for alarm or celebration. *Journal of the American Medical Association, 284*(11), 1432–1433.

Optimal Calcium Intake. (June 1994, 6–8). *NIH consensus statement online; 12*(4), 1–31. http://consensus.nih.gov/cons/097/097_statement.htm#CDC97T1 // (Also in *Journal of the American Medical Association* (1994), *272*(24), 1942–1948).

Reid, I. R., Ames, R. W., Evans, M. C., et al. (1993). Effect of calcium supplementation on bone loss in postmenopausal women. *New England Journal of Medicine, 328*(7), 460–464.

CHAD DEAL

Cancer Around 400 BC, Hippocrates described the long, bulky veins spread around some breast tumors as resembling the limbs of a crab, hence its name—*karkinoma* in Greek and, later, its Latin equivalent *cancer*. Although cancer is not one disease, all cancers share one characteristic and it is the uncontrolled growth of cells.

Cancer

Our normal body is built of 30 billion cells. Each healthy cell while restrained to a defined space—with the exception of blood cells circulating in the body—reproduces (proliferates) and dies (apoptosis) in a meticulous concord with itself and other cells to keep the body as a whole. Tumors arise when the process of reproduction loses its harmony. Thus, cells proliferate without control and form tumors. Tumors are called benign or in situ if they remain in the assigned boundaries (tissue). If tumor cells acquire an additional capacity of breaking the tissue in which they belong, they become malignant and further capable of invading other tissues. Offspring of malignant cells travel through blood or lymph vessels and lodge in a distant site. Invasion of distant sites by cancer cells originated in other sites (primary sites) is called metastasis. Most cancer deaths are the result of metastasis.

The process of cell reproduction is complex yet controlled mainly by two groups of genes, proto-oncogenes and tumor suppressor genes. These genes together with all the other genes are carried in the DNA molecules in the core of each cell (nucleus). Proto-oncogenes are responsible for the stimulation of growth and their activities result in reproduction and cell division. Mutation of these genes therefore will result in overgrowth of cells. *Ras* and *myc* gene families are examples of proto-oncogenes involved in cancers of breast, lung, colon, and leukemias. Tumor suppressor genes, in contrast, are an obstacle to improper cell division. Nonfunctional tumor suppressor genes will allow inappropriate cell reproduction. *BRCA1, BRCA2,* and *P53* are examples of tumor suppressor genes involved in breast and ovarian cancers. Although mutation in these two groups of genes contributes remarkably to the development of cancer, involvement of other muted genes together with other, yet unknown, mechanisms may also be important for tumors to become malignant and further detach from its residence and spread to other sites.

In contrast to infectious disease where the time between exposure to the infectious agent and the occurrence of disease (incubation period) is usually measured in days, weeks, or months, the latency period—the time from exposure to agents causing or contributing to cancer (carcinogens)—for cancer can be estimated up to decades. Transformation of normal cells to cancerous cells requires a relatively long process of accumulation of several muted genes over time. Individuals with inherited (carried from parents to children) muted genes develop cancer at a younger age because they require less time for the carcinogenic process to be complete.

Apart from cancers caused by inherited mutations in genes, which accounts for about 5% of all cancer deaths, most cancers are caused by factors related to individuals' environment and lifestyle and are hence modifiable. Epidemiological studies investigating cancer occurrence in relation to the migration of human populations have delineated the relative importance of these factors on cancer occurrence. While genetic compositions remain constant upon migration, environmental and lifestyle factors are subject to change. One evidence of the major role of environmental and lifestyle factor in cancer is the observed variation in the risk of several cancers across socioeconomic groups. Cancers of the breast, prostate, colon, and melanoma are more common in affluent than in underserved populations. Some of the factors associated with differences in cancer incidence across socioeconomic groups are reproductive behavior (i.e., late age at complete pregnancy and less number of children associated with increased breast cancer risk) and nutrition (i.e., consumption of red meat and saturated fat increase risk for colon cancer). The opposite is true for cancers of the cervix, stomach, liver, esophagus (throat), and lung, which affect people of lower socioeconomic status at a disproportionately higher rate. The prevalence of some unhealthy lifestyle factors such as smoking (cancer of the cervix, lung, and esophagus), heavy alcohol consumption (liver cancer), unsafe sexual behavior (cancer of the cervix), and infection with cancer-causing viruses and bacteria (*Helicobacter pylori* and stomach cancer) associated with several cancers seems to be higher in less affluent populations.

Preceded only by heart disease, cancer is the second leading cause of death in the United States. It was estimated that in 2003, over 1.3 million new cases would be diagnosed with cancer, and over half a million deaths would occur as a result of cancer. Leading sites of new cancer cases are prostate (33% of all new cases), lung and bronchus (14%), and colon and rectum (11%) in men; and breast (32%), lung and bronchus (12%), and colon and rectum (11%) in women. In both men and women, lung and bronchus is the leading site for cancer-related deaths. The cancer-related economic burden to the society is substantial, with over $189 billion in direct medical costs and lost productivity due to the disease and to premature death, as estimated for 2002.

CAUSES OF CANCER

Examples of external factors that contribute to accumulation of muted genes leading to cancer are: physical inactivity, tobacco and alcohol, nutrition, radiation and chemicals, bacteria and viruses, medications, and reproductive factors. Although the exact biological mechanism for some of these factors by which they contribute to cancer remain elusive, results from epidemiological studies provide clear evidence of their major role in cancer causation.

Physical Activity

There is sufficient evidence of the role of physical activity on the prevention of breast (see Breast cancer) and colon cancer and probably cancers of the endometrium (lining of the uterus) and prostate.

Tobacco and Alcohol

More than 25% of all cancer deaths could be prevented in the United States if people did not smoke. There is clear evidence not only that smoking causes lung cancer but also that passive smoking is a major cause of developing lung cancer. Tobacco consumption is the main cause of cancers of the upper respiratory tract, esophagus, bladder, and pancreas as well. As a result, the tobacco industry and its practices of marketing addictive products to targeted populations have come increasingly under scrutiny in the United States in recent years. This has led to litigation and multi-billion-dollar settlements by the tobacco industry. Communities have turned to policymakers as a strategy to control both youth's access to tobacco products and the general population's exposure to environmental tobacco smoke.

While antitobacco efforts have led to a decrease in the prevalence of smoking in some populations in the United States and many other developed countries, we are observing a rapid rise in rates of smoking in developing countries. Consequently, an increased risk of smoking-related cancers in these populations in one or two decades is well expected. Since alcohol and tobacco consumption are closely correlated habits, investigating their association with cancer has been difficult in small studies. However, this difficulty has been overcome by pooling the data from 53 studies, with findings indicating increased risk of liver and breast cancer with higher consumption of alcohol.

Nutrition

Overall, abundant and routine consumption of fruits and vegetables contributes significantly to the prevention of many cancers. In contrast, consumption of red meat and saturated fat is associated with various cancers. These associations are established for cancer of the colon and rectum. Overnutrition during childhood that leads to disproportionate growth may lead to increased risk of cancer through adulthood. This has clearly been shown in epidemiological studies of breast cancer. Women who spent their childhood in a food deprivation period (e.g., during World War II) had a decreased risk for breast cancer when compared with women growing up in periods of abundant food.

Radiation and Chemicals

Ultraviolet radiation (sunlight) can damage DNA and cause melanoma—the most lethal form of skin cancer. Individuals with fair skin are more susceptible to the carcinogenic effect of sunlight. Radon, another naturally occurring radiation from the earth, is shown to be related to lung cancer. The risk is accelerated among smokers. Exposure to high-dose ionizing radiation causes various types of cancer. Demonstrated carcinogenic effect of some chemicals used in industries has led to a remarkable decrease or banning of these chemicals in many industrialized countries, while they are still available and used extensively in developing countries. Examples of these chemicals and their effects are asbestos (e.g., used in brake lining of vehicles and insulation material) causing lung cancer and more drastically among exposed smokers than nonsmokers, benzene in painting material causing leukemia, use of hair dyes causing bladder cancer, arsenic used in pesticides and insecticides associated with both lung and skin cancer depending on the mode of exposure.

Viruses and Bacteria

The only known type of bacteria that has been linked to cancer is *H. pylori*, which is associated with stomach cancer. Several viruses are established as main risk factors for cancer. Human papillomaviruses are associated with cancers of the cervix (see Cervical cancer), anus, and other genital organs. Hepatitis B and C are causally related to liver cancer. Despite the high prevalence of infected individuals with these bacteria and viruses, for some yet unknown reason, only some eventually develop cancer.

Reproductive Factors and Medications

Late age at first pregnancy, nulliparity (never giving birth), early age at menarche, and late age at menopause are factors associated with breast, endometrial, and ovarian cancer (see Breast cancer and Endometrial cancer). Hormonal replacement therapy (HRT) used for menopausal symptoms increases risk for breast and endometrial cancer. Estrogen alone HRT is associated with increased risk for endometrial cancer and estrogen plus progesterone HRT increases risk for breast cancer. Use of combined oral contraceptives (estrogen plus progesterone) decreases risk for endometrial and ovarian cancer and may slightly increase risk for breast cancer among younger women (see Breast cancer). Similarly, fertility drugs may increase risk for ovarian cancer. Children using growth hormones may be at increased risk for leukemia, and some drugs administered for lowering cholesterol may increase risk for cancers of the colon and rectum.

Low-dose aspirin has been shown to moderately prevent adenomas (polyps) in the large bowel. Adenomas are possibly always prerequisites for development of colon cancer. A significant reduction in the remission of colorectal adenomas in patients with previous colorectal cancer has been observed among those who use aspirin on a daily basis.

Cancer stage is the most important predictor of prognosis; diagnosis at early stages of cancer implies increased chances of survival, and in the case of many cancers, cure. Similarly, adequate cancer treatment and follow-up care are important to enhance chances of survival, and even chances of cure. Many cancers, including some of the most common cancers, such as prostate, colon and rectum, breast, and cervix of the uterus, are amenable to screening. Despite the high-visibility media campaigns, however, screening rates have remained relatively low. Financial barriers and lack of knowledge, among others, have contributed to disparities in cancer-related outcomes. The uninsured and underinsured, for example, are at an increased risk for being diagnosed at later stages of cancer, and for receiving disparate cancer treatment and follow-up care, further contributing to poor outcomes.

The profound effects of lifestyle and behavior modifications on cancer risk imply a greater ability to prevent cancer. In addition, the availability of and access to effective screening, therapy, and follow-up care are likely to greatly influence prognosis through early cancer detection, increased survival, and even cure. Together, these elements constitute the foundation in our fight against cancer. With significant strides in the science of genetics and its epidemiology, further progress is to be expected through that venue as well.

SEE ALSO: Access to health care, Agricultural work, Breast cancer, Cervical cancer, Disparities in Women's Health and Health Care (pp. 13–20), Health insurance, Health maintenance organizations, Smoking, Women in the Workforce (pp. 32–40)

Suggested Reading

International Agency for Research on Cancer. (2002). Weight control and physical activity. *IARC Handbooks of Cancer Prevention, 6.* Lyon, France: Author.

Kogevinas, M. (1997). *Social inequalities and cancer.* Lyon, France: International Agency for Research on Cancer.

Moradi, T., Delfino, R. J., et al. (1998). Cancer risk among Scandinavian immigrants in the US and Scandinavian residents compared with US whites, 1973–89. *European Journal of Cancer Prevention, 7,* 117–125.

Schottenfeld, D., & Fraumeni, J. F. Jr. (1996). *Cancer epidemiology and prevention.* New York: Oxford University Press.

Suggested Resources

Cancer Facts & Figures, 2004. American Cancer Society. www.cancer.org

TAHEREH MORADI

Cancer Screening Screening and prevention play a key role in the management of cervical and endometrial cancer, and have a more limited role in ovarian cancer. Breast cancer screening is covered in the entry on Mammography.

OVARIAN CANCER

Ovarian cancer is the fifth leading cause of cancer deaths among American women and has a very high mortality rate. The 5-year survival rate is 75% if the cancer is confined to the ovaries and decreases markedly in women in whom the disease has spread. Unfortunately, this cancer is frequently diagnosed later in the course of the illness, after the tumor causes compression of surrounding structures or ascites develop (fluid in the abdominal cavity). As a result, two thirds of women with ovarian cancer have advanced disease when they are diagnosed.

The screening tests for ovarian cancer have not been proven to be of benefit to average-risk women. Ultrasound is a potential screening modality and is very sensitive. However, it carries a very large false-positive rate that results in unnecessary invasive procedures. Likewise, neither the measurement of serum tumor markers (blood tests) nor pelvic examination are good tests to look for ovarian cancer due to their lack of precision in making the diagnosis. The pelvic examination can occasionally detect cancers, however, the early cancers are often not felt on examination because they are very deep in the pelvis and rather small. Pap smears may, on occasion, show malignant ovarian cells, but this is not a screening test for ovarian cancer. Routine ultrasound testing of women without symptoms has a very low yield in detecting ovarian cancer and generates a large number of false-positive results that require invasive procedures.

In summary, routine screening for ovarian cancer by ultrasound, serum tumor markers, or pelvic examination is not routinely recommended. Women who are at increased risk of developing ovarian cancer should discuss their situations with their health care providers.

CERVICAL CANCER

Cancer of the cervix is the most common cancer of the reproductive organs after endometrial and ovarian cancers. Nearly 13,000 new cases of cervical cancer are diagnosed every year in the United States, with over 4,000 deaths attributed to this illness. Pap smears have resulted in significant reductions in deaths due to cervical cancer. Interestingly, the incidence of cervical cancer is increasing in younger women. For example, in 1981, women less than 50 years of age accounted for 21% of all the deaths. By 1997, women under the age of 50 accounted for almost 44% of all the deaths. This increase is felt to be a result of an early onset of sexual activity.

Cervical cancer begins in the lining of the cervix, which is the lower part of the uterus. It develops over many years. The first stage of development is called dysplasia. Dysplasia is defined by the cellular change that occurs when the cells go from the normal state to the precancerous state. This occurs most often in women in their late 20s and early 30s. These precancerous changes can resolve without treatment or they may progress into the next phase, which is called carcinoma in situ. From this phase, the cancer cells may spread locally to nearby tissues or can enter the bloodstream or the lymph glands and travel to other organs. This more advanced form of cervical cancer is found in women generally older than the age of 40.

Several of the risks related to cervical cancer are related to sexual activity and include multiple sexual partners, early onset of intercourse, and infection with the human papillomavirus (HPV). Smoking increases the risk of dysplasia. Low socioeconomic status is another risk factor. Women infected with HIV have a higher incidence of HPV infection and their lesions are more aggressive. In fact, cervical cancer in a woman with HIV is an AIDS-defining illness.

HPV DNA can be found in more than 90% of all cervical cancers. Women who are infected with HPV before the age of 25 are 40 times more likely to develop cervical cancer than those who are not infected.

Cervical cancer screening is performed by means of Pap smears. A screening Pap smear should be done under optimal circumstances. Specifically, the Pap smear should not be obtained if a woman has douched, used any vaginal medications, or inserted a tampon within the previous 24 hours. Cells can be inadvertently removed as a result and yield a falsely negative interpretation. The health care provider uses a speculum to perform this test. The cervix is located and a cervical spatula is placed firmly against the cervix and swept around 360°. The purpose is to recover the cervical cells from within a certain area of the cervix called the endocervix. There are specific methods of preserving the cells once they are placed on the slide. The U.S. Preventive Services Task Force (USPSTF, which is an independent group of experts that weighs the evidence for making clinical decisions) found poor evidence to determine whether or not the newer technologies, such as liquid cytology or computerized screening, are more effective than the conventional Pap smear in reducing death from cervical cancer. These methods are new and are commonly used. However, it is important to note that the task force found the evidence insufficient to recommend for or against the routine use of these newer technologies.

As is common in medicine, controversy does exist with regard to how frequently women should be screened for cancer, at what age they should be screened, and what should be done to follow up the abnormal

133

tests. As reported in the media, there can be a false-negative reading of 10–30% on Pap smears. This means that they may be reported as normal when an abnormality does exist.

In 2003, the USPSTF presented an update of recommendations for screening for cervical cancer. The task force found good evidence from multiple studies that screening does reduce the incidence and deaths from cervical cancer. Evidence suggests that the benefit can be obtained by beginning the screening within 3 years of onset of sexual activity or the age of 21, whichever comes first. The screening should take place at least every 3 years.

The task force recommends against routinely screening women older than the age of 65 if they have had adequate recent screening with normal Pap smears and have no other risk factors for cervical cancer. It is important to emphasize that these particular women have had adequate recent screening. Women who have not had adequate screening with Pap smears should have regular screening at an interval to be decided in conjunction with her health care provider.

The USPSTF recommends against routine Pap smear screening in women who have had a total hysterectomy for a noncancerous disease. At the present time, the USPSTF concludes that there is insufficient evidence to recommend for or against the routine use of HPV testing as a primary screening test for cervical cancer.

The management of abnormal Pap smears is based on many factors. Up to 50% of patients have spontaneous resolution of borderline and low-grade lesions and do not require more invasive procedures. However, 20–50% of women with low-grade lesions have a more advanced lesion seen on colposcopy. Colposcopy is a procedure performed during the pelvic examination that uses an instrument similar to a microscope. It magnifies the cervix 8–10 times and allows for better visualization of the cervix, vagina, and vulva. The follow-up of abnormal lesions is based on many factors including history of prior positive Pap smears, HPV exposure, compliance with medical treatment, and sexual history. Women who are deemed to be at high risk may require more aggressive follow-up as compared to women who are at low risk.

In summary, for normal-risk women, Pap smears should be performed approximately every 3 years. She should make sure that she has not used vaginal medications, tampons, or douched during the last 24 hours. Women at increased risk, including previous abnormal smears, multiple sexual partners, early onset of intercourse, HIV-infected women, women of low socioeconomic status, and smokers, are appropriate candidates for more frequent screening. In contrast to the USPSTF, the American Cancer Society recommends screening beginning at the age of 18 years every year with the consideration of less frequent screening in low-risk women after three normal yearly examinations. Older women who have not had adequate screening should be specifically targeted for screening.

ENDOMETRIAL CANCER

Endometrial cancer begins in the endometrium, the inner lining of the uterus. Approximately 40,000 cancers of the endometrium are found each year. It is the most common gynecologic cancer; however, it has a relatively low death rate with fewer than 7,000 deaths every year. The peak incidence of endometrial cancer is between the ages of 55 and 65 years. Obesity, never bearing children (nulliparity), and a family history of endometrial cancer are risk factors. The other major risk factors are related to an abnormal balance between the hormones estrogen and progesterone. Estrogen causes growth of the cells that line the uterus and progesterone controls this growth. A prolonged period of stimulation of the lining of the uterus by high levels of estrogen results in more growth and a greater chance of cells changing into cancer. Therefore, any of the following may cause prolonged exposure of the endometrium to estrogen without the opposing effect of progesterone, thus increasing the risk for cancerous development. Age is a risk factor. The excessive use of estrogen alone without progesterones, tamoxifen use, late menopause, early onset of menses, and polycystic ovary syndrome can all result in more years of estrogen exposure, thus increasing the risk of the development of cancer. Hormone replacement therapy for women after menopause does result in some increased risk of endometrial cancer. The risk is very high when the estrogen is taken alone without the countering hormone progesterone. The addition of progesterone reduces the risk but does not eliminate it. Women who have a family history of breast or ovarian cancer are at increased risk, as are those who eat a diet high in animal fat. Women who are very obese may convert male hormones to estrone, a female hormone, in the fat cells, which can stimulate the endometrium and predispose it to cancer.

A woman's risk is reduced, as stated above, by the use of progesterone therapy to counterbalance the estrogen therapy. Combination oral contraceptives decrease the risk of endometrial cancer. Menopause before the age of 49, normal weight, and a history of having multiple pregnancies also decrease the risk of endometrial cancer.

Low-risk women without symptoms do not require screening for endometrial cancer. For women at high risk, however, endometrial biopsy, dilation and curettage (where the lining is removed from the uterus), or vaginal ultrasound are all potential screening modalities. There is no evidence to justify screening low-risk women with no symptoms. It is important to note that if endometrial cells are noted in a Pap smear report in postmenopausal women or atypical endometrial cells are noted in a women at any age, she should have further investigation. A major symptom that should prompt a woman to seek a medical evaluation is unexplained bleeding after menopause. Some women over the age of 30, but not yet menopausal, who have spotting between periods, prolonged periods, or extremely heavy periods, should also be evaluated.

SEE ALSO: Cervical cancer, Ovarian cancer, Uterine cancer

Suggested Reading

Barker, L. R., Burton, J. R., & Zieve, P. D. (Eds.). (2002). *Principles of ambulatory medicine* (6th ed.). Philadelphia: Lippincott, Williams & Wilkins.

Carlson, K. J., Eisenstat, S. A., Frigoletto, F. D., Jr. & Shift, I. (1995). *Primary care of women.* St. Louis, MO: C. V. Mosby.

Suggested Resources

The National Cancer Institute http://cancertrials.mci.nih.gov The National Guideline Clearinghouse Guideline Synthesis http://www.guideline.gov/COMPARISON/brscreen.5.asp

KATHLEEN WOLNER

Candidiasis *see* Yeast Infection

Cannabis *see* Marijuana

Capacity In the health care and legal settings, the term "capacity" is often used with respect to mental competence and the ability to make an informed decision regarding one's health care, personal matters, financial affairs, or legal matters. With respect to our youth, capacity is defined by age, and a minor is considered legally incapacitated until reaching the age of majority, which can vary from state to state. A youth's capacity to make a decision cannot be discussed independently of the context in which the decision is made—the subject matter involved, the governing law (whether state or federal), and the time in history. For example, the age one can enlist in the armed services without a parent's consent may differ from the age in which a young person can marry without a parent's consent, enter into a binding legal contract, or exercise the right to vote.

Even if a child has a mental or intellectual disability which continues beyond the age of majority and the individual does not have the ability to make reasoned decisions, he or she will be considered to have capacity or be competent in the eyes of the law simply because he or she is no longer a minor. Therefore, once he or she has reached the age of majority, a court proceeding must be initiated to have the individual declared incompetent in one or more areas of decision-making and a guardian appointed. Guardianship proceedings, which are referred to as conservatorship proceedings in some states, are a matter of state law.[1] Clear and convincing evidence is required to support a finding of incompetence or incapacity, because such a finding strips the individual (the proposed "ward") of his or her ability to make any binding legal decisions in the area, such as matters of person or estate (finances), in which he or she is declared incompetent.

In adulthood, an individual's capacity may come into question if he or she is diagnosed with a severe mental illness that is not controlled by medication—either due to lack of response to a medication regimen, lack of treatment, or lack of adherence to a treatment plan. One's capacity can also be diminished by an accident resulting in a brain injury, chronic drug and/or alcohol dependence, or an illness, which severely impairs awareness of the environment, intellectual functioning, and/or reasoning abilities. Electrolyte

[1] Understanding the terminology used in your state is very important; for example, some states have both guardianship and conservative proceedings, which are distinct and applicable in different situations.

Capacity

imbalances and even reactions to prescribed medications can lead to mental impairment and incapacity, but fortunately in many, if not most, of these cases, the symptoms are reversible if the cause is identified and treated.

A stroke which affects the areas of the brain which control the ability to receive and process information, or other conditions and diseases which interrupt or impair blood flow to the brain, may lead to diminished capacity or incapacity. Scientists are continuing to gain new insight into diseases of the brain and causes of dementia, such as Alzheimer's disease, which reduce an individual's ability to retain and process information accurately.

No individual should be judged to be incapacitated merely due to a disability, advanced age, or being diagnosed with even a progressive condition such as Alzheimer's disease. One's capacity or incapacity is a functional determination made in a particular context. Some areas of decision-making require a higher level of comprehension and reasoning than others. For example, in many states, the "test" of competence or capacity to make a will—for example, the required level of demonstrated knowledge and understanding—is lower than that to enter into a binding contract. Several instruments to measure capacity are presently available to clinicians, but there is no one tool that is universally embraced as a definitive measure of capacity, nor is it reasonable to expect that one reliable, practical, and feasible measure can become the definitive tool to address the many variables involved in a determination of capacity, which include variations in state law.

To some extent, the issues facing the parent of a child with significant disabilities will be different from those facing the family or caregiver of an individual who developed impairments as an adult or in later life. If the child is likely to need a guardian throughout his or her life, many states allow the parent to nominate individuals to serve as the guardian if neither biological parent is available. Many children diagnosed with disabilities may have enough cognitive ability to use other, less drastic legal means to designate surrogate decision-makers when they reach the age of majority. These include durable powers of attorney for finances and health care powers of attorney. Similarly, adults whose cognitive or reasoning abilities are diminished may have the understanding, insight, and willingness to take legal measures to appoint persons of their choosing to handle their affairs if they become unable to do so. While evaluating whether or not an individual has the ability and willingness to put some safeguards in place in the event that he or she does become incapacitated in the future, it is also important to pursue evaluation and treatment to determine if the individual's deficits are reversible or if further deterioration can be delayed or minimized.

Although, as stated earlier, a determination of incapacity alone should not be based on age alone, advanced age can be associated with a greater likelihood of incapacity. In 2001, women were approximately 58% of the population age 60 and older and 70% of the population age 85 and older. Since women have greater longevity than men, they are more likely to face a period of infirmity or incapacity. "Compared with men, older women are three times more likely to be living alone, spend more years and a larger percentage of their lifetime disabled, [and] nearly twice as likely to reside in a nursing home."[2] These statistics show how important it is for women to plan for their futures by formally designating surrogate decision-makers for both financial matters and health care while they have the capacity to do so.

When making the decisions of who to name or appoint in durable general powers of attorney, health care powers of attorney, and/or living wills, successors or alternates should also be named so that if the first individual named cannot serve, there is another person identified to act in his or her place. When making these very important choices, the "principal" or person putting these documents into place should make her decisions based on "who is best for the job" and whose value system is consistent with her own rather than automatically choosing her spouse, oldest child, or closest relative. Although it is difficult to contemplate being incapacitated and unable to control one's personal and financial affairs, by planning for the future, the individual is exerting more control over her future by appointing trusted individuals to act on her behalf.

SEE ALSO: Advance directives, Conservatorship

Suggested Reading

Bigby, C. (2000). *Moving on without parents: Planning, transitions and sources of support of middle-aged and older adults with intellectual disability.* Baltimore, MD: Brookes.

[2] Administration on Aging Fact Sheet: *Meeting the needs of older women: A diverse and growing population,* http://www.aoa.gov/factsheets/ow.html Retrieved May 31, 2003.

Kapp, M. B. (2000). Measuring client capacity: Not so easy not so fast. *NAELA Quarterly, 13*(3), 3–6.

Luisis, S. A. (2002). Living alone: When is the elder no longer safe? In Mark E. Williams, MD Peggy Keen PhD, RNC (Clinical Eds.), *American Geriatrics Society 2002 Annual Scientific Meeting CME. Medscape Conference Coverage.* http://www.medscape.com/viewprogram/1924_pnt.

Morris, V. (1999). *How to care for aging parents.* New York: Workman. National Academy of Elder Law Attorneys (NAELA). http://naela.org

Spar, J. E. (2000). Attorney's guide to competency and undue influence. *NAELA Quarterly, 13*(3), 7–11.

Suggested Resources

Association for Retarded Citizens (ARC). http://www.thearc.org/

JANET L. LOWDER
SANDRA J. BUZNEY

Cardiovascular Disease

Cardiovascular disease (CVD) is the major cause of death and disability for U.S. women—43.3% of all female deaths occur from CVD. Overall, one in five women have some form of CVD, but this proportion varies depending on age: only one in seven women have CVD at ages 45–64 years but almost one in three women have CVD at age older than 65. Although women develop coronary artery disease (CAD) on average 10–20 years later than men, because they constitute a much larger proportion of the population older than 65, more women than men die annually of myocardial infarction. In the United States in 2000, 505,661 women died of CVD, almost twice as many as combined death from all forms of cancer. Black women have a 71% greater death rate from CAD than white women.

Although the death rate from CVD in men has declined, the mortality rate has remained relatively constant for women. Several factors may be contributory. Because women were excluded from older research studies or their proportion was small, less information is available about optimal preventive, diagnostic, and therapeutic modalities. Second, women more often present with "atypical" symptoms of chest pain, which may appear noncardiac and because electrocardiographic stress testing is less accurate in women than in men, some physicians either disregard the symptoms or avoid offering the appropriate testing to diagnose CAD in women. Third, because CAD (the major contributor to

CVD) develops in women later than in men, some misperceive this as a protective mechanism. Women, even with documented CAD, are less likely than men to be evaluated for cardiovascular risk factors and to receive adequate counseling and treatment. Women are also less likely than men to be referred to or to enroll in cardiac rehabilitation programs, which provide education about risk factor modification.

Risk factors for CAD are comparable in women and men. The *risk factors shared with men* are: dyslipidemia (presence of abnormal, elevated lipid, or fat, levels in the blood), diabetes, hypertension, smoking, obesity, sedentary lifestyle, and family history. Risk factors increase with age and may worsen after menopause. More than 50% of women older than 45 have hypertension with black women having an 85% higher rate of ambulatory visits for hypertension than white women. Cigarette smoking is present in more than 20% of women >18 and more younger women are new smokers than young men. At age 55, more than 40% of women have elevated cholesterol, more than 55% are obese, and 25% of women report no regular physical activity. A recent study suggested that moderate-intensity physical activity such as walking is associated with a substantial reduction in risk of stroke when compared with physical activity done at an average pace. Diabetes is an increasing disease in women: 5–7% of women >20 years old have diabetes, 5–7% have prediabetes, and another 2–5% have undiagnosed diabetes according to the American Diabetes Association. Diabetes in women increases cardiovascular risk by three- to sevenfold compared with a two- to threefold increase for men. Risk factors must be identified and treated early because atherosclerosis develops over decades before it becomes clinically manifest. The American Heart Association/American College of Cardiology guidelines advise that pregnancy and the preconception period is the "optimal time to review a woman's risk factor status and health behaviors to reduce future cardiovascular disease."

A *risk factor unique to women* is the use of oral contraceptives. High-dose oral contraceptives of prior years increased the incidence of heart attack, deep venous thrombosis, and stroke. The main mechanism appeared to be stimulating clot (thrombus) formation in the heart or brain arteries and leg veins. The current oral contraceptives have much lower estrogen content and do not appear to increase the risk of myocardial infarction or stroke; however, there is still a twofold increased risk of deep venous thrombosis or pulmonary embolism. Women smokers who use oral contraceptives are more likely to develop hypertension, heart attack, and stroke than nonsmokers, a risk that increases with age. Therefore, oral contraceptives are contraindicated in female smokers older than 35 years.

MENOPAUSE AND HORMONAL THERAPY

Menopause is associated with a severe decline in estrogen levels that may worsen cardiac risk factors. Premenopausal women who had bilateral resection of their ovaries and did *not* receive estrogen therapy had twice the risk of myocardial infarction than those who took estrogen. Although menopausal hormone therapy was previously considered cardioprotective, a recently completed trial, the Heart and Estrogen/progestin Replacement Study (HERS I and II), showed no cardiovascular benefit in postmenopausal women with documented CAD. Risks included a two- to fourfold increased incidence of venous thromboembolism (vein blood clot) and more than 50% increase in the need for gallbladder surgery. Another major trial, the Women's Health Initiative (WHI) involving predominantly healthy menopausal women, had the estrogen/progestin component of the study stopped prematurely because of increased incidence of invasive breast cancer in hormone-treated women and an unfavorable global risk score. Therefore, current guidelines do not recommend hormone treatment for primary or secondary prevention of CAD in postmenopausal women.

PREGNANCY AND HEART DISEASE

Pregnancy imposes a 30–50% increase in the amount of blood pumped by the mother's heart to the uterus and the baby, especially after second trimester. Labor imposes extra effort on the heart because of large changes in the circulating blood volume. Normally, this increase in heart activity is well tolerated by the mother. However, certain patients with preexistent heart disease, such as valvular heart disease (mitral stenosis, MS), pulmonary hypertension (high blood pressure in the arteries of the lung), some forms of congenital heart disease, and patients with chronic heart failure, may not tolerate well the cardiac changes related to pregnancy. Therefore, in a few women with severe heart disease, pregnancy may be contraindicated because of high risk for both fetal and maternal morbidity and mortality.

Furthermore, some women even with milder forms of congenital heart disease have an increased risk of congenital heart disease in the baby. All women with preexistent cardiac disease should undergo cardiac counseling when pregnancy is contemplated. Most women with valvular or congenital heart disease will require antibiotic prophylaxis prior to delivery. Women with mitral valve prolapse and mild valvular heart disease tolerate pregnancy very well. (These are both conditions where the valves of the heart have abnormal shape/structure.)

A particular heart disease not well tolerated during pregnancy is rheumatic heart disease. Women constitute 75% of the population with rheumatic mitral valve disease. Women with moderate to severe rheumatic MS or aortic stenosis (AS) are at increased risk of worsening heart failure and fetal loss. These patients, usually with severe symptoms, are advised to undergo valve repair or replacement prior to pregnancy. In severe MS, the increased blood volume and tachycardia (rapid heart beat) associated with pregnancy and labor will aggravate the blood stasis (pooling or sluggish movement of the blood) in the lung, can aggravate pulmonary hypertension, and trigger atrial fibrillation (rapid/"fluttering" irregular heart rate) and acute pulmonary edema (fluid accumulation in the lungs), a potentially lethal complication of MS. In these situations, some women may be candidates for balloon mitral valvuloplasty (a procedure performed in the cardiac catheterization laboratory), which can increase the mitral valve opening and alleviate symptoms during pregnancy. Although surgery on the mitral valve can be performed during pregnancy, open-heart surgery increases the risk of abortion and fetal damage.

Another disease that poses an increased risk of cardiovascular manifestations in both the mother and the fetus is systemic lupus erythematosus (SLE). SLE can be exacerbated by pregnancy, can cause fetal death, and can trigger congenital complete heart block in the baby. Although it is debated whether SLE is triggered by pregnancy, clearly if the woman becomes pregnant during an active SLE flare, this can be a serious burden for both the baby and the mother. Most immunosuppressive therapy cannot be safely used due to serious fetal side effects; 20–30% of women with active SLE have miscarriage with fetal loss in up to 50%. The presence of high levels of specific antibodies during pregnancy confers a 5% risk of congenital complete heart block in the fetus; often the baby requires a pacemaker implantation immediately after delivery. One frequent complication of pregnancy in SLE is the development of pre-eclampsia (hypertension during the second half of pregnancy). This is more likely to occur in women who have history of renal disease, hypertension, diabetes mellitus, preeclampsia, and antiphospholipid antibodies. As a result of all these potential problems, women with SLE are encouraged to delay pregnancy until the disease has been inactive for at least 6 months.

WOMEN AND VALVULAR HEART DISEASE

Women have a higher incidence of mitral valve prolapse than men. However, most studies suggest that men are more likely to develop mitral regurgitation, the main complication associated with mitral valve prolapse. If mitral valve prolapse is associated with mitral regurgitation (backflow of blood through the mitral valve of the heart), guidelines recommend antibiotic prophylaxis for dental or other invasive procedures.

Women are preponderant in the very elderly population; they appear to have an increased incidence of calcific AS (narrowing and calcium deposition on the aortic valve), which is a disease of elderly age. Both in this condition and in aortic regurgitation (backflow of blood through the aortic valve), their heart remains smaller in size compared with men. In men, one of the criteria for replacing the valve is enlargement of the heart chamber. Women with aortic valve stenosis (narrowing) develop less ventricular hypertrophy (thickening of the heart ventricle muscle) than men and more often have preserved left ventricular function than men. Women who have even advanced severe aortic regurgitation often do not enlarge their heart at the same rate as men. Therefore, they rarely meet traditional heart enlargement criteria required for valve replacement. This results in operation at a more advanced stage and thus worse outcome. Thus, in women, the timing of surgical replacement of valve should be considered earlier than is often the norm, even if the size of the heart remains relatively small.

Endocarditis is an infectious or inflammatory disease of the heart valves that can lead to damage of the heart valves causing either thickening of the heart valves (stenosis) or backflow/incompetence of the valves (regurgitation). Bacterial infections of the heart valves occur more often in men than in women (1.7:1) and are often associated with injection-drug use, preexistent valve disease (most commonly mitral valve prolapse and artificial valves), older age, poor dental hygiene, long-term dialysis, and diabetes mellitus. However, women are affected twice as often as men with immune, noninfectious endocarditis. These patients usually have SLE, antiphospholipid antibody syndrome (APLAS), or, more rarely, rheumatoid arthritis (RA). SLE involves the heart valves in more than 50% of the patients and can cause valvular thickening, sterile vegetations (small growths on the valves/Libman–Sacks endocarditis), or valvular insufficiency. Once it affects the heart, lupus has a worse prognosis than if it does not involve the heart. Because of the high prevalence of valvular abnormalities in SLE, these patients should receive consideration for antibiotic (prophylactic) treatment for infective endocarditis.

CARDIAC ARRHYTHMIAS AND SUDDEN DEATH IN WOMEN

Sudden death can be the first manifestation of CAD in women. Because CAD is often the cause of sudden death, women develop this usually 10–20 years later than men in a pattern following the development of CAD. However, female survivors of cardiac arrest are less likely to have underlying CAD and more likely to have dilated cardiomyopathy (enlargement of the heart chambers), or a normal heart. Also, they are more likely to have valvular heart disease or abnormalities in heart rhythm as causal. They likely benefit as much as men from implantable defibrillators, a device that corrects heart rhythm abnormalities, but overall fewer women have been studied in the clinical trials involving these devices.

Women are more likely to have toxic effects from some antiarrhythmic drugs. Some of these drugs which result in ECG abnormalities predispose them to multiform ventricular tachycardia, a special form of ventricular tachycardia which is potentially life threatening. Because of this, women are more likely to be hospitalized for initiation of this drug therapy.

Less dangerous but more frequent are the supraventricular tachycardias (rapid heart rate initiated in the upper heart chambers). Women have more frequent supraventricular tachycardia than men (2:1 ratio) and their symptoms may be triggered by pregnancy or the particular phase (luteal phase) of the menstrual cycle. One frequent form of supraventricular tachycardia is atrial fibrillation (rapid, irregular activity/"fluttering" of the atria). The prevalence of atrial fibrillation is higher in men and increases with age, but because women survive longer, overall there are more women than men with atrial fibrillation. Atrial fibrillation in women is more frequently associated with valvular heart disease or cardiomyopathy (dilatation, meaning enlargement), while in men it is more often associated with CAD. Women who develop atrial fibrillation are more likely to die than men with the same condition. They tend to have faster heart rates than men when they develop atrial fibrillation and their risk of recurrence after cardioversion (regularization of rhythm) is somewhat higher. Their risk for stroke after age 55 is as high as in men and therefore they should receive long-term anticoagulation. This is, however, complicated by their higher risk of bleeding from the anticoagulation therapy; therefore, they need more careful follow-up and fine adjustment of their dosing.

STROKE IN WOMEN

The incidence of stroke increases with age. Because the average life expectancy is higher in women, each year 40,000 more women develop strokes than men. The long-term survival after stroke is better in women than men. Women make up to 60% of total deaths from stroke. Black women have higher death rates from stroke (78.1%) compared with white women, most likely due to a higher incidence of and more severe hypertension. Therefore, early treatment of hypertension, diabetes, and dyslipidemia (abnormal fats in the blood)—the major risk factors for stroke—can have great impact on prevention of stroke at older age in women.

PULMONARY HYPERTENSION

Normally, the pressure in the lung circulation is five times lower than blood pressure in the arteries. Any abnormal elevation in the arterial or venous pulmonary pressures can lead to pulmonary hypertension (elevated pressure in the lung circulation). Pulmonary hypertension is a multifactorial disease causing breathlessness on exertion, fatigue, and hypoxemia (lowered oxygen levels in the blood), and in severe forms is associated with high mortality and need for lung transplant. Because the pulmonary circulation carries blood between the right and the left heart, any disease of the left heart can lead to pulmonary hypertension and consequently any chronic disease of the lung or pulmonary

circulation will impose a strain upon and can lead to right-sided heart failure.

Primary pulmonary hypertension (PPH, also called idiopathic) is pulmonary hypertension of unknown cause. It is twofold more common in women than men and fourfold more frequent in blacks. Although the exact mechanism is not known, it has been hypothesized that the disease occurs in patients with a genetic predisposition for an abnormal proliferation of small pulmonary arteriole/capillaries and is triggered by certain environmental factors. Such factors include appetite suppressants, cocaine, and autoimmune connective tissue disorders such as SLE. Women comprise up to 75% of patients who have either taken appetite suppressive drugs or have systemic lupus. Anorectic drugs have been used for more than 30 years to help reduce weight in obese patients. The amphetamine aminorex led to an epidemic of pulmonary hypertension in late 1960s. The most recent ones, fenfluramine and dexfluramine, can cause pulmonary hypertension. These drugs have also been linked to aortic and mitral valvular disease (abnormality in aortic and mitral valves) and have been voluntarily withdrawn from the market.

Connective tissue diseases such as SLE, scleroderma, and phospholipids syndrome are also associated with pulmonary hypertension in women. The treatment of PPH consists of oral or intravenous vasodilators and anticoagulants (meaning blood thinners and warfarin). The oral vasodilators of choice are long-acting formulations of calcium channel blockers (such as nifedipine or diltiazem). However, only about one third of patients respond to this treatment. There are new therapies currently utilized, such as epoprostanol and bosentan.

AUTOIMMUNE DISEASES OF CONNECTIVE TISSUE AND CARDIOVASCULAR INVOLVEMENT

Connective tissue disorders are a cluster of autoimmune diseases in which antibodies are generated against certain cell proteins (part of connective tissue), which trigger a potent inflammatory response that particularly involves the arterial wall. Thus, cardiovascular involvement is very common in these patients. Because the autoimmune processes are stimulated by the high levels of estrogen in the childbearing years, diseases such as RA, SLE, sarcoidosis, systemic vasculitis (Takayasu and giant cell arteritis) much more often affect women than men.

The prototype of these autoimmune diseases is SLE. The cardiovascular involvement of SLE is ubiquitous and CVD is the most common cause of death in patients with longstanding lupus. Pericarditis, the inflammatory involvement of the pericardium (membrane surrounding the heart), is the most common cardiac problem in lupus (30% of patients have clinically significant disease), and can develop at anytime during the course of SLE. Although the clinical course of pericarditis is usually benign, it can acutely lead to hemorrhagic cardiac tamponade (compression of the heart by blood in the pericardium) requiring immediate removal or long-term consequences such as constrictive pericarditis (due to chronic thickening and calcification of the pericardium). Other than valvular involvement (discussed above), SLE can affect both the coronary arteries and the cardiac muscle itself. Middle-aged women with active lupus are more than 50 times more likely to develop myocardial infarction and this has been associated with disease duration, period of time treated with corticosteroids, postmenopausal status, and hypercholesterolemia. There is a high prevalence of subclinical CAD in women with SLE. It is due to accelerated atherosclerosis, inflammatory occlusion of the coronary arteries, and acute thrombosis, especially with high levels of autophospholipid autobodies. The cause of myocardial involvement of SLE is multifactorial but usually manifests as myocarditis (inflammation of the heart muscle by SLE). If SLE causes heart failure in the absence of CAD or valve disease, this may warrant a trial of corticosteroid therapy.

Antiphospholipid antibody syndrome (APLAS) can occur in the presence or absence of SLE. In the absence of other autoimmune diseases, APLAS does not cause myocarditis, pericarditis (inflammation of tissue around the heart), or conduction disease. APLAS may induce coronary artery thrombosis (blockage of the coronary arteries) with subsequent myocardial infarction and nonbacterial endocarditis.

RA and systemic scleroderma also produce an acute inflammatory pericarditis but more often are associated with chronic, small pericardial effusions (fluid around the heart) or calcification of the pericardium. Although RA has not been associated with myocarditis, rheumatoid nodules (tissue nodules which occur in RA) can localize to and destroy the cardiac conduction system causing heart block. Systemic scleroderma can involve the conduction system (system transmitting cardiac activity through the heart) but more often causes patchy microinfarcts (mini-infarcts). Individuals who

have a history of palpitations (very rapid heartbeat) or syncope (fainting spells) have a high risk of sudden death, warranting the prophylactic (preventative) implantation of cardioverter devices (devices that correct abnormal heart rhythm).

Takayasu arteritis is an inflammatory disease involving the aorta and its major branches. It is most often present in young women (women are affected 10 times more than men). The long-term consequences of this disease are hypertension, aortic aneurysm, and renal insufficiency due to renal artery stenosis (narrowing), and more rarely myocardial infarction due to coronary artery involvement. Giant cell arteritis is another inflammatory disease of the medium arteries, which affects older patients (usually over 70 years) and especially women (2–3:1 vs. men). The most common involvement is the temporal artery, near the eye, which manifests as severe headache or transient cerebral ischemic attacks (transient failure of blood flow to the brain). It responds very well to corticosteroids.

SEE ALSO: Acute myocardial infarction, Cholesterol, Coronary risk factors, Diabetes, Hormone replacement therapy, Hypertension, Oral contraception, Smoking, Stroke, Systemic lupus erythematosus, Venous thromboembolism

Suggested Reading

Mandell, B. F., & Hoffman, G. S. (2001). Rheumatic diseases and the cardiovascular system. In E. Braunwald (Ed.), *Heart disease, A textbook of cardiovascular medicine* (6th ed.). Philadelphia: W. B. Saunders.

Mosca, L., Manson, J. E., Sutherland, S. E., Langer, R. D., Manolio, T., & Barrett-Connor, E. (1997). Cardiovascular disease in women: A statement for healthcare professionals from the American Heart Association Writing Group. *Circulation, 96*, 2468–2482.

Mylonakis, E., & Calderwood, S. B. (2001). Infective endocarditis in adults. *New England Journal of Medicine, 345*, 1318–1330.

National Heart, Lung, and Blood Institute, NIH Office of Research on Women's Health, and Giovanni Lorenzini Medical Science Foundation. (2002). *International position paper on women's health and menopause: A comprehensive approach.* Bethesda, MD: Author.

Pearson, T. A., Blair, S. N., Daniels, S. R., et al. (2002). AHA guidelines for primary prevention of cardiovascular disease and stroke: 2002 update: Consensus panel guide to comprehensive risk reduction for adult patients without coronary or other atherosclerotic vascular diseases. American Heart Association Science Advisory and Coordinating Committee. *Circulation, 106*, 388–391.

Pearson, T. A., Bazzarre, T. L., Daniels, S. R., et al. (2003). American Heart Association guide for improving cardiovascular health at the community level: A statement for public health practitioners, healthcare providers, and health policy makers from the American Heart Association Expert Panel on Population and Prevention Science. *Circulation, 107*, 645–651.

Siu, S. C., Sermer, M., Colman, J. M., et al. (2001). Prospective multi-center study of pregnancy outcomes in women with heart disease. *Circulation, 104*, 515–521.

Smith, S. C., Jr., Blair, S. N., Bonow, R. O., et al. (2001). AHA/ACC scientific statement: AHA/ACC guidelines for preventing heart attack and death in patients with atherosclerotic cardiovascular disease: 2001 update: A statement for healthcare professionals from the American Heart Association and the American College of Cardiology. *Circulation, 104*, 1577–1579.

Wenger, N. K. (2002). Clinical characteristics of coronary heart disease in women: Emphasis on gender differences. *Cardiovascular Research, 53*, 558–567.

DAN SORESCU
NANETTE K. WENGER

Carpal Tunnel Syndrome

The carpal tunnel is formed within a bracelet of small bones located at the top of the wrist and a tough fibrous tissue known as the transverse carpal ligament located on the underside of the wrist. The median nerve and the tendons that flex and extend the fingers pass through this small tunnel. Carpal tunnel syndrome (CTS) is a musculoskeletal disorder that occurs when the median nerve, which runs from the forearm to the hand, becomes compressed or pinched at the wrist. This can cause pain, weakness, numbness, or tingling in the affected hand and fingers. CTS has been attributed to a combination of factors, including fluid retention from pregnancy, swelling of the tendon within the carpal tunnel, or from arthritis and certain hormonal disorders, such as diabetes, thyroid disorders, and during menopause. Repetitive bending and extending of the tendons in the hands and wrists, especially when done in a forceful manner for long periods without rest, can also increase pressure within the carpal tunnel. Such postures of the hands and wrists often occur in job-related circumstances in which the worker might perform repeated movements of the hands; hold the wrist in awkward postures, such as in a bent position; use forceful grips such as holding a tool too tightly because it is too big or heavy; or exert pressure on the wrist by using the palm of the hand as a hammer or by frequently resting the wrist on a hard surface. Frequent use of vibrating hand tools is also a risk for CTS. Individuals who work in assembly jobs using their hands, such as appliance manufacturing, meat, poultry, or fish preparation, sewing, grocery checking, carpentry, and other jobs where there is a combination of highly repetitive, forceful work have been found to be at increased risk for CTS. Frequent use of the computer keyboard has also been implicated in CTS. The highly repetitive and forceful work using awkward postures may also be encountered in certain hobbies, such as woodworking, knitting, or crocheting.

The most common symptoms of CTS include numbing, tingling, and pain on the palm side of the thumb and fleshy part of the palm near the thumb, the front and back of the index and long fingers, as well as the lateral side of the ring finger. In some cases, pain may also extend up the arm to the elbow and shoulder. Depending on the severity of the condition, symptoms may also involve hand weakness, the inability to grip items, and include changes in touch and sensitivity to temperature. The first symptoms, usually numbness and tingling, often happen at night.

It is estimated that approximately 3–4% of the general population in the United States has symptoms consistent with CTS. Although women are approximately three times more likely to develop CTS, it is also diagnosed in men. This increased prevalence of CTS in women may be due to the smaller size of the carpal tunnel or perhaps to jobs involving repetitive use of their hands. CTS is diagnosed through a combination of clinical examinations and specialized tests, usually involving electrodiagnostic testing of the median nerve in the wrist.

Treatments for CTS range from resting the limb and avoiding the activities that may be causing the nerve compression and symptoms, and immobilizing the affected hand and wrist at night using a rigid splint, to surgery to release the pinched median nerve. Recommendations for treatment are based on the judgment of the diagnosing physician and are dependent upon many considerations. More importantly, however, efforts should be placed on prevention, working collaboratively with employee–management teams in the case of factors related to the workplace to evaluate the work environment, including the workstation and the tools themselves; the repetitive movements involved in getting a task accomplished; and the possibility of incorporating rest breaks or rotating to different jobs.

SEE ALSO: Tendonitis, Women in the Workforce (pp. 32–40)

Suggested Reading

American Physical Therapy Association. (1996). *What you need to know about carpal tunnel syndrome: A physical therapist's perspective.* Alexandria, VA: Author.

Anderson, V. (Ed.). (1988). *Cumulative trauma disorders: A manual for musculoskeletal disorders.* New York: Taylor & Francis.

Suggested Resources

Mayo Clinic.com (2003). Rochester, MN. http://www.mayoclinic.com

NIOSH Facts: *Carpal Tunnel Syndrome.* (1997). Department of Health and Human Services, Centers for Disease Control and Prevention, National Institute for Occupational Safety and Health, Cincinnati, OH. http://www.cdc.gov/niosh

NINDS Carpal Tunnel Syndrome Information Page. (2001). Department of Health and Human Services, National Institutes of Health, National Institute of Neurological Disorders and Stroke, Washington, DC. http://ninds.nih.gov

MARIE HARING SWEENEY

Cataract A cataract is a clouding of the eye's natural lens. Depending on the degree of cloudiness, a cataract can cause a little blur in vision to near total loss of vision. The rate at which a cataract will progress is highly variable. A cataract is not a film over the eye that can be peeled away. A cataract is not visible in the mirror unless it is very dense. Vision can be restored only by surgical removal. Generally, waiting to have a cataract removed will not affect the outcome. A cataract need not be removed, as it is not usually harmful to the eye. The symptoms which patients experience will help to decide whether to proceed with surgery. The term "ripe" is an outdated term. Cataract surgery is necessary when diminished vision interferes with daily living patterns and removing the cataract is worth the rare risks involved.

The majority of cataracts are formed later in life as a part of the aging process. Some patients develop cataracts earlier than others. They are usually not inherited. Cataracts can develop as a result of injury, chronic eye disease, systemic diseases (such as diabetes), and side effects from drugs such as steroids. Exposure to sunlight has been implicated in causing cataracts. Rarely are babies born with cataracts. Cataracts are not caused by reading, watching too much television, sewing, or any other normal activity. Limiting visual activity will not slow down the progression of a cataract. Vitamins and herbal remedies have not been proven to prevent the progression of cataracts.

The only treatment now for cataracts is surgical removal. There are no medications that stop the progression of cataracts. Laser surgery at present is not used to remove cataracts. There are several ways to remove a cataract. In the past, the most common method was the intracapsular procedure, which involves removal of the entire lens and its supporting structures. Today, due to advances in medical instrumentation and surgical technique, an extracapsular cataract extraction is the preferred method in most cases. Through a 3.00- to 4.00-mm incision, a cataract is removed by breaking the cataract into pieces with what is called "phacoemulsification" or ultrasonic power and then the cataract is "sucked out." A cataract is like a grape. A circular opening is made in the front peel of the grape, the contents are sucked out, and the front and back part of the grape will remain. The technique leaves a membrane that helps protect the retina and supports the intraocular lens implant.

Once the natural lens is removed, a new one must replace it to focus the eye and provide clear vision. This can be done in three ways:

1. Spectacles (glasses) are worn obviously in front of the eye. This is the oldest method, and for quite some time, it was the only method. The glasses required after cataract surgery are thick; they give good central vision but the side vision is compromised. Objects are magnified by 25% which makes it difficult to become accustomed to these glasses. This is a very poor choice and almost never done presently.

2. Contact lenses are a better method. They can afford good central and side vision. Difficulty arises due to trouble inserting the lens, irritation caused by the lens, and maintenance of the contact lens.

3. Intraocular lenses are the best method. The lens is placed in the eye in nearly every cataract operation performed today. Excellent results have placed intraocular lenses well beyond the experimental stage. In the last 20 years, over 5 million intraocular implants have been placed in the United States. Under usual conditions, the lens need not be replaced. It does not have to be removed to be cleaned at any time. The intraocular lens affords vision that is the most natural.

Intraocular lenses that we use are placed in one of two locations. Most are placed behind the iris. These are termed *posterior chamber lenses.* This is the best place for the implanted lens as it is the position where the natural lens existed. The other location is in front of the iris. These are termed *anterior chamber lenses.* In some patients, this may be the only option if the membranes in the eye are weak.

Intraocular lenses may be inserted after a previous surgery when the patient did not originally have any implant inserted. Many surgeons feel that the placement of a lens as a second procedure is somewhat less satisfactory and more hazardous than placing it at the time of surgery, but many thousands of lens implants have been successfully placed secondarily.

In the "old days," cataract surgery involved prolonged hospitalization and "sand bags" for immobilization. Many people remember their grandparents undergoing this type of operation and are unnecessarily alarmed about surgery. With modern microsurgical techniques, cataract surgery has become safer and healing more predictable than in the past. The surgery is done on an outpatient basis.

The operation is performed under a local anesthesia, with monitoring of the patient's heart rate and blood pressure. Depending on the surgeon's preference, it can be performed with a "block" anesthesia injection around the eye or performed just with topical eyedrop anesthetic agents. This is called *topical anesthesia* and is becoming more popular. Injection is not required nor is a patch or shield as discharge. Generally, however, the patient will need to wear a protective shield at bedtime.

Patients will probably be examined the day after the surgery. Eyedrops are taken before and after the procedure. Normal daily activities can be resumed the day after surgery. Usually a new glass prescription is required and is given about 3 weeks after the operation.

As in any surgical procedure, an element of risk exists, and complications can occur during surgery or in the healing process in spite of the best of care (occlusion of a blood vessel, retinal detachment, corneal decompensation, macular edema, bleeding, and infection). It may be impossible to predict who may develop a problem.

A rare complication may be dislocation of the intraocular lens implant and it may need to be repositioned. Very rarely the implant may need to be removed. Infection is a very serious complication, which can significantly reduce vision after surgery. To help prevent this, eyelashes are draped and the face and eyes are washed with an antiseptic. Hemorrhage or bleeding is a complication that can range from mild to very serious. The worst bleed is called an expulsive hemorrhage and can leave the eye without vision. The hemorrhage occurs under the retina, away from the cataract operation, and is a random occurrence. Fortunately, this is very rare. A retinal detachment can occur in 1–2% of patients having cataract surgery. If a patient is very nearsighted or myopic, there is a greater risk of developing a retinal detachment. If a detachment

is detected early, it can be reattached surgically with usually little vision loss. Macular edema or swelling of the macula (the center of the retina) may occur in 20% of cases. Fortunately, in almost all cases, the fluid is absorbed and good vision returns. Glaucoma may occur after cataract surgery, but usually can be controlled with drops.

During surgery, the membrane that supports the implant may be too weak and part of the cataract may fall back into the eye. This has happened to nearly all cataract surgeons. The best method to handle this complication is usually to have a retinal surgeon remove the piece at a later time.

It should be emphasized that cataract surgery is very safe in the majority of cases. The patient is usually very happy with the results. Future developments will make the operation even safer and more rewarding for both the patient and the surgeon.

See Also: Aging, Diabetes, Glaucoma

Suggested Resources

The American Academy of Ophthalmology: www.aao.org
The American Society of Cataract and Refractive Surgery: www.ascrs.org
Facts About Cataract Surgery: http//www.nei.nih.gov/health/cataract/cataract_facts.htm

Kathleen Lamping

Cervical Cancer Cancer of the uterine cervix is an important worldwide health problem. The cervix is the opening of the uterus at the top of the vagina. Death rates in the developing countries from this disease are similar to death rates from breast cancer and lung cancer. In the developed nations, the widespread use of screening tests such as the Pap smear has both reduced the number of women getting the disease and improved the chances of surviving the disease. In this entry, we will review the risk factors for cervical cancer and its precursor, cervical dysplasia, the screening methods available, and the basics about the symptoms of cervical cancer and its treatment.

RISK FACTORS

Many women are not aware of the fact that cervical cancer is essentially a sexually transmitted disease.

Research has shown that a family of viruses called human papillomavirus (HPV) can infect the cells of the genital tract, and in some cases will lead to cancerous changes of those cells, particularly in the cervix. While almost all cervical cancers are caused by HPV, the great majority of women infected by HPV will *never* develop cancer.

The risk factors for cervical cancer are therefore the same as those for sexually transmitted infections such as: early age at first intercourse, multiple sexual partners, or having a partner with multiple sexual partners. Other risk factors may be due to impairment of the body's immune system from fighting the HPV infection such as: HIV infection or AIDS, immune suppressive drugs (such as those taken by patients who have undergone an organ transplant), and smoking.

HPV infections often occur without causing any symptoms. In some cases, a patient may develop small warts on the external genital area. Problems in the cervical cells leading to cervical cancer can take years to occur, or in many women will never occur at all.

CERVICAL DYSPLASIA

After a woman becomes infected with HPV, the virus can enter the cells of the zone of the cervix called the "transition zone." This is the area where lining-type cells of the vagina and cervix (squamous cells) join with the glandular cells in the inside canal of the cervix. This process can result in cervical dysplasia, which is the specific condition which is screened for with the Papanicolaou test, or Pap test. Although the Pap test is designed to look for dysplasia, it can also be read as "abnormal" due to other changes such as inflammation or the changes due to hormone shifts after menopause. For that reason, when a Pap smear is abnormal, an examination of the cervix with a microscope called a colposcope and actual biopsies of the cervix are done. Those biopsies will determine whether dysplasia changes are present, and whether they are mild, moderate, or severe.

Mild dysplasia, also called cervical intraepithelial neoplasia-1 (CIN-1), is often a temporary reaction to an HPV infection, and in 70% of cases will resolve with no treatment. Moderate dysplasia (CIN-2) and severe dysplasia (CIN-3) are less likely to resolve on their own, and therefore have the potential to progress to cancer. That process of progression takes 5–15 years, so the effective identification and subsequent treatment of CIN-2 and CIN-3 can prevent the development of cervical cancer in most women.

Treatment for cervical dysplasia often involves removal of the transition zone area of the cervix in an outpatient procedure called loop electrocautery excision procedure (LEEP), and is highly effective.

Another test that is used for screening is actually swabbing the cervical area and testing for the HPV virus. This test has been shown to be able to identify women who do not need to proceed with colposcopy and biopsies when the Pap smear has only a mild abnormality. In addition, it may be used in women over 30 in conjunction with the Pap test as a more effective predictor of risk for cervical cancer.

SYMPTOMS OF CERVICAL CANCER

Cervical dysplasia causes no symptoms in most women. In women with undetected or untreated cervical dysplasia over a period of time, those abnormal cells can develop the ability to invade other tissues and at that point are defined as a cancer. Invasive cervical cancer causes symptoms such as irregular vaginal bleeding, bleeding after sexual intercourse, or a bloody or foul-smelling vaginal discharge. Symptoms of more advanced disease include pelvic or back pain or swelling in the legs.

STAGES

All cancers are assigned a stage which is a representation of how advanced it is when it is diagnosed. The stage helps to determine both the treatment options and the prognosis. In cervical cancer, Stage I disease refers to cancer that has not progressed beyond the cervix. There are substages such as IA and IB to help differentiate between tumors that are microscopic in size versus tumors that may be very large, but still confined to the cervix. Stage II refers to cervical cancer that has spread off of the cervix onto the upper vagina or into the soft tissues that support the uterus and cervix at the sides, called parametria. Stage III applies when the cancer has spread farther down to the lower vagina, or out farther into the parametria to the side of the pelvis. Stage IV is the most advanced and applies when other organs such as the bladder or rectum, or distant from the cervix such as the liver or lungs, are involved.

Cervical Cancer

When a woman is diagnosed with cervical cancer, various tests will be performed to help determine the stage. These include a thorough pelvic examination, including a rectal examination, chest x-rays, blood tests, and often a CT scan of the abdomen and pelvic area. After her doctor determines her stage, the treatment options will be outlined. In some cases of advanced disease, surgery will be used to obtain more information prior to making a treatment plan. This may include cystoscopy (looking in the bladder with a telescope), proctoscopy (looking in the rectum with a telescope), or a more major surgery to remove lymph nodes that might be affected by the cancer.

TREATMENT

In the earliest cases of invasive cervical cancer, when there has been only minimal microscopic invasion of the cervix, the doctor may recommend a vaginal or abdominal hysterectomy (removal of the cervix and uterus, but not necessarily ovaries), or a cone biopsy, which is a cone-shaped removal of the outer cervix. Cone biopsy is usually used when a woman would like to preserve the possibility of childbearing. These are highly effective treatments and result in cure rates over 95%.

If the cancer is not microscopic, but is still confined to the cervix or upper vagina (Stages I and IIA), treatment options include radical hysterectomy with lymphadenectomy or combined pelvic radiation with chemotherapy. Radical hysterectomy involves removal of the uterus and cervix with the surrounding tissues of parametria and upper vagina together with the pelvic lymph nodes. Radiation includes external treatments to the whole pelvic area and internal treatments directly to the cervix, combined with a regular dose of chemotherapy to help the radiation work more effectively. Either of these treatments is effective in early stage disease, and one is generally selected based on other factors such as risks for surgery or radiation. In some centers in the United States, Canada, and Europe, an option to preserve fertility is available called the radical trachelectomy. This is a removal of the cervix with the parametria and upper vagina with the lymph nodes, but the remainder of the uterus is left behind, and can potentially be used for childbearing. This procedure may not be possible in all women with this stage of disease, but in selected women can be effective.

For all other stages of cervical cancer (Stages IIB–IV), the treatment that has been shown to be the most effective is radiation combined with chemotherapy. This is performed as was described for early stage disease, but may be given to a higher dose level or even to a wider area.

In some cases, a woman may undergo radical hysterectomy designed to be the definitive treatment, but then may require radiation after surgery due to findings at the time of surgery, such as cancer spread to the lymph nodes.

OUTCOME

Women with microscopic forms of cervical cancer have very high possibilities of survival—close to 100%. Once the cancer is visible, in the early stages (IB and IIA), the chances of surviving average about 85%. Stage IIB will have a 65–70% survival rate, whereas Stage III will have a 24–40% chance of survival, and Stage IV only 5%. Surgical options, the side effects from surgery and radiation, and the management of symptoms have all improved so that many women who undergo treatment for this disease are able to recover complete function and do not suffer from lasting side effects. The most important aspect of reducing the impact of cervical cancer, however, will be to detect and treat cervical dysplasia before it has the opportunity to progress. In the future, there may be a vaccine available to reduce the risk of infection with the HPV virus, or to help the immune system fight the HPV infection and decrease the risk of developing dysplasia or cancer.

SEE ALSO: Cancer screening, Colposcopy, Diethylstilbestrol, Genital warts, Human papillomavirus, Hysterectomy, Pap test, Pelvic examination

Suggested Reading

O'Meara, A. T. (2002). Present standards for cervical cancer screening. *Current Opinions in Oncology, 14,* 505–511.

Solomon, D., Schiffman, M., & Tarone, R. for the ALTS group. (2001). Comparison of three management strategies for patients with atypical squamous cells of undetermined significance: Baseline results from a randomized trial. *Journal of the National Cancer Institute, 93,* 293–299.

Wright, T. C., Cox, J. T., Massad, L. S., et al. (2002). Consensus guidelines for the management of women with cervical cytological abnormalities. *Journal of the American Medical Association, 287,* 2120–2129.

Suggested Resources

American Cancer Society website "What women should know about HPV and cervical health," http://www.cancer.org/docroot/NWS/content/NWS_2_1x_What_Women_Should_Know_about_HPV_and_Cervical_Health.asp? site area=NWS&viewmode

National Cancer Institute website: http://www.cancer.gov/cancerinfo/types/cervical/

ANNE O'MEARA

Cesarean Section

Cesarean section is the name of the abdominal operation used to deliver a baby. The most recent birth statistics from the Centers for Disease Control and Prevention (CDC) reveal that 24.4% of the 4 million births in the United States in 2001 were by cesarean section, meaning that 1 million cesarean sections were performed in 2001, making it the most commonly performed surgical procedure in the United States. This is also the highest national rate since 1989. The rate was 22.9% in 2000.

HISTORY

It is widely believed that the term cesarean refers to the birth of Julius Caesar, presumably by a surgical method. Historical documentation is rather sketchy about this subject, but there is evidence that Caesar's mother lived to hear of her son's invasion of England. This causes some question as to Caesar's birthing method because cesarean type births at that time were done only in an attempt to save the baby when the mother was dead or nearly so.

INDICATIONS

One of the most common indications, or reasons, for having a cesarean section is a history of a previous cesarean section. This is referred to as a "repeat cesarean." In 2001, 7.5% of all births were by repeat cesarean. This leaves 16.9% as the rate of primary, or first-time, cesarean sections. The most common reason for a primary cesarean is failure to progress in labor. Causes of failure to progress include the arrest of dilation of the cervix, arrest of descent of the head, or cephalopelvic disproportion (baby's head is too large to fit through the birth canal).

Other indications for cesarean section include breech presentation, twins (or higher order multiples such as triplets), fetal distress (the proper medical term is "fetal intolerance of labor" or "non-reassuring fetal status"), placenta previa (placenta blocking the birth canal), abnormal vaginal bleeding (possibly due to placental abruption which is when the placenta begins to detach from the uterine wall before the baby is born), and active herpes or HIV infection.

RISKS

Delivery by cesarean section is felt to be more risky for a woman's health than vaginal delivery and usually the recovery time is longer. Risks include postoperative infection (such as uterine infection or wound infection), hemorrhage, and associated blood transfusion, injury to other organs such as the bladder or bowel, and possible injury to the baby such as a cut during delivery. Additionally, having a first cesarean may increase the risk that subsequent deliveries will also be by cesarean. Cesarean section is also more costly than vaginal delivery.

PREVENTION

Some patients may be candidates for a vaginal birth after cesarean (VBAC). The success rate for attempted VBAC is about 75%. Furthermore, subsequent deliveries are also likely to be vaginal. However, subsequent trial of labor in the presence of a prior cesarean scar increases the risk for a tear in the uterine scar, referred to as a uterine rupture. The risk of uterine rupture is about 5 per 1,000 for spontaneous labor, but increases if labor is induced or augmented with oxytocin (a medication commonly used to make contractions more effective). A uterine rupture can lead to fetal oxygen deprivation or death, and possibly a maternal hysterectomy if the damaged uterus cannot be repaired.

Some ways to avoid a cesarean section include the turning of a breech baby to head down by a practitioner skilled in this procedure (called an external cephalic version). Limiting one's pregnancy weight gain to the normal range may help keep the baby's weight lower and possibly prevent a cesarean for failure to progress, although there are little data to support this statement.

IS THE RATE OF CESAREAN TOO HIGH?

Many authorities feel that the birth of one in four babies in this country by cesarean is too high. There are national efforts to try to lower the rate. One target that has been published is a cesarean rate of 15%. In general, there has a been a drop in the rates of VBAC over the last several years.

One reason cited for the sharp drop in the rate of VBAC may be due to a growing fear of the potential risk of uterine rupture, which though rare can occur suddenly without warning and be potentially catastrophic. This carries an increased risk of liability and may be a deterrent to some practitioners counseling patients to try VBAC.

Additionally, there is growing evidence that vaginal delivery may have long-term risks that can be minimized by cesarean delivery. For example, urinary incontinence, pelvic relaxation, and pelvic prolapse are conditions seen later in life that may require surgery or other treatments, and these conditions occur far more often in women who have delivered babies vaginally than by cesarean section. Some doctors feel that a woman should be able to request a cesarean delivery.

HOW MANY?

There is no consensus as to the maximum number of cesarean sections that a woman can safely undergo. Reports in the literature have been conflicting with the highest number reported as being 13.

Suggested Resources

www.drspock.com.

BRYAN S. JICK

Charismatic Healers For more than 2,000 years, charismatic healers have been healing people from mental, physical, and spiritual sickness. Common methodology used by charismatic healers includes: praying, laying of hands, anointing with oil, Biblical scripture, exorcisms, sacraments, and pilgrimages to holy places. However, specific methodology of healing can vary according to the beliefs of a denomination.

Charismatic healing is founded on the ministry of Jesus of Nazareth, the Son of God, who healed people from all forms of sicknesses. Jesus' healing ministry ushered in the charismatic movement, which acknowledges healing as an ordained gift from Jesus. In his name, charismatic healers miraculously heal people from colds, flus, asthma, cancer, and heart problems that are caused by sin, demonic spirits, or biological imbalances.

Generally charismatic healers are male, mainly because of the belief that the Bible forbids females from any form of ministry. However, some denominations believe that females can minister to people. Over time women charismatic healers have been known to miraculously heal people.

Charismatic healer methodology can vary for each individual healer depending on their denomination. Catholic charismatic healers rely more on prayers, sacraments, and pilgrimages to sacred sites. Protestant charismatic healers rely on prayer, laying of hands, exorcisms, and anointing the individual with oil. Protestant healers will begin by anointing an individual on the head with oil, which represents that the Holy Spirit is present. Once the Holy Spirit is present, the healer will lay hands on either an individual's head or on the area of sickness. While praying in Jesus' name, the healer will ask God to heal the individual and will cast out any demonic spirits causing sickness. The healing can occur spontaneously or require more visits with the healer until the healing is evident.

Although charismatic healers believe in their gift of healing, they cannot heal everyone. According to charismatic healers, people can only be healed if it is God's will. If a healing is unsuccessful, the charismatic healer will encourage the person to seek medical attention. While some hold that seeking man's help demonstrates a lack of faith in God's ability to heal, many charismatic healers believe that God uses physicians as instruments for healing as well.

Through religious techniques charismatic healers are responsible for countless miraculous healings. Although no solid scientific evidence exists to prove the validity of charismatic healers, their supernatural healings continue to occur around the world. Many people believe in their calling to heal and continue to seek the help of charismatic healers.

Suggested Reading

Anderson, A. (2002, October). Pentecostal approaches to faith and healing. *International Review of Mission, 91*(363), 523.

Suggested Resources

Faith Healing. January 26, 2003. http://www.wikipedia.org/wiki/Faith_healing

Faith healing. http://www.encyclopedia.com/html/f1/faithhea.asp

STEPHANIE CABRERA

Chemical Dependence

Chemical dependence is a primarily genetic, chronic progressive disease of the brain that is characterized by the intermittent inconsistent loss of control over the use of mood-altering drugs, resulting in repetitive adverse consequences to the user. The basic brain problem of this disease of chemical dependence or "addiction" appears to be an inability to consistently control the use of drugs that produce an acute or quick surge of dopamine in the brain. This surge of dopamine leads to a feeling of euphoria or "high."

Chemical dependence is an illness that affects 10–13% of Americans at some time in their lives. Surprisingly, rates are the same for all cultural groups, all socioeconomic groups, and even groups with different educational levels. Lifetime prevalence rates are lower than this only in elderly women. Women born before 1935 have a high rate (as high as 50%) of lifetime abstinence from even low levels of experimentation with mood-altering drugs, and thus many may have never activated a potential addictive disease. However, women born since 1950 experiment with mood-altering drugs at the exact same rate as their male counterparts, and are activating the disease of addiction at exactly the same rate. Therefore, being female is not a protective factor from the disease of addiction, but being abstinent is a protective factor for women or men.

Chemical dependence is one stage on the continuum of mood-altering substance use in our society. This continuum of use ranges from abstinence, to low risk or "social" use, to substance abuse, to the disease of addiction. A more full description of chemical dependence or addictive diseases and suggested readings are in the entry entitled Substance use.

SEE ALSO: Addiction, Substance use

Suggested Resources

A national service for addiction treatment and prevention education funded by the Robert Wood Johnson Foundation. www.jointogether.org

TED PARRAN JR.

Chest Pain

Chest pain is one of the cardinal manifestations of heart disease. However, chest pain can also occur due to various other disease states. It is very important for the patient and physician alike to differentiate chest pain due to cardiac causes from that due to noncardiac etiologies.

CHARACTERISTIC FEATURES OF CARDIAC CHEST PAIN

Quality

Cardiac chest pain is variously described as a constricting, squeezing, pressure-like, "heaviness," burning, "weight in the center of my chest," or "band-like feeling across my chest." Usually this pain is incited by exercise, cold weather, heavy meals, physical exertion, or emotional/mental stressors. Patients are sometimes awakened by early morning chest pain. This pain usually lasts between 5 and 15 minutes, but can last as long as 30 minutes. Patients with severe coronary heart disease can have pain at rest with the above characteristics; pain of that severity is worrisome for a myocardial infarction (heart attack).

Location

The pain is usually located in the center of the chest (substernal), radiating down either arm, up to the neck, jaw, teeth, or into the upper back (interscapular).

Associated Symptoms

Patients may note shortness of breath, choking sensation, diaphoresis, dizziness, nausea, vomiting, or palpitations.

DIFFERENTIAL DIAGNOSIS

Other disease states can be confused with cardiac chest pain.

Esophageal Pain

Usually this type of discomfort is substernal and epigastric in location, and is associated with food intake and acid reflux. It can be burning in character and can be brought on by lying down after meals. This pain can easily be confused with cardiac chest pain, but it usually occurs more predictably with food intake. Antacids help to alleviate the discomfort. The difficulty in differentiating cardiac pain from esophageal pain is confounded by the fact that these two conditions often coexist.

Peptic Ulcer Disease

Burning discomfort in the mid-epigastrium, relationship with food intake, and relieved by antacids are important differentiating features for this type of pain.

Acute Pancreatitis

The pancreas is an abdominal organ which releases digestive juices and hormones such as insulin. Inflammation of the pancreas may occur due to alcohol dependence or biliary disease, among other etiologies. Pain is usually described as a sharp or dull ache in the epigastrium; it may be similar to cardiac pain, but is position dependent and radiates to the back.

Pericarditis or Pleuritis

These conditions—inflammation of the lining of the heart or the lungs, respectively—can cause chest pain which is sharp, increases with respiration, and is positional. This discomfort is often associated with a cough or respiratory tract infection.

CAUSES OF CARDIAC CHEST PAIN

The most common cause of cardiac chest pain is an obstructive or flow-limiting lesion in the coronary arteries due to atherosclerotic (cholesterol) plaque. The accumulation of plaque causes slow narrowing in the lumen of the artery until complete obstruction occurs. These plaques can rupture or break, thereby compromising blood flow to the heart suddenly, and thus causing a myocardial infarction. For these reasons, risk factor modification is crucial in order to prevent the occurrence of atherosclerosis.

Less common, but seen in women more often than in men, is spasm of the coronary artery leading to reduced blood flow, thus causing chest pain. Treatment for this is different from the treatment for coronary artery obstruction.

In some patients (most commonly, but not limited to, those with diabetes mellitus), chest pain can occur due to small vessel disease rather than to atherosclerosis involving large coronary arteries. This disease entity,

called "microvascular angina," cannot be visualized with the angiographic techniques we have today, but will often respond to similar treatments as other forms of coronary artery disease.

WORKUP FOR CHEST PAIN

A detailed clinical history and physical examination help to differentiate most other etiologies of chest pain from cardiac chest pain. Further clues can be obtained from blood tests and from a 12-lead electrocardiogram (ECG). If indeed the discomfort is felt to be cardiac (related to the heart) chest pain, the patient will often undergo an ECG, stress test, and/or cardiac catheterization (coronary angiography). A cardiac catheterization is a procedure during which a special chemical that is highly visible on x-ray (contrast agent) is injected into the coronary arteries in order to visualize (opacify) them. In this manner, flow-limiting lesions can be imaged by fluoroscopy (x-ray movies), and treated by balloon angioplasty or stenting (both specialized procedures in which an instrument inserted into the blood vessel is used to remove/reduce the effect of the obstruction in the vessel), if suitable. In some cases, the individual may be referred for heart surgery (coronary artery bypass grafting) if the disease is severe and widespread.

TIME IS MUSCLE

Patients who experience cardiac chest pain should seek medical attention immediately. Chewing four baby aspirins can reduce mortality, if the cause of chest discomfort is indeed a myocardial infarction. Administration of other medications as quickly as possible will save more muscle from suffering and dying, and thus will reduce complications and mortality. Performing coronary angioplasty and restoring blood supply to the muscle as soon as possible is very important.

WOMEN AND CHEST PAIN

While the majority of women presenting with acute myocardial infarction do complain of chest pain, other, more nonspecific complaints such as upper abdominal pain, shortness of breath, fatigue, and nausea occur more frequently in female than in male patients. Furthermore, chest pain is a less specific finding in women than in men, a fact that has led symptoms of chest pain in women to be discounted frequently. A heightened level of awareness must be present among physicians in order to prevent delays in the diagnosis and treatment of myocardial infarction in women.

Furthermore, as discussed in the entry on "Coronary artery disease," the underlying pathology of myocardial infarction may differ in women when compared to men, and this difference may make the timely diagnosis of coronary artery disease more difficult in women.

Interestingly, women tend to have normal coronary angiograms in the presence of chest pain and/or abnormal stress tests more commonly than men, pointing to the likely presence of microvascular disease as a more frequent etiology of pain in women.

SEE ALSO: Anxiety disorders, Coronary artery disease, Mitral valve prolapse

Suggested Reading

Braunwald, E., Zipes, D., & Libby, P. (2001). *Heart disease: A textbook of cardiovascular medicine.* Philadelphia: W. B. Saunders.

Christie, L. G., & Conti, C. R. (1981). Systematic approach to the evaluation of angina-like chest pain. *American Heart Journal, 102,* 897.

Horvitz, L. D., & Groves, B. M. (1985) *Signs and symptoms in cardiology* (p. 506). Philadelphia: J. B. Lippincott.

KAMALA TAMIRISA
CLAIRE DUVERNOY

CARDIAC SYNDROME X

This syndrome was first described 100 years ago as "pseudoangina"; patients manifested chest pain, and had an abnormal stress test, but had normal coronary arteries by angiography. Kemp et al. coined the term "cardiac syndrome X" in 1973 for this clinical scenario. The incidence is higher in postmenopausal women. The underlying pathophysiology is unclear, but different authors have proposed several mechanisms. Problems with the release of endogenous vasodilators leading to spasm of the coronary arteries could be one of the reasons for this symptom complex. Therefore, women with normal coronaries are sometimes given ergonovine in the cardiac catheterization lab in order to induce coronary artery spasm and reproduce the symptoms. Another reason why these women have chest pain despite normal coronary arteries is due to "microvascular angina"—a disease of small vessels which cannot be seen clearly during cardiac catheterization, as mentioned above. Overall prognosis for this group of women patients is dependent on the underlying cardiac risk factors, especially diabetes mellitus. Some authors have suggested that postmenopausal estrogen therapy may be helpful in improving symptoms of cardiac syndrome X in postmenopausal women, although this therapy should be administered cautiously given new findings of overall harm associated with it. Though mortality is not higher, these patients suffer from significant morbidity. Physicians need to be aware of this clinical condition and work with patients to modify cardiac risk factors and offer reassurance.

Child Abuse
Child abuse or maltreatment occurs in many settings and places around the world. There are various kinds of abuse, and many times a child is the victim of more than one type of maltreatment. The spectrum of maltreatment includes physical abuse, emotional abuse, neglect, and sexual abuse. Issues of child labor and exploitation, lack of appropriate health care, food, shelter, and adequate sanitation pose big threats to the safety of children throughout the world. Any of these can have long-lasting negative psychological effects on a child.

The actual number of maltreated children in the world is unknown because many cases are never reported, and most countries do not have or do not enforce laws against child abuse. Estimates in the United States show that in the year 2000 there were 5 million children referred for investigation of potential abuse; 879,000 children were found to be victims of abuse. The rate of abuse was 12.2 per 1,000 children. (Reasons for not finding abuse were: no evidence of abuse or risk, or insufficient information available.) Sixty-three percent of these were neglect, 19% physical abuse, 10% sexual abuse, and 8% psychological abuse. About 1,200 children died in the year 2000 due to abuse. Forty-four percent of abuse victims were less than 1 year old, and 85% were less than age 6. Perpetrators of abuse are usually the parents or caretakers of a child.

Child abuse or maltreatment can occur in many different forms. Physical abuse is defined as an intentional act that causes harm to the body. Emotional abuse is verbal or behavioral actions that can impede a child's psychological development. Behavioral actions such as rejection, isolation, criticism, or terrorizing a child are examples of emotional abuse. Neglect is defined as failure to provide appropriate needs to a child, and this may include omission of physical or emotional needs. For example, physical needs include food, clothing, and shelter, and emotional needs include appropriate nurturing for healthy development. Sexual abuse is when an adult uses a child for his or her own sexual gratification. One of the negative effects of the Internet is exploitation of children via pornographic photos now available throughout the world.

Child maltreatment occurs in most cultures and societies. Internationally, there are some types of abuse or neglect that are related to poverty, disease, war, or global economics. Street children found throughout the world may or may not be homeless, but poverty and home abuse are primary reasons for their taking to the streets to find money and food. AIDS and other diseases have left many children homeless. War has also killed many parents, leaving children homeless or in unstable family situations. In some societies, certain disciplinary procedures or rites of passage procedures (such as circumcision) are not regarded as maltreatment. Yet these procedures may induce significant psychological distress. In Kenya, for example, many boys would be hospitalized for hysterical paralysis shortly before they reached puberty and were required to undergo ritual circumcision. (Due to the global distribution of resources, millions of children live in poverty, are homeless, and are desperate for food, water, shelter, and warmth. Millions have no access to health care or education.)

In 1989, the United Nations adopted the Convention on the Rights of the Child (CRC), which grants children rights relating to their civil, political, economic, and cultural lives. Although many countries passed laws regarding these rights, children continue to suffer violations of these rights. They continue to be the victims of child labor, neglect, sexual exploitation, physical and emotional abuse, and are subject to the effects of armed conflict and the lack of access to education, health care, safe water, and sanitation facilities.

Diagnosing or identifying abuse can be difficult. (It can be difficult to document maltreatment in many cases.) Legal definitions may vary from state to state. In the United States, professionals such as physicians, nurses, or teachers are mandated by law to report to the police or child protection services if they suspect a child is being maltreated. Certainly, abuse can sometimes be

obvious, but mistakes have been made about what appears obvious. For example, parents have been accused of abuse when their children developed "black eyes" related to an eye tumor or after they had used "coining" as a treatment for fever. In many circumstances, it is hard to know if a child is being maltreated or is at risk for abuse. If someone suspects a child is being abused, those accusations should be taken seriously. Definitions may vary, but there are some guidelines available to help identify the various forms of abuse. Physical abuse should be suspected in a child with an injury or repeated injuries that cannot be explained or when an injury is not likely to have occurred as explained by the caretaker. Emotional abuse should be suspected if a parent is repeatedly verbally attacking a child, or ignoring or rejecting the child. Neglect can be identified by noting inadequate clothing, poor hygiene, or nutritional deprivation. Other clues to potential abuse include a child who is acting out, who runs away from home, who attempts to hurt or kill him/herself, or who reports that he/she is being abused. As these children grow, they may develop psychological problems, such as depression, anger, and eating disorders. Substance abuse, criminal behavior, and suicide are increased in abused children. Behaviors such as these may also lead one to suspect that a child has been maltreated.

There are a number of theories about what factors place a child at risk for abuse. Parents who abuse their children have been reported from most ethnic, geographic, religious, educational, occupational, and socioeconomic groups. Poverty is a significant risk factor for abuse in children. This may be due to several factors, such as increased stress due to unemployment, overcrowding, lack of food, and other necessities. Other factors that contribute to the occurrence of child abuse in poverty-stricken families include limited social support, higher incidence of violence in their community, teenage and single parenthood, and substance abuse. Mentally retarded or handicapped children are at increased risk for abuse. Many abusive parents have experienced abuse as children.

Trying to identify risk factors for abuse is an important means for prevention, and is a focus of research today. Some studies are looking at parental attributions as characteristics of risk for child-abusive parenting. Some studies are looking at characteristics of children that may predispose to maltreatment. Parental attitude toward a child may be more significant than actual characteristics of the child.

Treatment for a child who is being or has been abused may require many modalities. In the United States, it is mandatory to report to the Child Protective Services any child suspected of being a victim of abuse. Assessment of and treatment for physical injuries must be addressed immediately. A caseworker is then involved to help decide how to protect the child. First, it is important to place a child in a safe environment. This sometimes involves removing parental rights. The usual goal is to keep a child with a parent or eventually return a child to his/her home if at all possible. This can be a very difficult decision if there is the potential for further abuse in the home. Many times a child is returned to a home where abuse continues, if the risks were not fully identified. Other times the child may be placed by the court with relatives or in a foster home. If a child is to return to his/her home, it is important that the parent perpetrator receive psychotherapy and that social services continue observation of the child for months or years after the return.

A child is traumatized by abuse, as well as by removal from his/her parent. Counseling is very important to an abused child. This may involve talking or play therapy, directed at helping a child cope with fears and anxieties. Some children feel responsible if a parent has been jailed and this issue must be addressed in therapy. Most hospitals have teams trained in managing child abuse. Members of these teams are on call to assist these children in the emergency room or hospital. As children of abuse grow to adulthood, the management of their "posttraumatic" psychological effects of abuse is ongoing.

Prevention of child abuse is also multifaceted. Identifying at-risk families is a major goal. Parenting classes may help inexperienced mothers learn appropriate behavior and nonviolent discipline techniques. Stress management skills for parents are helpful in reducing stress and anger in difficult life situations. Support groups, and support from family, friends, or others in the community can help. Members of the groups should be encouraged to ask for respite if they feel likely to abuse their children. Keeping weapons out of the home will also help. In many states, there are laws to inform communities when pedophiles are released from prison. Increased community awareness about the location of potential abusers is likely to increase safety of the children in that community.

See Also: Domestic violence, Sexual abuse

Suggested Reading

Dadds, M. R., Mullins, M. J., McAllister, R. A., & Atkinson, E. (1993). Attributions, affect, and behavior in abuse-risk mothers: A laboratory study. *Child Abuse and Neglect, 27*(1), 21–45.

Johnson, C. F. (2000). Abuse and neglect of children. In R. E. Behrman (Ed.), *Nelson textbook of pediatrics* (16th ed., pp. 110–119). Philadelphia: W. B. Saunders.

Mulinge, M. M. (2002). Implementing the 1989 United Nations' Convention on the Rights of the Child in sub-Saharan Africa: The overlooked socioeconomic and political dilemmas. *Child Abuse and Neglect, 26*, 1117–1130.

Sidebotham, P., Heron, J., & Golding, J. (2003). Child maltreatment in the "children of the nineties:" The role of the child. *Child Abuse and Neglect, 27*, 337–352.

Suggested Resources

American Academy of Pediatrics: http://www.aap.org/

Child Maltreatment and Neglect: http://aolscv.health.webmd.aol.com/content/healthwise/135/33513.htm

National Clearing House on Child Abuse and Neglect Information: http://www.caleb.com/nccanch/

Denise Bothe
Karen Olness

Child Care The decision to use child care is an important issue to consider prior to working or obtaining further education for parents/guardians. Other issues for consideration include general health and personality of the child/children, number of children to be enrolled in child care, hours child care will be needed, and distance to be traveled for child care and/or employment and education opportunities. Once child care utilization has been decided, understanding the various aspects of quality and types of child care are important factors.

CHILD CARE RESOURCES

There are many resources for locating child care. "Word of mouth" recommendations from other parents, friends, or neighbors are excellent starting points. Physicians, employers, religious groups, YMCAs, or college/university listings may also be a resource for child care information. Phone listings and state agencies that license and regulate child care centers may be other resources.

Child Care

The type of child care available in a community depends on many factors. Large urban/suburban communities may have a wider selection of types of child care due to the number of children and the demand of working parents. Early planning and a clear understanding of individual child/children's needs, in order to keep as many options available as possible, is a key component of successful child care.

The cost of child care varies widely and may be based upon factors such as number of children, hours of child care provided, location of child care, age of child (children), educational level and number of providers, the inclusion of meals and supplies, in addition to the community supply and demand for child care.

QUALITY OF CHILD CARE

There are many factors which determine quality of child care. Licensure or regulation by the state or accreditation by a national child care organization may be one measure of quality child care. While these measures may not be available for all child care environments, other factors to consider include the ratio of child care providers:children, taking into consideration the age of the children and experience level of the providers. In addition to the experience level, the educational level of the child care provider and opportunities for continuing education are other important considerations. Duration of staff retention is an important measure of child care consistency. Responsiveness of staff to the child/children is important with regard to child-appropriate activities, addressing needs and requests of children, and appropriate use of discipline and redirection depending on the child's age. Examination of the physical space for safe, clean areas for children and the presence of child-centered equipment are other important considerations.

Health policies regarding diapering and toileting techniques, separation of food preparation and toileting/diapering areas, and hand washing policies for children and staff should be investigated. Nutrition is another important aspect of child care, since children may spend a majority of their day in a child care center. Variety and types of food provided are important to consider, especially if children have allergies or other health problems. There are many agencies that have agreed upon and recommended nutritional standards for child care centers. Perhaps the most important factor is how

the parent(s)/guardian(s) and the child (children) feel about the child care environment, from the level of personal interactions to the physical surroundings.

TYPES OF CHILD CARE

Child care can range from in-home care, home provider child care, or large child care centers. In-home care often refers to a person coming to the child's (children's) home to provide care, such as a relative or a nanny. Nannies may/may not have had formal education and/or experience taking care of children. In-home providers are often not regulated by the state but nanny placement agencies may be regulated in some states. Foreign exchange student programs may also be another resource for in-home child care. Prior to hiring an in-home provider, criminal record and child abuse background checks should be completed. In-home child care usually involves only the child/children within one family. Families may choose in-home providers so that children have a consistent provider in a familiar surrounding and transportation is less complex for the parents/guardians. Children in in-home child care may have less exposure to other children for interactive play and illnesses. If the in-home provider is ill, alternative child care arrangements must be made. In-home child care is often the most expensive type of child care.

Home providers refer to child care in the residence of the provider. There may be several families that use the home provider for child care, and the children will vary in age and number depending on the home provider and state regulations. Home providers should have a criminal record and child abuse background check by the state prior to providing child care. Home providers may or may not be regulated depending on the state. Home providers usually provide consistent care for a slightly larger number of children than in-home child care. Illness of the home provider may create challenges for a family to arrange alternative child care options. Home providers may be the least expensive of all the child care options.

Large child care centers (day care) refer to large centers that have many families and children of various ages enrolled. Large child care centers are licensed by the states and need to meet health, safety, and caregiver guidelines in addition to submitting to at least annual inspections. Large child care centers may also be accredited by national organizations and meet requirements above minimum standards for state licensure. Children who attend large child care centers may be exposed to a more diverse group of people, but may also have more illnesses than children in smaller child care environments. The cost of large child care centers will vary depending on the community, but generally will be less expensive than in-home child care.

SEE ALSO: Adolescence, Adoption, Child abuse, Day care, Parenting, Pregnancy, Quality of life, Stress, Teen pregnancy

Suggested Resources

Child Care Aware. (2003). Washington, DC (NACCRRA, 2001): http://www.childcareaware.org

National Association for the Education of Young Children. (2003). http://www.naeyc.org (accessed on July, 2003)

National Association of Child Care Resource and Referral Agencies. (2003). Washington, DC (NACCRRA, 2003): http://www.naccrra.net

National Network for Child Care. (2003). Iowa State University (April 2, 2002): http://www.nncc.org

Parents Place. (2003). IVillage (disclaimer updated June 22, 2001): http://www.parentsplace.com

DEANNA DAHL-GROVE

Child Custody Child custody means the legal responsibility for a child. When the parents of a child are married and live with the child, questions of child custody are rare. But when parents separate from each other or divorce, or when parents live separately from their child, there is often a question as to who has custody of the child.

Custody itself can be divided in to two parts, physical and legal custody. Physical custody refers to providing the day-to-day care for the child. Legal custody refers to making important decisions about the child, like choosing schools and making medical decisions. Physical and legal custody can be arranged differently for the same child.

Custody can also be separated into two other categories, sole custody and joint custody. Sole custody means that one parent has the responsibility for the physical or legal custody or for both. Joint custody means that the parents share physical or legal custody or both. It is possible to have many combinations of these types of custody. For example, one parent could have sole physical custody of the child while the

parents have joint legal custody. Joint physical custody does not have to mean an even split of time between parents. In most joint custody arrangements, the child will spend more time with one parent than the other, particularly if the child is in school and the parents do not live close enough to exchange the child frequently.

Laws about custody are set by each state, rather than by the federal government, because of which there can be many differences in laws between one state and another. Some states have laws that favor joint custody while other states do not.

Child custody decisions used to be determined by gender. The first gender-based presumption was that the father should have custody of the children, since he was responsible for them and should be able to benefit from their labor. That presumption was replaced by one in the opposite direction. The "tender years" presumption gave custody of young children to mothers because of a belief that the mother was a better nurturer. Current child custody law does not contain any formal gender-based presumptions. Lingering gender-based stereotypes may play a role in a judge's custody decision. Those stereotypes may help a woman win a custody battle because a judge believes women care for children well. On the other hand, those stereotypes may be a hindrance to women who do not fit the female image that the judge has in mind. For example, if a mother and father share equally in infant care activities such as bathing, feeding, and changing an infant, the father may be seen as outstanding and the mother many be seen as usual, even though their roles are equal.

Most custody decisions are made by the agreement of the parents, with the parents having an understanding of how a judge might decide, if that were required. When courts are called upon to make a decision, they can take into consideration the physical and mental health of the parents, any history of violence, each parent's relationship with the child, the parents' abilities to work with each other, and many other factors.

The laws of most states favor custody decisions that are stable and reliable for the child. For that reason, it is often harder to get a court to change a custody decision once a decision has been made. There may be a requirement that the child be in danger in order to make a change in custody soon after a recent court order.

Divorces are not the only times that child custody decisions are made. Parents who have never been married may separate, requiring a custody determination.

And often there are others who are not legally or biologically parents, but who fill the role of a parent. Grandparents may care for children, stepparents may play that role, and unmarried partners of a biological parent may all have emotional ties that are equivalent to a parent. But these emotional ties alone are not enough to even ask for custody in court. To be able to seek legal custody, a person must have standing, which means a right to be able to go to court over an issue. Generally a parental equivalent will not have standing unless that person has cared for the child, without the biological parent being around, for an extended period of time.

When one parent gets custody of a child, whether by agreement or through a judge's decision, the other parent will likely get to have visitation with the child. Visitation arrangements can vary depending upon the needs and abilities of the parents and the child. Visitation can be limited or restricted if the visitation poses a risk to the child.

Custody and visitation decisions should not be confused with determinations of parental fitness or termination of parental rights. Courts often become involved in families where there is abuse or neglect of a child. If the situation cannot be made safe for the child, the parents' rights could be ended. These are situations where the state takes custody of the child, and ordinary child custody cases rarely turn into such situations.

Custody determinations can be arranged by agreement of the couple, and when the couple cannot agree, a judge makes the decision. In most cases the parents reach an agreement, the judge makes sure the agreement is fair, and the judge makes the parents' agreement a part of a court order.

Lawyers can provide important services in child custody cases. Lawyers can make sure that people who agree to a custody arrangement understand how the agreement will affect them and the child. Lawyers can also represent parents in negotiating an agreement, or in presenting a case to a judge for a decision. But lawyers can be expensive. Sometimes free legal assistance can be obtained through a local office of the Legal Services Corporation, or through other local agencies. Many people represent themselves in a child custody dispute, but this should be a last resort.

See Also: Adoption, Child care, Cohabitation, Day care, Divorce, Divorce mediation, Domestic partnership, Parenting

Suggested Reading

Damman, G. (1997). *Collecting child support: 12 effective strategies.* Bellington, WA: Self-Counsel Press.
Lyster, M. (1996). *Building parenting agreements that work.* Berkeley, CA: Nolo Press.
Peters, D., & Strom, R. (1997). *Divorce and child custody: Your options and legal rights.* Philadelphia: Chelsea House.
Watnik, W. (1997). *Child custody made simple.* Claremont, CA: Single Parent Press.

SHEILA SIMON

Chiropractic Care Anyone who has ever intentionally cracked her knuckles or stretched and popped her neck has an idea of the benefit of chiropractic, for it is a similar manipulation of the joints that is chiropractic today. Yet despite the many people who report benefiting from chiropractic treatment, chiropractic has a controversial history that goes back to its foundation before the turn of the 20th century.

Chiropractors derive their theories and techniques from the work of D. D. Palmer—a magnetic healer—who performed the first chiropractic adjustment. In 1895, Palmer manipulated a bump on the neck of a janitor in the building where he worked, and after one of these treatment sessions, the janitor reported being able to hear. From this incident and his study of magnetic healing, Palmer developed the idea that a vital force permeates every cell of the body and that misaligned joints (called *subluxations* in the jargon of the trade) press on the nerves and disrupt the flow of the vital force. He believed that this disruption is the cause of illness and that manipulation of the joints can restore flow of the vital force and thus allow the body to achieve health. It is important to note that Palmer believed that any decrease or increase of life-force flow caused by bones pressing on nerves results in disease and that chiropractic treatment restores normal flow.

These ideas developed and evolved at a time when conventional medical practice (sometimes called *allopathic medicine*) was dramatically different than it is today. Before the Flexner report, which was published in 1910 and which brought about dramatic reform in medical education, many physicians were either self-taught or had learned medicine at the hands of other physicians. Almost anyone could call himself a doctor. Many medical practices of the time were unpleasant, ineffective, or dangerous. In such an environment, alternative approaches to healing sprang up. Chiropractic was one of these alternative approaches.

Today, chiropractic is commonly considered as one of many complementary and alternative approaches to medicine. This designation reflects chiropractic's historical rejection of conventional scientific approaches to knowledge and practice. Allopathic medicine is a reductionist approach, focusing on symptoms and attempting to identify their root cause. Chiropractic focuses on symptoms as well, but takes a whole body approach to wellness. Chiropractic is built on the belief that a vital force infuses every cell in the body, and that this belief is not subject to scientific testing. The chiropractic tradition offers a series of principles that are philosophical statements, not testable hypotheses. Chiropractors have not usually subjected their methods to the kinds of scrutiny that are common in medical practice, and they use terms in ways that are not consistent with usage in conventional medical settings. For example, when a chiropractor talks about *dis-ease*, she does not mean illness. In chiropractic tradition, "disease" is both the cause and effect. In fact, one proponent of chiropractic, Frank DeGiacomo, maintains that the treatment of any classified disease cannot be chiropractic. Contrast this idea with the long list of diseases many chiropractors claim to treat or prevent, and the inconsistencies multiply rapidly. However, philosophical inconsistencies abound in conventional medicine as well. In fact, it is the process of questioning traditional practice that has been the engine of discovery that has led to new and better treatments in both chiropractic and conventional medicine.

Chiropractors believe that the vital force is self-evident and that their practices are the most effective way to help the body achieve health. In response to criticisms of their approach, chiropractors emphasize the idea that nothing outside the body can heal the body but that restoration of the life force can allow the body to heal itself. And, of course, they believe that they have the best techniques for helping the body to heal itself. Some chiropractors reject the use of antibiotics and surgery as inconsistent with their basic principles. Other chiropractors see their healing modality as one among many that individuals may choose to achieve wellness under specific circumstances.

Some chiropractors promote other approaches that they view as consistent with their field. It is not unusual to find chiropractors selling vitamins, herbs, and devices designed to promote health. It is rare, however, for chiropractors to subject their practices to close scientific scrutiny. They argue that it is unfair to judge one healing tradition by the standards of another that takes a different approach. Because of this, chiropractors have faced an uphill battle against the forces of mainstream medicine. For example, chiropractors won an antitrust suit against the American Medical Association in 1987. However, the victory was a validation of their right to practice chiropractic rather than a validation of chiropractic techniques. A study by the RAND Corporation suggested that chiropractic techniques are an effective mode of treatment. Nevertheless, this study has been criticized because chiropractic was not studied under the conditions in which it is usually practiced. Many of the procedures performed were not administered by chiropractors, and physicians screened most patients receiving the procedures to assure that the physical manipulations were safe. A study published in *Consumer Reports* claimed to demonstrate the effectiveness of chiropractic. Instead, it showed satisfaction with chiropractic. Satisfaction and effectiveness are not identical.

To say that chiropractic is ineffective would be erroneous. The proper statement would be that evidence supporting the effectiveness of chiropractic is limited. Some studies do show its effectiveness for the treatment of back and neck pain when compared to no treatment. It is important to note, however, that such studies do not test the basic premises on which chiropractic is built.

As with any profession, chiropractic is evolving. Some chiropractors eschew treatment of conditions other than those associated with nerves, muscles, and bones. A limited but growing number of chiropractors recognize the importance of rigorously testing the effectiveness of their techniques. Chiropractors have begun to examine the cost-effectiveness of their treatments. Through these changes, chiropractic may increase its acceptance in the mainstream medical community. Those who are committed to the highest standards of research welcome these changes.

SEE ALSO: Acupuncture, Back pain, Chiropractors, Complementary and alternative health practices, Energy healing, Massage, Physical therapy

Suggested Reading

Barrett, S., & Jarvis, W. T. (1993). *The health robbers: A close look at quackery in America*. Amherst, NY: Prometheus.

Collinge, W. (1996). *The American Holistic Health Association complete guide to alternative medicine*. New York: Warner.

Chiropractors

DeGiacomo, F. (1978). *Man's greatest gift to man ... chiropractic.* Old Bethpage, NY: LSR Learning Associates.

Gevitz, N. (Ed.). (1988). *Other healers: Unorthodox medicine in America.* Baltimore: Johns Hopkins University Press.

Homola, S., & Barrett, S. (Ed.). (1999). *Inside chiropractic: A patient's guide.* Amherst, NY: Prometheus.

Palmer, D. D. (1997). *The chiropractor: 1914.* Kila, MT: Kessinger.

Peterson, D. H., & Bergmann, T. F. (2002). *Chiropractic techniques: Principles and procedures* (2nd ed.). New York: Churchill Livingstone.

BRUCE HARTSELL

Chiropractors Chiropractors are practitioners of the complementary and alternative medicine approach known as chiropractic. (Chiropractic is both a noun and an adjective.) They trace their roots to September 18, 1895, when David Daniel Palmer—a magnetic healer—used his hands to thrust on a bump on the neck of his janitor and in the process cured the janitor's deafness. The apparent healing is especially miraculous when one examines the distribution of the cranial nerves and discovers that the auditory nerve does not extend to the neck. But chiropractors have not historically emphasized conventional scientific approaches to knowledge.

From the apparent healing of the janitor, Palmer developed chiropractic (see entry Chiropractic). Palmer based the practice of chiropractic on his belief that a vital force infuses every cell of the body, that nerves are the paths through which this life force flows, and that misaligned joints (*subluxations*) disrupt the flow of the life force. He further believed that using the hands to manipulate various joints of the body—especially those in the spinal column—could restore disruptions of the life force and thereby allow the body to heal.

Despite the Flexner report in 1910, which brought reform to traditional medical education in the United States, chiropractic education was caught in conflict among competing ideas until it was finally standardized in the late 1950s and early 1960s. Most chiropractic schools now require at least 2 years of undergraduate education and 4 years of chiropractic school. Chiropractic education is criticized by members of mainstream medicine, however, for its tendency to emphasize untestable hypotheses and techniques for building a successful business at the expense of basic science. Despite the standardization of chiropractic education, chiropractors are not trained in the same kinds of diagnostic tests and treatments that physicians and surgeons are taught to use. In fact, chiropractors would be practicing outside of their legal authority if they were to use many of the tests and procedures that are common in medical practice.

Chiropractors today usually belong to one of three associations according to their beliefs about illness and its proper treatment. Members of the International Chiropractors Association are often referred to as *straights*, because they adhere to Palmer's belief that almost all diseases are caused by misaligned vertebrae and that manipulation of the spine can prevent or cure most diseases. Members of the American Chiropractic Association are known as *mixers*, because they mix Palmer's ideas with other ideas about the causes of diseases. While they may acknowledge the influence of germs and other biological factors in disease, they still tend to consider disturbance of the life force as the underlying cause of disease. A third group, and the smallest, is the National Association for Chiropractic Medicine. This group requires members to sign a written pledge to openly renounce the foundational chiropractic idea that disturbance of the life force caused by misaligned joints is the cause of disease. The pledge also requires members to limit their work to neuromusculoskeletal conditions of a nonsurgical nature.

Chiropractors today often seek to be primary care providers, and they offer a wide range of prevention and treatment services. Due to the limitations of their training, however, they cannot provide the range of services offered by physicians, and patients who rely on them for primary care may be at risk for misdiagnosis and mistreatment. Despite claims to the contrary, evidence for the effectiveness of chiropractors in treating most medical conditions has yet to be demonstrated under conventional scientific standards. However, customer satisfaction appears strong. The right of chiropractors to licensure and their right to practice were established on narrow legal grounds, not on the scientific merits of their approach. As with other complementary and alternative medical practices, the potential chiropractic patient is best advised to learn about a chiropractor's approach to healing and obtain references before entering into a therapeutic relationship.

SEE ALSO: Chiropractic care, Complementary and alternative health practices, Healers, Occupational therapists, Physical therapy

Suggested Reading

Barrett, S., & Jarvis, W. T. (1993). *The health robbers: A close look at quackery in America.* Amherst, NY: Prometheus.

Benedetti, P., & Macphail, W. (2003). *Spin doctors: The chiropractic industry under examination.* Toronto, ON: Dundurn Press.

Haldeman, S. (Ed.). (1993). *Principles and practice of chiropractic* (2nd ed.). Norwalk, CT: Appleton & Lange.

Magner, G., & Barrett, S. (Eds.). (1995). *Chiropractic: The victim's perspective.* Amherst, NY: Prometheus.

Palmer, D. D. (1997). *The chiropractor: 1914.* Kila, MT: Kessinger.

BRUCE HARTSELL

Chlamydia

Infection with *Chlamydia trachomatis* is the most common sexually transmitted disease in the United States and the most frequently reported infectious disease; an estimated 3 million cases occur annually. Chlamydia can be transmitted by vaginal, anal, or, less commonly, oral contact. The symptoms of chlamydia, which usually occur within 7–21 days of infection, can be very mild. Up to 50% of men, and up to 75% of women may have no symptoms at all. Women may notice an abnormal vaginal discharge, and men may have a discharge from the penis, or pain while urinating. Chlamydia can also cause inflammation of the rectum. Although often asymptomatic in women, chlamydia infection can produce chronic low-grade inflammation leading to scarring of the fallopian tubes and infertility. Other complications are discussed below.

The diagnosis of infection with *C. trachomatis* is made by sampling the infected area, most often vaginal or anal secretions. It is difficult to grow *C. trachomatis* using standard culture techniques, and there are a variety of Food and Drug Administration (FDA)-approved methods to detect chlamydia based on antigen detection and amplification of genetic material.

While acute infection of the urethra or cervix with *C. trachomatis* is usually not associated with significant morbidity, complications of chlamydia can be very serious. In women, pelvic inflammatory disease (PID) occurs when the infection extends to the fallopian tubes. PID can cause severe pain, requiring hospitalization and intravenous antibiotics. PID may result in scarring of the fallopian tubes, causing infertility, ectopic pregnancy, and/or chronic pelvic pain. Of those with PID, 20% will become infertile; 18% will experience debilitating, chronic pelvic pain; and 9% will have a life-threatening tubal pregnancy. Undiagnosed PID caused by chlamydia is common, leading to screening strategies discussed below. In addition to those direct complications of infection, women infected with chlamydia have a three- to fivefold increased risk of acquiring HIV, if exposed to the virus. Men with untreated chlamydia infection may develop pain and swelling of the scrotum and testicles, known as epididymitis.

Women who develop chlamydia infection during pregnancy may transmit *C. trachomatis* to the fetus at birth. A newborn may develop conjunctivitis (a serious eye infection) and pneumonia. Because of this, it is recommended that all pregnant women be tested for chlamydia.

Uncomplicated infection which responds readily to several antibiotics. The most common regimens include doxycycline given for 7 days, or single-dose therapy with azithromycin. The latter drug offers the advantage of better compliance, but is more expensive. Because chlamydia and gonorrhea often occur simultaneously and have significant overlap in their clinical presentation, it is standard to test for and treat both when one is suspected in a patient.

Utilizing safe sex practices, including latex condoms, may prevent chlamydia. Women with risk factors such as multiple sexual partners, and those who are not consistently using barrier methods of birth control should be tested annually for chlamydia infection. The Centers for Disease Control and Prevention has developed recommendations for the prevention and management of chlamydia for all providers of health care. These recommendations call for screening of all sexually active females under 20 years of age at least annually, and annual screening of women aged 20 and older with one or more risk factors for chlamydia (i.e., new or multiple sex partners and lack of barrier contraception). All women with infection of the cervix and all pregnant women should be tested.

SEE ALSO: Condoms, Gonorrhea, Herpes simplex virus, Human papillomavirus, Safer sex, Sexually transmitted diseases, Syphilis

Suggested Reading

Gripshover, B., & Valdez, H. (2002). Common sexually transmitted diseases. In J. S. Tan (Ed.), *Experts guide to the management of common infectious diseases* (pp. 271–303). Philadelphia: American College of Physicians.

Suggested Resources

Centers for Disease Control and Prevention website: http://www.cdc.gov/nchstp/dstd/Fact_Sheets/chlamydia_facts.htm

KAREN L. ASHBY

Cholesterol

Cholesterol The leading cause of death in women in the United States is heart disease resulting from clogged arteries. Although heart attack and angina used to be thought of as a "male" disease, that is no longer the case. Over 500,000 women in 2000 died from heart disease while about 440,000 men died from the same cause in that year, according to the American Heart Association. It is estimated that one in five women has heart disease. Women who have had a heart attack have a death rate of 38%, compared with 25% in men. The chance of a second heart attack within 6 years of the first one is 35% for women but 18% for men. It is essential to understand these staggering statistics in order to grasp the importance of tackling the problem of high cholesterol in women, a major risk factor for heart attack.

DEFINITION

Cholesterol is oily in nature but is not the same as fat. It is an essential molecule for making cell membranes, steroid hormones, nerve sheaths, and much more. The liver makes most of the cholesterol in the body and the rest comes from the diet. Too much cholesterol in the blood is known as hypercholesterolemia. This leads to clogged arteries, which causes heart attack, stroke, loss of circulation in the limbs, and kidney failure. This process is called atherosclerosis (see below).

Cholesterol in the blood is carried by protein particles called lipoproteins. The two most important are low-density lipoprotein (LDL) and high-density lipoprotein (HDL). Elevated levels of LDL are usually associated with cholesterol deposits in the blood vessels, so LDL is known as "bad cholesterol." Elevated levels of HDL actually protect against heart disease by scavenging cholesterol and removing it from the arteries, so HDL is known as "good cholesterol." Because of this, total cholesterol is not always the best measure of cholesterol. High HDL makes the total cholesterol level look too high but is actually a good thing.

Although high LDL is the best known risk factor for heart disease, low HDL is also an important risk factor. Low HDL occurs in weight gain, inactivity, and smoking. Factors leading to higher HDL include regular exercise, moderate alcohol consumption (no more than one drink per day for women, two for men), and certain medications (see Treatment below).

Triglycerides are often measured along with cholesterol. Triglycerides are fats floating freely in the blood. If blood with a very high triglyceride level is allowed to sit in a tube, after a while a thick whitish layer of fat will rise to the top. Triglycerides are also a risk factor for heart disease, although the reason is not as well understood as it is for cholesterol.

ATHEROSCLEROSIS

Atherosclerosis is a slow progressive disease in which cholesterol deposits form within the wall of blood vessels. Atherosclerosis begins with damage to the inner lining of blood vessels. Such injury commonly occurs with high blood pressure and smoking. The tissue behind the inner lining is exposed, which makes blood platelets sticky and causes smooth muscle cells to grow and fill in the area of injury. A partial blockage of the artery begins to form. Cholesterol particles become part of the growing deposit and cause further blockage of the blood vessel. Cholesterol deposits can be crumbly and may break apart, which causes a clot to form, suddenly blocking the artery. Or, deposits may grow slowly over time, causing gradually worsening blockage. Cholesterol deposits may also break off and block arteries elsewhere in the body, or weaken arteries causing vessel walls to balloon out (aneurysm).

Atherosclerosis can affect any artery of the body. When the arteries that supply blood to the heart muscle are blocked, a heart attack occurs. When brain arteries are blocked, this causes a stroke. Blockage in arteries in the legs can lead to gangrene, and blockage of arteries to the kidneys leads to kidney failure. Atherosclerosis in the aorta, the main artery coming from the heart, can cause the aorta to balloon (aortic aneurysm) and eventually rupture.

CAUSES OF ELEVATED CHOLESTEROL

High cholesterol can be inherited, but it can also develop in people without a family history of high cholesterol. Two inherited conditions are familial combined hyperlipidemia (occurring in 1 in 100 individuals), and familial hypercholesterolemia (occurring in 1 in 500 people). People with these conditions are at very high risk of premature heart attack and stroke, and need aggressive medical treatment. Family members should be screened for high cholesterol so they can be treated as early as possible.

The two most common causes of noninherited cholesterol elevation are an unhealthy diet and diabetes. Consumption of large amounts of saturated fat, cholesterol, and too many calories will lead to high LDL cholesterol in most people. Low-calorie, low-saturated-fat diets cause significant reductions in cholesterol.

Diabetes leads to high LDL cholesterol mostly when blood glucose (sugar) levels are poorly controlled. Therefore, both type 1 and type 2 diabetics are at risk. Diabetic people have 2–6 times the risk for atherosclerosis compared to nondiabetics, and need to aggressively control other risk factors such as high blood pressure, obesity, diet, and smoking. Other causes of high LDL cholesterol include excessive alcohol intake, hypothyroidism (underfunctioning thyroid), kidney disease, HIV/AIDS, obstructive liver disease, hormones such as progesterone or steroids, and occasionally some medications like thiazide diuretics or beta-blockers (which are used to control blood pressure).

SYMPTOMS

Severe elevations in cholesterol as in familial hypercholesterolemia can lead to cholesterol deposits in the skin or on tendons called xanthomas. Unfortunately, most of the time hypercholesterolemia goes unnoticed until a catastrophe occurs, such as a stroke, heart attack, loss of circulation to a limb or to the kidneys, or ruptured aortic aneurysm. The consequences of these events include sudden death, chronic disability, long-term illness with frequent hospitalizations, and depression.

ASSESSMENT OF RISK FOR HEART DISEASE

The National Cholesterol Education Program (NCEP) has developed guidelines (ATP III guidelines) to help estimate the risk of disease due to high cholesterol, and guide efforts at prevention and treatment. Individuals can assess their personal risk for heart disease on the basis of their risk factors. The highest risk groups are people with diabetes, heart disease due to atherosclerosis (heart attack, bypass, or angioplasty), symptoms due to blockage of the carotid arteries, blockage of the arteries in the limbs, or who have an abdominal aortic aneurysm. These people should aim for an LDL less than 100 mg/dl.

For people without those conditions, add one point for each risk factor that they have:

- Age (males 45 years or older; females 55 years or older)
- Family history of early heart disease due to atherosclerosis such as heart attack, bypass, or angioplasty (father or brother affected before age 55; mother or sister affected before age 65)
- Current cigarette smoking
- High blood pressure or taking blood pressure medicine
- Low HDL ("good") cholesterol (less than 40 mg/dl)
- *Subtract* one point if the HDL is 60 mg/dl or higher

People with two or more points should aim for an LDL less than 130 mg/dl. People with zero or one point should aim for an LDL less than 160 mg/dl.

TREATMENT

Diet and Exercise

The initial step in treating high cholesterol is diet, increased physical activity, and weight loss. Reducing dietary intake of saturated fat and cholesterol is beneficial in lowering LDL cholesterol, and regular, sustained aerobic exercise increases HDL cholesterol. Weight loss in women may cause a decline in HDL cholesterol without much change in LDL cholesterol. Fat tissue in postmenopausal women produces estrogen, and therefore losing this source may reduce HDL cholesterol.

Medication

Estrogen therapy was traditionally offered to postmenopausal women as prevention for coronary artery disease. Estrogen raises HDL cholesterol and lowers LDL cholesterol. Because of this, scientists expected that estrogen would prevent heart attacks. However, the HERS study and more recently the Women's Health Initiative found this is not true. These studies showed that using estrogen and progesterone in postmenopausal women did not reduce the risk of heart attack. The Women's Health Initiative is continuing to study women who have had hysterectomies and take estrogen alone, to find out if the same is true.

Table 1. Common side effects of cholesterol-lowering medications

HMG CoA reductase inhibitors (statins)	Muscle and liver inflammation
Bile acid sequestrants	Bloating, constipation
Niacin	Flushing, high blood sugar, liver inflammation
Ezetimibe	Fatigue, muscle pain, diarrhea
Fibrates	Liver inflammation

Cholesterol-Lowering Medications

"Statin" drugs inhibit the major enzyme responsible for cholesterol production in the liver. These are the most effective medications for lowering LDL cholesterol, reducing it by 25–35%. Statins are proven to reduce the chance of death from heart disease in women. They are comparatively safe and have limited side effects. They also have other benefits like increasing bone density and reducing the risk of fractures. Because statins occasionally cause liver or muscle inflammation, regular blood test monitoring is required.

Other cholesterol-lowering agents include the bile acid sequestrants: cholestyramine and colestipol (Table 1). These are older drugs, and work by increasing the conversion of cholesterol to bile acids, which then leave the body in the stool. These medications lower LDL cholesterol by 15–20%, and increase HDL cholesterol by 3–8%. Niacin, or nicotinic acid (not related to the nicotine in tobacco), is particularly effective in raising HDL cholesterol levels by up to 30%. It also lowers LDL cholesterol. The newest drug is ezetimibe, which blocks cholesterol absorption in the intestines. It lowers LDL cholesterol by 18%. Fibrates are used to lower triglycerides, but have little effect on cholesterol.

SEE ALSO: Diabetes, Diet, Heart disease, Nutrition, Obesity

Suggested Reading

Basaria, S., Kermani, A., & Dobs, A. S. (2001). Treating dyslipidemia in women. *Women's Health in Primary Care, 4,* 377–383.

Duell, P. B., Illingworth, D. R., & Conner, W. E. (2001). Disorders of lipid metabolism. In P. Felig & L. A. Frohman (Eds.), *Endocrinology & metabolism* (4th ed., pp. 993–1075). New York: McGraw-Hill.

Expert Panel on Detection, Evaluation, and Treatment of High Blood Cholesterol in Adults. (2002, September). Executive Summary of the Third Report of the National Cholesterol Education Program (NCEP). Adult Treatment Panel III, Final Report. NIH Publication No. 02-5215. Available at www.nhlbi.nih.gov/guidelines/cholesterol

Suggested Resources

National Cholesterol Education Program website: www.nhlbi.nih.gov/chd. A summary of current guidelines is given at: www.nhlbi.nih.gov/guidelines/cholesterol/atglance.pdf

Women's Health Initiative website: www.nhlbi.nih.gov/whi

ASRA KERMANI

Chronic Fatigue Syndrome

Chronic fatigue syndrome (CFS) is defined as severe fatigue of 6 months or longer, with no medical explanation. Four or more of the following eight symptoms must also have been present over the past 6 months, starting after the fatigue: substantial impairment in short-term memory or concentration, sore throat, tender lymph nodes, muscle pain, joint pain without swelling or redness, headaches of a new type or pattern or severity, unrefreshing sleep, and malaise after exercise lasting more than 24 hours. Muscle weakness and proven psychological or physical disorders rule out the diagnosis of CFS.

CFS affects both genders, all races, ethnicities, and socioeconomic populations, and can begin as early as age 5. Women are twice as likely to be affected with CFS compared to men. It is estimated that a half million people in the United States have a CFS-like condition.

CAUSE

Nobody really knows what causes CFS. Proposed causes include neuropsychological abnormalities; viral infection; immune and endocrine abnormalities; and metabolic, vascular, or enzymatic problems.

The neuropsychological symptoms are distinct from typical depression or anxiety disorders. Depression in CFS may be a reaction to being sick for so long, but there is more depression in CFS compared to other chronic diseases. Some think that CFS begins as a psychiatric disorder with immune, neurologic, and endocrine abnormalities arising afterward.

Certain viruses are suspected of causing CFS, including Epstein–Barr virus, coxsackie B virus, cytomegalovirus, measles, enterovirus, rubella, retroviruses, human herpes virus type 6, and human T-cell lymphotropic virus. However, there are no consistent or conclusive data to say that any specific virus causes CFS.

The immune system may be involved in CFS, because more than 65% of those diagnosed with CFS have a history of previous allergies. Reported endocrine abnormalities associated with CFS include low levels of adrenalin and related chemicals. These findings could account for the decreased energy and mood in affected individuals. Other possible metabolic abnormalities such as abnormal levels of brain chemicals, lack of adequate cerebral blood flow, and increased lung enzyme levels remain unproven.

SYMPTOMS

Debilitating fatigue is the hallmark of this syndrome. Daily functioning is often impaired. Aside from those symptoms required for diagnosis, other symptoms of CFS include alcohol intolerance, bloating, chest pain, chronic cough, diarrhea, dizziness, dry eyes or mouth, earaches, irregular heartbeat, jaw pain, morning stiffness, nausea, night sweats, shortness of breath, skin sensations, tingling sensations, and weight loss. The onset of CFS is often associated with a viral-like syndrome consisting of extreme fatigue, lung and sinus ailments, fever, and swollen glands. Stresses such as physical exertion, headache, and sore throat tend to make the fatigue worse.

DIAGNOSIS

Since fatigue is a common symptom in many diseases, a search for the cause of the fatigue needs to be considered. However, avoiding unnecessary and expensive tests is also important. Before diagnosing CFS, a complete history and physical examination should be performed on all patients to exclude another illness. Laboratory tests should be limited to complete blood cell counts and tests specific for the patient's symptoms.

Depending on the results of the history and physical examination, illnesses that may need to be ruled out include fibromyalgia, chronic mononucleosis, Lyme disease, psychiatric disorders, sleep disorders, myalgic encephalomyelitis, irritable bowel syndrome, hormonal disorders, neurasthenia, chronic sinusitis, anemia, occult celiac disease, rheumatic disease, alcohol abuse, substance abuse, sick building syndrome, multiple

chemical sensitivities, reactions to prescribed medications, eating disorders, cancer, autoimmune disease, obesity, and other conditions.

TREATMENT

Patients with CFS should not expect a quick fix. Sometimes using ineffective and unnecessary treatments does more harm. The best treatment strategy includes education, pain control, exercise, optimal diet, appropriate sleep schedule and antidepressants (both for mood and for chronic pain), combined with cognitive-behavioral therapy. Treatment for allergies and stress reduction may improve the quality of life for persons with CFS. A multidisciplinary approach involving medical, psychiatric, behavioral, and psychological evaluation and therapy has demonstrated effective results by restoring the ability to work and keep a job.

SEE ALSO: Autoimmune disorders, Chronic pain, Sleep disorders

Suggested Reading

The Merck manual of diagnosis and therapy (17th ed.). (1999). Also at www.merck.com/pubs/mmanual/

Suggested Resources

Centers for Disease Control/National Center for Infectious Diseases. Chronic fatigue syndrome website: www.cdc.gov/ncidod/diseases/cfs/

National Institutes of Health/National Institute of Allergy and Infectious Diseases. Chronic fatigue syndrome website: www.niaid.nih.gov/publications/cfs.htm

GINA BELL
LORI B. SIEGEL

Chronic Obstructive Pulmonary Disease

Chronic obstructive pulmonary disease (COPD), the fourth leading cause of death in the United States, is a chronic, progressive disease encompassing both emphysema and chronic bronchitis that lead to severe airflow obstruction. Emphysema causes irreversible lung damage by weakening and breaking the air sacs (the alveoli) within the lungs. As a result, elasticity of the lung tissue is lost, causing airways to collapse and airflow obstruction. Chronic bronchitis is an inflammatory

Chronic Obstructive Pulmonary Disease

Table 1. Clinical development of COPD (American Thoracic Society)

Stage 1	Lung function (as measured by forced expiratory volume or FEV_1 in 1 s) is greater than or equal to 50% of predicted normal lung function. There is minimal impact on health-related quality of life. Symptoms may progress during this stage, and patients may begin to experience severe breathlessness, requiring evaluation by a pulmonologist
Stage 2	FEV_1 lung function is 35–49% of predicted normal lung function, and there is a significant impact on health-related quality of life
Stage 3	FEV_1 lung function is less than 35% of predicted normal lung function, and there is a profound impact on health-related quality of life

disease that begins in the smaller airways (bronchiolitis) within the lungs and gradually advances to larger airways. It increases mucus in the airways and bacterial infections in the bronchial tubes, which, in turn, impedes airflow. Both components of COPD vary in proportion between affected individuals.

The clinical development of COPD has been described by the American Thoracic Society based on lung function measured as the forced expiratory reserve volume in 1 s (FEV_1) as shown in Table 1. In addition, physicians diagnose and classify COPD based on pulmonary function testing stated in the global initiative for chronic obstructive lung disease (GOLD) criteria from the World Health Organization. Individuals affected with COPD also present with certain symptoms that vary in severity, such as chronic cough, chest tightness, shortness of breath, an increased effort to breathe, increased mucus production, and frequent clearing of the throat. Among smokers, the natural history of COPD is that smoking behaviors often start during youth, lung function decline becomes apparent when smokers reach age 40–50 years, hospitalizations begin when smokers reach an age of about 69, and deaths may occur when they reach age 60–79. Research has been targeted to determine the genetic and environment interactions that are involved in the development of COPD as well as gender-related differences associated with the onset of this lung disease.

Long-term cigarette smoking remains the major environmental risk factor (besides second-hand smoke or exposure to air pollution) for the development of COPD, accounting for 80–90% of all cases and establishing a smoker as 10 times more likely than a nonsmoker to die of COPD; however, mounting evidence now suggests that genetic factors likely influence the variable susceptibility among individuals to develop COPD.

In nonsmokers, the FEV_1 (volume of air expelled on deep exhalation in 1 s) normally declines at a mean rate of about 20–30 ml per year during adult life; however, in most smokers, this mean rate of decline is increased to 30–45 ml per year, but in the subset of cigarette smokers who are susceptible to developing COPD, the rate of decline is 80–100 ml per year. Therefore, even though there is evidence of a dose–response relationship between the severity of lung disease and the pack-years of cigarettes smoked (increased severity of lung disease with long-term smoking), only 15% of the variability in FEV_1 is accounted for by smoking history. In addition, only a minority of cigarette smokers develop COPD, and frequent clustering of COPD has also been found in families. Such observations and recent evidence suggest a genetic predisposition to this lung disease.

There are a number of genetic associations that are currently being examined to determine how various genotype–environment interactions (interaction between the environment and the specific genetic makeup an individual has) are likely to be essential contributors to the development of COPD.

Gender-related differences are also apparent in severe, early onset COPD. Men have higher prevalence rates of COPD than women, which have been attributed to the historically higher rates of cigarette smoking in males. However, the increased rates of cigarette smoking in females have been associated with increasing rates of COPD in women. In addition, by 2000, the number of COPD deaths among women surpassed the number of men, even though the population-based mortality rates are higher among men.

Results from recent studies suggest that women may be more susceptible to the development of COPD. More specifically, female first-degree relatives of early onset COPD probands (individuals with COPD) who smoke or have smoked cigarettes have increased susceptibility to severe airflow obstruction (but not of chronic bronchitis) and hence to the development of COPD. Determination of such gender-related differences in the development of COPD will enable better treatments for women and men.

SEE ALSO: Addiction, Adolescence, Lung transplantation, Nicotine, Smoking

Suggested Reading

Ali, J., Summer, W. R., & Levitsky, M. G. (1999). *Pulmonary pathophysiology*. New York: McGraw-Hill.

Lomas, D. A., & Silverman, E. K. (2001). The genetics of chronic obstructive pulmonary disease. *Respiratory Research, 2*(1), 20–26.

Mannino, D. M., Homa, D. M., Akinbami, L. J., Ford, E. S., & Redd, S. C. (2002). Chronic obstructive pulmonary disease surveillance: United States, 1971–2000. *Surveillance Summaries, 51*(SS06), 1–16; http://www.cdc.gov/mmwr/preview/mmwrhtml/ss5106a1.html

Sandford, A. J., & Silverman, E. K. (2002). Chronic obstructive pulmonary disease, 1: Susceptibility factors for COPD genotype-environment interaction. *Thorax, 57*, 736–741.

Silverman, E. K. (2002). Genetic epidemiology of COPD (Supplement). *Chest, 121*(3), 1S–6S.

Silverman, E. K., Weiss, S. T., Drazen, J. M., et al. (2000). Gender-related differences in severe, early-onset chronic obstructive pulmonary disease. *American Journal of Respiratory Critical Care Medicine, 162*, 2152–2158.

S. Franco
Marilyn Glassberg

Chronic Pain

Chronic pain is a complex medical syndrome. Any episodic pain problem, including low back pain, neck pain, and migraine headaches, as well as many common medical problems such as diabetes can cause chronic pain. Chronic pain is any pain that, despite appropriate medical and surgical treatment, persists for 6 months or longer. Acute pain denotes tissue damage or injury, whereas chronic pain can develop insidiously from an acute problem. Many times the cause of the chronic pain cannot be determined. In these instances, chronic pain becomes the disease itself. Many people cope well with chronic pain; however, oftentimes, a chronic pain syndrome may develop.

The chronic pain syndrome has been defined by the Social Security Administration as intractable pain of 6 months or greater duration, which is associated with depression and anxiety that affects every aspect of a person's life. Vocational, recreational, and family relationships become altered and there is a marked restriction in daily activities. Sleep disorders are common. There are frequent visits to physicians. Patients have a history of multiple tests, treatments, and surgeries without alleviation of the pain. There is excessive use of medications, and frequent use of a variety of medical services including emergency room services is common.

Back and neck pain are the most common causes of chronic pain syndromes and are associated with significant workers' compensation costs. Back-related disability approaches 2% of the workforce at any given time. Lifetime prevalence for a significant episode of low back pain is 30–90%. The duration of an individual episode of low back pain is 2 weeks or more in 13% of individuals. The lifetime prevalence of neck pain is 40–70%. There are currently 28 million migraine sufferers worldwide, with more than 12 million in the United States. Twenty-one million of these sufferers are women and seven million are men. One in four households has at least one migraine sufferer. Other chronic medical problems which can produce chronic pain include rheumatoid arthritis (1%), diabetes (6%), and osteoarthritis (7%) (U.S. statistics).

Why should a single episode of illness, episodic pain problems, and chronic medical problems produce a chronic pain syndrome? Chronicity is determined not by the disease state alone, but by psychological and social factors. Certain psychological factors which predispose to a chronic pain problem include "catastrophic thinking" with interpretations of pain as mysterious or life threatening. Correlations between avoidance of an unpleasant situation such as working in a low-paying job or monotonous job or trying to avoid an unhappy marriage can lead to illness behavior which increases without a direct correlation to the pain itself. Fear of repeat injury and kinesiophobia (fear of movement) lead to deconditioning, which then produces a cycle of prominent susceptibility to strains/sprains and reinjury. Psychiatric illnesses such as depression (10–83%) share a high comorbidity with chronic pain. Situational or reactive depression may be associated with the pain, but endogenous depression can also be exacerbated by an episode of illness. This can lead to a lack of response to rehabilitation since depressed individuals do not rehabilitate well. Anxiety increases pain by causing an increase in release of stress hormones. Muscle contraction which produces chemicals such as lactic acid is also increased during anxiety. This can lead to a vicious cycle of chronic pain/anxiety/depression. Addictive disorders can also lead to chronic pain. However, meditation dependency may not be the initial presenting problem; patients in their attempts to alleviate their pain may increase the amount and frequency of their pain medications so that a dependency syndrome is produced. Lastly, personality disorders may predispose to chronic pain. There is a significant association of prior physical, sexual, or emotional abuse in patients with chronic pain.

165

Chronic Pain

The medical evaluation of chronic pain includes taking an appropriate history and performing a detailed physical examination. An evaluation of the specific pain problem should be undertaken if not previously done to ensure that no further testing or surgery is indicated. In addition, management of chronic pain requires a psychological evaluation to decide if someone is appropriate for self-management. Once it has been determined that all tests are complete, that no further assessment is required, and that medication adjustment alone will not alleviate a patient's pain, a comprehensive self-management program is imperative. Patients should be both medically and psychologically appropriate. Individuals must be motivated for rehabilitation and be willing to be active participants in their own health care. Any type of active thought disorder or dementia will not allow a patient to participate in self-management. The goal of chronic pain management is just that, "management" and not a cure. Some pain relief may ascertained, but a cure, in most instances, is not possible. Individuals who are satisfied with their current sedentary lifestyle and inability to function in society will not benefit from active participation in a pain management program. In general, the best indication of a patient's suitability for any type of self-management program is compliance with treatment instructions. Daily diaries to assess levels of activity including ability to sit, stand, walk, or lift before pain increases, amount of "up time" (time doing daily activities), and amount of "down time" (time spent resting or in bed) must be documented. Family and friends should be encouraged to participate in treatment. Family members need to provide support without excessive caretaking.

MAJOR GOALS OF PAIN MANAGEMENT

There are three primary treatment goals for someone with chronic pain. These are: adjusting medication to suit one's individual needs, training in psychological pain and stress management techniques, and increasing daily activities and improving the quality of one's life.

The first goal is to appropriately adjust medications. Forty percent of patients with chronic pain take narcotic analgesics. They overuse their pain medications to try to give themselves some relief. Addicting medications should be discontinued. Rebound pain from taking short-acting narcotic analgesics continues a cycle of dependency on medication and escalation in use. By discontinuing narcotic analgesics, a "drug holiday" is given.

Although initially an individual may respond with an increase in pain, the body's ability to naturally fight pain with its own endorphins will begin and the pain will actually diminish as narcotics are discontinued. Narcotic analgesics and sedative medications interfere with our own natural ability to produce pain-relieving substances (endorphins) and thereby the ability to fight pain naturally is enhanced with discontinuation. Nonaddicting, long-acting medications appropriate for the problem such as nonsteroidal anti-inflammatory agents, antidepressant agents which work centrally in the brain by stimulating endorphin production and strengthening the descending or inhibitory pain pathways by blocking the reuptake of seratonin should be prescribed. Many of these agents can be sedating and when used at bedtime, can allow an individual with chronic pain to sleep. Other medications may be useful in managing chronic pain. These include nonnarcotic analgesics such as Tramadol; the antidepressant medications; atypical antipsychotic agents such as olazapine; anticonvulsants including carbamazepine, Topiramate, gabapentin, and others; antispasticity agents such as tizanadine and Baclofen, and miscellaneous agents such as Mexiletine, topical lidocaine, substance P inhibitors such as capsaicin; and other topical agents that can be purchased over-the-counter such as topical aspirin may be useful.

The second goal of comprehensive treatment is training in psychological pain and stress management techniques. Pain is subjective and can be mediated by cognitive, emotional, and environmental influences. To understand the role of psychological techniques in management of chronic pain, one can conceptualize pain as consisting of both primary pain and secondary pain. Primary pain is the pain a person experiences from the tissue injury and damage. It is the direct result of nerve damage, scarring, and is usually irreversible. Therefore, primary pain is the least amount of pain a chronic pain sufferer can experience given ideal circumstances. Secondary pain, however, is the frequent fluctuation in chronic pain that can be experienced when an individual participates in life. This may be exacerbated by emotional and physical factors such as deconditioning, overexertion, body position, weather changes, anger, stress, and "life in general." Simply, secondary pain is variable and is the fluctuation of pain as a person goes through his daily life.

Although primary pain can be influenced by medications, secondary pain, in general, is influenced by psychological pain and stress management techniques. These include relaxation training such as progressive muscle relaxation, guided imagery, and autogenic training, which promotes deep muscle relaxation. These techniques can be taught as preventive strategies as well as abortive strategies when the pain begins to escalate. Biofeedback is another commonly used technique. By "feeding back" certain information such as muscle tension, body temperature, heart rate, and peripheral blood flow, a person can learn to voluntarily control these bodily functions. Biofeedback is most commonly taught in conjunction with other relaxation techniques. There is no clear evidence that biofeedback is superior to relaxation training alone.

Hypnosis is a very useful technique which can promote deep, general, muscular relaxation; however, it is more effective in controlling acute pain such as dental pain, surgical and burn pain, and pain from childbirth. Chronic pain is best managed with awareness techniques that are better managed with relaxation training and biofeedback.

Stress and anxiety have a significant impact on an individual's pain. There are a variety of stress management techniques that can be used including stress inoculation, assertiveness training, and time management.

The third goal of chronic pain management is increasing daily activity levels and improving the quality of life. Chronic pain is incurable, but not untreatable. Many patients who have chronic pain can learn to manage and control their problem and lead productive lives despite their pain. Physical rehabilitation is essential in order for someone to return to a normal life. Prolonged periods of bedrest can result in deconditioning. Decreased functional levels lead to decreased endurance, which can contribute to weakness, muscle spasms, and a vicious cycle of pain. Physical therapy assesses a patient's motor skills, posture, and body mechanics. The physical therapist should ideally identify muscle weaknesses and provide a gradual program of muscle strengthening and endurance building. Assessment of activities of daily living and teaching one appropriate body mechanics and postures, which will avoid and correct asymmetries of the body, will improve an individual's pain. Heat, cold, and deep myofascial release are appropriate for certain conditions. Joint mobilization, improving flexibility, and in certain individuals, joint stabilization is indicated.

An ergonomic evaluation is essential. Proper ways of sitting, standing, walking, carrying, lifting, and performing other activities of daily living can be taught by an occupational therapist. Ergonomics is "the laws of work." Assessing someone's workstation or home

environment is essential. Proper positioning of computers, adjustment in chair and desk heights, use of head sets, and back, arm, and foot supports can improve a person's ability to return to the work environment safely.

Chronic pain patients usually base their activity level on the amount of pain they are experiencing. However, in the case of chronic pain, pain is a fact of life. Patients need to learn to plan their activities so that it is "task contingent," not "pain contingent." Once a baseline level of activity is set, patients should follow a very simple rule; every day they must perform at least the same amount that they did on the day before. It does not matter on day one it took an individual 10 minutes to perform a task. If on day two the pain level is higher, as long as the task is completed it can take all day. By doing this, an individual can learn to avoid the "good day, bad day" syndrome. This keeps a person active and helps prevent that cycle of disability, pain, anxiety, and depression. Gradually, pain can be worked through and an individual can begin to establish a more normal routine.

Chronic pain can be used as a coping response; by using pain to avoid an undesirable event (visiting one's in-laws), pain is used as a coping activity. However, over time it is reinforced. Just as in Pavlov's dogs, every time the dog saw a food dish, he began to salivate, every time an individual thinks of going to his in-laws, his pain increases. This becomes a vicious cycle and the patient may actually lose voluntary control. The individual will then react to that and other distasteful situations by an exacerbation of pain. Therefore, pain should never be used as a coping tool.

Successful management of chronic pain requires active family participation. These are "the forgotten sufferers." As a person becomes disabled with chronic pain, family members are forced to assume many of the responsibilities of the pain sufferer. This includes job responsibilities and family responsibilities. Families need to become involved so that successful management includes them. Family members should be educated as to the nature of the chronic problem and should be provided with treatment rationale. Families should learn to not be critical and should also be taught not to enable. Both of these can cause significant family dysfunction and may exacerbate the chronic problem.

CONCLUSION

Chronic pain is a significant problem, which affects an individual's ability to function and be productive.

Clinical Trials

Pain and disability is multifactoral and involves medical, emotional, and socioeconomic factors. It is a complex problem, which requires comprehensive treatment. Evidence is substantial that patients who have failed individual therapies will benefit from a comprehensive pain management program and have an excellent outcome with regard to ability to function within society.

SEE ALSO: Addiction, Anxiety disorders, Arthritis, Depression, Migraine, Osteoarthritis, Sleep disorders

Suggested Reading

Covington, E. C. (2001). A pain medicine approach to chronic low back pain. *Continuum, 7*, 112–140.

Kriegler, J. S. (1993). Medical management of chronic low back pain. In R. W. Hardy (Ed.), *Lumbar disc disease* (2nd ed., pp. 293–297). New York: Raven Press.

Kriegler, J. S. (2002). Fibromyalgia. In B. Katirji, H. Kaminski, D. Preston, et al. (Eds.), *Neuromuscular disorders in clinical practice.* Boston: Butterworth Heinemann.

Kriegler, J. S., & Ashenberg, Z. A. (1987). Management of chronic low back pain: A comprehensive approach. In D. Goldblatt (Ed.), *Seminars in neurology* (pp. 303–316). New York: Thieme Medical.

McQuay, H. J., Moore, R. A., Eccleston, C., et al. (1007). Systematic review of outpatient services for chronic pain control. *Health Technology Assessment, 1*, 1–135.

Nelson, D. A., & Landau, W. M. (2000). Intraspinal steroids: History, efficacy, accidentality, and controversy with review of United States Food and Drug Administration reports. *Journal of Neurology, Neurosurgery, and Psychiatry, 70*, 433–443.

Van Tulder, M. W., Koes, B. W., & Bouter, I. M. (1997). Conservative treatment of acute and chronic non-specific low back pain. A systematic review of randomized trials of the most common interventions. *Spine, 22*, 2128–2156.

Vingard, E., Mortimer, M., Wiktorin, C., et al. (2002). Seeking care for low back pain in the general population: A two-year follow-up study. Results from the MUSIC-Norrtalje Study. *Spine, 27*, 2159–2165.

JENNIFER S. KRIEGLER

Climacteric *see Perimenopause*

Clinical Trials Clinical trials are a form of medical research involving human participants. What follows is a brief overview about what clinical trials are and why they are done, important considerations for individuals considering participation in clinical trials, and a history of women and clinical trials.

The primary purpose of clinical trials is to determine whether promising new strategies for treatment and/or prevention of illness are safe and effective. Sometimes clinical trials also assess whether other factors—like subtype of illness, co-occurring illnesses, or differences in rates of metabolism in different individuals—influence how safe and effective various treatments and prevention strategies are.

Clinical trials might be testing an experimental drug or medical device that looks promising in laboratory studies and animal studies, but has not yet been tested in humans. Or, they might be testing a new system for delivering a medication already proven to be safe and effective for humans—for example, through an extended-action pill format, nasal preparation, or as an injection. Many clinical trials compare different treatment or prevention strategies to provide information about which is better. For example, a clinical trial may test how a combination of psychotherapy plus medication compares with psychotherapy alone and/or medication alone to help guide treatment decisions for clinical depression; another might compare prophylactic surgery with intensive monitoring and "watchful waiting" for women found to be at high risk for breast cancer to provide information to help guide decision-making related to preventing breast cancer.

Clinical trials are generally divided into four phases, or steps along the pathway toward determining safety and efficacy (Table 1). The four phases are most well defined for medication trials. However, research design has become so complex that many trials do not fit nicely into one of these four phases. Nevertheless, these four phases provide an overview of the processes involved in establishing new treatment and prevention strategies.

While there are many different types of clinical trials, one thing they have in common is their ultimate objective: to advance the scientific knowledge upon which treatment and prevention strategies are based. Sometimes, "new" and "promising" experimental treatments or prevention strategies are thought to be better, just because they are new. However, until well-designed and well-conducted clinical trials are completed, we cannot know if a promising experimental treatment or prevention strategy will be safe and effective. In the United States, companies seeking to market medications or medical devices must get approval from the Food and Drug Administration (FDA). In order to get FDA approval, these companies must provide data from clinical trials showing that the investigational drug

Table 1. Four phases of medication clinical trials[a]

Phase I	Phase I trials assess *safety* and *toxicity* of an experimental agent in healthy volunteers or sometimes in individuals with the medical condition of interest. Phase I trials are only conducted if there are adequate data from laboratory and animal studies to justify trying the experimental agent in humans. Phase I trials generally enroll a small number of research participants and last a relatively short period of time (weeks to months). Experimental agents must pass through each stage to get to the next one.
Phase II	Phase II trials test further for safety and start to look for *effective doses* and other preliminary evidence of efficacy. Phase II trials generally enroll 50 to several hundred individuals and can take up to a couple of years to enroll enough research participants.
Phase III	Phase III trials are designed to *test for efficacy* and also to further assess frequency and severity of side effects. Phase III trials are comparative trials and compare the result from a group of participants receiving the experimental agent with a group receiving a "control" agent, either a standard available treatment or a placebo (a sugar pill). They generally involve random assignment to these different groups—thus research participants do not get to choose which group they will be in. In addition, research participants and the researchers themselves are frequently not allowed to know which group they are in during the course of the trial—a research design aspect known as "blinding" or "masking." "Randomized, controlled, double-blind" clinical trials are the gold standard for minimizing bias and providing reliable evidence for efficacy. Phase III trials may enroll thousands of individuals and take up to several years to complete enrollment.
Phase IV	Phase IV trials are used to inform questions about *longer term effectiveness* of medications (e.g., how well they perform in regular clinical settings for long periods of time as opposed to the more controlled environment of a phase III clinical trial) and to assess *longer term and rarer side effects*. Phase IV clinical trials are much less standard in design and depend on the relevant questions being asked.

[a] Only phases I–III are required for FDA approval. Phase IV trials are not required for FDA approval. They are conducted after FDA approval to answer remaining important questions.

or medical device is safe and effective. However, just because a new medication or medical device is approved for marketing, does not mean that it is necessarily safer or more effective than other available treatments. For example, in many medication trials for agents seeking FDA approval, experimental agents are compared with placebo (a sugar pill used to decrease bias in the clinical trial) to show that the experimental agent is safe and effective. Other types of trials directly comparing treatments may be needed to help determine if one is safer or more effective than another and/or if different treatments work better for different individuals.

Even though the primary purpose of clinical trials is to generate new knowledge, individuals sometimes view participation in clinical trials as an important option for accessing promising, albeit unproven and uncertain, alternatives to available treatments. This is especially true for some illnesses for which no good treatments are available. For individuals seeking to participate in clinical trials because of the possibility of personal benefit, and for their loved ones and health care providers helping them to make decisions about whether to participate, it is crucial to understand that participation in a clinical trial may not provide the medical benefits one is hoping for. It is also important for

all involved to remember that even if there is a chance of receiving direct medical benefit from participating in a clinical trial, receiving care in a clinical trial is different from receiving treatment outside a clinical trial.

Regular medical treatment is meant to provide personalized help to the individual seeking treatment; clinical trials are designed to answer scientific questions. "Treatments" used in clinical trials are intended to benefit future patients and society as a whole by advancing medical knowledge. Individual research participants may or may not receive medical benefit from the experimental interventions and "treatment" administered as part of a clinical trial. Interestingly, however, some researchers contend that just being in a well-designed clinical trial is good for individuals because they receive better care than is available outside of a clinical trial, and clinical outcomes of individuals in trials are better than those of individuals receiving regular medical care—and there are studies trying to assess whether these contentions are supported by evidence. Nevertheless, while it may be true that some individuals do receive medical benefit from their participation in clinical trials, this certainly is not always the case. Thus, such benefit may best be thought of as a "side effect" of clinical trial participation that some participants experience. And it is important to remember that providing individualized medical benefit to each participant in a clinical trial is not the main purpose of the trial.

Many individuals participate in clinical trials because they see participation as providing hope for medical benefit, even with all of the uncertainty involved. Some participate because of the desire to contribute to medical science and help future patients. Others participate because they feel a sense of camaraderie from being with other individuals with the same medical condition being closely monitored and cared for by a team of experts: the research physicians and nurses. Most participants in research have multiple motivations for considering research participation; for example, some might hope to benefit, but also understand that their participation helps to advance science and may help future patients, even though they themselves may not directly benefit from being in the trial.

While it is natural for individuals to have many different motivations for considering enrollment in a clinical trial, it is crucial that individuals have enough information and time to make an informed decision about whether or not to enroll. Although research undergoes review for its science and its ethics, a clinical trial that is determined to be appropriate to conduct may not be appropriate for or acceptable to every individual. For example, it is widely held that in order to be ethical, clinical trials must satisfy a requirement known as "clinical equipoise"—that is, a genuine uncertainty and lack of consensus exists within the medical community about whether the investigational treatment is as good as or better than standard treatment or placebo, when no effective treatment is available. However, even clinical trials that comply with this ethical standard still have features that depart substantially from standard medical practice. To increase scientific rigor, treatment alternatives (or placebo) are frequently randomly assigned to participants, participants and the research team are typically blind to which alternative is received, and protocol-driven limitations may be placed on the types and doses of interventions. Clinical trials generally do not allow the flexibility for individualized clinical decision-making that patients might be used to in working with their own personal physicians.

In addition, clinical trials may include research procedures that impose discomforts or risks for harm to participants who are not compensated by personal diagnostic or therapeutic benefits; instead, they are justified by the importance of the knowledge from the study. For example, participation in some trials may include medication washout periods, biopsies, overnight hospital stays, imaging studies with radiation exposure, blood draws, and questionnaires—not because something will be learned that will benefit the participant, but because they are needed to generate data necessary to test study hypotheses. Individuals who participate in clinical trials are closely monitored by the research team for adverse events that might be linked to their participation in the trial, and it is expected that their participation will be stopped by the research team if it looks like they are experiencing significant adverse events as a result of participating in the research. However, despite the fact that clinical trials are designed and reviewed to minimize risks of harm and the fact that there is close monitoring of the participants, some individuals may be harmed by their participation in a clinical trial—either by a research procedure or by the experimental intervention itself. These risks are on top of the risk of not receiving medical benefit from participating in a clinical trial. After all, clinical trials are conducted to see how well the experimental intervention works and if it is safe in humans.

For all these reasons, individuals considering participating in a clinical trial are encouraged to find out as much information about what it means to participate in clinical trials generally and what it would mean to participate in the particular trial they are considering. This process of gathering information and making decisions is referred to as the "informed consent process."

During the informed consent process, individuals should carefully read the consent form and any other information the research team has available to give them. Individuals should feel free to ask any and all questions they have about the research study, including who is funding the study and whether or not the researchers have a financial stake in the outcome of the study, if they desire this information. Individuals should also feel free to consult with their own personal health care providers and their family and friends about this decision. Books and pamphlets are available that offer more information about clinical trials and suggestions for important questions to ask when considering participation in one. Two such general resources published in 2002 are: *Should I Enter a Clinical Trial? A Patient Reference Guide for Adults with a Serious or Life-Threatening Illness*, a report by the Emergency Care Research Institute (ECRI), a nonprofit health services research organization committed to improving quality, safety, and cost-effectiveness of health care; and *Informed Consent: The Consumer's Guide to the Risks and Benefits of Volunteering for Clinical Trials*, by Getz and Borfitz (full citations in Suggested Reading at the end of this entry).

Individuals who consider participating in clinical trials should know that the decision whether or not to participate should be voluntary and a decision against participation should not affect their ability to get the medical care that is available to them otherwise. Also, after enrolling in a clinical trial, individuals are free to decide at any time during their participation that they wish to leave the clinical trial for any reason and instead receive standard treatment from their own health care providers. It is important to remember that we all owe a debt of gratitude toward individuals who volunteer for clinical trials, for it is the only way to get the evidence that many of us rely on to assess how safe and effective various treatment and prevention strategies are.

The dual concerns of safety and effectiveness sometimes compete with one another and create a dilemma related to the question, "Who ought to be allowed to participate in research as a research subject?" The history of women as research participants in clinical trials highlights the dilemma. While there are many regulations governing research with human participants, this has only been the case for the past 30 years. Prior to this, many pregnant women took the medications thalidomide and diethylstilbestrol (DES) before it was discovered that these medications caused birth defects and other health problems for the children who were exposed to the medications in utero. In 1977, resulting in part from these discoveries, the FDA barred pregnant women and women of childbearing potential from participating in early phase clinical trials assessing medications. The reasoning behind this policy was that early phase trials rarely provide benefit and have the potential to seriously harm the fetus. Although the FDA policy was limited to early phase studies, concerns about possible harms and legal liability translated into clinical trials that routinely excluded pregnant women and, in many cases, women of childbearing potential. Similar concerns also seemed to sway investigators from studying illnesses or medical conditions primarily affecting pregnant women or women of childbearing potential. This led to a period of time in which most clinical trials included primarily men or postmenopausal women. And this practice continued because it was widely believed in the scientific community—a community made up largely of men—that potential differences between women and men were scientifically and clinically unimportant. Now, we know that there are important differences between women and men, for

example, in drug metabolism and in prevalence of various medical disorders. Thus, these guidelines—which were originally intended to limit the harm done in clinical research—had the ironic effect of limiting new knowledge about women and their health issues.

In the late 1980s and early 1990s, both the National Institutes of Health (NIH) and the FDA issued policies and guidelines requiring that women of childbearing age be included in later phase research and that analyses be conducted to assess differences between men and women with regard to safety and efficacy of experimental treatments. The NIH created an Office of Research on Women's Health to promote research aimed at improving the health of women and to oversee the implementation of the NIH policy on inclusion of women in NIH-supported research. The FDA also has an Office of Women's Health which funds research and educational efforts to enhance women's health. It also works to ensure that clinical trials over which the FDA has jurisdiction include sufficient numbers of women to assess safety and efficacy of medications and devices seeking FDA approval.

Even though clinical trials have started to include women in sufficient numbers to provide information about safety and efficacy of treatments for women, there are not always sufficient numbers of individuals with other characteristics that potentially affect the safety and efficacy of medications and medical devices. For example, there are differences in drug metabolism among various ethnic groups that may not be picked up in clinical trials because there are not enough individuals from an ethnic group participating in a trial. Also, many clinical trials exclude individuals with co-occurring illnesses or who are on other medications from participation in the trial, and thus there is no information about whether the medications and/or devices studied are safe and effective in individuals with these co-occurring illnesses or when taken with other medications. Postmarketing surveillance of FDA-approved medications and devices can help answer some of these questions that are left unanswered by the approval process. In addition, postmarketing surveillance may uncover information about safety that leads an approved medication to be pulled off the market because data in a larger number of individuals, some with characteristics that were not included in previous clinical trials, show that it is not as safe as it originally seemed.

While postmarketing surveillance provides important information, it cannot substitute for information gathered from well-designed clinical trials. However, most information about use of medications during pregnancy and breast-feeding is garnered from surveillance data from pregnant and breast-feeding women who take medication after it is approved, rather than from clinical trials due to continued worries about exposing fetuses and breast-feeding infants to risks of harm in clinical trials. The paucity of reliable information lead women and their physicians to shy away from using medications during pregnancy or breast-feeding, to use lower doses of medications when they are needed, and to use older medications which seem to be safer based on reasoning that they have been around long enough that serious problems would have already shown up. However, though concern over taking medication while pregnant and/or breast-feeding is understandable, in many cases, not treating or inadequately treating a medical condition is equally concerning and raises questions that are currently unanswerable. Various federal agencies are working together to gather better systematic data on outcomes from women who have taken medications while pregnant and/or breast-feeding as well as to promote clinical research aimed at answering these types of questions related to maternal health.

We are starting to see the benefits of the concerted steps taken to improve the situation generated by many years of neglect regarding women in clinical trials research. While there is still room for improvement, these policies and programs have contributed greatly to enhancing the medical knowledge base for women.

SEE ALSO: Diethylstilbestrol, Discrimination, Disparities in Women's Health and Health Care (pp. 3–13), History of Women's Health in the United States (pp. 13–20), Informed consent, Thalidomide, Women's Health Initiative

Suggested Reading

Chen, D. T., Miller, F. G., & Rosenstein, D. L. (2003). Clinical research and the physician–patient relationship. *Annals of Internal Medicine, 138*(8), 669–672.
ECRI. (2002). *Should I enter a clinical trial? A patient reference guide for adults with a serious or life-threatening illness. A report by ECRI commissioned by the AAHP.* Available on-line at http://www.ecri.org/documents/bctoc2.html#table
Getz, K., & Borfitz, D. (2002). Informed consent: The consumer's guide to the risks and benefits of volunteering for clinical trials. Boston: CenterWatch. http://www.centerwatch.com

Suggested Resources

FDA Office of Women's Health: http://www.fda.gov/womens/default.htm
NIH Office of Research on Women's Health: http://www4.od.nih.gov/orwh
Women's Health Initiative: http://www.nhlbi.nih.gov/whi/index.html

DONNA T. CHEN

Club Drugs Also known as *designer drugs*, club drugs are a group of manufactured, psychoactive substances. While club drugs can differ substantially in their effects and pharmacologic classifications, they are subsumed under the category of *club drugs* because they are often abused in the context of dance clubs or raves (all-night parties). There is some disagreement as to which drugs are club drugs; however, the National Institute on Drug Abuse (NIDA) classifies the following as club drugs: methylenedioxymethamphetamine (MDMA, also known as Ecstasy), ketamine (Special K), methamphetamine (speed, ice, or glass), gamma hydroxybutyrate (GHB, Liquid G), and flunitrazepam (Rohypnol or Roofies). It is important to note that, while these drugs can be used recreationally, GHB and Rohypnol are also commonly called date-rape drugs because they are known to be used as a means of incapacitating a victim with the intention of sexual assault.

Perhaps the most widely used and quintessential club drug, MDMA is a synthetic drug with both hallucinogenic and stimulant properties. It is also referred to as an entactogen, which means that it can have the effect of making a person feel interconnected with, and empathic toward, others. First developed in 1914 as a weight-loss aid, MDMA was never marketed for that purpose. However, in the United States in the 1970s, the drug gained some popularity among clinical psychologists as an aid to psychotherapy and marriage counseling. In 1985, the use of MDMA was banned and placed on the list of scheduled drugs by the U.S. Drug Enforcement Agency. However, the popularity of the drug remained unchecked, and its use has since been associated in the United States mainly with youth subcultures. It is generally packaged in a tablet or capsule form, often with imprints of cartoon characters or popular corporate logos. While there is some disagreement in the scientific community regarding the long-term effects of MDMA, current research suggests that MDMA use results in the overproduction and then the depletion of serotonin which may result in depression. Other potential adverse effects can include dehydration, overheating (hyperthermia), tooth damage caused by jaw-clenching (bruxism), and possible effects on memory.

While MDMA has been associated with a number of deaths worldwide, tablets sold as MDMA often contain other substances which are harmful and even deadly, such as paramethoxyamphetamine (PMA).

Another club drug is GHB, a sedative-hypnotic which was formerly sold as a nutritional supplement in the United States before becoming a controlled substance. GHB is distributed as highly potent, colorless liquid with a salty taste. Doses are calibrated by water-bottle capfuls, and the difference between a recreational and a deadly dose can be very small. Taken alone or in conjunction with alcohol, GHB can be the cause of death. Deaths have occurred from the aspiration of vomitus during a GHB-induced coma or from the depression of the respiratory center in the brain stem. The reputation of GHB as a date-rape drug has been substantiated by numerous cases in which individuals, particularly women, were surreptitiously drugged and then sexually assaulted. Its effectiveness as a date-rape drug is compounded by its effect on memory; victims often cannot recall what has occurred during a GHB-induced coma.

A third popular club drug, used primarily by adolescents and young adults, is ketamine, which is sold in either a powder (white or yellow) or liquid form. It is generally snorted in small amounts, although it can be injected or smoked. This drug, which is primarily used in the United States for veterinary purposes, is a dissociative anesthetic, and it is related to phencyclidine (PCP). Users of ketamine often describe an out-of-body experience which they call a *k-hole*. While in this state, users often experience visual and tactile hallucinations, are unable to move, and are insensitive to pain. The adverse effects of recreational ketamine use can include depression, delirium, amnesia, respiratory problems, and death. There is also the danger of seriously injuring oneself due to the lack of pain sensation and an impaired ability to react quickly. There have also been reports of ketamine being used as a date-rape drug.

A final club drug, flunitrazepam (Rohypnol, Roofies), is also considered a date-rape drug, and its popularity as a recreational drug has waned considerably in some areas. Regular users can become addicted to Rohypnol. This powerful tranquilizer comes in the form of a tablet which is not produced in the United States. Rohypnol has a sedative-hypnotic effect in sufficient doses, and it can cause temporary amnesia. When mixed with alcohol or other depressant drugs, Rohypnol can render an unsuspecting victim powerless to defend herself; such a mixture can also cause death.

While the popularity of club drugs has increased, many users of Ecstasy, ketamine, GHB, and Rohypnol are unaware of the short- and long-term dangers associated with these drugs. When mixed with alcohol or other drugs, these dangers multiply. Most importantly, neither alcohol nor club drugs should ever be used by pregnant or nursing woman, as these substances can result in an assortment of severe problems for all concerned.

SEE ALSO: Depression, Sexual abuse, Substance use

Suggested Reading

Beck, J., & Rosenbaum, M. (1994). *Pursuit of ecstasy: The MDMA experience*. Albany, NY: SUNY Press.
Cole, J. C., Sumnall, H., & Grob, C. (2002, September). Sorted: Ecstasy (and following peer commentary). *The Psychologist, 15(9)*, 464–474.
Hinchliff, S. (2001). The meaning of ecstasy use and clubbing to women in the late 1990s. *International Journal of Drug Policy, 12*, 455–468.
Holland, J. (2001). *Ecstasy: The complete guide. A comprehensive look at the risks and benefits of MDMA*. Rochester, VT: Park Street Press.
National Institute on Drug Abuse. (2001, March). Hallucinogens and dissociative drugs including LSD, PCP, ketamine, dextromethorphan. *NIDA research report series* (NIH Publication No. 01–4209). Washington, DC: U.S. Department of Health and Human Services.
Nicholson, K. L., & Balster, R. L. (2001). GHB: A new and novel drug of abuse. *Drug and Alcohol Dependence, 63*, 1–22.
Siegel, R. K. (1986). MDMA: Non-medical use and intoxication. *Journal of Psychoactive Drugs, 18(4)*, 349–354.

Suggested Resources

National Institute on Drug Abuse. *NIDA. Infofacts: Robypnol and GHB*. (NIH). U.S. Department of Health and Human Services. Available at: http://www.nida.nih.gov/Infofax/RohypnolGHB.html

JILL ADAIR MCCAUGHAN

Cocaine Cocaine is a mood-altering drug in the stimulant or "amphetamine-like" class. As a consequence, it tends to produce euphoria or "high" feelings by directly blocking the reuptake of dopamine in the brain. The resulting increases of dopamine produce an elevation of mood and euphoria. Cocaine has two additional effects, which are to block the sodium–potassium pump in nerve cells of the skin and tissues, and to

Cocaine

increase the circulating levels of a hormone called norepinephrine or noradrenaline.

The effect of blocking the sodium–potassium pump in peripheral nerve cells is to cause those cells to lose their ability to transmit sensation. This results in a local feeling of numbness, and the use of cocaine as a local anesthetic for the past century. The increase in norepinephrine or noradrenaline is responsible for the "stimulant" effects of cocaine including: increased heart rate, blood pressure, alertness, coordination and reflexes, and decreased fatigue, need for sleep, and appetite. In summary, the three major effects of cocaine—euphoria, stimulant effects, and local anesthesia—are each due to a separate action of the drug.

Like many organic molecules, cocaine comes in two forms—an acid form named cocaine hydrochloride or cocaine HCl, and a base or alkali form named cocaine-carbonate or "crack," "base," or "rock" cocaine. The only clinically important difference between the acid and base forms of cocaine is a change in the vapor point of cocaine base. As a consequence, cocaine base (or "crack" or "rock" cocaine) can be smoked, whereas cocaine HCl burns rather than vaporizes when heated and therefore cannot be smoked. As it turns out, smoking a mood-altering drug is the quickest way to get the highest concentration of that drug to the brain, followed closely by using the drug I.V. Since the addicted or chemically dependent brain tends to seek the highest level of dopamine-trigged euphoria possible, there has been a tendency for individuals addicted to cocaine to move toward either I.V. use or smoking the drug.

HISTORICAL USE OF COCAINE

Cocaine is a naturally occurring substance found in the leaves of the coca tree. This substance has been used for as long as 2,000–3,000 years by peoples in the mountainous regions of Central and South America. The use of cocaine by humans for many hundreds of years was primarily by the chewing route of administration or the brewing of a weak coca leaf tea-like beverage. These two routes of delivery, across the oral cavity mucous membrane or through the absorption of the stomach and small intestine, are characterized by their slow gradual rate of absorption and thus delayed gradual onset and mild intensity of euphoria or "high." The concentration or amount of cocaine in coca leaves is quite low and therefore the "historical" use of cocaine was characterized by slow rates of absorption, very low

potencies or amounts of cocaine, and a gradual mild degree of mood-altering effect. The physical effects of cocaine even at these "historical" low doses were significant, however, producing an increase in energy, decrease in fatigue or tiredness, increased stamina, decreased appetite, and improved concentration and coordination. So for tens of centuries cocaine was used as a performance enhancer in the workplace, and as a mood-altering beverage in social or religious settings.

In the 1800s, cocaine was identified as a possible treatment for some psychiatric illnesses, notably depression or "melancholia," and recognized for its local anesthetic effects. As a consequence, the extraction of cocaine from the coca leaf (much like the extraction of digitalis from the fox-glove leaf during the same period) became widespread and thus the purity and potency of cocaine dramatically increased. Cocaine emerged in the late 1800s for the first time in history as a potentially very potent stimulant and euphoria-producing drug.

COCAINE USE PATTERNS

Conviction for possession or use of any amount or form of cocaine in this country constitutes a felony. As a consequence, it is difficult, if not impossible, to truly discuss low risk or "social" use of cocaine at present. Thus for practical purposes, all cocaine use in American communities must be viewed as being cocaine abuse. From historical reports, experience of other countries, and even National Institutes of Health (NIH) research, it is clear that not all cocaine users develop addiction to the drug. In fact it appears that a minority, perhaps as low as 15–20%, of cocaine abusers in our community develop cocaine addiction, while the majority remain abusers or move toward abstinence. Estimates are that as many as 40 million Americans have experimented with or intermittently used cocaine.

There is a qualitative and quantitative difference between a cocaine abuser who *does not* have chemical dependence and a cocaine abuser who *is* addicted. Abusers tend to use occasionally, in social settings, for brief periods and in low amounts. They fail to meet three (or usually even one) of the *Diagnostic and Statistical Manual of Mental Disorders*, fourth edition (DSM-IV) criteria for addiction. I.V. use or smoking of "crack" or freebase is generally not seen among abusers and is a strong indicator of addiction. Individuals with cocaine addiction demonstrate intermittent repetitive loss of control over their cocaine use resulting in adverse consequences in their lives. They tend to use it in a pattern of escalating binges—sometime using cocaine for up to 4 days at a time with little to eat, drink, or sleep during that period. Cocaine-dependent people will primarily either smoke the cocaine or use it I.V.

Typically chemical dependence or addiction with cocaine as the drug of choice involves a binge–crash–"honeymoon"–binge–crash … pattern. This is due to the pharmacology of the drug cocaine and complex interactions with the brain of an addicted person. This pattern involves the binge phase: several hours to a few days of compulsive repetitive self-administration of cocaine. Because of the development of tolerance during a binge, patients experience less and less euphoria or "high," and increasing amounts of dysphoria or "low" feelings—often progressing to frank paranoia. This binge is followed by a crash phase: a period of several hours to up to a day and a half of marked increase in sleeping, eating, depressive feelings, and remorse for the actions during the binge. In fact, the behaviors during the crash phase are really the opposite of those during the binge phase. The crash phase is followed by the "honeymoon" phase where people can go for a few to several days promising to never binge again and being relatively unaffected by the drug. Unfortunately, this phase is routinely followed, often on the next payday, by another binge–crash cycle. Many patients who are well into this pattern think that they are not addicted since they do not use every day. Nothing could be further from the truth.

Sadly, judgment is exceedingly sensitive to cocaine effects. As high doses are ingested during a binge, the erratic behavior associated with cocaine addiction can become horrifying, with unspeakable family, legal, and job-related consequences. During a cocaine epidemic, there is typically a marked community rise in violent crime, drive-by shootings, domestic violence, child abuse and neglect, sexually transmitted disease, and unanticipated pregnancy.

TREATMENT OF COCAINE DEPENDENCE

The treatment of addiction in general and cocaine in particular requires a focus on eliminating all use of cocaine *and* all other mood-altering drug use. Abstinence is the treatment goal. The reason for abstinence from other mood-altering drugs in addition to cocaine is the common pattern of initially quitting cocaine only to continue to use alcohol or marijuana, with the rapid relapse back to cocaine use. The disinhibition associated with other drug or alcohol use, combined with a rapid intense escalation of cocaine cravings, frequently results in a relapse. For more information on general principles of addiction treatment and the maintenance of abstinence, see the entry Substance use—"Abuse" and "Dependence."

Cocaine addiction can involve a high degree of physical dependence—primarily affecting the brain. Cocaine withdrawal symptoms are virtually all mediated by brain changes and thus have historically been termed "psychological or psychiatric," but given that the brain is a physical organ, it is most appropriate to consider these physical effects. The symptoms include mood swings, depression, irritability, difficulty concentrating, vivid dreams and intrusive thoughts about using cocaine, sleep disorder, periodic increased heart rate and hand tremor and sweating, and a persistent urge to use cocaine. Detoxification from cocaine frequently involves physical removal from "using" opportunities, provision of a supportive therapeutic sober environment, and treatment of psychological or psychiatric symptoms that may precipitate relapse. In addition, a trial of detoxification medications is common, including possibly beta-blockers or alpha agents, and medications used to treat Parkinson's disease. Medications are in clinical study that may be able to block cocaine's effect, or even work like an anticocaine immunization or vaccine.

Rehabilitation refers to an inpatient residential or outpatient program that commonly lasts a month or more and entails daily counseling to develop skills to avoid cocaine and all drug and alcohol use for life. Maintaining abstinence can be quite difficult when faced by cocaine cravings and dreams, especially in a society where the majority of people are social or low-risk users of alcohol. There are special self-help meetings specifically developed for cocaine dependence called Cocaine Anonymous or "CA." For more information regarding self-help "12-step" meetings, see the entry Substance use.

SEE ALSO: Addiction, Addiction ethics, Chemical dependence, Heroin, Injection drug use

Suggested Reading

American Psychiatric Association. (1994). *Diagnostic and statistical manual of mental disorders* (4th ed.). Washington, DC: American Psychiatric Association.

Cognitive-Behavioral Therapy

American Society of Addiction Medicine. (2003). *Principles of addiction medicine* (Vol. 3). Washington, DC: American Society of Addiction Medicine.

Mooney, A. (1992). *The recovery book.* New York: Workman.

Suggested Resources

National Center for Substance Abuse Treatment website, with much cocaine treatment information: www.samhsa.gov/csat/csat.htm

National Institute on Drug Abuse website, the preeminent website for drug addiction research in the world. The "epidemiology" section of this site contains links to the two surveys evaluating drug use patterns in the United States: the National Household Survey and the National High School Survey: www.drugs.gov

This is a national service for addiction prevention education funded by the Robert Wood Johnson Foundation, with much information on cocaine problems: www.jointogether.org

TED PARRAN, JR.

Cognitive-Behavioral Therapy Cognitive-behavioral therapy (CBT) is a family of interventions used to help people recognize and overcome a wide variety of problems. It is based on the theory that how a person thinks about a situation affects how he/she feels about it and ultimately affects how he/she reacts or behaves as a result. The therapist teaches the person to recognize these cognitive distortions ("irrational thoughts") and their result. Once the distortion is recognized, the person can restructure her/his thoughts and change the emotional and behavioral result.

For example, you are at home waiting for a friend to come over for dinner and he is an hour late. There are several ways you can think, feel, and react to this situation. You can think, "maybe he's been in an accident." If you think this, you may feel nervous or scared. As a result, you may bite your nails, pace, call all the hospital emergency rooms and the police to check for accident victims, or maybe ruminate to the point of getting a stomachache. When he does arrive, you may cry, hug him tight, and tell him how worried you were.

You can think "he's blowing me off, he doesn't care about me." If you think this, you may feel angry. As a result, you may pace, call his house or office and leave nasty messages, or maybe tear up his picture or things he has given to you. When he does arrive, you may yell and scream at him, start a physical altercation, or slam the door in his face without giving him the opportunity to explain.

You can think "he's with another girl, I'm not good enough, smart enough, pretty enough, etc." If you think this, you may feel worthless or unsure of yourself. As a result, you may cry, make a mental list of all of your "faults," or maybe even think no one will ever like you or want to be with you. When he does arrive, you may be quiet, distant, or even tell him he could do better.

You can think "he's late, now I have some extra time to get something done until he gets here." If you think this, you may feel content or even relieved that you have the extra time. When he does arrive, you may continue with your evening as planned and have a good time.

In each of these scenarios, you had "automatic, irrational thoughts" based only on conjecture and not based on fact.

Some people get confused and think CBT is trying to have people turn everything into a positive, "look for the silver lining." CBT is more sophisticated than that. It teaches people to recognize the result of irrational thoughts and to change the thoughts, emotions, and resultant behaviors. In the above example, if your friend was late because he was inconsiderate and did not care that you were waiting, CBT may help you to see that this is not a reflection on you and your self-worth but more a function of his attitude and behaviors.

CBT is not one specific intervention but a family of interventions based on the underlying theory. You and your therapist will discuss your particular problems and tailor the intervention to address those needs. The interventions are geared at identifying the irrational thoughts and resultant problematic feelings and behaviors and then teaching you how to replace those with more healthy coping techniques.

CBT is short-term, structured therapy that involves active participation on both the therapists' and the clients' parts. Depending on the target problem, you may have as few as 2 or 3 sessions or up to 15–20 sessions. In addition, most CBT requires "homework" between sessions. The homework assignments are geared to practicing the skills learned in therapy by applying them to the "outside" world. The next therapy session will usually address the homework assignment and how it worked or did not work, reshaping the exercises, and trying again.

CBT has been shown to be effective in helping with a wide variety of problems. Issues such as depression, anxiety, phobias, and eating disorders as well as being nervous in public speaking, resolving issues that come up in adjusting to new situations (job, relocation, marriage, divorce, parenthood), and grief are all problems that can be helped with CBT interventions.

CBT has been subjected to the rigors of scientific research. Because of the structured nature of the interventions, it is particularly suited to being delivered consistently across therapists to be able to study its effectiveness. Studies have shown CBT to be as effective as medications in treating psychological problems and in some cases better than medication. The combination of CBT and medications is consistently helpful over medications alone.

As with any treatment, it will only work if you follow through on the therapy. CBT is an effective family of interventions that can make a significant, long-term impact on the lives of those who engage in it.

SEE ALSO: Anxiety disorders, Depression, Mood disorders

Suggested Reading

Beck, A. T. (1979). *Cognitive therapy and the emotional disorders.* New York: Meridian Books.

Burns, D. D. (1999). *The feeling good handbook.* New York: Plume.

Padesky, C. A., & Greenberger, D. (1995). *Mind over mood.* New York: Guilford Press.

Suggested Resources

www.nacbt.org

DEBRA R. HROUDA

Cohabitation
Cohabitation means living together in an intimate relationship. Cohabitation implies a relationship that is like a marriage, but without any legal ties. People may choose cohabitation because they do not wish to have the formal legal ties of a marriage, including financial ties. For example, a person may lose eligibility for some federal income and health care benefits if they marry someone who has an income. Other couples may choose cohabitation because they are not legally permitted to marry. Lesbian couples, or couples where one partner is separated but not legally divorced, do not have marriage as an option.

Cohabitation can lead to a marital relationship in a small number of states. These states recognize what is called "common-law marriage" when people have lived together for a required time period and held themselves out as a married couple. Most states do not recognize common-law marriage.

Since cohabitation is not, in most cases, a marriage, the couple cannot use the divorce process to resolve issues in the event that they separate. Disputes over who can keep what possessions are often difficult. Because the law does not recognize cohabitation, a court would award property to the person who has title, such as the title holder to a car or piece of real estate. Often this leads to unfair results when both parties contributed to the purchase but only one has title.

People who cohabit can construct many legal ties that ordinarily come from marriage. They can have wills that leave possessions to each other. They can give each other a "power of attorney" which allows one person to make important decisions about health care or finances if the other is unable to do so. If the couple has children, the father can establish his legal relationship with the child.

SEE ALSO: Child custody, Divorce, Domestic partnership

Suggested Reading

Curry, H., et al. (1999). *A legal guide for lesbian and gay couples.* Berkeley, CA: Nolo Press.

Ihara, T. L., & Warner, R. (1997). *The living together kit: A legal guide for unmarried couples.* Berkeley, CA: Nolo Press.

Samuelson, E. (1997). *The unmarried couple's legal survival guide: Your rights and responsibilities.* Secaucus, NJ: Carol.

Stanley, J. (1999). *Unmarried parents' rights.* Naperville, IL: Sphinx.

SHEILA SIMON

Colonoscopy
see Colorectal Cancer

Colorectal Cancer
The lifetime risk of developing colon cancer is about 60% and is slightly higher in men than in women. Half of those affected persons will die of the disease. It is rare before the age of 50 years and the incidence increases thereafter. Death caused by colon cancer has decreased over the last 20 years. Colorectal cancer death rates are rising in African Americans. The overall 5-year survival rate for colorectal cancer is 60%.

Colorectal Cancer

DIGESTIVE SYSTEM ANATOMY

The digestive system consists of the esophagus, stomach, small bowel, colon, and rectum. The colon and the rectum store the waste until it is evacuated from the body. The colon and the rectum form a long muscular tube about 6 ft long also known as the large intestine. The rectum is the specific name for the last 8–10 in. of the colon.

RISK FACTORS FOR COLORECTAL CANCER

Multiple factors can increase the risk for colon cancer. Being born in North America or Western Europe is a risk factor. A diet that is high in fat, red meat, and sucrose may contribute to colorectal cancer. Alcohol consumption, smoking, obesity, and a history of pelvic radiation are also risk factors. Colorectal cancer occurs as people age and those with a longstanding history of ulcerative colitis are at high risk. Persons with first-degree relatives, that is, parents and siblings with colorectal cancer, are at increased risk to develop it. In general, it is recommended that the latter group start to have colorectal cancer screening 10 years before the age that the relative was diagnosed. On the other hand, those born in Africa or Asia are at lesser risk for colorectal cancer. Diets that are rich in fruits, vegetables, and fiber, along with high intake of calcium appear to decrease the risk for colorectal cancer. There is a suggestion that postmenopausal hormone replacement in women, long-term aspirin, or nonsteroidal anti-inflammatories and vigorous activity are also protective against colorectal cancer.

HOW DOES CANCER DEVELOP?

It is felt that colorectal cancers arise from polyps, specifically adenomatous polyps. Of Americans over the age of 50, 30–50% will develop these polyps. One in 20 adenomas will progress to cancer and this occurs over a period of over 10 years. The cancer risk is related to specifics of the adenomas including their size, number, architecture, and abnormalities seen at the cellular level on microscopic examination. It is based on this understanding that screening for colorectal cancer is done.

DEFINITIONS

1. A fecal occult blood test (FOBT) is a test used to look for small amounts of blood in the stool that cannot be seen with the naked eye.
2. A sigmoidoscopy is an examination of the rectum and the lower colon, using a lighted instrument called a sigmoidoscope. These scopes are usually 60–70 cm (24–28 in.) in length.
3. A colonoscopy is an examination of the rectum and the entire colon, using a lighted instrument.
4. A double contrast barium enema (DCBE) is a series of x-rays of the colon and rectum. The patient receives an enema with barium, which outlines the colon and rectum. This also defines masses and other abnormalities of the lining of the colon.

SCREENING FOR COLON CANCER

Screening for colon cancer can be done in many ways. The choice of which screening is best for the patient should be based on his/her preferences and the available resources for testing and follow-up. The physician or health care provider should explain the benefits and potential risks associated with each option before deciding on the screening process.

The frequency of screening is based upon the test. If the FOBT cards are used, three cards must be collected every year. There may be false-positive results where the test can indicate the presence of blood when there is nothing wrong with the colon. The U.S. Preventive Services Task Force is a body of experts that evaluates the effectiveness of screening tests based on the clinical evidence, the magnitude of benefit, and potential risks. The task force strongly recommends that clinicians screen men and women at the age of 50 years and older for colorectal cancer.

The method of screening is still under debate. There are different options and different benefits of each option. There is good evidence that periodic FOBT reduces mortality from colorectal cancer and fair evidence that sigmoidoscopy alone or in combination reduces mortality. The standard in practice is three stool cards collected yearly and sigmoidoscopy performed every 5 years, beginning at the age of 50. Recent studies have suggested that colonoscopy, which is a full examination of the entire colon, can find more cancers because there is direct visualization of the entire colon. Colonoscopy is the most sensitive and specific test for finding cancer in polyps (meaning that most of the cases it detects are really cancer and most of the ones it says are not cancer are really not cancer), but does come with higher risk than the other screening tests. The risks are small, but include a risk of bleeding and perforation, usually related to removal of polyps or biopsies. The colonoscopies require an overnight bowel cleansing preparation, mild sedation, highly trained personnel to do the test, and a longer recovery time. At this point, the task force feels that it is not certain whether the potential added benefits of colonoscopy, relative to the other screening alternatives, are large enough to justify the added risks, cost, and inconvenience for all patients. This is an area that will continue to be evaluated. A colonoscopy for screening purposes need only be done every 10 years.

The age at which colorectal cancer screening should be stopped is not known. In general, screening has been done in patients younger than 80 years of age. In theory, the yield should be higher in older persons, that is, we should find more cancers in older persons. However, the benefits may be limited as a result of the other medical conditions of the patient that may affect the treatment of any cancer that could be found. It is appropriate and reasonable to stop screening in patients whose age or comorbid conditions limit their life span.

The FOBT requires three consecutive stool samples be obtained at home and brought into the clinic. It has not been established whether the patient should avoid certain foods or medications. However, adding water to the specimens before testing them, does increase the sensitivity of finding blood. It is important to remember that three different stool cards from spontaneously voided stools are the standard and that neither a rectal examination nor the testing of a single specimen obtained during a rectal examination is considered adequate screening. A combination of both FOBT and sigmoidoscopy may detect more cancers. It is highly recommended that the stool cards, that is, FOBT cards, be returned before the sigmoidoscopy. A positive test on an FOBT is an indication for a colonoscopy. The sigmoidoscopy should not be performed in the presence of a positive stool card.

IF I NEED TO HAVE A SIGMOIDOSCOPY, WHAT SHOULD I EXPECT?

The actual sigmoidoscope is between 60 and 70 cm long. It is a flexible tube, especially the first few inches where the light is located. Within the scope there are channels for air to be put into the patient to open up the colon. There is a suction channel to pull out extra fluid and small bits of stool. It has the ability to remove a biopsy from the lining of the colon (a small piece of tissue usually is removed). The colon is a soft tube that when empty of stool after laxatives and enemas, collapses and is very flat. In order to visualize the lining of the colon, the person doing the examination usually has to put in some air to open this area up so he/she can see the mucosa. At the beginning of the examination, the scope is inserted into the patient. The main examination of the colon occurs as the scope is withdrawn from the patient and air can be removed at the same time. The test takes about 15 minutes and patients tolerate the test very well. One risk of the procedure is the gassy feeling the patient may feel from the air. There is a small risk of bleeding if a biopsy is taken and there is a very miniscule risk of perforation if a biopsy is removed. The test overall is very well tolerated, especially in the hands of experienced endoscopists. This test is done every 5 years, in association with three stool cards every year.

WHAT IS A COLONOSCOPY?

A colonoscope is a similar scope with much greater capabilities for removal of polyps because the scope allows examination of the entire length of the intestine. This scope allows the physician to evaluate for inflamed tissue, growths, ulcers, bleeding, and spasm. The main differences between the sigmoidoscopy and the colonoscopy are that the latter examines the entire colon and requires a sedative and a more extensive bowel-cleansing regimen.

The patient lies on his/her left side for the procedure and is given some medication to relieve the discomfort of the examination. The scope is inserted and slowly guided through the entire length of the colon. The physician examines the colon and the result is given to the patient at the end of the examination. If anything abnormal is found, the physician can remove a piece of it (biopsy), which is sent to the lab for further evaluation. Possible complications of colonoscopy are bleeding and puncture of the colon; however, these complications are very uncommon. This procedure takes between 30 and 60 minutes. The sedatives and pain medications protect the patient from feeling any discomfort during the examination. The patient generally needs to wait for 1–2 hours for the sedative to wear off. It is most safe for the patient if he/she brings someone to drive him/her home.

SEE ALSO: Cancer, Pain, Preventive care

Suggested Reading

Barker, L. R., Burton, J. R., & Zieve, P. D. (Eds.). (2003). *Principles of ambulatory medicine* (6th ed.). New York: Lippincott, Williams & Wilkins.

Carlson, K. J., Eisenstat, S. A., Frigoletto, F. D. Jr., & Shift, I. (1995). *Primary care of women*. St. Louis, MO: C. V. Mosby.

Suggested Resources

The National Cancer Institute: http://cancertrials.mci.nih.gov

The National Guideline Clearinghouse Guideline Synthesis: http://www.guideline.gov/COMPARISON/brscreen.5.asp

KATHLEEN WOLNER

Colposcopy

Colposcopy is the examination of the female genitals (cervix, vagina, or vulva) with an instrument called a colposcope. It is usually done to evaluate any lesions suspected of representing abnormal tissue growth or cancer. This may be an abnormal Pap smear or any lesion which does not resolve spontaneously in a reasonable amount of time as decided by the clinician. The colposcope is an instrument which permits magnification of lesions of the genital tract. A mild solution of acetic acid is applied to areas of the genital tract and abnormal areas turn white enhancing the quality of the colposcopic examination. All surface (epithelial) lesions become more distinct and structures including the cells on the wall of the cervix become more distinguishable using this method. After gross microscopic examination of the affected tissue for acetowhite changes and blood vessel patterns, tiny samples of tissue (biopsies) are removed and sent to pathology for histological (microscopic) evaluation. Colposcopy of the cervix can either be deemed satisfactory or unsatisfactory based upon the visualization of an area where

the different types of cervical wall cells (squamous and columnar epithelium) of the cervix interface, called the transition zone (T zone) and all margins of any visible lesions. Sampling of the endometrium and endocervix may be necessary depending on the original abnormality noted upon cellular (cytological) examination of the Pap smear and the findings at colposcopy. If colposcopy is deemed unsatisfactory or if any high-grade lesion is suspected or diagnosed, a diagnostic excisional procedure (small tissue sample cutting) may be scheduled. This tissue is then examined for the characteristics of abnormal growth/cancer and for involvement of the margins. Techniques for excision include cervical conization (special type of tissue removal technique) using the laser or scalpel, loop electrosurgical excision (LEEP), or loop electrosurgical conization.

Usually biopsies are painless; however, a local anesthetic may be used during a diagnostic excisional procedure. Once performed, colposcopic evaluation is usually followed closely for at least 1–2 years.

During pregnancy, abnormal Pap smears are also evaluated by colposcopy and biopsies are necessary if the lesions appear high grade. Occasionally, a pregnant patient may need to undergo the surgical excision of a high-grade cervical lesion. The cervix is more vascular (increased blood supply) in pregnancy and there is an increased risk of bleeding. This risk is managed by performing the procedure in the hospital setting.

SEE ALSO: Pap test, Pregnancy

MARGARET L. MCKENZIE

Comfort Women

Sexual exploitation has always been a part of war. However, the Japanese military not only exploited women sexually, but also actually enslaved them. Hundreds of thousands of women were either tricked or forced into sexual slavery during the Japanese occupation of Korea, from 1910 to 1945, and during World War II. These women were called *Jungun Wianbu* in Korean or *Jugan Inafu* in Japanese, meaning military comfort women. Now, some advocate using the term "military sex slaves" or MSS, because the term "comfort women" is too innocuous to reflect accurately the situation of the women.

The majority of comfort women were Korean, but women from the Philippines, China, Burma, Taiwan, and Indonesia were also forced to become sex slaves for the Japanese military. Some Dutch and Australian women, mostly nurses, also became comfort women. The few Japanese women to become comfort women were Japanese prostitutes.

In the beginning, Japan tricked the majority of the young girls into becoming comfort women by promising factory-type jobs. The opportunity for work was appealing to many young women and their families, because the economy in Korea had steadily declined due to Japanese colonialization. The colonialization primarily affected farming families because Japan took the crops to feed their soldiers. The depressed economic state of Korea allowed Japan to lure these young women away easily. This was called *Kunro Jungshindae*, or virgin recruitment. Some women received draft notices, whereas others were simply promised work. However, as the supply of young women ran short, Japanese police and "recruiters" began kidnapping younger girls, some as young as 13; even married women were not safe. Many were abducted right off the street and were not even allowed to say goodbye to their families. Once taken, these women were transported to many different locations, such as China, Japan, Rabaul, Hong Kong, Indonesia, and Taiwan. Some women went to privately operated comfort houses, while others were taken to military-run comfort houses on the front line. The conditions of these "comfort stations" were appalling. Many had no heat and only thin straw mats on the floor. They were partitioned off into small rooms only big enough for the mats. It was here that the comfort women would receive the soldiers, almost continuously.

Comfort women were given regular checkups by military doctors to prevent venereal diseases. Women who became infected were given injections of a drug called 606, which also caused miscarriages. If a woman became too sick to perform her "duties," she disappeared and was not heard from again. Due to the repeated venereal diseases and frequent miscarriages, many former comfort women were never able to have children; few women ever married. This had serious repercussions for the women, as status and security in Asian countries is often based on marital ties and children.

Why did Japan establish these comfort houses? The purported reasons for the establishment of comfort houses were to protect the local women from rape, to prevent the soldiers from being infected with venereal diseases, and to encourage the soldiers by providing a "necessary" comfort.

Former comfort women were silent until recently, perhaps due to shame and fear that society would judge them for the atrocities of the Japanese military. A few made attempts to reveal the plight of former comfort women, but were largely ignored. There was tension between Japan and Korea after the war and during the postcolonial period; it was feared that any mention of the comfort women issue would destroy the delicate economic relations between the two countries. Therefore, those who wanted to go public were quietly encouraged to remain silent.

The silence was broken in 1991, when one former Korean comfort woman came forward publicly. Kim Hak Soon filed a lawsuit against the Japanese Government seeking reparations. Other former comfort women also joined the lawsuit, but remained anonymous; again, the fear of stigmatization prevailed. Former comfort women want a formal apology from Japan and reparations. Japan has established a private fund for payment to former comfort women, but has not provided any official acknowledgment. Few women have accepted moneys from the private fund, believing that the use of private funds instead of government money is just another way for Japan to avoid official recognition of the sexual enslavement.

The issues involving former comfort women are becoming recognized around the world. The Korean Counsel for the Women Drafted for Military Sexual Slavery by Japan, The Comfort Women Project at San Francisco University, and the Washington Coalition for Comfort Women Issues are just a few of the organizations that have raised the issue of Japan's subjugation of comfort women in international forums.

SEE ALSO: Rape, Violence

Suggested Reading

Hicks, G. L. (1995). *The comfort women: Japan's brutal regime of enforced prostitution in the Second World War.* NSW, Australia: Allen & Unwin.

Howard, K. (Ed.). (1995). *True stories of the Korean comfort women.* New York: Cassell Academic.

Kim-Gibson, D. S. (1999). *Silence broken: Korean comfort women.* Parkersburg, IA: Mid-Prairie Books.

Schellstede, S. C., & Soon, M. Y. (Eds.). (2000). *Comfort women speak: Testimony by sex slaves of the Japanese military.* New York: Holmes & Meier.

Yoshimi, Y. (2001). *Comfort women: Sexual slavery in the Japanese military during World War II.* New York: Columbia University Press.

TAMBRA K. CAIN

Complementary and Alternative Health Practices

Complementary and alternative medicine (CAM) is a group of health-related practices that are generally viewed as falling outside of mainstream medicine. CAM is the term currently utilized by the National Institutes of Health. However, semantics used to describe this area of medicine can often be confusing. The term that people are most familiar with in the United States is "alternative" medicine. However, this term is not favored by some, as it seems to imply abandoning conventional care in favor of a nonconventional or alternative approach. "Complementary" medicine is the term most frequently used in England. It implies that the nonconventional therapies will be used to complement the conventional care that a person is receiving. A more current term is "integrative" medicine. Integrative medicine is considered by most to describe an approach to health that incorporates considerations of mind, body, and spirit with an openness to look beyond mainstream medicine. The National Institutes of Health has categorized CAM into five main areas. They include alternative medical systems, mind–body interventions, biologically based therapies, manipulation and body-based methods, and energy therapies.

Alternative medical systems are complete systems of medicine which differ from the dominant medical system in the United States, frequently referred to as Western medicine or biomedicine. These systems, such as traditional Chinese medicine and Ayurvedic medicine from India, have their own unique way of viewing health, disease, and treatment. However, in any culture, there is always a dominant medical system and multiple alternative or nondominant systems. All of these systems have various strengths and weaknesses, as well as similarities and differences.

Mind–body interventions are a category of treatments that recognize and utilize the connection between the mind and the body. They include such modalities as hypnotherapy, biofeedback, guided visualization, and progressive relaxation, to name a few. Recognizing the connection between physical health and emotional or mental state can often lead to significant improvement in symptoms or even cure of various conditions.

Biologically based therapies such as dietary supplements, including vitamins, minerals, and herbs, as well as the use of foods to treat or prevent disease, are popular as they are usually readily accessible by the general population. Many of these therapies are effective; however, some may interact with medications or be otherwise potentially harmful. It is important to review potential dietary supplement–drug, dietary supplement–dietary supplement, or even food–drug interactions when considering biologically based therapies. A complete list of one's dietary supplements should be included when disclosing medication use.

Manipulation and body-based methods include therapeutic massage, of which there are over 80 techniques, chiropractic manipulation, and osteopathic manual therapy. These methods in general can be particularly effective for musculoskeletal-related disorders, including relief of pain, spasm, and stiffness. Although additional non-musculoskeletal-related conditions may respond to manipulation or body-based therapies, further research is needed to clarify the most appropriate indications.

Energy therapies utilize an individual's or nature's healing energy to bring about relief of symptoms or treat disease. These therapies include such modalities as therapeutic touch, healing touch, Reiki, Chi Gong, and polarity. Electromagnetic or magnet therapy is also included in this category. Again an area with great potential, energy medicine is gaining recognition, and some have suggested is the next great frontier for medicine.

In 1993, David Eisenberg published the results of a research survey which showed that approximately 38% of the U.S. population had used some form of CAM during the previous 12 months. This realization stunned many and led to an increased interest in CAM on the part of not only consumers, but health care providers, health care systems, insurers, and developers of health-related products. When Eisenberg repeated his study in 1997, he found that use of complementary medicine had increased to 42% of the population. Total number of visits to CAM providers had gone from 427 to 629 million visits, a number larger than all visits to U.S. primary care physicians during the same year. It was also reported that people were spending an estimated $27 billion out of pocket on CAM-related services and products.

It is important to point out that another discovery of the Eisenberg surveys was that less than half of consumers were telling their physician about their use of CAM. This is particularly concerning given the recognition that while many CAM treatments are likely effective, many also have the potential to interact with conventional medical therapies.

The growing interest in CAM has clearly been consumer driven. Researchers such as John Astin have investigated the reasons that people seek CAM therapies. What Astin and others have discovered is that the vast majority of individuals do not abandon conventional care but use CAM as an adjunct to the conventional care they are receiving. Most people who use both conventional and nonconventional therapies do so because they believe the combination to be superior to either alone. Many people pursue CAM therapies because they are looking for a more holistic orientation to health. Some have suggested that in this era of "high tech," many also desire the "high touch" frequently offered by CAM providers.

Investigators have also looked at CAM use within specific populations. Multiple studies have confirmed that patients with cancer, rheumatologic, and other chronic conditions utilize CAM at an even higher rate than the general population. In a paper written by DiGianni, it was reported that 63–83% of women with breast cancer used at least one type of CAM. The reasons for CAM use among these populations vary but include not only the hope that the CAM modality will help treat a medical condition, but also the desire for an increased sense of control that often comes from the ability to incorporate CAM into one's plan of care.

It is perhaps not surprising that more women than men utilize CAM. Women are typically the primary health care decision-makers within a family. As one begins to seek information about health, it is hard not to come across various recommendations on CAM either from friends, health professionals, literature, or the Internet. However, one must look at all sources of information with a critical eye in order to make a truly informed decision. Much of the information available on CAM has been supplied by companies that provide the service or product. This information is often presented in such a way as to make the potential product appear supported by scientific studies, when in fact it is often not the case. For that reason, it is advisable that women discuss their use of CAM with their physician or other health care providers.

In the past, many people had the correct perception that most health care providers were not open to a discussion on CAM. However, that has changed. The conventional medical community now clearly recognizes that the general public desire access and increased information on CAM modalities. Many medical, nursing, and allied health schools have responded by adding some training on CAM into their curriculum. This is leading to a generation of health care providers with a more open attitude toward CAM. The federal government has also recognized the increased utilization of CAM and, in response, has established the National Center for Complementary and Alternative Medicine (NCCAM) under the NIH. With a budget of $113 million in 2003, NCCAM, as well as other institutes at the NIH, is funding significant research in the area of CAM. As more of this research becomes available, health care providers, and in turn the general public, will be better able to make evidence-based decisions regarding the use of CAM.

It has become increasingly apparent that CAM is, and will continue to be, an important component of our health care system. For women concerned with their own health or the health of loved ones, consideration of select CAM modalities in conjunction with conventional care is essential when considering a comprehensive plan of care. Multiple resources should be consulted when determining which CAM modalities to incorporate and discussion with one's health care provider is strongly recommended.

SEE ALSO: Chiropractic care, Energy healing, Massage, Meditation, Yoga

Suggested Reading

Domer, A., & Dreher, H. (1996). *Healing mind, healthy woman: Using the mind–body connection to manage stress and take control of your life.* New York: Henry Holt & Co.

Hudson, T. (1999). *The women's encyclopedia of natural medicine.* Los Angeles: Keats.

Murray, M., & Pizzorno, J. (1998). *Encyclopedia of natural medicine.* California: Prima Health.

Northrup, C. (1998). *Women's bodies, women's wisdom: Creating physical and emotional health and healing.* New York: Bantam Doubleday Dell.

Pelletier, K. (2000). *The best alternative medicine: What works? What does not?* New York: Simon & Schuster.

Weisman, R., & Berman, B. (2003). *Own your health: Choosing the best from alternative and conventional medicine.* Deerfield Beach, FL: HCI Books.

ADAM I. PERLMAN

Comstock Laws

Comstock Laws In 1873, the U.S. Congress passed what became known as the "Comstock" laws. The act made it illegal to import, mail, or transport in interstate commerce obscene materials, including contraceptive devices and information on birth control. The act was named after Anthony Comstock, a Union Army veteran of the American Civil War. He also assisted in forming the New York Society for Suppression of Vice, of which he was also named the secretary. That organization mounted a campaign to regulate morality, resulting in the Comstock Laws. The Comstock Law was quickly adopted by many states in the sexually repressive environment of the 1800s. After the passage of the so-called Comstock Laws, Anthony Comstock became an inspector for the U.S. Postal Service and brought about over 2,000 convictions under this law. His writings include *Frauds Exposed* (1880) and *Traps for the Young* (1883).

In 1916, Margaret Sanger opened the first birth control clinic to be operated in the United States. Sanger opened her clinic in Brooklyn, New York, with the intention of testing the constitutionality of New York's version of the Comstock Law. Under the New York version of the law, a physician could prescribe contraceptives to prevent or cure a disease. Sanger and her staff were arrested and Sanger served a 30-day sentence at a women's prison. When Sanger's case came before the U.S. Supreme Court, the Court held that under the statute, the phrase "prevent or cure a disease" should be read broadly enough to include pregnancy. This meant that the New York Comstock Law was overturned.

Largely due to Sanger's efforts, a bill was introduced in 1923 to remove birth control from the Comstock Law. This bill failed. A "doctor's only" bill introduced in 1930 which would have permitted the distribution of contraceptives through doctors also failed. The bills were strongly opposed by the Catholic Church, whose official stance was against birth control.

While the Comstock Law has been trimmed extensively, a version is still valid law. Title 18 U.S.C. Sec. 1462(c) still makes the importation or transportation of obscene material by way of "express company or other common carrier or interactive computer service" illegal.

SEE ALSO: Birth control; Sanger, Margaret

Suggested Reading

Bates, A. L. (1995). *Weeder in the garden of the Lord: Anthony Comstock's life and career*. Lanham, MD: University Press of America.

Beisel, N. (1997). *Imperiled innocents: Anthony Comstock and family reproduction in Victorian America*. Princeton, NJ: Princeton University Press.

Chesler, C. (1993). *Woman of valor: Margaret Sanger and the birth control movement in America*. New York: Anchor Books.

Moore, G., & Moore, R. (1986). *Margaret Sanger and the birth control movement: A bibliography, 1911–1984*. Metuchen, NJ: Scarecrow Press.

TAMBRA K. CAIN

Condoms

Condoms are one of the oldest forms of contraception and the best recognized forms of protection against sexually transmitted infections (STIs), including human immunodeficiency virus (HIV). The continued high prevalence of STIs has resulted in a substantial increase in condom use over the past decades. The 1995 report from the National Survey of Family Growth (NSFG), a survey of women 15–44 years of age, found that condom use at first intercourse increased from 18% in the 1970s to 36% in the late 1980s to 54% in the 1990s. The NSFG noted that 7.9 million women, 15–44 years of age, use condoms for pregnancy prevention and an additional 4.2 million women use condoms for protection from STIs. Research indicates that about a third of women have partners who use condoms consistently, a third use condoms occasionally, and a third never use condoms for protection against STIs. Understanding factors associated with noncondom use is essential for the design of effective condom promotion efforts.

Considerable research has examined factors that are associated with the use and nonuse of condoms. Several studies have demonstrated an association between nonuse of condoms and having personal attitudes and beliefs that were not supportive of safer sex, consuming alcohol, using noninjection drugs, being unemployed, and having a limited education. Numerous studies have examined relational barriers associated with condom nonuse. Having poor communication skills, having an older male partner, a male partner who abuses drugs or alcohol, or is abusive significantly increase women's risk of STIs. Research has also demonstrated that condom use is dependent on women's relationship status. Specifically, women in committed relationships are significantly less likely to use condoms compared with women in casual or new relationships. These studies highlighted that women's risk for HIV is largely attributed to the attitudes and behaviors of their male partner.

An estimated 1–3% of the general population is allergic to latex, the material from which condoms are traditionally made. To address complaints regarding allergies to latex and decreased sexual enjoyment from use of latex condoms, a male condom made of polyurethane was developed. Polyurethane is a strong, impermeable material with good heat transfer that is less susceptible to deterioration during storage than latex. Subjectively, users express greater preference for the polyurethane condom over latex in regard to appearance, lack of smell, comfort, sensitivity, and natural look and feel. If preference translates to greater use, the male polyurethane condom may address important barriers that have been linked with nonuse of condoms.

A novel development in condoms is the female condom. The Reality female condom was approved by the Food and Drug Administration (FDA) in 1993 as a method to protect against unplanned pregnancy and STIs, including HIV. The Reality female condom is a silicon-lubricated, intravaginal barrier consisting of a soft, loose-fitting polyurethane sheath with a flexible ring at each end. The device is inserted similar to a diaphragm, the inner ring is compressed and is pushed into the vaginal cavity. The external ring and 1–2 inches of the sheath remain outside the vagina, partially covering the labia. Although the female condom requires male cooperation, it does not require male initiative. Notable features of the female condom are: (a) the fact that women can place it autonomously and can trust that it is not torn or taken off by the male partner, (b) the high level of protection it can afford when used correctly, and (c) the increased sexual pleasure it affords women. Since the outer ring of the female condom partially covers the external genitalia, the female condom may be particularly beneficial in preventing infections. Unlike the male condom, women are more likely to use the female condom with a steady partner, compared to a new or casual partner. The less desirable features of the female condom are: (a) the need to touch one's genitalia to insert the female condom, (b) the need to practice insertion and to use the device several times before mastering it, (c) the fact that it can be seen by the partner, (d) the disagreeable look of the device, (e) the occurrence of vaginal bleeding (nonmenstrual), (f) the discomfort as experienced by the male and/or female partner, and (g) the noise made by the female condom. Moreover, female condoms cost about $2.75 each in the U.S. retail stores and $0.63 for the public sector. By comparison, the wholesale price per male condom is $0.04.

Significant research has been conducted to examine the effectiveness of condom promotion efforts for women. These programs often emphasize enhancing women's sexual communication skills, promoting attitudes that are supportive of condom use, enhancing healthy relationship norms, mastering condom application skills, and identifying *triggers* that make using condoms challenging. However, maximally effective condom use promotion programs need to go beyond enhancing women's attitudes, intentions, and skills, and foster change in social structures or policies that affect condom use practice as an innovative method of reducing women's risk of unplanned pregnancy and STIs, including HIV.

SEE ALSO: Acquired immunodeficiency syndrome, Birth control, Lubricants, Safer sex, Sexually transmitted diseases

Suggested Reading

Breitman, P., Knutson, K., & Reed, P. (1994). *How to persuade your lover to use a condom…and why you should* (2nd ed.). New York: Prima.

Jukes, M., & Tilley, D. (1996). *It's a girl thing: How to stay healthy, safe, and in charge.* New York: Knopf.

McIlvenna, T. (1999). *The complete guide to safer sex* (2nd ed.). New York: Dembner Books.

CHRISTINA M. CAMP
GINA M. WINGOOD

Confidentiality

Confidentiality In the course of providing care, health care professionals routinely learn very personal, intimate information about their patients. As professionals, they begin with a fiduciary or trust duty to hold in confidence all personal patient information entrusted to them. This ethical obligation is enforced legally through civil damage suits based on both statutory and common law (judge-made precedent), and is embodied in the licensing provisions of virtually all state professional practice acts and accompanying regulations. Federal regulations promulgated in 2002 to implement the Health Insurance Portability and Accountability Act (HIPAA) impose on health care entities very specific requirements regarding the handling of personally identifiable medical information contained in patient records, and impose severe sanctions for unauthorized disclosures.

There are, however, a number of exceptions to the general confidentiality rule. One is that a patient may voluntarily and knowingly waive, or give up, the right to confidentiality of particular information. This is done daily to make information available to third-party payers (for instance, Medicare or private health insurers), quality of care auditors (such as surveyors of the Joint Commission on Accreditation of Healthcare Organizations), and other public and private entities (like patients' powers of attorney). Additionally, the usual confidentiality obligation may be outweighed when there is jeopardy to innocent third parties, such occurs when a patient with serious sensory or cognitive impairments insists on driving a motor vehicle or a dangerous psychiatric patient threatens to kill a specific victim and appears to have the present ability and intent to make good on that threat. State laws vary regarding the health care provider's obligation to report a threat to public health or safety authorities.

Third, the patient's expectation of confidentiality must yield when the physician is mandated by state law to report to specified public health or safety authorities, the physician's reasonable suspicion that certain conditions (e.g., domestic violence, elder mistreatment or neglect, certain infectious diseases, birth, and death) are present. Mandatory reporting laws represent the state's exercise of its inherent police power to protect the general health, safety, welfare, and morals of the community or its *parens patriae* authority to protect individuals who are not capable of protecting themselves.

Further, the physician may be compelled to reveal otherwise confidential patient information by the force of legal process, that is, by a judge's issuance of a court order requiring such release. This is a possibility in any lawsuit involving a factual dispute about a patient's physical or mental condition.

Since the delivery of health care today frequently is a team endeavor, each patient implicitly gives permission for the sharing of certain otherwise private information among the members of the treatment team. Such information sharing is essential to optimal care. However, only information that is directly relevant and necessary to facilitate the contribution of each team member should be available beyond the physician, and each team member who is privy to patient information is bound by the same legal and ethical constraints regarding confidentiality that apply to the physician.

SEE ALSO: Medical malpractice, Patients' rights

Suggested Reading

Final Rules implementing the Health Insurance Portability and Accountability Act, 67 *Federal Register* 53181–53273 (August 14, 2002).

Humber, J. M., & Almeder, R. F. (Eds.). (2001). *Privacy and health care*. Totowa, NJ: Humana Press.
Saunders, J. M. (1996). *Patient confidentiality*. Salt Lake City, UT: Medicode.

MARSHALL B. KAPP

Congestive Heart Failure Heart failure is an increasingly common disease because of the improved survival rates of patients after coronary heart disease events. About 4.6 million persons are being treated for heart failure in the United States, and 550,000 new cases are diagnosed each year. The prevalence of heart failure increases with age; approximately 80% of all heart failure admissions occur in persons older than 65 years of age. Heart failure has a tremendous impact on U.S. health care costs, disability, and loss of employment.

Heart failure is a disease state in which the heart is unable to pump blood at a rate required by the body's metabolism. This can result either from a diseased heart (myocardial failure), or because of excess load placed on the normal heart due to various other disease states. Heart failure is usually the end point for all forms of heart disease.

Heart failure can result from two causes:

1. Inability to pump blood due to defective heart contractility and/or filling and emptying. The type of heart disease in which the predominant problem is a defect in contractility is called "systolic" heart failure. In contrast, a defective or impaired filling/emptying state resulting in heart failure is called "diastolic" heart failure.

2. Heart failure due to other disease states like systemic infections, severe anemia, thyroid disease, and the like. In these conditions, the heart may be structurally normal, but due to increased load, the heart fails to keep up with the demand.

FORMS OF HEART FAILURE

1. Heart failure can be right heart failure, left heart failure, or a combination of both. Right heart failure occurs in people with lung diseases like emphysema, in which increased blood pressure in lung arteries (pulmonary vessels) results in right ventricular failure. Left heart failure is the failure of left ventricle, which is

Table 1. Causes of heart failure

Low-output heart failure (systolic or diastolic heart failure)	High-output heart failure (other disease states)
• Congenital heart disease • Valve diseases (most commonly aortic or mitral valve disease) • Rheumatic heart disease • Hypertension (high blood pressure) • Diabetes • Coronary heart disease • Viral cardiomyopathy[a] • Drug-induced cardiomyopathy (such as adriamycin)[a] • Peripartum cardiomyopathy[a] • Sarcoidosis • Alcoholic cardiomyopathy[a] • HIV cardiomyopathy[a] • Other infiltrative and metabolic diseases (rare) • Familial (rare) • Idiopathic (unclear etiology)	• Severe chronic anemia • Thyrotoxicosis (severe hyperthyroidism) • Beriberi disease (vitamin B1 deficiency—rare) • Bone diseases like Paget's and multiple myeloma • Blood disorders like polycythemia vera • Pregnancy • Tumor-like carcinoid syndrome • Arteriovenous fistulas (as in hemodialysis patients) • Congenital arteriovenous fistulas

[a] Cardiomyopathy: weak heart muscle.

responsible for pumping blood throughout the body, and eventually leads to right ventricular failure also.

2. Acute or chronic heart failure: As described above, related to the time of onset of symptoms.

3. Low-output heart failure is due to weak and defective heart as mentioned above, whereas high-output heart failure is due to other diseases where the demand on the heart is very high (Table 1).

4. Systolic and diastolic heart failure: Problems with contractility or forward pumping function of the heart, or impaired filling (e.g., due to a thickened ventricular wall due secondary to hypertension) of the heart.

SYMPTOMS OF HEART FAILURE

Patients with heart failure can develop these symptoms either suddenly over hours (acute heart failure or flash pulmonary edema) or over days and months (chronic heart failure) by progressively becoming short of breath and manifesting slow weight gain.

1. Shortness of breath or dyspnea on exertion.
2. Orthopnea: Dyspnea that develops in the recumbent position and is relieved by elevation of the head with pillows.
3. Cough: Usually with clear sputum or nonproductive. However, pink frothy sputum is characteristic of pulmonary edema (lungs filled with fluid).
4. Paroxysmal nocturnal dyspnea: Attacks of dyspnea occurring at night that awake the patient from sleep suddenly. Associated with anxiety and suffocation due to bronchospasm and lung congestion.
5. Edema: Usually dependent in lower extremities, ankles, and sacrum if the patient is recumbent most of the time.
6. Weight gain: Patients gain weight progressively or suddenly due to fluid buildup and edema.
7. Right upper abdominal pain: Due to congestion of the liver because of fluid backup and edema.
8. Ascites (abdominal distention due to fluid accumulation) or pleural effusion (fluid accumulation around the lungs).

CLINICAL AND LABORATORY FINDINGS

1. On physical examination, patients with heart failure can have tachycardia (fast heart rate), low or

high blood pressure, increased respiratory rate due to shortness of breath, low blood oxygen levels, increased neck vein distention (increased jugular venous distention due to increased right atrial pressure), cardiomegaly (large heart), murmurs or gallops (extra heart sounds), edema, hepatomegaly (distended liver).

2. Laboratory data: Elevated kidney function tests (serum creatinine, blood urea nitrogen), liver enzymes (due to congestion of the liver), and abnormal electrolytes (serum sodium, potassium, and chloride). Electrocardiogram, echocardiogram, and heart catheterization may be performed depending on the patient's clinical status.

SURGICAL TREATMENT

1. If a combination of the above medications (Table 2; optimal medical therapy) does not improve the individual's condition, or if the person is admitted to the hospital because of severe heart failure and is on life support, he or she may qualify for certain devices called ventricular assist devices (VADs) that can be surgically implanted into the failing heart. These devices are temporary for the most part, but recently are being evaluated for long-term use at some centers. These devices work as an auxiliary pump; patients may be discharged home with these devices in place, or may go on to wait for heart transplantation.

Table 2. Treatment

Class	Some examples	Use	Common side effects
Diuretics	• Furosemide (Lasix™) • Bumetanide (Bumex™) • Hydrochlorothiazide • Dyazide™ • Spironolactone	Increase urine output Reduce vascular volume and congestion	Electrolyte abnormalities (particularly serum potassium levels) Kidney problems
Vasodilators	• Nitroglycerin (Imdur™, Isordil™) • Hydralazine • Calcium channel blockers	Reduce fluid return to the heart Reduce blood pressure and reduce load on heart	Low blood pressure Headache
ACE inhibitors	• Lisinopril • Fosinopril • Ramipril • Monopril • Captopril	Reduce blood pressure and increase the forward blood flow	High serum potassium Kidney problems Dry cough
Beta-blockers	• Carvedilol • Metoprolol	Reduce heart rate and thus reduce oxygen demand on heart	Slow heart rate Fatigue
Inotropes	• Digoxin	Increase contractility	Avoid electrolyte abnormalities Avoid dehydration and overdose Side effects include rhythm problems, heart block
Others	• Aspirin • Cholesterol-lowering medications • IV medication for sicker patients	Used in some patients depending on etiology	Refer to particular medication side effects in reference manual (PDR)

2. If medical therapy fails in reaching symptomatic goals and patients are good candidates for heart transplant, those less than 60 years of age and without other contraindications may qualify for cardiac transplantation. Many factors including other medical illnesses and social history (tobacco smoking, alcohol dependence, and lack of social support) can preclude listing the individual on a transplant waiting list. There is a marked shortage of donor organs, and waits can be as long as 2–5 years. After transplant, close follow-up is mandatory because of the need for immunosuppressive therapy and the constant monitoring that is entailed.

3. Biventricular pacing is a new modality which has shown benefit in individuals with NYHA IV (Table 3) heart failure in whom maximal medical therapy has been instituted and symptoms continue. Both ventricles of the heart are paced in order to increase synchronized pumping of the heart muscle, and thus optimize forward blood flow and reduce congestion.

WOMEN AND HEART FAILURE

Several studies have shown that current state-of-the-art therapy has similar benefits for both men and women with heart failure. There is no evidence for sex-specific differential outcomes in women with heart failure when compared with men.

Pregnant women with heart failure should be closely followed by a cardiologist specializing in heart failure along with a high-risk obstetrician. Medications like beta-blockers and ACE inhibitors may be contraindicated, and extreme volume shifts occur during pregnancy, requiring adjustment of medications by experienced physicians. Similarly, beta-blockers should be used during nursing only after consulting a cardiologist and obstetrician.

PERIPARTUM CARDIOMYOPATHY

Peripartum cardiomyopathy is a form of heart disease in which left ventricular systolic dysfunction results in signs and symptoms of heart failure. Symptoms usually occur during the last trimester of gestation, and the diagnosis is usually made in the early peripartum period. The incidence of this condition is estimated to be approximately 1 in 15,000 in the United States. Other causes of heart failure should be ruled out before diagnosing peripartum cardiomyopathy. The illness can occur as late as 6 months after delivery, and is more likely to occur in multiparous women, those with twin pregnancies, those with preeclampsia, and in women

Table 3. New York Heart Association Classification (NYHA Class)

Class	Symptoms	Specific activity
NYHA I	Ordinary day-to-day activity is well tolerated without any limitation due to heart failure symptoms	Patients can do outdoor work, recreational activity, and work. Only prolonged recreation and strenuous activity precipitates symptoms
NYHA II	Slight limitation of ordinary activity due to symptoms	Daily activity as mentioned above brings on fatigue, shortness of breath, or chest tightness
NYHA III	Marked limitation of daily activity. Comfortable at rest	Less than ordinary activity causes symptoms
NYHA IV	Inability to carry on any activity and symptomatic even at rest	Nocturnal dyspnea and dyspnea at rest. Unable to perform activities of daily living

Note: This classification is used to assess the severity and physical limitation related to the heart condition. This classification is used for patients with heart disease and heart failure only.

older than 30 years of age. The etiology for this disease is not clearly understood. A majority (50–60%) of patients recover ventricular function rapidly within 6 months of delivery. Peripartum cardiomyopathy tends to recur with subsequent pregnancies. Individuals who do not improve and recover function usually deteriorate (20–30%) and require transplantation in order to avoid death or persistent heart failure. The remaining 20–30% of women with peripartum cardiomyopathy stabilize on medical therapy.

MANAGEMENT

Acute heart failure is treated with oxygen, diuretics, digitalis, and vasodilator agents. Other medications of proven benefit in heart failure patients must be used with extreme caution. Because of the increased incidence of strokes associated with this disease, patients also require anticoagulation. VADs and transplantation are other options for severe cases which are refractory to medical therapy. Early delivery of the fetus may be recommended depending on the severity of the disease. Subsequent pregnancies should be considered high risk due to the propensity for recurrence of this form of cardiomyopathy. In many, if not most cases, women are counseled to avoid further pregnancies because of the risk to themselves.

SEE ALSO: Chronic obstructive pulmonary disease, Hypertension, Pregnancy, Systemic lupus erythematosus

Suggested Reading

American College of Cardiology/American Heart Association Guidelines and Recommendations: Management of Heart Failure. www.acc.org—refer to clinical guidelines.

Braunwald, E., Zipes, D. P., & Libby, P. *Heart disease: A textbook of cardiovascular medicine* (6th ed.) (chapters on Heart Failure).

Lang, R. M., Lampert, M. B., et al. (1998). Peripartum cardiomyopathy. In U. Elkayam & N. Gleicher (Eds.), *Cardiac problems in pregnancy* (3rd ed., pp. 87–100). New York: Wiley-Liss.

Pearson, G. D., Veille, J. C., Rahimtoola, S., et al. (2000). Peripartum cardiomyopathy: National Heart, Lung, and Blood Institute and Office of Rare Diseases (National Institutes of Health) Workshop Recommendations and Review. *Journal of the American Medical Association, 283*, 1183–1188.

KAMALA TAMIRISA
CLAIRE DUVERNOY

Conservatorship

Ordinarily the person who will be most directly affected by any specific decision about health care, finances, residential issues, or other personal matters is the person who gets to make that choice. There may be times, however, when the individual is not intellectually and emotionally capable of making and announcing difficult personal decisions. In those cases, the legal system may need to intervene on behalf of the incapacitated individual. This may be accomplished through a variety of legal devices that vary in terms of their intrusion into personal autonomy. One of these legal devices is guardianship/conservatorship.

Every state has enacted statutes that empower the courts to appoint a surrogate with the authority to make decisions on behalf of a mentally incompetent ward. The terminology for the court-appointed surrogate decision-maker varies among jurisdictions; although "conservator" and other terms are used in some states (e.g., California), "guardian" is the more commonly employed term.

Guardianship/conservatorship statutes are an example of the state's inherent *parens patriae* power to protect those who cannot take care of themselves in a manner that society thinks is appropriate. The origins of some form of guardianship based on the state's benevolence toward the dependent can be traced back beyond 13th-century England.

The terms "capable" or "having capacity" usually are used to describe individuals who, in a health care clinician's professional judgment, have sufficient capacity to make their own choices. The terms "incompetent" or "incompetence" refer to a court's formal ruling on the decision-making status of an individual in the context of an official guardianship proceeding, although some modern guardianship statutes use the term "capable" to refer to a judicial judgment.

Every adult is presumed to be legally competent to make personal decisions in life. This presumption may be rebutted, and a surrogate decision-maker may be appointed, only on a showing by clear and convincing evidence that the individual is cognitively and/or emotionally unable to participate authentically (i.e., consistent with previously held values) and self-sufficiently in a rational decision-making process.

State guardianship statutes contain a two-step definition of competence. First, the person must fall within a particular category such as old age, mentally ill, or developmentally disabled. Next, the individual must be found to be impaired functionally—in other words,

190

actually unable to care appropriately for person or property—as a result of being within that first category. The requirement of functional impairment is emphasized in those states, such as California, whose statutes restrict eligibility for guardianship to those who are "gravely disable" or the equivalent.

In disputed, adversarial guardianship proceedings, medical and psychological experts are usually called on to testify by each side about the proposed ward's categorical problem and its impact on the proposed ward's functional abilities. In practice, this medical and psychological testimony frequently becomes the primary, if not the exclusive, basis for adjudicating incompetence.

A court appoints a guardian or conservator as substitute decision-maker for an incompetent person. The incompetent person for whom a guardian is appointed is a "ward," and the relationship created between the guardian/conservator and ward is called "guardianship" or "conservatorship."

The guardian who is appointed ordinarily is a private person (relative, friend, or attorney) or institution (bank or trust company). The majority of guardians are relatives of the ward. Some states have developed "public guardianship" systems under which a government agency, acting either directly or through contract with a private not-for-profit or for-profit organization, functions in the guardian role for a ward who has no one else. Elsewhere, some private corporations and organizations offer their services as guardians directly to the courts, either for a fee or on a voluntary, pro bono basis.

A guardianship may be discontinued when it is no longer needed; in some states, appropriateness must be reviewed at least annually. The party arguing for termination bears the burden of proving that competence has been restored.

See Also: Advance directives, Informed consent, Probate

Suggested Reading

Schmidt, W. C., Jr. (1995). *Guardianship: The court of last resort for the elderly and disabled*. Durham, NC: Carolina Academic Press.

Smyer, M., Schaie, K. W., & Kapp, M. B. (Eds.). (1995). *Older adults' decision-making and the law*. New York: Springer.

Zimny, G. H., & Grossberg, G. T. (Eds.). (1998). *Guardianship of the elderly: Psychiatric and judicial aspects*. New York: Springer.

MARSHALL B. KAPP

Constipation

Constipation is a condition in which the waste matter in the bowels is too hard to pass easily, or in which movements are so infrequent that discomfort or uncomfortable symptoms result. It also refers to a sense of incomplete evacuation. There is no right number of daily or weekly bowel movements. Regularity may mean bowel movements three times a day for some people or three times a week for others. Constipation is a symptom, not a disease, and can be caused by different conditions.

CAUSES

The most common cause of constipation is poor diet. A diet high in animal fats and refined sugar, but low in fiber causes constipation. People who eat a lot of convenience foods or fast foods, which are low in fiber, may suffer from constipation. Some studies have suggested that high-fiber diets result in larger stools and more frequent bowel movements. Inadequate fluid intake can also cause constipation. Water and other fluids add bulk to the stools, making bowel movements easier. Poor bowel habits resulting from frequent travel, lack of exercise, or lengthy bed rest due to an accident or illness may also cause constipation.

Irritable bowel syndrome (IBS), also known as spastic colon, is a common cause of constipation. Some people develop spasms of the colon that slow the movement of intestinal contents through the digestive tract, leading to constipation. Pregnancy is another cause for constipation. The reasons may be mechanical due to the pressure of the heavy womb, which compresses the intestine, and hormonal due to the hormonal changes during pregnancy. A less common cause of constipation may be a stricture or obstruction that prevents wastes from being passed through the intestines, as in the case of hernia, tumor, or cancerous growth. Thyroid hormone deficiency can cause constipation and is more common in women than in men. Constipation can be a warning sign of a serious condition such as cancer. Other uncommon causes may include certain hormonal disturbances, medications, mechanical compression, diseases such as scleroderma or lupus, and certain neurological or muscular diseases, such as multiple sclerosis, Parkinson's disease, and stroke. Injuries to the spinal cord and tumors pressing on the spinal cord may cause neurological problems resulting in constipation.

Contraception

Constipation in children is usually due to poor bowel habits. Some children find it inconvenient to use toilets outside the home. Severe emotional stress at home and or at school may cause children to withhold their stools. When the periods between bowel movements become too long, children may develop fecal impaction, in which stool is packed so tightly in the bowel that the normal pushing action of the bowel is not enough to expel the stool spontaneously.

Prolonged constipation can cause uncomfortable symptoms such as nausea, heartburn, headache, or distress in the rectum or intestines, which may last until the stool is passed. These symptoms are a reaction of the nerves when the waste matter in the rectum causes pressure and stretching. Constipation can occasionally lead to complications, such as hemorrhoids (caused by extreme straining) or fissures (caused by the hard stool stretching the sphincters). Years of constipation and straining can weaken pelvic muscles, causing the bladder or rectum to bulge into the vagina and leading to urinary incontinence or increased difficulty with bowel movements. After many years of chronic constipation, diverticulosis and diverticulitis can develop. In diverticulosis, the wall of the colon weakens and develops small pockets or outpouchings. In diverticulitis, these outpouchings become obstructed and inflamed, and serious infection can result. Hospitalization and bowel surgery may become necessary.

PREVENTION AND TREATMENT

First, determine the cause of the problem. A physician can sometimes identify the likely cause by talking with you and doing a physical examination. If abnormalities or a blockage of the intestines are suspected, blood tests, stool tests, sigmoidoscopy, or colonoscopy may be recommended. If the test results show that there is no disease or blockage, evaluate your dietary habits. The goal of treatment is regular bowel movements and stools that are formed but not hard. Establish a regular routine for elimination. It is important to avoid unnecessary tensions and worry, including concern over constipation itself. Do not expect to have a bowel movement everyday. Regularity differs from person to person. If your bowel movements occur regularly without pain you are probably not constipated.

A well-balanced diet that includes fiber-rich foods, such as whole-grain bread, and fresh fruits and vegetables helps in preventing constipation. Dried beans, broccoli, and green leafy vegetables are rich in fiber. Drink at least eight glasses of fluid daily and exercise regularly to help to stimulate intestinal activity. Laxatives should be the last resort for treating constipation. Preventing constipation will help you feel better now and also reduce the risk of serious complications later in life.

SEE ALSO: Laxatives, Nutrition

Suggested Reading

Cantor, A. J. (1962). *Control of constipation.* New York: J. Messner.
Jensen, B. (1999). *Dr. Jensen's guide to better bowel care.* New York: Avery.
Ratnaike, R. N. (Ed.). (1999). *Diarrhoea and constipation in geriatric practice.* New York: Cambridge University Press.
Yasny, K. (1997). *Put hemorrhoids and constipation behind you* (2nd ed.). East Canaan, CT: Safe Goods.

RAJKUMARI RICHMONDS

Contraception   *see* Birth Control

Cori, Gerty

Gerty Cori discovered her interest in biochemistry during her first year of medical school. At that time, however, she probably never imagined this interest would culminate in the honor of being the first American woman to win the Nobel Prize in physiology or medicine.

Gerty Cori was born Gerty Theresa Radnitz in Prague, Czechoslovakia (now the Czech Republic), on August 15, 1896. She was the oldest of Otto and Martha Radnitz's three daughters. Her family was a wealthy Jewish family, allowing Gerty to be privately tutored at home until age 10. When Gerty turned 10 years old, she was sent to a girls' finishing school to learn about culture and social grace. By the age of 16, however, Gerty, perhaps influenced by an uncle who was a professor in pediatrics, decided to attend medical school. Since the training she received during her years of finishing school did not include lessons in math and science, Gerty found herself facing a huge challenge. Before Gerty could enter medical school, she had to master 8 years of Latin and 5 years of mathematics, chemistry, and physics.

Gerty began to educate herself the summer of her 16th year. While on summer vacation with her family, she met a high school teacher who offered to tutor her in Latin. By the end of that summer, Gerty had mastered 3 years of Latin. That fall, Gerty enrolled in a Realgymnasium in order to study the remaining courses she would need to enter medical school. She graduated from the Realgymnasium in 1914, and passed the entrance exam for medical school at the age of 18.

Gerty enrolled in the medical school at the German branch of the University of Prague, one of the oldest and most distinguished of European universities. There Gerty discovered both a love for biochemistry, and a 17-year-old named Carl Cori. Gerty and Carl met in anatomy class, and teamed up for laboratory research in biochemistry. They quickly found that they also shared an interest in the outdoors, literature, music, and art. Gerty and Carl worked well as a team, jointly publishing the results of their collaboration on an immunological study. In 1920, Gerty and Carl graduated from medical school, and were married within the year.

The couple moved to Vienna, where Gerty took a job working for the Karolinen Children's Hospital. During her employment there, Gerty studied and published papers on cretinism (congenital thyroid deficiency). The couple soon decided, however, to leave Europe. By 1922, Carl had accepted a biochemist position at the New York State Institute for the Study of Malignant Diseases (now known as the Roswell Park Memorial Institute). Carl secured an assistant pathologist position for Gerty, and she joined him in America 6 months later. The couple worked at the Institute for the next 9 years, during which they published more than 50 papers. In addition, Gerty published another 11 on her own. The Coris became American citizens in 1928.

During their 9 years at the Institute, the couple became increasingly interested in how the body transfers energy from one place to another. By 1929, the couple could explain how mammals get their energy for heavy muscular exercise. The couple discovered that energy moves in a cycle from the muscle to the liver, and then back to the muscle. When a mammal uses a muscle, glycogen, a starch-like substance, in the muscle is converted into a sugar called glucose. The muscle extracts energy from the glucose, but some glucose remains as lactic acid. The body, using the liver, recycles the lactic acid back into sugar. The sugar then returns to the muscle, where it is converted into glycogen. Although the Coris called the cycle "the cycle of carbohydrates," the world has come to know it as the "Cori cycle."

As this research had little to do with research on cancer, the Coris began to look for opportunities with other institutions. Due to nepotism laws, universities were only willing to offer a position to Carl. Refusing job offers if both Carl and Gerty could not be hired, in 1931, the couple finally accepted two positions at Washington University in St. Louis, MO. Carl was hired as chairman of the Department of Pharmacology, while Gerty was only given a research assistant position. Gerty would hold this position for 13 years, until she was made an associate professor in 1944. In 1947, Gerty was finally made a full professor.

During their employment at Washington University, the Coris continued their research. They not only discovered a new glucose compound, glucose-1-phosphate (or Cori ester), but that this compound was the product of the first step in a three-step process of breaking glycogen into sugar. By 1938, the Coris began research on enzymes, discovering phosphorylase, an enzyme involved with the carbohydrate cycle. It was this discovery that led to both Carl and Gerty being awarded the Nobel Prize in 1947. The Coris shared the Nobel Prize with Bernardo A. Houssay, an Argentinean researcher who had conducted research on a hormone in the carbohydrate cycle.

In 1947, Gerty Cori learned she was suffering from a disease of the bone marrow. Surviving the next 10 years through continuous blood transfusions, Gerty expanded her research with enzymes. She eventually demonstrated that four inherited diseases that usually killed the patient in early childhood, resulted from a lack of certain enzymes in the carbohydrate cycle. Her discovery marked the first time an inherited disease was shown to result from a lack of certain enzymes, and opened up for study the entire field of genetic diseases.

Before Gerty Cori succumbed to her disease on October 26, 1957, she had published 200 scientific papers, had become the fourth woman to be made a member of the National Academy of Sciences, was appointed by President Truman to the board of the National Science Foundation, and received numerous awards in recognition of her contributions to science.

SEE ALSO: Women in the Health Professions (pp. 20–32), Discrimination, Genetic counseling

Suggested Reading

McGrayne, S. (1993). *Nobel Prize winning women in science: Their lives, struggles, and momentous discoveries.* New York: Birch Lane Press.

Opfell, O. (1986). *The lady laureates: Women who have won the Nobel Prize.* Metuchen, NJ: Scarecrow Press.

Reynolds, M. (1999). *American women scientists: 23 inspiring biographies, 1900–2000.* Jefferson, NC: McFarland.

Yost, E. (1959). *Women in modern science.* New York: Dodd, Mead.

Young, L. (1999). *A to Z of women in science and math.* New York: Facts On File.

BRANDY GLASSER

Coronary Artery Disease

Cardiovascular disease is the leading cause of death in women in this country, claiming the lives of over half a million women each year. Women present with coronary heart disease (CHD) events on average 10 years later than men, but have a steady rise in the incidence of myocardial infarction (MI) or "heart attacks" as they reach and go through menopause. In fact, cardiovascular disease death rates for women have outstripped rates for men every year since 1984, with continued widening of the gap each year. Some of the reasons for this increase are tobacco addiction, untreated hypertension (high blood pressure), obesity, high dietary fat intake, and lack of regular exercise. Furthermore, new evidence suggests that in addition to continued differences in the way men and women are treated after an MI, differences exist in the basic structure of the arterial walls and "clot formation" when compared to men. These differences may be especially grave in younger women; mortality rates after acute MI are twice as high in women less than 50 when compared to men in the same age group. Women greater than 75 years show mortality rates equal to their male counterparts.

ARTERIAL DISEASE

Cholesterol-rich particles are deposited inside arterial walls. The arteries become occluded due to the progressive buildup of plaque (cholesterol and blood particles such as platelets) inside artery walls. This plaque can then rupture and erode, compromising blood flow to the heart muscle and resulting in acute MI. Plaque erosion has been more commonly found in women younger than 50 years, and is highly associated with cigarette smoking. In contrast, plaque rupture has been found to be more common in older women, and is associated with significantly higher total cholesterol levels than in patients dying with plaque erosion. Along with plaque rupture and erosion, vascular spasm is more common in women than in men, and can result in heart attacks and chest pain.

RISK FACTORS

The significant risk factors for CHD include tobacco smoking, hypertension, diabetes mellitus, high LDL ("bad cholesterol"), low HDL ("good cholesterol"), and also family history of premature CHD (<55 years of age). Female patients are more likely than men to have a history of hypertension, diabetes, angina, and congestive heart failure.

Tobacco smoking remains the most common reversible cause of CHD. There is evidence for a relative estrogen deficiency in female smokers, as documented by earlier onset of menopause, higher rates of osteoporosis, and lower endometrial cancer risk. The majority of infarcts, which occur in middle-aged women, can be attributed to tobacco use.

Female diabetics have a three- to sevenfold increase in heart disease risk, compared with a two- to threefold elevation in risk in men with diabetes. The deadly interplay between diabetes and other risk factors in women is particularly important; diabetics have more unfavorable lipid profiles, with higher LDL, triglycerides, and lower HDL levels. Diabetics are more likely to be hypertensive and obese than nondiabetic women. One possible explanation for this excess risk is that diabetes may impair estrogen binding in the vasculature. The presence of diabetes as a risk factor greatly magnifies the adverse effects of other factors such as cigarette smoking, elevated cholesterol levels, and hypertension.

SYMPTOMS

Common symptoms suggesting acute MI are chest pain, along with shortness of breath, nausea, and diaphoresis. Several factors make accurate recognition of MI more difficult in women than in men. While the majority of women presenting with acute MI do complain of chest pain, other more nonspecific complaints such as upper abdominal pain, dyspnea, fatigue, and nausea occur more frequently in female than in male patients. Significantly fewer women present to emergency rooms in less than 2 hours—the golden time period for reperfusion therapy—underscoring the need for education of both patients and providers.

TREATMENT

There are also conflicting data with respect to treatment strategies for women diagnosed with acute MI.

While some authors have suggested that the gender gap for mortality is due to underutilization of proven strategies such as acute coronary intervention, more recent data have shown no difference in rates of cardiac catheterization and intervention after diagnosis.

Proven treatment strategies during acute MI for women are similar to those for men.

Aspirin has been shown to be of benefit in females. Other agents shown to be of benefit in a female as well as male population include beta-blockers, cholesterol-lowering medication, clopidogrel (potent clot inhibitor at the level of the platelet), and angiotensin converting enzyme (ACE) inhibitors. Acute treatment of MI includes thrombolytic agents (these agents dissolve the clot) as well as primary angioplasty (trying to open the diseased artery immediately in the cardiac catheterization laboratory). Both strategies have shown benefit in women and men.

However, procedural complications and mortality rates are significantly higher in women, according to data from 1985 to 1986 National Heart, Lung and Blood Institute Coronary Angioplasty Registry. Complications occurred at a rate of 29% in women versus 20% in men, while procedural mortality was 2.6% for women and 0.3% for men. Some authors have related the gender difference in outcomes after both angioplasty and coronary artery bypass surgery to smaller vessel size in women, greater age of female patients, greater number of comorbid conditions, and generally poorer functional status.

Mortality for women may be higher after thrombolytic therapy due to intracranial bleeding, a relatively more frequent event in female patients. Women continue to show higher death rates, higher transfusion rates, and higher rates of vascular complications after percutaneous intervention. Furthermore, women were less frequently given intravenous blood thinning agents such as GP IIb/IIIa inhibitors as adjunctive therapy during interventional procedures, despite data showing benefit for their use. Furthermore, women less frequently received stents than their male counterparts.

PREVENTION

Lifestyle change, regular exercise, weight loss, and quitting cigarette smoking are very important in preventing heart attacks. An aspirin a day has been proven to be of benefit in patients with risk factors for coronary artery disease and in those with coronary artery disease.

HORMONE REPLACEMENT THERAPY (HRT)

Finally, no benefit for primary or secondary prevention has been demonstrated for HRT in post-menopausal women. In fact, recently published randomized, placebo-controlled trials including the Heart and Estrogen/Progestin Replacement Study (HERS) and Women's Health Initiative (WHI) found either no benefit or slight increase in risk of CHD events for women taking HRT versus those on placebo.

In women with known heart disease, taking hormones after menopause does not protect against heart attack or stroke, and increases the risk of dangerous blood clots and gallbladder disease. Furthermore, long-term HRT also does not appear to prevent cardiovascular events in healthy women. Basic research suggests that younger, nondiseased vascular tissue may be more likely to respond to the effects of HRT, and future clinical studies may address this. HRT is very effective in the amelioration of menopausal symptoms such as hot flashes and vaginal dryness; current knowledge favors short-term, targeted use of HRT only for women with troubling menopausal symptoms who do not have contraindications to their use.

PREGNANCY AND CHD

While cholesterol plaque accounts for the vast majority of heart attacks in women, there are a few rare etiologies that may cause CHD in pregnant women. Acute MI during pregnancy occurs at a rate of 1 in 10,000 pregnancies, with slightly less than half the cases being caused by cholesterol plaque. Spontaneous coronary thrombosis (clot formation) without underlying plaque does occur. Possible mechanisms include the presence of a relative hypercoagulable (tendency to clot easily) state during pregnancy, with decreased availability of factors which dissolve blood clots. Increased vascular reactivity during pregnancy may also be a factor, with a greater propensity toward vascular spasm and constriction. Use of oxytocin (Pitocin), which is used to induce labor, may play a role as well. Spontaneous coronary dissection occurred in 16% of the cases described. This ominous complication of pregnancy is thought to occur because of hormonally mediated biochemical and vascular changes occurring in arterial walls during pregnancy. These same factors may also play a role in rare cases of acute MI that have occurred in young women taking oral contraceptives.

Rare causes of MI in young women, such as pregnancy or oral contraceptive, must not be ignored. Diagnosis of MI in a female requires heightened suspicion because of the often nonspecific nature of the presenting complaint. Clinicians should strive toward aggressive, early treatment of MI in women just as in men, with accepted strategies including thrombolytic therapy and primary angioplasty or stent implantation. Primary percutaneous revascularization may be especially efficacious as an initial treatment strategy in females because of the increased risk of hemorrhagic stroke associated with thrombolytic therapy in women. Secondary prevention after MI should include proven medical therapy such as aspirin, beta-blockers, ACE inhibitors, and lipid-lowering therapy with statins; HRT no longer has a meaningful role to play.

SEE ALSO: Acute myocardial infarction, Chest pain, Cholesterol, Congestive heart failure, Diabetes, Hormone replacement therapy, Hypertension, Menopause, Oral contraception, Pregnancy, Smoking

Suggested Reading

Duvernoy, C. S., & Eagle, K. A. (2001). Acute myocardial infarction in women. *Women's Health in Primary Care, 4,* 542–556.

Duvernoy, C. S., & Mosca, L. (1999). Coronary heart disease in women: What are the gender differences? *Journal of Critical Illness, 14,* 209–216.

Duvernoy, C. S., & Mosca, L. J. (2002). Hormone replacement therapy trials: An update. *Current Atherosclerosis Reports, 4,* 156–160.

Mosca, L., Collins, P., Herrington, D. M., et al. (2001). Hormone replacement therapy and cardiovascular disease: A statement for healthcare professionals from the American Heart Association. *Circulation, 104,* 499–503.

KAMALA TAMIRISA
CLAIRE DUVERNOY

Coronary Risk Factors

Despite many recent advances in therapy, coronary artery disease (CAD) remains the major contributor to death and premature disability in developed countries. This condition accounts for one third of all deaths in women. Furthermore, it is predicted that cardiovascular disease (CVD), due mainly to atherosclerosis (disease of the arteries), will become the leading cause of total disease burden in the world by the year 2020. Understanding the reasons for this increasing prevalence and studying methods for prevention of CAD is therefore of tremendous importance. Over the past several decades, we have learned a great deal about the process of atherosclerosis and now appreciate the concept of "coronary risk factors," or factors that are associated with an increased likelihood of developing CAD. Much of our understanding of these factors comes from prospective, observational studies of large populations of patients such as the Framingham Heart Study and the Seven Countries Study. The Framingham Heart Study is particularly useful because, unlike many other older medical studies, it included women from its beginning in 1948.

There is a widely held misperception that CAD is mainly a disease of men and is a killer of men. In fact, CVD is as likely a cause of death in women as men over their lifetime. This is particularly the case given the longer life expectancy of women in the United States. While it is true that premenopausal women have a lower risk of CVD, it appears that women lag 10–15 years behind men with regard to risk of CVD. After menopause, coronary risk accelerates in women and begins to approach that of men as age advances. The reasons for the "female advantage" remain unclear but cholesterol levels appear to play some role. After menopause, levels of high-density lipoproteins (HDL, the good cholesterol) begin to decline. Levels of low-density lipoproteins (LDL, harmful cholesterol), on the other hand, begin to rise and this rise is sustained at least to age 80. The changes in the lipid profile are not sufficient to fully explain the female-to-male advantage, however. Recent medical studies of the effects of postmenopausal estrogen therapy have yielded surprising results. While hormone replacement therapy (HRT) with estrogen has been shown to raise HDL and lower LDL, large medical studies have not demonstrated any protective role of HRT with regard to CAD events. The Heart and Estrogen/Progestin Replacement Study (HERS) was a large medical study that evaluated postmenopausal women with known CAD and another study, the Women's Health Initiative, evaluated hormone replacement in predominantly healthy women. Not only was there no protective benefit to hormone replacement, but there appeared to be a trend toward increased CAD mortality. This appears to be particularly the case in the first years of therapy. At this point, there is a lack of evidence that HRT is useful to prevent CAD events.

HYPERTENSION

Considerable data from epidemiological studies support a link between hypertension (high blood pressure) and atherosclerosis. This makes hypertension the most prevalent of risk factors with over 80 million Americans defined as having high blood pressure (traditionally defined as a reading of 140/90 mm Hg as measured with a blood pressure cuff). Prevalence of hypertension is higher in men than in women until age 60 at which time it becomes more prevalent in women. This fact combined with the longer life expectancy of women leads to a higher number of hypertension-related complications in women than in men after age 65. In addition to increasing the risk of coronary atherosclerosis, hypertension also increases the risk of stroke and heart failure. Data from another landmark medical study, the Framingham study, show that hypertension causes more strokes in women than men (59% vs. 39%). The same study also showed that women with hypertension are more likely than their male counterparts to develop congestive heart failure (hazard ratio 3.21:2.04). Control of blood pressure with medications appears to reduce the risk of subsequent cardiovascular events. Initial medical studies of antihypertensive treatments clearly demonstrated a benefit of treatment in men as well as elderly women with insignificant effect in younger women, particularly white women. This was likely because most trials did not include sufficient numbers of women to come to a reliable conclusion. In fact, 3 of the 10 major older clinical trials (a type of medical study) excluded women. It was not until more recent studies that clear benefit for women was demonstrated. The Treatment of Mild Hypertension Study (TOMHS) studied 557 men and 345 women aged 45–69 with mild hypertension. Treatment resulted in equal risk reduction of major cardiovascular clinical events in women and men. Similar results were obtained from the large Systolic Hypertension in the Elderly Program (SHEP) trial.

LIPID DISORDERS

Perhaps the most well-established and well-studied risk factors for CHD are abnormalities in blood cholesterol and lipid levels. The typical diet consumed in Western societies contains between 50 and 100 g of fat and 0.5 g of cholesterol. These fats are not water soluble and are transported in the blood in association with lipoproteins. Abnormalities in the metabolism of these lipoproteins lead to elevated levels of cholesterol and triglycerides in the blood. While some individuals have genetic abnormalities that lead to impaired metabolism

of lipids, the majority of cases of elevated levels of cholesterol result from lifestyle factors. These include sedentary lifestyle, obesity, and diets high in total and saturated fats.

The National Cholesterol Education Program Adult Treatment Panel III (NCEP III) recommends that adults 20 years of age and older should undergo fasting lipid profile evaluation once every 5 years. This blood test includes measurement of total cholesterol, LDL, HDL as well as triglycerides. The primary contributor to CHD risk is the LDL level. However, elevated triglyceride and decreased HDL are also significant risks and appear to be stronger predictors of risk for CAD in women than men.

Current NCEP guidelines apply the same cholesterol targets for women as men but recognize certain differences particularly with regard to HDL. Each 1% decrease in HDL level confers a 2–3% increase in risk of CAD. HDL cholesterol is generally higher in women than men. The most recent guidelines define a low HDL as less than 40 mg/dl for men but a level less than 50 mg/dl is considered a marginal risk factor for women and frequently is a marker of the metabolic syndrome.

Dietary modification by reducing fat intake and increasing fiber content is often the first step in therapy for those with elevated cholesterol levels and should be used in conjunction with drug therapy when this is needed. Highly effective and potent medications, namely, the "statin" class of drugs, are now available that have been demonstrated in large clinical trials to be very effective in lowering LDL as well as moderately raising HDL. These agents have been shown to significantly reduce the risk of CHD events in those with as well as those without known coronary disease. The Cholesterol and Recurrent Events (CARE) trial, for example, studied 576 postmenopausal women 3–20 months after myocardial infarction (MI, heart attack). These women had average cholesterol levels. Women in the study who were treated with pravastatin (a statin drug) had a 43% reduction in fatal CAD or recurrent MI. This result is similar to that from pooled data from other trials using statins, which showed an average reduction of 29% in CAD events as compared with 31% in men.

Most recently, the Heart Protection Study enrolled over 20,000 patients with history of CVD or diabetes who were between the ages of 40 and 80. This study included over 5,000 women. Patients treated with simvastatin had a 27% reduction in major coronary events. This benefit was similar in both sexes and was, interestingly, irrespective of initial cholesterol level.

Coronary Risk Factors

Treatment with this class of medication to aggressively lower cholesterol levels in high-risk female and male patients can significantly reduce cardiovascular complications.

DIABETES MELLITUS AND THE METABOLIC SYNDROME

Diabetes mellitus, a condition marked by fasting blood glucose (sugar) levels of 126 mg/dl or higher, is not only a well-established risk factor for CHD but also a disease that is becoming more prevalent at an alarming rate. This is largely due to the increasing prevalence of obesity as well as the aging of the population. The morbidity and mortality of diabetes is mostly due to atherosclerosis. In fact, having diabetes places one at the same CAD risk as someone with known CAD. It appears that diabetes confers a higher degree of risk on females than males. In other words, women with diabetes have an absolute risk for coronary events similar to diabetic men.

The metabolic changes in diabetes are complex and a major reason for the increased risk is the alteration in the lipid profile. Those with diabetes characteristically have elevated triglyceride (a specific type of lipid) levels and depressed levels of HDL. Women with diabetes have a more abnormal lipid profile, which may explain their particular susceptibility to atherosclerosis. As a result of this increased risk, a very important aspect of the care of those with diabetes should focus on optimizing their overall risk of CAD. This includes tight control of elevated blood sugars and a hemoglobin AIC (a compound in the blood that is measured with laboratory testing) of 7.0 or less. Along with aggressive control of the blood glucose level, other risk factors such as hypertension and lipid abnormalities should be optimized. The target blood pressure in a patient with diabetes is no more than 130/80 mm Hg as measured with a blood pressure cuff.

A syndrome in which multiple cardiac risk factors are present, so-called "syndrome X" or "insulin resistance syndrome," is marked by truncal obesity (waist of 35 in. or more in women), hypertension, and glucose intolerance or frank diabetes, as well as plasma lipid abnormalities. The lipid profile in those affected by this syndrome typically is characterized by low HDL, elevated triglyceride, as well as elevated LDL. A recently conducted survey in those over 20 years of age estimates this syndrome to be present in 22.6% of women,

with the highest prevalence in Mexican American women, a rate of 27.2%. As is the case in patients with diabetes, management of those with the metabolic syndrome should consist of aggressive measures targeted at reducing the multiple risk factors for CAD. This includes weight reduction, blood pressure control, management of the lipid abnormalities, as well as management of the elevated blood glucose levels.

SMOKING

Cigarette smoking is the most important preventable risk factor for CHD. It remains the major preventable cause of early death, disability, and health expense in the United States accounting for over 400,000 deaths each year. Estimates suggest that 11% of deaths in women are attributable to smoking and that one in four women smoke. The number of cigarettes smoked per day is directly related to cardiovascular events. Smoking as few as 1–4 or 5–14 cigarettes a day increases the risk of coronary events two- to threefold. Women in the Nurses' Health Study who smoked more than 25 cigarettes a day had 5.5 times the risk of a fatal coronary event as women who did not smoke. In addition, smoking is a major contributor to the incidence of stroke and peripheral vascular disease (a disease of the blood vessels in the legs and arms). Nonetheless, it is estimated that 24% (48 million) American men and women continue to smoke and there has been an alarming trend toward an increase in the proportion of women smokers, particularly young women.

The need and benefits of smoking cessation cannot be overemphasized. Stopping cigarette smoking is a difficult task and often requires a multifaceted approach including patient education, pharmacologic agents as well as a close partnership between the patient and the health care provider. This is particularly important since data suggest that smoking cessation techniques are less effective in women and that women have higher relapse rates. There is a very important interaction between cigarette smoking and oral contraceptive (OCP) use. The risk of coronary disease in women who are smokers as well as users of OCPs is increased approximately 20- to 30-fold above baseline and is 6–8 times higher than for those who smoke only. For that reason, use of OCPs should be avoided in smokers over the age of 35.

OBESITY AND SEDENTARY LIFESTYLE

Obesity is a risk factor for CAD and one particular type of obesity is a particular indicator of risk in women. This is the so-termed "male fat pattern" of weight distribution which is characterized by weight that is mostly distributed around the trunk. A good measure of this is the waist-to-hip ratio with higher ratio correlated with increased risk for CAD (e.g., waist 46 in. and hip 38 in. ratio 1.2:1). This type of obesity appears to be closely linked to the abnormal lipid profile seen in the metabolic syndrome.

Closely related, sedentary lifestyle has been consistently shown to be a risk factor for CAD. The National Institutes of Health Consensus Panel on Physical Activity and Cardiovascular Health recommends that a person accumulate at least 30 minutes of moderate intensity physical activity on a daily basis. The Nurses' Health Study, initiated in 1976, prospectively followed 121,700 female nurses. A study of 72,488 patients from this cohort who did not have CVD, aged 40–65, showed interesting results with regard to exercise. There was an inverse association between physical activity and the risk of CAD. Women who walked the equivalent of three or more hours per week at a brisk pace had a lower risk when compared to women who walked infrequently. This reduction was similar in women who reported regular, vigorous exercise, suggesting that both types of activities significantly reduce the risk of coronary events.

HOMOCYSTEINE

Homocysteine is a naturally produced chemical in the body which may accumulate in the blood as a result of genetic abnormalities in certain enzymes or due to deficiencies in the vitamin folic acid. Data show a link between elevated levels of homocysteine in the blood and the risk of abnormal clotting (thrombosis), as well as CAD. It appears that dietary supplementation with folic acid can lower the level of this chemical; however, trials are needed to show whether this is effective in reducing the risk of coronary events.

INFLAMMATION

Much effort has been expended toward finding a possible infectious cause for the CAD. While there are no convincing data linking any specific microbe to an elevated risk of CAD, it is widely accepted that inflammation plays an important role in the atherosclerotic process. For this reason, blood levels of markers that rise in the presence of inflammation have been studied looking for a correlation to CAD. Elevated levels of high-sensitivity C-reactive protein (hs-CRP), a naturally occurring protein in the body, can predict the risk for future heart attack as well as outcomes in those with varying extents of CAD. hs-CRP appears to be a more important and predictive risk factor in women than men. However, the mechanism by which hs-CRP confers a higher risk is not fully understood. It is possible that this protein serves simply as a marker of the presence and extent of atherosclerosis instead of playing a causative role. Some of the same medications used in the treatment of elevated cholesterol levels also reduce levels of hs-CRP. These include the statin drugs pravastatin, simvastatin, and atorvastatin as well as ciprofibrate, which belongs to the fibrate class of cholesterol-lowering medication.

SUDDEN CARDIAC DEATH AND RISK FACTORS

Sudden cardiac death (SCD) is defined as death within 1 hour of onset of symptoms. While SCD is more common in men than women, it is still a considerable public health problem with 120,000 cases occurring annually. Analysis from the Nurses' Health Study shows that 69% of women who suffered SCD had no reported history of CAD prior to the event. This highlights the need to identify factors associated with increased SCD risk. The NHS found that risk for SCD is closely associated with risk for CAD with 94% of women reporting at least one coronary risk factor. Smoking, hypertension, and diabetes were associated with a 2.5- to 4-fold increase in SCD risk which is similar to the risk conferred by having had a history of prior MI. This finding suggests that aggressive modification of CAD risk factors may decrease the risk for SCD. CAD is the major contributor to morbidity and mortality in women. Some risk factors are modifiable with changes in lifestyle or with medications, while others are unmodifiable such as age and genetics. Reducing the risk of CAD is achieved through a healthy lifestyle of diet, exercise, and smoking cessation while aggressively controlling disease processes that increase the risk of atherosclerosis.

Cosmetic Surgery

SEE ALSO: Acute myocardial infarction, Cardiovascular disease, Cholesterol, Diabetes, Exercise, Hormone replacement therapy, Hypertension, Nutrition, Smoking

Suggested Reading

Albert, C. M., Chae, C. U., Grodstein, F., et al. (2003). Prospective study of sudden cardiac death among women in the United States. *Circulation, 107*, 2096–2101.

Barrett-Connor, E. (1997). Sex differences in coronary heart disease—why are women so superior? The 1995 Ancel Keys Lecture. *Circulation, 95*, 252–264.

Expert Panel on Detection, Evaluation, and Treatment of High Blood Cholesterol in Adults. (2001). Executive Summary of the Third Report of the National Cholesterol Education Program (NCEP) (Adult Treatment Panel III). *Journal of the American Medical Association, 285*, 2486–2497.

Grady, D., Herrington, D., Bittner, V., et al. for the HERS Research Group. (2002). Cardiovascular disease outcomes during 6.8 years of hormone therapy. Heart and Estrogen/progestin Replacement Study Follow-up (HERS II). *Journal of the American Medical Association, 288*, 49–57.

Hayes, S., & Taler, S. J. (1998). Hypertension in women: Current understanding of gender differences. *Mayo Clinic Proceedings, 73*, 157–165.

Heart Protection Study Collaborative Group. (2002). MR/BHF Heart Protection Study of cholesterol lowering with simvastatin in 20536 high risk individuals: A randomised placebo controlled trial. *Lancet, 360*, 7–22.

Kannel, W. B., & Wilson, P. W. F. (1995). Risk factors that attenuate the female coronary disease advantage. *Archives of Internal Medicine, 155*, 57–61.

Manson, J. E., Hu, F. B., Rich-Edwards, J. W., et al. (1999). A prospective study of walking as compared with vigorous exercise in the prevention of coronary heart disease in women. *New England Journal of Medicine, 341*, 650–658.

Writing Group for the Women's Health Initiative Investigators. (2002). Risks and benefits of estrogen plus progestin in healthy postmenopausal women. Principal results from the Women's Health Initiative Randomized Controlled Trial. *Journal of the American Medical Association, 288*, 321–333.

GEORGE M. SOLIMAN
NANETTE K. WENGER

Cosmetic Surgery Cosmetic surgery (also called plastic surgery) is used both to correct true deformities and improve undesirable appearances. In our culture, there is a tremendous emphasis placed on our personal appearance, both in the workforce and in social situations. Television and magazines play a large role in this by showing mostly young, thin people who do not have sagging skin or unpleasant features. No one ever sees a person with "saddle bags" on the cover of a fashion magazine. This could be one of the major reasons why people seek plastic surgery. Both men and women feel the pressure to look their best, and more men are seeking plastic surgery because of this very fact.

Another reason to consider plastic surgery is self-consciousness about a certain part of the body (e.g., a large nose) that may have been a source of ridicule in childhood. For some people, dislike of a body feature causes real distress and is a constant source of self-consciousness during daily life. How we feel about ourselves affects how we relate to others. However, some people with great looks have a poor self-image, and many people who might be considered homely are perfectly satisfied with their appearance.

Individuals with realistic expectations are more likely to be satisfied with the results of cosmetic surgery. Not every real or imagined cosmetic flaw can be corrected. One should not undergo cosmetic surgery just to please someone else. Cosmetic surgery can help with one's self-image and allow healthy self-confidence to flourish, but surgery will not automatically improve one's social life and will not correct any psychological problems that may exist. When there is a question of an underlying emotional or psychological problem, a psychological evaluation may be suggested prior to surgery.

Finding a good plastic surgeon is extremely important. The choice of surgeon can be the most important step in the entire process. Look for a physician who is board certified by the American Board of Plastic Surgery (ABPS). If the plastic surgeon is "board eligible," it means that he/she has completed education, but is yet to take the board examination. The surgeon should also belong to the American Society of Plastic Surgeons (ASPS), which has stringent rules for membership. ASPS has a website with a wealth of information regarding plastic surgery. In addition, a lot of the plastic surgeons have their own webpage, which can educate you about that particular person. Developing confidence in your plastic surgeon is very important. You may be able to speak to one of his or her patients. Asking other patients about your surgeon can provide very valuable information. Insurance policies often do not cover cosmetic surgery, so checking with your insurer is very important as well.

Every surgical procedure carries some risk, including infection, a poor cosmetic result, scarring, and, very rarely, death. These risks are very small, but one should carefully consider the risks and benefits before undergoing any procedure. Undergoing cosmetic surgery involves a large commitment on the part of both the patient and the physician. One should carefully consider the options before making this decision.

SEE ALSO: Body image, Liposuction

Suggested Resources

Website: www.plasticsurgery.org

JANET BLANCHARD

Couples Therapy All individuals have a basic need to form attachments and develop meaningful relationships. At the same time, we also have a basic need to be separate and develop our individual potential. Balancing these conflicting needs is the central issue of intimate relationships and helping couples establish or reestablish that balance is the central issue for couples therapy. This is addressed by understanding how the couple manages, respects, and accepts differences. Accepting differences supports individual development and frees partners to be truly intimate by reducing the inevitable power struggles which emerge when changing a partner takes precedence over acceptance.

Couples therapy can address the needs of married couples, same-sex couples, premarital couples, or couples in a committed relationship who have chosen not to marry. It is indicated when one or both partners feel their needs are not being met in the relationship, yet want to see if their relationship can succeed. Couples therapy is not indicated if domestic violence is an issue. The issues that couples bring to therapy can include finances, sex, infidelity, addiction, parenting, communication, difficulty in resolving conflict. They can also be related to external events such as job loss, illness, or family crisis. Often couples come for counseling at transition points in their lives such as the birth of child, job change or move, or midlife crisis.

There are many models of couples therapy. Most couples therapists operate from a primary theoretical model but draw on other practice models to meet the needs of a particular couple. Structural Therapy developed by Salvadore Minuchin views a couple as a system that operates by its own rules and repetitive patterns. Structural therapists describe the conflict between attachment and individuality as an issue of boundaries and assess how strong the boundaries are around the couple and around each individual. A boundary that is too rigid around a couple does not allow for individual growth. Boundaries that are too rigid around each partner undermine attachment. The goal of the therapy is to help the couple shift the rules and patterns of their system that keep their boundaries rigid and prevent a balance that meets each partner's needs.

Intergenerational Therapy as developed by Murray Bowen considers the impact of extended family across generations on the couple relationship. How families historically have managed togetherness and individuality affects succeeding generations' ability to couple. Goals of therapy are to help the couple through insight, understand their family of origin issues so they are less likely to repeat them.

Cognitive Behavioral Therapy as developed by such theorists as Albert Ellis and Neil Jacobson focuses on cognitions and beliefs. The cognitive therapist helps the couple pinpoint how they act toward each other to try to control each other in order to get their needs met. The goals are to increase cognitive awareness of their destructive behavior and the beliefs that support that behavior and to improve their problem-solving skills.

Solution-Focused Therapy as developed by Steve DeShazer and his colleagues proposes that a couple does not need to understand a problem to develop a solution for it. The focus of the work is identifying strengths and resources to be adapted to create a solution. Goal setting is central to the approach and is accomplished by identifying specific behaviors and interactions that the couple would like to increase. These behaviors are determined by examining the couples' previous attempts at developing solutions and focusing on what has worked.

Object Relations Therapy as described by Rubin and Gertrude Blanck views becoming a couple as a developmental phase with the goals of establishing sexual relations, establishing a new level of intimacy, separating from parents, and increasing the opportunity for developing autonomy. Object relations therapists focus on what each partner internalized about significant relationships in their families and how/what they learned impacts how they interact with and attach to their intimate partner. Understanding and insight are necessary to meet the goal of separating what was previously internalized from the present relationship.

Couples therapists may be licensed social workers, counselors, psychologists, or psychiatrists. Because couples therapy is a subspecialty of therapy, couples therapists should have additional training and experience in working with couples. The American Association of Marriage and Family Therapists (AAMFT) provides referral information.

Insurance does not generally pay for couples therapy. One partner must usually be identified as a patient with a mental health diagnosis in need of therapy. The other partner then participates in the therapy which is billed as conjoint therapy. Each partner in couples therapy needs to be prepared to examine his or her own role in the relationship problems.

SEE ALSO: Cognitive-behavioral therapy, Divorce mediation, Psychoanalysis

Suggested Reading

Blanck, R., & Blanck, G. (1968). *Marriage & personal development.* New York: Columbia University Press.

Bowen, M. (1985). *Family therapy in clinical practice.* New York: Jason Aronson.

DeShazer, S. (1985). *Keys to solutions in brief therapy.* New York: Norton.

Ellis, A. (1962). *Reason and emotion in psychotherapy.* New York: Lyle Stuart.

Gerhart, D. R., & Tuttle, A. R. (2003). *Theory based treatment planning for marriage and family therapists.* Pacific Grove, CA: Brooks/Cole-Thomson Learning.

Minuchin, S. (1974). *Families and family therapy.* Cambridge, MA: Harvard University Press.

PHYLLIS D. HULEWAT

Crystal Methamphetamine

Crystal methamphetamine, also known as "meth," "crystal," "crank," "glass," "ice," and "speed," is a powerful stimulant that can be inhaled, injected, smoked, or taken orally. Methamphetamine is the most potent in the class of stimulant drugs called amphetamines. Chemically similar to epinephrine (adrenaline), amphetamines are synthetic drugs that produce stimulation of the central nervous system, inducing decreases in appetite, increased libido, feelings of euphoria, alertness, and physical competence, as well as anxiety and insomnia. Amphetamine was first produced in 1887; methamphetamine was first synthesized from ephedrine (the active ingredient in the herb ephedra) in 1893.

In the mid-20th century, physicians began to prescribe amphetamines for a variety of conditions, ranging from asthma and narcolepsy to attention deficit disorder and obesity. Use of amphetamines increased throughout the 1940s and 1950s; they were regularly distributed to soldiers fighting on all sides during World War II to enhance physical endurance and overcome fatigue. In the postwar period, many women in the United States and the United Kingdom used amphetamine as a means of combating depression, losing weight, and as an aid to the monotonous daily completion of household chores, hence the label "mother's little helper." In Japan, epidemic abuse of methamphetamine left over from World War II eventually resulted in the passage of the Stimulants Control Law in 1951. In the United States, amphetamine and methamphetamine increased in popularity throughout the 1960s and a substantial black market emerged in California. Its growth was given an unintended boost by the Controlled Substances Act of 1970, which greatly constricted the legal means of obtaining amphetamines.

In the 1970s, the distribution of illegal methamphetamine in the United States was largely associated with motorcycle gangs. However, methamphetamine is no longer associated solely with gangs. Since the late 1990s, hundreds of methamphetamine labs have been raided by local and federal law enforcement in both urban and rural areas, where poverty, unemployment, and the demands of industrial and agricultural jobs contribute to a demand for stimulant drugs. Methamphetamine has also become integrated into gay culture and the "rave" scene, where it is commonly used to power all-night dancing sessions and to boost sexual performance. Because methamphetamine can be readily produced from commonly available ingredients, it does not require import networks (although such networks are frequently involved with large-scale distribution). All methods of making methamphetamine employ toxic chemical agents and some source of ephedrine, such as over-the-counter cold medicine. Methamphetamine labs vary greatly in size and efficiency, from "mom and pop" outfits that cook the drug for personal use and local sale, to large-scale factories that turn it out for mass distribution. Due to the volatile chemicals involved, all of these pose potential health hazards, not only to the individuals involved in production, but also to the surrounding community and the natural environment.

Like cocaine, amphetamines produce an initial pleasant feeling, or rush, caused by increased production of dopamine in the brain. This is followed by an elevation of mood and energy, and a subsequent steep decline. Methamphetamine use can result in drug dependence. Unlike cocaine, which tends to be very short-acting, the euphoric effects of methamphetamine may last for 6–24 hours depending on the dose. Unfortunately, the drug does not provide the energy that the user feels while under its influence; this is drawn from the limited stores of the body itself. As a result, people using the drug "come down" with their energy drained. Chronic users become accustomed to chemically elevated moods and energy levels, and cessation of use results in a severe "crash," which may be accompanied by deep depression and intense craving for more of the drug. This, in turn, may lead to another "binge" of drug use. Methamphetamine addicts are sometimes called "tweakers" because of their compulsive and paranoid behavior.

Methamphetamine appeals to poor and working women because of its relative cheapness. The drug promises to fill the gap between the multiple expectations placed on women and the limited resources available to them, and growing numbers of women are using methamphetamine as a means of keeping up with work and household tasks, losing weight, and combating depression. However, abuse and/or dependence may result in many more problems: unhealthy weight loss, insomnia, impaired memory, cardiovascular damage, psychosis, prenatal complications, congenital deformities, and neglect or abuse of children. There are also substantial legal ramifications for the manufacture, use, and sale of the drug. The association of methamphetamine with intravenous injection and heightened sexual activity raises the risk of acquiring sexually transmitted diseases including HIV/AIDS, and blood-borne diseases such as hepatitis. Since methamphetamine use can produce confusion, impair judgment, and heighten aggressiveness, it may also contribute to sexual victimization. Barring effective prevention and treatment efforts or a lessening of the societal pressures placed on women in the United States methamphetamine abuse and dependence will continue to threaten the health of the women who use it for years to come.

See Also: Club drugs, Depression, Substance use

Suggested Reading

Anglin, M. D., Burke, C., Perrochet, B., Stamper, E., & Dawud-Noursi, S. (2000). History of the methamphetamine problem. *Journal of Psychoactive Drugs, 32*(2), 137–141.

Joseph, M. (2000). *Speed: Its history and lore.* London: Carlton Books.

McCrady, B. S., & Epstein, E. E. (Eds.). (1991). *Addictions: A comprehensive guidebook.* New York: Oxford University Press.

Murphy, S., & Rosenbaum M. (1999). *Pregnant drug users: Combating stereotypes and stigma.* New Brunswick, NJ: Rutgers University Press.

National Institute on Drug Abuse Research Report. (1998). *Methamphetamine abuse and addiction* (NIH Publication No. 98–4210). Washington, DC: U.S. Dept. of Health and Human Services.

Rawson, R. A., Washton, A., Domier, C. P., & Reiber, C. (2002). Drugs and sexual effects: Role of drug type and gender. *Journal of Substance Abuse Treatment, 22*, 103–108.

PAUL J. DRAUS

Curanderos

Curanderos During colonial Spain, curanderos emerged as spiritual and physical healers. The word *curandero* comes from the Spanish word "curar," which means to heal. Curanderismo, healing by curanderos, is a combination of Greek medicine, Judeo-Christianity, European witchcraft, ancient Arabic medicine, and Indian herbal medicine. With roots throughout Latin America, curanderos have significantly shaped the role of medicine in countries with large Hispanic populations.

Relying on spiritual and herbal remedies, curanderas (male) and curanderos (female) heal individuals in three realms: physical, spiritual, and emotional. Curanderos can specialize in different types of healing: (a) yerberas, are herbalists; (b) sobadoras, are folk chiropractors; and (c) parteras, are midwifes. Yet, curanderos are most notable for "limpiadas," which are cleansings for an individual's spirit. Curanderos profess that most sickness is the result of unclean spirits. Through prayers and rituals, a curandero deciphers the cause of an individual's unclean spirit. Usually, curanderos discover that the patient's illness was triggered by a spell. After the limpiada, the evil spirits leave and the individual is healed.

Curanderos continue to practice healing in Mexico, South America, and the southwestern United States. Despite their popularity, curanderos maintain low profiles and restrain from publicizing their services. Consequently, curandero services are often spread by word of mouth, which often attracts patients from other regions.

Generally, curanderos may be preferred over medical doctors for two major reasons. First, a curandero charges a substantially lower fee than a medical doctor. Further, in rural areas, many patients do not have health insurance so that cost-conscious patients are more likely to visit curanderos. Second, curanderos can be more accessible than medical doctors because curanderos are more prevalent in suburbs and rural communities.

Curanderos have been healing people from sickness and evil spirits for centuries; thus, the level of confidence Hispanics have in curanderos has not wavered. Although not all Hispanics believe in curanderismo, a large majority of the Hispanic community considers curanderos as their only source of healing from sickness and evil spirits. As a result, curanderismo continues to be passed down from generation to generation, influencing healing and medicine.

SEE ALSO: Latina

Suggested Reading

McClain, C. S. (1989). *Women as healers cross cultural perspectives.* New Brunswick, NJ: Rutgers University Press.

Suggested Resources

Linan, L. (2000). Curanderismo: Holistic Healing. http://www.dpsk12.org/programs/almaproject/pdf/Curanderismo.pdf

Salinas, I. Curanderismo. http://nexus.colum.edu/user/iverson/opp/archives/Latin_Sanctuary/Curahis.htm

STEPHANIE CABRERA

Curie, Marie Marie Curie lived from 1867 to 1934 and made enormous contributions to science. She won two Nobel Prizes (in 1903 for physics and in 1911 for chemistry) and had a daughter, Irene, who also won this high honor of science in 1935. Born in Warsaw during the time that Poland was under Russian rule, Marya (nicknamed Manya) Sklodovska was first in her high school class and later studied in the "Floating University," an outlawed night school. She worked as a governess to earn money to allow her to further her studies, then moved to Paris, adopting the French form of her name, Marie.

In Paris, Marie enrolled in the Sorbonne and was the first woman to earn a degree in physics in 1893. In 1894, she earned a degree in mathematics. Also in 1894, she met Pierre Curie, a French physicist whom she married the following year in a small civil ceremony. Two years later, their first child, Irene, was born.

Toward the end of 1897, Marie began work on her doctoral thesis, with the goal of earning her PhD. She and Pierre had become intrigued by the discovery of x-rays by Wilhelm Roentgen; the rays were called "x" rays since it was not understood where they came from.

Roentgen had made a photographic image of the bones in his wife's hands using the rays. A colleague of the Curies, Professor Henri Becquerel, began a search for the source of the rays and discovered that uranium salts emitted rays.

Marie used a piezo-quartz electrometer to test mineral samples, and quickly discovered that the strength of the rays was directly related to the amount of uranium in the sample. She also found that another element, thorium, produced rays similar to those produced by uranium. From these discoveries, she postulated that the ability to give off rays was an atomic property, which she called "radioactivity."

She examined hundreds of compounds and found that two uranium ores, pitchblende and chacolite, were more strongly radioactive than pure uranium. Marie and Pierre directed their efforts at studying pitchblende, which is uranium oxide (a compound of uranium, oxygen, and other elements). They hypothesized that pitchblende must have another component that was responsible for the increased radioactivity. They found a new element, which they called "polonium" in honor of Poland. Six months later they added the discovery of a second element previously unknown in pitchblende. They called this element "radium," and it was the more strongly radioactive of the two new elements.

The Curies chose to focus their efforts on extracting radium and studying its properties. Because radium is a very small component of pitchblende, the couple spent a great deal of time in physically intensive labor refining and purifying pitchblende to yield radium. During this period, Marie also began to work as a teacher at a girls' school.

In 1903, Marie earned her "doctor of physical science" degree. In November 1903, the Curies along with Henri Becquerel were awarded the Nobel Prize for physics for their work on radioactivity. In 1904, Pierre received a promotion to Professor of Physics at the Sorbonne and was given funds to hire three assistants for his laboratory. Marie became a laboratory chief, thus starting her first paid research position.

The Curies had a second daughter in December 1904, whom they named Eve. Tragedy befell the family on April 19, 1906, when Pierre was killed while crossing a busy street. Eve Curie later wrote in her biography of her mother that Marie became a "pitiful and incurably lonely woman" when she was widowed. Refusing a pension, she later assumed the chair given to Pierre with the title of Assistant Professor, becoming the first woman to take a position in French higher education.

Marie's second Nobel Prize, this one in chemistry for the preparation of a gram of pure radium, came in 1911. Several years later, during World War I, Marie became the Director of the Red Cross' Radiological Service. In this position, she worked tirelessly to establish x-ray installations in the field to aid diagnosis and treatment of the war-wounded. She conceived of radiological cars as portable x-ray units; these were nicknamed "les Petites Curie," or "the little Curies." Marie and her daughter Irene worked during the war establishing radiological services and training men to run the equipment.

Following the war, Marie set up the Curie Pavilion of the Institut du Radium. Her later years were spent directing the laboratory and raising money to allow further studies. Throughout her time working with radioactive substances, Marie had been plagued with health problems, including cracked hands, fatigue, cataracts, and kidney problems. In 1934, she died; the doctor's report listed the cause of death as "an aplastic pernicious anaemia of rapid, feverish development." Despite radiotherapy's multiple uses in medicine, the long-term unprotected exposure to radiation had done irreparable damage to Marie Curie's own health.

SEE ALSO: Cancer, Women in the Health Professions (pp. 20–32), Women in Health: Advocates, Reformers, and Pioneers (pp. 40–48)

Suggested Reading

Curie, E. (1937). *Madame Curie: A biography by Eve Curie.* Garden City, NY: Doubleday.
Giroud, F. (1986). *Marie Curie: A life.* New York: Holmes & Meier.
Pflaum, R. (1993). *Marie Curie and her daughter Irene.* Minneapolis, MN: Lerner.

Suggested Resources

The Center for the History of Physics. (2000). A division of the American Institute of Physics: http://www.aip.org/history/curie/contents.htm (accessed July, 2003)

PAULA L. HENSLEY

Daily Living *see* Activities of Daily Living

Day Care Day care is the care, on a continuing basis, of a child by someone other than the child's parents. Day care can come in many forms, and it is not limited to daytime. Parents who work evenings and nights often need "day care" for children at night.

Center-based day care is provided in a place that is built or made to suit the purposes of caring for many children. Center-based day care is usually regulated by the state. The regulations can require qualifications for the staff of the day care, the physical properties of the facility, and the ratio of staff to children. Center-based day care can be run by a not-for-profit group or by someone who is working to make a profit. The not-for-profit centers are often associated with religious groups and they may share space. Not-for-profit centers typically have a board of directors or advisors that allows for parent input into how the center is run.

Home-based day care is an alternative to center-based day care. Home-based day care may also require state licensing by the state, depending on the number of children that are cared for. Even less formal than home-based day care is the provision of care for a child or children by a relative, friend, or someone employed for the purpose of child care. These arrangements are not regulated, with the exception of laws that apply to employing and paying people.

Parents choose different forms of child care for different reasons. Each form has its advantages and disadvantages. Center-based care offers children an opportunity to meet and play with other children, and offers parents reliability and reassurance that more than one adult is involved in the care of the child. Home-based day care offers a comfortable environment and a smaller number of children. Hiring an individual to provide day care allows the caregiver to focus on the individual child. Different day care providers have different ways of working with children. Some day care providers offer structured learning opportunities for the children, while others may offer less structured opportunities.

Finding good day care can require some work. Many areas have child care referral resources that can identify center-based and home-based day care services. The state licensing agency may be a good place to start to get this information. Asking other parents may be the best way to get information about the quality of various day care options.

The use of day care may be an issue if parents divorce or separate. Our national constitution requires people to be treated equally and laws that treat men and women differently must have a valid reason for doing so. Still, men and women are often treated differently. Child care is one of those areas where the historical separation of roles by gender may have an influence. Men who work outside the home are regarded as typical. But women who work outside the home may be considered less typical and this may be to their disadvantage in a child custody dispute.

SEE ALSO: Child care, Child custody, Divorce, Parenting, Quality of life

Suggested Reading

Brazelton, T. B., & Greenspan, S. (2000). *The irreducible needs of children: What every child must have to grow, learn, and flourish.* Cambridge, MA: Perseus.

SHEILA SIMON

---

de Beauvoir, Simone

Simone Lucie-Ernestine-Marie-Bertrand de Beauvoir was born in Paris on January 9, 1908, the eldest of two daughters of Françoise and Georges de Beauvoir. She graduated from the Sorbonne in 1929. de Beauvoir was a philosopher, novelist, and essayist. Until 1943, de Beauvoir taught philosophy at several colleges, before devoting herself completely to writing.

It was at the Sorbonne that Simone met Jean-Paul Sartre, the famous French existentialist. Simone de Beauvoir and Jean-Paul Sartre became lifelong friends and companions. They did not marry and never lived together, yet they were a couple and spent 51 years together in intellectual companionship. Many of de Beauvoir's writings were reflections on either Sartre or his philosophical views. *She Came to Stay* (1943), one of de Beauvoir's first writings, deals with a romantic love triangle, a situation de Beauvoir experienced in her relationship with Sartre. It is also considered to be a representation of the existentialist theory of "being and nothingness" attributed to Sartre.

Existentialism is a philosophy centered on individual existence and personal responsibility for acts of free will in the absence of certain knowledge of what is right and wrong. Other writings by de Beauvoir that echo existentialist theories are *All Men are Mortal* (1946), *The Blood of Others* (1946), and *The Mandarins* (1955). The novel that made Simone de Beauvoir famous is *The Second Sex*, first published in 1949, in which she analyzes the role and status of women, and examines the history of the oppression of women. It is in *The Second Sex* that de Beauvoir proclaimed women in a patriarchal society to be the "other" and that one is not born a woman, but rather "becomes" one. Some consider the book to be an application of Sartrean existentialism to the situation of women.

In addition to these works, de Beauvoir also wrote fiction, philosophy, manifestos, and coedited a monthly review with Sartre. de Beauvoir's autobiographies include *Memoirs of a Dutiful Daughter* (1958), *The Prime of Life* (1962), *Force of Circumstance* (1963), *A Very Easy Death* (1964), and *All Said and Done* (1974). In 1981, 1 year after his death, Simone de Beauvoir wrote a farewell tribute to her lifelong companion, entitled *Adieux: A Farewell to Sartre.* She also edited Sartre's letters to her, although they were not published until after her death, *Quiet Moments in a War: The Letters of Jean-Paul Sartre to Simone de Beauvoir 1940–1963* (1993).

On April 14, 1986, in Paris, Simone de Beauvoir died, leaving a great literary legacy. Recently, Sylvie Le Bon de Beauvoir, Simone's adopted daughter, discovered her 1927 diary, written while at the Sorbonne. Scholars hope that her diary will shed some light on her thinking and her pre-Sartre philosophical views.

SEE ALSO: Feminism; Greer, Germaine

Suggested Reading

de Beauvoir, S. (1993). *The second sex.* New York: Alfred A. Knopf.

Evans, M. (1985). *Simone de Beauvoir: A feminist mandarin.* London: Travistock.

Felder, D. G. (1996). *The 100 most influential women of all time.* New York: Carol.

Merriam-Webster Dictionary (1st ed.) (1997). Existentialism. Springfield, MA: Merriam-Webster.

Moi, T. (1990). *Feminist theory and Simone de Beauvoir.* Cambridge, MA: Blackwell.

Schwarzer, A. (1984). *After the second sex: Conversations with Simone de Beauvoir.* New York: Pantheon Books.

Simons, M.A. (1999). *Beauvoir and the second sex: Feminism, race, and the origins of existentialism.* Lanham, MD: Rowman & Littlefield.

TAMBRA K. CAIN

Dementia

Dementia, a devastating syndrome of multiple etiologies, probably affects up to 4 million people in the United States. The cost of the dementia syndromes to the United States has been estimated at up to $140 billion per year in caregiving costs, lost productivity, and medical and institutional care. Because the risk of dementia increases with age, and as the proportion of the U.S. population over 65 is rapidly increasing, dementia is emerging as a major public health problem of the 21st century. The dementia

Dementia

syndrome refers to a group of symptoms related to a sustained decrease in intellectual function from previous levels. Memory decline is always a part of this syndrome along with combinations of other impairments such as problems with judgment, language, recognition, or performing tasks. Personality change can also occur as a component. The dementia syndrome usually begins gradually, although in some cases it can occur suddenly, depending on the underlying cause. Some studies have suggested that dementia is more common in women than men, especially after age 85, while other studies have shown no gender differences.

There are multiple causes of the dementia syndrome, with over 60 disorders having been associated with dementia. However, the most common causes are: (1) Alzheimer's disease, (2) vascular disease, and (3) diffuse Lewy body dementia. Other less common, but debilitating causes of the dementia syndrome include Parkinson's disease, Huntington's disease, and progressive supranuclear palsy. Potentially reversible causes of dementia include depression, medication effects, thyroid disease, vitamin deficiencies, and syphilis.

Alzheimer's disease also known as dementia of the Alzheimer's type (DAT) is the most common type of dementia, accounting for 50–60% of cases. The risk of DAT is age related with the risk over age 65 about 5–8% and the risk over age 85 increasing to 25–50%. Other risk factors for developing DAT include Down's syndrome, history of head injury, and a family history of dementia. While the risk for DAT appears inherited in some cases, in other cases, there is no family history. The cause of DAT is not known, but is currently thought to be related to the genetically determined overproduction of abnormal brain proteins ("beta amyloid") or abnormal brain protein processing and deposition. Microscopically, the brains of DAT sufferers show abnormal "plaques" and "tangles." The impact of DAT on brain chemistry is a prominent degeneration of systems involving the neurotransmitter acetylcholine that is critical to intact cognitive function, although other neurotransmitters are also involved. The clinical picture of a typical patient with DAT is a description of a gradual decline that may not have been noted by family members until difficulties became obvious several years after onset (i.e., getting lost while driving, leaving the stove burners on).

Vascular dementia accounts for 10–20% of dementias. The major risk factor for this type of dementia is high blood pressure or hypertension. The clinical picture of vascular dementia differs from that of DAT; in vascular dementia, it is more common to see a stepwise decline. Treatment of high blood pressure or other cardiovascular disease can sometimes halt the progression of the illness but will usually not reverse symptoms. Often, a clue to vascular dementia is an association in time with a stroke and the onset of sustained memory problems. Strokes are not always obvious in terms of their symptoms and neuroimaging (such as magnetic resonance imaging or MRI) can detect strokes that were clinically silent.

Dementia with Lewy bodies (DLB) likely occurs in 15–25% of elderly patients with dementia. In DLB, patients have both cognitive impairment as well as symptoms of Parkinson's disease (muscular rigidity, shuffling gait when walking, tremor in the hands, limited facial expression, and so forth). In addition, other symptoms such as falls, hallucinations, false beliefs (delusions), fluctuations in alertness or cognition, as well as fainting episodes may be present. Importantly, patients with DLB are very sensitive in terms of side effects to medications called neuroleptics or antipsychotics which are often used to treat behavioral symptoms in dementia.

Behavioral or neuropsychiatric symptoms commonly occur in dementia of all types and include depression, apathy, agitation, delusions, hallucinations, and sleep problems. A recent study found that 80% of participants exhibited at least one of these symptoms at some point after the onset of the memory disturbance. These symptoms, as opposed to the core cognitive symptoms of dementia, tend to be the ones that create problems for patients, families, and caregivers, and can lead to earlier placement in nursing homes.

The assessment of a person suspected of having dementia should include careful history, physical/neurological examination, as well as selected laboratory testing. On examination, focal neurological problems should be identified and the patient should be screened for depression as well as memory problems. The latter is usually screened for with the Mini-Mental State Examination (MMSE), a cognitive screening test that can be easily performed by physicians during an office visit. Importantly, the MMSE neither confirms nor rules out the presence of dementia; however, scores below a certain cutoff indicate the need for further workup and attention. Laboratory screening for thyroid disease and vitamin B12 deficiency is also recommended. Imaging of the brain, such as a noncontrast computerized tomography (CT) or MRI scan, is often appropriate. Neuropsychological testing is a helpful adjunct both to examine patterns of cognitive impairment that may be helpful to distinguish among the types of dementia as well as to establish a baseline of cognition for the individual patient.

Treatment of dementia includes both psychosocial and pharmacological treatments. Psychosocial treatments may include therapy to help the patient come to terms with their diagnosis as well as to work with the caregiver and family system in maintaining good activity levels for the patient and reducing the burden on caregivers. Referral to dementia support groups and resources is especially helpful for patients and their families. Pharmacological treatment includes treatment of: (1) the core cognitive symptoms as well as (2) secondary behavioral complications. Currently, the mainstay of treatment for the core cognitive symptoms in DAT (also used in DLB and, to a lesser extent, vascular dementia) are a class of drugs known as the "cholinesterase inhibitors" (donepezil, rivastigmine, galantamine). Notably, while these agents do not reverse the underlying illness of dementia, they slow its speed of decline and, in some cases, may improve problematic behaviors. Side effects of these medications include nausea, diarrhea, and loss of appetite. Vitamin E and selegiline may also reduce the rate of decline in patients with DAT. Ultimately, it is thought that actual disease modification in DAT will occur from preventing accumulation of abnormal brain protein (beta amyloid). For vascular dementia, treatment of underlying vascular risk factors (smoking, hypertension, diabetes, heart disease) is important. Treating the behavioral complications of all types of dementia is another very important part of treatment. Behavioral approaches can be effective in decreasing problem behaviors. Medications should be tailored to both the individual patient and the accompanying constellation of symptoms and may include: neuroleptics or antipsychotics (used to treat hallucinations, paranoia, or delusions), antidepressants (used to treat depression and anxiety), anticonvulsants (used for mood stabilization and for agitation), and trazodone or Desyrel (used for sleep difficulties and for agitation). Benzodiazepines (diazepam or Valium, alprazolam or Xanax, lorazepam or Ativan, and so forth) should generally be avoided or minimized due to concern of side effects (worsened cognition, falls) and especially of "paradoxical disinhibition" (reaction of agitation/worsened behaviors as opposed to the desired calming effect).

The vast majority of people with dementia are cared for at home by family or other informal caregivers.

Even when placement is needed in alternative living settings, family and informal caregivers continue to provide vital care to their loved ones with dementia. While caregivers can derive great satisfaction from this role, they also face chronic stress that can result in a variety of health problems. Caregivers need to cope with changes and losses in their relationship with the affected patient. The role of parent and child may be reversed, and the intimacy and companionship shared by spouses or parents may be lost. In some cases, caregivers may find themselves caring for family members with whom they have had a difficult relationship. Friends may not know how to behave or how to help. Siblings may disagree on treatments or living situations for the affected family member. All of these changes can contribute to the stress of caregiving. The warning signs of "caregiver stress" include exhaustion, insomnia, irritability, problems with concentration, physical health problems, impatience, low mood, excessive worry, feelings of isolation or loneliness, resentment, and guilt. Caregiver stress can be reduced by getting respite from caregiving including regular physical exercise, a healthful diet, learning relaxation techniques, getting regular medical care, and using respite opportunities to socialize and get rest. Support and education groups provide caregivers knowledge about particular conditions, helpful resources in the community, and techniques for handling difficult behaviors. Groups also provide a safe and encouraging place to express fears and celebrate successes. Future planning for legal, financial, and medical situations can also relieve stress and improve well-being.

See Also: Alzheimer's disease

Suggested Reading

American Psychiatric Association. (1997). *Practice guideline for the treatment of patients with Alzheimer's disease and other dementias of late life.* Washington, DC: American Psychiatric Association.

Knopman, D. S., DeKosky, S. T., Cummings, J. L., Chui, H., Corey-Bloom, J., Relkin, N., et al. (2001). Practice parameter: Diagnosis of dementia (an evidence-based review). Report of the Quality Standards Subcommittee of the American Academy of Neurology. *Neurology, 56,* 1143–1153.

Lyketsos, C. G., Lopez, O., Jones, B., Fitzpatrick, A. L., Breitner, J., & DeKosky, S. (2002). Prevalence of neuropsychiatric symptoms in dementia and mild cognitive impairment. *Journal of the American Medical Association, 288,* 1475–1483.

Mintzer, J. E., Lewis, L., Pennypacker, L., Simpson, W., Bachman, D., Wohlreich, G., et al. (1993). Behavioral intensive care unit (BICU): A new concept in the management of acute agitated behavior in elderly demented patients. *Gerontologist, 33,* 801–806.

Depression

Ross, G. W., & Bowen, J. D. (2002). The diagnosis and differential diagnosis of dementia. *Medical Clinics of North America, 86,* 455–476.

Ruitenberg, A., Ott, A., van Swieten, J. C., Hofman, A., & Breteler, M. M. B. (2001). Incidence of dementia: Does gender make a difference? *Neurobiology of Aging, 22,* 575–580.

Small, G. W., Rabins, P. V., Barry, P. P., Buckholtz, N. S., DeKosky, S. T., Ferris, S. H., et al. (1997). Diagnosis and treatment of Alzheimer disease and related disorders. Consensus statement of the American Association for Geriatric Psychiatry, the Alzheimer's Association, and the American Geriatrics Society. *Journal of the American Medical Association, 278,* 1363–1371.

Suggested Resources

Alzheimer's Association. (800) 272-3900; www.alz.org

American Association for Geriatric Psychiatry. www.aagpgpa.org

National Family Caregivers Association. (800) 896-3650; www.nfcacares.org

HELEN C. KALES
KARYN S. SCHOEM
SUSAN M. MAIXNER

Depression This widely used term may be referred to as a symptom, a syndrome, an illness, or a disorder. A depressive symptom refers to a temporary, subjective sense of sadness that everyone does experience at one time or another and it may be related to any condition. A depressive syndrome is defined as a collection of signs and symptoms, objective and subjective, that taken together is recognized as a condition that is less severe than a clear illness or disorder. A mood is a sustained emotion that one experiences subjectively but can be observed by others, while an affect is an emotion seen and noted by others only. Disturbances of mood and affect are very common and much of psychiatry is concerned with trying to define when a syndrome reaches a threshold for becoming an illness and requires treatment. Depressive illnesses require a certain severity and duration of the symptoms in order to qualify for a diagnosis. Many persons suffer a great deal from conditions that have not met formal diagnostic criteria. This situation is often referred to as "sub-syndromal" depression. Depressive illnesses are among the most underdiagnosed and unrecognized conditions yet are the most treatable of major health conditions.

Depressive disorders are the most common mental illnesses and are the second leading cause of disability in the Western world after heart disease. The diagnosis of major depressive disorder requires a certain severity and duration of the symptoms for more than 2 weeks including mood changes, which are defined in the *Diagnostic and Statistical Manual of Mental Disorders,* fourth edition (DSM-IV) as "a depressed mood most of the day nearly every day as indicated by subjective (e.g., feels sad or empty) or observations made by others (e.g., appears tearful)." Other disturbances include signs of biological (somatic) dysfunctions such as appetite changes, increased or decreased sleep, diurnal variation, and diminished interest in sex; also other symptoms such as problems with concentration and memory, anhedonia that is a lack of pleasure in one's usual activities, fatigue, increased or decreased physical activity, and often suicidal or homicidal ideation. The latter is of special concern since suicidal persons are often depressed and have visited a health care provider prior to their attempt to act on those thoughts. Other subtypes of depression include bipolar (presence of mania or hypermania), atypical (unusual features such as increased sleepiness and hyperphagia), delusional (presence of psychosis), dysthymia (less severe and chronic for more than 2 years), geriatric (older ages), and comorbid (presence of other psychiatric illnesses). In making these diagnoses one must exclude those that may be caused by other medical conditions and substance or alcohol use.

The causes of mood disturbances are the subject of considerable research with yet much still to be done. It is known that mood disturbances are associated dysregulation of biogenic amines, the best studied of which are the neurotransmitters, norepinephrine, serotonin, and dopamine. There are neuroendocrine factors (hormones), neurotransmitters, genetic factors, and psychosocial factors, all of which interact in vulnerable individuals to produce disease. Treatments have been based on the newer knowledge about causes, especially in the area of development of new medications as well as the refinement of many psychotherapies.

Mental disorders affect both men and women equally, but the patterns and presentations are often different between men and women. Much of what we know and much of the current research are not yet sufficient to completely understand why these differences exist nor to fully understand the variations in incidence, prevalence, etiology, clinical presentation, treatment responses, and prevention strategies.

Starting in adolescence and extending through menopause, women experience twice the rates of depressive disorders (major depressive disorder, dysthymia, rapid cycling bipolar disease, and seasonal affective disorder) compared to men. Women also experience a higher incidence of anxiety disorders such as phobias, agoraphobia, panic disorder, generalized anxiety disorders, and posttraumatic stress disorder. Women often have other mental disorders that accompany the depressive ones, such as anxiety problems or alcohol and substance abuse. Men tend to have higher rates of alcohol and drug abuse. While schizophrenia, obsessive–compulsive disorder, and bipolar disorders occur at similar rates in men and women, there are different patterns that characterize the onset, course, and treatment responses.

The fact that women experience twice the rate of depressive disorders as men do, does not in any way suggest that they are weaker or have a greater susceptibility to mental illnesses. While the causes for gender differences remain unclear some theories have been suggested, such as, these variations may be a mistake in sampling and/or women may recall past episodes of depression better than men. However, the most likely explanation is that biological and psychological factors may be involved. Since differences appear between men and women in the likelihood of developing depression at puberty in women and not in men, there are probably hormonal and genetic influences. Women are most likely to experience mood changes during their reproductive years, especially at times related to menses, pregnancy, after pregnancy, or weaning a baby. Ten to fifteen percent of women experience major depression in the postpartum period and these figures may be even higher during the pregnancy.

Psychological and cultural factors may also contribute to the gender differences in the rates of depression between men and women. Women may face more social and economic difficulties, more physical and sexual abuse, different role expectations, and responsibilities for balancing child care and careers. In cross-cultural research women's social status contributes to their well-being. Women with young children at home have an increased risk for depressive disorders. Some of the best predictors for depressive disorders are a past personal history of depression, a family history of depression, a lack of social supports, loss of close family or friends, and other major life stressors.

Diagnosis of major depression includes a history of mood change lasting for more than 2 weeks with accompanying signs and symptoms of changes in sleep, appetite, weight, concentration, memory, sexual interest, anhedonia, fatigue, and possibly ideas of self-harm

or harming others. The latter is characterized by feelings of helplessness, hopelessness, and being "trapped" in some situation. Dysthymia is a more minor mood change lasting for 2 years or more. Seasonal affective disorder is a mood change that occurs during times of the year when there is less light. Rapid cycling bipolar disorder refers to a manic depressive illness where there are four or more episodes of mania or depression in a given year.

Menstrual related depressive and anxiety symptoms are quite common. Premenstrual syndrome (PMS) occurs in about 70% of normal women and is characterized by a collection of physical and psychological symptoms that may include depression, irritability, lability, or less often elation that starts a few days to a week or more before the onset of menses and are usually relieved with bleeding. The physical symptoms include breast tenderness, water retention, edema and bloating, and occasional headaches. Many women can function throughout these periodic times. However, about 4–5% of women experience much more severe symptoms that can interfere with their functioning at school, work, or with interpersonal relationships. This condition is called premenstrual dysphoric disorder (PMDD). It is important to note that about half of the women who experience PMS or PMDD may be experiencing the worsening of another condition such as depressive illnesses, anxiety disorders, substance abuse, alcoholism, or psychosis. It is helpful to keep a prospective diary in order to find out if the woman does have PMS or PMDD. The causes of PMS and PMDD are not clearly known except for their relation to sex hormones. Research is under way to clarify the relationship of ovarian hormones to brain neurotransmitters, adrenal hormones, thyroid function, and psychosocial variables. Mild PMS does not require treatments, while more severe reactions have been managed with diet, vitamins, exercise, relaxation training, group support, use of antidepressants especially the selective serotonin reuptake inhibitors or antianxiety medications. There has not been good support for the use of ovarian hormones.

DEPRESSION AND PREGNANCY

Many women while pregnant or in the period that follows the delivery of a baby may be more emotionally stressed without meeting the criteria for any mental

Depression

illness. Some of the normal psychological changes include anxiety, mood lability, and concerns about bodily changes and well-being of the fetus. Women are more likely to suffer mood and behavioral changes during this time than at any other part of the life cycle. Following are some of the most prevalent conditions:

The blues, often referred to as postpartum blues, postnatal blues, or 3-day blues, happen to as many as 70% of women, occur within 48 hours of delivery, last 2–3 days to 2 weeks, and are experienced by women cross-culturally. The most common symptoms are emotional lability, elation or tearfulness, sadness, anxiety, irritability, insomnia, and fatigue. These feelings come as a surprise to many women who are so pleased to have a baby, but are not expecting those feelings. Often, rest is helpful but no other special treatments are needed.

Postpartum depression (PPD) is defined as a major depressive disorder that occurs during or after pregnancy or a pregnancy loss. It has similar symptoms to depressive illnesses occurring at other times, except for more feelings of guilt and possible obsessional thoughts of harming the baby after it is born. PPD may occur up to 9 months after birth, usually within the first 3 months, affects 10–15% of women giving birth to healthy babies with a higher incidence with babies who are ill or have congenital malformations. Adolescent mothers have a higher incidence of PPD. Risk factors for having PPD are past history, family history, inadequate social supports such as family and friends, perinatal loss, and birth of multiple babies (twins, triplets, or more). Milder forms of depressive illnesses are called adjustment reactions with depressed mood. Evaluation by health care staff should always include a careful physical exam plus laboratory tests for thyroid function. Alcohol and drug use may complicate these disorders.

Treatment of PPD includes psychotherapy, usually interpersonal or cognitive behavioral, group therapy, self-help groups such as Depression After Delivery (DAD), and medications. Light therapy has been helpful. At this time there are no conclusive data about the use of ovarian hormones such as estrogen and progesterone. Since these hormones drop precipitously after delivery, their role is being studied. It is important to weigh the risk benefits of use of medications in the pregnant and postpartum woman who is nursing. Some medications can be used safely and should be carefully considered. Untreated depressive illnesses may last as long as 9 months or longer. About 50% of women with PPD may have a recurrence in subsequent pregnancies or within 4 years. Recent studies have shown the effectiveness of preventive treatment by giving medications during pregnancy or right after delivery.

Peripartum psychosis is the most severe mental illness associated with pregnancy and afterward and occurs in about 1 per 1,000 deliveries. More than half of these women have depressive illnesses, while others may have schizophrenic or other causes. The symptoms, in addition to those already mentioned, include hallucinations, delusions, a loss of reality, confusion, distractibility, and inability to focus attention. There is often danger of suicide or harming the baby. Usually, hospitalization is indicated plus treatment with antipsychotic medications as well as psychotherapy. Such individuals should not be left alone until they show marked improvement. Electroconvulsive therapy (ECT) is also an effective, rapidly acting, and safe treatment for peripartum psychosis.

MENOPAUSE-RELATED DEPRESSION

While there has not been good evidence to suggest that menopause (no menstrual periods for a year) is associated with any increase in depressive illnesses for those women who have not had any psychiatric problems before, some newer epidemiologic information suggests there is a small increase. The perimenopause, however, those years preceding the final menstrual period, which is a major hormonal transition like puberty, may present women with more depressive and irritable symptoms. Treatment is symptomatic. Recent work interestingly suggests that women with major depression may have an earlier onset of menopause.

In summary, depressive symptoms and disorders are very widespread. Unipolar major depression is the number one cause for burden of disease in the world according to the World Health Organization (WHO) in 1990. The conditions are hard to diagnose but are very treatable.

SEE ALSO: Bipolar disorder, Dysthymia, Postpartum disorders, Pregnancy

Suggested Reading

Sadock, J. B., & Sadock, V. S. (2000). *Comprehensive textbook of psychiatry* (7th ed.). Philadelphia: Lippincott, Williams & Wilkins.

MIRIAM B. ROSENTHAL

Dermatitis

Dermatitis, also referred to as eczema, is an inflammation of the skin. This is a common condition that has a variety of different causes and presentations. It may be acute or chronic and extent of involvement may be localized or generalized. Depending on the specific features, various types of dermatitis have been classified. Itching is a common feature.

Atopic dermatitis is most common in infants and children and is often seen in individuals with family members who have asthma or hayfever. It begins in infancy and many children outgrow it by adolescence. It is characterized by red and itchy patches with a predilection for skin folds such as behind the elbows or knees as well as the neck, wrists, and ankles. The areas also have a tendency to become infected due to introduction of bacteria from scratching. Over time, the skin in these areas becomes thickened with a leathery appearance. It is most commonly treated with topical corticosteroids or newer nonsteroid prescription medications called topical immunomodulators. Oral antihistamines are often required to reduce the itching that can be so severe as to interfere with sleep and daily activities. Antibiotics may be required for secondary infection. Moisturization with bland emollients and avoidance of overly drying the skin such as bathing too frequently are also helpful.

Contact dermatitis arises as a result of an allergic or irritant reaction due to substances touching the skin. Examples include poison ivy, costume jewelry, or perfumes in soaps or laundry detergent. Signs and symptoms include redness and itching, and depending on the severity there can be significant swelling and formation of blisters. These skin changes are limited to the site of exposure to the substance that elicits the allergic or irritant reaction. Treatment consists primarily of identifying the cause and avoiding it; however, resolution can be hastened with topical corticosteroids and, in severe cases, oral corticosteroids. If the condition is chronic and the inciting substance is unclear, skin patch testing may be performed to identify the causative allergen.

Seborrheic dermatitis is characterized by greasy yellowish scaling on the scalp and, in severe cases, the face. It is more common in adults, but can be seen in infants in the form of cradle cap. The presence of yeast is thought to play a role in its development. It may occur during times of stress or in people who have neurologic conditions. It is treated with medicated dandruff shampoos, topical corticosteroids, and antiyeast preparations.

Stasis dermatitis usually occurs on the lower legs and is characterized by itchy red and scaly patches. Over time, it leaves behind brown patches that are generally asymptomatic. The cause is attributed to fluid accumulation in the tissues beneath the skin, and is often seen in association with varicose veins or ankle swelling. Improving the condition that is causing fluid buildup in the legs is the most beneficial treatment, and topical corticosteroids are often used if the situation is chronic. Because stasis dermatitis is usually asymptomatic, it often goes untreated and can result in eventual ulceration of the skin, which can be difficult to heal.

SEE ALSO: Adolescence, Asthma

Suggested Reading

Bergstresser, P. R. (1989). Contact allergic dermatitis. *Archives of Dermatology, 125,* 276–286.

Rietschel, F. L., & Fowler, J. F. (1995). *Fisher's contact dermatitis* (4th ed.). Philadelphia: Williams & Wilkins.

MARY GAIL MERCURIO

Diabetes

Diabetes mellitus is a disease in which blood glucose (sugar) levels rise out of control. Insulin is the hormone that regulates blood glucose levels by signaling cells to take glucose out of the bloodstream and by signaling the liver not to put more glucose into the bloodstream. Insulin is made in the pancreas, an organ that lies in the upper abdomen, just below and behind the stomach. Diabetes occurs either because the pancreas fails to produce enough insulin (type 1 diabetes) or because cells do not respond normally to insulin (type 2 diabetes). Type 2 diabetes accounts for the vast majority of diabetes. Only about 5–10% of all diabetes is type 1.

Diabetes is the most common hormone disorder. About 17 million people in the United States have diabetes, accounting for 6.2% of the population. Another 6 million or so cases are undiagnosed. In 1999, diabetes was the sixth leading cause of death. In general, people with diabetes are twice as likely to die as those without diabetes. For women and young adults, diabetes increases the death rate by fourfold. According to the American Diabetes Association, in 1997, diabetes cost the United States $98 billion. Direct medical costs were $44 billion. Indirect costs related to disability, loss of work, and premature death were even higher, accounting for $54 billion.

Type 1 diabetes, in which the pancreas does not produce enough insulin, used to be called juvenile-onset diabetes because it is usually diagnosed in children and young adults. However, type 1 diabetes can also develop later in life. Type 1 diabetes is an autoimmune disease in which the body's immune system destroys insulin-producing cells in the pancreas, called beta cells. Usually a viral infection provokes this abnormal immune reaction. There seems to be an inherited predisposition to type 1 diabetes. If one identical twin has type 1 diabetes, the other twin has a 50% chance of developing it.

After type 1 diabetes starts, there may be a short period when insulin is not required, called the "honeymoon period." However, when beta cell destruction is complete, patients must take insulin to stay alive. Glucose is the preferred fuel for organs and tissues. In the absence of insulin, cells cannot take in glucose for fuel, and blood glucose levels rise out of control. Instead, the body makes ketoacids as an alternate fuel. High levels of ketoacids in the blood can lead to acidification of the blood, which can be fatal.

Type 2 diabetes accounts for 90–95% of all diabetes. Insulin resistance is the hallmark of type 2 diabetes, although type 2 diabetes can also involve reduced insulin production. In insulin resistance, cells are insensitive to insulin, and do not take up glucose as fast as they should when exposed to insulin. Abdominal obesity seems to predispose people to insulin resistance. In turn, insulin resistance leads to elevated cholesterol and triglyeride levels, high blood pressure, clogged arteries (as in coronary artery disease), kidney stones, and polycystic ovary syndrome.

Risk factors for developing type 2 diabetes include increasing age, obesity, family history of type 2 diabetes, personal history of gestational diabetes, impaired glucose tolerance, and inactivity. There is a strong genetic basis for type 2 diabetes, likely due to multiple genes. If one identical twin is affected, the other has a 95% chance of developing type 2 diabetes. Certain ethnic groups are also at higher risk. These include African Americans, Hispanic Americans, American Indians, Asian Americans, and Pacific Islanders. Most patients develop type 2 diabetes after the age of 40; however, there are increasing numbers of younger type 2 diabetic patients. Glucose levels usually are high for 4–7 years

before type 2 diabetes is diagnosed, because classic symptoms do not occur until glucose levels become extremely high.

DIAGNOSIS

Classic symptoms of diabetes are increased urination, excessive thirst, and blurry vision as well as unusual weight loss, increased hunger, and fatigue. Usually, however, diabetes is diagnosed based on blood tests. Diabetes mellitus can be diagnosed by any of the following three criteria: (1) fasting glucose greater than 126 mg/dl on two or more occasions, (2) random blood glucose of 200 mg/dl or higher in the presence of symptoms (excessive urination, excessive thirst, weight loss), or (3) two glucose readings over 200 mg/dl during a 2-hr oral glucose tolerance test after drinking a solution containing 75 g of glucose. Gestational diabetes, or diabetes developing in pregnancy, is defined with slightly different cutoff values and is diagnosed with a 3-hr oral glucose tolerance test that uses a 100-g glucose load.

"Prediabetes" involves glucose levels that are above normal but not high enough to be called diabetes. Impaired fasting glucose (IFG) refers to fasting glucose between 100 and 125 mg/dl. Impaired glucose tolerance (IGT) is defined as glucose values between 140 and 200 mg/dl during a 2-hr glucose tolerance test, with normal fasting glucose levels. In either case, the diagnosis should be confirmed by repeat testing.

SHORT-TERM COMPLICATIONS

Diabetes can cause medical emergencies in both type 1 and type 2 diabetics when blood glucose levels rise extremely high. This can occur if a diabetic patient does not take her insulin or pills or does not follow a diabetic diet. Infection, heart attack, and other physical stresses can also cause high glucose levels. Extremely high glucose levels lead to loss of glucose in the urine, which pulls water along with it, leading to excessive loss of water from the kidneys. This results in dehydration, which further concentrates glucose in the blood causing glucose levels to rise. Weight loss occurs both as a result of water and calorie loss.

In type 1 diabetes, this scenario can occur abruptly when insulin is severely deficient. A condition called ketoacidosis develops. Blood glucose levels rise to 300–600 mg/dl. Since the cells are now unable to use glucose for fuel, the body starts to break down fat to produce ketoacids. When ketoacid levels rise, the blood becomes acidic, which impairs enzymatic reactions throughout the body. This results in abdominal pain, nausea, and vomiting. Ketones can be detected in the urine and produce a fruity odor on the breath. Brain cells do not use ketones, so they starve in the absence of insulin, producing coma. Diabetic ketoacidosis was universally fatal prior to the discovery of insulin. Now, about 2% of patients with this condition die.

In type 2 diabetes, insulin resistance is the main problem and insulin is not as severely deficient. Therefore, ketoacidosis does not occur. Instead, glucose levels continue to rise to 1,000 mg/dl or more. This produces a condition known as nonketotic hyperosmolar state. With such high glucose levels there is simply too much "stuff" in the blood and water is pulled out of cells to try to dilute the blood back to a normal range. This water is then lost in the urine. Such severe dehydration causes drowsiness, delirium, coma, or seizures. The elderly are more vulnerable, but overall about 20–40% of people with this condition die.

LONG-TERM COMPLICATIONS

Improved medical care has made diabetes a chronic disease. Mildly elevated glucose levels can be tolerated in the short term, but over many years damage is done to small blood vessels (microvascular disease) or to large blood vessels (macrovascular disease).

Microvascular complications include blindness from damage to the retina, kidney failure, and nerve damage (neuropathy). Diabetes is the leading cause of blindness in people aged 20–74 years. Diabetes is also the leading cause of kidney failure requiring dialysis, accounting for 43% of new cases. Nerve damage affects 60–70% of diabetics and causes an inability to sense trauma. Because of this, diabetics are prone to unnoticed skin breaks, which can become infected. Diabetic feet especially heal slowly if at all, and many diabetic foot infections ultimately require amputation. Diabetes accounts for more than 60% of all nontraumatic lower limb amputations.

Macrovascular complications include heart disease and stroke. These complications are exacerbated by high blood pressure and high cholesterol, which often go along with diabetes. Heart disease is the leading cause of death in diabetes, occurring 2–4 times more often in diabetics than in nondiabetic individuals. Stroke is also 2–4 times more common in diabetes.

PREGNANCY-RELATED COMPLICATIONS

Diabetes can cause many problems in pregnancy. In the first trimester, about 5–10% of fetuses develop major birth defects and 15–20% of pregnancies end in miscarriage. During the second to third trimesters, excessive fetal weight gain (macrosomia) occurs, especially in poorly controlled gestational diabetes. This leads to complications during delivery for both the mother and the baby. The goal of diabetic treatment in pregnancy is tight control of glucose levels to reduce the chance of these problems. In gestational diabetes, if glucose levels are not controlled with diet and exercise, then insulin (or sometimes oral medication) is used. Women with preexisting diabetes who become pregnant also need intensive monitoring and treatment.

INFECTIONS

Patients with diabetes are prone to certain infections in the urinary tract or skin and soft tissue and fungal infections such as vaginal yeast infections. Good glucose control helps prevent infections and may also help with wound healing. About 30% of patients with diabetes also have severe periodontal disease.

TREATMENT

Type 1 diabetes must be treated with insulin. There are different types of insulin and different schedules and modes of delivery. Generally speaking, type 1 patients need a long-acting or intermediate-acting insulin to cover them for a 24-hr period regardless of food intake, plus a short-acting insulin to take care of glucose swings during meals. Examples of long-acting insulins are ultralente and glargine; intermediate-acting insulins are NPH and lente; and short-acting insulins are regular and lispro.

An insulin pump may be used in cases involving type 2 diabetes that does not respond to treatment or type 1 diabetes in which a patient does not follow her prescribed regimen. The insulin pump acts as a continuous insulin infusion. This is a device in which fast-acting insulin is stored in a reservoir, and is connected by tubing to a needle inserted under the skin, usually in the abdomen. The pump is programmed to provide different basal rates of insulin infusion throughout the day and night. Patients have to monitor their blood glucose before meals and exercise and make adjustments over and above the basal rate (*boluses*). They also have to make adjustments by taking extra calories for low sugar reading (corrections). The insulin pump can provide smoother glucose control, but patients have to be extremely motivated in order to check their glucose up to 6–8 times daily. There is higher risk of low blood sugars because of tighter blood sugar control.

Currently, researchers are working on pancreatic islet cell transplantation for the treatment of type 1 diabetes. When successful, the procedure cures diabetes, but immune-suppressing drugs are required and can have toxic side effects. Sometimes the transplanted cells just do not last or they may be destroyed by the same autoimmune reaction that made the person diabetic in the first place.

Treatment of type 2 diabetes includes oral medication and/or insulin. The medication chosen depends on a variety of factors, such as how long the person has been diabetic, whether she is overweight or lean, and how high the blood glucose rises. There are different classes of oral medications. In general, there are medications that cause increased insulin output from the pancreas, such as the sulfonylureas (glyburide, glipizide, and others). Nateglinide also increases output from the pancreas but is shorter acting and may be helpful in patients with high blood sugars after meals. These medications can cause low blood glucose and weight gain.

A treatment known as metformin may help obese patients with insulin resistance and helps muscles use glucose while also reducing glucose output by the liver. It must be used with care in patients with kidney problems and congestive heart failure. Common side effects include gas and diarrhea, which are minimized when metformin is taken with meals. Weight gain is not a side effect, and some patients might lose some weight. Medications of the group thiazolidinediones (pioglitazone, rosiglitazone) are also effective in reducing insulin resistance. With these drugs, liver function must be monitored with blood tests. Weight gain and edema are common side effects so these medications cannot be used in severe heart failure. Finally, insulin remains an important medication in the treatment of poorly controlled type 2 diabetes, either when oral agents have failed *or at any time* that patients develop insulin deficiency.

TREATMENT GUIDELINES

The goal of diabetes treatment is to achieve optimal control of blood glucose, cholesterol, and blood pressure.

Table 1. Diabetes monitoring goals

HbA1c (%)—reflects 3-month average glucose	≤7%
Glucose before meals (mg/dl)	80–120
Bedtime glucose (mg/dl)	100–140
Blood pressure (mm Hg)	≤130 systolic, ≤85 diastolic
LDL cholesterol (mg/dl)	≤100
HDL cholesterol (mg/dl)	≥45
Triglyceride (fat) (mg/dl)	≤150

Regular exercise, attention to the feet and nails, and annual eye exams are excellent preventive measures. Regardless of what medication is used, the mainstay of diabetes treatment is always diet and exercise.

The American Diabetes Association dietary recommendations are as follows: carbohydrates should comprise 50% of daily calories, fat less than 30%, and cholesterol should be less than 300 mg daily. Of the fat, less than 10% of calories should be derived from saturated fat and greater than 10% from monounsaturated fat. Protein intake should be 0.8 g/kg body weight and dietary fiber intake should be between 20 and 35 g daily.

The care of diabetes often involves several team members: patient, physician, diabetes educator, nutritionist, podiatrist (foot doctor), ophthalmologist (eye doctor), and/or psychologist. Patients are required to monitor blood sugars by using a glucometer, a machine that uses special strips on which a drop of capillary blood is obtained by pricking the fingers or arm with a lancet (tiny needle). Capillary blood monitoring lets patients and their care providers assess glucose control and make adjustments in diet, exercise, or medications. See Table 1 for treatment guidelines.

PREVENTION OF COMPLICATIONS

Two major studies in both type 1 and type 2 diabetes have shown that tight control of glucose reduces complications. The Diabetes Control and Complications Trial (DCCT) was a study of type 1 diabetic patients. It conclusively showed that intensive glucose control reduces microvascular complications. The DCCT showed a 60% reduction in the risk of developing neuropathy, 27% reduction in the risk of retinopathy, and 54% risk reduction in developing kidney damage. The United Kingdom Prospective Diabetes Study (UKPDS) was a large study of patients with type 2 diabetes. The UKPDS trial showed that intensive glucose control led to a 25% reduction in retinopathy and cataracts and 30% reduction in risk of early kidney damage. In patients with high blood pressure and type 2 diabetes, intensive control resulted in 30% reduced risk of stroke and 46% reduction in death.

PREVENTION OF DIABETES

The Diabetes Prevention Program was a study of persons at risk of developing type 2 diabetes. It showed a 58% reduction in diabetes with 30 minutes a day of moderate physical activity along with a 5–10% reduction in body weight. Metformin, too, reduced the risk of diabetes by 31% but was less effective in persons older than 45 years and in those with a body mass index greater than 35. There is no definite evidence that anything can be done to prevent type 1 diabetes. The Diabetes Prevention Trial used insulin in subjects at risk for type 1 diabetes, based on family history and other parameters, but this was not effective. In women with polycystic ovary syndrome, metformin taken before and throughout pregnancy reduces the occurrence of gestational diabetes from 31% of pregnancies to 3%. Metformin appears to be safe to for use in pregnancy. More research is being done on all forms of diabetes.

SEE ALSO: Cardiovascular disease, Cholesterol, Diet, Hypertension, Nutrition, Obesity

Suggested Reading

Brotman, D., & Girod, J. P. (2002). The metabolic syndrome: A tug-of-war with no winner. *Cleveland Clinic Journal of Medicine, 69,* 990–994.

Haffner, S. (2002). Metabolic syndrome, diabetes and coronary heart disease. *International Journal of Clinical Practice* (Suppl. 132), 21–37.

Nathan, D. M., & Cagliero, E. (2001). Diabetes mellitus. In P. Felig & L. A. Frohman (Eds.), *Endocrinology & metabolism* (4th ed., pp. 827–926). New York: McGraw-Hill.

Suggested Resources

American Diabetes Association. (2003). www.diabetes.org

ASRA KERMANI

Diaphragm The diaphragm is a dome-shaped, flexible device inserted into the vagina that covers the cervix and prevents conception by blocking live sperm from entering the uterus and tubes. The diaphragm is a reversible, prescription, barrier method of contraception.

The most frequently used diaphragms are made of latex, but a silicone diaphragm is now on the market for those with latex sensitivity. It is designed to be used with spermicidal jelly.

Obtaining a diaphragm requires a medical appointment for proper fitting and a prescription. The device may be purchased at a pharmacy for $15–50. The cost for the medical appointment will add additional expense unless covered by insurance. In addition, the over-the-counter spermicidal jelly used with the diaphragm must also be purchased at additional cost. The diaphragm should be refitted following a full-term pregnancy, abdominal or pelvic surgery, a miscarriage, or abortion after 14 weeks of pregnancy, and/or weight gain or loss of 10 pounds or more.

The diaphragm is an excellent method of contraception for women who do not wish to or cannot use hormonal contraception. However, the use of the diaphragm is somewhat complicated and requires forethought to have supplies on hand. It may interrupt spontaneity if it is used at the time of intercourse, though it may be inserted up to 6 hours prior to having sex. About 20 out of 100 women will become pregnant using the diaphragm for one year of typical use, 6 out of 100 with perfect use. Therefore, those for whom unintended pregnancy may present serious consequences may wish to consider a more effective method of birth control. If a woman is not comfortable touching her genitals or has difficulty with placing the diaphragm correctly, she may wish to consider another method. The diaphragm should not be used:

- following recent cervical surgery
- less than 6 weeks after childbirth
- following recent second trimester abortion
- by those with uterine prolapse
- by those with allergy to the spermicide or latex
- by women who have had toxic shock syndrome

While it is not contraindicated entirely, women who have frequent urinary tract infections or have poor vaginal muscle control may wish to avoid using the diaphragm.

The diaphragm is used with spermicidal jelly and inserted prior to intercourse. Inspection of the diaphragm prior to placement ensures that it has no holes or tears. It is left in place for 6 hours following intercourse to assure that all sperm have been immobilized prior to removing the barrier. It may be left in for as long as 24 hours. However, if the initial act of intercourse occurs more than 6 hours after insertion or if there are multiple acts of coitus, more spermicidal jelly must be inserted into the vagina prior to each act of intercourse. Oil-based lubricants should not be used with a latex diaphragm as this may weaken the latex and decrease the effectiveness of the method. Following removal, the diaphragm is cleaned with plain soap and water and allowed to dry thoroughly before replacing in the case. There is no need to use any type of powder or cornstarch on the diaphragm.

The diaphragm is often overlooked when considering methods of birth control. Diaphragms are inexpensive and an immediately reversible form of contraception. In addition, they may also provide some protection from cervical infections such as gonorrhea and chlamydia as well as human papillomavirus. Diaphragms are not considered as effective in this way as condoms. They are not as effective as hormonal or surgical methods of contraception but may be a wise choice for those who are not frequently sexually active, would not be devastated by an unintended pregnancy, need protection from infection, or who are unable or unwilling to use hormonal methods.

See Also: Birth control, Condoms, Pelvic organ prolapse, Toxic shock syndrome, Urinary tract infections

Suggested Reading

Hatcher, R., Trussel, J., Stewart, F., Cates, W., Stewart, G., Guest, F., et al. (1999). *Contraceptive technology* (p. 400). New York: Ardent Medica.
What's in store for non-latex barrier methods. (1998). *Contraceptive Technology Update, 19*(3), 40–41.

Suggested Resources

Planned Parenthood Federation of America. (2000). *Facts about birth control: The diaphragm and cervical cap.* Retrieved October 2000, from http://www.plannedparenthood.org/bc/bcfacts10.html

Nancy Myers-Bradley

Diet   Prevention of disease is the cornerstone of a healthy life and what you eat has an enormous impact on your chances of avoiding disease. A poor diet is one of the major causes of problems such as heart disease, diabetes, and obesity. Diet is defined as the amount and kind of food and drink that a person takes in a day. It also refers to food selections planned to meet specific requirements of the individual, by including or excluding certain foods.

Eating practices are influenced by taste and food preferences, the body's ability or inability to process various foods, concerns about nutrition and weight control, lifestyle, availability of food in the environment, food product safety, the social situation, and the emotional meaning attached to foods and eating. Eating is an important source of pleasure and an occasion for social interaction. In our society, extralarge servings of food and snacking on high-calorie snacks have replaced the three-meal pattern of the olden days. We all know that obesity is on the increase. Obesity can lead to chronic disorders such as diabetes, heart disease, arthritis, stroke, and cancer, which have an enormous impact on overall health costs.

The United States Department of Agriculture (USDA) and the Department of Health and Human Services (DHHS) recommend eating a variety of foods; maintaining a healthy weight; choosing a diet low in fat, saturated fat, and cholesterol; choosing a diet with plenty of fruits, vegetables, and grain products; and using sugars and salt in moderation. If you drink alcoholic beverages, do so in moderation. Moderate drinking is described as no more than one drink a day for women and two drinks per day for men. Pregnant women should not drink alcohol.

A balanced diet is a diet that provides the amount of energy, protein, vitamins, minerals, and other nutrients that a person needs, consistent with the dietary guidelines for Americans. A balanced diet is different at different ages. The aim of the diet is to maintain a healthy life without any nutritional deficiencies, while avoiding excesses and minimizing the risk of diet-related diseases. A balanced diet can be achieved by planning the meals based on "The Food Guide Pyramid," in which all five food groups are arranged in the form of a pyramid along with the number of recommended servings. Foods are placed in the pyramid to show the need to eat more foods from the bottom of the pyramid and fewer from the top. Foods in one group cannot be replaced by food from another. Planning your diet based on the food pyramid will help you reduce the intake of total fat, saturated fat, and sugar.

A vegetarian diet excludes meat. Some people prefer to eat only plant-based foods due to religious and cultural practices, environmental concerns, and ethical reasons. There are three types of vegetarian diets: vegan or strict vegetarian, lacto-vegetarian, and lacto-ovo-vegetarian. Vegans exclude all animal foods such as meat, fish, egg, dairy products, honey, poultry, and fish. This diet is deficient in vitamin B12, riboflavin, calcium, and iodine. It is not suitable for pregnant women, nursing mothers, and children due to the increased needs for calcium in these groups. Leafy green vegetables are good sources of calcium, but this calcium is not absorbed well because it is bound to oxalic acid. Lacto-vegetarians include dairy products but exclude eggs. Lacto-ovo-vegetarians include eggs and dairy products in their diet. Vitamin B12 is usually lacking in vegetarian diet. Foods like tofu and breakfast cereals are fortified with vitamin B12. If these foods are not eaten, supplementation is recommended.

A modified diet is based on a normal diet, but altered in its consistency, texture, nutrients, and caloric value to meet the needs of certain diseases or conditions. For instance, people with swallowing difficulties may require thickened liquids to avoid accidentally inhaling what they drink. People with heart disease may require a low-sodium diet to avoid retaining fluid.

The majority of weight loss diet plans use a low-carbohydrate diet for rapid weight loss. People lose weight and keep it off only for a short time. Glycogen, the body's carbohydrate reserves, is stored with water. When low-carbohydrate dieters use up their carbohydrate reserves, about 3 g of water is lost for every gram of glycogen that is used. This produces rapid weight loss, which is regained after a short period of time. When the stored glycogen is depleted, the body uses fat reserves for its energy needs and chemicals called ketones are produced. Ketosis, a condition in which ketones are found in the blood and urine, can produce undesirable effects such as nausea, gout, dehydration, muscle weakness, and kidney failure. Weight-reducing diets can be effective only if the calorie intake is less than the calories required by the individual. Excluding one group of foods and indulging in another food group will result in nutritional deficiencies but not in weight loss. The best bet to win the weight control battle is to eat less and burn more calories by exercising.

See Also: Body mass index, Calcium, Cholesterol, Nutrition

Suggested Reading

Bender, A. E. (1985). *Health or hoax?: The truth about health foods and diet.* Buffalo, NY: Prometheus Books.
Messina, M., & Messina, V. (1996). *The dietitian's guide to vegetarian diets: Issues and applications.* Gaithersburg, MD: Aspen.
Wescott, P. (2000). *Diet and nutrition.* Austin, TX: Raintree Steck-Vaughn.

Suggested Resources

Medline Plus: nutrition webpage: www.nlm.nih.gov/medlineplus/nutrition.html

RAJKUMARI RICHMONDS

Diethylstilbestrol Diethylstilbestrol (DES) is a synthetic form of estrogen, which was prescribed to millions of women from 1940 to 1971. It was thought to prevent miscarriage and ensure a healthy pregnancy. Its use declined in the 1960s after studies showed that it was not effective in preventing the complications of pregnancy that it was prescribed for. It was also found that when given during the first five months of pregnancy, DES can interfere with the development of the reproductive system in a fetus. The females whose mothers took DES while pregnant are referred to as "DES daughters."

While there may be no obvious signs of DES exposure, there are health risks. All DES daughters have a risk of about 1 in 1,000 for a rare cancer of the vagina or cervix called clear cell adenocarcinoma. It usually occurs after age 14, with most cases found at age 19 or 20. Some cases have been reported by women in their 30s or 40s. This cancer is practically nonexistent in non-DES-exposed women.

A link has been found between DES exposure in utero and an increased risk of developing abnormal cells in the tissue of the cervix and vagina. Terms used to describe this condition are dysplasia, cervical intraepithelial neoplasia (CIN), and squamous intraepithelial lesions (SIL). Although these abnormal cells resemble cancer cells in appearance, they do not invade nearby healthy tissue as cancer cells do. These abnormal cellular changes usually occur between the ages of 25 and 35, but may appear at other ages as well. Although this condition is not cancer, it may develop into cancer if left untreated.

DES daughters are at increased risk of infertility, ectopic pregnancy, miscarriage, and preterm labor and delivery. DES daughters have an increased incidence of structural changes in the vagina, uterus, or cervix, which may or may not be linked to pregnancy problems. Most DES daughters can become pregnant and carry their babies to term, but because of the known risks, they require high-risk obstetric care and early confirmation of pregnancy.

Dilation and Curettage

Women exposed to DES may also need to consider appropriate contraception. Although studies have not shown that the use of birth control pills or hormone replacement therapy is unsafe for DES daughters, some doctors believe these women should avoid these medications. Structural changes in the vagina or cervix should cause no problems with the use of diaphragms or spermicides.

Women who used DES may have a slightly increased risk of breast cancer. DES mothers should practice monthly breast self-exams, have regular breast cancer screening, and yearly medical checkups that include a pelvic examination and a Pap test.

There is some evidence that DES-exposed sons may have testicular abnormalities, such as cysts on the ducts behind the testicle, undescended testicles, or abnormally small testicles. The risk for testicular or prostate cancer is unclear. A DES son should practice regular testicular self-exams and inform his physician of his exposure and be examined periodically.

Researchers continue to study DES exposure as daughters move into the menopausal years. The cancer risks for exposed daughters and sons are being studied to determine if they differ from the unexposed population.

In addition, researchers are studying possible health effects on the grandchildren of mothers who were exposed to DES during pregnancy. They are referred to as third-generation daughters or DES granddaughters. There are two published studies. One done in 1995 found that the age menstruation began was not affected by the mother's exposure to DES. A 2002 study concluded that third-generation effects of in utero DES exposure are unlikely.

Individuals born between 1940 and 1971 should ask their mothers or other relatives who might know of the mother's pregnancy history if she took any medication during her pregnancy, or if she had any problems during her pregnancy. If a woman used DES while pregnant, it is advisable that she tell her children about her DES exposure. Even if they have not had health problems, they need to know so they can get the health care they may need now or in the future. The need for an annual pelvic exam is critical and is slightly different from a routine exam.

For a list of resources including books, support groups, organizations, and attorneys see DES Action USA (510-465-4011; desaction@earthlink.net; www.desaction.org).

SEE ALSO: Cancer, Cervical cancer, Miscarriage, Pregnancy

Suggested Resources

DES Action USA. *Health risks and care for DES daughters.* Retrieved March 6, 2003, from http://www.desaction.org

DES Cancer Network. *Health care guidelines for DES-exposed women and men.* Retrieved March 6, 2003, from http://www.des-cancer.org

National Cancer Institute. Med News. (2002, November 6). *DES: Questions and answers.* Retrieved March 6, 2003, from http://www.med.uni-bonn.de/cancernet/600034.html

POLLY HAMPTON
JUDITH TRENTMAN

Dilation and Curettage

Cervical dilation and uterine curettage (D&C) is a procedure done for both diagnostic and therapeutic reasons. D&C is one of the most commonly performed operations in the United States. Dilation entails enlarging the cervical opening or "os" with instruments specifically for this purpose called dilators. Dilation may be done alone for problems of cervical stenosis (scarring and/or narrowing of the cervical os), for placing of IUDs, or for dysmenorrhea (menstrual cramps) due to a narrowed cervical canal. It may also precede procedures such as hysteroscopy, use of a scope to visualize and/or photograph the inside of the uterus for diagnosis of structural conditions such as polyps or fibroids in the uterine cavity. Minor treatments such as removal of polyps can be done through the hysteroscope. Cervical dilation may be performed under paracervical, epidural, spinal, or general anesthesia depending on the reason for the procedure.

After the cervix is dilated, curettage may be performed using a curette, a sharp instrument for scraping. Curettage is the partial or complete scraping of the uterine wall to obtain representative tissue samples for diagnosis of uterine cancer or precancerous conditions, to remove retained tissue remnants of a pregnancy following miscarriage or birth, or for termination of pregnancy (abortion). Curettage is also indicated for treatment in the occasional case of uterine bleeding that does not respond to medical therapy, generally hormones, or bleeding that is life threatening. The tissue obtained during the procedure is sent to the pathology laboratory for analysis.

Complications of a D&C include perforation of the uterus, infection, bleeding, or reactions to medications used for anesthesia. Perforation of the uterus means that a surgical instrument goes through the uterine wall. This occurs in less than 1% of patients. In those instances when perforation occurs, the outcome is usually not life threatening nor is surgical intervention required. The patient may be observed for several hours after the procedure to assure that there is no life-threatening bleeding or infection requiring further treatment. Laparoscopy that allows for inspection of the abdomen and pelvis through small incisions in the abdominal wall may be used if the patient is stable but there is concern about serious organ damage to uterus, blood vessels, or bowel. Severe cases of bleeding may lead to hysterectomy. Another complication of D&C is called Asherman's syndrome. This complication is rare and involves the formation of scar tissue in the uterus. Aggressive curettage or an abnormal reaction to this scraping can cause Asherman's syndrome. Thick scars can result, which may partially or completely obliterate the uterine cavity. This scarring can cause menstrual bleeding to stop and cause infertility if further hysteroscopic surgery is not successful. Abscess, infection, or hemorrhage can complicate the postoperative course in a very small percentage of patients.

In summary, D&C can be very helpful for the diagnosis and treatment of abnormal uterine bleeding in the nonpregnant woman. It can be the method used to evacuate the uterus for a woman with a miscarriage or unintended pregnancy.

SEE ALSO: Abortion, Hysterectomy, Miscarriage, Sexual organs, Uterine fibroids

Suggested Reading

Pernol, M. L. (Ed.). (1991). *Obstetrics and gynecologic diagnosis and treatment* (7th ed., pp. 900–902). Norwalk, CT: Appleton & Lange.
Youngkin, E. Q., & Davis, M. S. (1998). *Women's health: A primary care clinical guide* (p. 146). Englewood Cliffs, NJ: Prentice-Hall.

Suggested Resources

Williams, C. E., & McNamara, R. M. (2001). Dilation and curettage. Retrieved April 2001, from http://www.emedicine.com/aaem/topic156.htm

NANCY MYERS-BRADLEY

Disability Individuals with disabilities, the currently preferred term used to describe disabled or handicapped persons, refers to those whose physical or mental impairments so interfere with life's activities, including working, that they are set apart from those without disabilities.

Disability, like beauty, is in the eyes of the beholder. Whether the beholder is the Social Security Administration, an employer, an insurance company, a retail business, the bureau of motor vehicles, a doctor, or a partner, an individual may or may not be considered disabled.

Insurance companies and health professionals sometimes measure disability in terms of how many activities of daily living (ADLs) a person can perform independently. The Mayo Clinic separates ADLs into Basic ADLs required for an individual to care for themselves in a limited environment: Dressing, Eating, Ambulating, Toileting, Hygiene (acronym DEATH, ironically), and Instrumental ADLs, the higher level abilities required to function in the community: Shopping, Housework, Accounting, Food Preparation, Transportation (SHAFT). For people with physical, developmental, and age-related disabilities, and their advocates, these are the concepts that help identify appropriate housing and resolve placement issues.

Another touchstone is the Social Security Administration's definition of disability, focused more on an individual's ability to work and make a living in our competitive world. Social Security assessment proceeds through a five-step sequential evaluation. To be disabled, a claimant must (1) not be working at a level known as substantial gainful activity, (2) suffer from severe medically determinable impairment that lasts more than 12 months, (3) either meet a listed impairment or suffer from an impairment so severe that it (4) prevents return to past relevant work performed in the last 15 years and (5) prevents entry into other jobs existing in significant numbers in the national economy.

A blind or paraplegic person may meet a listing, and be what we would all call disabled, but if she is gainfully employed, she is not disabled under the first step of the Social Security definition, and would receive no benefits.

For private long-term disability insurance coverage, and even short-term disability coverage, a distinction is often made between own occupation and all occupation coverage. Whether a person's impairments prevent her from performing the duties of her own occupation is one measure of disability. Sometimes after a period of a year or two, the policy will require the disabled person to prove that she is not unable to go back to her old job, but unable to go to work at *any* job. Since there

Discrimination

is still no parity legally required between physical and mental disabilities, long-term disability insurance coverage sometimes has a 2-year limit on coverage for mental impairments.

The workers' compensation system differentiates among permanent partial, temporary total, and total permanent disability, and may assign a percentage disability for the loss of a limb or the loss of use of a body part or organ.

Under the Americans with Disabilities Act, disability refers to the inability to perform the bona fide occupational qualifications (BFOQs) required to perform all the duties of one's job.

Who makes these decisions? On what medical evidence are such findings of disability based? Sometimes the opinions of one's own treating physicians or other health care professionals are given the most weight; sometimes it is the opinion of the independent medical examiner or panel of physicians employed by the company or government that is determinative of the claim. It is important that each individual find out whether his or her employer's disability coverage is provided through an insurance company, regulated under state law, or through a self-funded or Employment Retirement Income Security Act (ERISA) plan that is exempt from state insurance regulations and is governed instead by the U.S. Department of Labor.

More women (20.7%) than men (18.6%) suffer disabling conditions, and while bad backs are the leading cause of disability for both genders, women are twice as likely as men to suffer from arthritis. While fewer women suffer from mental disorders (not mental retardation and learning disabilities) than men, women are twice as likely to struggle with depression.

As Tolstoy put it, all happy families resemble one another, but each unhappy family is unhappy in its own way. Healthy people do not typically gather in support groups focused on peculiar ways in which they are healthy, unless you consider a bowling league or an investment club as a celebration of physical or mental health. Disabled people and their families often connect with other disabled people and their families, linked by the disease or impairment that has changed their lives. Syndromes and symptoms, diseases and diagnoses give disabled people something in common that goes beyond shared suffering, an unspoken language that only the victims, and perhaps their caregivers, understand. Undoubtedly, for better or for worse, a disability shapes a person's day and life in ways the rest of us can only read about and try to imagine.

SEE ALSO: Activities of daily living, Americans with Disabilities Act, Capacity, Health insurance, Social Security disability benefits

Suggested Reading

Asch, A., & Fine, M. (Eds.). (1988). *Women with disabilities: Essays in psychology, culture and politics.* Philadelphia: Temple University Press.

Beisser, A. (1988). *Flying without wings: Personal reflections on loss, disability, and healing.* New York: Bantam Books.

Jans, L., & Stoddard, S. (1999). *Chartbook on women and disability in the United States. An InfoUse Report.* Washington, DC: U.S. National Institute on Disability and Rehabilitation Research.

Mathews, G. F. (1983). *Voices from the shadows: Women with disabilities speak out.* Toronto, Ontario, Canada: Women's Educational Press.

National Institute of Mental Health (NIMH). (2001). *Women hold up half the sky, fact sheet on women and mental health research* (NIH Publication No. 01-4607). Betlesda, MD: Author.

JANET L. LOWDER
MARY B. MCKEE

Discrimination

Women face discrimination on a variety of fronts in health today ranging from the battle to include contraceptives in basic health plans, to biases inherent in the male-dominated medical establishment. This has created an atmosphere of growing resentment that has spawned a campaign toward a better understanding of the critical issues women face when making medical choices. Identifying and drawing attention to the problem areas is the first step to overcoming gender bias in medicine. Sexism in research, insurance, diagnosis, and treatment has created a situation where women make uninformed decisions, receive inferior care, and in some instances endure downright neglect.

One of the most difficult and troubling examples of sexism is in medical research. Women are often excluded from participating in research into new drugs, medical treatments, and new surgical techniques. There is a widespread practice in the medical community of using exclusively male subjects in the study of disease. The raw data garnered from these studies are then "interpreted" to include women. Using males as experimental subject not only ignores the fact that females may respond differently to the drugs and mechanisms tested, but may ironically lead to less accurate models even in the male. One glaring example of this can be found in the study of heart disease. Physicians consider research into heart disease as primarily addressing men; it is considered applicable to older women only. This is despite the fact that the incidence of heart disease has steadily increased among women since at least the 1950s.

Research has also provided one of the most frightening instances of the total disregard by the medical establishment of women's unique vulnerabilities while pregnant. From the early 1940s till 1971, obstetricians prescribed the drug known as diethylstilbestrol (DES) to pregnant women who were suspected of being prone to miscarriages. Some women, who took the drug experimentally, were not told the truth about what they were taking and were instead told that they were taking a vitamin. DES is now known to be a carcinogen and has left a time-bomb legacy in the daughters and, in some cases, sons of DES mothers. Their daughters suffer vaginal and cervical cancer at a rate far in excess of the rest of the female population in their age range. Worse still, there may be no way to tell how many more will develop cancer later in life.

Research, however, has also given us a glimmer of hope with one of the most positive and visible examples of the changes women are instituting in medical research. Women have been primarily responsible for the increase in funding for research relating to breast cancer. Until recently breast cancer research received less funding and study than AIDS, despite the fact that breast cancer kills twice as many people. In the early 1990s women pushed for a national policy shift that culminated in congressional mandates to increase funding for breast cancer research by 40% annually.

Women's efforts have impacted other areas characterized by blatant sexism. When the removal of mammography screenings from Medicare coverage was threatened in 1989, women successfully lobbied Congress to prevent this action. The importance of providing adequate coverage for breast cancer screenings has led to 39 states requiring at least some form of third-party coverage for mammography screenings at some level.

Medical institutions and practices are not the only areas where discrimination has impacted women's health. Insurance companies have bitterly contested and fought the inclusion of prescription contraceptives and related medical visits and exams in their basic health care packages. As a result, women are sometimes denied vital and basic health access and coverage, which seriously compromises and endangers their health. Half of all fee-for-service health plans do not cover any contraceptive methods at all, and only a third cover oral contraceptives. Of the five leading Food and Drug Administration (FDA)-approved reversible contraceptives, only 39% of health maintenance organizations (HMOs) cover all five. This discrimination has been recognized by the U.S. Equal Employment Opportunity Commission that issued a ruling in its December 2000 findings that the exclusion of the costs of prescription contraceptives from health care packages (while at the same time covering vasectomies and Viagra prescriptions) amounted to discrimination based on sex.

When diagnosing women, doctors (primarily men) many times fail to thoroughly examine female patients and often disregard important and useful information that female patients provide to them. Women constantly have to fight against the assumption that their ailments are "all in their head." Male doctors frequently tend to dismiss women's complaints as psychosomatic, but there is a deeper reason for this than is readily apparent. This is because so little direct research is done focusing on women and how to best treat the ailments that afflict them. Frequently, women with symptoms similar to those of men are taken less seriously; the women's examinations are less extensive than a comparatively performed exam on a male. In addition, women may not be provided with information on how to best diagnose and treat the symptoms.

These shortcomings can be contrasted with the overdiagnosis and overtreatment of women as obstetrical and as gynecological patients. In this setting, women undergo humiliating and often unnecessary exams and procedures. Pelvic exams, in particular, are a major source of anxiety among women of all ages. One major problem in properly diagnosing women is that women many times have very little direct knowledge of their own bodies and as a result completely defer their judgment to their doctor. This can have terrible repercussions on their personal health choices because medicine has the potential to become an institution of dogmatic social control. An example of this can be found in obstetricians–gynecologists who are official and legitimate experts in the female reproductive tract. Some of these doctors have broadened their influence beyond the scope of their training and experience and now advise women on the female sex role, psychology, and sexuality, notwithstanding a lack of expertise in these fields and their tendency to interpret their findings from a primarily male point of view.

Treatment is perhaps the domain in which women endure the most harsh and terrible form of discrimination. One of the most commonly recommended breast cancer treatments is the removal of the entire affected breast (a mastectomy) despite the fact that over 90% of women may be eligible to receive lumpectomies instead. As a result, many women needlessly undergo the more radical treatment when a viable alternative is often readily available. Often, a male physician does not understand the psychological and emotional impact of the loss of such a vital part of a woman's body and, consequently, may provide no assistance in dealing with the trauma that is associated with the loss.

Similar issues arise with respect to two other surgical procedures: hysterectomy and removal of the ovaries. The frequency with which hysterectomies are performed may be due to gynecologists' perception of the uterus as an expendable organ, useless for purposes other than childbearing. Ironically, one of the reasons given for performing a hysterectomy at a gathering of the American College of Obstetricians and Gynecologists was that it reduced the frequency of unpleasant, humiliating pelvic exams and tests. This underscores a complete lack of understanding and empathy on the part of the medical community toward women. It is very difficult to imagine any group of doctors ever recommending the removal of a male's reproductive system simply to save him the humiliation of having to cough twice for his doctor. As stunning as all of these revelations about sexism in medicine are, it should be noted that the problems and issues confronted here address only a small fraction of the problems that women face in the health care industry today as patients and consumers.

It is critical that women inform themselves about their own bodies, and their treatment options and fight against the traditional sex-role learning, which encourages women to be passive and dependent on male doctors. As a nation we need to push the insurers to fairly cover women. While this may sound simple, implementing it will not be due to the general lack of information or understanding in the greater medical community and the reluctance of insurance companies to provide adequate affordable care to women. There is hope that these issues will be addressed more thoroughly because an increasing number of women are choosing a career in medicine. We must ensure that discrimination in women's health becomes the subject of discussion among historians, and not debate among legislators.

See Also: Affirmative action, Birth control, Pelvic examination, Sexual harassment, United States Civil Rights Act of 1964

Suggested Reading

Corea, G. (1977). *The hidden malpractice: How American medicine mistreats women.* New York: Jove.

Dan, A. J. (Eds.). (1994). *Reframing women's health.* Thousand Oaks, CA: Sage.

Laurence, L., & Weinhouse, B. (1994). *Outrageous practices: The alarming truth about how medicine mistreats women.* New York: Fawcett Columbine.

Mendelsohn, R. S. (1981). *Male practice: How doctors manipulate women.* Chicago: Contemporary Books.

Rakusen, J., & Davidson, N. (1982). *Out of our hands.* London: Pan Books.

Scully, D. (1980). *Men who control women's health.* Boston: Houghton Mifflin.

ROBERTO HERNANDEZ

Dissociative Identity Disorder

Dissociative identity disorder (DID), formerly known as multiple personality disorder, is one of five dissociative disorders recognized by the *Diagnostic and Statistical Manual of Mental Disorders*, fourth edition (DSM-IV). Of the dissociative disorders, DID is associated with the most chronic and severe symptomatology.

Dissociation is a process wherein a person mentally separates oneself from reality. There are common, everyday dissociative experiences such as daydreaming or "losing oneself" in a good book, for example, but with DID, an individual has typically experienced dissociation during a traumatic event such as physical, sexual, or emotional abuse, or during times of perceived harm (e.g., invasive medical procedures, natural disasters, and so forth). The dissociation appears to serve as a protective defense mechanism and as a means of self-preservation.

The DSM-IV defines DID as follows:

1. The presence of two or more distinct identities or personality states (each with its own relatively enduring pattern of perceiving, relating to, and thinking about the environment and self)
2. At least two of these identities or personality states recurrently take control of the person's behavior
3. Inability to recall important personal information that is too extensive to be explained by ordinary forgetfulness
4. The disturbance is not due to the direct physiological effects of a substance or a general

medical condition (American Psychiatric Association, 1994)

Most individuals who develop DID have likely been exposed to childhood trauma (usually between the ages of 3 and 9), during which time he or she mentally separates from the experience in an effort to avoid emotional and/or physical pain. The different personalities evolve over time as a means of coping with future traumas and feelings of being threatened. It seems the more severe the trauma, the greater the number of personalities that develop.

The prevalence of DID is approximately 1% of the population, although about 90% of those with the disorder are completely unaware they have it. It is more frequently diagnosed in women than men, but some data support equal gender prevalence (men may be in treatment for other comorbid diagnoses, and the DID is overlooked). And not all children who are abused or traumatized dissociate or even go on to develop DID; that seems to depend on individual predisposition and has been observed more frequently in first-degree biological offspring of persons with the disorder.

Symptoms and characteristic features include the following: time loss and inconsistencies, amnesia for events, being recognized by "strangers," hearing voices within one's head, flashbacks, nightmares, hypervigilance, distinct and abrupt changes in one's behavior/personality (often forgotten by the person), finding unaccountable objects in one's personal belongings, and referring to oneself by another name or in the third person. Also observed are depression, mood lability, anger, panic attacks, phobias, eating disorders, relational difficulties, suicidal thoughts, feelings of worthlessness, and self-injurious behaviors.

The various personality states of DID can manifest as many very different identities within one individual; "alters," to which they are often referred, can be of both sexes, have varying ages, and even display differing medical conditions, perceived physical attributes, and unique voice and handwriting structure.

Because the disorder can be very destabilizing to one's life and functioning, there are several recommended treatment options. Individual psychotherapy seems to be the most widely accepted and effective intervention, often supplemented with hypnosis, art and group therapies, and pharmacotherapy. Once a person with DID understands and accepts the diagnosis, the goal becomes reintegration (or unification) of the various personality states. This usually requires

identification of individual personalities, with eventual communication between them. Antidepressant or anxiolytic medications are used adjunctively if necessary, as is hospitalization if self-injurious or other destructive behavior warrants such. Although the healing process can be longstanding, and at times quite painful, reintegration appears to be a vital element in facilitating recovery for the person with DID.

SEE ALSO: Depression, Eating disorders, Psychotherapy, Sexual abuse

Suggested Reading

American Psychiatric Association. (1994). *Diagnostic and statistical manual of mental disorders* (4th ed.). Washington, DC: American Psychiatric Association.

Haddock, D. B. (2001). *The dissociative identity disorder sourcebook.* New York: McGraw-Hill.

Kaplan, H. I., & Sadock, B. J. (1997). *Synopsis of psychiatry* (8th ed.). Baltimore: Williams & Wilkins.

Sinason, V. (Ed.). (2002). *Attachment, trauma and multiplicity: Working with dissociative identity disorder.* New York: Brunner-Routledge.

Steinberg, M., & Schnall, M. (2000). *The stranger in the mirror: Dissociation, the hidden epidemic.* New York: Cliff Street Books.

GRETCHEN K. GARDNER

Diverticulum *see* Pelvic Pain

Divorce
Divorce is the undoing of a marriage. In some states it is called a dissolution of marriage. No matter what the label, this is a way to formally end legal ties between a husband and a wife, and resolve other issues that may connect them, such as child custody, child support, property division, debt division, and spousal support. Divorces are granted by courts, and most of the laws regarding divorce are made by the states, rather than the federal government.

Divorces can be arranged by agreement of the couple, and when the couple cannot agree, a judge makes the decisions. In the majority of divorces, the couple reaches an agreement, the judge makes sure the agreement is fair, and the judge makes the couple's agreement a part of a court order.

To obtain a divorce there must be a reason or "grounds" for the divorce. Early in the history of our country the grounds for divorce were very limited, often requiring proof of adultery. Current divorce law includes many more grounds, including physical cruelty and mental cruelty. Most states now also have grounds for divorce that are called "no fault." To obtain a divorce using "no fault" grounds one may be required to show that the couple is living separately, the marriage has broken down, and there is little possibility that the marriage could be repaired.

Couples who divorce often have children in common. When these children are minors or have special needs, the divorce must address how the children will be cared for and how they will be supported financially. The arrangement of who will care for the children is called child custody. Custody can be further divided into physical custody and legal custody. Physical custody refers to who provides daily care for the child. Legal custody refers to who makes important decisions in the child's life. In a divorce, one parent can get custody and the other parent can have visitation rights, or the parents can share custody. Shared custody is often called joint custody, but does usually involve a perfectly equal division of time spent with each parent. At one time, a presumption existed in favor of the mother retaining custody, but this is generally no longer the case.

Along with child custody come decisions about financial support of the child or children. There is an expectation that each parent will contribute to the financial support of the children. Most often the parent who does not live with the child full time will be required to provide more financial support. The parent who houses the child supports the child directly through housing, food, clothing, and similar expenses. There are many variations in how states calculate a parent's responsibility for child support. Some states consider only the nonresident parent's income while other states consider the income of both parents. Some states use a simple percentage of income to calculate the amount of support, while other states have more complex formulas. In each state there is an office, funded by the federal government, which can help people get and enforce child support orders.

Divorces also divide the things that a couple owns. Things like a home, automobiles, furniture, appliances, and clothing are distributed either by agreement or by a judge's decision. Other nontangible things can also be divided. Retirement savings plans and business interests can be divided as well, and it is often difficult to estimate the value of these items. If parties cannot agree as to how to divide their possessions, the court can make the division, or the court could order a sale and have the proceeds divided. A small number of states use a system called "community property" in which the possessions are divided equally between the wife and husband. Most states' laws require a judge to divide property in a way that is fair, which sometimes, but not always, means an even split.

Many couples who divorce have debts, and a divorce can help to resolve who is responsible for which debts. Dividing debts is different from dividing property because debts involve someone who is not a part of the marriage. It can be harder to separate from a credit card company than it is to separate from a spouse. A court can order one person to pay a particular bill, but if both people agree to be responsible for the debt originally, both people will still be responsible. This becomes important if the person who promised to pay a bill can no longer pay it, decides not to pay it, or tries to discharge the debt in bankruptcy. Protecting yourself in these situations can be tricky.

In some divorce cases one former spouse makes payment for the support of the other. This used to be called alimony, and is often called maintenance now. Maintenance payments are not based on gender, as they used to be in the past, so either spouse may have to support the other. Maintenance is more often a part of a divorce where the marriage has been long and where the parties do not have equal abilities to support themselves. Maintenance can be awarded on a permanent basis, or it can be for a specific time period. Maintenance is often limited in time when it is for the purpose of giving one spouse the opportunity to get an education that will increase that person's ability to support herself or himself.

Divorce can be both a financial loss and an emotional loss. Living expenses will increase because the couple will maintain separate housing. At the same time expenses are increasing, income may decrease. Unless some kind of spousal support is awarded, each former spouse will take home his or her own paycheck, which may be less than that of the other. Emotionally, divorce can mean loss of support and companionship of the spouse, and even relationships with friends can be affected. People experiencing this kind of loss may be able to find a support group through a local social service agency.

Lawyers can provide important services to people who want a divorce. Lawyers can make sure that people who agree to a divorce understand how the agreement will affect them. Lawyers can also represent a spouse in negotiating an agreement, or in presenting a case to a judge for a decision. But lawyers can be expensive. Sometimes free legal assistance can be obtained through a local office of the Legal Services Corporation, or through other local agencies. Many people represent themselves in a divorce, but where there are complicated issues about children and finance, this should be a last resort.

Finally, divorce is only available to married people. While this may sound obvious, it affects a large number of people who establish a relationship without being married. Such people cannot use the process of divorce to help make decisions about which person should receive which belongings, and how children should be cared for. Other legal processes may be available, but those processes rarely cover the wide variety of issues that come up when people end relationships.

SEE ALSO: Adultery, Child custody, Cohabitation, Day care, Domestic partnership, Domestic violence, Marital status, Prenuptial agreement

Suggested Reading

The American Bar Association guide to family law: The complete and easy guide to the laws of marriage, parenthood, separation and divorce. (1996). New York: Times Books/Random House.

Lyster, M. (1996). *Building parenting agreements that work.* Berkeley, CA: Nolo Press.

Mercer, D., & Pruett, M. K. (2001). *Your divorce advisor: A lawyer and a psychologist guide you through the legal and emotional landscape of divorce.* New York: Simon & Schuster.

West, R. P. (1997). *How to find the right divorce lawyer.* Chicago: Contemporary Books.

SHEILA SIMON

Divorce Mediation Divorce mediation is a process in which two people who have made the decision to separate or divorce meet with a neutral mediator to negotiate the terms of their separation or divorce. It is appropriate for married couples, same-sex partners, or any couples who have been in a committed relationship that has involved shared financial resources or parenting. Success in mediation does not depend on the partners being friendly or even liking each other. Very angry couples can mediate. Success depends on a willingness to settle and to make a fair plan. Contraindications to mediation include domestic violence, impaired judgment due to active substance abuse or mental illness, and a history of dishonest or illegal behavior.

The traditional alternative to mediation for married couples is an adversarial legal system in which each partner hires an attorney to negotiate for them. The attorney must zealously represent his or her client, which can lead to an emotionally and financially costly battle. Mediation was developed as an alternative that allows partners to stay in control of their process, the results of which will affect their lives for years to come. The legal system does not provide any alternative for same-sex couples or live-in partners.

Divorce mediation is a structured process. Once partners have agreed to explore mediation, an initial appointment can be scheduled. The primary goal of this appointment is to learn about the mediation process and come to an agreement about whether or not to proceed with mediation. Once a decision is made to mediate the partners will be asked to sign a mediation agreement that identifies the rules that govern the mediation process. While each mediator designs his or her own agreement, the following are usually included:

1. The cost of mediation, which is shared by the parties, is stated.
2. The mediator will not act as an attorney or represent either of the parties. The parties are advised to retain separate counsel to act as their consultants during the mediation process.
3. The parties may not dispose of any joint assets without prior agreement.
4. The parties agree to full disclosure.
5. The parties agree not to take legal action during the mediation.
6. The mediation process is confidential and should the parties find themselves in litigation they may not call the mediator or his or her records into that litigation.
7. At the conclusion of the mediation, the mediator will write a memorandum of understanding detailing all of the agreements.

At the conclusion of the initial session, the partners and the mediator set an agenda for the negotiations. Items on the agenda include developing a childcare plan, division of assets, division of personal property, and monthly support. A childcare plan involves making decisions about custody of the children, where the children will live, and how each parent will be spending time with the children. It can also include how decisions such as schooling, discipline, enrichment, and medical care will be made. In addition, decisions about how the parents will share in the financial support of the children will be made. Many states have guidelines for setting child support amounts. Because parents are in control of developing a childcare plan, they can adapt the plan to meet the unique needs of their children in a way that attorneys or the court could never do.

Most mediators will have forms for the parties to fill out that will list all of their assets and debts and their income and expenses. To ensure full disclosure, documentation for all assets, debts, and income will need to be provided. A plan is developed to equitably share available resources to maximize each partner's ability to get on with their lives. At the conclusion of the mediation, the mediator will write a memorandum of understanding. If the parties have retained counsel, they will each be given two copies; one for themselves and one for their attorney. This is not a legal document so it will have to be implemented into a formal separation agreement and filed with the court.

The critical role of the mediator is to facilitate the negotiations. This requires that they help develop options, consider the consequences of their choices, balance the power, ensure that no party agrees to anything they feel intimidated into or that they do not understand, and help to unblock impasses. The agreements are the couples' agreements not the mediator's who does not act as an arbitrator or a judge but as a neutral facilitator guiding a couple through the painful process of ending a relationship.

Divorce mediators can have an advanced degree in a mental health field or be an attorney. They should have at least 40 hours of mediation training. Mediators are not licensed as yet but local courts often have referral lists as does the Association for Conflict Resolution.

See Also: Child custody, Couples therapy, Divorce, Prenuptial agreement

Suggested Reading

Haynes, J. M. (1981). *Divorce mediation: A practical guide for therapists and counselors.* New York: Springer.

James, P. (2001). *The divorce mediation handbook: Everything you need to know.* San Francisco: Jossey-Bass.

Lemmon, J. A. (1985). *Family mediation practice.* New York: The Free Press.

PHYLLIS D. HULEWAT

Domestic Partnership

Domestic partnership is a description of a status of an intimate relationship between two people. Domestic partnership that can also be called a civil union is often used by same-sex couples who cannot obtain a marriage license due to gender restrictions in state laws. Such partnerships are increasingly being recognized by employers, local governments, one state, and some countries outside the United States. The processes for establishing such a relationship vary.

Domestic partnerships allow couples to enjoy some benefits of marriage. For example, an employer that recognizes domestic partnerships will likely cover both the employee and the partner in a group health insurance plan. Civil unions also provide recognition of the status of the relationship and the partners' commitment to each other.

Domestic partnerships do not provide all the benefits associated with marriage and the types of benefits associated with such unions may vary from location to location. Because of this, domestic partners may wish to pursue other methods to establish other legal connections. Wills can distribute property to partners and their families. Couples can give each other a "power of attorney" that allows one person to make important decisions about health care or finances if the other is unable to do so. Establishing legal ties to a child through what is often called "second parent adoption" may be an option in some states.

See Also: Child custody, Cohabitation, Divorce, Marital status

Suggested Reading

Curry, H., et al. (1999). *A legal guide for lesbian and gay couples.* Berkeley, CA: Nolo Press.

Ihara, T. L., & Warner, R. (1997). *The living together kit: A legal guide for unmarried couples.* Berkeley, CA: Nolo Press.

Samuelson, E. (1997). *The unmarried couple's legal survival guide: Your rights and responsibilities.* Secaucus, NJ: Carol.

Stanley, J. (1999). *Unmarried parents' rights.* Naperville, IL: Sphinx.

SHEILA SIMON

Domestic Violence

Domestic violence, or intimate partner violence, is defined as a pattern of assaultive and coercive behaviors, including physical, sexual, and psychological attacks as well as economic coercion that adults or adolescents use against their intimate partners. Other terms used to describe intimate partner violence include domestic abuse, spouse abuse, courtship violence, battering, marital rape, and date rape. Some professional fields use the term domestic violence to refer to any type of interfamilial violence.

Domestic violence has been widely recognized as an international problem. Worldwide, the United Nations International Children's Emergency Fund (UNICEF) reports that a quarter to half of women around the world experience some form of violence from an intimate partner over their lifetime. The World Health Organization (WHO) estimates that worldwide, between 10% and 69% of women are physically assaulted by an intimate partner at some time in their lives and that 40–70% of female murder victims are killed by an intimate partner. While there is less information about the frequency of male victims, they are generally considered to be at lesser risk of both victimization and severe injuries from victimization.

It is very difficult to ascertain the number of domestic violence victims because many victims may try to hide their experiences with abuse. Factors that hinder reporting of abuse include a societal stigma of being a victim, fear of retaliation by the perpetrator, fear of lost income, or fear of isolation from family. Because of these barriers, many victims are never identified.

The National Crime Victimization Survey is conducted annually to estimate the incidence of violent victimizations. This survey estimates that there are 960,000 incidents of domestic violence annually, with 85% of the victims being women. This translates to eight in every 1,000 women and one in every 1,000 men aged 12 or over being a victim each year. Another large national survey conducted by the Commonwealth Fund (1999) estimates that 3.9 million women are physically abused each year. Variation in estimates may be due to different samples, different definitions used in surveys, or different questions used to solicit information about abusive events.

Intimate partner violence is a repetitive phenomenon. Nearly a third of female victims reported that they had been victimized at least twice in the previous 6 months. Violence is also considered to be cyclical and often escalating, so that periods without abusive events may be followed by intensified abuse.

Intimate partner violence leads to many short- and long-term adverse health outcomes. About half of women who report being a victim of abuse report that they were physically injured and among victims treated in Emergency Departments approximately a third require hospital admission. Over half of women who are victims experience mental health effects, including depression, anxiety disorder, symptoms of post-traumatic stress disorder, and suicide attempts. Victims are also at high risk for stress-related physical conditions, such as gastrointestinal disorders and chronic pain syndromes. Abuse has been linked to pregnancy complications such as low weight gain, anemia, and infections as well as to adverse pregnancy outcomes such as premature labor and low infant birthweight.

Economic costs related to intimate partner violence are high. The annual cost for direct medical treatment of battered women is estimated at approximately 1.8 billion. The total costs of intimate partner violence as a crime are estimated at $67 billion.

Although there is no specific profile for a domestic violence victim, there are several risk factors that have been identified consistently in the existing research. These include young age of the victim and/or partner, low income and educational status, low self-esteem, isolation, and experiences with violence as a child.

Similarly, perpetrators of domestic violence share some common characteristics. Among the strongest predictors of abusive behavior is witnessing domestic abuse in the childhood home. This research suggests that abuse is largely a learned behavior and that abusive patterns begin in childhood. Personality characteristics such as insecurity, low self-esteem, controlling behavior, extreme jealousy, aggressive personalities, borderline personality, narcissistic behavior, and antisocial personality disorders have also been linked to abusive behavior.

Societies that have marked gender inequality and rigid gender roles, which support a man's right to inflict violence and which do not have strong sanctions against violence, render women particularly vulnerable. Women are also less likely to report abuse and seek help in such societies.

Prevention of abuse largely focuses on identification and support for victims, legal reform, and treatment programs for perpetrators. Clinical screening of abuse in Emergency Departments and clinics has helped identify victims and has increased referral to support systems. It is important for clinicians to recognize that victims of abuse may present with stories that are inconsistent with their diagnoses. Many women try to hide their abuse, in some cases because the abusive partner is with them during treatment. An inconsistent story, especially when accompanied by old injuries, is an indicator of abuse. Victims may also present to clinicians with nonspecific symptoms. Because many of the physical consequences of abuse are stress related, clinicians should routinely screen for abuse when treating these conditions.

Several states have mandatory reporting laws for health care providers, although these laws are controversial. Women's crisis centers and battered women's shelters are important components of prevention. These centers offer such services as protected and anonymous shelter, job training, counseling, and assistance with legal matters.

Legal reforms include better definitions of domestic violence in the court system and more rigorous prosecution and sentencing. Victimless prosecution is one example. In victimless prosecution, the state can prosecute the perpetrator in the absence of a formal victim complaint so that the victim does not need to be the primary accuser. This approach was enacted because many women recanted their reports of abuse to police because of fear of retaliation or fear of losing financial support for themselves and their children. Most police jurisdictions have implemented training to better prepare police officers to recognize and respond to domestic disputes. Some jurisdictions have also implemented mandatory arrest at the scene and this is thought to reduce physical consequences from violent events. Wider use of restraining orders has been implemented throughout the United States, although evaluations of their use have shown various levels of effectiveness.

Treatment programs for batterers offer an avenue for perpetrators to understand and reduce their abusive behaviors. Group counseling is the most common approach and programs focus on discussion of gender roles, communication skills, and skills to solve problems. When men voluntarily seek help and actively participate in such programs they are thought to be effective. However, many men who attend these programs do so based on a court order or by referral and often do not complete the program.

There is great need for evaluation of prevention measures to determine which are most appropriate for victims and which are most successful at reducing violent events.

SEE ALSO: Homicide, Sexual abuse, Stalking, Violence

Suggested Reading

The Commonwealth Fund. (1999). *Health concerns across a woman's lifespan: The Commonwealth Fund 1998 Survey of Women's Health.* New York: Author.

The National Center for Injury Prevention and Control. (2001). *Intimate partner violence fact sheet.* Atlanta, GA: Centers for Disease Control and Prevention. http://www.cdc.gov/ncipc/fact-sheets/ipvfacts.htm

National Research Council. (1996). *Understanding violence against women.* Washington, DC: National Academy Press.

Straus, M., Gelles, R., & Smight, C. (1990). *Physical violence in American families: Risk factors and adaptations to violence in 8,145 families.* New Brunswick, Canada: Transaction.

United States Department of Justice. (1998). *Violence by intimates: Analysis of data on crimes by current or former spouses, boyfriends, and girlfriends.* (NCJ-167237). Washington, DC: U.S. Department of Justice, Bureau of Justice Statistics Factbook. http://www.ojp.usdoj.gov/bjs/

CORINNE PEEK-ASA

Douching
Douching is the irrigation or flushing of the vagina with plain water, vinegar and water, or other name brand prepared or medicated products. The fluid is allowed to run into the vagina from a bag connected to tubing or is flushed into the vagina from a premixed squeeze bottle. Many women feel this is necessary for good hygiene, "to feel fresh," or to treat a problem without visiting a medical provider.

Douching has been shown through numerous studies to increase the risk of developing a bacterial infection of the vagina (called bacterial vaginosis or BV). Women who douche increase their chances for developing this infection by 40%. BV is a vaginal infection caused by a loss of lactobacilli, the normal vaginal bacteria that produce hydrogen peroxide and provide protection against other, less healthy bacteria. Symptoms of BV are a creamy gray to yellow, malodorous discharge. BV is a sexually associated condition but is not sexually transmitted. Many women do not realize they have this infection. Those who are not pregnant do not require treatment if they are asymptomatic. However, BV during pregnancy has been associated with preterm birth and low-birthweight infants.

Douching has also been linked in studies to HIV acquisition, ectopic (tubal) pregnancy, and pelvic inflammatory disease, a serious infection of the upper reproductive tract including the uterus, tubes, and pelvic cavity. For these reasons, it is not recommended as a healthy practice. Women who have an odor, discharge, or other gynecological or pelvic symptoms are encouraged to see a health care provider for appropriate diagnosis and treatment. The use of douching can cause or exacerbate their symptoms as well as make them more at risk for more serious complications.

SEE ALSO: Ectopic pregnancy, Pelvic pain, Sexual organs

Suggested Reading

Fiscella, K., Franks, P., Kendrick, J. S., Meldrum, S., & Kieke, B. (2002). Risk of preterm birth that is associated with vaginal douching. *American Journal of Obstetrics and Gynecology, 186*(6), 1345–1350.
Hatcher, R., Trussel, J., Stewart, F., Cates, W., Stewart, G., Guest, F., et al. (1998). *Contraceptive technology* (pp. 191–192). New York: Ardent Medica.

Suggested Resources

Warner, J. (2002). *Douching linked to vaginal infections: Largest study to date confirms risks. WebMD* (On-line): http://my.webmd.com/content/article/51/40784.htm?lastselectedguid={5FE84E90-BC77-4056-A91C-9531713CA348}

NANCY MYERS-BRADLEY

Dowry

In most societies, marriage plays an important role for men and women alike. In the past few decades there has been much research on the institution of marriage and the family among economists and anthropologists. One of the most intriguing and contested issues is the dowry.

A dowry, in its simplest form and structure, is the "property that a woman brings to her husband at the time of marriage. The dowry apparently originated in the giving of a marriage gift by the family of the bridegroom to the bride and the bestowal of money upon the bride by her parents." There have been many cultures that had some form of dowry. It was most familiar in propertied cultures such as Ancient Greece and Rome, India, and Medieval Europe. According to the *Columbia Encyclopedia*, the dowry system in England and the United States, except Louisiana, is not recognized as law. However, in civil-law countries the dowry is still recognized as an important form of property. The current status of the dowry has complex repercussions, and

is not as altruistic as the definition above seems to purport. The regions that practice dowries, legally or illegally, are primarily in South Asia (India, Nepal, Pakistan, and Sri Lanka) and the Middle East. There are also a few remote areas of Africa that recognize the practice.

If a dowry is merely a gratuitous payment from the family of the bride to the family of the groom, why are virtually all nations trying to stop the dowry? The most recognizable impact and repercussion of a dowry system can be found in remote parts of India. In India, the groom and the groom's family, either directly or indirectly, sets the amount of the dowry. The dowry can be in various forms such as cash, clothes, jewels, wedding and/or reception expenses, honeymoon expenses, travel expenses, fees for education (virtually always for the groom), and often times the marital home. If the family of the bride is opulent or the groom and his family are sufficiently mollified, the wedding and dowry are considered successful. However, if either the groom or his family is dissatisfied with the dowry or the bride's family is destitute, the dowry may be considered insufficient with sometimes devastating results.

An informative and progressive movement entitled "India Together" lists possible treatment of the bride if the dowry is insufficient. The first case is labeled "Extreme": "the bride will be subjected to extreme forms of torture, both physically and emotionally, which may include beating and infliction of physical pain, that may result in her death or permanent physical handicap." The second is "Severe": "the bride will be threatened with dismal consequences including divorce and physical abuse, and will have to bear the insults slung at her parents." The last is "Harsh, but Standard": "the bride is reminded of her inadequacies and faced with complaints about her parents. In some cases, pressure is created on her and her parents to meet the demand subsequently."

If the family of the bride is unable to give a sufficient dowry due to financial problems, the impact becomes a national problem. Dowry is closely linked to many crimes against women in India; to list a few: female infanticide, domestic violence, neglect of a girl child, denial of educational and career opportunities to daughters. The persuasive use of statistics provided by India Together regarding the present-day trend of higher mortality rates among females, the growing illiteracy rates among women in India, and the National Crime Bureau of the Government of India are evidence of the growing rate of dowry deaths. Although in 1961 the Indian government passed the Dowry Prohibition

Act that outlawed dowry payment, according to Roy and Singh, the legislation is purely symbolic and virtually impossible to enforce, especially in remote parts of India.

India is not alone in combating dowries. In Bangladesh, the Grameen Bank is a group fund and major small-scale credit program that provides production credit and other services to the poor. Production credit is a private-lending system where a person can receive a loan from a financial institution to produce certain foods, clothing, and other profit-making endeavors. The loans are paid back with a minimal, if any, interest rate. Founded in 1976 by Muhammed Yunus, the Grameen Bank provides financing for nonagricultural self-employment activities to 2 million borrowers, 94% of whom are women. In order to participate in the microloan program, an eligible woman must memorize, chant, and follow the "Sixteen Decisions." These decisions include "We shall not take any dowry in our sons' wedding, neither shall we give any dowry in our daughters' wedding," and "We shall educate all of our children."

With the work of progressive ideology such as India Together and the Grameen Bank, many may be able to reduce the discrimination and abuse that accompanies a dowry. Although the dowry seems like an offering, more and more it is a sale of a loved one into domestic slavery. Slavery is always an unwelcome and uninvited wedding guest.

See Also: Child abuse, Discrimination, Divorce, Domestic violence, Feminism, Slavery, Violence

Suggested Reading

Dowry. (2002). *Columbia encyclopedia* (6th ed.). New York: Columbia University Press.

Dowry. (2003). *Merriam-Webster's collegiate dictionary* (Electronic ed., version 1.5, 1996).

Pitt, M. M., & Khandker, S. R. (1998). The impact of group-based credit programs on poor households in Bangladesh: Does the gender of participants matter? *The Journal of Political Economy, 106*(5), 958–996.

Roy, A., & Singh, S. (2003). The dowry campaign launched and the dowry campaign pledge. *India Together.* Retrieved May 2002, from http://www.indiatogether.org/women/dowry.html

NATHAN A. CRAIG

Drugs for street drugs *see* name of specific drug, for example, Heroin. For prescription medications, *see* name of specific illness or disorder, for example, Hypertension

Durable Power of Attorney for Health Care

The standard power of attorney (POA) is a written legal instrument authorizing a person (named an agent or attorney-in-fact) to sign documents and conduct transactions on behalf of the principal or maker who has delegated away that authority. The principal can delegate as much (for instance, a general or complete delegation) or as little (such as a delegation specifically delineating what types of choices the agent may and may not make) power as desired. The principal may end or revoke the arrangement at any time, as long as the principal remains mentally competent to do so.

The POA in its traditional form does not work well as a method for dealing with medical decision-making authority on a voluntary, prospective basis. The ordinary POA ends automatically when the principal who created it dies or becomes mentally incompetent. The underlying theory is that, because a deceased or incompetent person no longer has the physical or mental ability to revoke the POA, the law should exercise that right immediately for the principal. Thus, a person who establishes a standard POA to help in managing medical affairs would be cut off from such assistance at precisely the time when assistance is needed the most, namely, when the principal cannot act personally.

In an effort to get around this practical problem, every state legislature has enacted legislation authorizing citizens to create (or execute) a durable power of attorney (DPOA). In contrast to the ordinary POA, the effect of a DPOA may endure or continue beyond the principal's later incapacity as long as that continuing authority is what the principal intended in executing the DPOA.

To remove any ambiguity about the applicability of the DPOA concept to the area of medical decision-making (including choices about life-sustaining medical treatments such as mechanical ventilators or antibiotics), almost every state has passed legislation that explicitly authorizes the use of the DPOA in the medical context. Some statutes use terminology such as *health care representative, health care agent,* or *health care proxy.* In addition, a number of states use a single, comprehensive advance directive statute to expressly authorize competent adults to execute both proxy and instruction directives; other states have separate statutes for each type of advance directive. Under most state laws, in order to avoid a real or apparent conflict of interest from materializing, the health care providers for the principal who has executed a DPOA are disqualified from serving as agents under the DPOA. The agent may, but need not be, a family member of the principal.

Proxy directives provide the advantage, for both patients and their health care providers, of legally empowering a live advocate for the patient who can enter into discussions and make decisions regarding the patient's medical treatment based on the most current information and other considerations, most importantly the agent's interpretation of the patient's previously expressed and implied wishes. The DPOA is irrelevant, however, for people who do not have available to name as a potential agent someone else whom they can trust to make future medical decisions for them.

SEE ALSO: Advance directives, Capacity, Informed consent, Living wills

Suggested Reading

Bishop, S. (1999). Crossing the decisional abyss: An evaluation of surrogate decision-making statutes as a means of bridging the gap between post-Quinlan red tape and the realization of an incompetent patient's right to refuse life-sustaining medical treatment. *Elder Law Journal, 7*, 153–183.

Dubler, N. N. (2001). Creating and supporting the proxy-decider: The lawyer–proxy relationship. *Georgia Law Review, 35*, 517–538.

Sabatino, C. P. (1999). The legal and functional status of the medical proxy: Suggestions for statutory reform. *Journal of Law, Medicine & Ethics, 27*, 52–68.

MARSHALL B. KAPP

Dysmenorrhea

Primary dysmenorrhea is painful menstrual cramping in the absence of pelvic pathology (disease of the pelvis). The pain occurs only in relation to ovulation. The pain involves the uterus and can also radiate to the lower back and thigh area. The painful period can also be accompanied by sweating, tachycardia, headaches, nausea, vomiting, diarrhea, and tremors. Dysmenorrhea is more common in younger women, declining after 30 years of age. The symptoms are induced by the hormone prostaglandin and are mediated within the lining of the uterus (endometrium) that is the primary site of prostaglandin production during menses. The pain is thought to be caused by (secondary to) reduction in blood flow (ischemia), which accompanies the uterine contractions in menstruation. The treatment of primary dysmenorrhea includes prostaglandin inhibitors to reduce uterine contractions and intrauterine pressure. Common medications include fenamates, aspirin, and nonsteroidal anti-inflammatory drugs such as Motrin, Naprosyn, Anaprox, and indomethacin. Other effective treatments include oral contraceptives that inhibit ovulation and suppress prostaglandin production in the lining of the uterus (endometrium). A specialized procedure to cut specific nerves causing the pain (laparoscopic uterosacral nerve ligation) has been used in patients who have not been helped by standard medical therapy. However, this is not a routine practice. Dysmenorrhea has been reported to be increased among mother and sisters of women with painful periods.

Secondary dysmenorrhea is painful menstrual cramping due to pelvic pathology. This may occur at any age after menarche and before menopause and is usually seen in women over 20 years of age. A complete history and physical examination along with diagnostic tests such as laparoscopy, hysteroscopy, ultrasound, and hysterosalpingography (specialized imaging test to examine the uterus and tubes going out from the uterus) may assist in the diagnosis of this condition. Common causes of secondary dysmenorrhea (menstrual pain related to another medical condition) include cervical stenosis (cervical closure/narrowing), endometriosis (abnormal uterine tissue), pelvic infections due to sexually transmitted diseases, adhesions from having prior pelvic surgery, pelvic congestion syndrome, stress, and use of an intrauterine device (IUD). In addition, secondary dysmenorrhea may occur in patients with psychological issues. Many causes of secondary dysmenorrhea require surgical management but some patients may benefit from a referral to a chronic pain management clinic where a multidisciplinary approach to their pain is planned.

SEE ALSO: Endometrial polyps, Endometriosis, Menstrual cycle disorders, Uterine fibroids

Dyspareunia

Suggested Reading

Emans, S. J. H., & Goldstein, D. P. (1990). *Pediatric and adolescent gynecology*. Boston: Little, Brown.

Herbst, A., Mishell, D., Stenchever, M., & Droegemueller, W. (1992). *Comprehensive gynecology*. St. Louis, MO: Mosby-Year Book.

Mishell, D. R., & Brenner, P. F. (1994). *Obstetrics and gynecology*. Boston: Blackwell Scientific.

Stenchever, M. (1991). *Office gynecology*. St. Louis, MO: Mosby-Year Book.

DIANE YOUNG

Dyspareunia Pain during or after sexual intercourse is called dyspareunia. Women with dyspareunia may experience pain in the labia, clitoris, vagina, or deep in the pelvis. There are many causes of dyspareunia, and most can be treated successfully. The pain of dyspareunia can vary from superficial pain at penile entry of the vagina, to deeper pain with full penetration or penile thrusts. Some women experience painful spasms of the vaginal muscles with intercourse known as vaginismus.

Some common causes of dyspareunia include vaginal dryness, skin conditions, endometriosis, infections, and psychological trauma. Vaginal dryness occurs because the normal increase in vaginal lubrication during sexual stimulation may be diminished at certain times in a woman's life such as during breast-feeding or at menopause. This is caused by a lowered level of the female hormone estrogen. Certain medications can also cause vaginal dryness, including tamoxifen and antihistamines.

Certain chronic skin conditions, such as eczema and lichen planus, can cause irritation to the labial area. Similarly, allergic reactions to clothing or chemicals (such as bath preparations, laundry products, feminine hygiene products, contraceptive jellies and foams, or condoms) can lead to irritation and dyspareunia. A condition called vulvar vestibulitis is a chronic irritation of the tissue at the opening of the vagina.

In endometriosis, the cells in the lining of the uterus migrate up through the fallopian tubes and grow abnormally inside the pelvis. This may lead to pain with intercourse, painful menses (dysmenorrhea), and/or infertility. Infections such as urinary tract (bladder) infections, vaginal infections, and sexually transmitted diseases can all lead to pain during or after intercourse. Women who have experienced psychological trauma such as previous sexual abuse or sexual assault may later develop sexual difficulties, including dyspareunia.

A thorough history and physical examination will sometimes pinpoint the specific cause of dyspareunia. The physician will seek to understand the timing and circumstances of the pain, type of pain (superficial or deep, at penile entry or later during intercourse), and any improvements with changes in positions. The woman seeking evaluation for dyspareunia should have an accurate record of her current medications and previous medical and surgical history. The sexual history will be important to discuss, including any previous abuse, the onset of the symptoms, and whether any remedies have been tried (such as lubricants if vaginal dryness has been experienced).

The physical examination will require a thorough evaluation of the female genitalia, including the labia, clitoris, vagina, and pelvic organs (uterus, ovaries, and supporting tissues). Depending on the suspected cause of the pain, the physician will obtain cultures to detect infection or biopsies of chronically irritated tissue. If endometriosis is suspected, a surgical procedure known as laparoscopy may be necessary to look inside the abdomen in order to make an accurate diagnosis.

TREATMENT

The treatment should be aimed at the cause of the pain. Conditions leading to vaginal dryness can usually be successfully treated with lubricants (such as Astroglide) or estrogens in either oral or vaginal forms. Labial skin conditions are generally treated with medicated creams to reduce inflammation and by the avoidance of any clothing or chemicals leading to an allergic reaction. Vaginal and urinary tract infections are almost always successfully treated with the appropriate antibiotic or antifungal medication, either topically or orally. Endometriosis may require treatments that are either medical (medications to reduce or suppress growth) or surgical (to remove the abnormal growths).

Dyspareunia that results from previous psychological trauma or pain that remains undiagnosed after a

234

medical evaluation, often requires psychological counseling. Therapists with specific training and interest in dyspareunia and other sexual disorders can provide effective treatment leading to improvement.

PREVENTION

To prevent the more common causes of dyspareunia, women should consider the following:

1. If vaginal infections are a problem, avoid tight clothing. Wear cotton underwear and change to dry clothing immediately after swimming.
2. To avoid urinary tract or bladder infections, wipe front to back after urinating, and urinate soon after intercourse.
3. When vaginal dryness is noted, use lubricants to minimize further irritation.

SEE ALSO: Endometriosis, Sexual organs, Vaginismus

Suggested Reading

Eyler, A. E. (2000). Sexual function and dysfunction in women. In R. Rakel (Ed.), *Saunders manual of medical practice* (pp. 631–635). Philadelphia: W. B. Saunders.

Gabbe, S. G. (Ed.). (2002). *Obstetrics: Normal and problem pregnancies* (4th ed.). New York: Churchill Livingstone.

Johnson, R. V. (Ed.). (1994). *Mayo Clinic complete book of pregnancy and baby's first year.* New York: Morrow.

KEITH A. FREY

Dysthymia   Dysthymic disorder is a chronic mood disorder characterized by depressed mood (extreme irritability in children and teenagers) almost every day for most of the day for at least 2 years in adults and 1 year for children and teenagers. Most individuals with these disorders complain that they have been depressed for as long as they can recall. Other symptoms that accompany these feelings are at least two of the following: appetite abnormalities, changes in sleep patterns, excessive tiredness, poor self-esteem, difficulties with memory and concentration, and feelings of hopelessness and helplessness. Although the term "dysthymia" was first used in 1980 in order to bring a clearer understanding of depressive disorders that did not meet the criteria for major depression, were more chronic and less severe, and implied a temperamental dysphoria, the term is often imprecise. Perhaps a good definition is that of a chronic, low-grade depression that lasts more than 2 years.

Using the best definition possible, as outlined in the *Diagnostic and Statistical Manual of Mental Disorders*, fourth edition, this is a common condition affecting about 3% of the population in the United States. Women have about 1.5–3 times more such conditions than men from adolescence through menopause. They occur more often in unmarried persons, those with low income and more health and other psychiatric illnesses. In fact about 75% of those with dysthymic disorder have another psychiatric diagnosis, the most common of which is major depressive disorder. Other common disturbances that exist with dysthymia are anxiety disorders such as panic and substance abuse, attention deficit disorder, conduct disorders, and personality disorders.

Causes of dysthymia are not clearly known, but some of the same factors that cause major depression have been implicated so that biological, psychological, and social factors are most likely involved. Some of the biological factors seen in major depression also occur in dysthymia such as rapid eye movement (REM) latency and decreased REM density. Those with dysthymia are much less likely to have positive results on tests of the adrenal axis (abnormal levels of hormones in the blood) such as the dexamethasone-suppression test (DST). Psychological theories relate to early developmental problems while cognitive theories revolve around diminished self-esteem and sense of helplessness. In helping make the diagnosis one must take care to be sure that the person does not have major depression, and if one does, it is known as double depression. Also, it is important to note that there is no mania or hypomania. About half of those with dysthymia have gradual onset prior to age 25. They are at increased risk for major depression or for bipolar I or II. Women with dysthymia are also at risk for premenstrual syndrome (PMS), premenstrual dysphoric disorder (PMDD), and pregnancy-related depressions.

While the outlook for those with this disorder used to be quite dismal with only about 15% achieving a complete remission, newer treatments have raised this to about 75%. Newer treatments include some of the

Dysthymic Disorder

medications that raise serotonin levels of the neurotransmitters such as the antidepressants Prozac, Zoloft, Celexa, and others. Psychotherapies also have proven effective with and without medications. These include cognitive-behavioral, interpersonal, insight-oriented, family, and group therapies. Hospitalization is not usually indicated.

SEE ALSO: Anxiety disorders, Depression

Suggested Reading

Sadock, J. B., & Sadock, V. S. (2000). *Comprehensive textbook of psychiatry* (7th ed.). Philadelphia: Lippincott, Williams & Wilkins.

MIRIAM B. ROSENTHAL

Dysthymic Disorder *see* Dysthymia

Eating Disorders

Eating disorders (ED) are classified in the *Diagnostic and Statistical Manual of Mental Disorders,* fourth edition (DSM-IV) on the basis of symptom clusters, characterized by severe disturbances in eating behavior and excessive concern about body shape or weight. Patients generally deny symptoms, are reluctant to seek help despite significant medical and psychiatric comorbidity, and are brought to care by family worried about their severe weight loss.

Anorexia nervosa (AN) includes an intense fear of gaining weight, refusal to maintain a normal weight, disturbed perception of one's own shape or size, and, if female, amenorrhea of at least three consecutive cycles. AN is subcategorized as (a) restricting (severe diet/low intake) or (b) binge eating/purging type (self-induced vomiting, misuse of laxatives, diuretics, or enemas). Comorbid symptoms include depression or sadness, social withdrawal, irritability, insomnia, or decreased sexual interest. Depression may be secondary to the physiological sequelae of semistarvation and resolve only after partial or complete weight restoration. Obsessive–compulsive features like frequent thoughts of food, hoarding food, picking/pulling apart small portions of food or collecting recipes, and concerns of eating in public are common.

Bulimia nervosa (BN) includes recurrent episodes of out-of-control, excessive or binge eating (occurring on an average, at least twice a week for 3 months), and self-evaluation, unduly influenced by body shape and weight. Individuals are typically ashamed and binge eat in secrecy. Unlike AN, BN patients are typically within normal weight range and restrict their total caloric consumption between binges. Patients with BN may have difficulties with impulse regulation and substance abuse.

Many patients, particularly in younger age groups, have a combination of ED symptoms that cannot be easily categorized as either AN or BN and are technically diagnosed as eating disorders—not otherwise specified (ED-NOS). The Eating Attitudes Test, Eating Disorders Inventory, or Body Shape Questionnaire may be helpful in assessing ED.

AN often begins in the midteens and affects up to 4% of adolescents and young adults. In females, the lifetime prevalence of AN ranges from 0.5% to 3.7% when more broadly defined while BN ranges from 1.1% to 4.2%. Both are 6 to 10 times more common in females, and are more prevalent in industrialized societies. Rates are rising in countries like Japan and China, where women are increasingly exposed to cultural change and modernization. In the United States, eating disorders are common in young Hispanic, Native American, and African American women, but are still less frequent than in Caucasian women. Female athletes involved in running, gymnastics, or ballet, and male bodybuilders and wrestlers are at greater risk.

Biological and psychosocial factors are implicated in the pathophysiology, but exact mechanisms remain unknown. Endogenous opioids may reduce hunger in patients with AN, while endorphin levels increase after purging and initially induce feelings of well-being. Diminished neurotransmitter (norepinephrine) turnover and activity are suggested by reduced 3-methoxy-4-hydroxyphenylglycol in the urine and cerebrospinal fluid of some patients with AN. Antidepressants often benefit patients with AN or BN and implicate a role for the neurotransmitters serotonin and norepinephrine. Starvation from AN or BN results in hypercortisolemia (elevated blood cortisol), nonsuppression of dexamethasone, suppression of thyroid function and amenorrhea (absence of menstrual periods). Computerized tomographic (CT) studies of the brain may show enlarged sulci and ventricles (abnormal brain structure), a finding that is reversed when patients with AN gain weight. Positron-emission tomography (PET) scan indicates higher metabolism in the caudate nucleus (a structure in the brain) during the anorectic state than after hyperalimentation (enriched tube or intravenous feeding). First-degree female relatives and monozygotic (identical) twins of patients with AN have higher rates of AN and BN. Children of patients with AN have a lifetime risk for AN which is 10-fold that of the general population (5%). High levels of hostility, chaos, and isolation and low levels of nurturance and empathy are reported in families of children presenting with ED. Some believe self-starvation develops as adolescents struggle to be unique and independent, yet respond to societal pressures to be slender.

Any medical illness like malignancy, brain tumors, epilepsy, gastrointestinal disease, or AIDS that is associated with weight loss can simulate AN and sometimes BN. Likewise, patients with major depression may have a decreased appetite but no associated fear of obesity or body image disturbance, unless a comorbid ED exists. Patients with somatization disorder do not generally express a morbid fear of obesity, and are less likely to have severe weight loss or amenorrhea. Patients with schizophrenia may have delusions about food being poisoned but rarely are concerned with caloric content. Kluver–Bucy syndrome is a rare condition characterized by hyperphagia (excessive eating), hypersexuality, and compulsive licking and biting. Klein–Levin syndrome, another uncommon disorder, is more frequent in men, and consists of hyperphagia and periodic hypersomnia (excessive sleeping).

Medical Comorbidity of Eating Disorders. Complications are related to weight loss and purging (vomiting and laxative abuse).

TREATMENT

A comprehensive treatment plan includes a combination of nutritional rehabilitation with behavior changes, psychotherapy, and medication. Treatment guidelines are readily available with an abridged, up-to-date version at www.guidelines.gov/index.asp.

Indicators for hospitalization include weight less than 75% of the estimated healthy weight, serious electrolyte or metabolic abnormalities, significant vital sign abnormalities, failure of intensive outpatient intervention, or comorbid psychiatric illness, particularly suicidality. Nutritional rehabilitation supports 2–3 lb/week weight gain for a hospitalized patient and 0.5–1 lb/week for an individual treated as an outpatient. Intake levels should start at 30–40 kcal/kg per day in divided meals. Inpatient treatment includes monitoring daily morning weights, vital signs, fluid intake and output, and frequent physicals to detect circulatory overload, refeeding edema, or bloating. Monitoring low potassium or phosphorus levels and obtaining an electrocardiogram will help to detect medical complications. Stool softeners and not laxatives are preferred for treatment of constipation, while vitamins and mineral supplements replenish deficiencies. Praising positive effort yet restricting exercise and purging are important behavioral strategies. Close supervision and restricted access to bathrooms for at least 2 hr after meals may be necessary.

Psychosocial treatments are required during hospitalization and after discharge. Commonly used models include dynamic expressive-supportive therapy and cognitive behavioral techniques. Planned meals with self-monitoring as well as exposure and response prevention can strengthen gains. Support or therapy groups or 12-step programs like Overeaters Anonymous may provide adjunctive treatment and diminish relapse. Family therapy and marital therapy is helpful with dysfunctional family patterns and interpersonal distress.

Medications for treatment of AN can be initiated before or after weight gain. Individuals can maintain normal eating behaviors as well as treat associated psychiatric symptoms. Antidepressants like serotonin-specific reuptake inhibitors, for example, fluoxetine (Prozac) are commonly considered, particularly if, depressive, obsessive, or compulsive symptoms persist in spite of or in the absence of weight gain. Tricyclic antidepressants should be used with caution due to greater risks of cardiac arrhythmias or hypotension. Occasionally, low doses of antipsychotics can be used for marked agitation with psychotic thinking. Antianxiety medications like benzodiazepenes can be helpful for extreme anticipatory anxiety before eating. Estrogen replacement alone does not generally appear to reverse osteoporosis or osteopenia, and unless there is weight gain, it does not prevent further bone loss. There is no evidence regarding efficacy of biphosphonates in treatment of associated osteoporosis. Agents which encourage bowel motility, such as metoclopramide are commonly used for bloating and abdominal pains due to gastroparesis and premature satiety ("fullness") but require monitoring for drug-related extrapyramidal side effects.

Antidepressants are also used to reduce the frequency of disturbed eating behaviors and treat comorbid depression, anxiety, obsessions, and impulse-disorder symptoms in BN. Fluoxetine is currently approved by the Food and Drug Administration for BN, but other antidepressants like sertraline (Zoloft), paroxetine (Paxil), citalopram (Celexa), imipramine, nortriptyline, desipramine, and monoamine oxidase inhibitors (MAOI) have also been used. Doses of tricyclic antidepressants and MAOI antidepressants parallel those used to treat depression, but higher doses of fluoxetine (60–80 mg/day) may be needed to treat BN. Bupropion is contraindicated in purging bulimic patients, who have greater risk of seizures. Lithium remains an adjunct for comorbid bipolar disorders or treatment resistance.

As a general guideline, it appears that one third of individuals fully recover, one third retain subthreshold symptoms, and one third with higher psychiatric comorbidity remain chronically eating disordered. Long-term follow-up of AN shows recovery rates ranging from 44% to 76% with prolonged recovery time, but mortality up to 20% is primarily from cardiac arrest or suicide. Short-term success with BN is 50–70%, with relapse rates between 30% and 50% after 6 months. Although there are little long-term data on BN, patients generally fare better as compared to AN patients.

See Also: Adolescence, Anorexia nervosa, Binge eating disorder, Body image, Bulimia nervosa, Depression

Suggested Reading

American Psychiatric Association. (1994). *Diagnostic and statistical manual of mental disorders* (4th ed.). Washington, DC: American Psychiatric Association.

American Psychiatric Association. (2000). Eating disorders measures. *Handbook of psychiatric measures* (pp. 647–673). Washington, DC: American Psychiatric Association.

American Psychiatric Association Work Group on Eating Disorders. (2000). Practice guideline for the treatment of patients with eating disorders (revision). *American Journal of Psychiatry, 157*(Suppl. 1), 1–39.

Becker, A. E., Grinspoon, S. K., Klibanski, A., et al. (1999). Eating disorders. *New England Journal of Medicine, 340,* 1092–1098.

Kay, J., Sansone, R. A., et al. (2001). Eating disorders. *Hospital Physician Psychiatry Board Review Manual, 5*(2), 1–12.

Keel, P. K., Mitchell, J. E., Miller, K. B., et al. (1999). Long-term outcome of bulimia nervosa. *Archives of General Psychiatry, 56,* 63–69.

Kathleen N. Franco
Rashmi S. Deshmukh

Ectopic Pregnancy

Ectopic pregnancy occurs when the blastocyst (embryo) implants at locations other than the endometrium, or lining of the uterine cavity. The most common site of occurrence is in the fallopian tube. Other sites include the cervix, the cornual portion of the uterus, the ovary, and the abdominal cavity. The incidence of ectopic pregnancy has been steadily increasing. In the United States, about 2 out of every 100 pregnancies end in an ectopic pregnancy. The increased incidence of ectopic pregnancy is thought to be due to the increased incidence of salpingitis (infection of the fallopian tubes), due to chlamydia or other sexually transmitted diseases. The delay in childbearing to the 30s, the use of progestin-only contraception, and tubal surgery including tubal sterilization also contribute to the increased incidence seen. Other causes include a congenital or acquired abnormality of the fallopian tube, hormonal imbalances, ovulation induction medications, and abnormality of embryonic development. In some social groups, the incidence of ectopic pregnancy is higher. In African American women and unmarried women, the risk of death from a ruptured ectopic pregnancy is higher than in the general population. Although the rates of ectopic pregnancies have increased, the percentage of ectopic pregnancies that become fatal has decreased.

The most common presenting symptoms of an ectopic pregnancy are abdominal pain, absence of menses, and irregular vaginal bleeding. The diagnosis of ectopic pregnancies is made with a thorough history and physical examination, and a variety of specialized tests including obtaining serial serum HCG levels (serial levels of substance in the blood produced by the developing fetus), performance of a transvaginal ultrasound (sound wave visualization of the structures around the vagina), culdocentesis looking for internal bleeding (examination of fluid to determine presence of blood), and laparoscopy (specialized examination using a small tube). Ninety percent of women with ectopic pregnancies have an abnormal pattern of serially obtained quantitative HCG levels.

Edema

Management of ectopic pregnancies includes surgical and nonsurgical management. Current surgical treatment includes laparoscopy or laparotomy. Nonsurgical management includes medical therapy with methotrexate or expectant management where the patient is closely observed. The rate of repeat ectopic pregnancies after a single ectopic pregnancy is about 15%. The subsequent conception rate in women with an ectopic pregnancy is about 60%.

SEE ALSO: Infertility, Pregnancy

Suggested Reading

Emans, S. J. H., & Goldstein, D. P. (1990). *Pediatric and adolescent gynecology.* Boston: Little, Brown.

Herbst, A., Mishell, D., Stenchever, M., & Droegemueller, W. (1992). *Comprehensive gynecology.* St. Louis: Mosby-Year Book.

Mishell, D. R., & Brenner, P. F. (1994). *Obstetrics and gynecology.* Boston: Blackwell Scientific.

Stenchever, M. (1991). *Office gynecology.* St. Louis, MO: Mosby-Year Book.

DIANE YOUNG

Eczema *see* Dermatitis

Edema Edema, commonly referred to as swelling, is a widespread finding with multiple potential etiologies. Weight gain generally occurs prior to edema formation as the body's total water stores increase. In most cases, edema first occurs symmetrically in the lower extremities. This is due to gravity's role in increasing the hydrostatic (fluid) pressure in the lower extremity veins and is referred to as dependent edema. However, edema can be generalized (referred to as anasarca), asymmetric, or it can be localized to the lungs (pulmonary edema), peritoneal cavity (ascites), or pleural cavity (hydrothorax).

The regulation of the body's water stores is complex. One third of the total body water is extracellular, of which three quarters is extravascular. This relationship is governed by a complex interaction of fluid pressure, proteins, and vessel wall permeability referred to as the *Starling forces.* The hydrostatic (fluid) pressure in the vasculature and the colloid oncotic (protein) pressure in the interstitium promote efflux of fluid from the vascular to the extravascular space. The hydrostatic interstitial pressure and the intravascular colloid oncotic pressure sustain intravascular volume. Intact lymphatic drainage and capillary endothelial integrity are essential for maintaining fluid homeostasis. Any changes in this delicate balance favoring increased extravascular fluid accumulation lead to the formation of edema.

Congestive heart failure is a common cause of edema. The weakened heart results in an increase in hydrostatic pressure in the lungs and venous vasculature in left and right heart failure, respectively. Additionally, as blood flow to the kidneys is reduced, neurohormonal changes take place that lead to fluid and sodium retention increasing the body's total water stores. The combination of increased venous capillary pressure and increased total body water leads to an egress of fluid to the extravascular space. Edema develops as interstial fluid accumulation outpaces the lymphatic system's ability to drain. Additionally, patients with constrictive pericarditis or restrictive cardiomyopathy may develop peripheral edema via similar mechanisms. In these conditions, the heart's ability to relax and fill during diastole is impaired. This leads to systemic venous hypertension (i.e., increased hydrostatic pressure).

Chronic venous insufficiency is another frequent cause of edema. This occurs as a result of venous valvular incompetence. It is most often secondary to the sequelae of deep venous thromboses (blood clots). Lower extremity edema develops, usually asymmetrically, then varicosities, induration, pigment changes, and fibrosis. In severe cases, venous stasis ulcers can develop around the medial malleoli (ankle).

Hypoproteinemia, low blood protein, leads to edema because the decreased intravascular protein concentration shifts the Starling forces in favor of interstitial fluid accumulation. Hypoproteinemia can occur through a variety of mechanisms. These include severe nutritional deficiency, severe liver disease with decreased protein synthesis, protein-losing gastrointestinal diseases, and nephrotic syndrome.

Cirrhosis, end-stage liver disease, results in edema by many mechanisms. Portal hypertension increases venous hydrostatic pressure and decreases the "effective" circulating volume thereby leading to decreased kidney perfusion. This stimulates neurohormonal changes that result in increased renal sodium and water retention. Additionally, protein synthesis is often impaired and decreases plasma oncotic pressure.

Initially, fluid accumulation in cirrhosis develops in the peritoneal cavity with ascites.

Lymphedema results from impaired lymphatic drainage. Secondary lymphedema is usually caused by lymph node surgery, radiation, or cancerous invasion. Primary lymphedema is most commonly lymphedema praecox (10:1 female-to-male ratio). It is usually limited to the foot and calf and it occurs in young women often at the time of menarche or first pregnancy.

Pregnancy is a unique situation. Edema is the norm occurring in approximately 80% of all pregnancies. Most weight gain occurs after 20 weeks with approximately 70% due to water. Total body water increases from 7 L to 9 L. This occurs secondary to neurohormonal changes associated with pregnancy. Postpartum the fluid is quickly eliminated once the neurohormonal milieu returns to the prepregnancy state.

Edema in menstruating females in the absence of cardiac, hepatic, or renal disease is referred to as idiopathic edema. Initially, it occurs premenstrually, but often becomes persistent. The exact etiology of this phenomenon is uncertain, but it is felt to be caused by exaggerated volume depletion with standing secondary to venous pooling. This increases hydrostatic pressure and promotes extracellular fluid accumulation. The neurohormonal milieu then shifts to favor sodium retention further promoting edema. Additional potential etiologies for idiopathic edema include refeeding and diuretic-induced edema. In refeeding edema, weight-conscious individuals drastically reduce caloric intake for a period of time. At the end of the diet, increased caloric intake increases insulin release promoting sodium retention. In diuretic-induced edema, minor ankle edema leads to initiation of a diuretic. This activates neurohormonal changes favoring edema formation. Once diuretics are withdrawn, edema develops secondary to these neurohormal changes, which take some time to resolve. The mistaken assumption is then made that long-term diuretic therapy is necessary.

Many medications are well known to cause edema. Common culprits include calcium channel blockers, minoxidil, diazoxide, thiazolidinediones, estrogens/progesterones (including oral contraceptives), corticosteroids, and nonsteroidal anti-inflammatory agents. Cessation of the offending agent results in resolution of the edema. Other etiologies of edema include allergic reactions, angioedema, severe burns, and idiopathic edema where edema formation is secondary to altered capillary endothelial permeability. Myxedema occurs most commonly in hypothyroidism and its genesis is not fully understood, but altered capillary endothelial permeability is known to play a role.

The treatment of edema depends upon the etiology. The mainstays of therapy generally include sodium restriction and diuretic therapy. Support hose is an important and often overlooked tool to aid in the management of lower extremity edema particularly in patients with venous insufficiency. Edema in pregnancy is treated primarily with sodium restriction and support hose. In myxedema, correction of the underlying endocrine abnormality is necessary to eliminate edema.

SEE ALSO: Cardiovascular disease, Chest pain, Chronic obstructive pulmonary disease, Congestive heart failure, Hepatitis, Pregnancy, Thyroid diseases, Weight control

Suggested Reading

Braunwald, E. (1998). Edema. In A. S. Fauci, E. Braunwald, K. J. Isselbacher, J. D. Wilson, J. B. Martin, D. L. Kasper, et al. (Eds.), *Harrison's principles of internal medicine* (pp. 210–214). New York: McGraw-Hill.

Chou, S., & Atwood, J. E. (2002). Peripheral edema. *American Journal of Medicine, 113*, 580–586.

Davidson, J. M. (1997). Edema in pregnancy. *Kidney International, 51*(S59), S90–S96.

Rose, B. D. (1999, October 18). Idiopathic edema. *Up To Date.* Version 11.1.

W. LANCE LEWIS
NANETTE K. WENGER

Education   This entry will address both education and literacy since they are closely linked concepts, albeit with very different meanings. The *Merriam-Webster Dictionary* defines education as "the action or process of providing schooling for" or "to train by formal instruction and supervised practice especially in a skill, trade, or profession." Literacy is defined as the quality or state of being able to read and write. Often these terms are used interchangeably; however, although one might be educated, it does not ensure that one is literate. In a review of the literature, some studies used the terms interchangeably, others discussed education but measured literacy, while still others distinguished between general literacy and health literacy.

EDUCATION

The National Institutes of Health report associations between education and health across a broad range of illnesses, including coronary heart disease, many types of cancer, Alzheimer's disease, some mental illnesses, diabetes, and alcoholism. In addition, many important health risk factors for disease, such as use of cigarettes, have been linked to educational attainment. For most diseases, segments of the population with lower levels of education have higher risks of these diseases.

Education appears to be a protective factor in health. In some studies of clinical treatments, those with lower levels of educational attainment demonstrated poorer outcomes. In studies of chronic diseases such as HIV or diabetes, the effectiveness of self-management and adherence to medical treatment appear related to educational attainment. However, there is little research on what specific aspect of the educational process or experience is linked to health.

Several different types of biological, psychological, and social pathways have been proposed as possibly explaining the association between education and health. Examples of possible psychological or social pathways include the following:

1. Education leads to higher income, which allows the purchase of more health insurance, better housing, and other goods and services.
2. Education might lead to greater optimism about the future, self-efficacy, or sense of control, which might alter health behaviors or adherence to medical treatments or ability to self-manage chronic illnesses.
3. Education might improve important cognitive skills including literacy, enhanced decision-making, and analytical skills, which allow individuals to be more successful in managing their health problems, in interacting with the health care system, or in preventing future health problems.

IMPLICATIONS FOR WOMEN'S HEALTH

Domestic Violence

According to results from the National Violence against Women survey, couples with status disparities (e.g., educational level, income) experience more intimate partner violence than do couples with no status disparities; however, women were significantly more likely to report violence by a current partner if their education level was greater than their partners. In a study of pregnant Mexican women, women with less than a primary education were 1.78 times more likely to be victims of domestic violence.

Preventive Care

Regardless of race and ethnicity, women of color who had a regular doctor were at least twice as likely as those who did not to receive preventive care. However, women with less than a high school education were less likely to seek preventive care.

LITERACY

In its 1991 National Literacy Act, Congress defined literacy as "an individual's ability to read, write, and speak in English, and compute and solve problems at levels of proficiency necessary to function on the job and in society, to achieve one's goals, and develop one's knowledge and potential." Literacy was redefined in the Workforce Investment Act of 1998, as "an individual's ability to read, write, and speak in English, compute and solve problems at levels of proficiency necessary to function on the job, in the family of the individual and in society." This new definition is a broader view that recognizes literacy as more than just an individual's ability to read. As information and technology have increasingly shaped our society, the skills we need to function successfully in it have gone beyond reading, and literacy has come to include the skills listed in the updated definition.

Measuring Literacy

When literacy was simply a synonym for reading skill, it was typically measured in grade-level equivalents. In other words, an adult's literacy skill was described as equivalent to reading at a specific grade in the U.S. educational system of kindergarten through twelfth grade. A more complex and realistic conception of literacy that emphasizes its uses in adult activities helped create momentum for new forms of literacy measurement. To determine the literacy skills of American adults, the 1992 National Adult Literacy Survey (NALS) used test items that resembled everyday life tasks involving reading prose, understanding common legal and governmental documents, and using quantitative skills. The NALS classified the results into five levels that are now commonly used to describe adults' literacy skills.

Almost all adults in Level 1 can read a little but not well enough to fill out an application, read a food label, or read a simple story to a child. Adults in Level 2 usually can perform more complex tasks such as comparing, contrasting, or integrating pieces of information, but usually not higher level reading and problem-solving skills. Adults in Levels 3 through 5 usually can perform the same types of more complex tasks on increasingly lengthy and dense texts and documents.

The NALS found a total of 21–23%—or 40–44 million—of the 191 million American adults age 16 or older at Level 1, the lowest literacy level. Although many Level 1 adults could perform a number of tasks involving simple texts and documents, all adults scoring at Level 1 displayed difficulty using certain reading, writing, and computational skills considered necessary for functioning in everyday life. Rather than classifying individuals as either "literate" or "illiterate," NALS created three literacy scales: prose literacy, document literacy, and quantitative literacy. Each scale reflects a different type of real-life literacy task.

Many factors help to explain why so many adults demonstrated English literacy skills in the lowest proficiency level defined (Level 1). Twenty-five percent of the respondents who performed in this level were immigrants who may have been just learning to speak English. Nearly two thirds of those in Level 1 (62%) had terminated their education before completing high school. A third were age 65 or older, and 26% had physical, mental, or health conditions that kept them from participating fully in work, school, housework, or other activities. Nineteen percent of the respondents in Level 1 reported having visual difficulties that affected their ability to read print.

In the executive summary of the 1993 report, "Adult Literacy in America: A First Look at the Results of the National Adult Literacy Survey," the National Center for Educational Statistics reported that individuals surveyed who demonstrated higher levels of literacy were more likely to be employed, work more weeks in a year, and earn higher wages than individuals demonstrating lower proficiencies. Adults in the lowest level on each of the literacy scales (17–19%) were far more likely than those in the two highest levels (4%) to report receiving food stamps. Nearly half (41–44%) of all adults in the lowest level on each literacy scale were living in

poverty, compared with only 4–8% of those in the two highest proficiency levels.

HEALTH LITERACY

The term *health literacy* was first used in a 1974 paper titled "Health Education as Social Policy." In discussing health education as a policy issue affecting the health care system, the educational system, and mass communication, Simonds called for minimum standards for health literacy for all school grade levels. This early use of the term shows there is a link between health literacy and health education. The President's Committee on Health Education defined, in 1973, health education as "...a process which bridges the gap between health information and health practices." Failures in health education have certainly contributed to poor health literacy, but the roots of health literacy problems in the United States are not just in the history of our system of education. Health literacy problems have grown as patients are asked to assume more responsibility for self-care in a complex health care system. Patients' health literacy, then, can be thought of as the currency needed to negotiate this complex system.

A 1999 report of the Council of Scientific Affairs of the American Medical Association refers to functional health literacy as "the ability to read and comprehend prescription bottles, appointment slips, and the other essential health-related materials required to successfully function as a patient." The National Institute on Deafness and Other Communication Disorders defines health literacy as incorporating "...a range of abilities to read, comprehend, and analyze information; decode instructions, symbols, charts, and diagrams; weigh risks and benefits; and, ultimately, make decisions and take action...specifically associated with disease prevention and health promotion." Therefore, health literacy is essential to health promotion, defined as "the science and art of helping people change their lifestyles to move toward a state of optimal health," particularly as we address issues of primary prevention. A health literate individual is more apt to know how to answer the question "How do I keep myself well?" Adequate health literacy may be of even greater importance in secondary prevention (prevention of complications or after effects of existing disease), as ineffective communication between health providers and patients can result in medical errors due to misinformation about medications and self-care instructions.

Education

According to Healthy People 2010, an individual is considered to be "health literate" when he or she possesses the skills to understand information and services and use them to make appropriate decisions about health. Alarmingly, these skills and strategies are absent in more than half of the U.S. population. This fact is more disturbing when one considers that these are the very skills and strategies that often lead to longer life, improved quality of life, reduction of both chronic disease and health disparities, as well as cost savings.

IMPLICATIONS OF EDUCATION LEVEL AND LITERACY FOR WOMEN'S HEALTH

A woman's health reflects both her individual biology and her sociocultural, economic, and physical environments. These factors affect both the duration and the quality of her life. For example, the average life expectancy for a woman varies considerably according to her race. In 1997, the average life expectancy for white women was 5 years longer than that of African American women (80 vs. 75 years). Women who live in poverty or have less than a high school education have shorter life spans; higher rates of illness, injury, disability, and death; and more limited access to high-quality health care services.

Historically, women have also been the primary health care providers and health decision-makers for their families. Nearly two thirds of women polled in a recent national survey indicated that they alone were responsible for health care decisions within their family, and 83% had sole or shared responsibility for financial decisions regarding their family's health. Women are also the primary caregivers for ill or disabled family members. Of the estimated 15% of Americans who are informal caregivers, an estimated 72% are women—many of them sandwiched between caring for an ailing relative and caring for their own children.

In a recent review article on literacy and women's health, Tomlinson found that literacy, rather than ethnicity, was more strongly associated with risks for poor health, except in the case of childbirth outcomes and smoking habits. In some studies where formal education was high and health literacy was low, she found that this was due to a lack of specific information, misconceptions, or misinterpretations. These findings led

to the conclusion that formal education neither assures health literacy nor eliminates genetic or environmental predisposition for disease since traditional beliefs, values, and religion influenced health knowledge and perceptions.

In a study by Shimouchi and colleagues, literacy was identified as a predictor of infant mortality in 97 developing countries. In Nicaragua, a survey of women and infants found fertility and infant mortality declining over 30 years; the former explained by an increase in the level of education, the latter by targeting socioeconomically disadvantaged women with interventions to reduce infant mortality.

IMPACT ON HEALTH CARE PRACTITIONERS' EDUCATION AND PERCEPTIONS

Health care practitioners' efficacy in delivering services and disseminating information regarding women's health is influenced largely by formal education, cultural beliefs and perceptions about health, and access to health care information and resources. Reports of traditional practices (ways of protecting and restoring health that existed before the arrival of modern or Western medicine) often reflect patient and provider relationships based on common links, informal literacy, and perceptions. Tomlinson reports that traditional providers are the preferred health care provider for many women, regardless of provider level of literacy or training.

The impact of literacy on women's health illuminates the measure of responsibility providers must assume in educating their patients, and the magnitude of the need to provide systematic support. Health communication professionals must consider education and literacy and all their facets when developing health materials and communication strategies for a range of diverse audiences—each with differing abilities, experiences, levels of knowledge, and cultural beliefs and practices.

The National Literacy and Health Project of the Canadian Public Health Association has conducted numerous surveys that confirm that low literacy has a major negative impact on health and that literacy is a major factor underlying other determinants of health. They report that poverty, low literacy, and health problems are interrelated in a number of ways, for example, literacy affects people's access to decent jobs and decent incomes. Low-literacy workers are more likely to have unskilled jobs that tend to be more dangerous, leading to a higher than average rate of workplace injury. Low literacy limits the opportunities, resources, and control that people have over their lives, which may lead those individuals to have limited opportunities to make informed choices about their lifestyle resulting in unhealthy lifestyle practices. Literacy and health goals have a better chance for success when pursued together, and people working in health and adult education fields should form partnerships, using literacy as a channel for health promotion among low-literacy populations.

SEE ALSO: Cancer screening, Gender, Life expectancy, Preventive care

Suggested Reading

Canadian Public Health Association. (2003, July). National literacy and health program. Ottawa, Canada. http://www.nlhp.cpha.ca

Castro, R., Peek-Asa, C., & Ruiz, A. (2003). Violence against women in Mexico: A study of abuse before and during pregnancy. *American Journal of Public Health, 93*, 1110–1116.

Cornelius, L., Smith, P., & Simpson, G. (2002). What factors hinder women of color from obtaining preventative health care? *Journal of Public Health, 92*(4), 535–538.

Simonds, S. K. (1974). Health education as social policy. *Health Education Monograph, 2*, 1–25.

Tomlinson, L. (2003). Patient and practitioner literacy and women's health: A global view from the closing decade 1990–2000. *Ethnicity and Disease*, 248–258.

Suggested Resources

Kirsch, I., Jungeblut, A., Jenkins, L., & Kolstad, A. (1993). Executive summary of *Adult literacy in America: A first look at the results of the National Adult Literacy Survey.* Washington, DC: U.S. Department of Education, National Center for Education Statistics. http://nces.ed.gov//naal/resources/execsumm.asp

National Center for Education Statistics. (2003, July). U.S. Department of Education, Washington, DC. http://nces.ed.gov

National Institute on Deafness and Other Communication Disorders. (2003, July). National Institutes of Health, Bethesda, MD. http://www.nidcd.nih.gov/health/education/news/improving_health_literacy.asp

National Violence Against Women Prevention Research Center. (2003). Research. http://www.nvaw.org

Selden, C., Zorn, M., Ratzan, S. C., & Parker, R. M., compilers. (2002). Health literacy. National Library of Medicine, Current Bibliographies in Medicine, no. 2000–1 (online). Bethesda, MD (2003, July). http://www.nlm.nih.gov/pubs/resources.html

U.S. Department of Health and Human Services, Office of Women's Health. (2003, July). Washington, DC. http://www.4woman.gov/owh

GAIL E. SOUARE

Endometrial Polyps Endometrial polyps are noncancerous (benign) growths found within the uterine cavity. Usually they are asymptomatic and remain undetectable for decades. In women without symptoms, they are often found coincidentally when pelvic ultrasound is performed for unrelated problems. However, in women with abnormal uterine bleeding, investigation of the bleeding may lead to their detection.

The symptoms most often related to uterine polyps include abnormal bleeding, postcoital staining (bleeding after intercourse), chronic vaginal discharge, painful periods (dysmenorrhea), or infertility. Generally, the abnormal bleeding associated with polyps is characterized by: intermenstrual (bleeding between periods) or premenstrual spotting, or heavier menstrual flow, or increased clotting at the time of menses. Additionally, one fourth of women with polyps in the tube leading from the vagina to the uterus (endocervical polyps) will have an endometrial polyp.

Luckily, 99% of polyps removed by hysteroscopy (surgical removal via small tube) are benign (noncancerous). In women who are experiencing symptoms, however, hysteroscopic removal is imperative to evaluate the histology (microscopic evaluation) of the endometrial polyps. Endometrial cancer and excessive growth/numbers of cells of the endometrium (hyperplasia) rarely occur within an endometrial polyp. In fact, only 1% of endometrial polyps may have a coexisting malignancy present. Even though cancer is rarely found within an endometrial polyp, the surgical removal of the polyps in patients who have abnormal bleeding is imperative for two reasons. The first is to treat menstrual dysfunction and the second is to reliably exclude premalignant or malignant disease.

Recent advances in imaging techniques have allowed for noninvasive (without surgery) detection of polyps in the uterus and cervix. These include specialized diagnostic procedures called transvaginal ultrasound (TVUS) and saline infusion sonography (SIS). Ultrasound is frequently requested for the evaluation of pelvic pain, infertility, screening purposes, and in cases where a standard pelvic exam does not provide a full clinical assessment. The ultrasound is often particularly helpful in imaging/visualizing the endometrium. Ultrasonographers can reliably determine the endometrial thickness and texture. When the endometrial is thickened, then gynecologists can better ascertain the causes of thickening by performing simple procedures like SIS or office hysteroscopy. These quick office-based procedures can reliably determine the presence of endometrial polyps.

Patients who have symptomatic uterine polyps can be offered minimally invasive treatment with removal of polyps using a small tube inserted in the uterus (operative hysteroscopy). This technique permits rapid, safe, and effective removal of the polyp with minimal anesthesia as an outpatient procedure. Because the tube is inserted into the vagina for access to the uterus, conventional abdominal surgery can be avoided. Fortunately, polyps rarely reoccur when removed completely at hysteroscopy.

SEE ALSO: Dysmenorrhea, Menstrual cycle disorders

Suggested Reading

DeWaay, D. J., Syrop, C. H., Nygaard, I. E., et al. (2002). Natural history of uterine polyps and leiomyomata. *Obstetrics and Gynecology, 100,* 3–7.

Gebauer, G., Hafner, A., Siebzehnrubl, E., & Lane, N. (2001). Role of hysteroscopy in detection of endometrial polyps: Results of a prospective study. *American Journal of Obstetrics and Gynecology, 184,* 59–62.

Kamel, H. S., Darwish, A. M., & Mohamed, S. A. (2000). Comparison of transvaginal ultrasonography and vaginal sonohysterography in the detection of endometrial polyps. *Acta Obstetricia et Gynecologica Scandinavica, 79,* 60–64.

LINDA D. BRADLEY

Endometriosis

Endometriosis is the presence of tissue, which should exist only inside the uterus (endometrial glands and endometrial stroma), at sites outside the uterus. This disease affects many women in the reproductive age group, and chronic pelvic pain associated with endometriosis is one of the most common symptom complexes that gynecologists are required to treat. Although its etiology has not been conclusively identified, it is generally believed to involve abnormalities in the immune system. It is unclear whether this is causal or simply a response to abnormal implants.

Endometriosis is associated with painful periods (dysmenorrhea), painful intercourse (dyspareunia), noncyclical pelvic pain, and infertility. There are also a myriad of associated symptoms, especially those that involve the gastrointestinal tract. Chronic pelvic pain associated with endometriosis can be difficult to treat because of the large number of patients who have a relapse. The diagnosis of endometriosis can only be made by a specialized procedure involving a small tube that allows visualization inside the uterus/pelvis (laparoscopy). Blood (serum) markers and pelvic imaging techniques such as ultrasound lack sufficient sensitivity and specificity to allow a diagnosis.

Most endometrial deposits are found in the pelvis (ovaries, peritoneum, ligaments and structures around the uterus, vagina, and rectum). Deposits outside of the pelvis, including those in the umbilicus, and previous surgical wounds are uncommon. The physical appearance of endometriosis at laparoscopy can be quite varied. The diagnosis is usually made visually at laparoscopy, but cellular (histologic) analysis is important as well.

SYMPTOMS AND DIAGNOSIS

Patients with endometriosis can present with a wide variety of symptoms and signs. Typically, dysmenorrhea, dyspareunia, and noncyclic lower abdominal pain are common. Gastrointestinal symptoms such as constipation, diarrhea, and abnormal urge to defecate (tenesmus), similar to irritable bowel syndrome, are also common. Urinary symptoms are less common but pain with urination may occur. Patients with infertility may not have any pain that they consider manageable. The diagnosis in these patients is made at the time of diagnostic laparoscopy for infertility. Many diagnostic tests have been proposed. The most popular is a blood test called CA-125. Imaging modalities are generally not useful.

Intensive efforts are under way to develop noninvasive methods of diagnosing endometriosis. Recently, encouraging reports suggest that specialized tests of blood or fluid in the abdomen (serum and peritoneal fluid cytokines) might be helpful in the nonsurgical diagnosis of endometriosis.

LAPAROSCOPIC ASSESSMENT

Diagnosis of endometriosis can be suggested by history and examination, but definitive diagnosis can be made only by visualization with a small tube (laparoscopy) or conventional exploratory surgery (laparotomy). Endometriosis is a heterogeneous disease that ranges in severity from minimal to severe. The most commonly used classification of endometriosis is according to the American Society for Reproductive Medicine (formerly American Fertility Society). In this system, the surgeon assigns a certain number of points for disease identified at laparoscopy. This is based on the area and depth of endometrial implants in the abdominal cavity (peritoneum) or ovary, as well as the extent of fibrous growths (adhesions) on the ovaries, tubes connecting ovaries to uterus (fallopian tubes), and related tissues. The patient is then assigned a stage of I–IV. Definitive diagnosis of ovarian endometriomas should be confirmed by microscopic cellular (histopathologic) examination.

Endometriosis remains a difficult clinical enigma. The clinician has to rely on the clinical history and physical exam. Generally, diagnostic tests and imaging modalities are not useful and diagnostic laparoscopy is still the "gold" standard. However, empirical medical therapy for chronic pelvic pain is acceptable before diagnostic laparoscopy, in some circumstances. First-line treatment for painful symptoms could be medical or surgical. In infertility, surgery has been shown to be effective while medical suppressive therapy has not. Assisted conception has a primary role in moderate and severe disease.

In the hands of the experienced laparoscopic surgeon, advanced endometriosis can be managed effectively with short convalescence and excellent long-term results. The primary care physician can manage most endometriosis-associated symptoms. Consultation with a specialist is recommended in certain circumstances.

MANAGING PAIN ASSOCIATED WITH ENDOMETRIOSIS

In a double-blind randomized clinical trial, it was found that two thirds of patients will have significant relief from surgical management of endometriosis. More dramatic relief was found from surgical management of advanced endometriosis rather than early disease. Medical therapy has been found to provide a similar response rate.

MANAGING INFERTILITY ASSOCIATED WITH ENDOMETRIOSIS

It is well established that a relation exists between endometriosis and infertility. In advanced cases of endometriosis, fertility is affected as a consequence of the anatomical distortion of the pelvis caused by adhesions or ovarian cysts, or both. Unlike an infection, endometriosis does not damage the lining (luminal epithelium) of the fallopian tube and thus surgery is more likely to be successful. In minimal or mild cases of endometriosis, the exact nature of the relation between the disease and infertility is unclear. In a randomized clinical trial to assess surgical management of early stage disease in patients with infertility, it was found that the pregnancy rate can double. Medical suppressive therapy has not been shown to increase pregnancy rates. Pregnancy rates with endometriosis-associated infertility may be improved by laparoscopic surgery for moderate to severe disease. Advanced endometriosis is characterized by extensive pelvic distortion that can be corrected by surgical treatment.

SEE ALSO: Infertility, Laparoscopy

Suggested Reading

Al-Azemi, M., Bernal, A. L., Steele, J., Gramsbergen, I., Barlow, D., & Kennedy, S. (2000). Ovarian response to repeated controlled stimulation in in-vitro fertilization cycles in patients with ovarian endometriosis. *Human Reproduction, 15*, 72–75.

Bedaiwy, M. A., Falcone, T., Sharma, R. K., Goldberg, J. M., Attaran, M., Nelson, D. R., et al. (2002). Prediction of endometriosis with serum and peritoneal fluid markers: A prospective controlled trial. *Human Reproduction, 17*, 426–431.

Jerby, B. L., Kessler, H., Falcone, T., & Milsom, J. W. (1999). Laparoscopic management of colorectal endometriosis. *Surgical Endoscopy, 13*, 1125–1128.

Jones, K., & Sutton, C. (2000). Endometriomas: Fenestration or excision? *Fertility and Sterility, 74*, 846–848.

Ling, F. W. (1999). Randomized controlled trial of depot leuprolide in patients with chronic pelvic pain and clinically suspected endometriosis. Pelvic Pain Study Group. *Obstetrics and Gynecology, 93*, 51–58.

Lundorff, P., Hahlin, M., Kallfelt, B., Thorburn, J., & Lindblom, B. (1991). Adhesion formation after laparoscopic surgery in tubal pregnancy: A randomized trial versus laparotomy. *Fertility and Sterility, 55*, 911–915.

Marcoux, S., Maheux, R., & Berube, S. (1997). Laparoscopic surgery in infertile women with minimal or mild endometriosis. Canadian Collaborative Group on Endometriosis. *New England Journal of Medicine, 337*, 217–222.

Mol, B. W., Bayram, N., Lijmer, J. G., Wiegerinck, M. A., Bongers, M. Y., van der Veen, F., et al. (1998). The performance of CA-125 measurement in the detection of endometriosis: A meta-analysis. *Fertility and Sterility, 70*, 1101–1108.

Nezhat, C., Nezhat, F., Nezhat, C. H., Nasserbakht, F., Rosati, M., & Seidman, D. S. (1996). Urinary tract endometriosis treated by laparoscopy. *Fertility and Sterility, 66*, 920–924.

Nezhat, C. H., Seidman, D. S., Nezhat, F. R., & Nezhat, C. R. (1998). Long-term outcome of laparoscopic presacral neurectomy for the treatment of central pelvic pain attributed to endometriosis. *Obstetrics and Gynecology, 91,* 701–704.

Redwine, D. B. (1999). Ovarian endometriosis: A marker for more extensive pelvic and intestinal disease. *Fertility and Sterility, 72,* 310–315.

Singh, M., Goldberg, J., Falcone, T., Nelson, D., Pasqualotto, E., Attaran, M., et al. (2001). Superovulation and intrauterine insemination in cases of treated mild pelvic disease. *Journal of Assisted Reproduction and Genetics, 18,* 26–29.

Sutton, C. J., Ewen, S. P., Whitelaw, N., & Haines, P. (1994). Prospective, randomized, double-blind, controlled trial of laser laparoscopy in the treatment of pelvic pain associated with minimal, mild, and moderate endometriosis. *Fertility and Sterility, 62,* 696–700.

Tulandi, T., & al-Took, S. (1998). Reproductive outcome after treatment of mild endometriosis with laparoscopic excision and electrocoagulation. *Fertility and Sterility, 69,* 229–231.

Mohamed A. Bedaiwy
Tommaso Falcone

Energy Healing   There are many popular holistic modalities that work with the human energy system. One of the underlying principles they share is the belief that all living things have an energy field that surrounds them that is essential to life. Different cultures refer to this life force as *chi* (China) or *prana* (India) or *ki* (Japan). There are also energy centers in the body known as *chakras* (a Sanskrit word meaning spinning vortex). The third part of the energy system is a complex network of meridians, pathways of energy flowing throughout the body. It is believed that an open, flowing energy system is essential to maintaining good health. Pain, illness, and disease can be considered the result of some form of blockage or disruption in the flow of energy in the energy field, the energy centers, or the meridians. Different modalities work to clear and open this flow of energy and to restore harmony and balance in order to promote physical, emotional, mental, and spiritual well-being. Practices such as acupressure and acupuncture work to open the flow of energy in the meridians. Other practices such as Healing Touch, Reiki, and Therapeutic Touch work primarily with the energy field and energy centers. All three of these modalities are done with the client fully clothed and seated in a chair or lying on a table. There is research to support the use of these modalities for accelerated wound healing, pain management, and decreased anxiety. The research base continues to grow as these practices gain acceptance by the general public and traditional medicine. These three modalities will be explained in more detail.

Healing Touch is an energy-based therapeutic approach that uses touch to influence the energy system, thus affecting physical, emotional, mental, and spiritual health. Healing Touch is taught in a multilevel educational program that moves from beginning to advanced practice. It was developed by Janet Mentgen, RN, BSN, who has been practicing energy-based care since 1980 in Denver, CO. Healing Touch practitioners use their hands to assess and treat the energy system. Practitioners may work using physical touch although it is not required and at times practitioners work several inches and sometimes feet away from the body. The practices taught in the Healing Touch curriculum come from a variety of sources including well-known healers such as Alice Bailey, Brugh Joy, Rosalyn Bruyere, and Barbara Brennan. To learn more about Healing Touch, class schedules, and to locate a practitioner, contact Healing Touch International, Inc. at 303-989-7982 or on the web at www.healingtouch.net.

Therapeutic Touch was developed in the early 1970s by Dolores Krieger, PhD, a registered nurse and professor of nursing at New York University, and Dora Kunz, a noted healer. Therapeutic Touch is "a contemporary interpretation of several ancient healing practices" (Krieger, 1993, p. 11). Therapeutic Touch practitioners follow a sequenced procedure that includes centering, assessment of the energy field, smoothing or unruffling the energy field, and sending or modulating energy. This is done in an effort to assist the client to move to a state of energy balance. Therapeutic Touch practitioners complete basic levels of training including mentorship with experienced practitioners. To learn more or locate a practitioner, contact Nurse Healers-Professional Associates International at 801-273-3399 or www.therapeutic-touch.org.

Reiki is the Japanese word for "universal life energy." This energy-based, hands-on practice focuses on transferring or channeling energy into specific areas of the body. There are 12 standard hand placement sites on the body, but an experienced Reiki practitioner may also place his/her hands on other areas of the body to address painful or diseased areas. Reiki can also be done off the body. Reiki is taught or more correctly passed down in an oral tradition from a Reiki master to a student. For more information about Reiki, contact The Reiki Alliance at 208-783-3535 or on the web at www.reikialliance.com.

It is important that someone wishing to try one of these modalities be an informed consumer and ask about training, credentials, and expertise. All of these practices should be seen as complementing traditional medical care.

SEE ALSO: Complementary and alternative health practices

Suggested Reading

Barnett, L., & Chambers, M. (1996). *Reiki energy medicine: Bringing the healing touch into home, hospital and hospice.* Rochester, VT: Healing Arts Press.

Hover-Kramer, D. (2002). *Healing touch: A guidebook for practitioners.* Albany, NY: Delmar.

Krieger, D. (1993). *Accepting your power to heal: The personal practice of therapeutic touch.* Santa Fe, NM: Bear.

MARY M. DUENNES

Environment

Environment The effects of the environment on health have long been recognized. In the United States, industrial growth and increasing urban population centers in the mid-19th century resulted in concern about the water supply and sewage management. Furthermore, increasing use of coal-burning furnaces and the subsequent soot and cinders in the air led to public fear and, ultimately, organization of public policy to address these problems. State and local health boards were used to improve public sanitation with clean drinking water the first priority. Adequate sewage treatment was also a priority, although, due to economic limitations, strategies for sewage treatment were slower to be adopted.

In the latter part of the 19th century, the problems of air pollution were addressed by common councils of large industrial cities. States would authorize cities to regulate smoking nuisances (if the states were to do anything). The local ordinances developed took a variety of forms including modest fines for dense smoke emissions to responsibility of an owner to eliminate smoke emissions from his/her facility. Other ordinances prohibited the use or sale of coals with certain ash and sulfur content. The enforcement of these laws was difficult as the agencies had little resources for enforcement. As air pollution increased in the first half of the 20th century, county air pollution agencies replaced city smoke inspectors. Finally, in 1955, the federal government got involved through the Air Pollution Act of 1955.

In general, environmental protection up to the 1970s was largely left up to the states. However, public concern over national and international environmental conditions led to increasing federal government involvement and the development of statutory requirements. The states were allowed to develop more stringent standards, but were required to at least meet the standards set forth by the federal government. Policies enacted by the federal government include the National Environmental Policy Act; the Federal Insecticide, Fungicide, and Rodenticide Act; the Toxic Substances Control Act; the Clean Air Act; the Clean Water Act; and the Safe Drinking Water Act to name a few.

Environmental epidemiology, which is the study of the effect of the external environment on health, examines a broad range of factors. In addition to examining associations between water and air quality to health, environmental epidemiology is also concerned with diseases associated with vector-borne and soil-borne contaminants. Vector-borne illnesses are those that stem from a nonhuman carrier of disease organisms and are generally of greater concern in developing countries compared to industrialized countries. Mosquitoes, flies, rats, and mice can all spread disease to human populations. Of particular concern is malaria, which is spread by mosquitoes. Malaria is one of the most widespread vector-borne diseases. Soil-borne parasites also pose a health threat. Soil-borne parasitic diseases include ascaris (roundworm), hookworm, whipworm, strongyloides, and animal nematodes.

Environmental epidemiology can also examine how health is affected by people's work environment and living environment. Approximately 137 workers die each day from job-related diseases, more than eight times the number of workers that die from job-related accidents. These illnesses may be caused by a variety of substances including poisonous chemicals, dyes, metals, and radiation. Also, there has been increased attention to the association between place of residence and health. While some of this association can be attributed to factors such as air/water pollution and lead exposure, other factors related to place of residence are considered to have effects on health outcomes. For example, resources such as easy access to medical care, education, transportation, health and welfare services, and police protection are all expected to have important effects on health. In addition, networks of community support and the behavioral norms in an area are thought to play a role in health outcomes. The location of stores that sell nutritious foods, alcohol, and cigarettes can have an effect on health as can the amount of advertising for these products (i.e., billboards) in an area. Finally, for infectious diseases, the prevalence of diseased people in the area and the amount of contact with these people are important in predicting transmission of infectious disease.

Studies of the environment and health are complicated not only by traditional concerns in epidemiological studies such as confounding, but also by specific difficulties of environmental studies. Exposure assessment is a vital part of environmental epidemiology but exposure assessment is often inadequate. Sometimes there are no documented exposure data for individuals who are at risk. Even when exposure information exists, it is often not complete. For example, several different pieces of information on the exposure are often needed including the intensity and frequency of contact as well as routes of entry into the body. Studies of communities exposed to environmental contaminants are also problematic. Again, often the exposure is poorly defined. Furthermore, people living in the area around an exposure may be small in number thereby limiting the range of outcomes that can be studied. Similarly, often the endpoints of interest are rare and/or have a long latency period. Publicity of the situation may influence reporting of exposure and/or an atmosphere of fear or anger may make studying the effects difficult.

Many associations between environmental exposures and disease have been noted in spite of these limitations, although some of these associations are controversial. Cadmium, lead, and other heavy metals found in the environment have been associated with osteoporosis, which is characterized by fragility of the bones. Autoimmune diseases, such as multiple sclerosis, rheumatoid arthritis, scleroderma, and systemic lupus erythematosus (SLE), also have links to environmental exposures. These diseases, which are more common in women than in men, have been linked to certain pharmaceuticals and solvents. Specifically, lupus has been associated with both hydrazine (an industrial chemical) and tartrazine (a food additive). Certain cancers have been associated with radiation, natural and man-made chemicals, and sunlight. Black lung (or pneumoconiosis) occurs when particles such as asbestos, silica dust, graphite dust, coal dust, and the like damage sensitive areas of the lung, which subsequently leads to scar tissue. More commonly, pollutants and chemicals in the air are known triggers for asthma.

Uranium can damage living tissue and a single high dose can be fatal. While most people will not come into contact with uranium, miners and medical professionals who work with x-rays need to take precautions against uranium exposure. Finally, in the 1970s, scientists discovered that the use of diethylstilbestrol (DES) in pregnant woman could lead to cancer in the reproductive organs of the daughters of these women. Consequently, the use of DES and other synthetic hormones during pregnancy has ceased. However, there is concern that other chemicals and man-made pesticides may have similar effects.

While efforts at the local, state, and national level have addressed clean water, air, sewage management, and cleanup of hazardous waste sites, less money has been spent on addressing health risks from chronic low-level exposures to hazardous substances. Several low-level exposures are of particular concern. Pesticides are widely used in the United States, with more than 1 billion pounds of synthetic organic pesticides produced each year. Specifically, PBCs and DDT have been known to affect the immune system, the neurological system, and the endocrine system, and some researchers have speculated that these pesticides are a promoter of breast cancer. The use of PBCs has declined over the years, although concern about residual levels of PBC still remains.

Another pollutant of concern is mercury. Mercury is a widespread persistent air pollutant and organic mercury (a mercuric compound) has been found in the aquatic food chain. Both are of concern to pregnant women, since levels that would produce no or minimal symptoms in the mother have been found to have consequences for the fetus. Two other pollutants that have received increased attention over the years are asbestos and lead. Asbestos can be found in a variety of items including insulation, floor tiles, shingles, and fire-resistant dry wall. While it is rare for asbestos to be installed today, previous exposure or exposure during asbestos removal, renovation, or maintenance of buildings are of concern. Asbestos fibers enter the body through inhalation or ingestion of the fibers, which subsequently become embedded in the respiratory or digestive system. This inhalation or ingestion of the fibers may cause disabling or fatal disease.

Lead is another pollutant that has received increased attention. Lead is most commonly found in homes in lead paint chips that have separated from the wall, which may be pulverized into dust. Lead also exists in homes in lead pipes and some ceramic food containers with lead glazing. Lead exposures have been associated with negative reproductive effects in men and women and long-term exposure of lead in children has been associated with reductions in cognitive abilities and shorter attention spans. It has been suggested that levels of lead in children have been declining over the years, perhaps in part to increased attention to this issue.

The environment, defined in multiple ways, plays a major role in the health of the population. Air and water quality, containment of hazardous wastes, and vectors that transmit disease are all important environmental factors. Additionally, health is also affected by one's environment, more broadly defined, meaning "their work environment and their place of residency." There has been increased involvement in the monitoring of the safety of our environment and increased understanding of the specific aspects of the environment that are associated with detrimental health effects. It is hoped that continued study and monitoring of these factors will result in a healthier population overall.

SEE ALSO: Pregnancy, Women in the Workforce (pp. 32–40)

Suggested Reading

Blumenthal, D. S., & Ruttenber, A. J. (1995). *Introduction to environmental health* (2nd ed.). New York: Springer.

Macintyre, S., Ellaway, A., & Cummins, S. (2002). Place effects on health: How to conceptualise, operationalise and measure them? *Social Science and Medicine, 55*, 125–139.

National Research Council (U.S.). Committee on Environmental Epidemiology. (1991). *Environmental epidemiology.* Washington, DC: National Academy Press.

National Research Council (U.S.). Committee on Environmental Epidemiology. (1997). *Environmental epidemiology* (Vol. 2). Washington, DC: National Academy Press.

Nolan, L. (2001). Our environment, our health. *Association of Women's Health, Obstetric and Neonatal Nurses, 5*(6), 25–29.

Talbott, E. O., & Craun, G. F. (1995). *Introduction to environmental epidemiology.* Boca Raton, FL: Lewis.

WHO Commission on Health and Environment, and World Health Organization. (1992). *Our planet, our health: Report of the WHO Commission on health and environment.* Geneva: Author.

Suggested Resources

National Institute of Environmental Health Sciences. Retrieved 2/14/2003, from the World Wide Web: http://www.niehs.nih.gov/

NATALIE COLABIANCHI

Episiotomy

Episiotomy is a procedure designed to enlarge the vaginal opening at the time of delivery of the fetal head. It is performed when the baby's head is crowning (visible 3–4 cm). Options for pain relief during the procedure include local injection of an anesthetic such as lidocaine, epidural anesthesia, intravenous narcotics, or local nerve block. The procedure is performed by making a vertical incision at the midline directly below the vagina between the vagina and the anus ("midline" episiotomy) or creating an incision at a 30° angle from the vertical ("mediolateral" episiotomy). In the United States, the midline technique is most common.

Episiotomy was a routine obstetrical practice for many years. It was thought that routine episiotomy decreased the length of the second stage of labor ("pushing") and protected the baby's head, as well as protected the mother from damage to the anal sphincter and long-term problems with bowel and bladder incontinence. However, based on recent studies, it is clear that avoidance of episiotomy results in fewer and smaller tears, particularly in women undergoing their first vaginal delivery. Indeed, massaging or stretching the vaginal tissue daily for several weeks prior to delivery has been shown to decrease the rate of episiotomy and tears.

Current indications for episiotomy include shoulder dystocia (impaction of the baby's shoulder against the maternal symphysis pubis), breech delivery, and instrumented vaginal delivery (forceps or vacuum-assisted vaginal delivery). These are all circumstances in which additional room may be required for certain maneuvers in order to deliver the baby safely.

Episiotomy and perineal lacerations are classified based on the layers of tissue that are disrupted during the procedure. First- and second-degree episiotomy or tear both disrupt the vaginal wall but spare the anal sphincter (ring of muscles around the anus). A third-degree episiotomy or extension severs the anal sphincter (ring of muscles surrounding the anus). If the episiotomy extends from the vagina into the rectum, it is referred to as a fourth-degree extension, or if cut deliberately, a proctoepisiotomy.

Episiotomy and laceration (cut or tear) repair are generally performed using a continuous length of absorbable synthetic suture. This technique reduces pain in the postpartum period. The suture does not need to be removed at a later date.

Care of the perineum after episiotomy or perineal laceration includes the use of ice packs, nonsteroidal anti-inflammatory medication (i.e., ibuprofen), and topical sprays, all of which reduce swelling and pain. Infection and bleeding or the formation of a hematoma (collection of blood beneath the sutures) are possible complications. Infection is generally treated by removing the sutures and prescription of oral antibiotics. A hematoma may be evacuated by removing the sutures and allowing the tissues to heal openly. Occasionally, fecal (stool) incontinence can develop if the anal sphincter or its nerve are damaged. This may require surgery at a later date.

SEE ALSO: Labor and delivery, Urinary incontinence and voiding dysfunction

Suggested Reading

Baxley, E. G., & Gobbo, R. (2001). Episiotomy and repair of lacerations. In S. D. Ratcliffe (Ed.), *Family practice obstetrics* (2nd ed.). Philadelphia: Hanley & Belfus.

Carroli, G., & Belizan, J. (2003). Episiotomy for vaginal birth (Cochrane review). In: The Cochrane Library, Issue 1. Oxford: Update Software.

Eason, E., Labrecque, M., Wells, G., & Feldman, P. (2000). Preventing perineal trauma during childbirth: A systematic review. *Obstetrics and Gynecology, 95,* 464–471.

ANDREA DARBY-STEWART

Equal Rights Amendment

The Equal Rights Amendment (ERA) began as a proposed (but unratified) amendment to the U.S. Constitution. First introduced to Congress in 1923, it was not finally approved by the Senate and submitted to the states for ratification until almost 50 years later. The wording in the 1972 version, while not identical to its earlier incarnation, nevertheless adhered to the same basic premise: that sex should not determine the legal rights of both men and women. The meaning of this underlying principle underwent tremendous change as the nature and focus of the women's movement evolved during the 1960s. Unfortunately, the inability to carefully lay out a definite strategy to promote the proposed amendment helps explain why it ultimately failed to be ratified in the required 38 states.

The group most directly responsible for the development of the ERA in the early 1920s was the National Woman's Party (NWP), which was formed by Alice Paul. On the 75th anniversary of the 1848 Woman's Rights Convention, Paul introduced the first incarnation of the ERA which read: "Men and woman shall have equal rights throughout the United States and every place subject to its jurisdiction." The ERA was to be a vehicle for advancing women's rights beyond those already achieved with the passage of the 19th Amendment, which had given women the right to vote. The NWP proposed the ERA in order to draw attention to and eliminate the many inequalities that still deprived women of equal treatment in the eyes of the law and in society.

The NWP, as well as professional women and intellectuals, strongly supported the proposed amendment. However, support among women for the amendment was not universal. There was a split with some women's groups which feared that the labor laws that had been enacted to protect women would be jeopardized by the ERA. These reformers were not about to give up three decades of hard-won social and labor legislation aimed at protecting working women. Many strong women leaders on the left were openly suspicious because to them the ERA seemed to benefit professional women at the expense of wage-earning women. There was also open opposition by wage-earning women even in the early 1940s, when both the Republican and Democratic parties added their support of the ERA.

The civil rights movements of the 1960s fostered the second strong wave of political activism on the part of women in this century; this time women made equality, not suffrage, the central symbol of their struggle. Leading the way was the National Organization for Women (NOW). The intervening years had seen a radical shift in the support base of the ERA. Wage-earning women who had at first opposed the ERA now came to embrace it. This change of support reflected the changing political and economic atmosphere within the country. During the first half of the century, the disparity in the treatment of women ranging from long working hours and low wages required that women be protected through a series of gender-specific legislation. However, with the introduction of the Civil Rights Act of 1964, new and more powerful forms of protection supplanted the older protective laws. This, coupled with new economic opportunities, gave women wage-earners an incentive for promoting the ERA. This was primarily due to the fact that this period marked the first time it was economically possible for a full-time employed woman to support herself and two children.

Outside the women's movement, opposition to the amendment ranged from strong to openly hostile, and it was always better organized and financed. Phyllis Schlafly led intense opposition based on the same fears that had once been generated to oppose women's suffrage. The opposition claimed that the ERA would deny a woman's right to be supported by her husband, privacy rights would be overturned, women would be sent into combat, and abortion rights and homosexual marriages would be upheld. Intense opposition on these grounds from various conservative religious and political organizations effectively brought the Amendment's ratification to a standstill.

The ERA came very close to being adopted. Within a year of Senate approval, 30 state legislatures ratified the ERA and by 1977 the number had risen to 35. The states that opposed the ERA were primarily in the south and the Rocky Mountain regions of the country. The only non-ERA state outside these regions, Illinois was the site of a titanic struggle in the early part of the 1980s. Ultimately it, too, failed to approve the proposed amendment. Even if Illinois had approved it, the chance of it being adopted in two of the remaining fourteen states was remote at best.

The inability to respond effectively to the criticism or to establish the necessary grass-roots programs to promote the Amendment were the two main reasons the ERA was not ratified. These reasons, however, should provide a lesson to any future incarnation of the ERA because, whatever its failings, the ERA succeeded in fostering discussion on legal and social concerns relating to women's status as full and equal citizens.

SEE ALSO: Discrimination, Sexual harassment, United States Civil Rights Act of 1964

Suggested Reading

Berry, M. F. (1986). *Why ERA failed: Politics, women's rights and the amending process of the Constitution*. Bloomington: Indiana University Press.

Hoff-Wilson, J. (Ed.). (1986). *Rights of passage: The past and future of the ERA*. Bloomington: Indiana University Press.

Mansbridge, J. J. (1986). *Why we lost the ERA*. Chicago: University of Chicago Press.

Mathews, D. G., & De Heart, J. S. (1991). *Sex, gender, and the politics of ERA: A state and the nation*. New York: Oxford University Press.

ROBERTO HERNANDEZ

Ethnicity   The United States has long encompassed a large number of ethnicities, races, and cultures. This appears to be increasingly true. The country's recognition of this diversity and its recognition of the considerable strength that such variety brings to the country and its peoples also appear to be increasing. Many other nations are also having similar experiences of increasing diversity among people and a movement away from earlier tendencies to devalue cultural differences and to keep cultural and ethnic groups segregated. Diversity, and indeed even celebration of diverse ethnicities and other human characteristics, enriches a given culture, bringing a greater breadth of perspectives, ideas, values, attitudes, and contributions overall. The world over the later half of the 20th century has increasingly recognized, although certainly not fully accepted, the value of cultural and ethnic differences. This is true in spite of the fact that so-called ethnic strengths historically have been built upon by maintaining similar values and characteristics within a given ethnic or cultural group. However, increasing diversity may also lead to a blending of ethnic differences, thus risking the loss of unique aspects of various cultures and ethnicities over time.

This said, the complexity of the concept of ethnicity and its closely related concepts of race and culture are briefly explored below. First, ethnicity is "defined" and related to other concepts. Then, the observed relationship of ethnicity to some basic health status variables in the United States is outlined. Finally, some of the difficulties in the measurement of ethnicity and problems associated with the concept itself are discussed. At the end, key references are provided from which much of this material has been drawn and which will provide the interested reader many more details.

"Ethnic" usually refers to characteristics of a people, especially a group of people who share a distinct and common set of characteristics, such as culture, religion, language, race, or nationality. In comparison, "race" generally refers to biological factors that are the basis of group differences, especially observable physical features. "Culture" usually refers to shared elements that provide a basis for perceiving, believing, communicating, evaluating, and behaving within a common context. However, no consensus exists regarding precise definitions of ethnicity or race or culture, and it is very common (unfortunately) for people in general, and researchers in particular, to use the terms ethnicity, race, and culture interchangeably. The extensive list of possible central characteristics that may be used to define an ethnic group hints at the complexity of the concept itself and the varied ways in which it is used.

For many in the United States, ethnic group also connotes "minority group," that is, a smaller group within a larger dominant group. This, of course, is an ethnocentric application of the concept—wherein it is used to refer to those outside the larger group, but is not used to refer to those among the majority group. Furthermore, ethnicity often connotes "race" or "nationality" to many people, particularly so-called races or nationalities that are not among the majority population. Thus, by this usage in the United States, whites or Caucasians or non-Hispanic whites are not ethnic groups in the minds of most people, but Asians, blacks or African Americans, Hispanics or Latinos, American Indians and Alaskan Natives, and Pacific Islanders are—primarily because none of those latter groups represent a majority. In parts of various U.S. states, whites are not in the majority—for example, in the state of New Mexico, no traditionally labeled group represents a majority (Hispanics 44%, non-Hispanic whites 44%, Americans Indians 9%, and other groups about 3%). The absurdity of this ethnocentric usage and meaning of ethnicity as commonly applied in the United States thus becomes apparent.

More objectively, any group sharing a distinct and common set of characteristics would be considered an ethnic group, irrespective of its numbers relative to other groups, including so-called whites. But this suggests an additional problem in assessing and utilizing ethnicity/race as a means by which to predict or classify groups of people—whites, Hispanics, blacks, Native Americans, and other large groups are not homogeneous regarding culture, religion, language, or nationality—in fact, it is clear that each "group" is quite diverse in all these respects. Thus, although ethnicity is usually measured by simple broad self-labels, it is actually based upon a complex concept that reflects many dimensions.

In the United States, the assessment of ethnicity is usually done by simply asking a person in an interview or survey how they describe themselves. Historically, a variety of lists of ethnic groups have been used and have changed somewhat over time. Currently, the following list is increasing in use: Asians, blacks or African Americans, Native Americans (or American Indians) and Alaskan Natives, Pacific Islanders, white or Caucasian, and "Mixed" or "Other," this latter category recognizing

that many people do not distinctly fall into one of the others. Note that among that list, Hispanic is omitted because it is now recognized that "Hispanic" is a separate dimension relative to the larger list, which largely reflects what is usually described as "race." In this fairly recent assessment scheme, Hispanic status is measured with a separate question that precedes the one above, thus recognizing that Hispanics or Latinos or those of Spanish descent may be among white or black "races" and implicitly that Hispanics are not a homogeneous group. Of course, Hispanics are not homogeneous in many nonracial senses as well because Hispanics who "originate" from Spain, Mexico, the Caribbean, South America, and the United States (where some count their heritage back hundreds of years) often have quite distinct cultures and other characteristics.

The current U.S. categories used to assess "ethnicity" emanate from the U.S. Federal Office of Management and Budget, which announced this system in 1998 and encouraged other federal agencies to follow it for the sake of consistency in reporting. The Department of Health and Human Services and the U.S. Census Bureau among others have adopted this two-question approach to ethnicity. Those who use it, often to meet federal standards, are encouraged by governmental guidelines to consider making such ethnicity assessments at a finer grained level, but they are not required to do so. This too suggests that the sociopolitical systems that have evolved this scheme also recognize that ethnicity is more complex than what the simple categories or labels listed above imply.

Assessing ethnicity (or race) in a population usually serves one of two major purposes. The first is descriptive, wherein the percentage of people that can be attributed to a particular broad ethnic group is simply provided as information to characterize a population. The second is analytic, wherein differences in nonethnic characteristics or behaviors are reported to vary as a function of membership in an ethnic group. Below we will discuss some of the many problems with the analytic use of ethnicity, but first we will turn to a brief and simple review of the known general relationships of ethnicity to several major health status measures in the United States to illustrate the analytic use of ethnicity.

ETHNICITY AND HEALTH STATUS

Health Status Indicators (HSIs) were developed as a part of Healthy People 2000, a set of Department of

Health and Human Services objectives for the United States. A central goal for these objectives was to help reduce disparities in health care among various ethnic groups in the United States and to encourage significant improvement in the health indicators for the population overall. In addition to reporting the rates of various illnesses, an index of disparity was used to summarize ethnic/racial differences in the HSIs. Examination of trends for the period 1990–1998 showed that most of the 17 HSIs improved for most ethnic/racial groups, although the differences between ethnic groups did not change very much.

Infant mortality is often used as a principal measure of health status among groups and nations worldwide. In the United States, rates of infant mortality have long been much lower for non-Hispanic whites, Hispanics, and Asian/Pacific Islanders than for blacks and American Indians/Alaskan Natives, roughly by a factor of two times. During the 1990s, infant mortality decreased notably for all groups to 6.0/1,000 for whites, 5.8/1,000 for Hispanics, and 6.6/1,000 for Asians, and although declining by roughly 25%, remained much higher for black non-Hispanics (13.9) and American Indians/Alaskan Natives (9.3). Rates for low birthweight, however, showed a different trend, increasing by as much as 18% for some groups over the decade—whites (6.6/1,000), Hispanics (6.4), Asians (7.4), blacks (13.2), and American Indians/Alaskan Natives (6.8). The percentages of women with no prenatal care during their first trimester of pregnancy in 1998 showed marked declines of 24–35% compared to 1990.

The total death rate is also used as a prime HSI nationally and globally. The total death rate decreased over the 1990s roughly 10% for all groups except American Indians/Alaskan Natives, who showed a 4% increase in death rate between 1990 and 1998—whites (453/100,000), Hispanics (343), Asians (265), blacks (711), and American Indians/Alaskan Natives (458). The ratio of rates between highest and lowest groups (the disparity ratio) was 2.7 in 1998, the same as it was in 1990, indicating no reduction in overall health differences among groups.

Death rates by "violent" means showed substantial overall declines during the decade of the 1990s—homicide (28%), suicide (10%), and motor vehicle crash (15%). Percentages of decline across ethnic groups were roughly similar with two major exceptions: (a) the rate of suicide for American Indians/Alaskan Natives actually increased 8%, and the rates of decline of death by homicide (11%) and motor vehicle crashes (4%) were

much less than for the other groups; and (b) Asians showed a much lower decline in suicide rate (2%) than other groups, probably because their rate was already the lowest by far. The disparity ratio actually increased over the period for motor vehicle crash (2.6–3.7) and suicide (2.1–2.3), but it declined for homicide (9.7–8.2).

Death rates by major diseases are also used as important indicators of health status in the United States. For example, rates of death from heart disease declined overall by 16% over the 1990s, and this decline was uniform for all ethnic groups, except it was notably lower for blacks (11%) and American Indians/Alaskan Natives (8%). The disparity ratio among groups actually increased slightly from 2.7 to 2.8. The decline in stroke death rate was much lower overall (9%) than for heart disease and was not uniform among groups, with American Indians/Alaskan Natives actually increasing 3%. The disparity ratio was 2.2, down from 2.5 in 1990.

A number of other trends in major HSIs can be found that illustrate the substantial differences in health among the various major ethnic/racial groups in the United States. Comparison of disparity indices in 1990 to those in 1998 reveal that for 11 of 17 HSIs, ethnic difference has shown a decline, but statistically significantly so for only 6 of the indicators, while 5 indicators showed increases, 3 of them significantly. Thus, overall little decrease in health differences seems to have occurred over the decade of the 1990s, and for some groups on some measures, notable increases were revealed, particularly for American Indians/Alaskan Natives.

"MEASURING" ETHNICITY

Turning back to ethnicity/race as a means to measure a concept, much debate has focused on the appropriateness of using self-reported ethnicity or race as a variable to predict or explain differences in health and other outcomes. A substantial scientific literature over the past two decades discusses the problems surrounding the use of "ethnicity" as an independent variable (i.e., a characteristic that influences other characteristics, but is not itself affected by those characteristics). A consensus among researchers is not apparent, but ethnicity (and gender) continue to be used as if they are potential causes in a wide range of health outcomes. This, in spite of the fact that many experts in scientific research methods agree that measuring and using ethnicity for this purpose may produce nothing more than descriptive results at best, and onereous ones at worst. Some argue that ethnicity and race are simply sociopolitical concepts that have little, if any, basis in scientific reality. Others, however, argue that underlying genetic differences exist among ethnic and racial groups (and other groups) and that these genetic differences may well be important factors that contribute to risks for both mental and physical illnesses. Knowledge about such factors might contribute to more effective diagnosis and better treatments. Still others argue that even if group genetic differences do matter, cultural and social differences between ethnic groups contribute greatly to behaviors that are causes of or associated with a variety of health factors.

It has often been argued that although genetic, behavioral, social, and cultural differences among ethnic groups may be predictors of average health status, it is much more important to examine differences within the ethnic group than to examine the differences between ethnic groups to gain an understanding of the health and illness and to increase effectiveness of diagnosis and treatment. Additional problems with using ethnicity to explain or predict health are substantial. Researchers often assume that individuals in an ethnic group all share some common characteristic associated with culture, and that the cultural characteristic is associated with mental or physical ill health. Two major problems are apparent with this thinking. First, as previously discussed, there is considerable variation among individuals within an ethnic group on almost all characteristics. Second, ethnicity usually serves as a substitute for some other concept of true interest, such as culture, and in particular specific features of culture. Thus, ethnicity is often used as a substitute measure for culture or attitudes or behaviors. These are usually much more difficult to measure, and thus researchers simply assess ethnicity instead.

The measurement of the variable that is directly associated with the outcome is easier to defend scientifically. For example, if a researcher were studying use of birth control and determined that those who identified themselves as "Hispanic" were significantly less likely to use birth control pills, it would be scientifically imprecise (some methodologists and theoreticians would say flat wrong) to say that being a member of an ethnic group "causes" use of specific birth control methods. A variable that might be closer to the outcome (here, use of a specific birth control method) might be "religious preference" because Hispanics predominantly identify themselves as Catholics, and the Catholic formal doctrine forbids use of birth control pills. But "religious preference" would still be a substitute variable since many Hispanics may express a Catholic religious preference, but not equally hold to the church doctrine about birth control, and thus use birth control pills. Probably closer characteristics of pill use would be attitudes about birth control or acceptance of Catholic religious doctrine or prior experiences with birth control or the lack of experience with birth control methods. Measures of these might well show much better ability to predict birth control use than simply having the status of "Hispanic ethnicity." Hence, rather than just using "ethnicity," researchers should carefully think about the likely causes of the outcome they are studying and measure those characteristics that are the most directly associated with the outcome, if possible. Commonly, that means measuring past behaviors or current attitudes or beliefs fairly directly rather than simply assessing ethnic group status.

Another serious problem in the assessment of ethnicity involves how to categorize individuals who are of "mixed" ethnicity or individuals who are not aware of their "full ethnicity." If the characteristic that was most closely associated with the outcome under study was assessed instead of the substitute characteristic ethnicity, this problem would disappear. Frequently the problem of great diversity within ethnic groups is compounded by researchers who "homogenize" so-called minority groups by comparing the responses of all minority ethnic groups to whites, as if all members of all minority ethnic groups share something in common.

Another problem is that in many research studies that detect differences across various ethnic groups, the ethnic groups vary in many ways other than underlying culture or attitudes or beliefs. For example, they differ in educational level, income level, age distribution, language fluency, general acculturation, and many possibly unknown ways. Researchers often attempt to "control" for such differences using statistics, but serious problems exist for interpreting such analyses that "equate" groups using various covariates. Simply put, real differences in groups cannot be meaningfully eliminated using abstract mathematical "corrections." Thus, nonequivalent ethnic groups are different in many ways, and statistical controls cannot disentangle such differences in any clear manner.

Recommendations for the application of several guidelines for using ethnicity in research have been made by many authors: (a) make clear the assumptions that are the basis for the use and assessment of ethnicity in a particular context; (b) test specific hypotheses about specific aspects of culture or other characteristics of ethnicity rather than using ethnicity as a substitute variable; (c) consider matching samples of different ethnic groups selected for study while retaining as much diversity within the group; (d) fully report in scientific manuscripts the sample characteristics and sampling methodology used in studies; (e) use sample sizes large enough to adequately detect the differences that are likely to be found in naturally occurring groups; (f) use several measures and several assessment methods, where feasible, to be sure that the concept being measured is actually the causal factor being studied (i.e., convergent validity); (g) work with cultural/ethnic experts to ensure appropriate translation of language and concepts of the measures being used; and (h) use study results to generate further research rather than assume findings are valid. Thus, use of the concept of ethnicity should entail careful thinking and planning to enable the collection of data of the highest quality and that most directly speak to the research questions.

It is clear that various "ethnic groups" as commonly assessed differ on many characteristics, including many measures of health status, but it is also true that such groups differ on many other characteristics, such as income, education, language use, general acculturation, attitudes, beliefs, and values, among many others. It seems unwise to attribute differences, such as differences in health status, purely to characteristics of ethnic status in any simple or direct manner. Different ethnic groups for many reasons experience the world in different ways, which are likely in turn to lead to differences among and within ethnic groups in many complex ways. Indeed, different ethnic groups express different cultures, and it is the more direct study of specific aspects of culture that may lead to greater understanding of the differential ethnic experiences, rather than stereotypically treating all members of the same ethnic group as the same. That is, it is not only important to recognize the diversity among the many ethnic groups in the United States and the world, but also to recognize the immense diversity with each of those groups and to attempt to understand how the greater diversity may or may not contribute to variation in health among individuals.

SEE ALSO: Acculturation, African American, Asian and Pacific Islander, Birth control, Cardiovascular disease, Education, Latinos, Socioeconomic status

Suggested Reading

Alvidrez, J., & Arean, P. A. (2002). Psychosocial treatment research with ethnic minority populations: Ethical considerations in conducting clinical trials. *Ethics and Behavior, 12*, 103–116.

Burchard, E. G., Ziv, E., Coyle, N., Gomez, S. L., Tang, H., Karter, A. J., et al. (2003). The importance of race and ethnic background in biomedical research and clinical practice. *New England Journal of Medicine, 348*, 1170–1175.

Cooper, R., Kaufman, J. S., & Ward, R. (2003). Race and genomics. *New England Journal of Medicine, 348*, 1166–1170.

Keppel, K. G., Pearcy, J. N., & Wagener, D. K. (2002). Trends in racial and ethnic-specific rates for the health status indicators: United States, 1990–1998. *Healthy People Statistical Notes, 23*, 1–16.

Nazroo, J. Y. (2003). The structuring of ethnic inequalities in health: Economic position, racial discrimination, and racism. *American Journal of Public Health, 93*, 277–284.

Okazaki, S., & Sue, S. (1995). Methodological issues in assessment research with ethnic minorities. *Psychological Assessment, 7*, 367–375.

Phinney, J. (1996). When we talk about American ethnic groups what do we mean? *The American Psychologist, 51*, 918–927.

Triandis, H. C. (1996). The psychological measurement of cultural syndromes. *The American Psychologist, 51*, 407–415.

U.S. Department of Health and Human Services. (2001). *Mental health: Culture, race, and ethnicity.* Washington, DC: Author.

Walsh, M. E., Katz, M. A., & Sechrest, L. (2002). Unpacking cultural factors in adaptation to type 2 diabetes mellitus. *Medical Care, 40*, 129–139.

Witzig, R. (1996). The medicalization of race: Scientific legitimization of a flawed social construct. *Annals of Internal Medicine, 125*, 675–684.

Zuckerman, M. (1990). Some dubious premises in research and theory on racial differences: Scientific, social, and ethical issues. *The American Psychologist, 45*, 1297–1303.

TEDDY D. WARNER

Examination *see* Pelvic Examination, Physical Examination

Exercise
Women can expect to maintain a youthful and independent life by establishing a regular exercise program. The multiple benefits of exercise for women are well documented in research conducted over the past 30 years. Exercise can reduce the risk of heart disease, prevent osteoporosis, maintain a healthy body weight, improve mental alertness, reduce fatigue, and eliminate stress. More recent studies even show a reduction in breast and colon cancer in women who lead an active, healthy lifestyle.

Exercise

According to the Centers for Disease Control, heart disease is the number one cause of death in women, with an estimated mortality rate of 500,000 women per year in the United States. A low aerobic fitness level is an independent risk factor for cardiovascular mortality in women who have coronary artery disease. Nevertheless, the death rate can be reduced by regular exercise. A recent study concluded that women who walked at least 3 hours per week cut their risk of dying of cardiovascular disease by 40%.

Exercise improves cardiovascular mortality by reducing the major risk factors for heart disease. This includes lowering high blood pressure, total cholesterol, low-density lipoproteins (LDLs) and triglycerides, and increasing high-density lipoproteins (HDLs). Exercise also promotes decreases in body weight and fat stores. It offers a nonpharmaceutical approach to ward off the expense, side effects, and morbidity and mortality of drugs and surgery. Regular exercise combined with a healthy diet is the best strategy for preventing heart disease.

A second major benefit of regular physical activity is strengthening bones, thereby reducing the risk of osteoporosis (loss of bone density). Osteoporosis affects in excess of 20 million postmenopausal American women. It leads to muscular weakness, bone fractures (primarily of the hip and spine), disability, and death. Less than one third of women who fracture their hip recover sufficiently to conduct basic life activities. Although osteoporosis can be a debilitating disease, the potential consequences are preventable by combining low-impact and resistance exercises with a calcium-enriched diet.

Regular activity that includes both weight bearing and resistance exercises also improves bone mineral density, and even when bone loss has already occurred, exercise can halt and may reverse bone loss. In addition to these benefits, exercise builds muscle that helps maintain strength, balance, and coordination—all of which play a key role in preventing bone-breaking falls. Many older women who fracture a hip or spine must depend on family members or long-term care facilities to aid in their daily living activities. Preventing osteoporotic fractures is a critical component of the quality of life for the growing population of older American women.

In addition to physical benefits, regular exercise improves mental well-being; it reduces emotional stress and alleviates bouts of anxiety and depression. Studies demonstrate that exercise stimulates the release of endorphins—the feel-good hormones. Psychologists have observed that walking or running has both physiologic and psychological benefits for people who are depressed. A study of women suffering from mild depression found that when they became involved in a fitness program, their symptoms decreased significantly compared to women placed on an antidepressant.

Physical fitness also leads to increased mental alertness and capacity; sleep quality improves and that leads to reducing fatigue. Research has shown that self-esteem and self-control increase with regular exercise, enhancing both mood and mental health. Self-confidence is also improved through regular exercise, and that contributes to better work performance and ability to better handle life's personal and professional challenges.

The benefits of exercise start when you begin. Recommendations to increase physical activity need not include formal regimens or gym memberships. Those beginning an exercise program, whether formal or informal, should strive to make it enjoyable, choosing a regimen that includes variety to work multiple muscle groups and to prevent boredom and sustain motivation. However, in order to enjoy all of the benefits of exercise, it is essential that beginners visit their doctor for a physical checkup and obtain medical clearance before starting any exercise program.

The American Academy of Sports Medicine (AASM) recommends at least 30 min of cardiovascular activity on most days of the week. The 30-min sessions can take place all at once, or they can be divided into 10- or 15-min sessions. Cardiovascular benefits are achieved by reaching and maintaining 60–80% of the target heart rate for the entire 30-min period. Your target heart rate is calculated by subtracting your age from 220 and multiplying that number by 0.6 or 0.8 (depending on your health status). Cardiovascular exercises include walking, running, aerobic dance, swimming, elliptical trainers, stair-climbers, and cross-country ski machines.

In addition to low-impact cardiovascular activity, an exercise regimen should include resistance/weight training to help maintain bone density. For example, free-weights or weight machines both contribute to bone health. Resistance training should be included 2–4 times in a weekly exercise program. Stronger bone is built by training the major muscle groups of both the upper and lower body. Work muscle groups on alternating days in order to prevent muscle damage. A reasonable target objective is two or three sets of 8–15 repetitions for each activity. Begin with lower weights, and then determine the proper amount by noting when a particular weight causes the muscle to fatigue during the last few repetitions.

Exercise should become a part of daily activity. Many women fail to exercise, citing family and career responsibilities as obstacles that prevent them from maintaining a regular program. However, when exercise becomes an integral part of daily life, women can better handle their many responsibilities. The physical and mental benefits of exercise are too numerous to ignore, especially as a means of promoting and maintaining a younger, healthier body. The benefits of exercise start when you begin.

SEE ALSO: Body mass index, Cardiovascular disease, Cholesterol, Coronary artery disease, Coronary risk factors, Depression, Hypertension, Osteoporosis and osteopenia, Sports injuries, Yoga

Suggested Reading

American College of Sports Medicine. (2000). *ACSM's guidelines for exercise testing and prescription* (6th ed.). New York: Lippincott, Williams & Wilkins.

American Heart Association. (1997). *American Heart Association fitting in fitness: Hundreds of simple ways to put more physical activity into your life.* New York: Times Books.

Kolata, G. (2003). *Ultimate fitness: The quest for truth about health and exercise.* New York: Farrar, Straus & Giroux.

Meeks, S. (1999). *Walk tall: An exercise program for the prevention and treatment of osteoporosis.* Gainesville, FL: Triad.

Thayer, R. E. (2001). *Calm energy: How people regulate mood with food and exercise.* New York: Oxford University Press.

Villepigue, J., & Rivera, H. A. (2002). *The body sculpting bible for women.* New York: Hatherleigh.

MARY ANTHONY

F

Falls Prevention

A fall is defined as an *unplanned descent to the ground with or without injury*. Risk factors for falls are described as *intrinsic* (having to do with an individual's condition and symptoms, or internal characteristics of the individual) or *extrinsic* (having to do with the environment, or characteristics that are external to the individual).

Examples of intrinsic risk factors are heart problems and sleep disturbances, postmeal blood pressure changes, neurological and muscle disease, urinary or bowel incontinence, dementia or mental confusion, and impulsivity. Examples of extrinsic risk factors include icy sidewalks, throw rugs, or poor footwear. Falls can happen to anyone anytime. Older women, especially Caucasian and Asian women, are at higher risk. Falls are the leading cause of death in people over age 75. Most falls occur in the home, and many occur either in the bathroom or when getting up to go to the toilet. Hip fractures are the most severe consequence of a fall, and 75% of people who suffer a hip fracture never recover completely. Half of all patients who suffer a fall causing serious injury will die within 1 year.

Older people are at higher risk of falling because the natural process of aging reduces eyesight, balance, and proprioception (the inner sense of the body's position in space). Osteoporosis is a major risk factor for falls among middle- to late-aged women, because it can affect strength, balance, and postural stability. Injury due to falls and the fear of repeat falls can cause elderly people to avoid physical activity, leading to reduced strength and deconditioning, putting them at even greater risk for falls. A history of previous falls, especially within the last 3 months, is among the strongest predictors of repeat falls.

Simple changes can reduce the risk of falls in the household, such as removing clutter, tripping hazards, and slippery surfaces. Throw rugs and electrical cords running across the floor should be eliminated. Carpet edges should be tacked or taped down. Bathrooms should have sturdy grab rails near the tub and toilet (towel rods are not strong enough). Elevated toilet seats can make it easier to sit and stand up again. In some cases, a bedside commode may be necessary to reduce the need to walk any distance or climb stairs at night. Lighting should be bright and easily accessible in all rooms of the house. Stairs should have handrails on both sides. Footwear should be practical, with nonskid soles and adequate support. Nighttime footwear should be nonskid, fit snugly, and not fall off. Alcohol intake should be minimized or avoided completely.

If assistive devices such as canes or walkers are needed, they should be used consistently. In the case of falls, false pride and unwillingness to use appropriate equipment can lead to life-threatening injury. Scheduled toileting can help avoid the urgent need to urinate and reduce the risk of falls. Drinking adequate fluids will help avoid lowered blood pressure from mild dehydration. People who become dizzy when arising from bed should sit on the bed for 1–2 minutes before walking. Balancing and strengthening exercises such as water exercise, tai chi, or yoga can reduce the risk of falls. If physical conditions such as urinary urgency or dizziness are a persistent problem, medical treatment may be helpful.

Some medications can increase the risk of falls. Sedating medications can cause grogginess. Blood pressure medications can cause dizziness. Appropriate use of these medications can minimize the risk of falls. Elderly people should ask their physician to review their medications with the risk of falling in mind. If an elderly person falls twice within 6 months, even without significant injury, a medical evaluation should be done to look for treatable causes.

SEE ALSO: Osteoporosis and osteopenia

Suggested Resources

AARP checklist for home safety: www.aarp.org/universalhome/check-list.html

EVANNE JURATOVAC

Fecundity

Fecundity It is clear that women's fecundity, or fertility, decreases with increasing age. By the age of 35, a woman has half the chance of becoming pregnant than a 25-year-old. An assessment of the ovarian capacity for fertility can be accomplished with some simple tests. These tests do not have a high sensitivity or a high specificity. An abnormal test is associated with a poor pregnancy rate but a normal test does not guarantee a successful outcome. The most commonly used test for ovarian reserve is to measure follicle-stimulating hormone (FSH) and the hormone estradiol on day 3 of a menstrual cycle. A more sensitive test is to measure a day 3 FSH and estradiol, followed by ovarian stimulation with the medication clomiphene citrate 100 mg from days 5 to 9 of the cycle. Another serum FSH is performed on day 10, after completion of the clomiphene citrate. An elevated serum FSH (generally 12 IU/L, but this varies according to the lab) or estradiol (greater than 80 pg/mL) is associated with a poor prognosis with assisted reproductive technology.

A variety of environmental factors have been associated with decreased fecundity. Reproductive toxins such as ethylene glycol and toluene are commonly found in the workplace. Smoking and heavy use of marijuana will decrease fertility in men and women. Alcohol in high quantities (more than five drinks per week) is also associated with decreased fertility as well as a variety of pregnancy-related complications, such as preterm deliveries. Some studies have linked high caffeine intake with delayed conception. Commercially available lubricants and saliva are also spermicidal.

SEE ALSO: Endometriosis, Infertility

Suggested Reading

Clark, A. M., Thornley, B., Tomlinson, L., Galletley, C., & Norman, R. J. (1998). Weight loss in obese infertile women results in improvement in reproductive outcome for all forms of fertility treatment. *Human Reproduction, 13*, 1502–1505.

Falcone, T., Goldberg, J. M., & Miller, K. F. (1996). Endometriosis: Medical and surgical intervention. *Current Opinion in Obstetrics and Gynecology, 8*, 178–183.

Hatch, E. E., & Bracken, M. B. (1993). Association of delayed conception with caffeine consumption. *American Journal of Epidemiology, 138*, 1082–1092.

Legro, R. S., Finegood, D., & Dunaif, A. (1998). A fasting glucose to insulin ratio is a useful measure of insulin sensitivity in women with polycystic ovary syndrome. *Journal of Clinical Endocrinology and Metabolism, 83*, 2694–2698.

Pagidas, K., Falcone, T., Hemmings, R., & Miron, R. (1996). Comparison of surgical treatment of moderate (stage iii) and severe (stage iv) endometriosis-related infertility with IVF_ET. *Fertility and Sterility, 65*, 791–795.

Rowe, P., Comhaire, F., Hargreave, T. B., & Mahmoud, A. M. (Eds.). (2000). *WHO manual for the standardized investigation, diagnosis and management of the infertile male.* Cambridge, UK: Cambridge University Press.

Sharara, F. L., Scott, R. T., Jr., & Seifer, D. B. (1998). The detection of diminished ovarian reserve in infertile women. *American Journal of Obstetrics and Gynecology, 179*, 804–812.

TOMMASO FALCONE
RAKESH SHARMA

Female Genital Mutilation

Female Genital Mutilation Female genital mutilation (FGM), also known as female circumcision or female genital cutting, is a common practice in most African and some Middle-Eastern countries. FGM can be classified into five types:

Type 1: Sunna (traditional)—removal of varying degrees of the clitoral prepuce.

Type 2: Intermediate—developed by a midwife in the early 1950s in response to an edict by the government of Sudan forbidding Pharonic circumcision (see below). This method includes the removal of the clitoris, labia minora, and parts of the labia majora.

Type 3: Pharonic—similar to the intermediate, but usually more severe and encompassing the removal of greater parts of the labia majora.

Type 4: Infibulation (sometimes used synonymously with the Pharonic circumcision)—after the Pharonic and intermediate forms of circumcision, the left and right raw edges of the female genitalia are sewn together using suture, string, thorns, silk, or whatever might be available.

Type 5: Incision—incising the clitoral prepuce, which is the technique for female circumcision in most parts of the world other than sub-Saharan regions of Africa.

Today the practice of FGM is primarily associated with certain ethnic groups and has no relation to political or religious boundaries. It is found across the African continent in a broad, triangular east–west band that stretches from Egypt in the northeast and Tanzania in the southeast to Senegal in the west. Infibulation occurs most frequently in the Horn of Africa, namely, Ethiopia, Djibouti, Somalia, and Sudan. The World Health Organization estimates that between 85 and 114 million girls and women have been subjected to this practice. There are many cultural beliefs surrounding FGM that vary by region and ethnic origin. Some of the more universally accepted beliefs include that FGM will decrease the woman's sexual desire, prevent promiscuity, and ensure chastity before marriage; that it enhances physical beauty; that it helps maintain cleanliness and health; and that it provides greater pleasure for men.

In addition to cultural beliefs, there are many religious beliefs surrounding FGM. Many relate the practice to the Islamic religion because of the wide use of the term "Sunna" for one type of circumcision, which means "following the traditions of the Prophet Mohammed." However, it is mistaken to believe that this practice is limited only to the Islamic religion. Some groups that practice Christianity also practice FGM. There are also a number of social commonalities associated with FGM, including tradition, rights of passage, ancestor worship, sacrifices to fertility gods, and protection of the family honor.

FGM presents several health risks. The most frequent complications include severe pain, blood loss, inability to empty the bladder, infection of the wound, and damage to adjacent tissues. More severe immediate effects are sepsis (severe infection sometimes called "blood poisoning"), shock, and tetanus. HIV and hepatitis may be passed through the use of unsterile instruments, especially when groups of girls undergo FGM at the same time. Long-term complications include chronic pelvic inflammatory disease, chronic urinary tract infection, sexual difficulties, infertility, and problems with labor and delivery. Menstrual and urinary blockages are very common. Urinary dermoid cysts are very common and can grow to the size of a grapefruit. Keloid scars, which commonly form on the vulval wound, can become so enlarged that they obstruct walking. However, they do not threaten health except during labor. It is estimated that 31% of circumcised women develop at least one, and more commonly several, of these complications.

Decircumcision, the splitting of the circumcision skin fold, is always necessary during labor. Despite the suffering, most women request recircumcision after delivery. Infibulation causes prolongation of labor and obstructed delivery, with increased risk of brain damage to the infant and stillbirth. Another problem related to childbirth is the development of a passage between the bladder and the vagina (vesicovaginal fistulae). This is caused when the head of the fetus exerts friction or pressure against the urinary bladder for a long time, which can occur for several hours as the infant's head slowly passes through the birth canal. As a result, the thin membranes between the vagina and bladder break down, leaving a hole. Postpartum blood loss is another concern due to the cutting of scar tissue, often by untrained midwives.

The World Health Organization has taken an active role in eliminating the practice of FGM, providing technical and financial support for grass-roots initiatives. In 1995, the 104th Congress of the United States passed Senate Bill 1030, the Federal Prohibition of Female Genital Mutilation Act of 1995, outlawing the practice of FGM of girls under the age of 18. Several states have implemented similar laws.

SEE ALSO: Immigrant health, Infertility

Suggested Reading

Lightfoot-Klein, H. (1989). *Prisoners of ritual: An odyssey into female circumcision in Africa.* New York: Harrington Park Press.

Toubia, N. (1994, September). Female circumcision as a public health issue. *The New England Journal of Medicine,* 712–716.

Toubia, N., & Izett, S. (1998). *Female genital mutilation: An overview.* Geneva: World Health Organization.

GAIL E. SOUARE

Female Trouble *see* Abdominal Pain, Menopause, Menstrual Cycle Disorders, Menstruation, Ovarian Cyst, Pelvic Pain, Sexual Organs

---

Feminine Ethics *see* Feminist Ethics

Femininity Femininity is defined in various dictionaries in either a circular manner as *the quality of being feminine* or indirectly as *qualities associated with the female sex.* This is because femininity is typically conceptualized as a constellation of multiple interacting elements that coalesce to yield an energy, an essence, or a state of being. We recognize femininity when it is encountered, but it is difficult to distill the interacting elements to a single, unifying definition that can be applied uniformly. Femininity also is often confused with gender role, which is a categorized distinction of activities and responsibilities deemed socially appropriate for females and males in a particular society (see Gender role). However, using a linguistic metaphor to illustrate the difference, gender role represents the parts of speech, whereas femininity and masculinity represent the grammatical rules of style under which the parts of speech can be combined to generate prose.

The dominant conceptualization of femininity in most modern societies is best described by sex-role theory, which proposes that humans unconsciously integrate archetypical ways of behaving that are appropriate to their assigned sex from society's institutions. Sex-role theory organizes women's behavior as passive, intuitive, submissive, and subjective, whereas men's behavior is classified as aggressive, rational, dominant, and objective.

Idealized versions of sex-role theory in which these qualities are alleged to complement each other in a balanced way can be found in the folklore of many cultures (e.g., yin/yang, sun/moon, and the like). However, sex-role theory fails to account for the fact that cultures do not value the characteristics of each sex equally. Women are not esteemed for their passivity to the same degree as men are for their aggressiveness.

Feminist scholars exposed the limitation of sex-role theory by emphasizing that different power levels exist in society's femininity/masculinity archetypes. In response, sociologists scrutinized sex-role theory and deemed it too rigid in several key areas. Primary among these is that it fails to recognize that women and men do not always embody their respective archetypes, other than to label this diversity as deviant. Furthermore, it does not address individual differences in behavior in various situations. Femininity, as it is characterized by sex-role theory, is an archetype that few, if any, women exemplify all of the time. Sex-role theory also fails to articulate how characteristics become assigned to feminine and masculine archetypes. For example, there may be no daily activity that requires more rational thinking than being the primary caretaker of a child, yet rationality is assigned as a characteristic of the masculine archetype. Additionally, the most successful figures in men's professional sports are those who are described as having an intuitive sense of the game, yet intuition is assigned as a characteristic of the feminine archetype. Sex-role theory also assumes that gender forms the core of a person's identity and ignores other key contextual factors such as race, ethnicity, class, and religion.

Regardless of how femininity is conceptualized, more often than not, it occupies a position of lesser value relative to masculinity, a reality all but ignored in sex-role theory. This is evidenced by the near universal and exclusive linkage of feminine worth with chastity. In fact, some theorists contend that femininity is portrayed in religious texts as a metaphor for immorality, whereas masculinity is depicted as righteous. For example, the Christian Bible—in particular the Old Testament—portrays femininity as treacherous, undisciplined, lascivious, deceiving, and manipulative—qualities that must be held in constant check by men. Consequently, in addition to archetypical representations of chastity, religious texts depict femininity as a rebellious spirit that can be redeemed only through obedience to men.

Responding to the inadequacy of sex-role theory to provide an accurate representation of how women and men relate to each other, sociologists developed a new theoretical framework that appropriately considers the structure of power, the sexual division of labor, and the social organization of sexuality and attraction. The Theory of Hegemonic Masculinity proposes that an archetypical form of masculinity exists in a given culture within a particular historical period, that masculinity always defines itself as different from and superior to femininity, and that social processes are organized to maintain masculine power by ensuring that subordinate groups view male dominance as fair, reasonable, and in the best interests of the society (see Masculinity). Thus, femininity is constructed around adaptation to male power. Its core component is attractiveness to men, around which revolve physical appearance, chastity, exclusive heterosexuality, sexual availability in the absence of sexual assertiveness, nurturance of children, obedience and deference to male authority, and ego-massaging (among others). In this respect, femininity could be construed as a social euphemism for female subordination to male dominance.

See Also: Body image, Feminism, Gender, Gender role, Latinos, Marianismo, Masculinity, Veils

Suggested Reading

Hofstede, G., & Arrindell, W. A. (1998). *Masculinity and femininity: The taboo dimension of national cultures* (Cross-Cultural Psychology, Vol. 3). Thousand Oaks, CA: Sage.

Trigiani, K. *Out of the cave: Exploring Gray's anatomy* (website). http://web2.iadfw.net/ktrig246/out_of_cave/index.htm

White, E. (2002). *Fast girls: Teenage tribes and the myth of the slut.* New York: Scribner's.

ANGELA PATTATUCCI ARAGON

Feminism To speak of *feminism* in the context of a set of overarching ideals that define a unified movement is a misrepresentation. It is more accurate to speak of *feminisms*, which highlights the fact that identifying oneself as a feminist can mean different things. Characteristic of any expanding movement, there are disagreements and overlap between feminists. This does not mean to suggest that feminism is fragmented, but rather to emphasize the diversity of feminist thought and belief that is respected.

Radical feminism is paramount among the many flavors of modern feminism. Often characterized as feminism's unappealing element, radical feminism has been the creative engine generating the theoretical development that has formed the foundation of contemporary feminist thought. Radical feminism was born out of the civil rights and peace movements of the late 1960s. Radical feminists view the oppression of women as the most fundamental form of oppression, one that cuts across boundaries of race, culture, and economic class.

Their goal is revolutionary social change. At the heart of radical feminism is challenging how gender is constructed and reified into gender roles. Radical feminism questions authority, including authority arising from within feminism, and as such has been responsible for spawning many of the other varieties of feminism.

As radical feminism splintered into several other groups, cultural feminism came into prominence. Although some claim that radical feminism simply evolved into cultural feminism, the fundamental approach of the two movements is quite different. While radical feminism seeks to transform society, cultural feminism is pessimistic about the possibility for sustainable social change and instead focuses on building alternatives. Cultural feminists rationalize that if changing the dominant culture is unrealistic, then at least they can avoid it as much as possible. The justification for abandoning social change as a goal emerges out of a collection of theoretical work that argues for the inherent superiority of the female sex (women are *kinder and gentler*). Regardless of whether it is biologically determined or socially constructed, cultural feminists believe that women's kinder and gentler nature is so thoroughly ingrained that it is intractable.

A second group that splintered from the radical movement of the 1960s consists of the separatists. Commonly but incorrectly labeled lesbians, these are feminists across all sexual orientations who advocate separation from men; in some cases it is total, whereas in others it is partial. The essence of separatism is that by separating from men, women are able to view themselves in a different context. Many feminists embrace this belief by participating in various forms of temporary separation for personal growth (e.g., all-women retreats). The difference is that separatists practice this philosophy as a lifestyle.

Marxist/socialist feminism is another branch that splintered from the radical movement. Marxist/socialist feminists argue that women are oppressed, and attribute that oppression to the capitalist/private property system. They advocate the overthrow of the capitalist system as the ultimate way of ending women's oppression.

Radical feminism and its numerous branches primarily represent a movement focused on issues defined by white women, rendering women of color invisible. However, out of the civil rights movement of the 1960s emerged a strong group of feminists of color who paralleled the philosophy and the dynamic nature of radical feminism in many respects but would not, because they could not, limit their focus to women's issues. Feminists of color maintain that women's oppression must be considered in a broader context than just a myopic focus on sexism.

Departing from the political and theoretical focus of other branches, ecofeminism is more spiritually oriented and in some circles is combined with Goddess worship and/or vegetarianism. The essence of ecofeminism is the belief that the exploitation of resources without regard to long-term consequences is the direct result of attitudes fostered by a patriarchal/hierarchical society. Thus, parallels are often drawn between society's oppression of women and its treatment of the environment. By resisting patriarchal domination, ecofeminists believe that they are also resisting the plundering and destroying of the Earth. Beyond its focus on socially conscious environmentalism, ecofeminism is a variation on Marxist/socialist feminism.

Liberal feminism is a variety of feminism that works within the structure of mainstream society to integrate women into that structure. It is basically a social justice movement that seeks equality for women and traces its roots back to the feminism of past centuries, such as the suffragist movement. The compromise and accommodation strategies of liberal feminists line up well with the *kinder and gentler* beliefs of cultural feminists. However, these methods have met with limited success. Although liberal feminists are associated with some of the most profound advances for women, more often than not, the advances were the result of a radical movement emerging out of dissatisfaction with the slow pace of progress that pushed the liberal feminist agenda to the left of center.

SEE ALSO: Femininity, Feminist ethics, Gender, Gender role, Lesbian, Lesbian ethics, Masculinity, Queer

Suggested Reading

Cott, N. F. (1989). *The grounding of modern feminism.* New Haven, CT: Yale University Press.
Hooks, B. (2000). *Feminism is for everybody: Passionate politics.* Cambridge, MA: South End Press.
Moraga, C. L., Tinker, J., & Anzaldua, G. E. (1984). *This bridge called my back: Writings by radical women of color* (2nd ed.). New York: Kitchen Table Press.

ANGELA PATTATUCCI ARAGON

Feminist Ethics

It cannot be said that there is one feminist perspective on issues related to health and health care. In fact, the perspective known as "feminist ethics" actually encompasses greatly divergent views and multiple schools of thought, including liberal feminism, Marxist feminism, radical feminism, psychoanalytic feminism, and socialist feminism. In addition, a distinction has been drawn between feminist and feminine ethics. Whereas feminist ethics is said to argue against patriarchal dominations, for equal rights, and a just and fair distribution of scarce resources, feminine ethics advocates on behalf of an ethics of care that encompasses nurturance, care, compassion, and networks of communications. The ethic of care rejects the cognitive emphasis of other approaches to ethical analysis and emphasizes the moral role of emotions. The detachment inherent in the cognitive approaches is criticized precisely because it fails to recognize the attachment inherent in relationships.

Feminist/feminine ethics accomplishes four tasks: (a) the provision of an emphasis on the importance of women and their interests; (b) the provision of a focus on issues especially affecting women; (c) the reexamination of fundamental assumptions; and (d) the incorporation of feminist insights from other fields into the field of ethics. Feminist medical ethics has been assigned the responsibility of developing conceptual models that will restructure the power associated with healing, to allow individuals to have the maximum degree of control possible over their own health.

EMPHASIZING WOMEN AND WOMEN'S ISSUES

Feminist ethics is often concerned with the content of the discussion, such as reproductive technologies and the rationing of medical care. For instance, while many ethicists approach the issue of abortion by weighing the relative importance of preserving life or protecting autonomy, feminist ethicists approach the issue of abortion by examining the difference that it will make in women's lives if they are free to decide to continue or not to continue each pregnancy. In general, feminist approaches to medical care have argued that increased reproductive technology generally means increased medical control.

Feminist ethicists have long argued that the medical research agenda in the United States is determined with reference to those who are white, upper and middle class, and male. The consequences of the resulting narrow perspective are troublesome: (a) hypotheses are developed and research conducted without reference to sex or gender, although the frequency of various diseases differs by sex; (b) some diseases which affect both sexes, such as coronary heart disease, are defined as male diseases, resulting in little research being conducted on women with those diseases; (c) research affecting primarily women has received a low funding priority; and (d) suggestions for research based on personal experiences of women have been ignored.

The exclusion of women from research results from a number of mechanisms, including eligibility criteria that specifically exclude women from participation in specific studies and reliance on gender-neutral eligibility that serve to exclude because they fail to take into account women's responsibility for the home and family. The exclusion of women has been defended with reference to the need for homogeneity among research participants to facilitate the research and statistical analysis, the potential liability that could result should a woman and/or her offspring be injured during the course of the research, and a belief that it is morally wrong to include women in studies because they may be, or may become, pregnant. The one notable exception has been the inclusion of women in contraceptive research.

Genetic research has been of particular concern for some feminist ethicists. Because women are already deemed to be responsible for reproduction and family life in general, it is feared that women's reproductive options will become fewer as physicians insist, based on newly acquired knowledge, that genetic testing constitutes the standard of care. Some theorists visualize a devaluation of motherhood, as women are denied the role of *the* mother of their children as a result of new technologies. One writer analogized the participation of women in such ventures to the trade of a prostitute who sells her womb, ovaries, and egg, instead of her vagina, rectum, and mouth. Because of these concerns, at least one ethicist has asserted that any ethical guidelines for preembryo research must involve women in their formation and in the formation of national policies relating to preembryo research and that the impact of proposed national policies on women as a group should be considered in their assessment.

SEE ALSO: Femininity, Feminism, Lesbian ethics, Patients' rights

Suggested Reading

Corea, G., et al. (Eds.). (1985). *Man-made women: How new reproductive technologies affect women* (pp. 38–51). London: Hutchinson.

Holmes, H. B., & Purdy, L. M. (Eds.). (1992). *Feminist perspectives in medical ethics* (pp. 8–13). Bloomington: Indiana University Press.

Larrabee, M. J. (Ed.). (1993). *An ethic of care: Feminist and interdisciplinary perspectives.* New York: Routledge.

Mastroianni, A., Faden, R., & Federman, D. (Eds.). (1994). *Ethical and legal issues of including women in clinical studies* (Vol. 2, pp. 11–17). Washington, DC: National Academy Press.

Tong, R. (1993). *Feminine and feminist ethics.* Belmont, CA: Wadsworth.

Tong, R. (1997). *Feminist approaches to bioethics: Theoretical reflections and practical applications.* Boulder, CO: Westview Press.

Wolf, S. M. (Ed.). (1996). *Feminism and bioethics: Beyond reproduction.* New York: Oxford University Press.

SANA LOUE

Fetal Alcohol Syndrome Fetal alcohol syndrome (FAS) is a pattern of birth defects resulting from drinking alcohol during pregnancy. FAS occurs in 1 out of every 750 births. It was formally recognized and named in the early 1970s and is currently the leading cause of mental retardation in the United States. Alcohol is directly responsible for up to 20% of cases of mental retardation with IQs in the 50–80 range (100 is considered normal); the average IQ for a child with full-blown FAS is 63. FAS is completely preventable if a woman does not drink alcohol during her entire pregnancy. Exactly how alcohol causes FAS is not well understood on a molecular level.

Symptoms of FAS are irreversible, and the brain damage caused by alcohol in a developing fetus is permanent. Children with FAS never "catch up" physically or mentally. Therefore, the best treatment for this condition is prevention. All women of childbearing age need to be screened for alcohol use disorders. Surveys estimate that 3.5% of pregnant women have a "frequent drinking" pattern, defined as two or more drinks per day or more than five drinks per occasion; 16.3% of pregnant women reported "any drinking," defined as at least one drink in the preceding month. Appropriate counseling techniques and referrals for ongoing treatment will help reduce or eliminate drinking before conception and during pregnancy.

Several factors help determine the effect alcohol will have on the fetus. Timing and dosage of alcohol exposure are important. Alcohol is most damaging in the first trimester of pregnancy. When the mother drinks, the fetus has the same blood alcohol level as the pregnant woman. However, because of its small size and immature liver, the fetus can stay drunk for 3–4 days even though the mother is only drunk for several hours. Binge drinking (defined as two or more drinks per hour) has been found to be more detrimental to the fetus than low-level, chronic drinking. However, because there is no proof that small amounts of alcohol are safe, the best advice is for women to completely abstain from alcohol during pregnancy.

Other factors that determine the effects of alcohol on the developing fetus include nutritional factors, metabolic factors, individual factors of the mother and child, and genetic factors. Among women who drink, risk factors for FAS include increased marital age, higher number of previous children, low socioeconomic status, other drug use, or a previous child with FAS.

Genetic factors can influence the incidence of FAS. One study reported that Southwest Plains Indians had an FAS rate of 9.8 per 1,000 live births, compared to a worldwide incidence of 1.9 per 1,000 live births. Southwest Plains Indians lack or have a reduced amount of an enzyme necessary to break down alcohol, causing higher and longer levels of alcohol exposure to the fetus.

The diagnosis of FAS is based on four criteria: prenatal alcohol exposure, growth retardation, facial malformations, and neurodevelopmental problems. The criteria for growth retardation include weight and height that fall below the 10th percentile. More than

one, but not necessarily all, of the following facial malformations must be present: short palpebral fissures, thin upper lip, indistinct philtrum, short nose, and flat midface. Other associated facial features may be present, but are not sufficient to determine the presence of FAS; these include epicanthal folds, a low nasal bridge, abnormal smallness of the jaw, and minor ear anomalies (Figure 1).

A wide variety of neurodevelopmental disorders are associated with FAS, including microcephaly (head circumference less than the 10th percentile), memory problems, impaired emotional attachment to caregivers, impaired motor skills, neurosensory hearing loss, learning disabilities, impaired visual/spatial skills, intellectual impairment, problems with reasoning and judgment, attention deficit disorder, and hyperactivity. More than one of these neurodevelopmental disorders may be identified, but not all conditions need to be present to diagnose FAS.

Children who do not meet all four criteria for FAS may still be injured by maternal alcohol use, in a condition that used to be known as fetal alcohol effects (FAE). In medical practice, FAE has been replaced by two terms, alcohol-related birth defects (ARBD) and alcohol-related neurodevelopmental disorder (ARND). ARBD includes abnormalities of the face, eyes, ears,

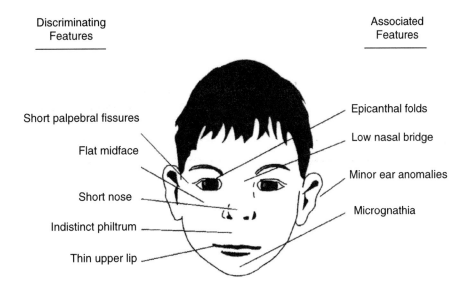

Figure 1. Facial features particularly characteristic of a child with fetal alcohol syndrome (FAS). Discriminating features (i.e., those considered definitive signs of FAS) are shown on the left side of the illustration; characteristics listed on the right side are associated with FAS but are not sufficient to determine the presence of the syndrome. Microencephaly (small head circumference) is not a facial feature per se, but a central nervous system characteristic. (Palpebral fissures = eye opening; philtrum = groove between nose and upper lip; epicanthal folds = skin folds covering inner corner of the eye; micrognathia = abnormal smallness of the jaw.) (*Source*: Streissguth & Little, 1994.)

heart, brain, kidneys, and limbs. Some examples of ARBD are atrial septal defect, ventral septal defect, bulging eyes (ptosis), low-set posterior rotation of the ear, poorly developed or absent kidneys, fusion of the radius and ulna bones in the forearm, and abnormal palmar creases. ARND includes changes in behavior, cognitive function, language, attention, memory, attachment, and fine motor skills.

SEE ALSO: Addiction, Alcohol use, Pregnancy, Substance abuse

Suggested Reading

Centers for Disease Control and Prevention. (1997). Alcohol consumption among pregnant and childbearing-aged women—United States, 1991 and 1995. *Morbidity and Mortality Weekly Report, 46*(16), 346–350.

Identification and care of fetal alcohol-exposed children: A guide for primary-care providers. (1999). NIH Publication No. 99-4369. Rockville, MD: NIAAA.

Identification of at-risk drinking and intervention with women of childbearing age: A guide for primary-care providers. (1999). NIH Publication No. 99-4368. Rockville, MD: NIAAA.

Stratton, K., Howe, C., & Battaglia, F. (Eds.). (1996). *Fetal alcohol syndrome: Diagnosis, epidemiology, prevention, and treatment.* Washington, DC: National Academy Press.

Suggested Resources

National Organization on Fetal Alcohol Syndrome (NOFAS): http://www.nofas.org

CHRISTINA M. DELOS REYES

Fetish The word *fetish* denotes both a magical charm and a fabrication or artifact. Most recently, the term has acquired a large repertoire of meanings and is often associated with fashion, sexuality, and/or power. In the context of eroticism, fetishism has been conceptualized along a spectrum ranging from Level 1, at which point there is only a slight preference for certain types of sexual partners, sexual stimuli, or sexual activity so that fetishism is not actually present, to Level 4, at which point specific stimuli may actually take the place of a sexual partner. Some fetishists are attracted to both the involved body part and its covering, while others focus on the covering only. Inanimate objects that are frequently the object of desire include, for instance, boots, stockings, body piercings, masks, and leather wear.

Some researchers have found that a degree of fetishism is extremely common among many men. For instance, some men may be fascinated with erotic lingerie or women in very high heels or wearing certain types of clothing. Although fetishism has often been associated in the media with sadomasochistic behaviors, fetishism does not require a dynamic of dominance and submission or sadistic–masochistic behavior or ritual.

In general, health care providers do not speak to their patients about the need to have "safer sex" when engaging in fetishistic sex. Sex toys, including whips and other devices, should be cleaned properly in order to avoid transmitting infections between individuals. This is especially true if any blood, semen, or vaginal fluid is involved.

SEE ALSO: Acquired immunodeficiency syndrome, Hepatitis, Libido and desire, Piercing, Safer sex, Tattoos

Suggested Reading

Gosselin, C., & Wilson, G. (1980). *Sexual variations: Fetishism, sadomasochism, transvestism.* New York: Simon & Schuster.

North, M. (1970). *The outer fringe of sex: A study in sexual fetishism.* London: Odyssey Press.

Steele, V. (1996). *Fetish: Fashion, sex & power.* New York: Oxford University Press.

DAVID VIDRA
SANA LOUE

Fibrocystic Breast Disease Fibrocystic breast disease, better called "fibrocystic changes," are common changes that affect most women, especially during the reproductive years. Approximately 60% of women will experience some symptoms related to fibrocystic breasts. Single or multiple benign tumors may be present, or a woman may just note general "lumpiness" in her breasts. Usually symptoms are worse prior to menses, but they may occur during any part of the cycle. After menopause, especially if women are not taking any hormone replacement therapy (HRT), symptoms usually lessen or disappear.

Fibrocystic changes are diagnosed primarily by history and physical examination. Breast cysts, which may be part of fibrocystic changes, may be noted on breast self-exam, or physical exam by a health care provider. A breast cyst is a fluid-filled space that is lined with glandular cells and may become large and painful. An ultrasound and/or breast aspiration can usually prove the diagnosis. In general, mammography does not have a role in diagnosing fibrocystic changes, and most importantly, fibrocystic changes do not increase a woman's risk of breast cancer.

Treatment of fibrocystic changes is aimed at relieving a woman's symptoms of pain and discomfort. Avoiding coffee, tea, caffeine, and chocolate is often recommended to relieve symptoms, but this is not supported by scientific data. Vitamins, calcium, birth control pills, diuretics, or "water pills" (particularly spironolactone), and a testosterone derivative, Danocrine, have all been used to relieve the symptoms of fibrocystic changes.

A woman with fibrocystic breast changes who finds a lump should still have the lump evaluated. A breast lump may be evaluated initially by fine needle aspiration. If the lump is aspirated and clear cyst fluid is obtained, then no further evaluation needs to be done. However, if a lump cannot be aspirated in the office, then often an ultrasound or ultrasound-guided aspiration will be attempted. If the lump is found to be solid, then it may need to be biopsied.

A solitary lump, particularly if found in an older woman, needs to be evaluated for possible breast cancer. If the breast biopsy is benign, in general, no further treatment is needed.

A solid lump, especially in a very young woman, is likely to be a fibroadenoma. A fibroadenoma is a solid, benign tumor that can grow very large, and is usually found in women who are in their teens or early 20s. They do not necessarily have to be removed, but many women choose to have these excised to avoid confusion about the possibility of cancer later in life.

While fibrocystic changes, per se, do not increase the risk of breast cancer, a biopsy showing hyperplasia, which is excessive cell growth, indicates a slightly increased risk of breast cancer. If these cells are both hyperplastic and atypical, then she has a risk of breast cancer that is higher yet.

As menopause approaches, many women who have had fibrocystic breast changes during their reproductive years may become more concerned about breast cancer. Even in women with fibrocystic changes, the recommendation for mammography remains the same. Mammography should be performed every 1–2 years during a woman's 40s and yearly after age 50.

In summary, it is important to emphasize that fibrocystic breast changes are not a disease and are common in most women of reproductive age.

SEE ALSO: Mammography

KAREN ASHBY

Fibromyalgia

Fibromyalgia syndrome (FMS) is a real illness with multiple symptoms that each need to be dealt with in order to achieve recovery. To treat FMS, one must understand what it is.

Most people with FMS report at least several, if not all, of the following symptoms:

1. Muscle and joint pain that can be severe at times and then let up
2. Decreased energy or feeling exhausted at times, and at other times feeling driven, which can lead to a vicious cycle of ups and downs
3. Tender points that are painful when pressed on, and generalized body aches
4. Mood problems, mostly depression, but also during pain-free times feeling pressured to make up for lost time
5. Insomnia or unrefreshing sleep: feeling unrested and fatigued on awakening
6. Mental cloudiness and confusion often referred to as "fibro fog," along with an excess of mental "noise"

The cause of these symptoms is uncertain. Normally, the brain filters out the "noise" of minor stresses such as the occasional body pains we all have. After undergoing a higher level of stress, the body seems to become hypersensitive to unpleasant sensations. A person with FMS then feels bombarded and overwhelmed.

Autoimmune dysfunction is often blamed because many people with FMS have abnormal rheumatological blood tests. Neurochemical abnormalities may play a role since depression is often a major part of the syndrome. FMS may be related to previous trauma such as a car accident or prior abuse. Probably, multiple causes combine to give rise to FMS. For example, a person may be genetically predisposed to FMS, but an event such as trauma or a viral illness may set off the cascade of symptoms.

FMS is a diagnosis of exclusion: that is, other causes must be ruled out before blaming FMS. The hallmark of FMS is pain and tenderness to touch in at least 11 of the 18 characteristic tender points. The tender points are best tested on a bad day, as the tenderness can come and go. Depending on the results of the medical history and physical examination, tests may be done to rule out autoimmune disorders, vitamin deficiencies (B$_{12}$, folic acid, or minerals), infections (such as Lyme disease or hepatitis C), or disease of various internal organs.

The cornerstone of FMS treatment includes moderate exercise and stretching. Overly vigorous exercise can make symptoms worse. Good dietary and sleep habits are important, as is minimizing physical and psychological stress.

Medications have a central role in treating symptoms but cannot cure FMS. Finding the right medication is often a matter of trial and error. For pain, over-the-counter and prescription nonsteroidal anti-inflammatory pain relievers are helpful. As with other chronic pain conditions, narcotics should be avoided. Antiseizure medications (including Neurontin, Tegretol, and Depakote) also help relieve pain, as well as stabilizing mood and helping the brain filter out pain "noise." Many people with FMS find antidepressants to be very helpful, both for pain and for mood symptoms. The serotonin reuptake inhibitors (SSRIs like Prozac, Paxil, Zoloft, and Celexa), tricyclic antidepressants, and others (such as Effexor, Remeron, or Wellbutrin) can help the brain deal with physical and psychological stress. Fibromyalgia syndrome patients often use muscle relaxants (such as Flexeril, Zanaflex, Soma, Skelaxin, and Norflex), usually along with anti-inflammatory medications, to treat muscle tightness and inflammation. Muscle relaxants are sedating, which can help FMS patients fall asleep. For initiating sleep, nonaddicting sleep medications (such as Ambien or Sonata) can be helpful. Tricyclic antidepressants (including amitriptyline, doxepin, or nortriptyline) can help bring about deep restorative sleep. Other medications used for sleep include Remeron or atypical agents such as Seroquel or Zyprexa.

Some clinicians recommend using a combination of medications from each category. Medications tend to help more than one symptom and different medications can have additive effects for the same symptom. It can take time to find the right mix, but eventually relief is possible.

See Also: Arthritis, Autoimmune disorders, Depression, Sleep disorders

Suggested Reading

Fransen, J., & Russell, I. J. (1996). *The fibromyalgia help book*. St. Paul, MN: Smith House Press.

Suggested Resources

National Fibromyalgia Association. 2238 N. Glassell St., Suite D, Orange, CA 92865; phone: (714) 921-0150. *Fibromyalgia aware*: www.fmaware.org

MARY C. SHEMO

Foot Care Lotions and exfoliants can be used to moisturize the area around the nails and dry skin on the feet. A pumice stone can be used to remove dead skin, particularly on areas that are callused. Individuals with dry skin may do so more frequently. Products containing aloe vera are often recommended to keep the skin moist.

Pain, swelling, and redness are signs that may indicate an infection or other problem, such as an ingrown nail. It is important to keep the area clean and to avoid "digging" into it in an attempt to cure the problem. In such situations, the individual may consult a podiatrist (doctor who specializes in the care of feet).

Pedicures can be relaxing and an enjoyable way of caring for one's feet. A pedicurist should be selected based on the cleanliness of the facility and his or her practice, rather than on the basis of price. Consider the following.

1. If the state requires a license to provide pedicures to the public, the license should be appropriately displayed and should be current.
2. All instruments used should be sterilized after each use or thrown away. Barbicide can be used to clean the equipment.
3. Cuts on the pedicurist's hand(s) should be covered to avoid possible transmission of infection to others.
4. The individual providing the pedicure should ask, or be informed if she does not, if the client has a particular medical condition that may predispose the client to a greater risk of injury or infection. For instance, individuals on blood thinners (such as Coumadin) may be at greater risk of seriously bleeding if they are cut by accident. Diabetic clients may be more prone to infection.

See Also: Diabetes, Skin care

Suggested Resources

http://www.cdc.gov/diabetes/pubs/complications/food.htm

MARA MEZA

G

Galactorrhea Galactorrhea is the spontaneous, nonobstetric production of bilateral white or clear nipple discharge. It is estimated to occur in 20–25% of women at some time in their life. Physiologic production of breast milk after pregnancy, or lactation, occurs after the breast has fully developed and been primed by numerous hormones including estrogen, progesterone, and thyroid hormone. The hormone prolactin is produced in the pituitary gland and promotes milk secretion. At the time of labor and delivery, there is a sharp drop in estrogen and progesterone levels, which in conjunction with a high prolactin level causes milk production (lactation). Prolactin is secreted continuously in nonpregnant women with normal blood levels of 1–20 ng/ml; levels increase to as high as 300 mg/ml during pregnancy and lactation.

The most common cause of galactorrhea is "idiopathic," in which the prolactin level is normal and there are no other identifiable causes of spontaneous nipple discharge. This accounts for nearly 35% of galactorrhea.

Prescription medications, herbal supplements, and illicit drugs account for 20% of all episodes of galactorrhea. The most common prescription medications that cause galactorrhea are antipsychotic medications and the selective serotonin-reuptake inhibitor antidepressant medications such as citalpram, fluoxetine, paroxetine, and sertraline. Antihypertensive medications including methyldopa, atenolol, and verapamil can also stimulate this condition. Any prescription hormones (i.e., oral contraceptive pills or hormone replacement therapy) or herbal estrogen or progesterone agent can contribute to this problem, which often develops after abruptly stopping the medication. The most common herbal supplements to cause galactorrhea are anise, fennel, red clover, and red raspberry. Marijuana, amphetamines, and opiates can also cause nonobstetric galactorrhea.

Eighteen percent of patients who present with galactorrhea are diagnosed with a tumor such as a prolactinoma or, rarely, lung or kidney tumors or a lymphoma. Prolactinomas, by far the most common tumors to cause galactorrhea, are nonmalignant growths of the anterior pituitary gland. They secrete high levels of prolactin, thus causing galactorrhea. Other symptoms of a prolactinoma include absence of menstruation and visual changes. Prognosis for these benign tumors is excellent. Breast cancer is generally not associated with galactorrhea.

In 13% of cases, systemic diseases including hypothyroidism, acromegaly (a disease characterized by excessive production of growth hormone), kidney failure, or Cushing's disease (a disease characterized by excessive steroid production) can cause galactorrhea. Other possible causes include chest wall irritation from skin conditions such as herpes zoster ("shingles") or eczema.

Diagnosis of the cause of galactorrhea includes careful questioning regarding symptoms and medications. Laboratory studies may include a pregnancy test, thyroid studies, and prolactin level. If the prolactin level is high, then the physician may order an imaging study of the brain such as a magnetic resonance imaging (MRI) to evaluate for pituitary gland abnormalities.

Treatment of galactorrhea is directed to its underlying cause. If medications are the culprit, then it may be beneficial to substitute another drug, if available. If a primary disease such as hypothyroidism is discovered, then initiation of appropriate treatment often eliminates galactorrhea. Patients discovered to have a prolactinoma may be offered surgical removal of the benign tumor, or medication to decrease prolactin production and tumor size. These include medications such as bromocriptine and pergolide.

SEE ALSO: Complementary medicine, Thyroid diseases

Suggested Reading

Harris, G. D., White, R. D., Carlson, B., et al. (2000, December). *Common breast problems* (Monograph, Edition No. 259, Home Study Self-Assessment Program). Leawood, KS: American Academy of Family Physicians.

Pena, K. S., & Rosenfeld, J. A. (2001). Evaluation and treatment of galactorrhea. *American Family Physician, 63*, 1763–1770, 1775.

ANDREA DARBY-STEWART

Gallbladder Disease

Gallbladder Disease The most common disorders affecting the gallbladder are consequences of gallstone formation. Gallstones are extremely common, occurring in up to 50% of women in their 70s. Factors associated with an increased risk of gallstone disease include being female, increasing age, race, with highest rates in Native Americans, Hispanics, and whites, obesity, Crohn's disease, pregnancy, occurrence in other family members, and rapid weight loss. The majority of patients with gallstones are asymptomatic. When symptoms do occur, patients most commonly present with biliary colic (pain in the cystic duct that drains the liver) or with acute cholecystitis (inflammation of the gallbladder).

Biliary colic results from continued contraction of the gallbladder while there is a stone in the cystic duct. Patients complain of pain, usually in the right upper quadrant or epigastrium (area over the stomach). The pain is classically described as being triggered by fatty foods, but pain may also occur with other foods or without a clear relationship to meals. The pain is constant, and may last from about 30 minutes to a few hours. In addition to pain, patients often complain of indigestion, bloating or belching, and nausea. Physical examination is usually unremarkable as are laboratory studies. After an initial attack about 50% of patients will suffer another attack within 1 year, while about 25% will be asymptomatic over the next 10 years.

Acute cholecystitis results from complete obstruction of the cystic duct, which then leads to inflammation of the gallbladder. The pain of acute cholecystitis usually starts more insidiously, with vague abdominal discomfort. As the degree of inflammation in the gallbladder increases, the peritoneum becomes inflamed and the pain localizes to the right upper quadrant or epigastrium. Unlike biliary colic, the pain persists and worsens over time. Patients may report radiation of the pain to the back or the right shoulder, or may describe the pain as "belt" like. Associated nausea and vomiting are common. Fever is also a frequent finding. On physical examination the right upper quadrant is tender, often with guarding and local peritoneal signs (marked tenderness upon touching the abdomen). A positive Murphy's sign, which is the sudden halt to inspiration with palpation of the right upper quadrant, is common. A mass or fullness may be appreciated, although this may be difficult to feel due to the tenderness of the abdomen. Laboratory studies usually reveal an increased white blood count.

The best imaging study for gallstone disease is ultrasonography. Ultrasound is more than 98% sensitive and more than 95% specific for gallstones. Sludge in the gallbladder may also be identified and can cause biliary colic. Ultrasound findings consistent with acute cholecystitis include thickening of the gallbladder wall and pericholecystic fluid (fluid around the gallbladder). Ultrasound can also show dilation of the biliary tree, which may result from obstruction of the common bile duct by a stone or a mass. Computed tomography is not nearly as sensitive or specific as ultrasound in diagnosing gallstones, although inflammatory changes around the gallbladder may be evident in acute cholecystitis. Biliary scintigraphy (also known as a "HIDA scan"—a test using radiolabeled material to image the gallbladder and associated structures) will show nonvisualization of the gallbladder in patients with acute cholecystitis due to gallstones.

The clinical scenario dictates treatment of gallstone disease. Patients with asymptomatic gallstones require no treatment since only about 10–20% of patients will develop symptoms. Several modalities have been described for dissolving gallstones. The bile salts chenodeoxycholic acid or ursodeoxycholic acid can be administered orally and, over the course of 6–12 months, can lead to complete dissolution of cholesterol stones, but up to 50% of patients will develop recurrent stones within 1 year. This modality may be considered for poor operative candidates. Direct dissolution and shock wave lithotripsy are considered experimental in the United States.

Patients with a single episode of biliary colic (gallbladder pain) may be observed. Recurrent episodes of colic tend to become more frequent and severe with time, so in these patients cholecystectomy (removal of the gallbladder) should be considered. Cholecystectomy is usually performed laparoscopically on an outpatient basis. Morbidity and mortality rates are low and most patients return to normal activities within a week or two.

Patients with acute cholecystitis should be admitted to the hospital for intravenous antibiotics. Cholecystectomy is usually performed within 24–48 hours. Patients who are poor operative candidates can be managed with antibiotics alone with success. However, in the presence of a palpable gallbladder or abnormal liver function tests nonoperative therapy usually fails. Persistence or worsening of fever or elevation in the white blood cell count despite antibiotic treatment are indications for immediate surgery. In most cases laparoscopic cholecystectomy will be successful. Conversion to open cholecystectomy is more likely in patients with acute cholecystitis.

While most patients report no consequence from cholecystectomy, some will complain of increased bloating or abdominal discomfort particularly with eating. These symptoms usually resolve with time.

Biliary colic can occur without gallstones. Biliary dyskinesia (abnormal contractions of the biliary tract) is an uncommon motility disorder of the gallbladder. Measuring a gallbladder ejection fraction using biliary scintigraphy makes the diagnosis. Cholecystectomy is indicated, although not all patients will have complete pain relief.

Other diseases of the gallbladder are quite uncommon. Polyps are occasionally identified on ultrasonography. In most cases cholecystectomy is indicated, although the incidence of progression to cancer appears to be small. Carcinoma of the gallbladder is rare and carries an extremely poor prognosis.

SEE ALSO: Abdominal pain

Suggested Reading

Barone, J. E., Bears, S., Chan, S., & Tsai, J. (1999). Outcome study of cholecystectomy during pregnancy. *The American Journal of Surgery, 177,* 232–236.

Harris, H. W. (2001). Biliary system. In J. A. Norton, R. R. Bollinger, A. E. Chang, S. F. Lowry, S. J. Mulvihill, H. I. Pass, et al. (Eds.), *Surgery: Basic science and clinical evidence* (pp. 553–584). New York: Springer.

Shea, J. A., Berlin, J. A., Bachwich, D. R., Staroscik, R. N., Malet, P. F., McGuckin, M., et al. (1998). Indications and outcomes of cholecystectomy: A comparison of the pre and post laparoscopic eras. *Annals of Surgery, 227,* 343–350.

Tabet, J., & Anvari, M. (1999). Laparoscopic cholecystectomy for gallbladder dyskinesia: Clinical outcome and patient satisfaction. *Surgical Laparoscopy, Endoscopy & Percutaneous Techniques, 9,* 382–386.

DEBRA J. GRAHAM

Gangs

Gangs Gangs have existed in this country for decades. What started out as a male-dominated phenomenon in the early 1930s has evolved into a non-gender-specific phenomenon. Adolescent females have become increasingly more involved in youth gangs and youth violence in the last 10 years, and as they engage in what is already considered high-risk behaviors, their likelihood for victimization and exposure to various health hazards increases.

Young women have been involved in gang-related behaviors since the 1950s. During the early years, their roles were primarily to manage the money that was generated by the illegal enterprises of the male gang members. These enterprises included drugs, illegal arms sales, and prostitution. At that time, the women were not viewed as actual members of the gang, but rather were more often the spouses or girlfriends of the male members. However, in the early 1990s there was a noticeable change in this trend. Young women began to form their own gangs, usually a subgroup of one of the male gangs, and in doing so, established their own code of membership, rules, and guidelines, and initiation rites.

There are many initiation rites in the gang culture. The two that are most often used are what is known as "jumping in" and "roll of the dice." In the jumping in process, the prospective gang member is placed in the center of a circle of established gang members and physically beaten. The beating is a timed process and the object is for perspective members to defend themselves to the best of their ability and to remain on their feet. If they fall down, they may be subject to being kicked and stomped, and subsequently not allowed to become a member. In the event perspective members remain standing, they are then allowed to become a peripheral or intermediate gang member. Peripheral members are allowed to follow and be an "apprentice" to established members of the gang before they are given any rank and status. Intermediate members are allowed to actively participate in the activities of the gang, and are granted some status in the gang. In the roll of the dice initiation, the perspective member becomes a sexual object. Several of the established male gang members roll a set of dice; the numbers that come up determine the number of established male gang members with whom the initiate must have intercourse. This method is used primarily with perspective female gang members. If the perspective gang member participates willingly she is admitted into the gang as an intermediate gang member. If the perspective gang member refuses to participate, she is usually forced. If she still wants to become a member, she is granted peripheral status in the gang, and after a period of time may be granted intermediate status.

Both of these methods present health risks to this population. The number of serious physical injuries during the jumping in initiations has been documented by the reports of increased numbers of young trauma patients, many of whom are adolescent females between the ages of 12 and 15 years, in the emergency rooms around this country.

The sexual acts performed during the roll of the dice initiation are unprotected. This places the adolescent female in the high-risk category for sexually transmitted diseases including HIV. This also places the adolescent female at risk for an unwanted pregnancy.

Another aspect of this alarming trend is the number of adolescent female gang members committing violent acts. There has been an increase in the numbers of adolescent and adult females being incarcerated for serious offenses ranging from aggravated assault to murder.

The two reasons adolescent females give for joining gangs and putting themselves at risk are their need to belong to a family and/or family unit and the sense of power they get from belonging to the gang. Their perception of external power gives them a sense of internal power and control.

A lot has been written about gangs and gang subculture, but little attention has been paid to the participation of females. As the trend in this area continues to grow, so does the need for more research.

See Also: Acquired immunodeficiency syndrome, Adolescence, Sexual abuse, Sexually transmitted diseases, Violence, Youth

Suggested Reading

Furr, A. L. (1997). *Exploring human behavior and the social environment.* Needham Heights, MA: Allyn & Bacon.

Molidor, C. E. (1996). Female gang members: A profile of aggression and victimization. *Social Work, 41*(3), 251–257.

Spergel, I. A. (1995). *The youth gang problem: A community approach.* New York: Oxford University Press.

PATRICIA M. HENRY

Gender There is controversy over how gender is defined and in the distinction between the terms gender and sex. The *Merriam-Webster Dictionary* defines gender as "the behavioral, cultural, and psychological traits typically associated with one's sex." Interestingly, the definition of sex encompasses "the sum of the structural, functional, and behavioral characteristics of living things that are involved in reproduction by two interacting parents that distinguish males and females." The definition of gender emphasizes psychological and cultural traits, whereas the definition of sex emphasizes structural and functional traits. Both definitions, however, include behavioral aspects.

The use of the term gender as something separate from one's sex is a fairly recent conceptual development. In American society, resistance to traditional gender role norms can be traced back to the suffrage movement of the 1920s and 1930s, although most chroniclers suggest that it was not until the mid- to late 1960s that gender took on a separate definition from sex. The rise of the feminist movement produced concerns about the traditional perspective on gender due to its unidimensionality and rigidness. At one extreme is the perspective that gender is solely made up of, and influenced by, one's biology. At the other extreme is the perspective that gender is unrelated to one's biology and completely determined by how individuals experience themselves. In between are researchers who argue that gender comprises varying degrees of biology, psychology, and culture. The traditional perspective on gender is that it involves two mutually exclusive categories, so that individuals who are high on masculine traits must be low on feminine traits. Many researchers now conceive of gender as involving multiple continuums, allowing for the possibility that one can be high or low on both *masculine* and *feminine* traits. Others take this a step further and emphasize that expression of masculine and feminine traits is dependent upon situational context. Still others argue that the entire conceptualization of sex-based traits is erroneous, calling attention to how these so-called traits are used to classify women as the *lesser sex* relative to men.

It would be erroneous to suggest that all biologists or all psychologists agree on how to define gender; however, there are some commonalities based on scientific discipline. Many biologists assert that gender is no different than sex, and is simply determined by the 23rd pair of human chromosomes. In this pair, females are designated *XX* and males are designated *XY*. Those who promote an essentialist perspective in psychology also endorse this definition, arguing that gender is nothing more than sex, decided at birth, and is unchanging. Evolutionary theorists also adhere to the essentialist perspective that gender is biologically based. These theorists focus on reproduction as the essential motive driving the behavior of all organisms. Evolutionary theories focus on women's and men's unequal investments in the care provided for their offspring and because of this, the differential adaptiveness of specific behaviors that help aid in the survival of these offspring. From this perspective, biological sex differences have produced environmental pressures that have led women and men to develop different gender roles. Because these gender differences are viewed as being evolutionarily adaptive, they are viewed as fixed, although presumably new environmental pressures could alter what types of gender displays are most adaptive.

There are other psychological theorists who adhere to the opposite view, suggesting that gender has nothing to do with one's sex, but rather involves the beliefs and feelings of one's experiences in a social and public environment. Psychologists who have adopted this view frequently describe the experiences of people who feel they are trapped in the body of the opposite sex (see Transsexualism) or people who have equal proportions of masculine and feminine attributes (androgyny). Although essentialists would focus their explanation of these individuals' experiences on their chromosomes and reproductive organs, social constructionists would focus their explanations on how masculine or how feminine these individuals feel throughout their daily lives and would use those guidelines rather than sex to describe their gender. Psychologists typically define gender identity as an individual's own sense of how *male* or *female* they feel, regardless of biological sex. It is in this identification that gender is realized.

Theorists who argue that gender is socially constructed focus on the different roles that women and men are expected to fulfill in a society. Anthropologists have documented the vast heterogeneity in the types of traits and behaviors that are viewed as masculine or feminine in different cultures. For example, in many nonindustrialized societies, men and women are expected to perform very different work roles, with men often being responsible for hunting and women for providing all other types of food as well as food preparation. In cultures in which women may haul heavy buckets of water for long distances, definitions of femininity and perceptions of what makes a woman attractive are very different from those in an industrialized urban culture that emphasizes a different set of roles and image of attractiveness. Such was also the case during frontier days in America and among low-status minority women who have been required to fulfill domestic and factory jobs. In contrast, among 21st century urban professional women, sweating may be acceptable at the gym, but not at the workplace.

If women and men express gender differently in different cultures, how do gender differences emerge? Social constructionists argue that gender roles are taught from birth through both implicit and explicit messages. The young boy who plays with his sister's makeup before going to school is frequently the object of ridicule by peers and adults and is unlikely to do so again. Many psychologists argue that children internalize these perceptions of what it means to be a girl or boy and that these traits become a part of their identity. Many sociologists have argued that gender emerges through the different ways in which men and women, as well as those of diverse ethnicities and classes, experience their bodies in a social and historical context. In addition to gender roles and gender identity, they emphasize the importance of gender stratification. Gender stratification is society's unequal distribution of wealth, power, and privilege between the sexes. Unlike essentialists, social constructionists do not believe that biology is destiny and therefore they do not view traditional gender roles as inevitable. However, they do believe that societies encourage men and women to adapt certain traits and roles and that most individuals internalize these messages. Thus, gender roles become an integral part of most people's sense of self.

Other theorists have argued that too much emphasis is placed on gender as an individual difference variable and instead suggest that gender may be more situationally dependent. Should a situation call for the display of more masculine attributes, most people are able to produce such characteristics. For example, an assertive leadership style may be viewed as masculine in American culture, but many women corporate leaders have adopted this leadership style. This belief that gender displays are based on situational demands and rewards challenges the assumption that gender is an integral part of an individual's personality and a core aspect of their self-concept. Postmodernist theorists go beyond the argument that gender roles are flexible and dynamic, instead arguing that gender is completely fluid and unrelated to stable aspects of the self, including personality and biology. These theorists argue that gender is not intrinsic to women and men, but instead represents a performance. In this light, an individual's performance can be viewed as either traditional or non-traditional with respect to society's expectations for their gender. Thus, everyone performs gender and can change how they perform it if they choose to do so.

See Also: Femininity, Gender role, Homosexuality, Lesbian, Marianismo, Masculinity, Queer, Transgenderism, Transsexuality

Suggested Reading

Butler, J. (1990). *Gender trouble: Feminism and the subversion of identity.* London: Routledge.

Diamant, L., & Lee, J. A. (2002). *The psychology of sex, gender, and jobs.* Westport, CT: Praeger.

Howard, J. A., & Hollander, J. (1997). *The gender lens: Gendered situations, gendered selves.* Thousand Oaks, CA: Sage.

Mackie, M. (1987). *Constructing women and men: Gender socialization.* New York: Holt, Rinehart & Winston.

Merriam-Webster Dictionary Online: www.m-w.com

Shaver, P., & Hendrick, C. (1987). *Sex and gender: Review of personality and social psychology* (Vol. 7). Thousand Oaks, CA: Sage.

Spence, J. T., Deaux, K., & Helmrich, R. L. (1985). Sex roles in contemporary American society. In G. Lindzey & E. Aronson (Eds.), *Handbook of social psychology.* New York: Random House.

Antonia Abbey
Christopher Saenz
Michele Parkhill
Lenwood W. Hayman, Jr.

Gender Role Gender roles are generally defined as sex-based categories that specify appropriate rules of conduct for males and females in a particular culture or society. Although grounded in *biological* differences between males and females, gender roles are *social constructs*. Simply put, based on the anatomical difference between men and women, each is prescribed varying and often stereotypical social roles that are reinforced at the individual level and by larger society. For example, a father may chastise his son for crying, judging such self-expression to be inappropriate for males. Similarly, young girls are often discouraged from playing football or other contact sports (even if they show promise) because the muscle development and aggressiveness associated with these activities are selectively encouraged for males and discouraged for females. This elaboration of gender role constructs is carried on into adulthood, at which point men are assumed to be self-reliant, emotionally distant, and the financial providers for their families, while women are viewed as the primary nurturers and emotional caretakers of the home and family.

The term *gender role* is often used interchangeably with terms such as *sex role* and *sex role stereotypes*. However, there is disagreement about the extent to which these terms are related. Sex role theory (see Femininity and Masculinity) suggests an innate or automatic process of integrating appropriate behaviors based on one's sex. Interestingly, evolutionary theorists view sexual selection as defining such a process. Using this theoretical framework, women are more invested in their offspring through pregnancy and childbirth and therefore choose mates carefully, based on their ability to provide for their offspring. In turn, men compete with each other for the attention of women and thereby thrive on combative, competitive behaviors with other men. These theories are grounded in the assumption of superiority of males over females; thus making the arguments less scientifically driven and more determined by social convention.

Gender roles are not only socially determined but also culturally upheld. In most countries, children are taught from birth to define themselves based upon the social demands placed upon them. Perhaps the most noticeable way is through their clothing. In many cultures, young boys wear hats and/or pants to define their gender while girls wear shawls or skirts. In various parts of Mexico, Ghana, and India, for example, infants are also identified as females by wearing earrings, bracelets, and other jewelry.

Complementing sex-specific attire, gender roles are introduced to children by the division of labor practices modeled and assigned by their parents. In many agrarian societies, girls are more often assigned to chores defined as female oriented, such as caring for younger siblings and performing household duties in the home or in the immediate vicinity of the home. Conversely, parents usually teach their sons to participate in caring for animals and similar tasks that may take them to surrounding pastures. Many parents in the United States also divide tasks for their children according to gender. Historically, boys have been relegated to tasks outside the home such as taking out the garbage and mowing lawns, while girls have been encouraged to be domestically inclined, performing tasks such as cleaning or cooking.

Gender roles are solidified in many cultures during early adolescence through rituals, or rites of passage ceremonies, held to establish their proper placement in society. These are usually public ceremonies, during which youth are recognized and formally acknowledged as adults, and emphasize gender as a predominant and defining part of the youth's adult status. For some cultures, the ceremonies may be in the form of celebrations to introduce the youth to the society (e.g., the Jewish Bar Mitzvah and Bat Mitzvah, Quinceañera in Spanish cultures, Debutante balls, and so forth). In other cultures, the ceremonies may include giving the youth permanent markings or tattoos. These events reinforce social demands of gender roles and through their participation, confirm the community's expectation that the youth will fulfill their necessary obligations according to their gender role.

Gender roles in families may differ according to race and economic status. For instance, economic pressures and constraints in many impoverished African American families often necessitate that sons and daughters share various household chores that cut across traditional gender lines. Additionally, many of these are single-parent families headed by females and exist in communities where there are shortages of males, which are often attributed to an inability to find work, homicide, or imprisonment. In this way, mothers perform duties stereotypically viewed as both male and female, and thereby teach their children to do the same. Some theorists relate this trend to African American women during slavery, who were required to maintain their homes as well as work alongside their male counterparts in field labor. Others have used this history to reference the pressures and challenges these women face in performing double duty, or functioning as the man and the woman in their homes. Still others view this history as a testament to the power and competence these women possess as matriarchs of their communities.

Over the past several decades, artificial distinctions based on gender have started to fade and in some cases even blend. In the United States and in other countries, there has been a significant pursuit toward addressing gender inequalities, thus allowing opportunities for both sexes to challenge preconceived notions of their functions in society. Researchers have determined that female college students hold similar job aspirations as men and place greater value on career attributes that have previously been viewed as male oriented, including power and leadership. This transition is perhaps most evident in the mass media's portrayal of heroes and heroines. In mainstream society, men are now encouraged to be both strong and emotionally available. They are socially sanctioned to pursue professions that were previously dominated by women (e.g., nursing, teaching) and to share household duties with women as evidenced in movies such as *Mr. Mom*. Similarly, women's roles have been expanded. They hold more professional positions of authority and power. In recent years, many movies have portrayed women as having the capacity to be militaristic, ruthless, and violent (e.g., *Lara Croft: Tomb Raider, GI Jane*). Therefore, the portrayal of the doting, submissive wife and mother in mid-20th-century television serials such as *Donna Reed* and *Father Knows Best* is viewed as antiquated under current standards.

Despite these advances in redefining gender roles, many countries have not successfully made such efforts to reform. In fact, women continue to be viewed as subordinate in many parts of the world, a convention that leads to serious health implications based largely upon their unequal status. With the rising worldwide concerns about the AIDS epidemic, women in some African and Latin American countries often are unable to refuse sex or to ask a man to use a condom even if she knows that her partner is infected. In these countries, men also subject women to physical and verbal abuse. Women's mistreatment is commonly ignored or assumed to be appropriate, given the roles of women in these cultures as being subservient, deferential, and powerless.

In many societies, married and single men are encouraged to have different sexual partners as part of a socially sanctioned masculine gender role construct, which places them at increased risk for contracting HIV/AIDS and other sexually transmitted infections. In Latin American cultures, the male gender role is conceptualized within the construct of *machismo*, which defines men as masculine within the confines of risk-taking behavior, such as proving their sexual drive and aggressive tendencies by having numerous sexual partners (see Masculinity and Marianismo). Thus, they are not only at greater risk for contracting a sexually transmitted infection and transmitting it to their female (or male) sexual partners but also are at greater risk for death from other risk-taking behaviors (e.g., homicides, accidents).

In many nonindustrialized countries, men are viewed as the gatekeepers of society and therefore hold the most powerful public positions. Because of this, they also relegate the access of information to women in society as well as uphold the stringently defined gender roles that maintain their status. In this way, many women are afraid to retaliate against the harsh treatment they suffer at the hands of men. They are also afraid to divorce abusive husbands for fear of being shunned by friends and relatives because, in many countries, women are not permitted to divorce their husbands. Consequently, for many women, gender role is a painful reminder of their secondary and paralyzed position in society.

SEE ALSO: Domestic violence, Dowry, Femininity, Gender, Marianismo, Masculinity, Sexual harassment

Suggested Reading

Amott, T., & Matthaeim, J. (1996). *Race, gender and work: A multicultural economic history of women in the United States.* Boston: South End Press.
Lorber, J. (1994). *Paradoxes of gender.* New Haven, CT: Yale University Press.
Whiting, B. B., & Edwards, C. P. (1988). *Children of different worlds: The formation of social behavior.* Cambridge, MA: Harvard University Press.

Suggested Resources

Drennan, M. *Gender and reproductive behavior.* http://www.jhuccp.org/pr/j46/j46chap4_3.shtml
University of Florida Counseling Center. *Male sex role: Changes and stressors.* http://www.counsel.ufl.edu/selfHelp/maleSexRole.asp

KRISTI Y. JORDAN

Genetic Counseling
Since the beginning of time, people have recognized the concept of inheritance—that is, traits are passed down from generation to generation. In most situations, those traits are looked at with pleasure. However, when there is a genetic condition in the family that causes disease or birth defects, there is usually great concern. Genetic disorders, while individually not very common, when combined as a group, comprise a significant portion of health care concerns. There are more than 6,000 genetic disorders. About 3–4% of all newborn infants have a genetic disease or major birth defect. Approximately 1% of live-born babies have a chromosomal abnormality such as Down's syndrome and birth defects or genetic conditions cause more than 20% of infant deaths. About 10% of adults and 30% of children in hospitals have a problem that is genetically related. Also, many common diseases such as cancer, diabetes, and heart disease have a genetic component.

Genetic counseling is the process of providing information, education, and support to individuals and families with a medical history or increased personal risk for a genetic condition. It also includes providing information, education, and support to those at risk for having a child with a birth defect or genetic condition. Medical geneticists and genetic counselors are health professionals with specialized training and experience in human and medical genetics and counseling. They provide diagnostic information, education, and supportive counseling concerning numerous birth defects, disorders, or abnormalities.

Nondirectiveness is the generally accepted philosophy of geneticists and genetic counselors. Genetic counseling is not about reducing the incidence of a genetic disorder, rather it is about helping patients and their families make informed decisions within the context of their own values, beliefs, goals, and personal circumstances.

A genetic evaluation and counseling is appropriate for any individual or family with concerns about the diagnosis, recurrence risk, treatment, or surveillance regarding a specific condition or birth defect. Families with concerns about any of the following may find it helpful to see a genetic counselor: (a) birth defects, such as congenital heart defects, spina bifida (open spine), or cleft lip and cleft palate; (b) genetic disorders affecting children and adults such as cystic fibrosis and muscular dystrophy and chromosomal disorders such as Down's syndrome, neurofibromatosis, and Huntington's disease; (c) mental retardation; (d) if there is more than one birth defect in a person, whether or not there is a known cause; (e) metabolic diseases such as phenylketonuria (PKU); (f) diseases that run in families, such as cancer, kidney disease, certain heart conditions, and mental problems such as bipolar disease and schizophrenia; (g) infertility, stillbirths, multiple miscarriages, or infant deaths; (h) marriage between close blood relatives; and (i) ethnic backgrounds known to have a higher chance of specific genetic conditions, such as Tay–Sachs disease in people of Jewish descent or sickle-cell anemia in African Americans.

Genetic counselors also provide information about concerns in future or current pregnancies including women who are in their mid-30s and older, prenatal tests such as maternal serum screening, amniocentesis or chorionic villus sampling (CVS), effects of infections, radiation, medications, drugs, or alcohol, and health problems such as diabetes, high blood pressure, or seizures.

At a genetic counseling session, families can expect that the genetic counselor will (a) gather information about their medical history, pregnancy history (e.g., any problems during pregnancy, drugs taken, illnesses, difficulties during delivery, and so forth), and developmental history (e.g., when a baby sits up, begins to talk and walk, how they did in school, and so forth); (b) ask the family to bring medical records, test results, or photographs to the genetics appointment; (c) ask about the family's history and draw a family tree (the pedigree); (d) discuss a specific diagnosis (if it is known) and how the diagnosis is managed, treated, and its prognosis—for example, discussing the use of folic acid prior to pregnancy to reduce the risk of neural tube defects; (e) discuss testing for specific diagnoses such as chromosomal disorders or single gene disorders; (f) discuss carrier testing, if appropriate (for example, testing for susceptibility genes for breast and ovarian cancer or disorders such as cystic fibrosis or sickle-cell trait); (g) discuss the chances of the birth defect or genetic disorder reoccurring in other family members (recurrence risk); (h) address the family's concerns in a supportive manner and encourage them to make decisions that reflect their own values and beliefs; and (i) make referrals to other health professionals or resources when needed.

Depending on the reasons for seeking genetic counseling, a family may only need to see the genetic counselor or genetics team once, or they may need to return for additional appointments to discuss test results or new information. In general, most genetic counseling appointments last 1–2 hours.

SEE ALSO: Alpha-fetoprotein screening, Preconception care, Pregnancy, Prenatal care, Ultrasound

Suggested Reading

Baker, D. L., Schuette, J. L., & Uhlmann, W. R. (1998). *A guide to genetic counseling.* New York: John Wiley & Sons.

National Society of Genetic Counselors. (1995). *Genetic counseling: Valuable information for you and your family.* Wallingford, PA: National Society of Genetic Counselors. www.nsgc.org

Nessbausm, R. L., McInnes, R. R., & Willard, H. F. (2001). *Thompson and Thompson: Genetics in medicine* (6th ed.). Philadelphia: W.B. Saunders.

ANNE MATTHEWS

Genital Development

Female genitalia consist of two main parts, the internal genitalia that includes the *uterus, fallopian tubes*, and *vagina* and external genitalia consisting of the *vulva.* Both internal and external genitalia develop in utero, that is, when the baby is still in the womb. In a series of experiments conducted in the 1950s, Alfred Jost demonstrated that the sex chromosomes (XX or XY) inherited determine whether the fetus will develop male gonads (sex glands) known as *testes*, or female gonads known as *ovaries*. In turn, the gonads determine the phenotypic sex (i.e., male versus female sexual/reproductive organs). An undifferentiated gonad develops during the fourth week of gestation, and for the first 2 months of growth, the two sexes develop identically. Starting around the eighth week of pregnancy, sexual differentiation begins when the testes first appear. In contrast, it is hard to observe the first appearance of ovaries and their development is determined based on the absence of testes rather than the presence of ovaries. Around the thirteenth week of pregnancy, however, the ovaries become apparent.

The "XX" sex chromosomes determine the growth of the ovaries. Ovaries produce the hormone estrogen that is essential for the further formation of the ovaries. Unlike in males, hormones are not required for the further genitalia development in females once the ovaries are fully formed. Rather, the internal urogenital tract develops from two sets of ducts present in both sexes: *Wolffian* and *Müllerian ducts*. In females, the Müllerian ducts give rise to the internal genitalia: fallopian tubes, uterus, and vagina. In the absence of testes the fetus' genital tubercle becomes the external genitalia, that is, the clitoris and the vulva. The development of internal and external genitalia is a continuous process starting in utero and continuing through puberty. Parts of the brain become sexually differentiated. One part of the brain secretes the gonadotropin-releasing hormone (GnRH) that is necessary for normal gonadal development. Changes to the structure and functioning of the brain are irreversible and take place during critical windows of human development.

VULVA AND VAGINAL ANATOMY

The word *vulva* means "covering," appropriately termed because it covers the openings to the urethra and the vagina. It includes the *labia majora, labia minor,* and the *vestibule.* The vulva begins at the top with the *mons,* or "mountain." The mons is the pad of fat covered by pubic hair. The first sign of puberty is the growth of pubic hair that grows thicker as girls go through sexual maturation. The pattern of pubic hair, called *escutcheon,* is an inverted triangle in females. The amount of pubic hair on the mons can vary depending on race; African American girls tend to have thicker and coarser hair compared to Asian women who have sparser growth. Caucasian women tend to be somewhere in between.

The *labia majora* are the outer folds of the vulva between the thighs and like the mons they contain a fair amount of fat. The labia majora has a large number of sweat glands and other glands that secrete sebum, a wax coating that provides lubrication and prevents friction during sexual intercourse. The labia majora surrounds the *labia minora* that are the thin flaps of skin without hair. The labia minora is filled with blood vessels that plump up with blood when a woman is sexually aroused. The labia minora and the mons come together at the *clitoris.* The clitoris has a large number of nerve endings and is easily sexually stimulated. The area between the labia minora is called the *vestibule.* Like the labia minora, the vestibule is also rich in blood vessels. The blood vessels, also called the *bulbs of the vestibule,* swell up and become firm when a woman is sexually aroused.

The *vagina* is a tube that extends from the vestibule to the *uterus,* also described as the womb. Most of the time the vagina is collapsed, but it stretches when penetrated. The vaginal lining is sturdy because it manages multiple activities including sexual intercourse, childbirth, and menstruation. These activities also create an increased vulnerability to bacterial infections. The cervical canal connects the vagina to the uterus. The uterus and fallopian tubes (also called uterine tubes) play a key role in fertilization and pregnancy. Every month the ovaries release one egg or *ovum* that travels through the fallopian tubes toward the uterus. Fertilization occurs if the ovum meets a male sperm in the fallopian tubes. The fertilized egg then proceeds down the fallopian tubes until it reaches the uterus, and it embeds itself in the lining of the uterus in preparation for gestation. The fertilized egg develops over the next 40 weeks into a baby. If the ovum remains unfertilized, it dissolves when it reaches the uterus, and the uterine lining plus blood that developed in preparation for nurturing a fertilized egg is shed. The process of discharging the blood and the uterine lining is called *menstruation.*

CHANGES IN THE VULVA AND VAGINA DURING CHILDHOOD AND PUBERTY

Newborn and Childhood

At birth the labia majora and mons are hairless. The labia majora is plump because of high estrogen levels at birth. However, as the estrogen levels decrease following delivery, the size of the mons and labia majora diminish. Low levels of estrogen cause the vagina in young girls to have a thin lining that lacks protective lactobacilli or "good" bacteria necessary for safeguarding the vagina from other bacteria. Therefore, young girls are often susceptible to irritations from chemicals such as those found in bubble bath or dyes.

Puberty

Girls' reproductive organs experience a growth spurt during puberty. The vagina doubles in length to about 3–5 in. long and the ovaries and fallopian tubes increase in size to about 3 or 4 in. in length. The uterus also grows in size, and in contrast to its upright position throughout childhood, the uterus begins to tilt during puberty. These changes are accompanied by hormonal shifts. Testosterone, primarily a male hormone but one that exists in females in small quantities, stimulates the growth of pubic and other bodily hair (e.g., armpits, legs). Girls typically develop body odor and acne as a result of increased testosterone during this period. Estrogen levels rise later in puberty giving way to breast development and menarche (see

Menarche). Menarche, or first menstruation, releases acid in the vagina, which in turn helps to fight off bacteria. During puberty, the *hymen*, which is a thin layer covering the vaginal opening, also undergoes change in preparation for adulthood. The hymen stretches thereby creating additional space for menstrual discharge and sexual activity. In some cases, the hymenal opening may be closed off completely (*imperforate hymen*) and may need to be surgically opened to allow for menstrual and sexual activity. By the end of puberty, the vagina and vulva are fully developed and girls are capable of sexual reproduction. Pregnancy and menopause bring about further structural changes in the lining of the vulva and vagina. Hormones fluctuate during these times and the stresses of childbirth often reshape the vaginal opening. Additional readings on these changes in later adulthood are provided at the end of the chapter.

GENITAL ABNORMALITIES

Turner Syndrome

Turner syndrome (TS) is characterized by the lack of development of secondary sexual characteristics (i.e., pubic hair and breast development). Other signs include growth retardation (somewhere between 4 ft, 6 in. and 4 ft, 10 in.), webbed neck, a broad chest with broadly spaced nipples, and cognitive difficulties, specifically a nonverbal learning disability. TS occurs in approximately 1 out of every 2,000–3,000 births of girls, and is the result of the absence or abnormality in the X chromosome from either parent. *Ovarian dysgenesis*, the massive loss of egg cells during fetal development and after birth, is implicated in the lack of development of the secondary sexual characteristics. The loss of eggs during development causes the ovaries not to develop in the fetus, and as noted earlier, ovaries are critical to the development of female genitalia during fetal development. Consequently, the absence of ovaries results in infertility in women.

Treatment for TS usually includes estrogen replacement therapy to stimulate the development of secondary sexual characteristics and a growth hormone to stimulate growth. If girls receive the treatment early enough in development, they can grow to a normal height. Unfortunately, TS is usually not diagnosed until late adolescence when the absence of typical pubertal processes becomes apparent.

Ambiguous Genitalia

Intersex condition or hermaphroditism (46, XX with bilateral ova–testis) is a blending or mix of male and female internal and external genitalia. It is estimated that 0.1–2% of the population have this condition. When infants are born with ambiguous genitalia, doctors typically decide which gender to assign, and then perform surgical procedures and administer hormonal treatments to reinforce that particular gender. Large numbers of infants with ambiguous genitalia are raised female. Genital surgery includes a clitoral reduction and vaginoplasty (reconstructing the vagina).

In some cases the intersex condition is not obvious until puberty. Early signs are ignored, but when the onset of puberty is delayed pediatricians and parents take notice. Even then, some pediatricians may regard delayed pubertal onset as a normal physiological process. Physicians may prescribe oral contraceptives for "girls" to stop virilization (e.g., facial hair growth) and stimulate menstruation and breast growth. The psychological impact of this late diagnosis can be devastating, particularly because it is damaging to adolescents' already vulnerable sense of self. Adolescents raised as girls may exaggerate their feminine characteristics to meet society's expectations but at the same time feel like they are living a lie. In addition, adolescents may get little support from family members who find it difficult to accept their offspring's new sexual status.

GENITAL MUTILATION

Genital mutilation, or female circumcision, involves the removal of external genitalia in women and may include partial or complete elimination of the clitoris, the labia minora, and/or partially stitching the labia majora together. This practice is highly prevalent in African countries. In Egypt, for example, 97% of women aged 15–49 were circumcised in 1995, with minimal variation in the percentage across age groups. Female circumcision is viewed as a universal sign of marriageability in Egyptian culture, and is maintained by people's fear of family dishonor if they eliminate the practice.

Public outrage in the Western world has spurred some change in the prevalence of female circumcision. A qualitative analysis comparing circumcision histories of women aged 15–54 and their daughters who were at least 5 years old found that educated women were less likely to have their daughters circumcised. One explanation offered was that education about the risks of clitoridectomy, including bleeding, infections, infertility, and urinary problems, served as a deterrent. However, this study also found that maternal decisions not to circumcise their daughters had more to do with women's resistance to beliefs about circumcision as a marker of purity and femininity, than to her knowledge of health risks. Circumcisions continue to take place in various countries across the world, but they are more likely to be performed by doctors than untrained professionals. Efforts to fully eradicate this practice will require careful attention to the social consequences of being ostracized and suffering family dishonor versus women's health.

SEE ALSO: Adolescence, Female genital mutilation, Puberty, Sexual organs

Suggested Reading

Brooks, N. A. (2001). Sexual differentiation and development of the reproductive organs. In R. Harding & A. D. Bocking (Eds.), *Fetal growth and development* (pp. 207–223). New York: Guilford.

Diamond, M. (1997). Sexual identity and sexual orientation in children with traumatized and ambiguous genitalia. *Journal of Sex Research, 34*(2), 199–211.

Powell, P. M., & Schulte, T. (1999). Turner syndrome. In S. Goldstein & C. R. Reynolds (Eds.), *Handbook of neurodevelopmental and genetic disorders in children* (pp. 277–297). New York: Cambridge University Press.

Stewart, E. G. (2002). *The V book: A doctor's guide to complete vulvovaginal health*. New York: Bantam Books.

Yount, K. M. (2002). Like mother, like daughter? Female genital cutting in Egypt. *Journal of Health and Social Behavior, 43*(3), 336–358.

C. BARVE
GERI R. DONENBERG

Giant Cell Arteritis Giant cell arteritis (GCA), also called temporal arteritis, is an inflammatory disease with predilection for the arms (upper extremity branches of the aorta) and head (cranial arteries). All the layers of the artery wall are affected. Microscopic examination reveals infiltration of the wall by inflammatory cells (lymphocytes and macrophages). One type of inflammatory cell, macrophages, can fuse together to form giant cells, thus the name giant cell arteritis. The disease follows a "skip" pattern, meaning that involved segments alternate with normal ones. The temporal artery located on the temple of the head can be hardened (indurated), tender, and can "roll" when touched (palpated).

Specific substances in the blood (antigens) involved in triggering the disease process have not been identified. Research has focused on increased prevalence in Caucasian people of northern European origin and possible seasonal variations suggesting as yet undetermined environmental agents as precipitating factors.

GCA is a relatively rare disease. It occurs almost exclusively in individuals older than 50 years. The average age of onset is 70 years. The disease incidence increases with age. Women are affected about twice as frequently as men. In Olmstead County, Minnesota, a prevalence rate of 1 per 500 persons aged 50 or older was reported.

The clinical features of GCA are extremely variable. The onset can be gradual over a few weeks, or abrupt. Characteristically, patients have pervasive bodily symptoms including progressive tiredness; decreased appetite and weight loss are common. Many patients describe new moderate to severe headache in the side (temporal region) or back (occipital region) of the head. Scalp tenderness is reported with combing, wearing eyeglasses, or sleeping on the affected side. In some cases, the headache can be reproduced by pressure over the temporal artery. More than half of the patients have low-grade fevers that oftentimes lead to extensive investigations aimed at ruling out infection or cancer. Other symptoms may include: pain in the masticatory muscles when chewing meat or solid foods, pain in the tongue precipitated by talking, and/or pain in one or more extremities with repetitive use. Some patients experience short episodes of visual loss; initially these episodes are short and vision is regained. Unfortunately, these episodes of loss of vision are warning signs for the irreversible loss of vision. Polymyalgia rheumatica (PR) can be associated with GCA. Patients affected by this condition report morning stiffness and pain in the shoulder, neck, and hip area, severe enough to limit their activities and oftentimes confine them to bed. Patients with GCA are more likely to have abnormal expansion of large blood vessels in the chest (dilatation of the thoracic aorta) than patients without the disease. As a consequence, routine chest radiographs (x-rays) to look for enlargement of the space between the lungs (mediastinum) should be performed yearly in GCA patients. If such a finding is noted, a computed tomography (CT) of the chest to evaluate the size of the aorta is indicated.

Laboratory data indicate inflammation. Tests indicating active disease process, the erythrocyte sedimentation rate (ESR), and the C-reactive protein (CRP) are usually markedly elevated. Anemia (low red blood cell count) is often present. Platelet count can be elevated. The liver function tests can be slightly abnormal. The artery in the temple area, the temporal artery, one of the most common affected areas, can be easily biopsied to confirm the diagnosis. Temporal artery biopsy should be done, if possible, before treatment is initiated. When transient visual symptoms are present, treatment should be initiated immediately.

Once the diagnosis of GCA is established, steroids, or a related medication, should be started at a dose between 40 and 60 mg per day. This dose can be reduced gradually in the following months as clinical response is attained. The ESR and CRP can be followed monthly. As markers of inflammation, these tests are expected to parallel the clinical improvement and tend to normal as the inflammatory process is under control. The majority of patients develop side effects from steroid therapy such as: osteoporosis with increased risk for fractures, diabetes, cataract, glaucoma, high blood pressure, obesity, acne, breakdown of the major hip-bone joint (aseptic osteonecrosis of the femoral head), and infections. Occasionally, in those who need prolonged therapy with high doses of steroid, the side effects from treatment may be worse than the disease itself. The goal is to gradually decrease the steroid to the lowest dose that controls the disease. The average duration of therapy is about 2 years and many patients are able to get off steroids completely. Although most patients initially do well, relapses occur and steroids should be restarted or increased and then tapered at a slower rate.

Addition of immunosuppressive medication such as methotrexate has failed to show a decrease in the number of relapses. Methotrexate can be an option in those who do not tolerate, or who develop significant side effects from steroids. There are a few promising case reports of resistant (refractory) GCA treated with the medications etanercept or infliximab. These drugs are biologic agents that target one of the mediators of the inflammatory process. At this time though, more studies are needed to confirm their usefulness in GCA.

SEE ALSO: Cardiovascular disease, Headache

Suggested Reading

Cantini, F., & Niccoli, L. (2001). Treatment of longstanding active giant cell arteritis with infliximab: Report of four cases. *Arthritis and Rheumatism, 44*, 2933–2935.

Hoffman, S. G., Cid, M. C., Hellman, D. B., et al. (2002). A multicenter, randomized, double-blind, placebo-controlled trial of adjuvant methotrexate treatment for giant cell arteritis. *Arthritis and Rheumatism, 16*, 1309–1318.

Hunder, G., & Valente, R. M. (2002). Giant cell arteritis: Clinical aspects. In G. S. Hoffman & C. M. Weyland (Eds.), *Inflammatory diseases of blood vessels* (pp. 425–441). New York: Marcel Dekker.

Salvarani, C., Cantini, F., Boiardi, L., & Hunder, G. G. (2002). Polymyalgia rheumatica and giant-cell arteritis. *New England Journal of Medicine, 347*, 261–271.

CARMEN GOTA

Gonorrhea

Gonorrhea Gonorrhea refers to infection caused by *Neisseria gonorrhoeae*, a bacterium that grows in the reproductive tract and moist mucous membranes, such as the mouth, throat, and anus. Gonorrhea is transmitted through sexual contact. Once a person is exposed to gonorrhea, symptoms may appear in several days, or may take up to 1 month. Symptoms of gonorrhea may vary greatly from person to person. Many women are asymptomatic. An abnormal vaginal discharge, burning upon urination, and occasionally pelvic pain may be the initial symptoms of gonorrhea infection. Men infected with gonorrhea, however, often note burning upon urination or a yellow-white discharge from the penis. Gonorrhea more often produces a purulent discharge from the cervix, compared to other sexually transmitted diseases such as chlamydia.

The diagnosis of gonorrhea is made by sampling the infected area, the cervix, urethra, rectum, or throat. Once gonorrhea is diagnosed, tests for other sexually transmitted diseases, including chlamydia, syphilis, and HIV, should be performed. Because gonorrhea and chlamydia have similar symptoms and may be transmitted together, it is appropriate to treat for both infections if one is diagnosed.

Untreated gonorrhea may cause serious morbidity. Gonorrhea may become a life-threatening, bloodborne infection and may spread to the joints producing septic arthritis. Gonorrhea is the leading cause of septic arthritis in young, sexually active adults. Usually only one or two joints are involved, and the joint infection may be accompanied by local inflammation of the tendons (tenosynovitis). Tenosynovitis due to *N. gonorrhoeae* can occur without joint involvement. The diagnosis of septic arthritis due to *N. gonorrhoeae* is made by aspirating the affected joint and finding characteristic changes in the synovial fluid. *N. gonorrhoeae* can be difficult to isolate from synovial fluid and a negative culture does not rule out the diagnosis.

Pregnant women with gonorrhea may pass it on to their fetus at the time of birth, causing newborn blindness or a bloodborne infection. Gonorrhea can cause pelvic inflammatory disease (PID) that can require hospitalization for intravenous antibiotics. Even a single episode of PID can significantly reduce a woman's fertility. PID may be further complicated by formation of a tubo-ovarian abscess. Treatment of tubo-ovarian abscess may require prolonged hospitalization or surgery. Chronic pelvic pain is a long-term complication of gonorrhea and may require prolonged pain management or surgery. Infertility and ectopic pregnancy are also serious possible complications of gonorrhea. Ectopic pregnancy may be life threatening.

A single dose of antibiotic will treat uncomplicated *N. gonorrhoeae* cervicitis or urethritis. Ceftriaxone 125 mg given intramuscularly is the standard therapy; single-dose oral therapy with quinolone antibiotics is also successful, but there is growing resistance of *N. gonorrhoeae* to this class of antibiotics worldwide. Therapy of septic arthritis or tubo-ovarian abscess requires a longer course of antibiotics. Reliably utilizing latex condoms and avoiding contact with partners who are infected may prevent gonorrhea.

See Also: Chlamydia, Herpes simplex virus, Human papillomavirus, Pelvic pain, Sexually transmitted diseases, Syphilis

Suggested Reading

Gripshover, B., & Valdez, H. (2002). Common sexually transmitted diseases. In J. S. Tan (Ed.), *Experts guide to the management of common infectious diseases* (pp. 271–303). Philadelphia: American College of Physicians.

Suggested Resources

http://www.cdc.gov/ncidod/dastlr/gcdir/gono.html

Karen L. Ashby

Greer, Germaine

Germaine Greer was born on January 29, 1939, in Melbourne, Australia. She was the first child of Margaret Mary "Peggy" and Eric Reginald "Reg" Greer. Germaine's younger sister Jane arrived 6 years later and her brother, Barry, was born 5 years after Jane.

In January of 1942, Germaine's father joined the Australian Imperial Forces and soon left for war. Germaine was just about to turn 3 and it would be almost 2 years before she would see her father again. During those 2 years, Germaine had all of her mother's attention for herself. Upon her father's return, this changed. Reg Greer returned from war a different man, cold and unaffectionate. Germaine was desperate for his affection, but he would reject any attempts she made. She also received less attention from her mother now that her father had returned. Her father's rejection and the decrease in maternal attention caused Germaine to become bitter.

Germaine's childhood was not the best. Her mother often resorted to corporal punishment to deal with the headstrong temperament of her oldest child and her father did nothing to stop the punishment. The Greer home was basically culturally devoid, absent the books that Germaine would later come to love.

Germaine was a bright but sickly child. She began school at St. Columba's, a small Catholic school attached to the church where her parents had married, in 1943. By all accounts, Germaine was a very bright, if somewhat reluctant, student. She left St. Columba's for Sacred Heart, then on to Holy Redeemer. In 1952 she went to Star of the Sea College. Germaine earned honors in English and French literature at the University of Melbourne, a master's degree at the University of Sydney, and in 1967 a doctorate in literature from Newnham College at the University of Cambridge in England. She then lectured at the University of Warwick in Britain.

In 1979 Greer taught poetry and directed the Center for the Study of Women's Literature at the University of Tulsa in Oklahoma. She soon left there and returned to writing. She is currently a Professor of English and Comparative Studies at the University of Warwick.

The *Female Eunuch*, first published in 1970, is Germaine Greer's most famous work and the one that launched her into history as a great feminist. The book deals with the systemic disempowerment of women, claiming that marriage is, in essence, slavery, and proposes that the way to regain power is through reclamation of women's sexuality. *The Female Eunuch* soon became a bestseller. Another of Greer's well-known publications is *Sex and Destiny: The Politics of Human Fertility* (1984). In this book, she criticizes the Western world for pushing Western birth control methods on Third World countries. Her opinions in this book brought her much criticism as being antifeminist.

Some of her other writings are: *The Obstacle Race: The Fortunes of Women Painters and Their Work* (1979), *The Madwoman's Underclothes* (1986), *Daddy, We Hardly Knew You* (1989), *The Change: Women, Aging, and the Menopause* (1992), *Slip-Shod Sibyls* (1995), and *The Whole Woman* (1999).

See Also: Birth control; de Beauvoir, Simone

Suggested Reading

Fraser, K. (1996). *Ornament and silence: Essays on women's lives from Edith Wharton to Germaine Greer.* New York: Alfred A. Knopf.
Greer, G. (1970). *The female eunuch.* London: MacGibbon & Kee.
Greer, G. (1989). *Daddy, we hardly knew you.* London: Hamilton.
Miller, L. (2003). *The impulsive, fatally naive diva of feminism made the world a better place in spite of herself.* Retrieved June 22, 1999, from http://www.salon.com/people/bc/1999/06/22/greer
Wallace, C. (1998). *Germaine Greer: Untamed shrew.* New York: Faber & Faber.

TAMBRA K. CAIN

Guardianship When a person is unable to fend for herself, whether because she is a parentless child or an adult who suffers from mental retardation, mental illness, substance abuse, or dementia, those around her may discuss the possibility of guardianship. Unlike voluntary measures short of guardianship, like setting up a joint bank account (where two people share control of funds), a representative payee (when one person looks after another person's government benefits), a conservatorship, a trust, or a power of attorney (voluntary arrangements that can be similar in scope to a guardianship), a true guardianship is rare and serious and may be established only by a court of law. This court, commonly called the county Probate Court, declares or appoints one person (the guardian) to protect the interests of another (the ward), whether the ward likes it or not.

A guardian of the person is authorized to only make medical decisions, including the ward's living arrangements, and to monitor closely the ward's needs and standard of living. (Legal documents called a durable *health care* power of attorney or a living will may alleviate the need for a guardianship of the person.) A guardian of the estate makes all financial decisions. (Again, legal documents called a durable *general* power of attorney or living trust may keep these matters private, out of court.)

The prospective ward has the right to resist the guardianship process and to have a say in who is appointed guardian, and next of kin are notified as well. Because such important rights are at stake, the process is a matter of public record and the ward's privacy (concerning medical and financial information that is usually confidential) is sacrificed for the sake of her safety and well-being. If the prospective ward cannot afford an attorney, one may be appointed for her by the court. Sometimes a parent is known as the natural guardian of a child, but someone (not always the natural parent) must be appointed guardian of the estate for a child who is to receive a substantial sum of money (usually around $10,000 or more) as an inheritance or personal injury recovery, to make sure that the funds are spent on the child or saved for the child's future. Some states have laws permitting or forbidding a person from applying for guardianship over a child just so the child may attend school as a resident of a particular school district. Sometimes a court will appoint what is called a guardian ad litem just for the purpose of protecting a minor or incompetent person's rights during the course of a lawsuit. A limited guardian or emergency guardian may be appointed for a one-time purpose: to make a critical medical decision or stop a person who is unable to control her spending habits.

The application and appointment process can be cumbersome and expensive. Legal paperwork often includes an application, a statement by a physician documenting the medical need for such an extreme measure, a court investigator's report, posting of a bond by the guardian (protecting the ward's funds if the guardian were to misuse or steal the funds), and oaths and affirmations promising the court that the guardian understands all the rights and responsibilities of serving in this position of trust (called a fiduciary relationship). The prospective ward as well as all of the ward's next of kin are notified of the impending guardianship hearing.

At the hearing, a probate judge or magistrate listens to all those who have gathered and decides not only whether to establish the guardianship at all, but also determines whether or not the prospective guardian, or an alternative, can be trusted to act in the ward's best interests. If the prospective ward, for example, an elderly person suffering from Alzheimer's disease, had named her preferred guardian in a power of attorney or other document, the court will take that expressed preference into consideration. Sometimes the court will appoint a relative to serve as guardian of the person and a bank to serve as guardian of the estate or a single person will be appointed to serve in both capacities.

During the course of a guardianship, the guardian asks the court for permission to spend or invest the ward's funds and makes periodic accountings to the court showing how much money comes and goes and for what kinds of purchases, as well as reports to the court confirming over time whether the ward still needs a guardian. A guardian must continually show the court that all decisions on the ward's behalf are in the ward's best interests, not merely convenient for the guardian, and that all funds are being spent on the ward or her dependents, designed to maintain the ward at a standard of living that matches the size of her estate and her medical and other needs.

If the ward has enough money, the court may allow the guardian reasonable compensation from the ward's estate. The guardian does not risk her own money by serving as a guardian and as long as she takes reasonable steps to protect her ward, should not be liable for the ward's actions that are out of her control.

Once a particular guardian is appointed (whether a person or an institution like a bank or a nonprofit group), it can be difficult to change guardians or have the entire guardianship terminated. Once a child turns 18, the guardianship ends and any funds held in her guardianship then belong to her outright. If a ward who had been declared incompetent regains her ability to take care of herself and manage her money, she may seek to terminate the guardianship. In extreme cases, where the court learns about a guardian's abuse of the ward or the ward's funds, the court may remove and replace the guardian. The Roman satiric poet Juvenal once wrote: *Sed quis custodiet ipsos custodes?* But who will guard the guardians themselves? We rely on our local county probate courts to keep an eye on those who serve as guardians for our society's most vulnerable members.

SEE ALSO: Conservatorship, Durable power of attorney for health care

Suggested Reading

American Bar Association. (1988). *Life services planning: Support services and alternatives to guardianship.* Chicago: American Bar Association.

Robertson, Edward D. Jr. (1991). *Personal autonomy and substituted judgement: Legal issues in medical decisions for incompetent patients.* Corpus Christi, TX: Diocesan Press.

Shmidt, Winsor C. Jr. (1995). *Guardianship: Court of last resort for the elderly and disabled.* Durham, NC: Carolina Academic Press.

Suggested Resources

National Guardianship Association. www.guardianship.org
Kansas Elder Law Network. www.keln.org

JANET L. LOWDER
CARMEN M. VERHOSEK

Hair Care Feeling positive about our appearance helps us to feel positive in other areas of our lives. Our hair speaks volumes about us—from the color to the cut and ultimately the style that we choose. Beautiful, healthy, chic hair can be a reality for everyone. It simply requires a little attention, the inclusion of a few easy details in our daily routine, and a good stylist.

Beautiful hair is achieved by using a shampoo that contains high concentrations of natural ingredients and essential oils and a minimum of synthetic additives. On a daily basis, rely on shampoos made with pure plant essence, provitamin B5, and antioxidants such as vitamin E. This choice is your first step in working toward the goal of healthy, beautiful hair. Additionally, a special detoxifying shampoo once a week may be helpful to remove any product buildup from accessory hair products or other toxins.

There are many variables that lend uniqueness to the appearance of our hair. One of these variables is the condition of the scalp; that is, whether it is oily, dry, or normal. Other variables include the thickness of the hair, including the actual density and diameter of each strand of hair. Finally, there is the texture, which influences how much straightness or wave the hair has.

Condition of hair is another factor. Hair that is damaged and has its cuticle sticking up tends to look dull. Proper conditioning in and out of the shower is important for promoting shiny hair. Combing conditioners through in a downward motion to smooth the hair cuticle is a key process.

Another important variable is the type of styling products used, which influence hair volume. Hair styling products may be oil- or water-based. Products are intended to either increase or decrease hair tensile strength. Hair oils, creams, sticks, pomades, and waxes are meant to decrease volume and smooth hair. Sprays, gels, and mousses are designed to increase hair volume and texture.

Individuals with fine or thin hair should take caution to avoid overconditioning. Alcohol additives, given a bad name by some companies, may be useful in adding volume to thin hair. Women with thick or medium-textured hair should use a shampoo with more active cleaning properties and a medium weight conditioner. Thick and medium-textured hair can tolerate leave-in conditioners and styling products that are either oil- or water-based. Hair that is curly and coarse, but fine, is prone to damage. This type of hair requires a very gentle shampoo and a heavy conditioner. Those with coarse hair may benefit from oil-based styling products that are geared toward decreasing volume. Try massaging jojoba mixed with essential oils for extra conditioning before a shower. Coarse, highly textured hair that is thick requires deep conditioning. Oil-based products should be used because thick coarse hair with texture is resilient and can take a highly active shampoo.

All types of hair should be cleaned periodically with a detoxifying shampoo. Those living in urban areas that are exposed to higher levels of pollutants should consider detoxifying once a week. The same is true for those using multiple styling products on a daily basis and for those swimming frequently in chlorinated pools or seawater. A good detoxifying shampoo with highly active cleansers can remove

Table 1. Hair care tips

Hair do's	Hair don'ts
• Use a detoxifying shampoo based on need, according to manufacturer's directions • Always condition especially longer hair • Cut your hair every 6–8 weeks (even growing out hair, trim ends 1/4 in. at least) • Brush your hair often • When using heat or chemical processes always use conditioner and other protective products	• Brush wet hair • Use uncoated rubber bands • Comb conditioners through hair • Sleep with rubber bands, barrettes, hair clips, hair combs, or bobby pins in hair • Subject hair to excessive heat from hair dryers and curling irons. Follow manufacturer's directions • Expose hair to the sun for long periods • Leave chlorine or seawater in hair after swimming

pollutants, oil buildup, and shampoo residue. However, overuse of a detoxifying shampoo can have negative effects, such as a loss of shine and pliability that may ultimately lead to breakage. Rely on a good detoxifying shampoo but avoid using it too often.

Our hair has a certain degree of resistance to damage. However excessive chemical use such as that involved in perming, bleaching, and double-process coloring can do irreparable harm. That is why it is so important to rely on a stylist who is knowledgeable about all hair types and who uses products considered least harmful to hair. Become knowledgeable about your specific type of hair and work within that framework (Table 1).

Most women rely on word of mouth when seeking guidance for hair care and styling. If such references are not readily available, choose a salon where the hair stylist seems adaptable to your aesthetic sensibilities and sense of fashion. Look for a stylist who has patience and who will help you articulate your hairstyle goals. Semantics and communication are important. It is unadvisable to ask for *a trim* or *a shaping*. This provides the stylist with little useful information. Instead, be as specific and direct as possible. A good stylist will be open to your ideas and will value pictures and sketches. Best results are obtained when you and the stylist work as a team to achieve your goals.

See Also: Calcium, Dermatitis, Diet, Hair loss, Hair removal, Iron supplementation, Nail care, Skin care

Suggested Reading

Ferrell, P., & Rackley, L. (1996). *Let's talk hair: Every black woman's personal consultation for healthy growing hair.* Washington, DC: Cornrows.
Janssen, M. B. (1999). *Naturally healthy hair: Herbal treatments and daily care for fabulous hair.* North Adams, MA: Storey Books.
Massey, L., & Chiel, D. (2001). *Curly girl.* New York: Workman.

Linda Agresta Sprinzl

Hair Loss The portion of hair that is seen is called the hair shaft. That which is below the surface of skin is the follicle. During our lifetime, each hair follicle undergoes repeated cycles of growth, rest, and regeneration. Hair loss can occur due to disturbances of the hair cycle, damage to the hair shaft, or disorders affecting the follicle.

DISTURBANCES OF THE HAIR CYCLE

Normally the majority of scalp hair is in the growth phase. A small percentage of hairs in the resting phase are shed each day (100–200 hairs shed daily). Under certain circumstances a higher percentage of hairs enter the resting phase and a woman may notice a sudden increase in hair shedding. Common causes include high fever, childbirth, severe infections, severe "flu," severe chronic illness, major surgery, thyroid disorder, crash diets, inadequate protein intake, and certain drugs. The shedding often starts months after the inciting cause but will stop after several weeks if the offending cause is removed or corrected.

DAMAGE TO THE HAIR SHAFT

Hair is composed primarily of the protein keratin, which is the same substance that forms fingernails and toenails. Sulfur crosslinks between hair proteins provide for the strength of the hair. Damage to the hair shaft by improper cosmetic techniques can cause hair breakage. There is little damage from normal dyeing, bleaching, waving, or straightening. However, breakage can occur from too much tension during waving, from waving solutions left on too long or improperly neutralized, from waving and bleaching on the same day, or from too frequent hair treatments. Other causes of hair breakage include excess tension in braids, ponytails, and cornrows, or excess friction due to helmets or orthodontic appliances. Hair breakage will stop if the cosmetic procedure is stopped and the hair is handled gently, but hairs already broken cannot be mended.

DISORDERS AFFECTING THE FOLLICLE

Hereditary hair thinning, or androgenetic alopecia, is the most common form of hair loss in humans. This condition is also known as male-pattern hair loss or common baldness in men and as female-pattern hair thinning in women. Onset may occur in either sex at any time after puberty. It is estimated that half of the population experiences hereditary hair loss by age 50.

The cause of hereditary hair thinning is a gradual shrinkage of the hair follicle, which occurs under the influence of androgens. The smaller hair follicle results in a finer and shorter hair shaft. Women with hereditary thinning usually first notice a gradual thinning of their hair, mostly on the top of their heads, and their scalp becomes more visible. Over time, the hair on the sides may also become thinner. The patient may notice that her "ponytail" is much smaller. This diffuse thinning of the hair can vary in extent but it is extremely rare for a woman to become bald. Extensive laboratory tests are usually not needed if the woman with hereditary thinning has normal periods, pregnancies, and hormone levels. Thyroid disease and iron deficiency are two causes of hair thinning that can easily be ruled out by laboratory tests. Treatment for women with hereditary thinning includes topical minoxidil solution that, when used regularly, can partially reenlarge the miniaturized hairs.

Alopecia areata is an autoimmune disease that affects almost 2% of the population in the United States. Inflammatory cells target the hair follicle, thus preventing hair growth. Typically a small round bald patch is noticed; this patchy hair loss may regrow spontaneously. In other cases there can be extensive patchy hair loss and in rare cases there is loss of all scalp and body hair (alopecia areata universalis). Alopecia areata occurs equally in males and females, at all ages, although young persons are affected most often. Alopecia areata typically has a relapsing and remitting course. Treatment is available when the disease is active but does not prevent future occurrences of hair loss.

SEE ALSO: Autoimmune disorders, Skin care, Skin disorders

Suggested Reading

Gummer, C. L. (2002). Cosmetics and hair loss. *Clinical & Experimental Dermatology, 27*(5), 418–421.

Olsen, E. A., Hordinsky, M., Roberts, J. L., & Whiting, D. A. (2002). Female pattern hair loss. *Journal of the American Academy of Dermatology, 47*(5), 795.

Price, V. H. (1999). Treatment of hair loss. *New England Journal of Medicine, 341*, 964–973.

Suggested Resources

American Academy of Dermatology: www.aad.org
National Alopecia Areata Foundation: www.naaf.org

PARADI MIRMIRANI

Hair Removal Excessive growth of facial or body hair (hirsutism) in women can be profoundly distressing, and is often perceived as loss of femininity. The psychological ramifications of excess hair growth in women cannot be overstated. Hirsutism is defined as the presence of excess hair growth in a male distribution including the chin, sideburns, and above the upper lip.

The diagnosis of hirsutism is somewhat subjective and there is clearly a cultural bias to what is perceived as "normal." The vast majority of female patients diagnosed with hirsutism have no underlying hormonal abnormality and have female relatives with similar hair growth. However, hirsutism may sometimes be a serious harbinger of underlying disease. If the hair growth is very significant or sudden in onset, or if there are other symptoms suggesting increased levels of male hormones (such as deepening of the voice, increased muscle mass, menstrual irregularities, decrease in breast size, or increase in genital size), then ovarian or adrenal abnormalities should be ruled out through laboratory testing. Occasionally women demonstrate increased hair growth in a distribution that is not solely in a male pattern, and this condition is referred to as hypertrichosis. This pattern of growth may be caused by certain drugs and inherited diseases.

Since male hormones (androgens) cause hirsutism, a common first-line approach to reduce the amount of hair is treatment with drugs that reduce levels of androgens. Combination oral contraceptives and antiandrogen drugs such as spironolactone (a mild water pill) are often used for this purpose.

Mechanical methods of hair removal are commonly used in women with varying degrees of undesirable hair growth. Depilatory creams and shaving remove hair at the surface of the skin, cutting the hair shaft by chemical or physical means, respectively. In contrast, tweezing or waxing removes hair from the root resulting in a longer delay in regrowth. Regardless of depth of the hair removal, all of these represent short-term hair removal methods that have the advantage of rapid results and the disadvantage of rapid regrowth. Electrolysis provides a more permanent form of hair removal by destroying the regenerative portion of the hair follicle with an electric current. Because a small needle must be introduced into the hair follicle, there is some discomfort associated with the procedure that can be minimized by using topical anesthetic beforehand. The most common side effects associated with the procedure are altered pigmentation, infection, and scarring. The success rate is highly dependent on the technical skill of the individual performing the procedure.

Lasers and other light-assisted methods are increasingly popular ways to remove hair that use the principle of selective photothermolysis. Varying wavelengths of light are used to target various skin or hair follicle substances, producing permanent hair reduction in a safe and effective manner. Currently, the more popular hair removal lasers target the pigment-producing cells in the hair, and for this reason, are most effective among patients with darker hair and lighter skin. Further research is needed to determine how permanently hair is removed with lasers.

One of the newest methods of hair removal is eflornithine cream. Its active ingredient blocks an enzyme ornithine decarboxylase that plays a critical role in the hair growth cycle. Rather than removing the hair, it slows its growth and therefore complements physical methods of hair removal by reducing the frequency of treatments. Side effects are mild and include treatment site discomfort and irritation.

Suggested Reading

Dierickx, C. C. (2000). Hair removal by lasers and intense pulsed light sources. *Seminars in Cutaneous Medicine and Surgery, 19*(4), 267–275.

Mercurio, M. G. (2001). Hirsutism: Diagnosis and management. *Journal of Gender-Specific Medicine, 4*(2), 29–34.

Moghetti, P., Tosi, F., Tosti, A., et al. (2000). Comparison of spironolactone, flutamide, and finasteride efficacy in the treatment of hirsutism: A randomized, double blind, placebo-controlled trial. *Journal of Clinical Endocrinology Metabolism, 85*(1), 89–94.

Wendelin, D. S., Pope, D. N., & Mallory, S. B. (2003). Hypertrichosis. *Journal of the American Academy of Dermatology, 48*, 161–179.

Mary Gail Mercurio

Harm Reduction Harm reduction is a set of strategies that encourages an individual to reduce the harm caused by a high-risk behavior. Harm reduction is not a new concept in public health since high-risk behaviors—also known as "bad habits," depending upon the era—have always existed and will continue to exist. What changes is how society views the behavior and societal responses to it.

Although harm reduction can be a very powerful means through which to modify high-risk behaviors and risk of disease, it is not without detractors who feel that harm reduction may undermine prevention and cessation programs. However, evidence of the success and long-term benefits, including cessation or abstinence, of harm reduction approaches for high-risk behaviors such as smoking, drinking and driving, and drug use is increasingly evident. While there has been little research devoted to the development and evaluation of their efficacy, the potential of microbicides to prevent the transmission of HIV and other sexually transmitted diseases has been described as a harm reduction approach for women with little control over whether their partner uses a condom. Again, fears have been raised that developing microbicides would reduce the focus on condom use, in spite of evidence that unprotected sexual intercourse continues to be a major risk behavior 20 years after AIDS was first described.

Harm reduction emphasizes the individual's input into the therapeutic process to ensure (a) that the client sets goals that are relevant to her/his social and environmental contexts and (b) that there is motivation to work toward reducing the harm caused by the behavior. The goal could be to reduce the harm experienced by the individual, the harm experienced by their families, or the harm experienced by the community in general. However, in order for harm reduction to be successful, barriers that inhibit individuals from seeking assistance must also be addressed (such as stigma, lack of access to services, lack of health insurance, fear of disclosure of the behavior), not just the behavior.

A very successful example of a harm reduction approach to a public health problem is the "designated driver" campaign targeting people who drink and drive. While it is against the law to drive a vehicle under the influence of alcohol (or other drugs), it is also recognized that people drink in social settings, that they on occasion drink too much, and that the person still needs to find a means to get home. The campaign encourages people to identify one member of the group to be the "designated driver," with this person preferably not drinking or drinking very little (one or two drinks over the entire evening). The designated driver is responsible for driving the other members of the group to their homes. While the designated driver campaign does not reduce individual harm resulting from alcohol intoxication, it significantly reduces the risk the drunk person faces should they get into a car and drive home. More importantly, the designated driver campaign reduces harm to the community should the drunk person be involved in an accident in which grievous harm (i.e., death or permanent disability) results to the drunk driver or an unsuspecting victim.

Another successful harm reduction approach has been the use of the nicotine patch to help smokers quit smoking or significantly reduce the number of cigarettes smoked when they are unable or unwilling to quit. The harmful effects of smoking are well documented. The challenges faced by smokers who wish to quit but are unable to do so are also better recognized and smoking cessation programs offer a variety of therapeutic approaches in order to manage both the physical dependency on nicotine and the psychological contexts that trigger a desire to smoke. One of these approaches is continued nicotine administration through a "patch" that is applied to the upper arm.

Using the nicotine patch allows the smoker to slowly reduce the amount of nicotine in their system over time, while dealing with the psychological contexts of their smoking habit. Thus, although there may be continued harm to the individual as a result of the ongoing exposure to nicotine, the harm to the individual is substantially reduced since the nicotine, along with tar, is not inhaled and it is expected that use of the nicotine patch will eventually cease. Harm to the individual's family and community is almost eliminated since exposure to secondhand smoke ceases. In some ethnic communities where rates of smoking for females are low, women could be the primary beneficiaries of harm reduction for smokers because their exposure to cigarette smoke would be significantly reduced; benefits would also accrue to children in the household.

HARM REDUCTION AND ILLICIT DRUG USE

Harm reduction, in the context of illicit drug use, has been defined as a "…pragmatic and humanistic approach to diminishing the individual and social harms associated with drug use," while others view harm reduction as "…a peace movement [that] is aligned with the humanistic values around which social work is organized." Although harm reduction has been successfully applied to reducing alcohol- and smoking-related harm, it becomes especially controversial when applied to reducing the harm caused by illicit drug use. The development of drug policies not founded on public health principles has resulted in long-term harm to women and their families, ethnic minority women in particular, by separating families through increased jail sentences for nonviolent drug-related crime. These communities often have the least access to drug treatment and other health and social service programs, and the greatest barriers to sustaining behavior change as a result.

SEE ALSO: Acquired immunodeficiency syndrome, Sexually transmitted diseases, Substance use, Violence

Suggested Reading

Brocato, J., & Wagner, E. F. (2003). Harm reduction: A social work practice model and social justice agenda. *Health and Social Work, 28*(2), 117–125.
Open Society Institute. (2002). *Harm reduction news.* New York: Author. http://www.soros.org

LINDA S. LLOYD

Headache Headache disorders can be divided into primary and secondary types. A secondary headache is one caused by an underlying disease or physiologic condition. Primary headaches are not symptomatic of another condition. They are among the commonest human afflictions. Tension-type headache has a lifetime prevalence of 78%, and migraine, 16%. Secondary headaches are much less common: post-traumatic headache has a lifetime prevalence of 4%, and headache caused by brain tumor, less than 0.5%.

The term *tension headache* is an old one that reflects two outdated, discredited ideas of pathophysiology: that the headache is due to emotional "tension" or to excessive "tension" (contraction) of pericranial muscles. Current thinking holds that abnormal sensitivity of brain nerve cells is the cause, but the old name, with a slight change, to tension-*type* headache, has been retained. Tension-type headache is more common in women, with gender ratios ranging from 1.04 to 1.4. Prevalence peaks between 20 and 50 years of age and then declines. The pain is dull, achy, pressure-like, and tight. It is mild to moderate in severity. It is located bilaterally, in the forehead, temples, back or top of the head, or all over the head, and often in a band-like distribution around the head. Unlike migraine, tension-type headache is not worsened by physical activity or associated with nausea, vomiting, photophobia (light sensitivity), or phonophobia (sensitivity to sound). Headaches typically last a few hours but can be as brief as 30 minutes or go on for years.

Tension-type headache sometimes responds to stress management, relaxation therapy, and exercise, but most patients require pharmacotherapy. The choice of an *abortive* medication, aimed at terminating a headache, depends on the severity and duration of the attack. Mild headaches often respond to over-the-counter (OTC) analgesic drugs, including acetaminophen, aspirin, and nonsteroidal anti-inflammatory drugs (NSAIDs), such as ibuprofen or naproxen, although four tablets rather than the traditional two may be required for effective treatment. A combination of simple OTC analgesics and caffeine may be more effective than a single drug. For more severe attacks, a similar combination including butalbital with or without codeine, available only by prescription, is more effective. Patients who use abortive medicines more than 2 days a week are at risk of developing *medication-overuse headache*. This takes the form of a chronic daily headache that responds to each dose of medicine for a short time but recurs soon afterward, creating a vicious cycle of rebound headaches. Avoiding this complication of treatment is the purpose of using medicines to reduce the frequency, severity, and duration of headache, that is, *preventive* therapy. Patients take a drug regularly, everyday, for months to years. Once their headaches have been under control for 3–6 months, the drug may be withdrawn. Amitriptyline, a tricyclic antidepressant, in a low dose, is the drug most often used, but other types of medication, including tizanidine, a muscle relaxer, and all the drugs used for migraine headache prevention are also effective.

Migraine is the second most common headache disorder; it is discussed elsewhere in this volume. *Cluster headache* is much less common, occurring in 15.6 men per 100,000 person-years and in 4 women per 100,000 person-years. It has a familial occurrence: The risk among first-degree relatives is 14 times higher than in the general population. The mean age of onset is 27–31 years. Its most characteristic feature is its temporal pattern. Episodes occur every other day to eight times a day for months, then they stop for months to years, then they start again; hence, the name "cluster headache." Sometimes headaches occur at the same time each day, often in the middle of the night. They are relatively brief, lasting 30 minutes to 3 hours, but usually less than 2 hours. The pain is strictly unilateral, and the side is the same in each episode of a cluster. It centers in the eye but may be more widespread and is very severe. Patients typically pace the floor during the headache, in contrast to migraine patients, who lie down. Cluster headaches are often associated with autonomic signs on the painful side of the head, including ptosis of the eyelid and pupillary miosis (Horner syndrome), conjunctival injection, lacrimation, and nasal congestion or rhinorrhea. Effective abortive treatments include inhaled oxygen, subcutaneous or intranasal sumatriptan, and intranasal lidocaine and preventive treatments include prednisone, verapamil, lithium, and valproate.

Pregnancy and breast-feeding have an impact on the treatment of headache. The formation of the organs of the body of the fetus takes place mainly in the first trimester of pregnancy. Some medicines are known to cause fetal malformations, and others are known not to do so, but there is no certain knowledge about most drugs. Most physicians advise women to take only medicines known not to cause fetal malformations during that period of pregnancy.

Acetaminophen, caffeine, NSAIDs, codeine, and other narcotics and probably sumatriptan are safe abortive agents, but only prednisone is safe as a preventive drug, for the types of headache discussed above. Amitriptyline is probably safe in the second and third trimesters. Late in pregnancy NSAIDs should be avoided, because they can impair closure of the fetal *ductus arteriosus.* Medicines taken by lactating women appear in their breast milk. The dose received by the infant is usually 1–2% of the maternal dose, which is safe for most drugs but not tricyclic antidepressants, butalbital, sumatriptan, or aspirin.

Secondary headaches may be due to physiologic states such as fasting, pathophysiologic states such as caffeine withdrawal, minor illnesses such as sinusitis, and serious diseases such as stroke and head trauma. Certain historical features may be regarded as "red flags," which indicate the possibility of serious underlying disease. A new severe headache of sudden onset may indicate subarachnoid bleeding, meningitis, or dissection of an artery in the neck or head. A headache that grows worse and worse over a period of days to weeks suggests the possibility of increased intracranial pressure or an intracranial mass lesion. Precipitation of a headache by exertion or sexual activity suggests subarachnoid hemorrhage or a malformation of the hindbrain. A headache disorder beginning late in life may be due to giant cell arteritis. A background of AIDS or cancer suggests that a new headache may be due to intracranial infection or tumor. A headache that remains localized to one part of the head for a long period of time suggests the possibility of a structural intracranial lesion there. Diseases that can present as a new headache and occur more commonly in pregnancy include subarachnoid hemorrhage, pituitary tumor and choriocarcinoma, preeclampsia, and intracranial dural venous sinus thrombosis.

SEE ALSO: Chronic pain, Giant cell arteritis, Neuropathy, Pain, Temporomandibular joint disorders

Suggested Reading

Dalessio, D. J., & Silberstein, S. D. (1993). *Wolff's headache and other head pain* (6th ed.). New York: Oxford University Press.

Lance, J. W. (1993). *Mechanism and management of headache* (5th ed.). Oxford: Butterworth-Heinemann.

Raskin, N. H. (1988). *Headache* (2nd ed.). New York: Churchill Livingstone.

Silberstein, S. D., Lipton, R. B., & Goadsby, P. J. (1998). *Headache in clinical practice.* Oxford: Isis Medical.

Silberstein, S. D., Stiles, A., Young, W. B., & Rozen, T. D. (2002). *An atlas of headache.* New York: Parthenon.

MARC D. WINKELMAN

Healers Why are women more numerous and important as healers in some medical systems and men in others? Do women healers have special attributes that differ from those of male healers?

Decades ago, I. M. Lewis offered the now classic thesis that women are healers where there are "cults of affliction," covert protest movements with rituals that feature possession/trance, which seek to compensate gender inequalities. Other anthropologists suggest that since men often suffer the same types of initiation illness as do women and also participate in possession cults, an explanation of why more women than men are healers in these cults can be found in the relationship between the gender system and systems of power and authority. More recently Lewis' notion has been critically reviewed by Janice Boddy (1989). Based on studies of the Zar cult in northern Sudan, she suggests that although the idea of status and power balancing may be accurate, it is too unidimensional to adequately explain Sudanese women's behavior. Boddy describes how men's and women's roles are complementary and suggests that this underlies women's involvement in the cult, expressed in Zar spirit possessions. In contrast to appealing to sociocultural factors, such as gender role constructs, Jeanne Achterberg suggests that certain gender-related, stereotypical personal attributes are found in women who become healers—subjectivity, receptivity, relatedness, and understanding—which are also attributes of the "wounded healer," an ideal type of healer.

Although the studies referenced above largely refer to women in developing countries, ritual healing cults are found in developed countries, particularly among immigrant and ethnic minority populations. The gender pattern in popular healing cults in the United States, such as Curanderismo, Espiritismo, Santería, and Vodun, seems to parallel that of their home country. Many more women than men are popular healers among Latinos (Mexican Americans, Puerto Ricans, Dominicans, and Cubans), African Americans, and South Americans. However, where the cult is large and status differences exist, then men often dominate as leaders. Similarly, in institutionalized religions that carry out healing rituals, there may be more men than women carrying out the healer role, and the men occupy higher status positions. This difference appears related to opportunities for social status in a community of believers, such as in the Catholic charismatic movement or the Pentecostal churches. Lawless describes how the relatively few women preachers in the Pentecostal churches in rural Missouri were considered illegitimate as religious leaders; this view seems to persist.

In the United States, the dominating presence of men in medicine began to change only in the mid-1970s. Prior to that time few women were admitted into medical training although many received training through apprenticeship or homeopathic schools. The Woman's Medical College of Pennsylvania was the exception as the only all-women medical school from 1910 to 1970.

Women as psychotherapists and physicians exhibit a deep commitment to their work, which assists them to endure the dilemmas and conflicts engendered in reconciling personal ("feminine") values (particularly those focused on home and family) with their vocations. The difficulties women experience in medical training and practice have been described for both the United States and Australia (Pringle, 1998; Wear, 1996). Currently many medical school classes have equal numbers of men and women but relatively few women hold leadership positions within the field of medicine. Psychology has been more open to women as practitioners yet, as in medicine, many more men hold high-status positions as chairs of academic departments or directors of clinics or other institutions. Although men dominate clinical psychology, women are predominant in the alternative routes for practicing psychotherapy, such as counseling psychology, psychiatric nursing, and social work.

CHARACTERISTICS OF WOMEN HEALERS

There are indications that women manage their distress more successfully than men when carrying out therapeutic work. One study of burnout among mental health professionals showed that although males and females reported the same numbers of job stressors, strong associations existed between stressors and burnout only for males; no clear associations were found for the women. Perhaps the emotional demands of mental health care are more compatible with women's ideas and self-expectations. The socialization of the traditional Spiritist healer into her healing role aims at protecting her from the "contagion" of malignant spirit-causes of a client's distress through sharing the healing process with a group and by working spiritually to attract spirit-protectors as personal guides. This suggests that enhanced relatedness among women mental health professionals (a professional "sisterhood") may serve as protective support against burnout.

Fewer malpractice claims are filed against women physicians. This suggests that because male physicians are more attached to the authority and power inherent in the physician's role, they are more affected when that role is attacked. Women practitioners worried more about responsibility than men, a parallel to popular healers in Peru as described by Glass-Coffin (1996). Several studies indicate that men attribute their successes to ability and their failures to luck, while women's attributions are exactly the opposite.

There are numerous studies comparing men and women physicians on patterns of provider–patient communication. Significant findings are that patients speak more, disclose more psychosocial and biomedical information, and make more positive statements to women physicians. In general, regardless of gender, patients of women physicians expressed greater comfort, were more engaged, disclosed more, and were more assertive.

WOUNDED HEALERS

Female psychotherapists report significantly higher rates of physical and sexual abuse in childhood, alcoholism and severe mental illness in parents, as well as death of a parent or sibling. Moreover, they experienced a relatively high prevalence of trauma and family dysfunction during childhood. These facts imply a "wounded healer" syndrome as motivation to enter mental health care or health professional careers, but discount the notion that women health professionals enter the field to resolve personal conflicts. One study showed that the women mental health professionals had significantly less anxiety, depression, dissociation, sleep disturbances, and impaired relationships than male professionals. Perhaps, like ritual healers, mental health professionals experience less distress because they have managed to overcome it (and utilize this capacity in their work).

THE LARGER PICTURE

A number of authors have argued that the mental health and medical professions are undergoing a process of "feminization." This view suggests the final piece in understanding the "why" and "how" of women as healers. It seems that a devaluation of psychotherapy and medicine as professional pursuits is occurring, in part due to the policies of managed care systems. This is related to the entry of growing numbers of women into medicine and mental health care professions, replacing men who begin to find these careers less attractive. This reasoning does not fully account for why women find health professional careers more attractive, or why women's participation in medicine has recently become more accepted (apart from the effect of the feminist movement). Medicine's dominant principles have objectified body-experience and have focused health care on the rational and on scientific achievements for restoring physical well-being, often to the neglect of subjectivity, satisfying communication, and the sharing of meaning and experience with patients. Healers in religious cults generally display these latter characteristics. It appears that growing dissatisfactions with modern medicine and mental health care have resulted in greater appreciation for these capacities in health care, which in turn has led to greater appreciation of women as healers.

SEE ALSO: African American, Asian and Pacific Islander, Charismatic healers, Complementary and alternative health practices, Cuanderos, Latinos. Physicians, Women in the Health Professions (pp. 20–32)

Suggested Reading

Boddy, J. (1989). *Wombs and alien spirits: Women, men, and the Zar Cult in Northern Sudan.* Madison: University of Wisconsin Press.

Bowman, M. A., & Allen, D. I. (1990). *Stress and women physicians* (2nd ed.). New York: Springer-Verlag.

Geis, R. E., Jesilow, P., & Geis, G. (1991). The Amelia Stern Syndrome: A diagnosis of a condition among female physicians? *Social Science and Medicine, 33*(8), 967–971.

Glass-Coffin, B. (1996). Male and female healing in Northern Peru: Metaphors, models and manifestations of difference. *Journal of Ritual Studies, 10*(1), 63–91.

Gross, E. B. (1992). Gender differences in physician stress. *Journal of the American Medical Women's Association, 47*(4), 107–114.

Hall, J. A., & Roter, D. L. (2002). Do patients talk differently to male and female physicians? A meta-analytic review. *Patient Education and Counseling, 48,* 117–124.

Koss-Chioino, J. D. (1992). *Women as healers, women as patients: Mental health care and traditional healing in Puerto Rico.* Boulder, CO: Westview Press.

Philipson, I. J. (1993). *On the shoulders of women: The feminization of psychotherapy.* New York: Guilford Press.

Pringle, R. (1998). *Sex and medicine: Gender, power and authority in the medical profession.* Cambridge, UK: Cambridge University Press.

Wear, D. (Ed.). (1996). *Women in medical education: An anthology of experience.* Albany: State University of New York Press.

JOAN D. KOSS-CHIOINO

Health Insurance

Health Insurance   Health insurance is a key factor facilitating access to health care services. Individuals without health insurance are often denied care, especially if the condition for which a patient is seeking care does not require any immediate attention and/or intervention. Uninsured and underinsured individuals tend to delay care and forego maintenance and/or routine health services to the extent that they can manage their symptoms. In addition, a large proportion of uninsured women do not see a medical specialist when needed and fail to fill prescriptions because of cost concerns.

Many studies have compared health care outcomes between insured and uninsured populations and invariably these studies have shown vast disparities by insurance status. Such disparities have been documented in the access, utilization, and outcomes pertaining to child care, prenatal care, cancer care, and a number of other clinical conditions. In comparing cancer-related outcomes, for example, studies have shown a greater likelihood of being diagnosed at later stages of disease among the uninsured, as compared to the insured. For cancers that are amenable to screening and prevention, such as breast and cervical cancer, such a finding reflects lack of access to cancer screening services.

To increase access to care among the near poor, state Medicaid programs have expanded their eligibility rules to provide coverage to pregnant women and children with household incomes exceeding the Federal Poverty Level (FPL). Similarly, there have been many programs in place to make it possible for elderly individuals with incomes higher than the FPL to enroll in Medicaid. Nevertheless, it has been estimated that approximately 14% of pregnant women (equating to over 450,000 women) remained without health care coverage when a substantial proportion may have qualified for Medicaid, and only half of the elderly potentially eligible for Medicaid actually enrolled in the program. Lack of knowledge of such programs, the stigma attached to welfare programs, and the long administrative process to enroll in Medicaid have been cited as possible reasons for low rates of participation in the program, especially in the elderly population.

According to recent census data, approximately 1 in 5 women 18–64 years of age is uninsured. Most uninsured individuals live in poverty or near-poverty, and many reside in rural areas. Eight percent of women receive health coverage through Medicaid; 40% through their own employment; 28% through their spouse's employment, as a dependent; 3% through other public sources such as the Veterans Health Administration System; and 4% purchase their own insurance policy. In the latter scenario, the insurance premium can be prohibitively costly, and individuals are closely scrutinized for preexisting health conditions, such as a chronic disease. They may be denied an insurance policy in the presence of such conditions. When the purchaser is the employer, however, the management is able to negotiate a more affordable rate with insurance companies because of large volume and employees are not screened for preexisting health conditions.

Health benefits constitute an increasingly significant proportion of the fringe benefits offered by employers. As part of cost containment efforts, many employers have limited the scope of services covered in their health benefits and/or increased the employees' share of health care expenses. Employers have also resorted to a wider base of part-time employees with limited or no fringe (health) benefits. Receiving coverage through a spouse's employer may also be problematic, as women's insurance status becomes dependent on their marital status, the spouse's employment, and the employer's decision to continue, discontinue, or limit health care coverage to the employees' dependents. It is of note that lesbian women represent a particularly vulnerable subgroup of the female population (estimated at 3–10%) with respect to barriers they face in receiving health care coverage through their partner's employer, as very few employers actually offer health insurance benefits to domestic partners. Even when the benefit is available, many are reluctant to let their sexual orientation be known to their employer for fear of discrimination.

Although most health plans provide coverage for various reproductive health services, such as pregnancy and childbirth, fewer plans actually provide coverage for contraceptives. According to the Henry J. Kaiser Family Foundation, only 13 states had enacted legislation as of October 2000 requiring coverage for contraceptive medication and supplies similar to other prescription medication. Nine other states had more

limited provision. Coverage for mental health services is often offered on a limited basis as well. It has been reported that 26% of insured workers have coverage for a restricted number of outpatient visits (20 or less), and only 11% have coverage for an unlimited number of outpatient visits. Similar restrictions apply to the use of inpatient mental health services.

In the absence of universal health care, insurance coverage remains a key element to timely and adequate access to and use of health services. Women must capitalize on political gains made in the last several decades to further advance their cause in providing coverage to the most vulnerable subgroups of the population and to expand coverage to services in reproductive care and mental health.

SEE ALSO: Access to health care, Disparities in Women's Health and Health Care (pp. 13–20), Medicaid, Medicare, Socioeconomic status

Suggested Reading

Ayanian, J. Z., Kohler, B. A., Abe, T., & Epstein, A. M. (1993). The relation between health insurance coverage and clinical outcomes among women with breast cancer. *New England Journal of Medicine, 329*, 326–331.

Conway, M. M., Ahern, D. W., & Steuernagel, G. A. (Eds.). (1999). *Women and public policy.* Washington, DC: CQ Press.

The Henry J. Kaiser Family Foundation. (2003). *The women's health data book.* www.kff.org

SIRAN M. KOROUKIAN

Health Maintenance Organizations

Health Maintenance Organization (HMO) is an all-encompassing term that refers to organizations that integrate the financing and delivery of health services, based on a prepaid, fixed fee per enrollee. This is different from the traditional fee-for-service (FFS) system in which a provider is reimbursed for a given service rendered to the patient. The prepaid aspect of the financing of services rendered by HMOs implies a certain level of efficiency as well as a special emphasis on prevention, early intervention/treatment, and health promotion, with the intention to reduce the occurrence of costly episodes of care because of delay in seeking and receiving care.

First initiated in the 1920s, HMOs expanded rapidly with the financial support of the federal government, which viewed the development of HMOs as a possible model that could lead to national health insurance. The 1973 Health Maintenance Organization Act defined the structural and design requirements that plans had to meet. HMOs experienced significant increases in market share in the 1980s, and further expansions followed the enrollment of Medicare and Medicaid beneficiaries in managed care programs. As of the mid-1990s, between 30% and 50% of the population in certain states were enrolled in some form of managed care programs.

HMOs operate under different structures. In staff-model HMOs, for example, physicians receive salary or incentive bonuses by the HMO or become partners with the HMO. In other models, such as group-model, network-model, and Independent Practice Association (IPA) model HMO, HMOs may contract with individual or groups of physicians that provide services to its members. Other arrangements include Preferred Provider Organization (PPO), where health services are purchased from a list of participating providers who may offer discounted rates in return for high volume. Beneficiaries may opt to use services by non-PPO providers, but at a higher rate of co-insurance and deductibles.

As its name implies, HMOs were initially developed with a strong commitment to health maintenance, including routine and preventive services. However, quality of care became an issue because of concerns that HMOs would limit enrollees' services as a measure of cost containment, given that health care providers would have to offer health services while operating on a fixed payment per enrollee. Furthermore, critics have argued that, as a cost containment strategy, HMOs may engage in a practice of marketing to healthy individuals, while discouraging sicker individuals from enrolling—a practice commonly referred to as "cherry-picking."

Numerous studies have compared quality of care between HMOs and traditional FFS systems. There appear to be no conclusive patterns of better or worse quality of care among HMO enrollees as compared with FFS beneficiaries. Findings from some studies have favored the FFS system, while other studies have shown that HMO enrollees used preventive and routine/health maintenance services at a higher rate than their FFS counterparts. In the case of cancer, for example, one study showed that HMO enrollees were more likely than their FFS counterparts to be diagnosed at earlier stages of cancers that were amenable to screening, suggesting more effective strategies of cancer screening in HMOs than in FFS settings. In addition, there are indications that the presence of HMOs in a given area may be associated with a dynamic in the local health care delivery system that favors higher use of preventive and screening services, as well as lower expenditures by FFS beneficiaries residing in that area. On the other hand, it has been shown that uninsured people experience more difficulty accessing care in areas with higher HMO activity than in areas with lower HMO activity.

The management and coordination of care by HMOs usually entail "gatekeepers," a term used to refer to the primary care physicians (PCPs) who attend to the patient's primary health care needs. The PCP is also the one to decide whether a patient should be seen by a medical specialist for a particular health problem. Such arrangements have been perceived by patients as being restrictive. Restrictions may also apply to certain tests, procedures, and medications, and in the absence of conclusive evidence of the benefits of a given intervention, the tendency has been to favor less intensive care. Such restrictions have been a source of dissatisfaction in the provider community.

Performance indicators, such as the proportion of women enrolled in an HMO to initiate prenatal care in the first trimester, and the proportion of enrollees to undergo a cancer screening program, are now published in report cards for each HMO by the National Committee for Quality Assurance, and such measures are used in the accreditation of HMOs. Women have vested interest in closely monitoring such measures, given the significant expansion of Medicare and Medicaid managed care programs, and the disproportionately higher representation of women and vulnerable subgroups of the population among Medicare and Medicaid beneficiaries.

SEE ALSO: Health insurance, Medicaid, Medicare, Patients' rights

Suggested Reading

Baker, L. C. (1999). Association of managed care market share and health expenditures for fee-for-service patients. *Journal of the American Medical Association, 281*(5), 432–437.

Gold, M. R. (Ed.). (1998). *Contemporary managed care. Readings in structure, operations, and public policy.* Chicago: Health Administration Press.

Riley, G. F., Potosky, A. L., Lubitz, J. D., & Brown, M. L. (1994). Stage of cancer at diagnosis for Medicare, HMO, and fee-for-service enrollees. *American Journal of Public Health, 84*(10), 1598–1604.

Suggested Resources

Health and Human Services Forum. *Building bridges across the department.* http://aspe.os.dhhs.gov/progsys/forum

National Committee for Quality Assurance: www.ncqa.org

SIRAN M. KOROUKIAN

Heart Attack *see* Abdominal Pain, Acute Myocardial Infarction, Chest Pain

---

Heartburn Heartburn is a symptom of gastro-esophageal reflux disease (GERD), which affects more than 60 million American adults at least once a month. About 25 million adults suffer daily from heartburn. Twenty-five percent of pregnant women experience daily heartburn. It is typically described as a burning sensation in the chest and throat. GERD is a digestive disorder that affects the lower esophageal sphincter (LES) that is a muscle around the bottom of the esophagus (food pipe). It protects the esophagus from the regurgitation or backup of acid and stomach contents into the esophagus during digestion. If acid backs up into the esophagus, the esophageal lining offers a weak defense, and heartburn and other symptoms can result.

There are multiple risk factors for the development of heartburn. These include eating patterns, pregnancy, alcohol, smoking, certain foods and medications, and anatomical factors. Eating pattern risk factors include lying down soon after eating or snacking at bedtime. Certain foods like chocolate, coffee and tea, carbonated beverages that can cause belching, peppermint, and fatty foods can contribute to the development of heartburn. Pregnant women can experience heartburn especially in the third trimester from pressure of the uterus on the stomach, impairing stomach emptying. Alcohol and cigarette smoke have both an irritant effect on the esophageal lining and an effect on the LES, impairing its function. Medications that can decrease the LES pressure and cause GERD include calcium channel blockers, anticholinergics, beta adrenergics, sedatives, nitroglycerine, nicotine, theophylline, and dopaminergics. Anatomical factors that contribute to heartburn include the presence of a hiatal hernia, motility disorders of the esophagus, and poor emptying of the stomach. Other symptoms that can be attributed to reflux include asthma symptoms, chronic cough, hoarseness, regurgitation of sour material into the throat, persistent hiccups, and, less commonly, nausea and vomiting in more severe cases.

The complications of GERD or heartburn include erosive esophagitis, or visible damage to the lining of the esophagus. Ulcerative esophagitis, or the development of ulcerations in an area or inflammation caused by acid reflux, can also occur. In a small percentage of patients with longstanding heartburn, a condition called Barrett's esophagus may eventually develop. Extended exposure of the esophagus to gastric contents causes a change in the lining of the esophagus, which is considered precancerous. It is not clear which individuals with GERD will develop Barrett's esophagus, but once it is discovered, lifelong surveillance for the development of cancer 'is recommended by some experts. Individuals at highest risk of developing cancer appeared to be Caucasian males over the age of 50 years. Strictures, or abnormally narrowed areas of the esophagus, can develop over time in patients with longstanding heartburn due to repeated injury and scarring of the esophagus. These can be treated endoscopically by inserting dilators into the esophagus to mechanically tear the fibrotic tissue and open the lumen of the esophagus.

Diagnosis of GERD or heartburn can be made if an individual's symptoms improve with medical therapy or lifestyle modification or both. If the diagnosis is uncertain, an upper endoscopy or EGD (esophagogastroduodenoscopy) can be performed to look at the lining of the esophagus and, if necessary, take biopsies. EGD requires placing a long flexible tube, with a light and a camera at its tip, into the patient's stomach, after the patient is given sedative medications for comfort. This examination can also detect Barrett's esophagus. If the EGD is normal, other tests such as a pH probe to monitor the acid in the esophagus, and manometry, to assess the pressures generated by the muscles of the esophagus, can also be performed. Individuals who develop alarm symptoms, such as difficulty swallowing, pain on swallowing, weight loss, anemia, or bleeding from the gastrointestinal tract, require immediate endoscopic evaluation, as these symptoms signal that a complication of heartburn has developed.

The management of heartburn starts with lifestyle modifications, including a change in diet to avoid foods that may contribute to heartburn, smoking and alcohol cessation, and staying upright after eating for at least 1–2 hours. Individuals should also avoid late-night snacks and consumption of large quantities of food at mealtimes. Medications such as over-the-counter antacids including ranitidine, famotidine, and cimetidine can be effective for patients with mild, intermittent heartburn. Individuals with more persistent or severe heartburn can benefit from more potent acid-suppressing agents, called proton-pump inhibitors, which can be prescribed by a physician. These medications, such as omeprazole, lansoprazole, rabeprazole, and pantoprazole, appear to be safe, have little in the way of side effects, and if taken daily can successfully eradicate heartburn symptoms.

Surgical treatments are also available for the treatment of heartburn that is well controlled with medical therapy in patients who do not wish to remain on life-long medication for heartburn, or for patients with persistent regurgtation. The standard surgical procedure is a fundoplication that can be done as an open surgery or more commonly, laparoscopically. In this procedure, the upper part of the stomach is wrapped around the esophagus to form a collar. Complications include excessive tightness of the wrap, which can cause bloating, inability to belch, and difficulty swallowing, or breakdown or slippage of the wrap, all of which are indications for reoperation. Long-term failure rates are reported at up to 63% after 10 years.

See Also: Alcohol use, Asthma, Chest pain, Pregnancy, Smoking

Suggested Reading

American Medical Association. (2002, July). *New considerations in the evaluation and management of gastroesophageal reflux disease (GERD).* Chicago: Author.

Kahrilas, P. J., & Pandolfino, J. E. Gastroesophageal reflux disease and its complications. In M. Feldman, M. H. Schlesinger, J. S. Fordtran, B. F. Scharschmidt, & L. S. Friedman (Eds.), *Gastrointestinal and liver disease* (7th ed., pp. 599–622). Philadelphia: Elsevier.

Scott, M. (1999). Gastroesophageal reflux disease: Diagnosis and management. *American Family Physician, 59,* 1161–1169.

ASHLEY FAULX

Hemorrhoids
Hemorrhoids, or enlarged veins in the anal area, represent one of the most common problems for which people seek medical advice. The actual incidence is unknown, but 10–25% of the adult population is thought to be affected. There appears to be a peak in middle age with a decline in the incidence after the age of 65.

Development of hemorrhoids is not completely understood, but seems to be more common in conditions such as chronic constipation, prostate enlargement, chronic cough, and pregnancy. All these conditions cause increased straining and increased intra-abdominal pressure. Contrary to popular belief, there is no evidence that prolonged sitting causes hemorrhoids.

Individuals can develop internal hemorrhoids, external hemorrhoids, or both types. Internal hemorrhoids can bleed or prolapse (protrusion of small tissue), but rarely cause pain. Bleeding is usually bright red in color, associated with defecation, and blood is seen on the outside of the stool, on the toilet paper, or dripping into the toilet bowl. Prolapse is recognized as a soft protrusion from the anus after defecation, which may resolve spontaneously or may require manual reinsertion into the anus. Prolapsed hemorrhoids that cannot be pushed back into the anus can become gangrenous and require emergency surgical intervention.

External hemorrhoids are usually seen as perianal skin tags, the result of thrombosed external hemorrhoids. Individuals can experience pain when external hemorrhoids thrombose, however there is usually no associated bleeding. Contrary to popular belief, hemorrhoids rarely cause itching. The itching can be attributed to poor hygiene, as the anal area may be more difficult to clean after defecation when hemorrhoids are present, or seepage of stool due to a prolapsed hemorrhoid.

Patients presenting with symptoms suggestive of hemorrhoids need a complete evaluation to be done before making the diagnosis of hemorrhoids, as other conditions can cause rectal bleeding and pain. After a thorough history has been completed, a physical exam including external anal inspection, digital rectal examination, and anoscopy (a small lighted scope inserted into the anus) should be done. For patients older than 40 years, evaluation with either flexible sigmoidoscopy or colonoscopy is indicated.

Most internal hemorrhoids can be treated successfully in the outpatient setting by primary care physicians. For patients with minor or infrequent symptoms, treatment begins with dietary modification and bulk laxatives. A high-fiber diet with plenty of raw fruits and vegetables, commercial fiber supplements, and increased fluid intake keep stools soft and decrease straining and irritation of existing hemorrhoids. The use of topical hydrocortisone creams is common, although there is little evidence of benefit in the scientific literature. Hydrocortisone creams may help decrease perianal itching, however, improved anal hygiene should be stressed. Hydrocortisone creams should not be used on a long-term basis as they may cause thinning of the perianal tissues.

If symptoms persist despite these measures, there are procedures that can be done in the doctor's office. The most common techniques employed are injection sclerotherapy and rubber band ligation. Using sclerotherapy a solution is injected into the hemorrhoid and causes scarring and obliteration of the vessel. Rubber band ligation, or placement of a very small rubber band around the base of the hemorrhoid, will cut off the blood supply to the tissue and cause the hemorrhoid to eventually slough off. Both procedures involve very little risk or discomfort to the patient. Patients may require more than one session for complete eradication of hemorrhoids. Other techniques include cryosurgery, laser hemorrhoidectomy, and various coagulation modalities, all of which may require repeat treatments for eradication of hemorrhoids.

Surgical excision of internal hemorrhoids is reserved for patients for whom the previously described procedures have not worked, or who have persistently prolapsing or nonreducible prolapsed hemorrhoids. This procedure is generally performed as same-day surgery and requires some form of anesthesia. Complications tend to be rare and recurrence of hemorrhoids is low.

Therapy for thrombosed external hemorrhoids varies depending on the severity of the patient's pain. If the pain is mild, a regimen of frequent sitz baths, stool softeners, and pain medications is followed, as the pain is generally self-limited and lasts for 7 days or so. If the pain persists beyond 7–10 days, despite these measures, excision of the external hemorrhoid can be performed. This procedure can be performed in the doctor's office, using injection of a local anesthetic and removal of the vein with a scalpel.

Patients with perianal skin tags from old thrombosed external hemorrhoids usually seek treatment because of problems associated with maintaining adequate anal hygiene. Unfortunately, excision of anal skin tags does not relieve the underlying problem of anal hygiene.

SEE ALSO: Constipation, Pregnancy

Suggested Reading

Hulme-Moir, M., & Bartolo, D. C. (2001). Disorders of the anorectum. *Gastroenterology Clinics of North America, 30*, 183–197.

Hussain, J. N. (1999). Office management of common anorectal problems: Hemorrhoids. *Primary Care, 26*, 35–51.

Pfenninger, J. L., & Zainea, G. G. (2001). Common anorectal conditions: Part II. *American Family Physician, 64*, 77–88.

ASHLEY FAULX

Hepatitis The word hepatitis is derived from the Greek word for liver and is defined as inflammation of the substance of the liver. Although hepatitis is usually thought of as caused by a viral infection, it might be a result of any number of injuries, including medications, alcohol, genetic diseases, or many other causes in addition to infectious diseases.

A large number of infections can involve the liver, causing hepatitis as part of their systemic effects, but there are five major viruses that specifically attack the liver. These are referred to as hepatitis A through E. Other hepatitis viruses have been described—including hepatitis G, for example—but their clinical importance is somewhat unclear. In the United States, the most important viruses are hepatitis A, B, and C.

HEPATITIS A

Hepatitis A infection usually results from the consumption of food contaminated with virus-laden feces of infected individuals. Foods that may be contaminated include shellfish, with many reports of outbreaks in people who eat raw clams or oysters; this is also because the virus is very hardy and requires cooking temperatures to be inactivated in foods or drinks infected by food handlers with poor hygiene. Shellfish are a notorious potential source of infection since, as filter feeders in shallow waters (and therefore, possibly exposed to water contaminated with sewage), they can concentrate a large amount of hepatitis virus. Because of its means of transmission, it frequently causes many people to become infected simultaneously. For example, an outbreak may result from a common source or from poor hygiene practices in an institutionalized setting (e.g., daycare centers or facilities housing the mentally retarded) leading to transmission from one infected person to another. Less commonly, people have acquired hepatitis A via infected blood transfusions, intravenous drug use, or sexually.

Hepatitis A is found worldwide. In developed countries, the rate of hepatitis A infection tends to slowly rise throughout childhood and early adulthood. In contrast, among developing countries, with crowded living conditions, inadequate sanitation, and contaminated drinking water, there is a very high rate of infection in the first few years of life. In the United States, it is estimated that 33% of the population has been infected with hepatitis A.

In children, hepatitis A often causes an illness with mild or even no symptoms. Because infected children often are not recognized as being ill, and because children may excrete virus for longer periods than adults, they play a major role in the spread of hepatitis A in both developing and developed countries. Among adults, however, it can cause much more substantial liver injury, including a violent hepatitis or even liver failure. It has been estimated that approximately 80% of adults who become infected with hepatitis A will develop symptomatic disease. Although it can cause extensive damage acutely, hepatitis A does not cause chronic liver disease.

The typical symptoms, like those of any hepatitis, include nausea, vomiting, vague abdominal discomfort, jaundice, fatigue, and generalized malaise. Laboratory studies are usually abnormal when patients are symptomatic and include rapid increases in liver enzymes reflecting hepatic necrosis (liver cell death), followed by a more gradual rise in serum bilirubin (a breakdown product of red blood cells normally processed and removed from the bloodstream by the liver) that is responsible for jaundice. The diagnosis is confirmed by a blood test revealing the presence of specific antibodies to the hepatitis A virus.

The typical presentation of hepatitis A includes a period without symptoms after initial exposure to the virus, usually lasting approximately 4 weeks, followed by a symptomatic period that may also last anywhere from 3 to 5 weeks. Rarely, this period can last up to 12 weeks, but then is usually followed by complete recovery. Very rarely, patients may develop an illness with a more prolonged jaundiced phase, lasting up to 3 months, or a prolonged relapsing hepatitis, with waxing and waning symptoms. This prolonged relapsing course can last up to as many as 12 months after initial presentation, but again, is typically followed by complete recovery. The last form of presentation, fulminant hepatitis, is very rare, but may cause so much damage as to require liver transplantation in as many as 50% of affected adults. Unfortunately, there is no other treatment option for patients with fulminant hepatitis A.

The risk of hepatitis A infection can be reduced by adequate sanitation, isolation of known or suspected infected individuals, and good hygienic practices particularly in restaurants, day cares, hospitals, and other institutions. In addition, groups at increased risk for hepatitis A, including health care workers, day-care workers, and travelers to endemic areas, such as missionaries and military recruits, should be vaccinated.

Individuals with other chronic hepatitis infections should also be vaccinated because of their reduced ability to tolerate additional injury to an already compromised liver. In addition, for people who have been exposed to hepatitis A, for example, family members of an infected individual, an immune globulin preparation (containing specific antibodies in high titers against hepatitis A) may prevent infection. Unfortunately, no specific treatment is available for patients with symptomatic hepatitis.

HEPATITIS B

Hepatitis B was the first hepatitis virus to be discovered, in 1967. Hepatitis B is the most common hepatitis virus worldwide with some estimates suggesting that half of the world's population may have been infected. In areas of high prevalence of infection, such as East Asia or sub-Saharan Africa, as many as 100% of the population may have been or may currently be infected with the hepatitis B virus. The most common mode of hepatitis B transmission is from mothers to their children around the time of childbirth. Other means of transmission include sexual transmission or via blood (e.g., needlestick injuries, intravenous drug use, or transfusions). In contrast, in low-prevalence countries such as the United States, the most common means of transmission is usually related to sexual contact with a chronically infected individual.

Unlike hepatitis A, which only has an acute form, hepatitis B infection may be acute or chronic. The age of acquisition of hepatitis B infection has implications regarding the likelihood of developing chronic infection. Infants who are infected shortly after birth may have a 90% chance of becoming chronically infected; in children between 1 and 5 years, the risk falls to 25–50%; and by adulthood, the risk falls to about 5%. Approximately 70% of patients with acute hepatitis B are either relatively asymptomatic or at least not jaundiced.

The time lag from an exposure to hepatitis B to the start of symptoms is usually between 1 and 4 months, and is accompanied by dramatic increases in liver enzymes, marking widespread destruction of the liver, then followed by jaundice. Over a period of several months, these enzymes gradually return to normal in the patients who recover completely. Less than 1% of patients will develop acute liver failure and either die or require a liver transplant.

Hepatitis

Chronic hepatitis B is the persistence of the virus in the liver and is detected by the presence of markers of hepatitis virus infection in the serum, such as the hepatitis B surface antigen (one of the proteins made in high titers in the liver of an infected patient) or hepatitis B viral DNA. Approximately 5% of the world's population is chronically infected, with the highest rates in the areas that have the highest rates of infection. In the United States or Western Europe, the overall rate of chronic infection is between 0.2% and 1%. The course of chronic hepatitis B is variable, depending on the age of acquisition of infection as well as other risk factors for liver disease (such as alcohol abuse) and the patient's immune response to the virus. Some patients are almost asymptomatic (the so-called "healthy carrier" state), whereas others, for example, from endemic areas such as China, may have progressive liver damage, leading eventually to cirrhosis or liver cancer in as many as 40–50%. In regions where hepatitis B is endemic, liver cancer is the leading cause of cancer-related death.

The course of chronic hepatitis B in North American patients generally can be divided into two phases—a so-called replicative phase in which the virus is actively multiplying and causing progressive liver damage, and a nonreplicative phase in which the virus lies dormant within the liver. Much of the variability of the course of hepatitis B stems from the duration of the replicative phase in which markers of active production of virus can be detected in the serum (such as the presence of envelope or E antigen). These markers are also an indication for higher infectivity and are usually accompanied by significant liver destruction. The clearance of E antigen, marked by the development of a specific antibody, results in a more quiescent phase of liver disease, often with lower or undetectable amounts of circulating virus and improvement in liver enzymes. These patients' liver disease can flare, however, if they develop an illness requiring treatment with steroids or other medications that suppress the immune system. A small percentage of these patients will eventually clear all signs of infection, losing markers of infection (e.g., the surface antigen) at a rate of 0.5–2% per year. The outcome for those who do not clear the virus varies, based on the length of time they have been infected. In addition, although the risk in North American patients is fairly small, if patients already infected with hepatitis B were to become infected with another hepatitis virus, including hepatitis A, C, or D (a rare form of hepatitis B), they are at increased risk

for developing severe liver disease or fulminant liver failure.

Several treatment options exist for hepatitis B patients. The first successful therapy was based on interferon and is effective in clearing markers of active disease from the blood in up to 40% of patients, but unfortunately has significant side effects.

More recently, several medications that interfere with the synthesis of hepatitis B viral DNA have been shown to reduce the damage of hepatitis B, causing loss of E antigen or seroconversion (i.e., development of an antibody to the E antigen) at similar rates. Although these drugs are much better tolerated, concern about the emergence of resistance has limited their use to patients with active disease.

HEPATITIS C

Hepatitis C is a virus with a worldwide distribution, infecting almost 3% of the world's population, including almost 4 million Americans. The virus is classified among the flaviviruses (a group which also includes West Nile virus, dengue, and yellow fever viruses). The genome of hepatitis C virus (HCV) codes for a long protein, about 3,000 amino acids in length, which is then processed into a number of structural proteins and enzymes necessary for replication. Based on sequence structure, an individual virus can be assigned to one of six different genotypes of hepatitis C; these have a varying geographic distribution. Most patients acquire hepatitis C infection via blood transfusion or blood exposures, such as needlestick injuries or intravenous drug use, or less commonly, from sexual exposure or in the perinatal period. Unlike infections with the other hepatitis viruses, HCV is much more likely to become chronic, typically in about 80% of patients who are exposed. The reason why some patients are able to clear the infection is unknown, but it is speculated that these patients may have more vigorous immune responses to the infection than those who do not clear the virus.

Although HCV infection usually becomes chronic, the likelihood that chronically infected patients will develop progressive liver disease is approximately 20%, typically occurring over a time period of about 20 years or more. Other factors that influence the rate of progression to cirrhosis (end-stage liver disease) include the amount of alcohol consumed, gender (disease in women tends to progress more slowly—possibly related to iron depletion), the age of acquisition (progression in younger patients may be slower), as well as some factors related to the virus type or the patient's underlying immune status.

Although some develop typical hepatitis symptoms, most patients who acquire the infection are asymptomatic, and often remain so for years. Patients are therefore often identified when abnormal liver tests are found on screening tests or alerted after donating blood to the Red Cross. Most screening tests detect specific antibodies to the virus; confirmatory antibody tests or very sensitive tests to detect the viral RNA can be used to confirm the presence of ongoing infection. Quality of life studies often detect an increase in nonspecific symptoms such as fatigue, weight loss, or abdominal discomfort, as well as anxiety and depression in patients with chronic HCV. Ultimately, with the onset of clinical cirrhosis, symptoms and complications of end-stage liver disease (such as liver cancer) become apparent. As in hepatitis B, a wide range of manifestations of HCV outside the liver has been found. Although somewhat uncommon, these include skin disease, rheumatologic disease, and endocrine and kidney diseases.

Treatment options for HCV are currently based on the use of interferon. These are derived from a family of naturally produced proteins that have direct antiviral effects as well as effects on the immune system, and are used in conjunction with a second antiviral medication, ribavirin. However, treatment side effects as well as low overall efficacy rates prevent the majority of patients from completely eliminating the virus permanently. New therapies on the horizon offer great promise for these patients; intensive efforts are also under way to produce a vaccine to prevent infection.

SEE ALSO: Immunization, Injection drug use, Quality of life, Safer sex

Suggested Reading

Koff, R. S. (2003). Hepatitis A and E. In D. Zakim & T. D. Boyer (Eds.), *Hepatology: A textbook of liver disease* (pp. 939–958). Philadelphia: W.B. Saunders.

Nair, S., & Perrillo, R. P. (2003). Hepatitis B and D. In D. Zakim & T. D. Boyer (Eds.), *Hepatology: A textbook of liver disease* (pp. 959–1016). Philadelphia: W.B. Saunders.

Younossi, Z. M., Ong, J. P., & O'Shea R. (2003). *Contemporary diagnosis and management of Hepatitis C.* Newton, PA: Handbooks in Health Care.

ROBERT S. O'SHEA

Hermaphroditism

The term hermaphrodite derives from Greek mythology. Hermaphroditus was the son of Aphrodite and Hermes, endowed with the beauty of both deities. One day, he was walking by a lake when the nymph Samalcis instantly fell in love with him. She pleaded for his love, which he soundly rejected. When he later disrobed and jumped into the lake for a swim, Samalcis followed and embraced him, but he tried to escape. Samalcis prayed to the gods that the two would never be separated. The gods answered her prayer by fusing Samalcis and Hermaphroditus into one body.

The medical establishment throughout history has used the term hermaphrodite (or in some cases *gynandromorphy*) to describe a cluster of genetic and physiological departures from the typical gestational sex development pathway that result in individuals born with variations in the appearance of external genitalia and/or incongruence between internal sex organs and external genitalia. Hence, the analogy to Hermaphroditus is clear. The term has largely fallen out of usage due to the action of intersex activists who feel that it sensationalizes and dehumanizes individuals who have suffered extreme physiological and psychological trauma stemming from surgical interventions to correct these conditions, but that in actuality are more akin to genital mutilation.

For purposes of classification, the medical establishment historically has made distinctions between *true hermaphrodites and pseudo-hermaphrodites*. True hermaphrodites, also known as *genetic mosaics*, are rare in occurrence. Although most people think of sex at the individual (or organism) level, each cell in the body also can be viewed as having a chromosomal sex—XX (female) or XY (male). Thus, genetic mosaic refers to individuals born with cell patches throughout the body that are XX and other patches that are XY. When a patch crosses through gonadal tissue, the typical result is an individual born with at least one *ovotestis* (a hybrid of ovary and testicular tissues) accompanied by varying degrees of genital virilization.

Pseudo-hermaphrodite refers to all other variations resulting from an absence or insufficiency of certain enzymes that act at points along the human sex determination pathway. The prefix *pseudo* is applied because these individuals are not genetic mosaics. Because the overall ground state for human sex development is female—or put another way, male is a biological modification of an elemental female form—a majority of the departures affect developing fetuses with an XY chromosomal constitution. Generally, depending on when the enzyme acts in the sex development pathway, XY gonadal tissue will cease its differentiation away from the female ground state (i.e., male development) and will instead follow a female developmental path from that point forward.

The most common examples are genetic variations in the testosterone biosynthetic pathway. Like many hormones in the human body, testosterone is derived from a cholesterol precursor molecule through a complex pathway involving the action of many enzymes. Changes in the levels or alterations in the capacity of any of these enzymes can ultimately influence the amount of active testosterone produced. The availability of high titers of active testosterone, coupled with the ability of this hormone to enter into cells through a receptor molecule, are necessary for elaboration of the external genitalia in XY fetuses. Without active testosterone and capable receptor molecules, or if quantities of either are insufficient, development will return to the female ground state and the individual will be born with either female genitalia or varying degrees of hybridization of female and male external characteristics. However, because male differentiation has occurred up to this point, the vagina is a blind pouch without a cervix. Uterus, fallopian tubes, and ovaries are also absent; instead, testicles are present in the abdomen where the ovaries typically would be located.

Androgen insensitivity syndrome (AIS), which affects the transport of active testosterone into cells, and 5-alpha reductase deficiency (5ARD), which affects the activation of testosterone, are among the best known examples. Congenital adrenal hyperplasia (CAH) is a genetic variation in the cortisol biosynthetic pathway (a branch of the testosterone pathway) resulting in insufficient production of cortisol and overproduction of testosterone. Developing XX fetuses are thus born with hybridization of female and male external characteristics, but the internal sex organs are female. Sex assignment at birth in all three examples is usually female, at times with corrective surgery to normalize the genitals to an idealized feminine appearance. But this practice has been strongly criticized by intersex activists, many of which liken the genital mutilation to child abuse.

If the condition remains undiagnosed for AIS and 5ARD newborns, it will manifest itself at puberty. Menarche will not occur. Those with complete AIS will also fail to develop ancillary and pubic hair, a process under the action of testosterone in both females and males. Girls with 5ARD or partial AIS will begin to undergo virilization at puberty, an occurrence that in some instances is traumatic and in others is welcome. Virilization will continue unless the testicles are removed from the abdomen and estrogens are administered.

Compared to the general population, rates of lesbianism are very high among the intersexed (hermaphrodites), which challenges us to rethink strict interpretations of postmodern theories based on social learning or essentialist theories grounded in psychobiology and evolutionary psychology for either gender or sexual orientation development.

SEE ALSO: Femininity, Gender, Gender role, Homosexuality, Intersexuality, Lesbian, Masculinity, Queer, Transgenderism, Transsexuality

Suggested Reading

Barbin, H., Foucault, M., & McDougall, R. (1980). *Herculine Barbin: Being the recently discovered memoirs of a nineteenth-century French hermaphrodite.* New York: Random House.

Dreger, A. D. (2000). *Hermaphrodites and the medical intervention of sex.* Cambridge, MA: Harvard University Press.

Fausto-Sterling, A. (2000). *Sexing the body: Gender politics and the construction of sexuality.* New York: Basic Books.

ANGELA PATTATUCCI ARAGON

Heroin

Revered by Sumerians, Egyptians, Greeks, and other ancient civilizations for its ability to ease pain, the opium poppy has yielded a number of chemical compounds that have revolutionized the control of pain as well as contributed to problems of addiction in modern societies. Morphine, one of the most powerful pain relievers known, was isolated from opium by a German pharmacologist in 1803. In 1874, a British chemist experimenting with morphine produced diacetylmorphine, a semisynthetic opiate marketed in 1898 by Bayer and Company under the name "heroin" (from the German word, *heroisch*, meaning "heroic" or "powerful") as a medicine for coughs, pneumonia, tuberculosis, and other ailments. Shortly after its introduction, the addictive nature of heroin became evident to the medical community.

Several waves of heroin addiction have been identified in the United States. For about the first two decades after its introduction, most heroin addiction was iatrogenic, sometimes associated with its prescription for morphine addiction. The Harrison Act of 1914 strictly regulated the use of heroin, and the legal sale of heroin was prohibited. Due to increasing problems surrounding heroin addiction, the U.S. Public Health Service opened narcotic hospitals in Lexington, Kentucky (1935) and in Fort Worth, Texas (1938). After World War II, African Americans and Hispanics in inner cities, in particular, were most affected by a second wave of heroin addiction. A third wave of heroin addiction began in the 1960s and continued throughout much of the Vietnam War era. The National Institute on Drug Abuse was established in 1973, partly in response to increases in heroin abuse during this period. Most data indicate that the United States is in the midst of a fourth wave of heroin addiction that began in the early 1990s in some areas of the country. In this latest wave, many new heroin users have been young (18–25) whites of middle-class background.

United Nations estimates suggest there were about 8 million heroin users worldwide in 2000, with almost 1 million "hard-core" (weekly use or more) users in the United States. Major sources of heroin in the United States include Mexico, Southeast Asia, Southwest Asia, and, more recently, Colombia and South America. While heroin typically is sold in powdered form, some Mexican heroin is a tar-like substance. Depending on its purity and form, heroin can be snorted (inhaled through the nasal passages), smoked, injected under the skin ("skin-popping"), or injected intravenously. Intravenous injection of heroin was rare until about 1930.

Whatever the route of administration, heroin produces a "rush" characterized by exhilarating feelings of euphoria, well-being, energy (at least initially), and power, followed by somnolescence—the "nod." This is why it is referred to on the streets as "boy," the "king" of drugs, in contrast to cocaine, or "girl," the weaker of the two. Use of heroin several times a day for several weeks results in physical dependence. Dependent heroin users experience painful, flu-like withdrawal symptoms when they cannot use the drug. Although not often life threatening, withdrawal symptoms are extremely unpleasant. At this stage, more frequent and/or larger doses of heroin are needed just to remain feeling "normal." The daily cost of a heroin habit can exceed $200. Physical withdrawal symptoms often motivate some heroin users to engage in illegal activities such as shoplifting, theft, fraud, prostitution, and other crimes to obtain the money needed to purchase enough

of the drug. Importantly, some people experiment with heroin and never become dependent, but the number of experimenters is unknown. In addition, some people use heroin occasionally over long periods of time without becoming dependent.

Since the early to mid-1990s, depending on geographic region, the purity and availability of heroin in the United States has increased significantly. Cost has decreased as well. Higher purity heroin can be administered efficiently by smoking or snorting. Although many recent, new heroin users initiated use of the drug by snorting or smoking, many users who become dependent eventually turn to injection. At least initially, dependent heroin sniffers can inject smaller quantities of heroin at a comparatively lower cost.

Heroin injectors are at risk for a wide range of health problems, including—but not limited to—infection at the injection site, endocarditis, hepatitis B and hepatitis C infection, HIV infection, overdose, and addiction. Women who inject heroin are often at greater risk of experiencing some of these health problems for a variety of reasons. For example, women often assume subordinate roles compared to men in injection settings. Consequently, women often inject after men and therefore may inject with syringes that have been used previously. In addition, given limited options for work, some women addicted to heroin may turn to prostitution to obtain the money necessary to buy daily supplies of the drug. Women heroin users who engage in sex work have a greater risk of being exposed to HIV and other sexually transmitted diseases. Heroin users who engage in prostitution are also at risk for experiencing violence, including sexual assault.

Substance abuse treatment modalities for heroin and other opioid dependence include the use of a number of therapeutic agents for detoxification and maintenance. The most widely used is methadone, a synthetic narcotic developed during World War II by the Germans as a substitute for morphine. In adequate doses, methadone that is taken orally can ease withdrawal symptoms and can block the physical craving for opiates as well as the euphoric effects. Women who use heroin often experience greater problems accessing drug abuse treatment services, particularly when they are mothers. Few drug abuse treatment programs provide child care services, thus creating a barrier to treatment access.

There is evidence that some women who abuse heroin may experience amenorrhea, anovulation, and infertility. It is not clear if this is due specifically to heroin or other lifestyle issues, such as poor nutrition. Finally, the fetus of a pregnant woman who abuses heroin is at substantial health risks, including dependence.

SEE ALSO: Acquired immunodeficiency syndrome, Addiction, Cocaine, Hepatitis, Injection drug use, Sexually transmitted diseases, Substance use

Suggested Reading

Carlson, R. G. (1999). "Boy" and "girl": The AIDS risk implications of heroin and cocaine symbolism among injection drug users. *Anthropology and Medicine, 6*(1), 59–77.

Inciardi, J. A., & Harrison, L. D. (Eds.). (1998). *Heroin in the age of crack-cocaine.* Thousand Oaks, CA: Sage.

Musto, D. F. (1987). *The American disease: Origins of narcotic control.* New York: Oxford University Press.

Rosenbaum, M. (1981). *Women on heroin.* New Brunswick, NJ: Rutgers University Press.

Stephens, R. C. (1991). *The street addict role.* Albany: State University of New York Press.

ROBERT G. CARLSON

Herpes Simplex Virus

Herpes simplex virus type I (HSV-I) and herpes simplex virus type II (HSV-II) are closely related viruses that cause two distinct clinical syndromes, with some overlap in the roles of the two viruses in each syndrome. Infection with HSV-I causes oral lesions ("cold sores," although not all cold sores are due to HSV-I) and is transmitted by saliva, most commonly by kissing or a shared drinking glass. HSV-II is a sexually transmitted virus that produces genital lesions. There is some overlap, with less than 5% of oral HSV caused by HSV-II and about 5% of genital HSV produced by HSV-I. In both cases, the signature lesions of infection are small vesicular (bubble-like) lesions filled with clear fluid that appear singly or in clusters. Like other members of the herpesvirus family, infection with HSV-I and II is lifelong, with dormant infection followed by recurrences common.

Genital infection with HSV is one of the three most common sexually transmitted diseases in the United States (with chlamydial infection and human papillomavirus infection). Genital herpes produces more emotional distress than significant medical consequences. Many cases are asymptomatic and the prevalence of infection in the general population approaches 25%.

Genital herpes is more common in women than men, infecting approximately one out of four women versus one out of five men. This difference in gender may be because male-to-female transmission is more efficient than transmission from females to males. About 26% of sexually active young women have evidence of exposure to HSV-II on blood tests of prior exposure to genital herpes.

Many individuals never have any signs or symptoms. When signs and symptoms do occur, they typically appear as one or more blisters on or around the genitals or rectum. The blisters break, leaving tender ulcers (sores) that may take 2–4 weeks to heal the first time they occur. The first episode usually occurs within 2 weeks after the virus is transmitted, and the sores typically heal within 2–4 weeks. Other signs and symptoms during the primary episode may include a second crop of sores or flu-like symptoms, including fever and swollen glands. Occurrences are not uncommon, but are almost always less severe and shorter than the first episode. The pattern of subsequent outbreaks of genital herpes is highly variable. Individuals may have no recurrences, one every year, or several per year. Although the HSV-II virus stays in the body indefinitely, the number of outbreaks tends to go down over a period of years. Individuals with frequent outbreaks of genital herpes can take prophylactic medicine to prevent outbreaks (see below). HSV-II infection can be severe in people with suppressed immune systems. Active genital HSV-II lesions can enhance the transmission of HIV, and may alter the progression of HIV disease.

HSV-II can produce potentially fatal infections in infants if the mother is shedding virus at the time of delivery. It is important that women avoid contracting herpes during pregnancy because a first episode during pregnancy causes a greater risk of transmission to the newborn. If a woman has active genital herpes at delivery, a cesarean delivery is usually performed. Fortunately, neonatal infection with HSV-II is rare.

Individuals with active lesions are very contagious and should avoid sexual contact during an outbreak. HSV-II is shed in very small amounts between symptomatic outbreaks and individuals with no active lesions can pass on the virus to a sexual partner, although the risk is very low. Even individuals with no symptoms of HSV-II can be contagious, but the risk per sexual encounter is very low. Occasionally one member of a monogamous pair will come down with a symptomatic case, having contracted the infection from his/her partner who may be an asymptomatic carrier. Because the risk per sexual encounter is low, this sometimes occurs after many into a relationship, and can lead to great consternation among the partners. When this occurs, it is essential for the health care provider to know and effectively communicate that HSV-II can be contracted from long-time asymptomatic partners.

The diagnosis of genital herpes can be made by visual inspection if the outbreak is typical, and by taking a sample from the sore(s). Blood tests can be used to confirm the diagnosis in atypical cases or in diagnosing asymptomatic infection.

There are a number of antiviral medicines that are effective in treating HSV-II, including acyclovir, valacyclovir, and famciclovir. These may be used in treating outbreaks; the benefit in terms of reducing the severity and duration of genital herpes is greatest for the first outbreak when patients are most symptomatic. The benefit in treating recurrences is more modest, but when the medicines are taken daily they are very effective in preventing recurrences.

The consistent and correct use of latex condoms can help protect against infection. However, condoms do not provide complete protection because the condom may not cover the herpes sore(s), and viral shedding may nevertheless occur. A vaccine for HSV-II is under development.

Oral lesions due to HSV-I have a similar natural history to genital lesions due to HSV-II and the therapeutic and preventive strategies are similar. Patients with many frequent recurrences may benefit from preventive therapy.

SEE ALSO: Gonorrhea, Human papillomavirus, Sexually transmitted diseases, Syphilis

Suggested Reading

Sinclair, G. I., & King, C. H. (2002). Herpes virus infections. In J. S. Tan (Ed.), *Experts guide to the management of common infectious diseases* (pp. 761–779). Philadelphia: American College of Physicians.

Suggested Resources

American Herpes Foundation: http://www.herpes-foundation.org/
Herpes Virus Association: http://www.herpes.org.uk/

KEITH B. ARMITAGE

High Blood Pressure *see* Hypertension

Hispanic *see* Latinos

HIV *see* Acquired Immunodeficiency Syndrome

Homelessness At any given night in the United States, approximately 600,000 people are without shelter while more than 2 million may have been homeless in any given year. Estimates put the number in the United States who have experienced homelessness and its health consequences at least once at about 12 million people. Most counts and studies define homelessness as being without stable housing and include those staying in shelters and sleeping overnight in their cars and doubled up with others in a temporary arrangement as well as those living on the streets.

An increase in the rate of homelessness beginning in the 1980s has been attributed to increases in the rate of poverty, decreases in cash and other public benefits, and decreases in the availability of affordable housing. Personal factors related to homelessness include mental and physical problems, a history of domestic abuse, substance abuse, and a lack of resources including social support. In fact, one extensive survey of a clinic population noted that health issues are at least a partial contributing factor to homelessness among the vast majority of those surveyed.

As well as being a reason for homelessness, mental and physical health problems may also be the result of homelessness. Overall, the total rates of illness and injury among the homeless are 2–6 times those of the general population. Homeless people lack the simple essentials for health including a good diet, daily hygiene, sleep, rest, and safety. The homeless are frequently forced to live in overcrowded, unsafe, or unsanitary conditions that expose them to communicable diseases, violence, and the outdoor elements as well as increase their stress. Some engage in risky behaviors such as substance abuse and unprotected sex, which increase the likelihood of disease.

Homelessness

Common health problems among the homeless include upper respiratory infection (about six times the rate as those who are housed); lacerations, fractures, and other outcomes of trauma (about three times the rate); skin ailments (including scabies, lice, and skin infections); chronic gastrointestinal problems; and peripheral vascular disease including cellulitis, leg ulcers, and phlebitis (the latter two found at rates 2–5 times higher). The most common reason for hospitalization is trauma and cellulitis. The rate of tuberculosis is anywhere from 25 to 300 times the rate of those who have regular housing, the rate of HIV infection is 3–4 times higher, the rate of other sexually transmitted diseases 2 times higher, and the rate of violence is 4 times higher than that of the general population. Over 50% of the homeless adult population have gross dental decay. Given these data, it is not surprising that long-term homelessness may result in about a 20-year reduction in life expectancy.

Studies tend to overstate the rate of mental illness because some mental health symptoms are also common reactions to a homeless situation and do not necessarily indicate a long-term diagnosable disorder. However, it is estimated that about 20–25% of the homeless have had a severe mental disorder at some time in their life. The most common disorders are schizophrenia, depression, personality disorders, and posttraumatic stress disorders. An analysis of ten studies showed that the rate of schizophrenia is about 4–16% with a mean of 11%.

Substance abuse also has a high prevalence among the homeless. Some studies estimate that half of those who are homeless had a substance abuse problem sometime in their lives. Those who are homeless may abuse drugs and alcohol in order to self-medicate for a mental illness or the stress of life on the streets. Substance abuse increases the risk of trauma, neurological problems, liver disease, and tuberculosis.

The serious health problems of the homeless are aggravated by poor access to health care. The homeless often lack the essentials needed to access care, such as health insurance or the money to pay for care, transportation to get to care, and documentation that is required by many facilities. Many in this population have language and cultural barriers and may fear and distrust the people and facilities that provide care or have little sense of time, which is needed to keep appointments. Even those who can get services can find it difficult to follow treatment since they cannot keep or store medications or get bed rest and must spend time on more critical survival needs. For example, in a study of over 1,000 people who had been prescribed medications, almost a third were unable to comply. The availability of treatment for women with children and those who are dually diagnosed (those with a mental and substance abuse disorder) is particularly limited.

Families are the fastest growing segment of the homeless population. Women are found in equal proportions to men in the under-20 population of homeless and comprise 25% of those who are homeless. Many have had a history of abuse in their past (reported rates of 31–60%) and continue to be vulnerable to abuse on the streets. Homeless women in one study had been robbed an average of 3 times, assaulted 14 times, raped 5 times, and shot once in their lives. One analysis found that 53% of the homeless women suffered from post-traumatic stress disorder and 60% from clinical depression. The related rate of substance abuse in homeless women has been reported from 16% to 67%. Homeless women have an unusually high pregnancy rate and their infants are more likely to die or be born with a low birthweight.

To address the health problems of the homeless, the Health Resources and Services Administration of the federal government administers the Healthcare for the Homeless Program under the Health Centers Consolidation Act of 1996. This program provides basic and preventive health services, street outreach, and critical case management services to over 500,000 people each year but cannot meet the huge demand for necessary and accessible medical care. Effective treatment programs require services that are comprehensive, accessible, and nonthreatening and address the other essential needs of the population, especially food and housing.

SEE ALSO: Access to health care, Domestic violence, Mental illness, Prostitution, Rape, Sexual abuse, Substance use, Violence

Suggested Reading

Harris, M. (1991). *Sisters of the shadow.* Norman: University of Oklahoma Press.

Kozol, J. (1988). *Rachel and her children.* New York: Crown.

Liebow, E. (1993). *Tell them who I am: The lives of homeless women.* New York: Free Press on Homelessness and Health Care.

McMurray-Avila, M. (1997). *Organizing health services for homeless people: A practical guide.* Nashvolle, TN: National Health Care for the Homeless Council.

Robertson, M. J., & Greenblatt, M. (1992). *Homelessness: A national perspective.* New York: Plenum Press.

Wright, J. D., Rubin, B. A., & Devine, J. (1998). *Beside the golden door: Policy, politics and the homeless.* New York: Aldine de Gruyter.

Suggested Resources

National Health Care for the Homeless Council: www.nhchc.org

BARBARA FISHER

Homeopathy

Homeopathy (pronounced home-ee-OP-a-thee, from Greek *homeo* "similar" and *pathos* "disease") is a form of alternative medicine that uses extremely dilute preparations of natural substances to treat disease, by harnessing the body's own healing energy and restoring balance in the patient's vital force. Homeopathy originated in Europe and the United States in the late 1700s and early 1800s and developed separately from conventional Western medicine.

Homeopathy is based on two main principles: (a) like cures like and (b) extreme dilution. Under the principle of "like cures like," diseases are treated with substances that cause the same symptoms as the disease. In fact, if the remedy initially causes worsening of the patient's symptoms, it is taken as evidence that the remedy is effective. The principle of "like cures like" is not entirely foreign to Western medicine. For example, allergy patients are sometimes injected with small amounts of the substance they are allergic to, in order to reduce the allergic response. Likewise, many of the medications used to treat abnormal heart rhythms can themselves cause abnormal heart rhythms.

The principle of dilution (or "potentization") is the most controversial aspect of homeopathy. This principle states that remedies become more effective when extremely diluted in water or alcohol. Homeopathic medications are repeatedly diluted and shaken after each dilution. Dilution is sometimes repeated to the point that no molecules of the active substance can be detected using modern methods of chemical analysis. Dilution is sometimes used in conventional Western medicine, as in allergy injections, but these treatments still contain detectable amounts of the active material. Theories about the structure of water and energy transfer have been offered to explain how extremely dilute homeopathic remedies could be effective, but these theories are not commonly accepted by the conventional medical community. It must be noted that even in conventional scientific medicine the mechanism of action for many treatments is not specifically known.

As with conventional scientific medicine, treatment studies are often contradictory. Many studies of homeopathy are considered inconclusive because of weaknesses in the design of the study. However, most homeopathic treatments have not been studied using modern scientific methods.

Homeopathic practitioners consider each individual patient's set of symptoms before choosing the appropriate remedy, which can be given in pill or liquid form. Homeopathic remedies are also sold over-the-counter. The label will give the dilution of the main ingredient, such as 6x, 12x, or 30x. The "x" represents a 10-fold dilution. The number indicates how many times the ingredient was passed through a 10-fold dilution. So, 6x means that one part of the medication was diluted in 10 parts of water (or lactose), and this dilution was repeated a total of 6 times. Preparations labeled with a "c" (6c, 12c, 30c) were passed through 100-fold dilutions, rather than 10-fold dilutions. More dilute preparations are considered more potent; for example, 12c is considered more potent than 12x, and 12x more potent than 6x.

Although homeopathic medications are generally considered safe, side effects from homeopathic medications may still occur. Because homeopathic remedies are so dilute, the Food and Drug Administration has not traditionally required testing for safety or effectiveness. Homeopathic remedies are allowed to contain more alcohol than other over-the-counter medications, but no problems caused by the alcohol content have been reported to the Food and Drug Administration. Homeopathic remedies probably do not interfere with other medications, but patients should always inform their health care provider of all the medications and herbs they use.

SEE ALSO: Complementary and alternative health practices

Suggested Reading

Stehlin, I. (1996, December 30). Homeopathy: Real medicine or empty promises? *FDA Consumer, 10*; also at http://www.fda.gov/fdac/features/096_home.html

Suggested Resources

Questions and Answers about Homeopathy. National Center for Complementary and Alternative Medicine (NCCAM) Publication

No. D183. (2003, April). http://nccam.nih.gov/health/homeopathy/index.htm

ALICIA M. WEISSMAN

Homicide

Homicide is the most extreme act of violence. Although all homicides involve death at the hands of another, homicide is in actuality a diverse group of events. Homicides can occur between strangers, acquaintances, and intimate partners; they involve a wide array of physical forces and weapons and they include many types of motivations and precipitating factors. Although diverse, homicides have some predictable characteristics that can be used to improve efforts to prevent their occurrence.

In the United States, homicide is the fourth leading cause of death for those aged 1–14, the second leading cause for those aged 15–24, and the third leading cause for those aged 25–34. In 2000, 16,765 people were the victims of homicide.

The homicide rate in the United States has fluctuated over time. After low rates in the 1950s, homicide rates reached an all-time high of 10.2 per 100,000 population in 1980. After decreasing until 1985, rates rose again to reach 9.8 per 100,000 in 1991. Since 1991, the homicide rate has continued to decline, but this decline has slowed since 1999.

Homicides have very distinct gender patterns. Men are more than 10 times more likely than women to perpetrate a homicide. Approximately 65% of all homicides involve a male offender and male victim and an additional 22% involve a male offender with a female victim. Only 12% of all homicides involve a female offender.

The relationship between the victim and perpetrator varies by gender. When a woman is murdered, the most likely perpetrator is an intimate partner. In contrast, men are more likely to be killed by strangers or acquaintances. Over 40% of homicides committed by women are against spouses or boyfriends and another 17% are against children or other family members. Only 7% of homicides perpetrated by women are against strangers compared to 25% of those perpetrated by men.

Furthermore, research has found that over half of the men who were killed by their wives had precipitated their own deaths through short- or long-term use of physical force or threats. Thus, domestic violence is an integral factor when examining the role of women as victims and perpetrators of homicide.

Risk factors for homicide and violent behavior are usually evaluated at the level of the social/community unit and the individual. At the social/community level, one of the fundamental factors in the rate of homicide is social disorganization. Social disorganization is defined as the inability of a community to realize the common values of its members and a lack of social control. Characteristics of communities such as high population density, a high percentage of the population between 15 and 34, tolerance for violence, income inequality, racial inequality, poverty, low levels of education, and high unemployment have consistently been linked to high homicide rates. However, the relative strength of these variables in predicting homicide rates has varied widely in different studies.

Individual characteristics vary greatly by the circumstances of the homicide. However, young, minority males are consistently identified as the most likely perpetrators of homicide. Individual characteristics such as living in poverty, low educational attainment, and unemployment are linked to homicide, but the interrelationship between these as individual or societal characteristics has not been thoroughly examined.

Prosecution and incarceration of homicide offenders has been the main societal response to homicide. The criminal justice system identified many levels and types of homicides. Criminal homicide includes murder, manslaughter, and negligent homicide, and each of these involves willful, intentional harm. Homicides can also be noncriminal, such as in the case of self-defense or legal intervention.

However, communities and law enforcements have recently increased their focus on preventing violence, including homicide. Such interventions include community policing, social programs to increase life skills training, employment training and placement, victim's support and advocacy groups, and improvements in the physical environment.

The World Health Organization has supported a science-based public health approach to reduce violence. The steps in such an approach include establishing national plans and policies for violence prevention, facilitating the collection of data to document and respond to the problem, building important partnerships with other sectors, and ensuring an adequate commitment of resources to prevention efforts.

SEE ALSO: Child abuse, Domestic violence, Mortality, Prison health, Sexual abuse, Violence

Suggested Reading

Fox, A., & Zawitz, M. W. (2003). *Homicide trends in the United States: 2000 update* (NCJ 197471). Washington, DC: Department of Justice, Bureau of Justice Statistics.

Gottesman, R. (Ed.). (1999). *Violence in America: An encyclopedia.* New York: Scribner's.

Smith, M. D., & Zahn, M. A. (Eds.). (1999). *Homicide: A sourcebook of social research.* Thousand Oaks, CA: Sage.

CORINNE PEEK-ASA

Homosexuality

Homosexuality is conceptualized in modern times as a *sexual orientation.* Individuals who are oriented toward romantic and sexual relations with members of the same sex are identified as homosexual, whereas those who are oriented toward the opposite sex are labeled heterosexual. These natural variations in human behavior can be found in all cultures throughout recorded history. Moreover, although the focus is typically on sexual behavior, homosexual and heterosexual also pertain to one's romantic/sexual attractions and fantasies.

Homosexual is also a sexual identity. However, people who define themselves as homosexual have rejected the term because it represents a label imposed from a medically oriented, heterosexual perspective. Instead, *gay* is preferred—in contrast to *straight* (describing heterosexuals). Additionally, while gay is an umbrella term that refers to both men and women, many homosexual women prefer to call themselves *lesbians.*

A number of scholars have taken the position that homosexuality as a sexual identity is a relatively recent phenomenon that emerged in the latter decades of the 19th century out of the convergence of two prevailing social trends. The first was the medicalization of homosexuality by European scientists such as Havelock Ellis, Magnus Hirschfeld, and Sigmund Freud. The process of studying homosexuality required that scientists define it in concrete terms and in opposition to heterosexuality. The second was the transition from agrarian to industrialized economies in Europe and the United States, which relocated many young men and women from farms to cities. Urban life offered a sense of anonymity and provided unique opportunities for gays and lesbians to meet each other. Although this explains the evolution of homosexual identities in the modern era, it may be naive to consider it a unique development. For

example, Plato's *Symposium,* written in 387 BC, includes a speech by Aristophanes, which offers what is probably the world's first recorded theory of sexual orientation. Aristophanes proposes that all human beings were originally similar to Siamese twins. After the gods split them apart, each yearned for his or her *lost half.* Those who had been male/female thus sought the opposite sex; those who had been male/male or female/female desired the same sex.

Plato's exceptionally progressive view that positioned homosexuality on equal plane with heterosexuality unfortunately did not persist in history. Instead, gays and lesbians have been the targets of hatred, violence, negative stereotypes, and discrimination. Today, homosexuals are a minority group in the United States and in other societies. However, unlike other minorities, the minority status of gays and lesbians is based on a departure from social norms centered on *heteronormativity* rather than on ascribed characteristics (see Queer for definition). This has made it difficult for homosexuals to secure, and most importantly maintain, the type of social gains that other minorities have been able to establish. In response to oppression, gays and lesbians have organized to press for civil rights that are currently denied.

In the early 1950s, a group of gay men led by Harry Hay in Los Angeles founded an organization called the Mattachine Society with the goal to liberate homosexuals from persecution. Shortly after, a group of eight women chartered a similar organization for lesbians called the Daughters of Bilitis. Both organizations published magazines—the Mattachine Society, *ONE,* and the Daughters of Bilitis, *The Ladder*—which defended lesbians and gays against entrapment, a common occurrence in those times. For example, a 1953 presidential executive order prohibited the employment of homosexuals (and bisexuals) in all federal jobs. The FBI investigated any government employee suspected of homosexual inclinations and in the process set a precedent for firms in the private sector to do the same. This created an oppressive work and social environment, where a mere accusation from an anonymous third party often provided sufficient cause for investigation and subsequent dismissal. Many people lost their jobs with little hope of finding work elsewhere.

When the Mattachine Society and Daughters of Bilitis were founded, every state had a sodomy law prohibiting sexual behavior between members of the same sex. Urban police forces routinely raided gay and lesbian bars. They arrested patrons for dancing, holding hands, or

311

simply being there. Newspapers often published the names of those arrested. Jobs were lost; lives were ruined. It was during one such raid at the Stonewall Inn in 1969, a popular gay nightspot in New York's Greenwich Village, that a group of gay men and lesbians defiantly challenged the police. Their act of rebellion set off three successive days of police confrontations with progressively larger contingents of protesting gay men and lesbians, an event that is commonly considered to be the spark that ignited the modern gay liberation movement. Each year, gay pride parades and celebrations occur in cities all over the world to commemorate the Stonewall Rebellion.

Since then, progress has been slow but steady. Many states have modified sodomy laws so that they no longer apply to consenting adults. Some cities and a few states have added sexual orientation to their civil rights codes to protect gay men and lesbians from job discrimination. Corporations extend benefit packages to the domestic partners of their lesbian and gay employees. In the year 2000, the legislature of the state of Vermont passed an historic law that created a new marital status called *Civil Unions* for same-sex couples and provided all state law benefits of marriage to couples joined in civil union. No longer hidden in the shadows of society, lesbians and gay men appear on television and in movies, and run for political office. High school students across the United States are forming gay–straight alliances and an expansive web of organizations and institutions exist that sustain a rich social, cultural, and civic life for gays and lesbians. However, violence and discrimination are still widespread. Gay men and lesbians can be denied housing and fired from their jobs in over 30 states with little legal recourse. Despite there being in excess of 2 million gay and lesbian parents in the United States, they still are not allowed to form families through legal, state-sanctioned marriage (with the exception of Vermont residents). Gay and lesbian organizations, along with others focused on civil rights, such as the American Civil Liberties Union and Greenpeace International, are working hard to end the violence and discrimination, and to afford gays and lesbians basic human rights.

SEE ALSO: Gender, Intersexuality, Lesbian, Lesbian ethics, Queer, Transgenderism, Transsexuality

Suggested Reading

Chauncy. G. (1995). *Gay New York: Gender, urban culture, and the making of the gay male world, 1890–1940.* New York: Basic Books.

D'Emilio, J. (1998). *Sexual politics, sexual communities: The making of a homosexual minority in the United States, 1940–1970* (2nd ed.). Chicago: University of Chicago Press.

Duberman, M. (1994). *Stonewall.* New York: Plume.

Vicinus, M., Chauncey, G., & Duberman, M. B. (1990). *Hidden from history: Reclaiming the gay and lesbian past.* London: Meridian Books.

ANGELA PATTATUCCI ARAGON

Hormone Replacement Therapy

Menopause is the cessation of menstrual periods. Women usually experience menopause at the age of 42–58, with the average age being 50–51 years. Menopause may occur slightly earlier in women who smoke or have a family history of early menopause. Otherwise, the age of menopause is unrelated to the age of the first menstrual period, use of oral contraceptive pills, pregnancies, or general nutrition. The term *perimenopause* refers to the entire time period of 3.5–4.5 years around menopause, when hormonal changes of menopause have begun.

Menopause is a time of significant hormonal changes. Since women today live one third of their lives after menopause, this health event also provides to women an opportunity to reevaluate life habits such as nutrition, exercise, and health surveillance.

The changes directly associated with menopause are related to the depletion of eggs from the ovaries. Women are born with more than a million eggs, which die or are ovulated during a woman's reproductive years. After menopause, estrogen production from the ovaries falls to one tenth of that before menopause and no progesterone is produced. Menstrual periods stop, often after months or years of irregular periods preceding the menopause. Both the early and later symptoms associated with menopause are related to the low levels of estrogen.

Fifty to seventy-five percent of women experience at least one symptom of menopause, with the most common being the hot flush (flash). Hot flushes are usually described as a sudden feeling of warmth from the chest upwards, associated with facial flushing and sweating. They may occur once or several times daily. Night sweats and hot flushes are considered to be *vasomotor symptoms*, related to the effect of falling levels of estrogen on the heat-regulating center of the brain. Sleep disturbances, often related to night sweats, and irritability are also associated with menopause.

Most studies have not shown an association between depression and menopause.

Lowered estrogen levels may also cause thinning of the vaginal wall, decreased lubrication and elasticity of the vagina, and changes in the bladder and urethra. In some women these changes lead to discomfort with intercourse or problems with urination. Estrogen contributes to the collagen content of a woman's skin, so the loss of estrogen may accelerate some of the skin changes usually associated with aging.

Osteoporosis and heart disease are later consequences of low estrogen levels. In the first years after menopause, bone may be lost at a rate of 1–5% per year. In some women, rapid loss of bone may result in fractures and chronic bone pain in as little as 10 years. Fractures of the vertebrae may cause loss of height, curvature of the spine, or back pain. Fractures of the hip are the most serious consequence of bone loss and can result in loss of independence or even death. Before menopause, women have a lower risk of coronary heart disease than do men, but after menopause the incidence of heart attacks increases rapidly until it approaches that of men in the same age group.

Some women may experience more symptoms than others after menopause. At least one quarter state that their symptoms are serious. These women may be the most likely to request some type of treatment for their symptoms. Conversely, some heavy women experience very few symptoms associated with menopause. Women make a type of estrogen in their fat cells, so heavy women may continue to have high levels of estrogen after menopause, even when their ovaries produce very little.

Lifestyle evaluation and changes should always be the first approach to relieving menopausal symptoms. A diet high in fiber and low in fat decreases the risk of heart disease, as does weight loss in overweight women. For some women, increased soy in their diet may improve vasomotor symptoms. Calcium and vitamin D intake should be optimized. A reduction in alcohol intake may decrease hot flushes and the risk of falls. Smoking cessation decreases the risk of heart disease and reduces the risk of osteoporosis. Exercise in general may improve mood, prevent weight gain, and improve sleep. Aerobic exercise reduces the risk of heart disease while weight-bearing exercise may decrease the risk of osteoporosis and falls. Vaginal lubricants and moisturizers can help vaginal dryness and regular sexual intercourse may prevent constriction of the vagina.

Whether or not to take estrogen replacement after menopause is one of the most confusing issues facing women today. Over the years there have been dramatic shifts in medical recommendations and public sentiment concerning the use of hormone replacement therapy (HRT). Accumulating information about risks and benefits of HRT suggests that emphasis should be placed on its use for the treatment of initial symptoms in the lowest possible dose for the shortest duration. In addition, there are now many alternatives to HRT that should be considered in the discussion of treatment options.

Estrogen is very effective in treating early menopausal symptoms. Hot flushes and night sweats are usually improved within days to about 2 weeks. Thinning and other changes in the vagina, bladder, urethra, and skin are usually reversible after one to two months of therapy. Women should take the lowest dose of estrogen that can relieve the symptoms.

In the past, many studies suggested that many women could benefit from taking estrogen after menopause for many years, even for the rest of her life. Long-term risks of estrogen treatment have been acknowledged for many years and include blood clots, a small increased risk of breast cancer, and endometrial cancer. The risk of endometrial cancer can be completely prevented by the addition of a progesterone-like medication to estrogen. This has become the standard approach for women who have not had a hysterectomy. Accumulated evidence suggested that HRT decreases the risk of heart disease by 50% as well as decreases the risk of osteoporosis and hip fractures. Several years ago, it was believed that these benefits so clearly outweighed any risks that most women should consider long-term HRT.

However, several excellent studies, including the Women's Health Initiative (WHI) and the Heart and Estrogen/Progestin Replacement Studies (HERS), showed recently that HRT does *not* prevent heart disease as was previously believed. Estrogen continues to be recognized as the most effective medication for the prevention of osteoporosis after menopause, but most health care providers do not now support its long-term use for prevention of heart disease or improvement of general health.

Many women seek herbal remedies to provide relief of menopausal symptoms. There are numerous herbal preparations marketed as dietary supplements to treat menopausal symptoms. Unfortunately, studies to evaluate their effectiveness, side effects, and interactions with other herbals and prescribed medications are extremely limited. Current data suggest that black cohosh and soy may be effective in some women, and a handful of other herbals such as red clover are promising. At least part of the action of these herbals is through the estrogen receptor. A woman should always inform her health care provider if she takes any dietary supplements.

Some nonestrogenic medications have also been shown to relieve menopausal symptoms. Progesterone-like substances and androgens (male-type hormones) when given without estrogen may provide some relief of hot flashes. A variety of nonhormonal medications may specifically inhibit hot flashes, including veralipride and gabapentin. A variety of medications are available to prevent or treat postmenopausal bone loss, including raloxifene and alendronate. Raloxifene belongs to a group of medications called selective estrogen receptor modulators (SERMs), which may act as estrogens or as "antiestrogens," depending on the cell type. For example, raloxifene acts like estrogen in bone cells by preventing bone loss, but it acts like an antiestrogen in the breast and brain by reducing the risk of breast cancer while worsening hot flashes.

For some women menopause is associated with very few symptoms and is in fact a welcome time point in the aging process. For many others, it is more troubling. Symptoms may be significant enough to require intervention with prescribed or nonprescribed medications. Because the study of menopause is so complex and is evolving so rapidly, women should seek many sources of information as they approach menopause.

SEE ALSO: Calcium, Cardiovascular disease, Coronary artery disease, Exercise, Menopause, Osteoporosis and osteopenia, Perimenopause

Suggested Resources

American College of Obstetricians and Gynecologists: www.acog.org
National Cancer Institute Website for patients: www.cancer.gov
National Osteoporosis Foundation: www.nof.org
North American Menopause Society: www.menopause.org

LORNA A. MARSHALL

Hospice
Hospice is the organized provision of care for the dying. Medically, the hospice approach focuses on pain medications in order to ensure comfort, rather than on invasive life-sustaining technologies such as respirators, resuscitation, and artificial nutrition and hydration. Hospice typically provides team support for the dying, including medical and nursing care, psychological counseling, and clinical pastoral care as requested. Hospice is the major alternative to death in a hospital, where the medical approach is generally more aggressive. Hospices usually have their own specially designed buildings to facilitate a "dying well," but most of their work involves teams that visit patients routinely in their homes to provide care. Hospice units are increasingly found in nursing homes.

The term "hospice" was coined by Dame Cicely Saunders, who was trained as a nurse, a medical social worker, and finally as a physician. Since 1948 she has been involved with the care of patients with terminal illness. She founded St. Christopher's Hospice in London as the first research and teaching hospice linked with clinical care in 1967. Dame Saunders understood the historical usage of the term "hospice" as a place where travelers in need of shelter and rest might spend the night before journeying on. It occurred to her that dying is "like a journey," and that people would need a special place of care before passing on. Thus, Dame Saunders applied the term "hospice" in this new context of journeying peacefully through death. Since her founding of St. Christopher's, the hospice movement has unfolded in many parts of the world.

In the United States, the first hospices were formed in the early 1970s, usually in churches and synagogues. Hospice care was deeply controversial because of its philosophy that people dying of various diseases—especially cancer—did not need to be forced into invasive or burdensome medical treatments. Often, oncologists in established medical settings were sharply critical of hospices. Most oncologists at the time were men, and almost all those involved in the early hospice movement in the United States and elsewhere were women. Elizabeth Pitorak, for example, a nurse, founded the Hospice of the Western Reserve in Ohio. Some women who founded hospices were subjected to legal action and a number were incarcerated for brief periods of time as they fought for the rights of the dying. Throughout the 1970s and into the early 1980s, hospice was ridiculed as "second level" care or as "only care." Many clinicians remained critical, asserting that hospice encouraged their patients to "throw in the towel" without fighting hard enough against death with every technology and drug available. Hospice was the center of the feminist ethics of care and it was pitted against the male-dominated "war against cancer." The tension between hospice and tertiary medical centers is nowadays less dramatic, but still exists. There are many who think that hospice care is a step down for their loved one and therefore resist it.

Hospice, reflecting its origins in the Anglican spirituality of Dame Saunders and in the spiritual traditions of others faiths, retains a distinct appreciation for the "whole" person on the journey toward death. Hospice teams usually consist of a nurse, a social worker, and an individual trained in clinical pastoral care. While all established hospices now have physician directors, it is still the devoted nurse—most often a woman—who has the major hands-on leadership role. While many hospitals now have palliative care units, these typically lack the team approach that is typical of hospice care.

More than any other aspect of modern health care, hospice is the creation of women, who continue to sustain it in many respects. It represents a context in which the feminist ethics of care was able to supercede legal casuistry, the "war" against disease that often meant war against the well-being of patients and the dehumanizing aspects of high-tech medical environments in the interests of comfort, care in the most basic and important sense of the word, and human dignity.

It remains a monument to the moral creativity of caring women.

SEE ALSO: Assisted living, Mortality, Nursing home, Patients' rights, Quality of life

Suggested Reading

Lynn, J. (Ed.). (1989). *By no extraordinary means: The choice to forgo life-sustaining food and water.* Bloomington: Indiana University Press.
Pohl, C. (1999). *Making room: Recovering hospitality as a Christian tradition.* Grand Rapids, MI: Wm. B. Eerdmans.
Volicer, L., & Hurley, H. (Eds.). (1998). *Hospice care for pateints with advanced progressive dementia.* New York: Springer.

STEPHEN G. POST

Human Papillomavirus

Human papillomavirus (HPV) infection may be the most common viral sexually transmitted disease (STD) in this country. As many as 30 million Americans are infected with HPV, and each year, an additional 1 million people become infected.

More than 80 distinct types of HPV have been identified; at least 20 of them can infect the genital tract. Infection due to HPV types 6 or 11 is usually associated with external genital warts, such as condylomata acuminata, whereas those due to HPV type 16 or 18 are associated with cancers of the genitals (cervical, vulvar, and anal carcinomas).

HPV infection likely begins with an abrasion or cut of the epithelium (skin, outside or inside). The wound provides viral access to the skin. During wound healing cell division accelerates, which may actually facilitate viral replication.

After introduction of the virus into the body (inoculation), an incubation period begins and lasts from 4 weeks to 8 months. The incubation is followed by an active expression phase. This phase is marked by rapid capillary proliferation (increase in small blood vessels) that usually persists from 3 to 6 months. It is during this phase that obvious growths (lesions) emerge or subclinical (one that cannot be seen) lesions develop.

Approximately 3 months after the initial proliferative phase and appearance of lesions (visible or not), an immune response can be detected. The result of the patient's immune response is a suppression of new lesions. This is known as the host containment phase. It is known that an intact immune system is at least as important as any available therapies for HPV infection in resolving the clinical manifestations of this disease.

After about 9 months, a latent phase begins. This phase is characterized either by continued clinical remission or by a continued active disease. If the active disease is continuing it may place the patient at risk for neoplasia (new growths or abnormal cell development (dysplasia) or cancer). In some patients, particularly younger women, the infection may resolve.

TRANSMISSION

Genital HPV infection is transmitted by intimate sexual contact. Early age at first intercourse, multiple sexual partners, and intercourse with a person who has external genital warts are risk factors for HPV infection. Smoking also increases risk. Although intra-anal warts are associated with anal (anoreceptive) intercourse, warts around the anus (perianal warts) are not.

Transmission of HPV from mother to infant is uncommon. Delivery by cesarean section, if not indicated for obstetrical reasons, is not recommended for infected women unless external genital warts are obstructing the birth canal.

DIAGNOSIS

Clinical exam has been proven a reliable method for establishing a diagnosis of genital warts; however, HPV can cause warts to form in the vagina, on the uterine cervix, and inside the urethra and anus. In many cases only cervical cytology (Pap smear) can pick up the characteristic cellular changes causing the Pap smear to be abnormal. It is the most common method of detecting subclinical disease. Sometimes biopsy should be performed when diagnosis is in doubt or when despite treatment, the disease worsens, or the patient has a weakened immune system (immunocompromised) or skin/warts are pigmented, feel hard, immobile, or ulcerated.

Women with HPV infection (and their sexual partners) should be examined for other STDs. Tests for the common STDs, syphilis, gonorrhea, and chlamydia; should be considered. Routine screening for cervical cancer should be performed annually; more frequent Pap tests are not required by a diagnosis of external genital warts, but should be performed if cervical dysplasia (abnormal cells) is noted on the Pap smear.

TREATMENT

The primary goal of treatment is to either remove symptomatic warts or destroy the dysplastic process actively or allowing patients' own immune system to destroy the lesions. It is important for the patient to understand that whether the external warts or dysplasia is resolved the HPV virus remains in the patient. This fact is a source of much consternation and must be understood. Although proper treatment may produce lesion-free periods, no evidence exists that any available therapy can eliminate the infection. As many as 21% of vulvar warts (warts on the outer parts of the vagina) resolve without treatment and up to 70–75% of Pap smears with mild dysplasia in the younger women will resolve in 1 year without treatment. The patient should be educated and involved in her treatment. No single therapy is ideal for all women or all lesions, warts, or abnormal Pap smears. Smoking cessation is strongly recommended.

If the patient is pregnant, external warts may be removed by bichloroacetic acid (BCA) or trichloroacetic acid (TCA) cryotherapy (freezing therapy) or surgical excision. If the patient is not pregnant, podophyllin,

imiquimod (Aldara), or interferon may be used. It is important to use these medications just as prescribed since soreness and pain commonly occur with overuse. Once lesions are gone, therapy may be stopped. For the abnormal Pap smear, mild dysplasia may be followed as it will be resolved in approximately 70–75% of the time after being followed over a year. If the patient is not comfortable with observation, cryosurgery may be used. If more advanced lesions are present, more advanced surgical removal techniques such as LEEP or cold knife conization may be utilized on a case-by-case basis depending on where the dysplasia is located. Discussion between the patient and physician is imperative.

A follow-up evaluation after visible genital warts have cleared is not necessary. Patients should be advised to watch for recurrences that develop most frequently during the first 3 months. However, follow-up visits may be useful for documenting a wart-free state, monitoring treatment compliance and complications, and providing patient education and counseling. The presence of external genital warts is not an indication for colposcopy (specialized examination procedure using a small tube) of the cervix or for more frequent Pap smears unless the patient has abnormal Pap smears.

Examination of the sex partners of HPV-infected women is not necessary for the management of their external warts because the role of reinfection in persistent disease is probably minimal. However, such examination is recommended to detect other STDs or previously unrecognized visible warts. Use of condoms can reduce but not eliminate transmission of HPV to uninfected partners. Patients should understand that they may remain infectious even after their visible warts have resolved.

SEE ALSO: Cervical cancer, Chlamydia, Colposcopy, Condoms, Sexually transmitted diseases

Suggested Reading

Eng, T. R., & Butler, W. R. (Eds.). (1997). *Confronting sexually transmitted diseases.* Report by a committee of the Institute of Medicine, Board on Health Promotion and Disease Prevention. Washington, DC: National Academy Press.

Suggested Resources

American College of Obstetricians and Gynecologists patient education: www.acog.org
Centers for Disease Control and Prevention. *Guidelines for treatment of sexually transmitted diseases.* http://www.cdc.gov

JAMES F. CARTER

Hypertension Hypertension (high blood pressure) is defined as a blood pressure of 140/90 mm Hg or higher when measured with a blood pressure cuff or being on medication for high blood pressure. The systolic pressure is the upper number of the reading, while the diastolic pressure is the lower number of the reading. Hypertension is a major risk factor for heart disease, which is the leading cause of death for women in the United States. Blood pressure increases with age with the increase in systolic pressure more pronounced in patients greater than 65 years old. Systolic hypertension is an elevated reading in the top number of the reading when measured by a blood pressure cuff. Sixty-five to seventy-five percent of hypertension in the elderly is isolated systolic hypertension, with the prevalence of isolated systolic hypertension higher in elderly women than men.

In the third National Health and Nutrition Examination Survey (NHANES III), although persons 65 years of age or older represented only 19% of the total population, they constituted 45% of persons with hypertension who were unaware of their condition, 32% of those who were aware of their condition but not being treated, and 57% of those who had treated but still had uncontrolled hypertension.

The prevalence of hypertension varies by sex and ethnicity. Compared with men, women under the age of 55 years have less hypertension, women aged 55–74 years have a similar prevalence of hypertension, and women over 75 years old have more hypertension. Blacks have higher rates of hypertension than whites for both women and men. Despite the equal occurrence of hypertension among women and men aged 55–74 and more hypertension in women more than 75 years old, until recently, little was known about the prevalence, treatment, and control of hypertension among older, postmenopausal women. Baseline data from the Women's Health Initiative (WHI) better define hypertension and its treatment in postmenopausal women.

In the WHI, the prevalence of hypertension was 37.8%. Older women (aged 70–79) had twice the prevalence rate (53.4%) of women 50–59 years (26.7%). Prevalence was higher in blacks than whites or Hispanics (59.3% vs. 35.5% whites and 33.4% in Hispanics) and in lower socioeconomic groups. The prevalence of hypertension was substantially higher among overweight women (body mass index [BMI]>27.3) than those not overweight (48.0% vs. 29.3%). Nondrinkers had a higher prevalence of hypertension than moderate drinkers

(46.2% vs. 31.6%) as did women who were sedentary compared with those who performed moderate exercise (45.3% vs. 31%). Women with one cardiovascular risk factor (family history of myocardial infarction [MI], hypercholesterolemia [elevated blood cholesterol], diabetes, or a history of MI, heart failure, or stroke) had higher rates of hypertension than those without such risk factors. Treatment rates did not differ by age, but black women had the highest treatment rates and Hispanic women the lowest (75.6% vs. 59.4%). Most hypertensive patients were treated with one drug (57.6%). The most commonly used drugs in monotherapy (a single drug is used to treat hypertension) were medications in the classes known as calcium channel blockers (16%) followed by diuretics ("water pills") and angiotensin-converting enzyme (ACE) inhibitors (14%). Beta-blockers (another type of medication used to treat high blood pressure) were used the least (9%). Of those treated, older nonwhite women were less likely to have their hypertension under control. Treatment patterns in WHI women did not follow accepted medical guidelines of the recent sixth Joint National Committee on Prevention, Detection, Evaluation, and Treatment of High Blood Pressure for the treatment of uncomplicated hypertension, which recommend diuretics and beta-blockers as preferred initial treatments. The WHI data suggest that these guidelines are not followed in the treatment of postmenopausal women, given that the most common drug class used as monotherapy was calcium channel blockers.

RESPONSE TO TREATMENT

The effectiveness of antihypertensive drug treatment in overall reduction in the risk of stroke and other cardiovascular disease events is well established. Large medical studies, such as the Systolic Hypertension in the Elderly Program (SHEP) and the Systolic Hypertension in Europe (SYST-EUR) trials, showed that treatment of isolated systolic hypertension with diuretics with and without beta-blockers (SHEP) and calcium channel blockers with or without ACE inhibitor or diuretic (SYST-EUR) reduced the rate of cardiovascular complications and cerebrovascular events in both women and men 60 years old or older—especially diabetics. It remains unclear whether the effect of antihypertensive treatment in reducing cardiovascular risk is dependent on sex. In the Treatment of Mild Hypertension Study, women and men assigned to treatment with antihypertensive drugs with lifestyle intervention versus lifestyle intervention alone experienced greater and generally similar benefits—a decrease in systolic and diastolic blood pressures and a reduction in cardiovascular events. In a review, the "Effect of Antihypertensive Drug Treatment on Cardiovascular Outcomes in Women and Men: A Meta-Analysis of Individual Patient Data from Randomized, Controlled Trials," women and men treated with antihypertensive medications had similar cardiovascular risk. Quantification of benefit in risk reduction shows that for women, the benefit is primarily in reducing the risk of stroke, whereas in men treatment prevented as many coronary events as strokes. The fact that statistical significance for coronary events or total mortality was not reached in women may have a simple explanation: The numbers of women participating in the study and their low rate of coronary events may have been too small to allow a proper statistical analysis.

Thus, 55- to 74-year-old women have the same rate of hypertension as men the same age and women older than 75 have more hypertension than their male counterparts. Hypertension is an important risk factor for the development of coronary heart disease and stroke in both sexes and there is good evidence that both women and men benefit from treatment of hypertension. There is no evidence that women respond differently to antihypertensive therapy than men, except that diuretics may be particularly useful in women. Some adverse effects of individual antihypertensive drugs may be more troublesome in women. ACE inhibitor-related cough is three times more common in women; swelling related to the use of some types of calcium channel blocking medications is more common in women; and hirsutism (excessive body hair) with the medication minoxidil is often intolerable among women.

HYPERTENSION WITH ORAL CONTRACEPTIVES

Oral contraceptive (OC)-induced hypertension affects about 5% of women using OCs. Age greater than 35 years old and obesity are the only known risk factors for OC-induced hypertension. It is not known whether the effects of OCs on blood pressure depend on the dose and type of estrogens and progestins (both "female hormones") that are used in the formulation of the OC tablets. The onset of OC-induced hypertension usually occurs within 4 months of beginning an OC, although the actual increases in blood pressure may be

related to the duration of treatment. Blood pressure usually returns to normal within 1 year after stopping the pill.

The cause of OC-induced hypertension is not well understood. The renin–angiotensin system (enzyme system in the kidney) is activated, but its role in causing hypertension has not been demonstrated; there does not seem to be a significant difference in changes in the renin–angiotensin system between OC users who remain normotensive (normal blood pressure) and those who develop hypertension. Most women on the pill develop renal vasoconstriction (constriction of blood vessels in the kidney); it has been suggested that those with the greatest propensity to develop renal vasoconstriction retain the most sodium and develop hypertension.

HYPERTENSION WITH PREGNANCY

Hypertension affects 10% of pregnancies in the United States and remains a leading cause of both maternal and fetal morbidity and mortality. Hypertension in pregnancy is defined as a systolic blood pressure ≥ 140 mm Hg or diastolic blood pressure ≥ 90 mm Hg; or systolic blood pressure increase of ≥ 30 mm Hg or diastolic blood pressure increase of ≥ 15 mm Hg over first trimester of prepregnancy values.

Chronic Hypertension

Chronic hypertension is hypertension that is present before pregnancy or diagnosed before the 20th week of gestation or that persists beyond 6 weeks postpartum. Most women have a benign (uncomplicated) course with an exaggerated decrease in diastolic blood pressure of as much as 20 mm Hg that often leads to normalization of blood pressure in midpregnancy. This drop in diastolic blood pressure may mask the diagnosis of chronic hypertension if prepregnancy values are unknown. The blood pressure usually increases to prepregnancy levels in the third trimester, leading to diagnostic confusion with preeclampsia (pregnancy-related hypertension). Proteinuria (protein in the urine) is absent in uncomplicated chronic hypertension; when it occurs for the first time in the third trimester, it is the best indicator of superimposed preeclampsia. Antihypertensive treatment should be initiated for a systolic blood pressure ≥ 150 mm Hg or a diastolic blood pressure ≥ 100 mm Hg unless there is evidence of renal

Hypochondriasis

Hypochondriasis is a psychiatric illness in which individuals experience anxiety about misinterpreted physical symptoms that they fear or believe indicate the presence of an undiagnosed medical disease. For example, a mark on the skin may be interpreted as cancer or a sign of AIDS, or sweating may be interpreted as a heart condition. This anxiety and associated behavior cause significant distress and/or impairment in work, social, or other areas of functioning for at least 6 months or longer. People with this disorder may seek frequent medical attention and diagnostic testing. Although tests may be negative, it is usually not enough to convince the person with hypochondriasis that nothing is wrong. The person with this disorder may be willing to acknowledge that their fears are exaggerated or that there is nothing seriously wrong with them, but in general fear and anxiety persist. Over time, the person with this disorder may focus almost exclusively on their fears of disease, which may limit their social conversations and interrupt their family and work lives.

One of the many somatoform disorders, hypochondriasis affects from 1% to 5% of the general population. Somatoform disorders are those disorders in which an individual complains of physical symptoms but the symptoms cannot be fully explained by any medical or other mental disorder. Other somatoform disorders include somatization disorder, conversion disorder, undifferentiated somatoform disorder, pain disorder, and body dysmorphic disorder. It is important to make the distinction between hypochondriasis and malingering. Individuals with hypochondriasis are not fabricating symptoms intentionally as are those who are malingering. Instead, they experience valid symptoms (usually amplified normal physical sensations) that cause them distress whether or not one is able to find a diagnosable disease.

Hypochondriasis affects both women and men of any race or socioeconomic status. It can occur at any time in the life span. Generally, this disorder arises in individuals who have had a serious illness or have witnessed a relative with a medical illness. Death in someone close to the patient or other psychosocial stressors are sometimes related to the onset of this disorder. Two thirds of patients with hypochondriasis have a co-occurring mental disorders such as anxiety, depression, or other somatoform disorders.

Primary care physicians are frequently the first to see these patients, with prevalence rates higher than in the general population ranging from 2% to 7%. Patients with hypochondriasis will usually "doctor shop" until they find one they feel understands their complaints and complies with their demands for medical testing. Physicians are often frustrated with these patients since they make frequent visits and efforts to reassure them go unheard. Patients usually resist referrals to mental health providers, believing that their symptoms are solely physical.

There are several strategies used in the treatment of hypochondriasis, although none are definitive. Cognitive–behavioral treatment has shown some promising results. Therapy is designed to target the dysfunctional beliefs and behaviors that accompany hypochondriasis. In the few studies that have been conducted, results suggest that cognitive–behavioral therapy leads to improvements in hypochondriasis symptoms, including reduction of fears of illness and somatic complaints.

There is a paucity of research on the pharmacotherapy of primary hypochondriasis. Pharmacotherapy to address common coexisting mental disorders (panic, obsessive–compulsive disorder, and depression) seems to help improve the symptoms of hypochondriasis. Medication should be started at subtherapuetic doses since patients with hypochondriasis are not likely to tolerate significant side effects.

Medical management of patients in the primary care office involves building a trusting doctor–patient relationship. It is recommended that visits be scheduled regularly whether current symptoms warrant it or not. Frequent visits coupled with attentive listening and examination are useful approaches to therapy. Tests and consultations are to be limited to those for which there is an obvious indication, not for reassurance sake. Referrals to a psychiatrist should be attempted to examine current psychosocial stressors.

The long-term prognosis of hypochondriasis is guarded. Symptoms of hypochondriasis sometimes dissipate if a bona fide medical disorder is uncovered, which validates the individual's experience. In some individuals, symptoms completely remit. More frequently, symptoms are chronic and of a variable nature. One study showed that two thirds of medical outpatients continued to receive the diagnosis of hypochondriasis after 5 years even though symptoms may have declined and role functioning improved during this time period.

See Also: Anxiety disorders, Depression, Psychosomatic disorder

Hysterectomy

Suggested Reading

American Psychiatric Association. (1994). *Diagnostic and statistical manual of mental disorders* (4th ed.). Washington, DC: American Psychiatric Association.

Barsky, A. J. (2001). The patient with hypochondriasis. *New England Journal of Medicine, 345*, 1395–1399.

Barsky, A. J., Fama, J. M., Bailey, E. D., & Ahern, D. K. (1998). A prospective 4- to 5-year study of *DSM-III-R* hypochondriasis. *Archives of General Psychiatry, 55*, 737–744.

Starcevic, V., & Lipsett, D. R. (Eds.). (2001). *Hypochondriasis: Modern perspectives on an ancient malady.* New York: Oxford University Press.

VIRGINIA E. AYRES

Hysterectomy Hysterectomy means the surgical removal of the uterus, or womb. According to the latest statistics from the Centers for Disease Control and Prevention (CDC; published in 2000), about 600,000 hysterectomies are performed annually, making it the second most common operation among women of reproductive age (cesarean section is first). Approximately 20 million U.S. women have had a hysterectomy. Half of all hysterectomies are in women under 45 years. The overall rate of hysterectomy is 5.5 per 1,000 women and half of all hysterectomies are accompanied by removal of the tubes and ovaries also.

ANATOMY

The internal female genitalia consists of the uterus, the fallopian tubes, the ovaries, and the supporting ligaments and blood vessels. The cervix, which resides in the upper vagina, is connected to the lower part of the uterus. The endometrium is the tissue lining the uterine cavity.

TERMINOLOGY

Commonly, a hysterectomy is referred to as either a "complete" or a "partial." These terms are nonmedical. A "complete" hysterectomy means that the uterus, the cervix, the tubes, and the ovaries have all been removed. There is no single medical term to describe this. Instead, the equivalent medical terms are a *total hysterectomy*, which means removal of the uterus and the cervix, combined with a *bilateral salpingo-oophorectomy*, which means the removal of both sets of tubes and ovaries. A "partial" hysterectomy means removal of just the uterus and the cervix, and the medical term for this is a *total hysterectomy*. If the uterus is removed but the cervix is left in place, it is called a *subtotal* or *supracervical hysterectomy*. If the hysterectomy is performed for cervical cancer, then a *radical hysterectomy* might be done. This is the removal of the uterus and cervix plus additional surrounding ligaments and lymph node tissue. This is a highly specialized procedure generally performed by gynecologic oncologists.

TECHNIQUES

There are many different ways that a hysterectomy can be performed, including abdominal, vaginal, laparoscopic, or a combination of these.

Most hysterectomies are performed using an abdominal incision. Removal of the uterus, cervix, tubes, and ovaries using an abdominal incision is a total abdominal hysterectomy and bilateral salpingo-oophorectomy.

A hysterectomy can also be performed entirely through the vagina. A total hysterectomy performed though the vagina is abbreviated *TVH* (total vaginal hysterectomy). If the tubes and ovaries are also removed, the procedure is called a *TVH-BSO* (total vaginal hysterectomy–bilateral salpingo-oophorectomy). The vaginal approach is sometimes combined with a laparoscopy. Laparoscopy is when small incisions are made, usually in the area of the belly button and the lower abdominal area. A narrow scope attached to a video monitor is inserted and very narrow instruments are used to perform surgery. If laparoscopy is combined with a vaginal hysterectomy, it is called a laparoscopic-assisted vaginal hysterectomy.

RISKS AND RECOVERY

Hysterectomy is considered major surgery and there are potential risks to keep in mind. These risks include, but are not limited to, risks from anesthesia, development of an infection, development of a blood clot in the circulation (an *embolism*), injury to another internal organ such as the bladder, intestines, or *ureter* (the tube connecting the kidney to the bladder), heavy loss of blood possibly requiring a transfusion, development of a *fistula* (connection between bladder and vagina or rectum and vagina), development of internal scar tissue that can lead to bowel obstruction (even years later), and complications during recovery, which may necessitate a second operation. Despite the variety of possible complications, in reality the risk of serious complications from hysterectomy is about 1%.

Another risk is that the procedure that is ultimately performed may not be the same that is begun. For example, some patients start out with a planned laparoscopic subtotal hysterectomy, but because of unanticipated developments end up with a total abdominal hysterectomy, considerably lengthening their expected recovery period.

Recovery from hysterectomy depends on the exact procedure used. In uncomplicated cases, generally expect full recovery to be 6–8 weeks for abdominal hysterectomy, 4–6 weeks for vaginal hysterectomy, 2–4 weeks for laparoscopic-assisted vaginal hysterectomy, and 1–2 weeks for laparoscopic supracervical hysterectomy. Keep in mind that these are average estimates and that individuals vary quite a bit in their recovery from surgery.

INDICATIONS

The most common indications for performing hysterectomy are fibroids, endometriosis, and uterine prolapse. These three indications account for almost 75% of all hysterectomies. Other indications are chronic pelvic pain, heavy menstrual bleeding, and uterine or ovarian cancer.

ALTERNATIVES TO HYSTERECTOMY

Depending on the medical problem, there are other procedures or treatments that can sometimes prevent the need for a hysterectomy. These include endometrial ablation, uterine artery embolization, and hormone therapy.

Endometrial ablation is a procedure that can be used when the problem is longstanding heavy menstrual bleeding and there are no fibroids. The endometrium is the lining of the uterine cavity. Menstrual bleeding occurs when this lining is shed during a menstrual period. Normally, this lining regrows every month. Ablation means that this lining is mostly or completely destroyed. Then it will not grow back, and very little menstrual bleeding will occur. There are many safe and effective techniques for performing

endometrial ablation. These include using a balloon inside the uterine cavity filled with hot water, irrigation of the uterine cavity with heated water, using electrical cautery, and using a freezing technique.

Uterine artery embolization (UAE) is a procedure that can be used when the problem is either large fibroids causing discomfort or heavy menstrual bleeding. UAE is performed by specially trained interventional radiologists and is usually an outpatient procedure. Using x-ray guidance, a narrow catheter is inserted into a blood vessel in the groin and then carefully advanced until it is in an artery directly providing blood to a fibroid. Then a substance is injected consisting of small synthetic particles (called microspheres) that cause the artery to become blocked. This cuts off the blood flow to the fibroids, resulting in their shrinkage (loss of blood causes the cells to die), which usually results in greatly reduced bleeding, often preventing the need for a hysterectomy.

Hormone therapy can be used when the main problem is longstanding heavy and/or irregular bleeding with or without fibroids or pelvic pain associated with endometriosis. In many cases women with irregular bleeding, even if they also have fibroids, can be placed on hormones (such as low-dose birth control pills) to regulate their bleeding, preventing the need for hysterectomy. Many insurance companies will not pay for hysterectomy if the indication is abnormal bleeding, unless the patient has been shown to have tried hormone therapy first and failed it. Some patients have conditions where they cannot safely take hormones, so this approach is not always feasible. Birth control pills can also help reduce the pain from endometriosis, in some cases preventing the need for hysterectomy.

MYTHS

Many people have misconceptions about hysterectomy. These are addressed below in a question and answer format.

Q: Doesn't hysterectomy always lead to menopause? After all, the periods are gone.

A: Hysterectomy does lead to elimination of menstrual periods. However, if the woman is not in menopause at the time of the hysterectomy, and if her ovaries are not removed, then she will not experience menopause after the hysterectomy. Menopause will occur naturally, when her ovaries stop producing estrogen, about age 51. If the ovaries are removed at the time of hysterectomy in a woman who is not yet in menopause, she will become menopausal, referred to as a *surgical menopause*. Estrogen therapy is usually given postoperatively to minimize the side effects of surgical menopause.

Q: I heard that after a hysterectomy, women lose interest in sex and no longer enjoy sex.

A: The capacity for female orgasm does not change after hysterectomy because the clitoris, which provides most of the nerve stimulation leading to orgasm, is not involved in the hysterectomy. Studies have shown that some women do have difficulties with their sex life after hysterectomy, but only a small percentage. Most women report that orgasm feels "different" due to the loss of the uterus, since the uterus does cramp with orgasm, but that overall the sensation is not less pleasurable. If the ovaries have been removed during the hysterectomy, then the woman's sex life may change because she has been abruptly placed into menopause. This risk can be greatly reduced if supplemental estrogen is begun shortly after the hysterectomy.

Q: My husband says that because of my hysterectomy, I am no longer a woman.

A: Your husband deserves a good, swift kick in the groin. Hopefully, a woman and her husband have discussed issues such as this prior to the surgery. Husbands need to go with their wives to the doctor before the surgery to ask questions, express concerns, and learn all that they can about the reasons for the surgery and what to expect afterward.

SEE ALSO: Cervical cancer, Dilation and curettage, Endometriosis, Laparoscopy, Menstrual cycle disorders, Sexual organs, Ultrasound, Uterine cancer, Uterine fibroids, Vaginal bleeding

BRYAN S. JICK

Suggested Resources

www.CancerSource.com

Hysteria Few topics in the world of psychoanalysis are as controversial as hysteria. There is no current consensus on whether or not hysteria exists today or whether or not it ever existed at any time at all. Explaining exactly what hysteria is and what it means has challenged and baffled many generations of physicians.

As an illness, hysteria has been associated with women even though male sufferers were at one time identified and discussed. It is commonly assumed that Hippocrates first used *hysteria* as a general descriptive term for the aliments of the womb. The word *hysteria* itself is derived from the Greek word for the uterus. There is also evidence that an identifiably corresponding disease is mentioned in ancient Egyptian manuscripts that predate the general Greek term by at least several centuries.

The problem with trying to apply hysteria in historical and cultural contexts is that the term refers to both an illness characterized by strange symptoms as well as to certain disturbing forms of behavior. Only as recently as 100 years ago it was thought that the physiological basis for female insanity existed in the reproductive organs. This may help explain why the ailment was said to cause the womb to "wander." But whether it was a malady or maladjustment, hysteria primarily involved the manifestation of many interchangeable outward symptoms without any tangible physical cause. It was a disease that made the victim appear irrational, untrustworthy, and difficult to control.

These are some of the reasons hysteria was also employed as a psychiatric label for the witchcraft writings of the 19th century. The label was applied to the historical findings of hysterical sensory disturbances, which were considered proof of witchcraft up until the 17th century. However, these "witches" were not seen as "hysterics" by their contemporaries. They were seen as willing servants of Satan, who deserved the harshest treatment and the most painful death imaginable.

During the 19th century a debate arose as to whether the illness was composed of symptoms or behaviors. Within the proper Victorian hierarchal view of the world, the hysteric came to embody femininity itself, both as a problem and an enigma. Modern historical analysis of Sigmund Freud's psychoanalytic approach has revealed a new view of this unique psychosomatic condition that hysteria was less of a clinical puzzle to be solved than a response to political intervention. Hysteria can be seen as a physical expression of a profound sense of discomfort when women tried to reach beyond their tolerable societal limits.

In modern times hysteria has virtually disappeared from our theoretical literature, diagnostic manuals, and training programs. The modern clinical symptoms of the disease are apt to be "mixed" forms where the illness is interspersed with other neurotic disturbances. The actual physical symptoms differ very little from those described in the 19th century. They range from complete paralysis to tremors, tics, amnesia, loss of speech or hearing, nausea, vomiting, and dramatic fits.

SEE ALSO: Feminism, Mental illness

Suggested Reading

Borossa, J. (2001). *Hysteria.* Toronto, Ontario, Canada: Totem Books.

Micale, M. (1995). *Approaching hysteria: Disease and its interpretations.* Princeton, NJ: Princeton University Press.

Micklem, N. (1995). *The nature of hysteria.* London and New York: Routledge.

ROBERTO HERNANDEZ

Idiopathic Environmental Intolerances

Idiopathic environmental intolerances (IEI), previously called multiple chemical sensitivities, is also known as environmental hypersensitivity (allergy) or environmental illness. IEI is an acquired condition in which a person repeatedly notices symptoms that seem triggered by exposure to a certain chemical substance(s) in amounts that are usually well tolerated by most people.

CAUSES

IEI is diagnosed mostly in adult women. Whether the condition is due to environmental exposure or a psychological disorder is controversial. No currently identified medical abnormalities explain why IEI occurs. Current theories include toxins leaking through the respiratory tract, toxins affecting the nervous system, or toxins affecting the immune system.

The list of environmental chemicals that may cause symptoms is very long. Many people with IEI are affected by smells, including any type of pollution, fumes, fragrances, or chemicals either in the house or workplace. Other possible triggers include certain foods, food additives, medications, electromagnetic fields, and mercury in dental fillings. There is no clear relationship between the symptoms reported and the known toxic effects of the specific chemicals. The symptoms occur at concentrations of the chemicals well below those expected to cause toxicity.

There are no symptoms that are diagnostic of IEI. The most common symptoms include malaise, tiredness,

sweating, nasal congestion, sore throat, hoarseness, cough, shortness of breath, chest pain, chest tightness, palpitations, nausea, abdominal pain, passage of a large volume of urine, joint aches, back pain, muscle aches, dizziness, headache, impaired thinking, poor memory, difficulty concentrating, tremor, tingling, anxiety, and irritability. Psychological reactions to IEI may include stress, anxiety, and panic at the thought that environmental exposure may have occurred. Patients may go to great lengths to avoid exposure to their triggers.

Physical examination and laboratory tests are not generally helpful. Measurements of environmental chemical levels or imaging studies do not help make the diagnosis. Because there are no diagnostic guidelines for IEI, the evaluation of a person with symptoms of IEI should include a medical history and physical examination and an evaluation of the environment. Treatable conditions should be ruled out. Overuse of diagnostic tests should be avoided.

Other diagnoses that may be considered include somatoform or conversion disorders, chronic fatigue syndrome (CFS), sick building syndrome (SBS), and fibromyalgia. Other possibilities include allergens, infectious microorganisms, irritants, and toxins.

The condition may develop slowly with a single environmental, or occupational trigger. Eventually the patient attributes a growing number of symptoms to an increasing number of common chemical stimuli under ordinary conditions. The person's occupational function and social life are often affected by IEI. Although IEI is not life threatening, it can be distressing and functionally disabling.

Some individuals with IEI have an underlying or concomitant psychiatric disorder that, when diagnosed, responds to medication. Avoiding exacerbating exposures should be considered. Prescription of unnecessary dietary, environmental, or occupational restrictions should be avoided.

There is no evidence from clinical studies that any treatment is effective. Some treatments can make the condition worse. Avoidance regimens can be extreme. Vitamin and mineral supplementation is not proven to help. Some other treatment programs include intravenous gamma globulin (to boost the immune system), or giving chemical and food extracts either by injection or oral drops to "neutralize" the reaction. None of these treatments are proven to be effective or safe.

SEE ALSO: Autoimmune disorders, Fibromyalgia

Suggested Reading

American Academy of Allergy, Asthma, and Immunology (AAAAI) Board of Directors. (1999, January). Idiopathic environmental intolerances. *Journal of Allergy and Clinical Immunology, 103* (1 Pt. 1), 36–40.

Staudenmayer, H. (2001, March 31). Idiopathic environmental intolerances (IEI): Myth and reality. *Toxicology Letter, 120*(1–3), 333–342.

LAURIE G. BROUTMAN
LORI B. SIEGEL

Immigrant Health

Immigrant Health As of March 2000, it was estimated that approximately 10.4% of the U.S. population, or 28.4 million individuals, were immigrants. Prior to 1965, the majority of immigrants came from European countries, such as the United Kingdom, Greece, Poland, Portugal, Germany, and Ireland. However, during the past 30 years, an increasing number of immigrants have come from Latin America, Asia, and Caribbean countries, such as El Salvador and Colombia, Vietnam and China, and Haiti and the Dominican Republic. Individuals may seek to enter the United States for any number of reasons, including a desire to reunite with family members, the acceptance of a new employment opportunity, or a need to leave one's country of origin due to persecution. The majority of individuals entering the United States from other countries do so legally, through established immigration procedures. Others enter illegally, oftentimes in search of a safe haven from persecutors.

Findings relating to the health of immigrants have been inconsistent, in part due to reliance on different definitions of "immigrant." For instance, some studies consider the health or illness of all foreign-born individuals, while others examine the health of those who are here legally or those who are here illegally.

The risk of morbidity and mortality varies by immigrant group and by disease. However, a number of studies have found that black and Hispanic immigrants experience lower rates of mortality than do blacks and Hispanics who were born in the United States. In addition, immigrants' risks of smoking, substance use, obesity, hypertension, and some forms of cancer are lower than the risks experienced by U.S.-born individuals of equivalent demographic and socioeconomic backgrounds. However, the risk of these illnesses appears to increase with increasing length of residence in the United States. In general, the risk of various infectious diseases, such as tuberculosis and parasitic infections, appears to be higher among various immigrant groups as compared to individuals born in the United States.

Immigrants seeking medical attention may face barriers as a result of language differences and the relative unavailability of competent interpreters, transportation difficulties, and providers' lack of familiarity with the healing beliefs and practices of their immigrant patients. In addition, the Personal Responsibility and Work Opportunity Reconciliation Act and the Illegal Immigration Reform and Immigrant Responsibility Act, which were both enacted in 1996, severely restrict the ability of even legal immigrants to rely on publicly funded medical services, apart from emergency medical needs and the diagnosis and treatment of specified infectious diseases. Many states have not adopted state legislation that would permit immigrants to rely on publicly funded care when they do not have privately funded health insurance. This is particularly problematic for women of childbearing age, who may not have the funds or the private insurance to cover the costs of prenatal care, labor, and delivery services, or care for their newborns. The legislation has engendered significant controversy because many of the immigrants who are denied publicly funded care, such as Medicaid, actually pay in to the system through their taxes.

Women who immigrate to the United States may experience a number of health-related difficulties that are gender-related. Women may suffer significant trauma during their transit to the United States; this may include sexual assaults and forced labor, sometimes in the form of sexual slavery. Once they arrive in the

Immunization

United States, they may confront additional problems that are gender-related. For instance, many immigrant women are more willing than their male partners to accept low-paying jobs in order to support themselves and their families. Once they become wage earners, they may be introduced to North American conceptualizations of gender roles. Their male partners may, as a result of their own unemployment, feel threatened by what appears to be a shift in the power structure within the family due to their inability to earn a living and their partners' newfound independence. For some women, these changes in their family structure have been associated with increases in domestic violence. Still other immigrant women may become subject to abuse by their U.S. citizen or legally permanent resident spouses or boyfriends, who have promised to file immigration papers on their behalf but have failed to do so. Specific provisions in our immigration law now permit abused immigrant women in such situations to file petitions on their own behalf so that they will not have to remain captive in abusive relationships.

SEE ALSO: Access to health care, African American, Asian and Pacific Islander, Discrimination, Domestic violence, Latinos

Suggested Reading

Fix, M., & Passel, J. S. (1999). *Trends in noncitizens' and citizens' use of public benefits following welfare reform 1994–97.* Washington, DC: Urban Institute.

Loue, S. (Ed.). (1998). *Handbook of immigrant health.* New York: Plenum Press.

Loue, S., & Bunce, A. (1999). *The assessment of immigration status in health research* (DHHS Publication No. PHS 99–1327). Hyattsville, MD: U.S. Department of Health and Human Services.

SANA LOUE

Immunization Adult immunization has not received the emphasis that has been directed toward vaccinating infants, children, and adolescents. Although vaccination is routine in pediatric practice, it is not commonplace in the practice of physicians who treat adults. Vaccines that should be considered in adult women include tetanus, influenza, MMR (measles, mumps, rubella), varicella-zoster, pneumococcus, meningiococcus, and hepatitis A and B. Indications for the specific vaccines and unique issues of vaccination in pregnancy are discussed below.

Adults should receive a booster dose of tetanus every 10 years. A primary series for unvaccinated adults is three doses: the first two doses given at least 4 weeks apart and the third dose, 6–12 months after the second.

Infection with the influenza virus produces more morbidity and mortality than any other infectious agent. Each year new strains of influenza circulate in the community, and protection requires annual vaccination. Influenza vaccination has long been strongly recommended for individuals over the age of 65 and those with chronic medical conditions. In recent years there has been increasing emphasis on vaccinating healthy adults less than 65 years of age. Recent studies have shown that vaccinating healthy working adults prevents illness and is cost effective. The traditional influenza vaccine is given by injection. The Food and Drug Administration (FDA) recently approved an influenza vaccine that can be administered by a nasal spray.

In the past few years, hepatitis B vaccination has become universal for all children, and is recommended for sexually active young adults. Childhood immunization with hepatitis B is relatively recent, and teenagers and young adults may not have been vaccinated. Hepatitis B vaccination is also recommended for health care workers, patients with chronic renal failure, and individuals whose job or lifestyle put them at increased risk for exposure to blood and body fluids. Hepatitis B vaccination requires three injections, the second and third given 1 and 6 months after the initial shot. Hepatitis A vaccine is most commonly given to travelers who will visit developing countries. Hepatitis A is by far the most common vaccine-preventable disease in travelers. A single dose of the vaccine provides full protection but only lasts 2–3 years. A booster given 6–18 months after the initial dose provides long-lasting protection. In addition to travelers, individuals with occupations known to be high risk for hepatitis A, such as intravenous drug users and, should receive the vaccine.

Vaccination against the bacteria *Streptococcus pneumoniae* with the pneumococcal polysaccharide vaccination is recommended for patients over 65 and those with specific chronic medical conditions such as renal failure, immunosuppression, liver disease, and cancer. Clinical trials have demonstrated that the pneumococcal vaccine is effective in preventing complications of *S. pneumoniae* such as sepsis, death, and meningitis in healthy elderly individuals. The benefit of preventing pneumonia is less clear. Patients who have had their spleen removed have an increased risk for sepsis due to *S. pneumoniae* and should receive the vaccine. The current recommendation is for a one-time vaccine with a booster after 5 years for patients over the age of 65, and every 5 years for the high-risk nonelderly.

Young adults are the most common age group that needs MMR vaccination. Measles and rubella are primary concerns in women. Adults born before 1957 may be considered immune to measles based on natural infection, which was almost universal prior to the introduction of the measles vaccine. A booster immunization with the live MMR vaccine after the first year and a half of life provides lifelong protection against measles. Routine use of the live vaccine began in the past decade and a half; and adults born after 1957 and before 1990 may not have received vaccination that will have long term protection. Adults born in or after 1957 should receive at least one dose of MMR unless they have a medical contraindication, documentation of at least one dose, or other acceptable evidence of immunity. A second dose of MMR is especially recommended for adults recently exposed to measles or in an outbreak setting, those who were vaccinated with an unknown vaccine between 1963 and 1967, are students in postsecondary educational institutions, work in health care facilities, or plan to travel internationally. One dose of MMR should be given to a woman whose rubella vaccination history is unreliable. Women should be counseled to avoid becoming pregnant for 4 weeks after vaccination. Women of childbearing age, regardless of birth year should have determination of rubella immunity. One lifetime dose of MMR should be adequate for protection against mumps.

Vaccination against the varicella-zoster virus (VZV), the causative agent of chickenpox, is recommended for all persons who do not have a reliable clinical history of varicella infection, or serological evidence of VZV infection, and have specific risks. Those at increased risk for VZV include health care workers and family contacts of immunocompromised persons, those who live or work in environments where transmission is likely (e.g., teachers of young children, day-care employees, and residents and staff members in institutional settings), persons who live or work in environments where VZV transmission can occur (e.g., college students, inmates, and staff members of correctional institutions, and military personnel), adolescents and adults living in households with children, women who are not pregnant but who may become pregnant in the future, and international travelers who are not immune to infection. Greater than 90% of U.S.-born adults are immune to VZV. Pregnant women or those planning to become pregnant in the next 4 weeks should not be vaccinated. Childhood vaccination against VZV is becoming routine; the duration of protection and the need for revaccination remain unknown.

The meningococcal vaccine protects against sepsis and meningitis due to the bacterium *Neisseria meningitides*. Young adults, particularly college students living in dormitories, are at increased risk for contracting *N. meningitides*, and should be considered for vaccination. It is becoming routine to offer meningococcal vaccination to students entering college. Others at increased risk include adults with terminal complement component deficiencies, with anatomic or functional asplenia (lack of a spleen). Travelers to countries in which disease is hyperendemic or epidemic ("meningitis belt" of sub-Saharan Africa, Mecca, Saudi Arabia for Hajj) should also be vaccinated. Vaccination requires one shot, but the duration of protection is only 4 years, and revaccination is required for continued protection.

Generally, live-virus vaccines are contraindicated for pregnant women because of the theoretical risk of transmission of the vaccine virus to the fetus. If a live-virus vaccine is inadvertently given to a pregnant woman, or if a woman becomes pregnant within 4 weeks after vaccination, she should be counseled about the potential effects on the fetus. However, live-virus vaccination during pregnancy is not ordinarily an indication to terminate the pregnancy.

Whether live or inactivated vaccines are used, vaccination of pregnant women should be considered on the basis of risks versus benefits, that is, the risk of the vaccination versus the benefits of protection in a particular circumstance. Neither killed nor live-virus vaccines affect the safety of breast-feeding for either mother or infant. Breast-fed infants can be vaccinated on a regular schedule.

SEE ALSO: Hepatitis, Preventive care

Suggested Reading

Keusch, G. T., & Bart, K. J. (2001). Immunization principles and vaccine use. In E. Braunwald, A. S. Fauci, D. L. Kasper, S. L. Hauser, D. L. Longo, & L. J. Jameson (Eds.), *Harrison's principles of internal medicine* (15th ed., pp. 780–789). New York: McGraw-Hill.

Suggested Resources

American College of Preventive Medicine webpage on vaccination: http://www.acpm.org/adult.htm

Incest

Family Medicine immunization webpage: http://www. immunizationed.org/

KEITH B. ARMITAGE

Incest "Incest" traditionally has been defined as sexual activity between close blood relatives who cannot legally marry. The definition has been expanded to include sexual contact in a kinship-type relationship where sexual activity is usually barred, this including non-blood family members, such as stepparents and stepsiblings. Fathers, stepfathers, uncles, and older siblings are the most frequent perpetrators. Girls are more likely to be victimized than boys. Father–daughter incest is the most frequently reported type of sexual abuse and mother–son abuse is the least common type.

Statistics vary on exactly how many girls have been abused. A 1979 study of 900 randomly chosen women in San Francisco showed that 38% had suffered childhood sexual abuse. A *Los Angeles Times* poll in 1985, involving all parts of the United States, found that 27% of women reported inappropriate sexual contact in childhood. In the same *Los Angeles Times* poll, 16% of men suffered childhood sexual abuse. The United States in 1997 reported 1 million substantiated cases of child abuse, 22% of these were sexual in nature; the majority of cases were incest as opposed to abuse by a stranger. Guilt and embarrassment by all members of an incestuous family make accurate reporting of cases difficult.

Sociologists often view the prohibition of incest as a means of socialization. Biological factors also support the incest taboo. Childbearing among close blood relatives may unmask hidden recessive genes, which may be harmful or lethal to progeny. Anthropologists state that a person's culture decides what forms of sexual contact constitutes incest.

Various factors contribute to the breakdown of the incest taboo. All socioeconomic groups are represented. Poverty, overcrowding, rural isolation, alcohol abuse, and mental health issues/mental retardation have long been associated with incest. Higher sociogroups tend to have less contact with reporting officials and may be more likely to conceal this type of sexual abuse.

Children who have suffered abuse may show symptoms that can produce lifelong effects. Anxiety, an overconcern with physical complaints, such as stomach pain and headaches, often becomes a difficulty. Formal posttraumatic stress disorder may develop with nightmares, flashbacks, and hypervigilance against perceived attacks, numbing, and increased startle reflex. Sexual preoccupation and aggression are common. Young children may display knowledge of sexual activity in play. Depression, low self-esteem, and suicidal behaviors are common as well. School performance may drop. A 1986 study by Browne and Finklehor demonstrated that 40% of adults with history of childhood sexual abuse had sequelae severe enough to merit therapy.

The diagnosis of incest can be a clinical challenge. The child may be fearful of the perpetrator, embarrassed, or ashamed and not disclose the needed information. Young children do not have the verbal or cognitive skills to relay information to health care or social workers. Physical signs and symptoms may be present, such as bruises, pain, genital itching, vaginal discharges, urinary tract infections, sexually transmitted diseases, as well as difficulty walking or sitting. Careful sets of interviews with the child, along with a thorough physical exam by a trained physician, are necessary for evaluation of suspected abuse.

Treatment of incest begins by providing protection for the child. Disclosure itself may be protective, as collusion and denial become more difficult. The child may need to be removed from her or his current environment, despite the potential for psychological trauma in doing so. After safety is assured, further psychiatric evaluation should follow. Psychotherapy for the child through play, artwork, or projective techniques can help the victim to come to terms with the trauma. The perpetrator's psychopathology and prognosis for change must be assessed. Family therapy may help in influencing restraint over inappropriate behaviors and establishing better functioning of the household. Legal agencies may be involved to help enforce appropriate behaviors of the perpetrator. On a larger scale, prevention and early detection programs may assist in lowering the numbers of sexually abused children and giving rapid treatment to those already affected by this common form of child abuse.

SEE ALSO: Child abuse, Depression, Posttraumatic stress disorder, Sexual abuse

Suggested Reading

American Psychiatric Association. (1994). *Diagnostic and statistical manual of mental disorders* (4th ed.). Washington, DC: Author.

Bass, E., & Davis, L. (1994). *The courage to heal: A guide for women survivors of childhood sexual abuse.* New York: Harper & Row.

Kaplan, H. I., Sadock, B. J., & Grebb, J. A. (Eds.). (1994). Problems related to abuse and neglect. *Kaplan and Sadock's synopsis of psychiatry: Behavioral sciences, clinical psychiatry* (7th ed., pp. 786–795). Baltimore: Williams & Wilkins.

McClendon, P. (1991). *Incest/sexual abuse of children.* www.clinical-socialwork.com/incest.html

SHARON ABEGG

Incontinence *see* Urinary Incontinence and Voiding Dysfunction

Infertility

Infertility is defined as the inability of a sexually active, noncontracepting couple to achieve pregnancy in one year, the time to which about 90% of couples succeed. Among couples of reproductive age, about 10% are infertile. Delayed marriage and childbirth is one of the main social factors that has resulted in increased infertility in society. Furthermore, sexually transmitted diseases still are the major cause of infertility in Western countries.

CAUSES OF INFERTILITY

The most common causes of infertility are: tubal disease, male disorders, lack of ovulation (anovulation), and abnormality of uterine tissue (endometriosis). The initial evaluation of infertility requires complete history of medical and surgical problems, a genetic history, a history of any sexually transmitted diseases, family history of early menopause, medication used, and allergies. Specific attention should be placed on details of potential occupational exposure to toxins as well as recreational drugs, smoking, and alcohol. All these questions apply to the male as well. Specific gender-oriented questions include menstrual abnormalities, history of milky discharge from the breasts (galactorrhea), abnormal, excessive body/facial hair (hirsutism), acne in women, and erection abnormalities and genital trauma in men.

Tubal Disease

Tubal disease that is a cause of infertility is the result of a sexual transmitted disease. It is generally accepted that tubal infertility developed in 12% of women after one episode of pelvic inflammatory disease (PID), 24% after two episodes of PID, and 48% after three episodes of PID. The most common organism involved is the bacterium *Chlamydia trachomatis*. In dealing with the reproductive health of a young woman, it is essential that the patient is informed of these risks and appropriately screened.

A specialized procedure to evaluate the health of the tubes leading to the uterus, the hysterosalpingogram (HSG), is used to assess the presence of tubal disease. It is performed in the follicular phase of the menstrual cycle. If the history suggests PID, a specialized blood test (sedimentation rate) should be performed. If elevated, the test should be postponed. If normal, then the patient should be given prophylactic antibiotic, doxycycline 100 mg twice a day, starting 2 days before the procedure.

The treatment of tubal disease depends on the severity. Mild disease can be treated surgically, More advanced disease is treated with in vitro fertilization (IVF). Treatment of tubal disease is associated with an increased risk of pregnancy outside of the uterus (ectopic pregnancy).

Anovulation and Ovulatory Dysfunction

Anovulation and other disturbances of ovulation are another important cause of infertility. There are several methods to evaluate ovulation. Basal body temperature charts are inexpensive and sometimes useful. Many patients find them cumbersome. There is a tendency to overinterpret data from these charts. A reasonable screening test would be a single blood progesterone (a type of hormone) level timed on the basis of a home urinary test. A serum level above 10 ng/ml is usually associated with normal ovulatory cycle. If anovulation is detected, then blood testing should be ordered to rule out thyroid disease, pituitary abnormality, and premature ovarian failure.

The most common cause of anovulation is polycystic ovarian syndrome (PCOS). This syndrome is defined as irregular menstrual periods associated with clinical or biochemical evidence of an abnormal endocrine state (hyperandrogenism). The onset is usually at the time of puberty. Many women with PCOS have insulin resistance that is independent of weight. These patients often have a family history of diabetes and are at greater risk to develop non-insulin-dependent diabetes at a younger age than the general

331

population. Obesity is a comorbid condition that accentuates the syndrome. Evaluation of these patients includes measurement of serum hormones (androgens and gonadotropins), exclusion of thyroid disease, and elevation in the hormone prolactin (hyperprolactinemia). These patients should have a simple measure of insulin resistance, such as fasting glucose and insulin.

The first treatment approach with PCOS patients is diet and exercise to modify insulin resistance. Many patients will achieve pregnancy spontaneously. If this is insufficient, oral glucose-lowering drugs such as metformin may be used. If this is unsuccessful, clomiphene citrate, a medication that is commonly used for ovulation induction, can be used.

Endometriosis

Endometriosis is the presence of abnormal uterine tissue (endometrial glands and stroma) at sites outside the uterus. This disease affects many women in the reproductive age group and is a common cause of infertility. Although its etiology has not been conclusively identified, it is generally believed to involve abnormalities in the immune system. It is unclear whether this is causal or simply a response to abnormal implants.

Endometriosis is associated with painful periods (dysmenorrhea), painful intercourse (dyspareunia), noncyclical pelvic pain, and infertility. Many patients with endometriosis-associated infertility do not have significant pain symptoms. The extent of disease is evaluated by a numerical system that involves the presence of endometriosis in the pelvis, or ovaries, and the presence of fibrous growths (adhesions). It is unclear how early stage disease can cause infertility. Advanced disease causes a significant distortion of the pelvic cavity that clearly results in infertility.

Medical suppressive therapy, such as with luteinizing hormone-releasing hormone agonist (LHRHa), does not improve fertility. However, surgical therapy for early stage disease has been shown in a randomized clinical trial to improve fertility. Advanced disease can be initially treated with surgery to restore normal anatomy. However, recurrent advanced endometriosis is best treated with IVF.

Leiomyomas

Leiomyomas are a type of benign tumor. They have a high prevalence in some ethnic groups, such as African Americans. Leiomyomas are not common causes of infertility. Investigation for infertility in patients with leiomyomas should proceed as in other patients with infertility. If there is distortion of the uterine cavity, then myomectomy (removal of abnormal tissue) may improve fertility. A woman should be counseled that adhesions may form and there may be an increased incidence of rupture of the uterus during pregnancy.

Male Infertility

Male factor infertility remains a significant problem contributing to approximately 50% of the cases attending infertility clinics. Male infertility involves a complex series of events, wherein abnormalities in one or more steps block the ability to initiate a viable pregnancy.

Male infertility is a multifactorial syndrome encompassing a variety of disorders. In more than half of infertile men, the cause of their infertility is unknown and could be congenital or acquired. The known causes of male infertility are quite numerous, including factors that prevent normal function of sex organs (pretesticular causes such as excess estrogen), disorders of the testicles such as abnormal maturation of the testes, and posttesticular causes such as abnormal sperm motility (movement).

LABORATORY EVALUATION

Laboratory testing provides additional insight into both the extent and mechanism of testicular dysfunction. The hormonal profile is essential in differentiating causes of infertility. Very low sperm counts can be associated with chromosomal abnormalities. These have been detected in about 10–15% of males with some types of sperm abnormalities.

In the majority of infertile men, detailed semen analyses are required to fully characterize their reproductive dysfunction. Conventionally, semen analysis includes measurement of sperm concentration, semen volume, percentage of motile sperm, and quality of forward progression of these motile sperm, viability, and morphology. Computer-assisted semen analysis (CASA) provides more sophisticated measures of sperm motion, such as velocity, linearity, and lateral head displacement.

THERAPY FOR INFERTILITY

The therapy for infertility has evolved immensely in the last 10 years. Ovulation induction drugs have not changed dramatically in the last 20 years. There are anti-estrogens such as clomiphene citrate and gonadotropins. The most recent change in gonadotropin therapy is that most of these drugs are now synthetic rather than derived from human products. Surgery does not have as dominant a role and has been supplanted by assisted reproductive technologies. The main indications for surgery are leiomyomas and endometriosis.

SEE ALSO: Endometriosis, Fecundity, Reproductive technologies

Suggested Reading

Clark, A. M., Thornley, B., Tomlinson, L., Galletley, C., & Norman, R. J. (1998). Weight loss in obese infertile women results in improvement in reproductive outcome for all forms of fertility treatment. *Human Reproduction, 13,* 1502–1505.

Falcone, T., Goldberg, J. M., & Miller, K. F. (1996). Endometriosis: Medical and surgical intervention. *Current Opinion in Obstetrics and Gynecology, 8,* 178–183.

Hatch, E. E., & Bracken, M. B. (1993). Association of delayed conception with caffeine consumption. *American Journal of Epidemiology, 138,* 1082–1092.

Legro, R. S., Finegood, D., & Dunaif, A. (1998). A fasting glucose to insulin ratio is a useful measure of insulin sensitivity in women with polycystic ovary syndrome. *Journal of Clinical Endocrinology and Metabolism, 83,* 2694–2698.

Pagidas, K., Falcone, T., Hemmings, R., & Miron, R. (1996). Comparison of surgical treatment of moderate (stage iii) and severe (stage iv) endometriosis-related infertility with IVF_ET. *Fertility and Sterility, 65,* 791–795.

Rowe, P., Comhaire, F., Hargreave, T. B., & Mahmoud, A. M. (Eds.). (2000). *WHO manual for the standardized investigation, diagnosis and management of the infertile male.* Cambridge, UK: Cambridge University Press.

Sharara, F. L., Scott, R. T., Jr., & Seifer, D. B. (1998). The detection of diminished ovarian reserve in infertile women. *American Journal of Obstetrics and Gynecology, 179,* 804–812.

TOMMASO FALCONE
RAKESH SHARMA

Informed Consent

Informed consent is the central ethical and legal practice standard in clinical care and human research. Informed consent, in its ideal form, should be viewed by clinicians, researchers, patients and their families as an opportunity to engage in a substantive, sustained dialogue that not only provides information but also helps all involved to clarify questions, preferences, and values, and gives rise to authentic decision-making. This process is an expression of the ethical principles of respect for persons, autonomy, justice, and truth-telling. Informed consent is sometimes signified in formal documents (e.g., "consent forms" for vaccinations, diagnostic tests, voluntary participation in research projects, or the release of health information), but is much more important and is not reducible to this bare exchange of paper and ink. It is for these reasons that informed consent serves as the practice that embodies the ideals of the profession of medicine and as a formal safeguard for individual rights in both clinical and research contexts.

Informed consent takes place in numerous contexts—professional relationships and personal situations with certain goals. For example, in preventive health contexts, an informed patient is most able to make the important choices that will optimize her well-being. This could mean choosing whether to have screening tests or making certain lifestyle decisions. In persons who become ill, the process of informed consent serves beneficent aims, with the goal of helping patients address their illness, obtain a diagnosis, and make informed and reasoned choices about treatment. For individuals who are considering participating in research studies, informed consent is at the heart of the relationship between the investigator and prospective volunteer; informed consent is vital *not* because it protects the investigator or institution in case something goes wrong (a popular misconception), but rather because it helps to clarify the balance between the scientific goals of the study (e.g., randomization and double-blind procedures) with respectful, beneficent, and just regard for the individual. In all of these contexts, as screening techniques, diagnostic tests and procedures, and treatment options become more varied—and often, highly technical and sophisticated—informed consent can be an intensely interactive, most human of enterprises. This view is becoming more widespread as empirical studies of informed consent highlight its importance and potential.

Informed consent is composed of three key components. The first, *information sharing,* requires that the patient or prospective volunteer be fully informed about the proposed test, treatment, procedure, or protocol. Full information includes the purpose of the treatment or study, the procedures involved, and the foreseeable risks and potential benefits. Careful exploration of information regarding all standard alternatives is essential in this process. For example, when considering whether to enter into a randomized clinical trial for cancer treatment, it is important to know what the usual standard of care consists of, how the patient can obtain access to standard treatment, and whether every arm of the trial is generally comparable to the usual standard of care. These specific pieces of information almost always involve probabilities and inherent uncertainty. Thus, patients and families must be encouraged to ask questions, and the process should be viewed as an iterative interchange, rather than a didactic session. In this regard, methods of sharing information are evolving, from the traditional paper-based consent form to interactive question-and-answer sessions, to augmentation with videotapes, multimedia, or web-based decision aids. At this time, research into the most productive methods for information sharing is progressing in treatment and research-related contexts, promising novel strategies and a bright future for this fundamental aspect of the informed consent process.

Decisional capacity, the second key element of informed consent, implies that the person making the decision possesses adequate decision-making capacity (the clinical term encompassing the legal concept of "competency"). Decision-making capacity itself, as defined by experts and legal authorities, consists of four related abilities: (a) communicating a stable preference regarding the decision; (b) understanding the information relevant to the decision; (c) reasoning rationally with the shared information; and (d) appreciating the significance of the choice and its consequences for one's own situation.

The third component of informed consent is the *capacity for voluntarism*. Decisions about clinical care or research participation must be free from coercion, and authentic, representing the wishes of the individual. One conceptual model of voluntarism proposes four domains of possible influence on an individual's ability to give consent voluntarily to treatment or research. First, developmental factors may make certain groups and individuals more or less vulnerable to coercion or to more subtle influences that decrease voluntarism. For example, some adolescents may be swayed by peer pressure while still forming their own set of values and preferences. A second domain of influence on voluntarism concerns illness-related factors. A person with a brain tumor, metabolic disturbances, or adverse reactions to medications (e.g., steroids) may experience distortions in their thinking, for instance, that cause them to feel hopeless and powerless. Yet another area of influence on the capacity for voluntarism is the broad category of psychological, cultural, and religious factors. For example, individuals who are not of the dominant culture may perceive causes of symptoms quite differently from more "mainstream" physicians. This disparity may affect the informed consent process and voluntarism in ways that we have yet to understand. Similarly, receiving a diagnosis of breast cancer may be such a traumatic event, for instance, that an individual may, even temporarily, be less able to assert herself in asking questions, gathering information, and considering all of her treatment options. Finally, external features and pressures (e.g., very rushed consent processes in an emergency situation or being institutionalized or physically or emotionally dependent) may result in subtle, or not-so-subtle, influences on voluntarism.

Numerous special considerations related to informed consent pertain to women's roles as patients or research participants. In this vein, it is important to note the history of exploitative practices involving women as patients and research subjects; these instances frequently involved, at least in part, the lack of informed consent. Enslaved African American women in our country were experimented on by surgeons during the 1800s; more recently, however, a research project in which Hispanic women seeking birth control medications were, without their knowledge, randomized into a trial where some women received placebo and pregnancy rates were tracked. With heightened attention to these cases, new restrictions on study enrollment, ostensibly designed to protect women, excluded categories of women (e.g., pregnant women and women of childbearing potential) from important clinical research. This in turn impeded the acquisition of new knowledge on which clinicians and patients could base their decision-making. On a positive note, this situation has been recognized and is being rectified; crucial work is now proceeding in many areas of women's health.

At present, women are participating in unprecedented numbers in clinical research and are increasingly proactive as patients and health care consumers, accessing as never before the wealth of information and opinions available online, in the media, and from family, friends, and health care professionals. With the innovations in experimental treatments for HIV, cancer, and mental illness, there is a growing sense of research participation as an opportunity and access to research as a societal right. As women gain stronger voices in clinical and research settings, it is important to keep in mind the role of psychological and cultural factors, as well as societal attitudes toward women. For many women, there exist potential barriers to informed consent, including socioeconomic or ethnic minority status, illiteracy, trauma, and illness itself. Many women face combinations of these factors.

Additionally, women generally speaking tend to emphasize relationship-related factors in their decision-making; this most likely applies as well to decisions about their own health care or research participation. Cultural factors can amplify this tendency, as interrelatedness and interdependence of one's family and cultural group are more highly valued in many ethnic groups. Another consideration is the possibility that some women may be more likely to view the physician or researcher as an authority figure—and therefore hesitate to ask questions or otherwise "question authority." An awareness of these subtle influences on the informed consent process can go a long way in making the process one that is meaningful and consonant with the individual's authentic wishes.

In clinical care and research settings, informed consent should be viewed as an essential part of any treatment or research-related decision, rather than merely as a legal requirement. Informed consent serves as a tool to maximize autonomous decision-making of every woman contemplating her own care or participation in a study. To this end, a number of positive and proactive approaches to the informed consent process are available. Physicians, investigators, and patients alike need more information about why informed consent is important (a number of tutorials regarding informed consent are available online and on videotape). In addition, informed consent needs to be conceptualized as an ongoing, iterative process, rather than a discrete occurrence. Several sessions can be scheduled to discuss a decision; this also serves to decrease any perceived pressure on the individual to reach a decision (in nonurgent situations) prematurely. Finally, informed consent is a process that is best conceptualized as a conversation, discussion, or exchange.

Enhanced consent procedures (including multimedia presentation tools and computer-based decision aids) are available as well as in development. A key point, however, is that these kinds of tools are meant to augment rather than replace the fundamentally human interaction that informed consent embodies. Even writing a simplified or more structured consent form can benefit patients. Overviews of studies and take-home information sheets are very useful, and some groups provide videotapes summarizing important aspects. Patients and research participants should be encouraged to ask questions during the informed consent process, be made aware of resources for learning more about informed consent or the particular treatment or protocol, and be supported and respected in their decision-making. Thus, some women may require more time, information, or explanation than others; these needs should be met nonjudgmentally. Sensitivity to the cultural needs, as well as educational or linguistic challenges, facing many women is also vital.

In summary, this brief overview points out the progress that medical ethics has made in recognizing the importance of informed consent. Thus, the emergence of informed consent as a cornerstone of medical ethics has been a major advance for women's rights and human rights in general. As medicine and biomedical research advance rapidly, the future is bright for women's participation in this progress; informed consent remains the fundamental scaffolding for their crucial participation.

See Also: Capacity, Clinical trials, Conservatorship, Discrimination, Durable power of attorney for health care, Patients' rights

Suggested Reading

Faden, R. R., Beauchamp, T. L., & King, N. M. P. (1986). *A history and theory of informed consent.* New York: Oxford University Press.

Gilligan, C. (1993). *Concepts of self and morality: In a different voice.* Cambridge, MA: Harvard University Press.

Grisso, T., & Appelbaum, P. S. (1998). *Assessing competence to consent to treatment: A guide for physicians and other health professionals.* New York: Oxford University Press.

Roberts, L. W. (2002). Informed consent and the capacity for voluntarism. *American Journal of Psychiatry, 159,* 705–712.

Stevens, P. E., & Pletsch, P. K. (2002). Informed consent and the history of inclusion of women in clinical research. *Health Care for Women International, 23,* 809–819.

Laura B. Dunn
Laura Weiss Roberts

Inhalant Abuse Inhalants are chemical compounds and gases that induce a mind-altering effect when inhaled. Inhalants can be found in hundreds of different household and industrial products. One classification system lists four general categories: (a) volatile solvents (e.g., paint thinners, glues, correction fluid, nail polish); (b) aerosol propellants (e.g., hair care products, deodorants, paints); (c) gases used in medical anesthetics (ether, chloroform, halothane, nitrous oxide) and household or commercial products (e.g., butane lighters, whipping cream dispensers, refrigerants); (d) volatile nitrites (e.g., amyl and butyl nitrites, the latter of which is sometimes sold as a room odorizer). Solvents, aerosols, and gases act as central nervous system depressants. Nitrites, in contrast, act on vascular smooth muscles and are sometimes used to enhance sex, primarily by gay men. As a result, nitrite abuse is sometimes classified as a different phenomenon from other inhaled substances.

Inhalants are administered via "snorting" directly from the container, "huffing" via a saturated rag, or "bagging" from a paper or plastic bag. The effects of inhalants are similar to alcohol but may include euphoria, delirium, and hallucinations. Acute adverse effects include loss of coordination and central nervous system depression. Depending on the particular substance inhaled, as well as the frequency and extent of use, long-term effects can include brain, liver, and kidney damage, short-term memory loss, hearing loss, limb spasms, and bone marrow damage. Users of solvents and aerosol sprays are also at risk of "sudden sniffing death syndrome," which can occur when the heart beats erratically.

Inhalant abusers are diverse but can be classified into three classes of users: (a) children and adolescents who are experimenting with inhalants; (b) adolescent polydrug abusers; (c) adult abusers. Unlike nearly all other classes of drugs, inhalant abuse is most common among younger adolescents and tends to decline with age. Early use may be related to the fact that many inhalants are inexpensive and readily available. The decline in use with age often reflects the fact that other drugs become available to older adolescents, who are also more able to afford them. Among older adolescents, inhalants may be abused in addition to other substances. Although inhalant abuse is generally seen as an adolescent phenomenon, sometimes it extends into adulthood. Adult abuse is an extremely underresearched phenomenon.

Since the 1970s, there has been a gradual increase of inhalant abuse among high school students in the United States. In 1975, lifetime prevalence among high school seniors was 10% and increased through 1994 to about 18%. Since then, there have been decreases with the 2002 hovering around 15%.

Inhalant abuse is differentially distributed across ethnic groups in the United States. African American youth have lower prevalence rates, compared to whites. In contrast, among some American Indian youth, inhalant abuse seems to be disproportionately high. In the 1980s, lifetime prevalence rates among high school students in some American Indian communities reached 32%. Recent research suggests that over the last decade there was a strong pattern of decrease in inhalant abuse in this population. Similarly, for a period of time there was a perception that Mexican American youth had much higher rates of inhalant abuse than non-Latino white youth. However, it was established that rates in this group are similar to those in the general population.

Earlier epidemiological data indicated that in the general population and among Mexican Americans, inhalant abuse was more common among males than females. Among Native Americans, this gender gap was much less significant. Recent studies report continued increase of inhalant abuse among females compared to males, a trend that has been observed in the use of other drugs.

Inhalant abuse is an understudied form of drug abuse. It presents a significant and particularly difficult challenge to drug abuse treatment providers since abusers comprise a very complex and dysfunctional group with high rates of delinquency and a wide range of psychological and social problems. Inhalant abusers are often found among individuals who have the fewest social resources and are the most marginal in a society.

Due to a persisting stereotype that most inhalant abuse occurs among males, there is little understanding of gender-specific health effects of inhalant abuse. It can be expected that inhalants, just like most other abused substances, have more adverse effects on women's health, compared to men, which presents additional challenge to the treatment services that are often oriented toward male substance abusers.

SEE ALSO: Chemical dependency, Substance use

Suggested Reading

Beauvais, F., & Trimble, J. (Eds.). (1997). *Sociocultural perspectives on volatile solvent use.* New York: Harrington Park Press.
Beauvais, F., Wayman, J. C., Jumper-Thurman, P., Plested, B., & Helm, H. (2002). Inhalant abuse among American Indian, Mexican American, and non-Latino white adolescents. *American Journal of Drug and Alcohol Abuse, 28,* 171–187.

Crider, R. A., & Rouse, B. A. (Eds.). (1988). *Epidemiology of inhalant abuse: An update* (NIDA Research Monograph No. 85). Rockville, MD: National Institute on Drug Abuse.

Kozel, N., Sloboda, Z., & De La Rosa, M. (Eds.). (1995). *Epidemiology of inhalant abuse: An international perspective* (NIDA Research Monograph No. 148). Rockville, MD: National Institute on Drug Abuse.

Sharp, C. W., Beauvais, F., & Spence, R. (Eds.). (1992). *Inhalant abuse: A volatile research agenda* (NIDA Research Monograph No. 129). Rockville, MD: National Institute on Drug Abuse.

RAMINTA DANIULAITYTE

Inheritance Although an inheritance need not come from a spouse's estate, many of the following issues are those faced by widowed women. Due to their greater longevity, women over age 65 are almost three times more likely to be widowed than men. If a woman has not been involved in financial planning with her spouse and is not aware of the marital assets or marital liabilities, in addition to dealing with her loss, she may face new financial realities very quickly. If her husband left her well provided for, there are still special considerations and concerns to face when coping with her new wealth, which are discussed below. However, if the wife was not left well provided for, she may be faced with creditors and the need to make a change in lifestyle, including entering or returning to the workforce if she is not employed outside the home.

Inheritance laws, which can be quite complex, are governed by state law. Most states are "noncommunity property" states. In community property states, each spouse has a claim for ownership of one half of the property acquired during the marriage. In noncommunity property states, the surviving spouse does not automatically have a claim on the marital assets. In most states, a surviving spouse who feels that the decedent's estate plan treated her unfairly has the right to elect to take under the laws of intestacy succession rather than under the will. This means that the surviving spouse will receive the share of the estate that she would have received if the decedent had died without leaving a will.

Individuals living in nontraditional relationships should also be aware that in all but a very few localities, estate planning is particularly important to protect their interests because otherwise they have no legal rights upon the death of the significant other. Unless assets are titled in joint names or the decedent has executed estate planning documents (e.g., a will and/or trust) naming his or her partner, the survivor will have no legal claim upon the decedent's assets. Many involved in deeply committed relationships suddenly find themselves literally forced to leave a shared home and treasured belongings when a death occurs.

As noted above, even being well provided for by an inheritance can be accompanied by various issues and challenges. Many people think that money will solve their problems, but that belief may not be realistic. For the woman who has not been involved in the family's money management, being faced with the new responsibility of financial management can be stressful and can place the woman at risk of exploitation. She may not have a relationship with reliable professionals who can help her soundly manage money or plan for her future. She is likely to be faced with advice from many different sources and recommendations or requests from individuals who are looking to benefit from her lack of experience. It may also be difficult to decide between purchasing some extras that she has always wanted, planning for her future, and providing financial assistance to children or other family members. It may be necessary to talk to several individuals to find the right fit for guidance for the future.

The death of a loved one is a stressful period. The receipt of inherited funds may occur at a time when the heir is also grieving her loss and is in a state of emotional turmoil. For example, there may be guilt that money has been received at the expense of a loved one. At this vulnerable time, making important financial decisions can be a struggle. Sorrow may be crippling and may impede one's judgment.

Sometimes, inheritance is unexpected. Many parents do not share their financial status with their children. Many others have not prepared an estate plan. Even with a well-written will, questions will need to be answered. Should the assets of the estate be disbursed right away? Should the family house be sold? What happens when one sibling wants to sell while the other wants to wait for various reasons? Should you give gifts or lend funds to friends or relatives? Should you buy a new house? A car? Should you take the vacation you have always dreamed of?

An inheritance may be the single largest sum of money that one receives in her lifetime. It may be significant enough to cause a reevaluation of one's goals in life and one's standard of living. Questions concerning career, retirement, providing for children's education and welfare, and considering charitable donations are all factors to be considered.

Financial advisers all agree on one basic rule when an inheritance is received. Do nothing for a while. Do not make any decisions immediately. It is important to deal with the emotional issues of inheritance before tackling the financial ones. A good rule of thumb is to wait 6 months to a year before making lifestyle changes. During this interim period, do not allow yourself to spend frivolously. If the inheritance is in cash, it might be held in short-term certificates of deposit, money market accounts, or other low-risk investments while a financial investment strategy is being developed and relationships with professional advisers are developed.

These advisers may include a lawyer, an accountant, a financial planner, and/or a money manager. The criteria used to select advisers should include honesty, integrity, experience, professional competence, and the appropriate credentials. References should be requested and the potential advisers should be interviewed. Quality of service should be more important than cost. An attorney can assist with probating the will and/or making distributions from a trust. Once the matters that need to be attended to immediately are resolved, you should consider your own estate planning needs. Even if you have estate planning documents in place, your estate plan should be reviewed if there has been a significant change in your family or in your financial status.

An inheritance will serve you best when used to build on your existing strengths. An individual plan must be developed. By taking a look at your entire financial situation and consulting with an estate lawyer and financial planner, you can utilize the money to your best advantage. Ask yourself these basic questions:

- Does your income exceed expenses?
- Are you saving at least 10% of your salary?
- Do you have money set aside for emergencies?
- Do you have adequate insurance?

Once these questions have been answered, you can think about investing your inheritance. Protect yourself. Preserve and conserve for your own future. Develop a plan for your retirement. If your employer offers a retirement plan, and even better, matches your contributions, your inheritance may enable you to establish an account or increase the contributions from your salary. If an employer-sponsored account is not available, or in addition to such an account, you might want to open an individual retirement account (IRA). For funds that are to remain readily accessible, compare the return on money market accounts to savings accounts and short-term certificates of deposit. Compound investments in mutual funds and stocks by reinvesting the dividends. If you divide your investments into a variety of categories and diversify interests, the risks will be varied and thereby increase your opportunity for profit.

Trust documents are an option in planning for your own financial future. A trust can protect assets from some creditors, provide for administration of your assets if you become incapacitated, and avoid probate administration upon your death. The trustee of a trust will fulfill two jobs—administration of the trust and money management. Again an attorney will be able to advise you best when it comes to this area. Making provisions for family members with special needs is a crucial issue, one best handled by a knowledgeable professional.

Improved financial planning will help you achieve lifetime goals. You should exercise caution and think of your long-term needs. Money can provide security, comfort, and convenience; like many things in life, the best plan will balance satisfying immediate needs and desires with preserving assets for the future.

SEE ALSO: Probate

Suggested Reading

Barney, C., & Collins, V. (2002). *Best intentions: Ensuring your estate plan delivers both wealth and wisdom*. Chicago: Dearborn Trade.

Plotnick, C. K., & Leimberg, J. D. (1998). *How to settle an estate: A manual for executors and trustees*. New York: Penguin Putnam.

Rottenburg, D. (1999). *The inheritor's handbook: A definitive guide for beneficiaries*. Princeton, NJ: Bloomburg Press.

Suggested Resources

Older Women's League (OWL): http://www.owl-national.org/reports.htm (Retrieved May 31, 2003).

JANET L. LOWDER
DEBORAH S. ROSSMAN

Injection Drug Use

The hypodermic syringe was invented in 1853 by a Scottish physician named Alexander Wood. For the first time, drugs could be injected under the skin, intramuscularly, or directly into the bloodstream to alleviate health problems. By the 1870s, the hypodermic syringe was widely used by American physicians to administer drugs, such as morphine, heroin, cocaine, and even strychnine. By 1885, however, the dangers of addiction as well as potential infection at the site of injection were recognized by medical professionals.

A wide range of psychoactive substances can be injected illegally for their euphoric effects. The most common intravenously injected illegal drugs include heroin, various pharmaceutical opioids (analgesics), cocaine, and methamphetamine. LSD, MDMA (ecstasy), and methylphenidate (Ritalin and others), among other drugs, are sometimes injected intravenously, although the number of people who administer these drugs in this way is comparatively small. Even crack cocaine can be injected when dissolved with an acid (e.g., vinegar or lemon juice), although the practice is not very common. While most illegal drugs are injected intravenously, some (e.g., ketamine and sometimes heroin and morphine) are injected just below the skin, a practice called "skin-popping."

Injection drug users are at risk for a wide range of health problems. The most common include infection at the site of injection, endocarditis, hepatitis B and C infection, human immunodeficiency virus (HIV) infection, overdose, and dependence. The emergence of HIV in the early 1980s has severely impacted injection drug users, particularly women. By June 1994, 64% of the AIDS cases among women were attributable to injection drug use. Of these, 48% were related to injection practices, and 20% were associated with sexual contact with a man who had injected drugs.

Injection drug users are at risk of infection with HIV and other bloodborne pathogens through a variety of mechanisms. The most well-known direct route of exposure to pathogens is through sharing contaminated syringes. Unless cleaned adequately with household bleach or another effective viricide, syringes used sequentially by more than one individual may contain small amounts of blood that enable the transmission of pathogens. Sharing syringes was initially perceived as a form of "ritual bonding" by public health professionals. However, ethnographic research demonstrated that syringe sharing is more directly related to difficulties in gaining access to sterile syringes. Sharing "cookers" (small containers used to mix drugs and water), "cottens" (material used to strain the solution while drawing it into a syringe), and rinse water is also recognized as potential routes of exposure to bloodborne pathogens. For example, water is used to rinse syringes to prevent clogging, thereby enabling syringes to be used multiple times. In a group setting, a number of individuals may share a common source of rinse water and potentially be exposed to pathogens through this process. Finally, various methods of mixing and distributing drug solutions, such as "backloading," have been recognized as forms of "indirect" sharing that put people at risk of exposure to bloodborne pathogens. In the case of "backloading," the drug solution is drawn up into one syringe and distributed to other injectors by flushing a measured amount of the solution into the back of other syringes. Injectors who receive the drug mixture could be exposed to pathogens in the syringe used to divide the solution.

New injection drug users are at increased risk of infection with bloodborne pathogens because they lack control of the injection process. Until people learn how to inject themselves, new injectors must yield control of the injection process to more knowledgeable injectors. Often, new injectors lack their own equipment and must use syringes provided by others, some of which may have been used previously. In some cases, new injectors may turn to "injection doctors" who specialize in performing injections for a fee in money or drugs.

For a variety of reasons, women who inject drugs may be at higher risk for infection with bloodborne pathogens. In some injection settings, women are at increased risk of exposure to pathogens because they often assume subordinate roles relative to men. Hence, women are often likely to inject after men, sometimes re-using the same syringe or other injection paraphernalia.

The complex relationship between injection drug use and sexual behavior sometimes places women at increased risk of infection with bloodborne pathogens and sexually transmitted diseases (STDs). At the most general level, women, as well as men, who inject drugs are often more likely to engage in riskier sexual behavior because the drugs injected alter consciousness and influence decision-making. As such, depending on the particular drug(s) injected, some users may be more likely to have sex with a higher number of people, with people less well known to them, and without using barrier protection. In the case of women who inject heroin, in particular, prostitution often becomes one of the few available means to make the money needed to purchase daily supplies of the drug. Women injectors who engage in sex work have increased chances of being exposed to HIV, hepatitis, and other STDs through high-risk sexual behavior (high number of anonymous partners; unprotected sex). In the case of other drugs, cocaine and methamphetamine injections are known to increase libido in many individuals and are often

339

associated with high-risk sexual practices. Delayed ejaculation associated with methamphetamine and cocaine use, for example, often leads to prolonged periods of vaginal or anal sex. This may place women as well as homosexual men at greater risk of infection with blood-borne pathogens due to the abrasion of tissues, if condoms are not used properly.

A variety of drug abuse treatment services are available for injection drug users. For opioid-dependent injectors, methadone detoxification or maintenance is one of the most common methods of treatment. Established therapeutic drugs for cocaine- and methamphetamine-dependent injectors are not available at this time. Women who inject drugs often have more difficulty accessing drug abuse treatment services compared to men. For example, women with children are often unable to participate in treatment services because they lack alternative child care resources. In summary, injection drug use affects women's health in multiple ways, depending in part on the drug(s) used.

SEE ALSO: Acquired immunodeficiency syndrome, Harm reduction, Heroin, Sexually transmitted diseases, Substance use

Suggested Reading

Carlson, R. G. (2000). Shooting galleries, dope houses, and doctors: Examining the social ecology of HIV risk behaviors among drug injectors in Dayton, Ohio. *Human Organization, 59*(3), 325–333.

Friedland, G. (1989). Parenteral drug users. In R. A. Kaslow & D. P. Francis (Eds.), *The epidemiology of AIDS: Expression, occurrence and control of human immunodeficiency virus type 1 infection* (pp. 153–178). New York: Oxford University Press.

Howard-Jones, N. (1971, January). The origins of hypodermic medication. *Scientific American*, 96–102.

Koester, S. (1996). The process of drug injection. In T. Rhodes & R. Hartnoll (Eds.), *AIDS, drugs and prevention: Perspectives on community action* (pp. 133–148). London: Routledge.

ROBERT G. CARLSON

Insomnia Sleep disturbances can have multiple causes. These can be organized into two broad areas, as primary sleep disturbances and secondary sleep disturbances. Primary sleep disturbances usually imply primary neurological sleep disorders, such as disordered breathing/breathlessness during sleep (sleep apnea), restless leg syndrome, and conditions of abnormal daytime sleepiness/"sleep attacks" (cataplexy and narcolepsy). Patients with sleep apnea may have significant daytime sleepiness as well as sleep disturbance. Sleep apnea may be both central (due to brain/central nervous system causes), obstructive (due to lung/airway causes), or mixed (both central nervous system and airway) disorders. The obstructive form of sleep apnea, which represents an anatomical obstructive process to the airways, has relatively good outcome compared to a central form of apnea. Treatment outcomes in these sleep disorders are directed to improving quality of sleep at proscribed times and optimizing the benefits of quality sleep. Treatment should primarily be driven by diagnosis rather than symptom-driven, which is often the mistake that results in compromised patient care. Patients presenting with primary neurological disorders causing insomnia need to have these entities identified with an appropriate workup which may involve a sleep lab evaluation. Treatment would be driven by the resulting diagnosis and treatments specific to the underlying disorder.

The broader and more common presentations of insomnia are due to other medical or psychiatric causes (secondary presentations). Medical causes of insomnia would be due to neurological disorders as well but not primary sleep disorders as described previously. Delirium (a medical disorder of disturbed consciousness/alertness) may result from primary neurological disorders or other medical problems (such as brain infection) that can impair brain function. Primary neurological diseases that can cause delirium include tumors, brain injury from many causes including stroke or bleeding (hemorrhage), and seizure disorders. Appropriate identification and treatment of these disorders with timely intervention are critical. Headache may present as a symptom and may occasionally indicate a serious process that needs to be identified and treated. Medical processes that impinge on the brain can cause delirious states or milder brain compromise. For example, a person with brain disease and compromised function from a dementia may have a urinary tract infection, which results in significant agitation and sleep disturbance. A person with a relatively intact brain but significant medical compromise such as significant untreated heart failure might find themselves unable to sleep. In each example, insomnia should not be treated with a sedative but rather by managing the acute medical problem.

Assuming that an individual's medical and neurological issues are not the cause of the sleep disturbance, then psychiatric illness could be the one contributing. Psychiatric disorders have many potential issues that need to be addressed. The mood disorders including depression and mania can have sleep disturbance as one of their principal symptoms. When this is not recognized, inappropriate interventions can lead to exacerbation of the illness, which often leads to further sleep disturbance. Even when the mood disorder is recognized, if the disorder is not well understood and managed, interventions can exacerbate the disorder and the sleep disturbance. Sleep disturbances occur in schizophrenia and anxiety disorders as well. When these disorders are not appropriately managed, the condition of the affected person can be significantly compromised. Sometimes, an individual with psychiatric illness and insomnia is in denial about the underlying illness and he or she may be unwilling to cooperate with appropriate treatment. In some cases, there are complaints of anxiety that are based on untreated psychotic illness. Interventions with sedative/anxiolytics can lead to complicating or compounding the illness of that person without fundamentally improving the condition. In a person with a dementing illness, insomnia as a sleep disturbance occurs. If the cause of the disturbance is not properly identified, then the course of that person's presentation may be significantly worsened.

Finally, there are persons who are relatively healthy but because of an acute stressor can experience a short-term symptom of insomnia. Such cases, in the absence of other issues, may be treated by sedative hypnotics provided they are limited to short-term use.

Further, stresses and maladaptive sleeping regimens often develop in a significant portion of the population. Sleep hygiene is an important ingredient in treatment. When insomnia occurs as in any other human symptom, there needs to be an understanding of the underlying causes that will determine the most efficacious intervention.

SEE ALSO: Mood disorders, Sleep disorders, Sleep hygiene

Suggested Reading

Cartwright, R. (1999). Sleep disorders: Diagnosis and treatment. *American Journal of Psychiatry, 156,* 493.

Nowell, P. D., Buysse, D. J., Reynolds, C. F., III, et al. (1997). Clinical factors contributing to the differential diagnosis of primary insomnia related to mental disorders. *American Journal of Psychiatry, 154,* 1412–1416.

Schnierow, B. J. (2000). The enchanted world of sleep. *American Journal of Psychiatry, 157,* 1190a–1191a.

PHILIP L. DINES

Intersexuality

Intersex is a blanket term used to describe individuals who possess bodies that the medical establishment cannot classify definitively as male or female. The occurrence is relatively frequent and is estimated at 1 in every 2,000 births.

The variations can be grouped into three major categories. The first encompasses people with chromosomal configurations other than XX (female) or XY (male), such as XXY, XXX, or a single X. Within this group are *genetic mosaics*—individuals with patches of XX and XY tissue (or other possible configurations) in their bodies. Also known as *true hermaphrodites* in the more archaic medical terminology, these individuals are born with both ovarian and testicular tissue. The second grouping is characterized by genetic variations in enzymatic pathways that affect the development of primary and/or secondary sexual characteristics independent of XX or XY chromosomal constitution. The final grouping is characterized by physiological variations that may or may not have genetic underpinnings, such as hypospadias (incomplete virilization of the penis), vaginal agenesis (absent vagina), cryptorchidism (undescended testicles), microphallus (less than 2.5 cm), and megaclitoris (greater than 0.9 cm), among others.

In prior generations, those born intersexed negotiated their way in society as best they could. However, advances in endocrinology and surgical techniques over the past 40 years have led to the alteration of intersexed bodies to conform to idealized male or female morphologies as a matter of standard medical procedure. This policy has been implemented in hospitals throughout industrialized countries beneath a cloak of secrecy and shame, where parents have often been coerced to make life-changing decisions about a newborn under extreme duress, and where there has been little consideration of how the child's gender will develop or of future sexual functioning. Instead, the elimination of so-called ambiguities in the appearance of external genitalia has been the primary concern.

The policy has been applied absent public scrutiny until only recently, largely due to the belief that gender is the logical outcome of sex assignment and is therefore shaped by social learning. Nevertheless, the celebrated case of identical twin boys, one that was reassigned a girl at 7 months of age following a circumcision accident, calls this mind-set into question. Doctors performed reconstructive surgery to make the victim's genitals appear female and administered female hormones at puberty to facilitate a typical female developmental trajectory.

If biology provides the canvas on which individual lives are painted, then one would expect identical twins to develop along similar gender pathways because they are genetic duplicates. However, if gender is shaped largely by social learning, then one would expect that the twin reassigned a girl at 7 months should adapt accordingly and with little difficulty, particularly with the help of castration to remove the masculinizing influence of androgens and the administration of female hormones at puberty. However, the reassigned twin mounted unfaltering resistance against attempts to guide her down a female developmental pathway. Estrogens prescribed at age 12 were frequently thrown away; surgery to extend the victim's rudimentary vagina and facilitate heterosexual intercourse was rejected. At age 14, the twin finally convinced physicians to halt their course of treatment and to assist her to live as a male. Additional surgeries were then performed, including mastectomy and phalloplasty (creation of a male sexual organ), along with initiation of a regimen of male hormones. The twin now lives as an adult man and is stepfather to three children.

Formation of the Intersex Society of North America (ISNA) in 1993 marked the beginning of a movement to educate the public with the goal of removing the secrecy, shame, and unwanted genital surgery associated with intersex status. Intersexed individuals came forward with testimonies of physical agony associated with repeated unsatisfactory surgeries, and emotional pain associated with genital mutilation as well as the isolation, secrecy, and shame with which they were forced to live. Out of this has emerged the five tenets of ISNA: (a) intersexuality is a basic problem of stigma and trauma, not of gender; (b) parents' distress must not be treated by surgery on the child; (c) professional mental health care is essential; (d) honest, complete disclosure is good medicine; and (e) all children should be assigned as boy or girl, *without* early surgery.

The intersex movement advocates providing the parents of intersexed newborns, as well as the intersexed children themselves, with honest and accurate information, including psychological counseling to address parental distress and referrals to other people dealing with the same issues. ISNA argues against using parental consent as a proxy for that of the intersexed child and believes that intersexed individuals should not be subject to surgeries designed to normalize their genitals without their explicit consent. They advocate

the assignment of sex at birth based upon the best information available but without surgery or other medical intervention unless it is to address a life-threatening condition.

The case of the twins, along with countless other testimonies from intersexed individuals, suggests that initial sex assignment is not always congruent with the intersexed child's subsequent gender development. For this reason and for reasons of social justice, ISNA advocates that only when the intersexed child is old enough to make an informed decision regarding the potential risks and benefits of genital reconstructive surgery should the option for surgical intervention be presented and considered.

SEE ALSO: Gender, Gender role, Hermaphroditism, Homosexuality, Lesbian, Queer, Transgenderism, Transsexuality

Suggested Reading

Colapinto, J. (2001). *As nature made him: The boy who was raised as a girl.* New York: Harper Perennial.

Dreger, A. D. (Ed.). (1999). *Intersex in the age of ethics.* Frederick, MD: University Press Group.

Kessler, S. A. (1998). *Lessons from the intersexed.* New Brunswick, NJ: Rutgers University Press.

ANGELA PATTATUCCI ARAGON

Intrauterine Device The intrauterine device (IUD) is a T-shaped plastic device that is placed into the uterine cavity. It provides a woman with a continuous method of contraception. The two types of IUD currently available in the United States are the copper-releasing device (ParaGard) and the hormone-releasing device (Mirena). The IUD prevents pregnancy by several different proposed mechanisms. The copper in the ParaGard IUD is a spermicide. The progesterone in the Mirena IUD causes thickening of the cervical mucus that sets up a barrier to sperm trying to enter the uterine cavity. All IUDs set up a sterile inflammatory reaction of the uterine lining, which also is lethal to sperm.

Throughout the world, the IUD is a very popular choice of birth control. It is not a commonly used contraceptive in the United States because of the fear that the IUD can cause serious pelvic infection. This fear stems from the history of problems associated with a particular type of IUD (Dalkon Shield™) which was used in the 1970s. The Dalkon Shield™ has been off the market since 1974 and had inherent design flaws which may have been the cause of the increased incidence of pelvic infection linked with its use. The IUDs that are available today are safe and effective. Although pelvic infection remains as a slight possibility with IUD use, the danger is more dependent on the user's risk factors than on the IUD itself.

The IUD is 99% effective in the prevention of pregnancy. It is as effective as a tubal ligation and creates less of a risk of ectopic pregnancy. Although the initial expense of this contraceptive is higher than other methods, the IUD becomes very cost effective with long-term use. The initial expense includes the cost of the device itself, any necessary laboratory testing, and the office visits for the screening for and insertion of the IUD. Since this device can be left in place for a considerable length of time, the ongoing cost is very low. The recommended length of use is 5 years for Mirena™ and 10 years for ParaGard™.

The IUD is a very "user-friendly" approach to birth control since it does not require the woman to have to remember to use her contraceptive method. It provides immediate contraceptive protection with insertion and its effect is completely reversible with the removal of the device. Even so, the IUD may not be the perfect choice for everyone. Some women may experience heavy bleeding and cramping with menstruation. This is much less common with the Mirena IUD. Mirena often causes a couple of months of irregular bleeding after insertion, followed by years of very light periods, or no periods at all. Increased bleeding and cramping with a ParaGard IUD can usually be managed with mild pain medications. Although the risk is small, the IUD use does have the potential for pelvic infection. This is mostly true of women who are not involved in a mutually monogamous relationship, as they are at most risk for sexually transmitted infections. Safe sex practices can decrease the incidence of infection within this group. Because pelvic infection can affect future fertility, the use of the IUD is generally not recommended for women who have not yet had children. This recommendation, however, is beginning to change with more information about how safe the IUD is. The ideal candidate for IUD use is a woman in a long-term mutually exclusive relationship, who has borne children, and desires a reversible method of birth control.

The IUD can also be used as a means of emergency contraception. If, after unprotected intercourse, an IUD is placed within 5 days, it can be a very effective abortifacient.

The IUD must be prescribed and inserted by a qualified health care provider. This birth control method can provide a woman with an extended, effective means of contraception. Women interested in using the IUD should have an honest and open dialogue with their health care provider about the risks and benefits of this method to determine if the IUD is the best contraceptive choice for them.

See Also: Birth control, Pelvic inflammatory disease

Suggested Reading

The Boston Women's Health Book Collective. (1998). *Our bodies, ourselves for the new century.* New York: Touchstone Books.

Hatcher, R., Trussel, J., Stewart, F., Cates, W., Stewart, G., Guest, F., et al. (1998). *Contraceptive technology* (17th rev. ed.). New York: Ardent Media.

Suggested Resources

Planned Parenthood Federation of America. (1998). *Understanding IUDs.* http://www.plannedparenthood.org/birth-control/iud.htm

Ruth Monchek

Iron Supplementation
Iron is a trace mineral that is vital for life but needed only in small amounts. Iron plays an important role in oxygen transport and energy production, and because of this, iron is a vital element in the daily diet. The average adult body contains about 4 g of iron, 3 g in active form and about 1 g in storage or transport form. About 70% of the active form of the iron is found in hemoglobin, myoglobin, and enzymes. The function of hemoglobin is to carry oxygen from the lungs to the other tissues and to take carbon dioxide back from the tissues to the lungs. The cytochrome enzymes help cells produce energy.

Iron in the oxidized or ferrous form is absorbed well compared to iron in the ferric form. Vitamin C (ascorbic acid) enhances iron absorption by converting ferric oxide to ferrous oxide, making it water soluble. Iron absorption increases with need, such as during periods of rapid growth in infancy, childhood,

Iron Supplementation

adolescence, and during pregnancy. When the body has enough iron, 10% of dietary iron is absorbed. This may increase to 12% or 13% when the body is iron deficient. Iron found in animal tissues is better absorbed than iron from vegetable sources. Tea and dietary fiber supplements slow iron absorption by forming insoluble iron compounds.

Iron deficiency results in anemia. Anemia is a condition in which the total hemoglobin content in the bloodstream is below normal. In anemia, the number of red blood cells may be low, or cell numbers may be normal if each red cell contains less hemoglobin than usual. Because of the reduced hemoglobin content, the blood carries less oxygen, which causes fatigue. A diet low in iron can cause iron-deficiency anemia, especially in infants, children, teenagers, and vegetarians. Iron deficiency can also be caused by chronic blood loss. Among women, heavy menstrual periods, closely spaced pregnancies, and breast-feeding can deplete the body's iron stores. Some people may become iron deficient because they cannot absorb enough of the iron in their diet. This occurs in Crohn's disease (an intestinal disease), or after surgical removal of part of the stomach. Certain drugs, foods, and caffeinated drinks interfere with iron absorption. Other dietary factors such as a lack of protein, calories, B vitamins, or vitamin C can lead to iron-deficiency anemia. At four times in the life cycle, iron intake is often inadequate: (a) infancy, (b) periods of rapid growth in childhood and adolescence, (c) reproductive age and during menstrual periods, and (d) pregnancy.

The symptoms of iron deficiency include fatigue, weakness, and pale appearance. Hemoglobin is red, and when iron deficiency causes the hemoglobin level to fall, the skin, nail, and mucous membranes become pale. Heart symptoms like rapid heartbeat, heart murmurs, and enlargement of the heart will appear if the anemia is severe. Another symptom that can occur with anemia is pica, in which the person craves and eats substances like paper, starch, dirt, or ice. Anemia can also cause upward curvature of nails, brittle nails, or ridges in the nails.

Anemia is diagnosed by measuring the amount of hemoglobin in the blood. However, having anemia does not mean that low iron is the culprit. Further tests are needed to diagnose iron deficiency. These include measuring the total serum iron, total iron-binding capacity, and the ferritin level. In iron-deficiency anemia, the hemoglobin, serum iron, and serum ferritin are below normal level, while the total iron-binding capacity is above normal.

Symptoms of iron-deficiency anemia are reversible by replenishing the body's iron stores. Prevention is the best treatment. Preventive measures for infants include iron supplements and introduction of fortified and enriched foods at the appropriate age. Pregnant women usually take iron supplement pills that contain ferrous sulfate until delivery. The supplements should be taken after meals. When iron deficiency is caused by poor absorption in the intestine, iron may be replaced through injections. The diet should be planned to increase iron intake and the intake of factors such as vitamins and animal protein that help in iron absorption. Avoid dietary factors that decrease iron absorption, like tea, phytates, and phosphates.

Even if symptoms of iron deficiency are present, do not take iron supplements without talking with your health care professional. If the iron loss is due to intestinal bleeding, taking iron pills may delay the diagnosis of a serious problem such as bleeding ulcer, or colon cancer. If the anemia is not due to iron deficiency, taking iron pills will not help the anemia, but may cause iron toxicity. Unnecessary iron supplements can also cause iron overload (hemochromatosis), in which iron is deposited in the liver and heart, causing liver and heart problems. It is difficult to overload with iron from food alone, because the intestines are usually effective in preventing excessive iron absorption. However, excessive amounts of iron can prevent the body from regulating iron absorption properly. Iron supplements are a leading cause of fatal poisoning in children. *Always store iron supplements in child-safe containers out of reach of children.* Iron supplements should only be used when tests show a deficiency of iron and a health care professional recommends what dose to take, and for how long.

SEE ALSO: Diet, Nutrition

Suggested Reading

Blashfield, J. F. (2002). *Iron and the trace elements.* Austin, TX: Raintree Steck-Vaughn.

Chopra, J. G., & Kevany, J. (1971). International approach to nutritional anemia. *American Journal of Public Health, 61,* 250–258.

Marsha, H. (1999). *Vitamins, minerals, and dietary supplements.* New York: John Wiley & Sons.

RAJKUMARI RICHMONDS

Irritable Bowel Syndrome
Irritable bowel syndrome (IBS) is a common condition characterized by abdominal pain or discomfort, bloating, and changes in bowel habits. An international consensus of IBS specialists has defined IBS as "a combination of chronic or recurrent gastrointestinal symptoms which are not explained by structural or biochemical abnormalities." Although causes of IBS are poorly understood, it is thought to result from a complex interplay of changes in intestinal motility, decreased tolerance for stretching of the intestine, psychological, and social factors.

An estimated 10–15% of the population in the United States is thought to have IBS. IBS has an enormous economic impact on society both in terms of work productivity and use of health care resources. IBS is responsible for a high rate of work absenteeism, with more than three times as many days missed annually by workers with IBS compared to workers without IBS. IBS patients have 2–3 times as many health care visits annually than non-IBS patients. IBS accounts for approximately 36% of patients seen by gastroenterologists and 12% of those seen by primary care providers. However, less than half of all IBS sufferers seek medical attention. The likelihood of seeking medical care is influenced less by the severity of symptoms and more by factors such as stress, psychiatric disorders (especially major depression and anxiety disorders), personality, and a history of abuse.

In the general population, up to two times as many women than men have IBS. However, among those seeking medical attention for their symptoms, there is a strong female predominance of up to 4:1. Similarly, although population studies reveal that IBS occurs equally across all adult age groups, young people in their 20s and early 30s are more likely to seek medical attention. Women are more likely to report constipation, bloating, nausea, and psychological symptoms.

DIAGNOSIS

Given the absence of any biochemical or structural abnormality in IBS, the diagnosis is made based on the symptoms listed as criteria for IBS. Laboratory testing is obtained to rule out other medical conditions, but tests should be chosen judiciously in order to avoid an unnecessarily expensive evaluation. The symptom-based criteria for IBS include 12 weeks or more (not required to be consecutive) of abdominal pain or discomfort within the previous 12 months, accompanied by two of the following three symptom patterns: (a) pain relieved by defecation; and/or (b) onset of pain associated with a change in stool frequency; and/or (c) onset of pain associated with change in stool form (e.g., hard, loose, watery). Other symptoms that are commonly reported include the sensation of urgent need to move one's bowels, sensation of incomplete emptying of the bowels, mucus passage, and abdominal bloating. Symptoms which are brought on or worsened by stress or meals are also frequently reported.

In general, a careful history, physical examination, and focused laboratory studies, including complete blood count, chemistry panel, albumin, thyroid function studies, and erythrocyte sedimentation rate should be performed. Patients with diarrhea should also have stool examined for ova and parasites. Other conditions that cause symptoms similar to IBS include colorectal cancer, inflammatory bowel disease, lactose intolerance, thyroid disorders, celiac disease, bacterial overgrowth, parasitic infection, and endometriosis. However, subjecting all patients with IBS-like symptoms to exhaustive testing in order to exclude these diseases is not recommended. In patients who meet IBS symptom criteria and who lack "alarm" signs or symptoms, the likelihood of discovering one of these diseases through an extensive evaluation (including endoscopy and radiology tests) is less than 1%. "Alarm" symptoms that do warrant extensive evaluation are weight loss, blood in stools, fever, abnormal physical examination, anemia, chronic severe diarrhea, nighttime diarrhea, a family history of colon cancer, symptoms of IBS developing for the first time in an elderly person, or symptoms that progressively worsen. Regardless of symptoms, all patients 50 years or more should be screened for colon cancer. Recent studies suggest that celiac sprue may be more common in those presenting with IBS-like symptoms. Therefore, in patients with diarrhea, laboratory tests for celiac sprue should be considered.

TREATMENT

Education about IBS and establishing a good relationship with a physician form the cornerstone of therapy. Instead of continued efforts to find a cause or "cure" for this chronic disorder, the goal should be the reduction of symptoms and development of coping skills. A diet history should be obtained to find out whether any foods or beverages (e.g., legumes, cabbage, broccoli, caffeine, lactose, sorbitol gum, and fatty foods) bring on or worsen symptoms. If a troublesome food is identified, the patient should try eliminating it from the diet to see whether symptoms improve. Most patients do well with education, reassurance, and dietary changes alone. For those who do not, a variety of medications may be used, either alone or in combination, and are chosen based on the individual patient's symptoms.

MEDICATIONS

A number of fiber-containing agents (e.g., psyllium and methylcellulose) are available and are used in IBS patients with either diarrhea or constipation. In diarrhea, the fiber gives bulk to the stool, and in constipation, the fiber helps intestinal contents pass through the colon more rapidly. Patients should be advised to start with a low dose and to increase gradually, as needed, in order to minimize the common side effects of bloating, excessive intestinal gas, and abdominal discomfort. For IBS patients with diarrhea who fail a trial of fiber, the antidiarrheal medication loperamide has been shown to be effective.

For the abdominal pain associated with IBS, there are a number of medications available to reduce symptoms. For pain exacerbated by meals, antispasmodic agents (dicyclomine and hyoscyamine), given 30–60 minutes before meals, will help to relax intestinal smooth muscle and thereby reduce cramping. Pain that is more frequent or severe is treated with tricyclic antidepressants (e.g., amitriptyline). Lower doses than those required to treat depression have been shown to improve abdominal pain in IBS. However, given that constipation is a common side effect of tricyclic antidepressants, they should be used with caution in IBS patients with constipation. Prozac-type antidepressants (serotonin reuptake inhibitors like sertraline) have also been tried for IBS pain, but have not been shown to be effective in randomized clinical trials to date.

Serotonin is a chemical or "neurotransmitter" found both in the brain and the intestinal nervous system that transmits messages from one nerve to another. Serotonin has been found to be involved in the regulation of intestinal motility and sensation. This observation has led to the development of two new IBS treatments, tegaserod and alosetron, which act by different mechanisms on serotonin receptors. Tegaserod, acting primarily by speeding up colonic transit and decreasing intestinal pain sensitivity, has been shown to be more effective than

placebo in relieving pain, bloating, and constipation in female IBS patients. Diarrhea is the most common side effect. Alosetron decreases gastrointestinal secretions and muscle contractions, thereby slowing colonic transit. It has been shown to be effective in improving stool frequency, stool consistency, and abdominal pain in female IBS patients with diarrhea. It is approved by the Food and Drug Administration (FDA) for "women with severe, diarrhea-predominant IBS who have failed to respond to conventional IBS therapy." Constipation, at times severe, is a common adverse event. In addition, there have been a number of reports of ischemic colitis (inflammation due to poor blood flow to the colon) in people who use alosetron. Therefore, the FDA advises that physicians not only educate patients regarding the potential risks, but also carefully weigh an individual patient's risks and benefits before prescribing. At this time, data do not support the use of either tegaserod or alosetron in men. Studies suggest that women have greater intestinal sensory perception, that is, increased sensitivity to bowel distention and peristalsis, and this may underlie the apparent difference in response to these new IBS treatments in men versus women.

BEHAVIORAL THERAPY

Because of the frequent association of symptoms with stress and the increased prevalence of psychiatric disorders among IBS sufferers seeking health care, a variety of behavioral therapies, including relaxation, biofeedback, hypnosis, cognitive therapy, and psychotherapy, have been tried in IBS. These behavioral therapies appear to be helpful in reducing chronic IBS symptoms by reducing anxiety and improving coping skills. If a psychiatric disorder is present, these therapies improve psychological symptoms as well. Severe refractory symptoms in women may signal a history of sexual or physical abuse.

Although IBS is a chronic condition, it is not life threatening nor does it lead to cancer or inflammatory bowel disease. Most people with IBS are able to minimize or even eliminate symptoms with dietary changes and stress reduction techniques. A few patients will also need prescription medications. When the diagnosis is unclear or when moderate to severe symptoms do not respond to therapy, a gastroenterologist should be consulted. IBS centers can help in difficult cases. For those patients in whom a psychiatric component seems likely, referral to a mental health professional is advised.

SEE ALSO: Diet, Nutrition

Suggested Reading

Brandt, L. J., Bjorkman, D., Fennerty, M. B., Locke, G. R., Olden, K., Peterson, W., et al. (2002). Systematic review on the management of irritable bowel syndrome in North America. *American Journal of Gastroenterology, 97* (11 Suppl.), S7–S26.

Cash, B. D., Schoenfeld, P., & Chey, W. D. (2002). The utility of diagnostic tests in irritable bowel syndrome patients: A systematic review. *American Journal of Gastroenterology, 97* (11), 2812–2819.

Chang, L., & Heitkemper, M. M. (2002). Gender differences in irritable bowel syndrome. *Gastroenterology, 123* (5), 1686–1701.

Heymann-Monnikes, I., Arnold, R., Florin, I., Herda, C., Melfsen, S., & Monnikes, H. (2000). The combination of medical treatment plus multicomponent behavioral therapy is superior to medical treatment alone in the therapy of irritable bowel syndrome. *American Journal of Gastroenterology, 95* (4), 981–994.

Irritable bowel syndrome. (2003, April). Bethesda, MD: National Institute of Diabetes and Digestive and Kidney Diseases (NIDDK). http://www.niddk.nih.gov/health/digest/pubs/irrbowel/irrbowel.htm

MARGARET F. KINNARD

J

Jacobi, Mary Putnam

Mary Putnam Jacobi (1842–1906) was a physician, women's rights advocate, writer, and medical educator; she is best known for her efforts to improve education for women and to advance the status of women in the medical field. Born in London, England, on August 31, 1842, Mary Corinna Putnam was the daughter of George Palmer Putnam, founder of the publishing firm of G. P. Putnam's Sons. Her younger brother, Herbert Putnam, was a librarian of Congress. The family returned to the United States in 1848, and Mary grew up in Staten Island, Yonkers, and Morrisania, New York.

Before Mary turned 18 years old, she had a story published in the *Atlantic Monthly* and she seemed headed for a literary career. However, her love of science led her to a medical career instead. She graduated from the New York College of Pharmacy in 1863 and the Female (later the Woman's) Medical College of Pennsylvania in 1864. After working for a few months at the New England Hospital for Women and Children in Boston, Jacobi decided in 1866 to seek further training in Paris. There she attended clinics, lectures, and a class at the École Pratique. She then sought admission to the École de Médecine in Paris, fighting to become one of the first women admitted to the school. She graduated in 1871 with high honors and a prize-winning thesis.

Jacobi returned to New York City, opened a practice, and began teaching at Dr. Elizabeth Blackwell's Woman's Medical College of the New York Infirmary for Women and Children. Frustrated by the lack of opportunities available to most women pursuing a medical career, in 1872, Mary organized the Association for the Advancement of the Medical Education of Women (later the Women's Medical Association of New York City). She was president of the association from 1874 to 1903. In 1873, she married Dr. Abraham Jacobi, generally considered the founder of pediatrics as a medical specialty in America. In the same year, she began a children's dispensary service at Mount Sinai Hospital. From 1882 to 1885, she lectured on diseases of children at the New York Post-Graduate Medical School, and in 1886, she opened a small children's ward at the New York Infirmary. In addition to clinical work and teaching, she found time for writing as well. She had over 100 medical articles and 9 books published, including the 1876 Boylston Prize winner entitled *The Questions of Rest for Women during Menstruation*. Jacobi also took an interest in social causes outside the medical field. She helped found the Working Women's Society and the League for Political Education. She died in New York on June 10, 1906.

SEE ALSO: Blackwell, Elizabeth; Discrimination

Suggested Reading

Encyclopaedia Britannica. (2003). Mary Putnam Jacobi. Chicago. http://concise.britannica.com/eb/article?eu=44171

Encyclopedia of world biography (2nd ed.) (1998). Mary Putnam Jacobi. Farmington Hills, MI: Gale Research.

Garnet, C. (2001). Portrait of a 19th century physician–writer. *The NIH Record, LIII*(8), 1.

The National Women's Hall of Fame. (1993). *Women of the Hall* (1998): http://www.greatwomen.org/women.php?action=viewone &id=86

The reader's companion to American history. (1991). The Society of American Historians. New York: Houghton Mifflin (2003):

http://college.hmco.com/history/readerscomp/rcah/html/ah_046800_jacobimarypu.html

NANCY MENDEZ

K

Kegel Exercises These are a series of exercises that strengthen the muscles surrounding the vagina. These exercises are easily learned and can be performed as convenient. Women who have strong vaginal muscles are less likely to suffer from urine incontinence or prolapse of the pelvic organs. Kegel exercises performed after childbirth promote healing of the vagina and help restore tone to the vaginal area.

The technique for Kegel exercises is simple. The woman firsts learns to contract her pelvic muscles by identifying the location of these muscles. A simple way to do this is to insert a finger into the vagina and attempt to squeeze the vaginal muscles around the finger. Another technique would be attempt to halt the flow of urine while urinating. This may be difficult at first but will become easier as the pelvic muscles become stronger.

At first, the muscles should be contracted for 2–4 seconds followed by a period of muscle relaxation. This exercise can be repeated five times. As the pelvic muscle strength increases, more repetitions can be performed and held for longer periods. Avoid holding the breath during the activity. These exercises can be performed without other people being aware of the activity.

SEE ALSO: Pelvic organ prolapse, Urinary incontinence and voiding dysfunction

Suggested Reading

The Boston Women's Health Collective (p. 274) (1998). New York: Touchtone.

Varney, H. (1997). *Varney's midwifery* (p. 156). London: Jones & Bartlett.

SUSAN WIEDASECK

Keloids Keloids are a benign skin tumor characterized by excessive proliferation of scar tissue. They usually arise at sites of trauma or prior surgery, but occasionally arise spontaneously in areas prone to high skin tension. They develop as a result of increased activity of fibroblasts, the cell type responsible for the production of scar tissue collagen protein. The incidence is most common in African American patients.

A keloid appears as a protuberant, shiny, firm plaque, or nodule on the skin surface. Newer keloids still in the formative stages are often associated with pain or itching, and older lesions are generally asymptomatic. They may form on any part of the body, although the upper chest, shoulders, upper back, and earlobes (where piercing has occurred) are especially prone to keloid formation.

The diagnosis of a keloid can generally be made on clinical grounds, particularly in the setting of prior trauma. If the diagnosis is in doubt, biopsy should be performed to rule out a dermatofibrosarcoma protuberans, a malignant tumor that may look like a keloid.

Treatment of keloids is very difficult. Surgical removal of a keloid is fraught with potential for recurrence of an even larger lesion because more scar tissue may be stimulated to form. This approach may, however, be warranted if combined with another modality to reduce likelihood of recurrence. Performing serial injections of corticosteroids with a small needle is a common approach for reducing symptoms and flattening the keloid. Silicone pads are of limited benefit in newer keloids. New approaches to keloid treatment that are still in the investigational stages include topical drugs that alter the inflammatory cell profile within the lesion, namely, cytokines. Evolving laser treatments may also be beneficial in reducing the size of keloids.

Without treatment, keloids continue to grow until they reach a steady state size, and regression without treatment is unusual. Tenderness and itching are the primary symptoms associated with a keloid, but the cosmetic disfigurement can be quite dramatic.

SEE ALSO: Piercing

Suggested Reading

Berman, G., & Bieley, H. (1996). Adjunct therapies to surgical management of keloids. *Dermatological Surgery, 22,* 126–130.

Tredget, E. E., Nedelec, B., Scott, P. G., et al. (1997). Hypertrophic scars, keloids, and contractures: The cellular and molecular basis for therapy. *Surgical Clinics of North America, 77,* 701–730.

MARY GAIL MERCURIO

Kleptomania

Kleptomania, the impulsive and irresistible urge to steal, may have been described as early as 370 AD by St. Augustine when he wrote in Confessions "Yet I lusted to thieve and did it compelled by no hunger, nor poverty." The term "kleptomania" is derived from the Greek words *klepto* meaning to steal and *mania* meaning insanity. Although kleptomania appears in the medical literature in the 19th century, current literature on the subject is limited.

Historically, kleptomania is an affliction associated with women. It gained widespread attention in the medical community in 19th century Europe. The rising status of medical science and the creation of the department store as a social arena for middle-class women were two strong influences on Victorian society's perception of theft among women. Shopping was then viewed as the female's natural arena and the department store offered women a place in urban society outside the home. Seen as the weak and unstable sex in that era, middle-class women were thought to be unable to control their shoplifting behavior due to the temptation of free access to merchandise the department store offered, in a way not previously known. Though the conception of kleptomania has changed and is now recognized in men as well as women, the ideas of the 19th century continue to influence contemporary views.

Kleptomania is currently understood by the medical community as a psychiatric disorder defined in the Impulse Control Disorders section of the *Diagnostic and Statistical Manual of Mental Disorders-IV* (Text Revision). The diagnostic criteria require that the affected individual exhibit a recurring failure to resist impulses to steal items, even though those items are not needed for personal use or for their monetary value. The individual also experiences a rising subjective sense of tension before the theft, and feels pleasure, gratification, or relief when committing the theft. Additionally, the stealing is not committed to express anger or vengeance, is not done in response to a delusion or hallucination, and is not better accounted for by another psychiatric disorder.

Kleptomania differs from criminal stealing in several important ways. In patients with kleptomania, the urge to steal is generally experienced as distinctly irresistible, intrusive, and often overpowering despite attempts to resist the urges. In addition, patients generally believe that stealing is wrong and most are embarrassed and ashamed of their behavior. The stealing is also often in response to emotional tension or anxiety which is relieved by the behavior. Often, the stealing behavior is impulsive and abrupt rather than premeditated and has an involuntary quality.

Kleptomania is presumed to be a rare disorder. Studies of groups of shoplifters usually yield a low rate of kleptomania ranging from 0% to 8%. The shameful nature of the disorder presumably prevents people from reporting it; thus, an accurate assessment of its prevalence is difficult to estimate. The available studies consistently find that kleptomania is more common in women and often begins in adolescence or early adulthood. Though little is known about the natural course of the disorder, it may follow an episodic or chronic course.

The presence of other psychiatric disorders in those suffering from kleptomania is very common. Some of the most frequent co-occurring diagnoses are those that are also more common in women. Mood disorders such as depression and bipolar disorder are seen most frequently. Other diagnoses include anxiety disorders such as obsessive–compulsive disorder, substance use disorders, and eating disorders such as anorexia

Kleptomania

nervosa and bulimia nervosa. The relationship between kleptomania and these other psychiatric disorders has been investigated in case studies. Individuals suffering from depression report that the act of stealing produces a "rush" or "high" that helps to temporarily alleviate their symptoms. Those diagnosed with anxiety disorders often reported a similar reduction in their anxiety after stealing.

The literature available on the treatment of kleptomania is limited. Case studies report some success with antidepressants such as Prozac and mood-stabilizing drugs such as lithium. Various forms of psychotherapy including behavioral therapy and psychoanalytic psychotherapy are found to be variably successful, but controlled studies are lacking. Some reports suggest that most people afflicted with kleptomania never seek formal treatment and simply disallow themselves to go shopping, thus avoiding the problem. Kleptomania is a diagnosis rooted in centuries of history but remains incompletely understood and infrequently studied in the modern medical community.

SEE ALSO: Anxiety disorders, Depression, Psychotherapy

Suggested Reading

Kaplan, H. I., & Sadock, B. J. (1997). *Synopsis of psychiatry* (8th ed.). Philadelphia: Lippincott, Williams & Wilkins.

NANCY K. MORRISON

Labor and Delivery The process by which a child is born is both simple and intricate. From the moment of conception, it is inevitable that the growing fetus will need to develop, grow, and eventually pass from its uterine environment either by a vaginal delivery or a cesarean section delivery. The cardinal signs of labor or mechanisms of labor describe the basic stages through which a fetus must pass to be delivered vaginally. The cardinal mechanisms are: (a) engagement defined as the lowest portion of the presenting part at or below the maternal ischial spines; (b) descent; (c) flexion; (d) internal rotation; (e) extension; (f) external rotation; and (g) expulsion. These seven stages vary slightly from patient to patient and labor to labor.

Labor can be both difficult to diagnose, difficult to initiate, and difficult to stop. Labor is classically defined as regular uterine contractions resulting in cervical change. However, labor can start with amniorhexis or ruptured membranes (breaking the bag of water). Cervical change can also occur prior to or without labor as in the case of prelabor cervical changes or incompetent cervix. In fact, the diagnosis of the initiation of labor is often made retrospectively.

Labor is divided into three or four stages. The first stage is defined as the period of time from the beginning of labor until complete cervical dilation. The second stage of labor is defined as the period of time from complete dilation of the cervix until delivery of the fetus. The third stage of labor is defined as the period of time from the delivery of the fetus until the delivery of the placenta, and the fourth stage of labor has been defined by some as the 1-hr period of time after the delivery of the placenta.

The first stage of labor is a process that is divided into two phases, latent and active, and results in the eventual complete dilation. It can be difficult to diagnose the initiation of the first stage of labor as well as the transition from the latent to the active stage. This transition is marked by an increase in the rate of cervical dilation. Typically this occurs at approximately 4 cm dilation. The average length of the active phase of labor ranges from 4.6 to 7.7 hr for nulliparous (women having their first babies) and 2.4 to 5.7 hr in multiparous (women having subsequent babies) patients. The second stage of labor (the pushing stage) ranged from 57 to 66 min for primaparous patients and from 17 to 24 min in multiparous patients. The use of epidural anesthesia can increase the length of the pushing stage. These average durations of the different stages of labor are used to help diagnose labor abnormalities and qualify treatments for them.

One of the dystocias (abnormalities) of the first stage of labor is a prolonged latent phase. Typically 20 hr is considered the cutoff in the primaparous patient, and 14 hr is the typical cutoff in the multiparous patient. Therapies for a prolonged latent phase include no intervention, analgesia (pain control), and augmentation of labor (helping the labor progress more efficiently). An example of analgesia commonly used is 10–20 mg of morphine. Oxytocin (more commonly referred to by its trade name Pitocin) is typically the drug of choice for labor augmentation. Oxytocin is an eight-amino-acid peptide hormone that is stored and released from the posterior pituitary.

Labor and Delivery

In addition, a prolonged latent phase, defined by greater than 12 hr for primaparous patients and greater than 6 hr for multiparous patients, has been associated with an increased risk of cesarean section, increased rate of more serious vaginal and perineal lacerations, and increased fever and bleeding.

Abnormalities of the active phase of labor are protraction and arrest disorders. A protraction disorder is defined by rates of dilation at less than the expected rates for nulliparous and multiparous patients. There is a usual expectation that a rate of 1.2 cm/hr change for nulliparas and a rate of 1.5 cm/hr change for multiparas are the outer limit of normal. There are, of course, many exceptions to these rules. Treatment is oxytocin augmentation.

Arrest of active phase is defined by the absence of dilation over a 2-hr period with adequate uterine contractile force. Assuming that oxytocin has already been administered for the preceding protraction disorder, the treatment for the arrest of active phase is cesarean delivery.

Dystocias or abnormalities of the second stage of labor include: protraction or arrest of descent of the presenting fetal part. Treatments for these disorders again are oxytocin and operative vaginal delivery or cesarean section delivery. These disorders were associated with a higher rate of cephalopelvic disproportion (CPD—baby will not fit through the birth canal), macrosomia (a large baby), and cesarean delivery. CPD, however, is a difficult diagnosis to make and is often an overused diagnosis. In general, it implies that either the fetus is too large or the maternal pelvis is too small to accommodate one another. Of course position or presentation can also affect this diagnosis and therefore each labor is unique regardless of any absolute measurement of the maternal pelvis or fetal size. In fact, after a cesarean for the diagnosis of CPD, the chance that a woman will be successful in having a vaginal birth after cesarean (VBAC) is approximately 83% after one prior cesarean and 75% after two prior cesarean deliveries.

MALPRESENTATION

Ninety-five percent of deliveries occur with a fetus in the vertex (head down) presentation. Malpresentation defines a presentation that is not in an occiput anterior (the baby is facing toward the mother's back) vertex presentation. This includes occiput posterior (the baby is "sunny-side up," i.e., facing upward as it delivers) and transverse presentation (looking sideways), breech (buttocks or legs presenting), transverse (the baby's side is facing down), or oblique lie. Although breech presentation is not an absolute contraindication to a vaginal delivery, meaning that it does not absolutely prohibit a vaginal delivery, it has fallen out of favor recently after the publication of a large multicenter European study that reported an increased risk of neonatal morbidity after breech vaginal birth. The delivery of a second twin that is in the breech presentation, however, is still a safe and acceptable mode of delivering a second twin in the right circumstances.

Abnormalities of the third stage of labor include issues involved in placental separation from the uterus. Removal of the placenta can be spontaneous (comes out on its own with just some gentle traction by the obstetrician or midwife) or manual (the obstetrician or midwife reaches in to the uterus to remove it). Spontaneous expulsion of the placenta results in fewer infections, less risk of uterine inversion (when the uterus turns inside out), and less blood loss. However, manual extraction may be necessary, with the proper anesthesia, in cases of cord evulsion (when the umbilical cord tears off the placenta), hemorrhage, or retained placenta.

Induction of labor (IOL) is a common procedure in the practice of obstetrics and can be challenging. It has the potential to be extremely successful and beneficial to the patient, but alternatively can increase the risk of a cesarean delivery. In general there are three things to consider when planning an induction: the indication, the chance of success, and the mode of induction. Indications for induction include both maternal and fetal.

Clear maternal indications for induction include most cases of severe preeclampsia, chorioamnionitis (infection of the fetal membranes), and intrauterine fetal demise (death). Fetal indications include prolonged pregnancy greater than 42 weeks, poorly controlled diabetes mellitus, severe intrauterine growth restriction (fetus is not growing as we hope and expect it to), premature rupture of membranes (the bag of water breaks before labor begins), and other conditions that would compromise fetal health and not benefit from prolongation of in utero existence.

The success of induction depends on many factors including the gestational age (how far along in pregnancy the patient is), parity (how many children the patient has had), and the cervical "ripeness." Inductions are more likely to be successful in the term pregnancy and in a multiparous patient. The term "cervical ripeness" is used to describe the cervical receptivity to induction agents. The classically described five cervical characteristics (dilation, effacement, station, consistency, and position) are combined to comprise what is now referred to as the Bishop score. A multipara with a Bishop score of greater than or equal to nine has a 100% chance of a successful induction with oxytocin and/or amniotomy.

The two common agents used are oxytocin and prostaglandins. Additional agents are also used for cervical ripening and/or dilation such as laminaria or Foley balloon catheters placed within the cervical os. High doses or rapid infusions of oxytocin have potential side affects including hypotension (low blood pressure) and water intoxication.

Prostaglandins are used for IOL as well. These medications can be of particular use in the induction of a patient with a poor Bishop's score or "uninducible" cervix on exam. The mode of action is both at the level of the cervical collagen as well as uterine muscle receptors.

Hyperstimulation syndrome is a disorder of labor that can occur during spontaneous or induced labors. Hyperstimulation syndrome occurs when contractions are too frequent and/or too long in duration. As a result of these frequent contractions, the fetus may experience distress and exhibit fetal heart rate abnormalities. Treatment is aimed at improving fetoplacental perfusion and decreasing uterine tone. Typical maneuvers used to increase oxygen supply to the fetus include repositioning the mother onto her left side to increase cardiac output, oxygen administration, giving medications that will slow contractions, and, on occasion, urgent cesarean delivery is required.

Cesarean delivery is the transabdominal surgical removal of the fetus from the uterus. The primary cesarean rate in the United States ranges from 8% to 18% on average and the total cesarean rate (including repeat cesarean sections) ranges from 16% to 22%. Typically, a Pfanensteil or vertical skin incision is used to start and the abdomen is opened in layers. The uterine incision is most commonly used in the term gestation is the low transverse incision which is considered to be the strongest in healing and least hemorrhagic. Other potential uterine incisions are the low vertical, the T-incision, the J-incision, and the classical incision. The average blood loss at the time of cesarean delivery is 1,000 ml versus 600 ml for a vaginal birth. There is also a higher incidence of febrile morbidity with cesarean delivery.

Assisted vaginal deliveries or instrumental deliveries include vacuum and forcep deliveries. An assisted delivery may be indicated when there is a prolonged second stage (it is taking too long for the mother to push out the baby), there is suspicion of fetal compromise, or when there is a need to shorten the second stage in instances of certain maternal ill health. Several prerequisites need to be met before an instrumental delivery is begun. Both forceps and vacuum deliveries are associated with an increase in neonatal and maternal morbidities. Some of these morbidities include: damage to the maternal soft tissue; maternal pain; neonatal subgaleal and cephalohematomas (blood clots in or around the brain); neonatal retinal hemorrhages (bleeding in the back of the eye); neonatal hyperbilirubinemia (increase in bilirubin, which causes jaundice); and neonatal facial nerve and/or ocular (eye) damage.

Despite a short-term morbidity of as high as 5%, the long-term morbidities do not appear to be increased.

Labor typically occurs at full term which is defined as a pregnancy at greater that 37 weeks gestation. However, up to 10% of all viable pregnancies are delivered before term. Depending on the exact gestational age at delivery, there can be serious morbidity and mortality rates in the neonate related only to prematurity. Some of the common risks of prematurity include: intracranial hemorrhage, respiratory distress syndrome, sepsis, necrotizing enterocolitis, retinal hemorrhage, auditory dysfunction, and jaundice.

Modern science has yet to understand the natural process for the initiation of labor at term and has only some ideas and associations for what causes preterm labor. The true biochemical process by which labor is initiated has yet to be described, and similarly the cessation of labor is hard to achieve. The cessation of labor or tocolysis has been attempted with several types of medications including: beta mimetics, oxytocin antagonists, nonsteroidal anti-inflammatories, magnesium sulfate, calcium channel blockers, progesterone, and even ethanol. There are varying successes with these drugs and varying side effects. Perhaps the most progress in preventing prematurity has been the use of maternal steroid administration, which may not be without its own side effects. Modern medicine continues to research potential therapies for preterm labor, yet the best medicine may continue to be prevention.

SEE ALSO: Cesarean section, Episiotomy, Pregnancy, Prenatal care, Teen pregnancy, Ultrasound

Lactation

Suggested Reading

Simkin, P. (1989). *The birth partner.* Boston: The Harvard Common Press.

Simkin, P., Whalley, J., & Keppler, A. (1984). *Pregnancy, childbirth, and the newborn: A complete guide for expectant parents.* New York: Meadowbrook.

Suggested Resources

www.drspock.com

JANET M. BURLINGAME

Lactation   Producing milk follows pregnancy and birth as inevitably and naturally as pregnancy follows conception. It is a normal function in all mammals and each species produces milk, which is the best specific food for its own newborn.

During pregnancy, under the influence of hormones such as estrogen and progesterone, the female breast undergoes noticeable changes. The blood vessels on the surface of the breast increase in size and become more visible. The nipple enlarges and the area around it, the areola, becomes larger and often darker. Small nodules often appear on the areola. The breast also becomes larger due to the increase in the milk glands and ducts that will carry the milk to the nipple after the baby is born. Even before birth, the milk glands will start to produce a clear yellow substance called colostrum. These changes often start early in pregnancy and will continue until after delivery when true milk production will start.

About 3 days after the birth of the baby, the mother will feel her breast filling up. For some, it is quite sudden, for others, it is more gradual. The baby will have been sucking at the breast regularly since birth and will have received colostrum, which is very rich and nutritious. A hormone called prolactin regulates the production of milk. It occurs any time after the birth. A different hormone called oxytocin produces the ejection of milk. Oxytocin is stimulated by the baby sucking at the breast. The release of oxytocin is also dependent on the relaxation of the mother. If there is too much tension, such as that caused by pain, fatigue, depression, or nervousness, the production of oxytocin will be inhibited and the milk will not let down as easily.

Breast milk contains a combination of protein, fat, enzymes (help in digestion), immunoglobulins (provide immunity from some diseases), leukocytes (help fight infections), hormones, and growth factors.

As well as being easily digestible and perfectly suited for the human infant (just as cow's milk is perfectly suited to the calf), breast milk is known to prevent infections in the infant. Breast-fed babies have fewer episodes of diarrhea, ear infections, and gastrointestinal problems.

The amount of breast milk needed by a baby is regulated by how much and how frequently the baby sucks at the breast. It is a wonderfully well-tuned mechanism of supply and demand. The more often the baby empties the breast, the more signals will be sent to the pituitary gland to increase production of prolactin and hence milk.

Just as immunity is passed from the mother through the breast milk, various food substances, infections, and medications can be transmitted. Under certain circumstances, such as when the mother has hepatitis, tuberculosis, or is HIV positive, it may be preferable for a baby to be formula fed. Medications taken by the mother will also be secreted in her milk. This is usually in very small amounts, but this is why it is very important to weigh carefully the need to take any medications during breast-feeding, and to always consult your midwife or doctor before taking any medications. It is important to remind whoever is prescribing a medication that the mother is breast-feeding.

When breast-feeding a baby, it is ideal to offer the breast whenever the baby appears to be hungry. If this in done consistently, the quantity of milk produced will equal what the baby needs. A breast-fed baby should have several wet diapers a day, and frequent bowel movements. Most babies after the first couple of days of life will breast-feed every 1–3 hours. If this does not occur, the new mother can call for assistance. The hospital where she had her baby will often have a lactation consultant, or she can contact her local chapter of La Leche League. Breast-feeding can be continued as long as both the mother and the baby feel comfortable doing so. Solid food is usually introduced between 4 and 6 months. The baby's pediatrician can assist the mother in making these choices.

Stopping breast-feeding is called weaning. It is best done very gradually in order to minimize discomfort of full (engorged) breasts and avoid mastitis, which is an infection of the breasts, which can occur when breasts become engorged.

Pregnant women should be strongly encouraged to breast-feed their babies. It is a very healthy and satisfying experience for both and helps create a strong bond between mother and child.

SEE ALSO: Breast-feeding, Pregnancy

Suggested Resources

http://www.breast-feeding.com
http://www.cdc.gov/breast-feeding
http://www.lalecheleague.org
lactation@juno.com

GINETTE LANGE

Laparoscopy

Laparoscopy is a medical procedure which can be utilized to treat a variety of gynecological disorders. A small tube (endoscope) is introduced into the affected organ. The medical practitioner can visualize the organ, and if indicated, perform surgery/treatments via the endoscope. Laparoscopy is often done to diagnose (by direct visualization) and treat the common condition of endometriosis (abnormal uterine tissue). Laparoscopic treatment of endometriosis can be either conservative or radical. Conservative surgery aims to retain the patient's fertility. However, such surgery may involve dissection of the urinary tract, the bowel, and the tissue around the vagina and rectum (rectovaginal septum). A wide range of laparoscopic procedures can be performed on patients with endometriosis. These include treatment of peritoneal lesions (endometrial tissue in the abdomen), the ovaries, the intestines, and the urinary tract.

The ovary is one of the most common pelvic organs to be affected with endometriosis. Ovarian involvement may be as simple as superficial implants to deeply infiltrating endometriosis. Two approaches have been proposed for the treatment of ovarian endometriosis: fenestration versus excision. Fenestration consists of simply opening the capsule of the cyst ovary and irrigating ("washing out"). No excision of endometriosis occurs. Excision requires removal of the ovarian cyst itself or at least its destruction by coagulation or laser techniques. The recurrence rate and the long-term outcome on ovarian function are unknown.

In the past, intestinal endometriosis diagnosed at laparoscopy has generally required conventional surgery. However, in our experience, laparoscopic treatment of colorectal endometriosis, even in advanced stages, is safe, feasible, and effective in nearly all patients.

Severe endometriosis of the bladder and the ureter (tubes leading from the kidney to the bladder) may be asymptomatic and can cause gradual kidney (renal) impairment. The efficacy of the laparoscopic approach for the diagnosis and treatment of severe urinary tract endometriosis has been thoroughly evaluated in the literature. Laparoscopic repair is the primary treatment of advanced endometriosis. However, superficial implants can be treated by simple excision (cutting away of abnormal tissue). Laparoscopic approach is safe and effective in the diagnosis and treatment of early as well as advanced urinary tract endometriosis.

Laparoscopic cutting of specific affected pelvic nerves (presacral neurectomy) is infrequently used as a last resort in the treatment of intractable endometriosis-associated pelvic pain. The pattern of pelvic pain improves dramatically after the procedure in the majority of cases. The procedure seems to be associated with an acceptable rate of long-term side effects.

Many studies compared laparoscopy and laparotomy (conventional surgery of the pelvis) in the management of endometriosis. It has been found that laparoscopy causes less postoperative growths (adhesions) and reduces impairment of reproductive function compared to laparotomy. Pregnancy rates with laparoscopic treatment and laparotomy are probably similar, although no randomized trial has been performed. Postoperative recovery has clearly been shown to be better with laparoscopy compared to laparotomy.

SEE ALSO: Endometriosis, Infertility

Suggested Reading

Al-Azemi, M., Bernal, A. L., Steele, J., Gramsbergen, I., Barlow, D., & Kennedy, S. (2000). Ovarian response to repeated controlled stimulation in in-vitro fertilization cycles in patients with ovarian endometriosis. *Human Reproduction, 15,* 72–75.

Bedaiwy, M. A., Falcone, T., Sharma, R. K., Goldberg, J. M., Attaran, M., Nelson, D. R., et al. (2002). Prediction of endometriosis with serum and peritoneal fluid markers: A prospective controlled trial. *Human Reproduction, 17,* 426–431.

Jerby, B. L., Kessler, H., Falcone, T., & Milsom, J. W. (1999). Laparoscopic management of colorectal endometriosis. *Surgical Endoscopy, 13,* 1125–1128.

Jones, K., & Sutton, C. (2000). Endometriomas: Fenestration or excision? *Fertility and Sterility, 74,* 846–848.

Ling, F. W. (1999). Randomized controlled trial of depot leuprolide in patients with chronic pelvic pain and clinically suspected endometriosis. Pelvic Pain Study Group. *Obstetrics and Gynecology, 93,* 51–58.

Lundorff, P., Hahlin, M., Kallfelt, B., Thorburn, J., & Lindblom, B. (1991). Adhesion formation after laparoscopic surgery in tubal pregnancy: A randomized trial versus laparotomy. *Fertility and Sterility, 55,* 911–915.

Marcoux, S., Maheux, R., & Berube, S. (1997). Laparoscopic surgery in infertile women with minimal or mild endometriosis. Canadian Collaborative Group on Endometriosis. *New England Journal of Medicine, 337,* 217–222.

Mol, B. W., Bayram, N., Lijmer, J. G., Wiegerinck, M. A., Bongers, M. Y., van der Veen, F., et al. (1998). The performance of CA-125 measurement in the detection of endometriosis: A meta-analysis. *Fertility and Sterility, 70,* 1101–1108.

Nezhat, C., Nezhat, F., Nezhat C. H., Nasserbakht, F., Rosati, M., & Seidman, D. S. (1996). Urinary tract endometriosis treated by laparoscopy. *Fertility and Sterility, 66,* 920–924.

Nezhat, C. H., Seidman, D. S., Nezhat, F. R., & Nezhat, C. R. (1998). Long-term outcome of laparoscopic presacral neurectomy for the treatment of central pelvic pain attributed to endometriosis. *Obstetrics and Gynecology, 91,* 701–704.

Redwine, D. B. (1999). Ovarian endometriosis: A marker for more extensive pelvic and intestinal disease. *Fertility and Sterility 72,* 310–315.

Singh, M., Goldberg, J., Falcone, T., Nelson, D., Pasqualotto, E., Attaran, M., et al. (2001). Superovulation and intrauterine insemination in cases of treated mild pelvic disease. *Journal of Assisted Reproduction and Genetics, 18,* 26–29.

Sutton, C. J., Ewen, S. P., Whitelaw, N., & Haines, P. (1994). Prospective, randomized, double-blind, controlled trial of laser laparoscopy in the treatment of pelvic pain associated with minimal, mild, and moderate endometriosis. *Fertility and Sterility, 62,* 696–700.

Tulandi, T., & al-Took, S. (1998). Reproductive outcome after treatment of mild endometriosis with laparoscopic excision and electrocoagulation. *Fertility and Sterility, 69,* 229–231.

MOHAMED A. BEDAIWY
TOMMASO FALCONE

Latinos

As of 2003, Latinos are the largest minority group in the United States, outnumbering even African Americans. There are over 32 million Latinos in the United States, with an average age of 25 years. To put this into perspective, approximately one in eight people in the United States is Latino, which places the United States fifth among nations with the largest number of Latino inhabitants, behind Mexico, Spain, Colombia, and Argentina. Furthermore, within the last 5 years, 37.5% of the population growth in the United States was attributable to Latinos. Notably, the vast majority of this growth was not due to immigration but rather increased Latino births in the United States. In California, for instance, over 40% of births are Latino. For these reasons, learning more about the Latinos in the United States is essential. Issues ranging from ethnic terms, nationalities, traditions, demographics, and health provide insight regarding this growing segment.

Whether to refer to this growing population as Latino, Hispanic, or Chicano can be confusing. The word *Latino* generally refers to someone who moved from Latin America to the United States or whose first language is Spanish. *Hispanic* refers to those whose descent is from Spain or Latin America. Most of the controversy regarding which term is politically correct stems from personal preference. Those who prefer Latino argue that it has a strong linguistic connection to Latin America, and thus encapsulates ethnic pride. On the other hand, those who find Latino less favorable argue that since Latino refers to those who moved to the United States from Latin America, it does not apply to those born in the United States. Conversely, avid supporters of the word *Hispanic* use it because it allows them to declare their Spanish decent and imply they were born in the United States. Those who find Hispanic less favorable argue it is a term coined by Anglos and thus lacks the same cultural depth as the word Latino. Nonetheless, many use both terms interchangeably because neither term is right or wrong. From time to time, regions will show a particular preference. For instance, currently, Latino is preferred in California while Hispanic is preferred in Florida and Texas. Adding to the list of choices is the word *Chicano,* another ethnic term that applies only to Mexican Americans living in the United States. The word *Chicano* is not only a word of ethnic pride but is also associated with certain political views that not every Mexican American may share and thus is not used by everyone in this group.

The term Latino or Hispanic encompasses a variety of nationalities that are often combined into one group or considered one nationality; however, this is an incorrect assumption. Latinos represent an array of different races, which include Indians, black Latinos, whites, or mestizos, which is a combination thereof or of Indian and European or black Latinos and European. Furthermore, there are over 20 different Latino nationalities which hail from different parts of the world such as Central, South, and North America, the Caribbean, Spain, and Puerto Rico. These nationalities are represented in the Latino population of the United States. Mexicans account for 66% of the Latino population, while Central and South America account for 14.5%, Puerto Ricans 9%, Cubans 4%, and other Latinos 6%. Despite political, social, and cultural differences among these different nationalities, the Spanish language and often religion tie them together. By and large, Catholicism has been the predominant religion in Latin

America; however, the Protestant Christian faith has made significant inroads.

Latino demographics by the U.S. Census supplies details on family, age, education, finances, and place of residence. Most Latino families have at least five persons and such large families tend to be Mexican. Also, remarkably, only 5% of the Latino population is over the age of 65 and over 35% is under the age of 18.

Even so, education among Latinos is very low. Less than 44% have a high school diploma, which indicates that at least two out of every five Latinos did not graduate from high school. Consequently, Latinos are more likely to work in service-related industries rather than in professional trades. Another result is that only 23% of Latinos earn over $35,000 and approximately 23% are living below the poverty level. Nonetheless, over 31% of Latinos continue to send money back to their country of origin. Furthermore, unemployment is substantially high among the Latinos at 6.8% compared to only 3.4% among non-Latinos.

Usually, Latinos live in the city or metropolitan area in regions such as the West, South, or the Northeast. Remarkably, California, Texas, New York, Florida, and Illinois account for 70% of all Latinos in the United States. Moreover, 45% of Latinos are geographically concentrated in only five cities: Chicago, New York, Miami, Los Angeles, and San Francisco.

The Latino culture is well known for particular cultural traditions such as *machismo, familismo, marianismo*, and *personalismo*. Cultural traditions are values, beliefs, and ways of life of a particular group. At an early age these traditions are learned and often emulated in adulthood. *Machismo* has both positive and negative connotations but unfortunately, the media often only portrays the negative aspects. *Machismo* is observable in a man who takes charge, possesses sole authority for decision-making, and retains certain rights for himself and his sons. Since these characteristics are often synonymous with sexism in American culture, *machismo* is often considered ethically wrong in the United States. Fueling this negative sentiment are cases of *machismo* that lead to domestic violence. On the other hand, the positive quality of *machismo* is evident in how the men care and provide not only for their immediate but extended family as well. *Machismo* can also be traced in many Latino men's pursuit to be good sons, fathers, and husbands.

Familismo is another cultural norm shared by the Latino community. The core of Latino society is the family. Generally, Latinos derive their identity, purpose,

and sense of belonging from the family. A typical family nucleus includes the immediate family, the extended family, and other adopted family such as compadres, which are essentially the equivalent of godparents but with a much more active role. High esteem for the family leads a Latino to base his or her decision-making on what will benefit the family and its future. Members of the family are considered an extension of support and are expected to help the family progress forward. Loyalty, sacrifice, and hard work are further qualities engrained in *familismo*. As the cornerstone of the family, Latina women nurture, preserve, and keep the family connected with the extended family.

The idealization of Mary, the mother of Jesus, is known as *marianismo*. According to Catholicism, Mary is the perfect role model for all women and mothers. Thus, Latina women are encouraged to pursue the pureness of mind, body, and soul; generosity; and hard work and sacrifice for the benefit of their family. Unfortunately, in the past, this burden restricted the role of Latina women; however, *marianismo* has somewhat relaxed among modern Latina women, enabling them to become more integrated in the workforce, business, and other roles in society. Despite these subsiding burdens, certain qualities of *marianismo* remain strong such as the importance of family, the dignity with which a Latina must carry herself, and the respect she must command from men.

In addition, *personalismo* embodies the significance placed on interpersonal relationships. Latinos prize friendship, camaraderie, and hospitality. A level of *confiaza*, mutual trust, cultivated in a relationship is cherished and the opportunity to *servir*, to help someone, is an honor. Other attributes stemming from *personalismo* are *respeto* and *dignidad*. *Respeto* means respect and for Latinos it encompasses courtesy, humility, and obedience. Also, respect for elders is strongly enforced and dignified conduct communicates self-respect. In addition, *dignidad*, dignity, highlights the importance of self-worth, which is often demonstrated by a hard work ethic.

A common phenomenon regarding the preservation or eroding of cultural traditions is referred to as acculturation. Acculturation is the result of keeping one's culture intact while adapting to another culture. Varying degrees of acculturation include partial, complete, and unacculturation. Partial acculturation refers to Latinos who have been in the United States at least for 11 years and are bilingual but speak Spanish at home; this represents 59% of the Latino population.

Latinos

Complete acculturation refers to Latinos who were born and raised in the United States and do not speak Spanish but identify with other Latino traditions, which accounts for 13% of the Latino population. In the United States, Latino traditions are easily preserved because of the close proximity of Latin America, the large number of Latinos in the United States, and the mainstream media, which keeps the music and culture popular. Lastly, a lack of acculturation refers to Latinos who were born outside of the United States and have spent little time in the United States, accounting for 28% of the population.

Significant health problems affect Latinos in the United States. These include HIV and AIDS, diabetes, cardiovascular disease, tuberculosis, and breast and cervical cancer.

Diabetes among Latina women has risen substantially, affecting over 25%. The number of deaths diabetes causes among Latina women has doubled in the last 30 years and now causes 33% of all their deaths. Risk factors which make Latina women susceptible to diabetes include genetics, obesity, impaired glucose resistance, and higher insulin resistance levels. While Mexicans in particular have higher incidences of glucose and insulin resistance, an alarming 46% of all Latina women are overweight. The health of the eyes and kidneys often deteriorate due to the debilitating effects of diabetes. Among Latina women compared to non-Hispanic white women, (a) retinopathy, an eye disease, is twice as high; (b) kidney disease leading to kidney failure is also twice as high; and (c) ketoacidosis which leads to diabetic coma is 50% higher. Moreover, vascular problems, which impede the flow of blood in the veins, are 7.6 times more likely to occur in Latinas. Further, an overwhelming four times as many Latinas will suffer from a stroke or heart disease due to diabetes. Since diabetes is more prevalent among Latina women, gestational diabetes is another cause of concern because it can lead to toxemia causing health problems for both the baby and mother.

In the United States, Latinos have been facing an HIV and AIDS crisis since 1983 when Latinos accounted for 14% of all AIDS cases. This crisis reached a critical level in 1999 when Latinos accounted for 20% of new HIV infections reported in the United States. Of the total new HIV infections among women in the United States, Latinos comprise 18%; Latinos account for 20% of the total new infections among men. In order for an HIV prevention program to be effective it must be tailored toward the different Latino cultures within the community. These different nationalities have varying customs, perceptions, and amounts of information which affect their risk behaviors. These risk behaviors affect the method of transmission such as injected drug use or unprotected sex among homosexuals, bisexuals, or heterosexuals.

Many of these preventable diseases are left untreated among Latinos due to lack of access to health care. Health care access includes information, screenings, basic health services, and medicines. Access to health care in rural areas for Latinos is difficult due to lack of transportation to medical centers. Affordability of health care services is another barrier for Latinos, especially for those who do not have health insurance. However, the primary barrier to health care access is language. If a Latino cannot communicate or understand English, he or she will be unable to utilize the health care systems and often does not have information regarding available health services. Furthermore, a health provider or center that is not culturally sensitive may make Latinos feel uncomfortable, causing them to not return.

Latinos are the most likely ethnic group to not have health insurance. Accordingly, only 43% Latinos have health insurance, compared to 73% of Caucasians. Often this is because the employer does not offer a health insurance plan and, even if they did, a Latino will usually waive the benefit because it is too expensive. An additional fear that deters Latinos from enrolling in a health plan is that it may affect their ability to obtain citizenship. However, Latinos who do not qualify for Medicare or Medicaid may still be able to receive care under the Hill–Burton Act. This federal law allocates money to hospitals to provide health care to persons without health insurance. Furthermore, there are local programs which will provide free breast and cervical screenings.

In conclusion, Latino traditions of family, respect, and hard work are values which can benefit every community. However, in order to improve education, jobs, and health care for communities across the United States, Latinos must be an integral part of the solution. Likewise, health problems such as diabetes, HIV and AIDS, and lack of health insurance among Latinos must be addressed in order for our communities to be healthy.

Latinos have changed the demographics of the United States dramatically. U.S. Census statistics indicate that Latinos are no longer a minority group that can be ignored. Hence, Latinos are not just a fundamental part of the United States' past and future but a significant part of our present.

SEE ALSO: Access to health care, Acculturation, Acquired immunodeficiency syndrome, Agricultural work, Cancer, Cardiovascular disease, Diabetes, Health insurance, Immigrant health, Marianismo, Rural health

Suggested Reading

The American Heritage Dictionary of the English Language (4th ed.) (2000). Boston: Houghton Mifflin.

Centers for Disease Control and Prevention, National Center for HIV, STD and TB Prevention. (2000, July). *Protecting the health of Latino communities; Combating HIV/AIDS.* http://www.cdc.gov/nchstp/od/nchstp.html

Krauss, N. A., & Weinick, R. M. (2000, November). *Access to care: Lack of English ability creates a substantial barrier to Hispanic children's access to health care.* Agency for Healthcare Research and Quality. http://www.ahrq.gov/research/nov00/1100RA3.htm

Manduley, D. (2000, August). Diversity at work. *Latin American and Caribbean.* http://www.diversityatwork.com/news/nov00/news_latin_ac.html

Monheit, A. C., & Vistes, J. P. (2000). *Health care costs and financing: Gap in health insurance coverage for Hispanic men widened between 1987 and 1996.* Agency for Healthcare Research and Quality. http://www.ahrq.gov/research/nov00/1100RA14.htm. (Last accessed January 12, 2004)

Therrien, M., & Ramirez, R. R. (2000, March). *The Hispanic population in the United States.* Current Population Reports, U.S. Census Bureau. http://www.census.gov

United States Department of Health and Human Services. (2001, April). *Diabetes and Hispanic American women.* http://4women.gov/faq/diabetes-hispanic.htm

United States Department of Health and Human Services. (2001, May). *Health care access and Hispanic American women.* http://4women.gov/faq/hca-ha.htm

Suggested Resources

Hispanics in the United States, Tri-City Herald. http://archive.tri-city-herald.com/newmajority/hispanics.html

The Latino Coalition. *About the Latino coalition.* (2001). http://www.thelatinocoalition.com/aboutus/

NCLR Health: *NCLR's Institute for Hispanic Health (IHH).* http://www.nclr.org/policy/health.html

ELIZABETH M. VALENCIA

Laxatives

Laxatives A laxative is a medicine that loosens the bowel contents and encourages evacuation. A laxative with a mild or gentle effect on the bowel is known as an aperient; and one with a strong effect is known as a cathartic or purgative. Laxatives facilitate evacuation by increasing the stool volume and stimulating the large intestinal muscle by increasing the intestinal pressure. This in turn triggers evacuation.

Signs of constipation are bowel movements that are difficult, painful, or less frequent than normal. Constipation can be prevented by drinking adequate amounts of water about 6–8 glasses per day, getting sufficient fiber by eating fruits, vegetables, and grains, and exercising regularly. Fiber is important because it provides the media for the bacteria to multiply and grow. A good bacterial action results in a larger volume of stool and smooth bowel movement. Laxatives should be used only as the last resort to treat constipation. A physician is best qualified to determine when a laxative is needed and which type is best.

A differential diagnosis should be done before recommending laxatives. A chronic constipation may be one of the symptoms of a serious problem like diverticulitis or when it develops in the later decades as a new complaint may herald colon cancer. Complaints of chronic constipation may also be due to obsessive–compulsive disorder. Laxative should not be used for these conditions. Normal bowel movements are variable, and may vary from two times daily to two to three times weekly. There are many reasons why a doctor may prescribe a laxative to empty the contents of the bowel. A laxative may be prescribed for preparation for a medical examination such as colonoscopy, preparation for a surgery, prevention of constipation secondary to drug therapy, to prevent straining during defecation after a surgery, and as a prophylactic measure for patients recovering from myocardial infarction.

Laxatives are classified according to the mechanism of action. There are five main types of laxatives, but some laxatives act in more than one way. Bulk-forming laxatives increase the volume of the stool. They also soften the stool and stimulate the bowel in a natural way by forming a bulky mass. Psyllium (Metamucil) and methylcellulose (Citrucel) belong to this group. They absorb water and expand as they pass through the digestive tract. Psyllium is one of the rich sources of fiber. Fiber is the indigestible material in plant foods. Psyllium should be taken with adequate amounts of water to avoid choking and obstruction of the esophagus, throat, and intestines.

Stimulant laxatives increase the peristaltic movement of the intestine. Dulcolax, Ex-lax, and Senecot are examples of this type. These agents can be used if bulk-forming laxatives have no effect. Check with your doctor before taking them. They are the most habit forming and should not be taken everyday. Do not take these with milk. They may cause cramps and abdominal pain.

Stool softeners act as detergents, moisturizing and breaking up the feces. Docusate (Colace) belongs to this group. It holds water within the fecal mass, and thus provides a larger, softer stool. Docusate is not recommended for acute constipation. In order to be effective, this should be taken before the fecal mass is formed. This is suitable for recurrent constipation and to prevent constipation caused by certain medication.

Lubricant laxatives include mineral oil, castor oil, and olive oil. They act by reducing intestinal absorption of fecal water and help with easy passing of stool. They are usually taken with other laxatives. Mineral oil is not recommended for long-term use.

Osmotic laxatives are glycerin and lactulose. They prevent the bowel from absorbing water so that the bulk volume increases. Lactulose may also increase peristaltic action of the intestine.

DANGERS OF LAXATIVES

Laxatives should be taken only with the advice of a physician. Chronic use of laxatives may result in a fluid and electrolyte imbalance, steatorrhea, osteomalacia, diarrhea, cathartic colon, and liver disease. Bulk-forming laxatives may delay the absorption of some medications taken at the same time as the laxative. Insulin-dependent diabetics may need to reduce insulin dosage while taking psyllium products. Mineral oil taken regularly leads to deficiency of fat-soluble vitamins. Minerals and docusate should not be taken together because docusate will absorb the mineral oil.

Some people take laxatives to promote weight loss. Laxatives do not promote weight loss. When laxatives are overused, they create dependency and worsen constipation. Laxatives lead to the loss of body fluids, and the body, in turn, compensates for dehydration by retaining water, which results in bloating. Children and pregnant women should not take laxatives without consulting their physician.

SEE ALSO: Constipation, Diet

Suggested Reading

Cummings, M. (1991). Overuse hazardous: Laxatives rarely needed. *FDA Consumer, 25,* 33–35.
Friedman, G., Jacobson, E. D., & McCallum, R. W. (Eds.). (1997). *Gastrointestinal pharmacology.* Philadelphia: Lippincott-Raven.
Fuchs, C. S., Giovannucci, E. Colditz, G. A., et al. (1999). Dietary fiber and the risk of colorectal cancer and adenoma in women. *New England Journal of Medicine, 40,* 169–176.
Lehne, R. A. (2001). *Pharmacology for nursing care.* Philadelphia: W. B. Saunders.

RAJKUMARI RICHMONDS

Lesbian There is no standard definition of lesbian. The term generally refers to a female sexual orientation that may involve one or more of the following components: behavioral, affective, or cognitive understandings of lesbian. The behavioral definition of lesbian emphasizes current or lifetime sexual activity with other women. The affective definition considers the subtleties of sexual or emotional desire and/or attraction for other women (in real time or in fantasy), regardless of whether or not these desires are acted upon. Rounding out the three conceptualizations, the cognitive definition refers to adopting a lesbian identity. Typically, women who self identify as lesbians will also fit the behavioral and/or affective understandings of the term. Nevertheless, some women may identify as lesbian for political reasons as an expression of solidarity with women, but neither experience desire and attractions for other women, nor have a history of lesbian sexual behavior.

Lesbians are a demographically diverse group. Women whose sexual orientation is directed toward other women exist in all cultures and societies. There are lesbians of every race, culture, religion, nationality, ability level, age, socioeconomic status, size, and so on. However, it is important to note that there are wide variations in lesbian social/political definitions and acceptability across various cultures and racial/ethnic groups. In fact, the meaning of the word lesbian has fluctuated over time in lesbian circles, in the feminist movement, in popular culture, and in the scientific community. These shifts reflect the range of lesbian identities and the political and social climates in which they live. Thus, it is difficult to make generalizations about lesbians, just as it is with any diverse group, including heterosexual women.

The term lesbian was not coined until 1868. The scientific community, in particular, the emerging fields of sexology and psychiatry, first used the term to describe women with *masculine* attributes and attractions for other women. Thus, the image of the *mannish lesbian* became popularized and medical professionals quickly decided that a lesbian sexual orientation represented pathology in search of a cure. This belief persisted for over 100 years, until the American Psychiatric Association removed homosexuality as an *illness* from the *Diagnostics and Statistical Manual*, a handbook used by mental health professionals, in 1975.

The concept of a lesbian *identity* crystallized in part through the gay and lesbian liberation movement, which began in the United States in the mid-20th century. In 1955, a group of eight women formed the Daughters of Bilitis, the first lesbian organization in the United States, to promote civil rights and provide an alternative method of meeting other lesbians through their newsletter, *The Ladder*. The emerging working-class lesbian bar culture was also a source of immense support and community building for the early lesbian liberation movement. Working-class women frequently found each other through coded articulations of gender called *butch* and *femme*. Although the lesbian feminist movement in the 1970s criticized such gender expressions as reinforcing heterocentric norms, several contemporary scholars point to the way the gender identities helped lesbian women survive in working-class society and find other lesbian women.

The problematics of assuming similarity among lesbians is well illustrated by the term's contested meaning within the feminist movement. Lesbian visibility increased considerably during the 1970s in the United States due to the lesbian feminist movement. Feeling overlooked by the male-dominated gay liberation movement and unwelcome in the women's movement, lesbian scholars and activists formed their own organizations—such as the Furies and the Radicalesbians—and published revolutionary lesbian feminist theory. Lesbian feminists examined scientific, popular culture, and feminist understandings of sexual orientation and gender to formulate concepts such as *compulsory heterosexuality*, and to advocate for the elimination of all oppressions in order for true equality to emerge. Lesbian feminist activists pointed out that the concept of lesbian references a woman's relation to a man and is only possible in a patriarchal society. In a sexist society, an independent woman is labeled a lesbian and is not considered a *real woman*. Thus, several lesbian feminists in the 1970s advocated for a broader understanding of lesbian as a *woman-identified woman*, that is, a lesbian is a woman whose primary identification is with other women, regardless of whether or not that identification is sexually based. Lesbian feminist politics sometimes also advocated temporary or complete separatism from men and patriarchal society as a means for women to reconnect and find their own language.

In the late 1970s, lesbians who practice butch/femme, bondage/domination, or sadomasochism (BDSM), and other representations emerged to critique the lesbian feminist utopian ideals of equality and mutuality. These groups criticize the lesbian feminist movement as being antisex with an agenda to *desex* the term lesbian. Additionally, lesbians of color and working-class lesbians have noted that much of the lesbian feminist work has come from a decisively white, middle to upper class perspective that cannot claim to represent the needs and perspectives of all lesbians. The lesbian feminist call for separatism has also been critiqued because it denies the importance of men in the lives of lesbians.

Lesbian history has been a process of uncovering evidence of women with same-sex attractions or experiences. Actually, lesbian historians, following lesbian feminist interpretations of lesbian as encompassing an emotional attachment to another woman, have uncovered strong evidence that romantic friendships between women have likely existed throughout time. Sappho, the famous poet from a Greek island called Lesbos around the 6th century BCE, and from which the term lesbian is derived, is such an example. Some scholars consider it problematic to label romantic relationships between women in history as lesbian, since sexual orientation was not categorized according to gender until the late 1800s. However, historians point out parallels to women in modern society. For example, same-sex attractions or relationships among women in history likely would have been devalued in relation to heterosexual, procreative sex.

Despite the wide variety of lesbian lives, all lesbians are susceptible to discrimination based on their sexual orientation. *Homophobia*, the belief that homosexuality is wrong or repulsive, is something all lesbians experience on some level during their lifetime. For example, in many areas of the United States, it is legal to discriminate against an individual based on their sexual orientation in housing and employment, as well as in marital and parental rights and privileges.

Along with discrimination, many lesbians become victims of *hate crimes*, a type of social terrorism that is usually violent and is committed against people because of their minority status. The perpetrator's homophobic beliefs lead him/her to irrational actions such as physical or verbal violence toward the minority group or individual. Some U.S. states have enacted hate crime legislation to address these irrational responses, but lesbians and gay men are still susceptible to homophobic violence.

Lesbian Ethics

Although lesbians share the same health risks all women do, there is some evidence that lesbians may be at a higher risk of certain health conditions. For example, some studies have found higher breast cancer mortality, mental health problems, and substance abuse in lesbian populations compared to heterosexual female populations. There is disagreement, however, over the etiology of health concerns specific to lesbians. While some have argued that nulliparity (lack of childbearing) may leave lesbians susceptible to certain cancers, there are also numerous obstacles to adequate health care. Lesbians' access to health care may be affected by the lack of culturally competent health care providers, the presence of homophobia in the health care system, and limited access to health insurance. This can be exacerbated by the lack of domestic partner benefits, or being economically disadvantaged, which includes being unable to afford health insurance and/or health care. Furthermore, some lesbians may hold false assumptions about their own health care needs. For example, many believe that they do not need routine gynecological exams because they do not have sex with men.

Lesbians are faced with similar mental health and developmental challenges that all women experience. However, lesbians face the unique challenge of *coming out*—accepting and deciding whether to make their lesbian identity public. Coming out is a process that can occur throughout the life span. Some lesbians come out as teenagers, young adults, in middle age, or late in life. Regardless of the age that this milestone is confronted, the stress of enduring the process, particularly if it is confounded by threats of violence and discrimination, can result in co-occurring conditions such as depression, substance abuse, internalized homophobia, and other mental health difficulties.

In recent times, lesbians have begun to own, define, and create new opportunities for themselves in our society despite adversity. The most noticeable trend has been embracing motherhood. Although lesbians have always enjoyed the option of motherhood, a surge in the rates of women choosing motherhood either as single women or in the context of same-sex relationships has been witnessed since 1980. These opportunities, along with greater public acceptance, have allowed lesbians to participate more fully and openly in society and to experience a greater range of themselves as women.

See Also: Feminism, Feminist ethics, Gender, Gender role, Homosexuality, Intersexuality, Lesbian ethics, Queer, Transgenderism

Suggested Reading

Nestle, J. (1987). *A restricted country.* Ithica, NY: Firebrand Books.

Panati, C. (1998). *Sexy origins and intimate things.* New York: Penguin Books.

Solarz, A. L. (Ed.). (1999). *Lesbian health: Current assessment and directions for the future.* Washington, DC.: Institute of Medicine.

Stein, A. (Ed.). (1993). *Sisters, sexperts, queers: Beyond the lesbian nation.* New York: Penguin Group.

Vida, G. (Ed.). (1996). *The new our right to love: A lesbian resource book.* New York: Touchstone.

Sarah A. Smith
Julianne M. Serovich

Lesbian Ethics A branch of ethics that cultivates the development of individual moral agency and integrity, lesbian ethics distinguishes itself from the focus on social control of traditional ethics. The centerpiece of the theoretical framework is that lesbians are oppressed in all societies. It also acknowledges that lesbians are agents of oppression, because sanctioned moral choices in societies uphold patriarchal oppression and are constrained by it. Lesbian ethics argues that in order to resist oppression, lesbians must create new value that supports thinking, which undermines its credibility.

Traditional ethical thought is bankrupt for lesbians because its function is social organization and control rather than individual integrity and agency. The dominance and subordination values around which traditional ethics revolve are antagonistic. Consequently, individual moral ability and agency is undercut rather than advanced. Taken together, traditional ethics legitimizes women's oppression by redefining it as social organization.

Within a traditional paradigm, *woman* derives its meaning from its relationship to *man*—the one who dominates—and as long as this context prevails, domination of women by men will seem natural and desirable. Consequently, patriarchal society formally denies lesbian existence because its very connotation implies a woman who thrives outside the sphere of male dominance. Instead, a lesbian is discounted as a confused heterosexual woman who is passing through a phase, a heterosexual woman who cannot get a man, a man in a heterosexual woman's body, or a man-hater. In patriarchal conceptualization, the notion of a woman loving another woman is impossible, or at the very least a man-hating monstrosity. Thus, the source of concern about lesbians is that they represent the potential for a reality in which male dominance does not exist, where women appropriate men's access to women. It destabilizes the foundation on which society is constructed. Indeed, lesbian reality renders men insignificant. Lesbian existence therefore carries the potential to effect a transformation of consciousness—the promise for autonomous female agency.

Lesbian ethics criticizes traditional ethical paradigms as fostering an illusion that all problems can be solved by an appeal to rules and principles. It notes that ethical principles are not applied in an egalitarian context, but rather in a reality of asymmetrical power. The ethical virtues that are lauded in society are therefore framed as master/slave virtues. Lesbian ethics argues that a majority of what passes for ethics in societies is not founded in the integrity and moral capability of an individual, but rather the extent to which individuals participate in the structural hierarchy of a social group or organization by adhering to its rules. Traditional paradigms mandate principles or rules of obligation to those occupying upper levels of hierarchical frameworks and corresponding rules of responsibility for those occupying lower positions, typically *for their own good*. Therefore, traditional ethics functions to promote social organization and control at the expense of individual integrity and agency.

A fundamental premise of lesbian ethics is that the driving force behind dominance and subordination is the institution of heterosexuality, and that women's oppression will remain a reality as long as social interactions are governed by its suffocating paradigm. Thus, rather than prove false a patriarchal structure that revolves around socially enforced dominance and subordination, lesbian ethics seeks to work outside the existing framework, to pursue a transformation of consciousness that strips the meaning from existing values, those which make oppression credible and acceptable, and renders them nonsensical.

Much of lesbian ethics focuses on language as a tool of oppression. For example, *woman* is more than a mere descriptive category, because imbedded within this concept are perceptions of normal female behavior and what qualifies as a woman. In other words, there is value attached to *woman*, value that is organized around a patriarchal dominance and subordination modality. However, if the values of oppression cease to be normalized—if they are no longer affirmed without question and cease to be integrated into lesbian lives—then lesbians will end the tyranny of patriarchal rule

and their interactions will be less apt to result in destruction.

Often erroneously characterized as founded on a utopian philosophical framework, lesbian ethics is anything but that. The fact that lesbians live and interact within the current oppressive patriarchal schema accents the need for creating new value. Contrasting the escapism of utopian paradigms, lesbian ethics is a framework for action. It emphasizes that through examining and questioning the foundation of patriarchal oppression and how it permeates every aspect of social interaction, one discovers that it is possible to engender individual moral agency and integrity that exists outside of it. Lesbian ethics therefore seeks to generate ways in which lesbians can weave a different locus of value, one where lesbian choices, actions, and reactions lead away from the path of oppression, and one where lesbians become an energy field capable of resisting oppression.

SEE ALSO: Femininity, Feminism, Gender, Gender role, Homosexuality, Lesbian, Masculinity, Queer

Suggested Reading

Allen, J. (1990). *Lesbian philosophies and cultures*. Albany: State University of New York Press.

Hoagland, S. L. (1989). *Lesbian ethics: Toward new value*. Palo Alto, CA: Institute of Lesbian Studies.

Mohin, L. (1995). *An intimacy of equals: Lesbian feminist ethics*. Binghamton, NY: Haworth Press.

ANGELA PATTATUCCI ARAGON

Libido and Desire

Libido and Desire   Few people can forget the impassioned romance between Julie Christie (Lara) and Omar Sharif (Yuri) in the film *Doctor Zhivago*, the palpable sexual tension between Kathleen Turner and William Hurt in *Body Heat*, or the fervent desire expressed by Meg Ryan while faking an orgasm in *When Harry Met Sally*. Anais Nin's (1990) erotic stories in *Delta of Venus* and D. H. Lawrence's (1968) *Lady Chatterley's Lover* explore other aspects of women's libido and desire. We remember these stories and films because we identify and resonate with the various components of the characters' sexuality, sometimes stimulating our own desire. The concept of desire has expanded considerably since Freud (1963/1923) introduced "libido": the biologic, instinct-based sexual

Libido and Desire

force driving human growth and development. Now by desire we also mean to include the psychologically based motive and the socially based wish (Levine, 1992).

Biologic drive is individually determined and fluctuates over the lifespan. Freud noted sexual feelings and behaviors in children that heighten, expand, and become more focused during puberty and adolescence, eventually becoming a motivating force for adult behavior. The complex neurobiological changes of puberty, commonly referred to as "raging hormones," stimulate sex drive. This hormonal fluctuation tends to stabilize in young adulthood. A man's sex drive tends to remain higher than a woman's. Women may note variability in their drive with the different stages of the menstrual cycle. The reproductive years and pregnancy pose biologic challenges to women that influence drive significantly. With advancing age, sexual drive usually declines in both sexes and is partially attributed to the gradual lowering of testosterone levels.

The literature on the neurobiology of sex drive which is reviewed by Meston and Frohlich (2000) and summarized here, focuses on the hypothalamic region of the brain which is thought to be the sexual drive center. It is a complex group of nerve cells with connections to the limbic system and the cerebral cortex. The limbic system is crucial to emotional experience and regulation; the cortex is vital to cognitive and thinking processes. These neuroanatomic connections suggest that sexual drive is a product of these brain regions operationalized through a delicate balance of neurotransmitters. These neurotransmitters include dopamine, serotonin, histamine, norepinephrine, and epinephrine, which can be influenced by many medications and street drugs. Drive tends to increase with higher levels of dopamine and lower levels of histamine. Epinephrine and norepinephrine appear to stimulate motivation but have little effect on drive itself. The effect of serotonin on drive and motivation is complicated due to its multiple roles in brain function via stimulation of receptors. Stimulation of some receptors results in the improvement of biologically based depressive symptoms, which increases sexual drive. Stimulation of other receptors directly impairs both sexual drive and function. This has become especially apparent with the increased use of antidepressant medication in the selective serotonin reuptake inhibitor category (e.g., fluoxetine [Prozac], sertraline [Zoloft], paroxetine [Paxil]) and others. Frequently, these medications will raise serotonin levels and stimulate both types of receptors. This simultaneously results in the improvement in a person's depression or anxiety such that they once again would like to have sex but impairs their intrinsic drive and other sexual functions. Different antidepressants stimulate dopamine and enhance drive or have no effect (e.g., bupropion, Wellbutrin). Not infrequently, elderly patients with low levels of dopamine due to Parkinson's disease or high prolactin levels (see below) have no sex drive, but will become much more sexual when dopamine-stimulating drugs are given.

Hormones, particularly testosterone and prolactin, significantly influence sexual drive, although hormones alone do not regulate human sexual desire. Testosterone makes a significant contribution to the sexual upheaval of puberty but tends to steady in early adulthood. As a man's sex drive is highly testosterone dependent, supplementation may restore his drive when drive and testosterone levels are low. Although testosterone supplementation in women with low desire and low testosterone levels may increase drive, it is not usually done because of the risk of masculinization (Meston & Frohlich, 2000). Due to controversy in the field, women considering testosterone, DHEA (a testosterone precursor), or other chemical replacements for low desire should first consult medical personnel knowledgeable in sexual medicine. High levels of prolactin appear to inhibit sex drive in both sexes. In women, a prolactin blood level high enough to decrease drive is caused by pregnancy, antipsychotic medication, prolactin-secreting pituitary tumors, and, more commonly, by lactation and breast-feeding. Prolactin has an inverse relationship with dopamine, such that increased levels of dopamine in the brain may lower prolactin levels and increase drive. Estrogen and progesterone are believed to have little direct influence on sex drive (Meston & Frohlich, 2000). Nonetheless, drying and increased fragility of the vaginal lining due to estrogen decline and deficiency causes discomfort that interferes with desire. Estrogen levels decline with aging or with early menopause due to medical factors (e.g., chemotherapy). The resulting vaginal symptoms can be ameliorated with lubricants or, if warranted, with hormone replacement therapies. However, estrogen replacement therapy can further suppress an already low testosterone resulting in a further decline in drive.

Biologic drive establishes "horniness," a base for the development of the arousing, emotional richness of real sexual life as portrayed in the films and books above. The richness is created by the more potent elements of desire: motive and wish. Levine (1992) describes *motive* as *the psychological aspect of sexual desire* and is a person's *emotional willingness to act sexually*. The *wish* includes the social factors that influence and form *personal expectations about sex*: how does the person's religion, philosophy, finances, degree of socialization, education, national or territorial origin, culture, employment, and political point of view influence sexual desire? The most successful books and movies examine the complexities of both motive and wish in the context of their storytelling. In *Doctor Zhivago*, Lara's and Yuri's passionate concordance of personalities, as if they were predestined to be together, fosters mutually intense desire. The pressures of the social environment created by the war heightened the desire, despite the social taboo of adultery. Turner's dark motives for seduction in *Body Heat* meshed perfectly with Hurt's mesmeric infatuation, blinding him to the realities of his situation. Sally's and Harry's inability to endorse their mutual attraction, and their hurtful interactions were clear de-motivators of desire. In *Lady Chatterley's Lover*, Constance Chatterley's affair with the gamekeeper on her husband's estate was motivated by unfulfilled emotional and sexual longings in her sterile marriage. Today this book is a classic but at the time it was written, it was scorned as pornography and labeled as offensive to society. Anais Nin's frank erotica speaks to women's ability to acknowledge, experience, and enjoy their sexuality and particularly their lusty desires. To this day, she is seen as a licentious, sexual outlaw by social and political conservatives. Defiantly challenging social taboos is a powerful aphrodisiac for the sexually adventurous.

Despite the almost daily discoveries in neuroscience, we should not underestimate the power of the nonscientific qualities determining a woman's sexual desire. When a woman's biologic drive, motive, and wish are consonant, her sexuality is a remarkable manifestation of her essence.

SEE ALSO: Masturbation, Sexual dysfunction

Suggested Reading

Freud, S. (1963/1923). The libido theory. In P. Rieff (Ed.), *General psychological theory: Papers on metapsychology* (pp. 180–184). New York: Colliers Books.

Lawrence, D. H. (1968). *Lady Chatterley's lover* (The Unexpurgated 1928 Orioli Edition). New York: Bantam Books.

Levine, S. B. (1992). *Sexual life: A clinician's guide.* New York: Plenum Press.

Meston, C. M., & Frohlich, P. F. (2000). The neurobiology of sexual function. *Archives of General Psychiatry, 57,* 1012–1030.

Nin, A. (1990). *Delta of Venus.* New York: Pocket Books.

Suggested Resources

Body Heat, Doctor Zhivago, Henry and June, When Harry Met Sally, White Castle

GARY MARTZ

Life Expectancy The mortality experience of a population can be summed up by the measure of life expectancy, which is the average age at death for a hypothetical group of people born in a particular year and being subjected to the risks of death experienced by people of all ages in that year. It is the average number of years to be lived either from birth or from some other specific age. Thus, the age to which the average person in a population will live is the number behind the concept of life expectancy. Life expectancy has two important applications to issues surrounding the broader topic of women's health. First, life expectancy is sex differentiated; that is, there is a well-established difference in longevity between the sexes. Simply stated, women live longer than men: the mortality of men is greater than that of women at *every age* of life thereby creating a resulting advantage in life expectancy for women over men at *every age*. Even taking into account changeable, nongenetic behavioral and lifestyle practices such as exercise, smoking, engaging in risky behavior, and the use of health resources, there still remains a persistent biological basis for this sex difference in longevity. This increased longevity can impact and influence many diverse aspects associated with women's health ranging from insurance rates to social security benefits to late-life migration decisions.

Second, life expectancy can be a barometer of the overall standard of living of a particular place on the surface of the Earth. For instance, since the 1950s, much of the developing world has seen sharp improvements in life expectancy due to improved nutrition, public health, and medical care, all of which have the effect of reducing the level of infant mortality and also reducing the risks associated with childbirth, which, in the past, might otherwise have endangered the health and welfare of the mother. However, life expectancy for women in sub-Saharan Africa (as just one example) is still considerably lower than that of women in the United States, Europe, or other industrialized nations. This important fact says much regarding not only the state of living conditions in sub-Saharan Africa but also about the status of women in this region. The rapid rise in heterosexual AIDS and the higher fertility rates found in the area influence the life expectancy of African women. They are indicative of cultural and societal conditions that keep women in subservient positions in relation to their male counterparts. The higher fertility rates experienced by women in less developed countries contribute to lower life expectancy: repeated pregnancies and childbirth increase the probability of dying of complications related to them. The difficulties associated with obtaining even low levels of educational attainment keep female illiteracy high, especially in hard-to-reach rural areas, thus depriving women of access to potentially lifesaving knowledge regarding contraception and other important women's health (and women's rights) issues.

For the world as a whole, average life expectancy has risen from about 30 years in 1900 to around 68 (for females) in 2000. The great variation in female life expectancy from nation to nation (from a low of 40 in the Central African Republic to a high of 83 in Japan) can be directly related to the level of economic development, which, in turn, affects everything from health care to literacy levels. Life expectancy is generally derived from what are known as *life tables*, which represent a set of tabular calculations showing the probability of surviving from one age to any subsequent age, according to the age-specific death rates prevailing at a particular time and place.

The concept of life expectancy can be explained by reference to women born in the United States. The expectation of life at birth for females born in the United States in 1998 was 79.5 years. This does not mean that the average age of death in 1998 for females *was* 79.5, because the life table calculations are based on a hypothetical population since it is not possible to follow people for their entire lives to calculate the pattern of dying. The life table starts with a hypothetical group of 100,000 babies born in a specific year and then subjects those babies to the probabilities of death implied by the death rates that prevailed in that year that the babies were born. Thus, if all the females born in the United States in 1998 experienced the risks of dying throughout their lives as reflected in death rates in the year they were born, then their average age at death *would be* 79.5. Some might die young and others might live past 100 but the average age at death for the entire population of females born in 1998 *would be* 79.5 years if the death rates remained unchanged over the entire lifetime of

babies born in that year. In fact, it is very likely that the average age at death will be higher, since there almost certainly will be improvements in health and mortality as those babies born in 1998 mature through time.

Of course, not all females have the same risk of dying and, in addition to the sex differential discussed above, differentials in occupation, status, and role can contribute to the life expectancy differential between male and female and among female populations in different areas of the world. As stated above, there seems to be an inherent genetic biological component that contributes to the longer life expectancies found in female populations. This goes hand in hand with the fact that the risk of death appears to be greater for males at all ages, even among fetal deaths. Among adults, males tend to be employed in more hazardous occupations; military deaths, for example, are primarily male. Males are believed to be under greater stress although this is changing in developed countries as females move into more stressful occupations. Males tend to smoke and drink more. Males drive more and are more often murdered. These are all factors that raise male mortality rates thereby lowering male life expectancy. At the same time, women in different societies may also benefit differentially because fewer childbirths increase the probability of living longer while more childbirths have the opposite effect. Pregnancy puts women at risk and that risk is higher in developing nations. Marital status is also important in this respect: married people live longer than unmarried people and, as women in developed countries tend to marry later in life, thus delaying childbirth, overall fertility rates decrease as do the risks associated with childbirth. The social status of women is also related to life expectancy although this relationship will vary according to the different types of political, cultural, and economic systems. In countries where women are especially affected by a patriarchal male culture (especially South Asian countries such as Bangladesh), the life expectancy differential is almost eliminated. Women who cannot access education (or who are prohibited from doing so) are at a severe disadvantage in making lifestyle alterations that may lead to increased life expectancies.

Differences in life expectancy from society to society tend to be due to social status inequalities. As social status and prestige increase (as evidenced by higher incomes and higher levels of educational attainment), death rates go down and life expectancies at birth increase. In essence, rich people tend to live longer than poor people due to any number of factors associated with improved living conditions brought about by higher incomes. In contrast, societies (and minorities within developed societies) suffering from social and economic disadvantages often have lower life expectancies. In the United States, for example, African American women have five times the risk of dying in childbirth as do white women, a clear indication of the differential access to health care. Indeed, current research suggests that socioeconomic status is more important than lifestyle factors in explaining the racial differences in mortality and thus life expectancies. However, the significant improvements in mortality rates in developed nations (across all groups) have considerably raised life expectancies—more than 31 years for females in the United States since 1900. In turn, this has more than doubled the proportion of female babies surviving from birth to age 65, which has led to the increase in the number of older persons in developed countries such as the United States. As the status of women improves in all parts of the world, life expectancy for women can be expected to improve as well.

SEE ALSO: Ethnicity, Maternal mortality, Morbidity, Mortality, Socioeconomic status

Suggested Reading

Gribble, J. N., & Preston, S. H. (Eds.). (1993). *The epidemiological transition: Policy and planning implications for developing countries.* Washington, DC: National Academy Press.

Livi-Bacci, M. (2001). *A concise history of world population* (3rd ed.). Oxford: Blackwell.

Murphy, S. (2000). Deaths: Final data for 1998. *National Vital Statistics Reports, 48*(11).

Siegel, J. (2002). *Applied demography.* San Diego, CA: Academic Press.

Weeks, J. R. (2002). *Population: An introduction to concepts and issues* (8th ed.). Belmont, CA: Wadsworth Thomson Learning.

JAMES CRAINE
JOHN R. WEEKS

Light Therapy Light therapy, also referred to as phototherapy, has been a unique form of treatment for individuals suffering from a depressive disorder that has seasonal patterns. In the majority of cases, these individuals develop an episode of depression in the fall or winter with remission of the episode in the spring. Light therapy requires that the individual be exposed to a bright artificial light source on a daily basis during the course of treatment.

The mechanism of action is based on the human circadian rhythm, which exhibits two distinct phases, a diurnal phase and a nocturnal phase. The diurnal phase is one of active engagement in the environment with increased body temperature and a decrease or cessation of the secretion of certain hormones including melatonin. The nocturnal phase is one of rest, sleep, a decrease in body temperature, and the augmentation of the secretion of these hormones.

The body's endogenous pacemaker for the establishment of this rhythm is the hypothalamus. It responds to the changes in light as detected by the retina of the eye. As a result of this light/dark cycle, a "phase–response curve" (PRC) is established. The PRC is a graphic representation of the relationship of light exposure or restriction on the circadian rhythm.

RHYTHM

Light exposure in early morning or dawn advances the curve or shifts the rhythm earlier. Light applied at dusk would delay or shift the rhythm later. Light applied in the middle of the day would be predicted to have minimal effect on the circadian rhythm.

In addition to understanding the significance of light and its effect on the circadian rhythm, it is also important to understand the role of melatonin and its effect on animal behavior. The pineal gland, located in the brain, is responsible for the nocturnal secretion of melatonin. The retina shares an axis with the hypothalamus and the pineal gland. Decreased light to the retina, as noted in the diurnal phase, causes secretion of melatonin. The seasonal pattern of animal behavior has been widely studied and has been associated with variations in melatonin secretion. With an increase in nocturnal (night time) secretion of melatonin, as would be expected in the fall and winter months, animals become less active and aggressive, eat less, sleep more, lose interest in sex, and withdraw from the environment. The opposite effect is noted with decreased melatonin secretion which occurs in the spring and summer months.

The most accepted theory for the efficacy of light therapy is based on the observation that exposure to bright artificial light in the morning causes a phase advancement of biological rhythms. This advancement has, in many cases, effectively treated the delayed circadian rhythm associated with major depressive disorders with seasonal patterns. The theory that light therapy works by effecting melatonin secretion has not been adequately supported in the literature.

Although the type of artificial light may vary (artificial bright light vs. fluorescent; green light vs. red light), an artificial light source without ultraviolet radiation with sufficient intensity is recommended for treatment. The more intense light sources, 10,000 lux, have been shown to be superior to less intense ones, 2,500 lux. In addition, the more intense the light source, the less time is required for therapy. Thirty minutes spent in a light box supplying 10,000 lux may be equivalent to 2 hours spent in front of a light source of 2,500 lux. The individual is exposed to the light source within 10 minutes of awakening. Although individuals are cautioned not to stare into the light source directly, occasional glances at the light are necessary to obtain full benefit of treatment. Individuals have reported improvement in depressive symptoms within the first week of treatment. Usually treatment lasts from 10 to 14 days. Artificial bright light is supplied through a light box or with a portable, head-mounted light visor.

Indications for light therapy are in the treatment of mood disorders associated with a seasonal pattern. This disorder is referred to as seasonal affective disorder (SAD). This depressive disorder is seen predominantly in women, affecting up to 80% of reported cases. The mean age of onset is 40 years.

Subsyndromal symptoms, meaning that symptoms are present without having the full syndrome, of SAD, often referred to as the "winter blues," have also shown response to light therapy. Other disorders have either equivocal results or anecdotal (not established by systematic research) reports of benefits. They include nonseasonal depression, antepartum depression, late luteal phase dysphoric disorder, bulimia nervosa, delayed sleep phase syndrome, early morning awakening, insomnia in the elderly, and jet lag.

Side effects of light therapy have included headache, eyestrain, nausea, insomnia, and hyperactivity or jitteriness.

In conclusion, light therapy has been shown to be of benefit to individuals suffering from a depressive disorder with a seasonal pattern. Other disorders listed above, including nonseasonal depression and antepartum depression, have fewer reported success rates but have also been noted to benefit in some cases.

SEE ALSO: Depression, Mood disorders

Suggested Reading

Boulos, A. (1998). Bright light treatment for jet lag and shift work. In R. W. Lam (Ed.), *Seasonal affective disorder and beyond* (pp. 253–287). Washington, DC: American Psychiatric Press.

Eastman, C. I., Young, M. A., Fogg, L. F., et al. (1998). Bright light treatment of winter depression: A placebo-controlled trial. *Archives of General Psychiatry, 55,* 883–889.

Parry, B. L., Gerga, S. L., Mostofi, N., et al. (1989). Morning versus evening bright light treatment of late luteal phase dysphoric disorder. *American Journal of Psychiatry, 146,* 1215–1217.

Schwartz, P. J., Brown, C., Wehr, T. A., et al. (1996). Winter seasonal affective disorder: A follow-up study of the first 59 patients of the National Institute of Mental Health Seasonal Studies Program. *American Journal of Psychiatry, 153,* 1028–1036.

ELAINE A. CAMPBELL

Liposuction Today, there is a great deal of pressure on women to conform to an ideal look and body proportion. But no matter how hard they diet and exercise, many women cannot reach this goal. There are areas of fat deposits that just do not seem to disappear. Looking for a solution to this problem, some women turn to liposuction. Liposuction, also known as lipoplasty, is a procedure that can help remove unwanted fat deposits.

It must be emphasized that liposuction is not a substitute for diet and exercise and should not be used as a quick fix. The American Society of Plastic Surgeons has found that several criteria can help predict who will have the best results from liposuction. A woman should be reasonably close to her ideal body weight, have relatively good skin tone, and have few stretch marks. However, these are ideal conditions and many women who do not fulfill these criteria can have good results from liposuction.

Liposuction can be performed on almost any area of the body: cheeks, chin, neck, upper arms, breast or chest area, back, abdomen, waist, hips, buttocks, thighs, inner knee, calves, and ankles. For example, liposuction may be performed to bring the hips and waist into better proportion, to reduce a bulging stomach, or remove excess fat from the upper arms.

Liposuction is one of the most popular cosmetic procedures performed today and has been given a lot of attention in the media. Some advertisements give the impression that liposuction is a simple procedure without any downtime. This certainly is not true and the decision to undergo liposuction should not be taken lightly. The procedure is performed in an operating room with a general anesthetic or sedation, on a same-day surgical basis.

Women seeking liposuction should make certain that it will be performed in an accredited facility under sterile conditions. The procedure involves making one or more small incisions near the area to be suctioned. A wetting solution is then placed in the opening which helps make suctioning easier and reduces the amount of blood lost. In ultrasound-assisted liposuction and power-assisted liposuction, sound waves or a vibrating tube are also used to break up the fat before removing it. A tube connected to a vacuum or suctioning machine is inserted into the opening and the fat is literally suctioned from that area. How much fat is removed is left to the judgment of the plastic surgeon. More than one area can be suctioned at one time. The maximum amount of tissue that may be removed in one procedure is 6 L (about 6 quarts).

The procedure causes bruising and swelling afterward. A mild pain pill is prescribed, and sometimes an antibiotic as well. If more than one area is suctioned, very limited activity is advised for 2–3 days. In addition, a compression garment is worn for 3–4 weeks to control swelling and fluid accumulation and exercise is avoided during that time. The swelling and bruising subside after 1–4 weeks. There is usually some numbness in the suctioned areas, which will also subside within 1–4 weeks. After the first week, the result of the procedure becomes noticeable, but it takes about 3 months before the final appearance is evident.

There are complications associated with any procedure and these must be discussed in detail with your surgeon before undergoing liposuction. Five to fifteen percent of patients experience cosmetic complications such as bumps or dents, wrinkles, discoloration, or small areas of numbness in the treated area. Surgery itself carries some risk, including infection and, very rarely, death. Patients should read about the procedure before talking with the surgeon so that informed questions can be answered. In addition, speaking to someone who has had the procedure is very helpful. Sometimes the surgeon will offer this. If not, do not be afraid to ask. Your surgeon should also have "before and after" photos to give a better idea of the results that can be expected.

One of the most commonly asked questions relates to weight gain. If a woman gains weight after liposuction, she will gain weight proportionately, that is, the weight should distribute evenly. Another question relates to cellulite. Liposuction will not treat cellulite and may in some cases make it look worse. Liposuction can provide good cosmetic results for carefully selected patients. All the risks and benefits should be discussed in detail with your surgeon at the first visit so that you can make an informed decision about whether this procedure will benefit you.

SEE ALSO: Body image, Cosmetic surgery, Obesity, Weight control

Suggested Reading

Medem. (2002). *Plastic surgery: Liposuction.* Arlington Heights, IL: American Society of Plastic Surgeons, Plastic Surgery Educational Foundation.

Pitman, G. H. (Ed.). (1993). *Liposuction and aesthetic surgery.* St. Louis, MO: Quality Medical.

Teimourian, F. (1987). *Suction lipectomy and body sculpturing.* St. Louis, MO: C.V. Mosby.

Suggested Resources

http://www.plasticsurgery.org/surgery/body/liposuction/liposuction.cfm

JANET BLANCHARD

Liver Spots

Solar lentigines, also known as "liver spots," "age spots," or "sun spots," are among the most common benign, pigmented lesions of the skin. These light tan to dark brown colored spots develop in areas of the greatest sun exposure of the skin, especially the face, backs of hands, forearms, and upper trunk in elderly persons. They differ from ordinary "freckles," which often start in childhood and may fade or even disappear with avoidance of sunlight. Solar lentigines (singular form: lentigo) occur in over 90% of those over 70 years of age, and become more common with age. However, they may also develop in younger persons with high exposures to sunlight or tanning beds, especially people with fair complexions.

Although harmless, solar lentigines result from high-intensity or cumulative sun exposure and may be associated with other signs of sun damage to the skin, including skin cancers. In addition, because solar lentigines often have irregular borders, and can be greater than 1 cm in diameter, occasionally they may appear similar to cutaneous melanoma, a form of skin cancer. Cosmetic treatments, including topical creams, chemical peels, liquid nitrogen, and laser therapies, may improve the appearance of solar lentigines. Protection from the sun, including avoidance of direct sunlight and use of sunscreens with high ultraviolet sun protective factors, will help prevent the recurrence of lentigines. Protection from sun exposure also plays an important role in the prevention of sun-damaged skin, especially when started early in life.

SEE ALSO: Melanoma, Skin disorders, Wrinkles

Suggested Reading

Bolognia, J. L. (1993). Dermatologic and cosmetic concerns of the older woman. *Clinics in Geriatric Medicine, 9*(1), 209–229.

Rhoades, A. R. (1999). Benign neoplasias and hyperplasia of melanocytes. In I. M. Freedberg, A. Z. Eisen, K. Wolff, K. F. Austen, L. A. Goldsmith, S. I. Katz, et al. (Eds.), *Fitzpatrick's dermatology in general medicine* (5th ed., pp. 1047–1051). New York: McGraw-Hill.

ANDREA WILLEY
PARADI MIRMIRANI

Living Wills

Beginning with California in the 1970s, all but a couple of states have enacted legislation regarding advance instruction directives for health care. These directives are commonly known as living wills, even though they have nothing to do with the distribution of property and deal with dying rather than living. Living will statutes often are termed natural death legislation. Specific legal provisions vary from state to state. However, the common theme of natural death legislation is support of an adult patient's right, while the patient is still mentally competent, to sign a written directive concerning the patient's wishes about the use of life-sustaining medical treatments in the event of later serious illness and an incapacity to make and communicate autonomous decisions at that future time. Compliance with such a directive protects or immunizes involved health care professionals and treatment facilities against possible civil or criminal liability for withholding or withdrawing medical treatments under the conditions specified in the directive.

Ordinarily, the principal or maker of the document is presumed to have the present mental capacity to execute a living will and to revoke it, absent substantial evidence to the contrary. The legal force of an instruction directive goes into effect only when the patient, after signing the document, later becomes intellectually and/or emotionally incapable of making medical decisions personally. In most cases, it is left to the individual's personal physician to clinically determine when that person has become incapable of making decisions and, therefore, when the advance directive becomes effective.

Most living will statutes and forms embody one of two approaches, either check-off options for particular types of treatment (e.g., "I do/do not want to be given antibiotics if I have a life-threatening infection") or extremely general, amorphous standardized language to express preferences regarding particular forms of medical treatment (such as, "If I become terminally ill, do not use any extraordinary or heroic medical measures to keep me alive longer"). Although we usually think of living wills as instruments for limiting life-sustaining medical treatment in the future, in some states, the living will statute permits a person to specify in an instruction directive that he or she requests the provision of particular medical interventions under certain enumerated circumstances (e.g., "I want my life to be extended through any available medical interventions to the greatest extent possible").

A handful of states have taken the legislative approach of providing a more open-ended format for documenting health care instructions prospectively. This creates an opportunity for individuals to write directives (often referred to as "Values Statements") that express their values, beliefs, and preferences in their own words by responding to questions such as, "What would be your most important goal if you were critically ill, to stay alive as long as possible or to be made as comfortable and pain-free as possible?" Some living wills incorporate personal religious considerations that are especially significant to the individual executing the directive.

SEE ALSO: Advance directives, Capacity, Durable power of attorney for health care, Informed consent

Suggested Reading

Hanson, L. C., & Rodgman, E. (1996). The use of living wills at the end of life. *Archives of Internal Medicine, 156*, 1018–1022.

King, N. M. P. (1996). *Making sense of advance directives* (rev. ed.). Washington, DC: Georgetown University Press.

Ulrich, L. P. (1999). *The patient self-determination act: Meeting the challenges in patient care.* Washington, DC: Georgetown University Press.

MARSHALL B. KAPP

Long-Term Care Long-term care (LTC) typically refers to *settings* in which individuals reside for ongoing care. Long-term care also refers to heath care needs or supervision that an individual may require for an undetermined time, or even lifelong. Long-term care can be acquired in one's home or more typically in sheltered care or independence-supporting settings described as continuing care retirement communities. In retirement communities, three levels of care are often described: independent living, assisted living, and nursing home.

On average, women live longer than men, and advanced age is associated with greater likelihood to experience disability, hence the greater need for LTC in women than in men. In fact, as reported by the American Association of Retired Persons (AARP), 72% of nursing home residents are women. About one in three women 65 years of age or older experiences a disability or a limiting illness, such as heart disease, diabetes, cancer, arthritis, or hypertension. In 1997, women accounted for more than 70% of individuals 75 years of age or older who required help with daily activities, including preparing meals, eating, bathing, or taking medications. Furthermore, women are more likely than men to be economically disadvantaged, raising many important questions as to the affordability of LTC by women. In 2001, the annual costs of nursing home care were estimated at $55,000 annually. Home health care ranged from an hourly rate of $18 for a home health aide to $37 for a licensed practical nurse. Income is associated with marital status, race, and ethnicity. As such, widows—representing 45% of women 65 years of age or older in 2001—have substantially lower income than married couples. Similarly, African American or Hispanic women are more likely than their white counterparts to have incomes below the Federal Poverty Level.

The decision to place an individual in an LTC setting is postponed until all efforts to care for that individual in the home environment fail. Maintaining normalcy of the environment and routine in the familiarity of the home is thought to contribute to improved quality of life. What is often overlooked is the burden that an undersupportive physical and emotional environment places on the individual's functioning, which can result in failure-to-thrive or decompensation of the individual. The decision to place an individual in an LTC setting is based not only on an individual's care needs, but also on the caregiver's abilities and desires.

According to the AARP, the vast majority of individuals with disabilities are cared for in their homes, by informal caregivers—usually wives or adult daughters. In 1997, 20% of such caregivers attended to the disabled individual's needs at least 40 hours a week, and one out of five caregivers who were employed gave up on their work either on a temporary or a permanent basis; half needed to incorporate flexibility to their working hours (going to work late or working fewer hours) in order to accommodate caregiving.

Caregiver burden, a term used to describe the impact of providing care on the caregiver, can present in two aspects: physical and emotional. This is observed frequently, as nearly one third of caregivers suffer from physical and/or mental problems of their own. Examples of physical burden are activities and responsibilities involved in the day-to-day care of the patient. Emotional burden refers to the feelings the caregiver has toward the patient, or the care receiver, that are the consequence of giving care. Burnout is a term that is used when the caregiver has exhausted the usual supports or when the care receiver's needs outweigh the ability of one individual to provide care 24 hours a day, 7 days a week. Burnout is suggested when a caregiver's health suffers or when his/her problem-solving abilities are diminished. The goal of selecting a nursing home is to do this before the caregiver is too exhausted to participate in finding solutions to day-to-day problems or in making decisions about placement of the patient in an LTC setting. Burnout can manifest itself through the deterioration of the caregiver's physical health, and a change in the quality of the caregiver–patient relationship. Discussions regarding placement in an LTC facility can have a psychological impact on both the patient and the caregiver, mainly because of the implied permanence and deterioration of the patient's independence. When the caregiver realizes that decisions regarding the course and site of care are made based on the individual's condition and functional abilities, the discussion can become emotionally less charged. Assisting the individual and support persons proceed in planning for LTC involves an evaluation of the individual's functional abilities and ability to afford an environment that is ideally most supportive and least restrictive.

Postponing placement to preserve funds is a realistic part of planning for LTC. Placement decisions involve the site and duration of care. Medicare is an age- and/or disability-based entitlement and typically only covers short-term care that is restorative, or rehabilitative, or "skilled" in nature. Even if an individual

373

has had the foresight to own a liberal LTC insurance private policy, there may be limitations on the site of care, such as institutional versus home. Medicaid is a payer for individuals with low incomes, and typically covers basic care at the nursing home level that is custodial or "nonskilled" in nature. In the event that an individual's income exceeds Medicaid income eligibility levels, the individual should *spend down* the excess amount to the Medicaid income eligibility level in order to become eligible to enroll in Medicaid.

There has been an increase in the number of LTC insurance policyholders in later years. These policies vary widely in the scope of covered services, as well as in cost. For example, some policies require that the beneficiary suffer severe cognitive impairment, or to need assistance with at least two activities of daily living, or to demonstrate "medical necessity" before providing coverage for LTC services, and reimburse a fixed amount for daily care ($100 per day in nursing home and $50 per day for home care). The mechanisms of LTC financing and service delivery have been evolving with the rapidly increasing proportion of the aging population.

Population statistics suggest that as the present "baby boomer" generation ages, health care services must cover the entire spectrum—from wellness programs, to meet the needs of healthier individuals, to skilled nursing and rehabilitative care for individuals with chronic illness and functional limitations. Currently, 5% of the elderly population live in LTC facilities; however, an increase of this population even by a few percentage points could strain resources both in terms of available facilities and available funding.

SEE ALSO: Activities of daily living, Assisted living, Medicaid, Medicare, Nursing home

Suggested Resources

American Association of Retired Persons at www.aarp.org
Resource for long-term care information at www.ltclink.net

EVANNE JURATOVAC

Lubricants During the course of sexual arousal, the walls of the vagina secrete a lubricant or mucus to facilitate coitus. Inadequate lubrication, a persistent problem for 40% of women in the United States, can cause vaginal intercourse to be painful. Inadequate lubrication can be facilitated by extended foreplay, and hormonal changes which can occur during the course of menstrual cycles, menopause, and breast-feeding. Water-based lubricants can both alleviate the problem of vaginal dryness and increase sexual stimulation for both partners. However, most importantly, it should be noted that lubricants improve the efficacy rate of condoms, thus reducing the risk of sexually transmitted infections (STIs), including human immunodeficiency virus (HIV).

In general, latex condoms are most effective when used in conjunction with water-based lubricants. Examples of water-based lubricants include KY Jelly and Astroglide. Water-based lubricants can protect latex condoms (barriers) against friction that may otherwise tear them during intercourse. Alternatively, oil-based lubricants should not be used with latex condoms, dental dams, or any other product made of latex. Examples of oil-based lubricants are petroleum jelly, massage oils, or creams. When latex comes in contact with oil-based products, a chemical reaction occurs which degrades the latex. This process can ultimately cause holes to develop in condoms, influence condom breakage, and reduce the amount of protection overall. For example, in a study conducted to assess the impact of lubricants on latex condoms during vaginal intercourse, researchers determined that the use of oil-based lubricants increased breakage in new and aged latex condoms, while water-based lubricants did not impact the breakage rate of new condoms and decreased the breakage rate in aged condoms.

Additionally, condoms lubricated with spermicides are not likely to be more effective than condoms used with other water-based lubricants. Most specifically, in recent times, nonoxynol-9 (N-9), a spermicidal in concentrations of 18% in some sexual lubricants, and lubricated condoms have been noted to contain detergents that disrupt cell membranes. Frequent use of N-9 as a contraceptive has been associated with an increased risk of epithelial infections in the vagina, cervix, and rectum. Such opportunistic infections have been demonstrated by a series of researchers to enhance the transmission of HIV. For example, one study has demonstrated that HIV incidence was greater in a high-risk population using N-9 than in a comparison population using a placebo.

In another study, researchers found that N-9 used without condoms was ineffective against HIV transmission. This study also showed evidence that N-9 increased the risk of HIV infection. It was further noted that this study was conducted among commercial sex workers in Africa who are at an increased HIV risk and used N-9 gel on a frequent basis. As a result of this study, the Centers for Disease Control and Prevention concluded that, given that N-9 has been proven ineffective against HIV transmission and heightens the possibility of risk, with no benefits, N-9 should not be recommended as an effective means of HIV prevention.

Moreover, a similar randomized study of women sex workers revealed a slightly higher risk for gonorrhea, a slightly lower risk for chlamydia, and no change in risk for HIV among women using film with 70 mg of N-9. Taken together, these findings speak the importance of the timely development of a safe, effective microbicidal spermicide that can reduce the transmission of HIV.

Lastly, couples experiencing infertility should avoid the use of all commercial lubricants. Even lubricants that are spermicide free contain ingredients that can inhibit sperm. The reduction of sperm motility and viability after exposure to commercial lubricants in vitro may be related to glycerin contained in lubricants. Researchers have demonstrated significant and immediate inhibition in motility and forward progression when sperm were incubated with 16.7% glycerin. Some natural food products useable as lubricants have proven to be less detrimental to sperm. Of the products tested, canola oil shows the least adverse effect on sperm motility and viability. Overall, studies examining the motility of sperm when exposed to lubricants suggest that when selecting a lubricant couples should consider one that has a minimal effect on pH, demonstrates low spermicidal activity, and has minimal effect on motility. Canola oil satisfies these criteria and has yielded support from several studies.

SEE ALSO: Condoms, Reproductive technologies, Safer sex, Sexually transmitted diseases

Suggested Reading

Foley, S., Kope, S. A., & Sugrue, D. P. (2002). *Sex matters for women: A complete guide to taking care of your sexual self.* New York: Guilford Press.

Stewart, E. G., & Spenser, P. (2002). *The V book: A doctor's guide to complete vulvovaginal health.* New York: Bantam Doubleday Dell.

Wingood, G. M., & DiClemente, R. J. (2002). *Women's sexual and reproductive health.* New York: Plenum/Kluwer.

CHRISTINA M. CAMP
GINA M. WINGOOD

Lumpectomy   *see* Breast Lumps

Lung Cancer

Lung cancer, a largely incurable disease, remains the leading cause of cancer deaths among women each year in the United States, exceeding annual breast cancer mortality in women and accounting for 12% of all new female cancer cases (Table 1). Although lung cancer has always been and continues to be more prevalent in men than in women, lung cancer mortality patterns now reveal that the rate of rise of such cancer deaths among men has slowed and begun to decline since 1990, whereas in women it has continued to rise. Several studies suggest that women are more susceptible than men to lung cancer and to conditions, like chronic obstructive pulmonary disease, that predispose to this cancer; hence the question has been raised as to whether lung cancer is a different disease in women than in men.

Overall smoking remains the most important risk factor for the development of lung cancer in both women and men, and the smoking trends have changed in women over the years to parallel an increase in the number of female lung cancer cases. "Although there has been a large decline from the peak female smoking rate of 34.2% seen in 1965, smoking among teenage girls has increased dramatically over the past decade. Among high school students, cigarette use (defined as at least one cigarette in the past 30 days)

Table 1. Estimated cancer deaths from the 10 leading sites in males and females: All ages, 1999

Females	%	Males	%
Lung and bronchus	25	Lung and bronchus	31
Breast	16	Prostate	13
Colon and rectum	11	Colon and rectum	10
Pancreas	5	Pancreas	5
Ovary	5	Non-Hodgkin's lymphoma	5
Non-Hodgkin's lymphoma	5	Leukemia	4
Leukemia	4	Esophagus	3
Uterine corpus	2	Liver/Intrahepatic Bile Duct	3
Brain and other nervous system	2	Urinary bladder	3
Stomach	2*	Stomach	3
Multiple myeloma	2*	All other sites	20
Other sites	21		

Note: Excludes basal and squamous cell skin cancers and in situ carcinomas except urinary bladder.
*These two cancers received a ranking of 10 (they have the same number of deaths and contribute to the same percentage).
Source: Landis, S. H., Murray, T., Bolden, S., et al. Cancer Statistics. *CA Cancer J Clin.* 1999, *49*, 8–31.

Lung Cancer

has increased from 21% in the 1980s to about 35% of both boys and girls in 1997" (Siegfried, 2001). In 2001, the U.S. Surgeon General issued a new report, *Women and Smoking*, in which the 600% increase since 1950 in female lung cancer death rate was described as "a full-blown epidemic," wherein smoking is now the leading cause of preventable death and disease in women.

Although research has been unable to determine whether the association between smoking and lung cancer is stronger for women than for men, studies now suggest that lung cancer induced by smoking, environmental factors, and the like follows a different pattern in women than in men; hence, there might be important differences between women and men that influence lung cancer risk. Reports have indicated that women smokers have a greater risk of developing small-cell lung carcinoma (smaller risk of squamous cell carcinoma) than men smokers (who have a similar risk for small-cell carcinoma and squamous cell carcinoma). In addition, studies report that for a given amount of smoking, women may be up to twice as likely to develop lung cancer as men, and nonsmokers who develop lung cancer are two and a half times more likely to be female than male.

Adenocarcinoma of the lung, more common among nonsmokers than smokers, is found predominantly in women, whereas men are more likely to be diagnosed with squamous cell carcinoma. This suggests that women may be more susceptible to adverse effects of tobacco due, in part, to female hormones, namely, estrogen-mediated effects. Taioli and Wynder found that early age at menopause (40 years or younger) is associated with a reduced risk of adenocarcinoma of the lung, whereas the use of estrogen-replacement therapy is associated with a higher risk of lung adenocarcinoma (Figure 1). In addition, the study revealed a positive interaction between estrogen-replacement therapy, smoking, and the development of adenocarcinoma of the lung. Estrogens may have a role in directly causing cancer (direct-acting carcinogens) and may enhance the metabolic activity of cigarette smoke cancer-causing components (carcinogens). Estrogen receptors have been reported in lung tumors when studied using special diagnostic microscopic stains, and lung tumors from women are more likely to express estrogen receptors than those from men.

Women may not only be more susceptible to the adverse effects of tobacco but also more prone to lung diseases that predispose to lung cancer. A history of pneumonia (especially in childhood), tuberculosis, asthma, chronic bronchitis, and chronic obstructive pulmonary disease/emphysema have all been associated

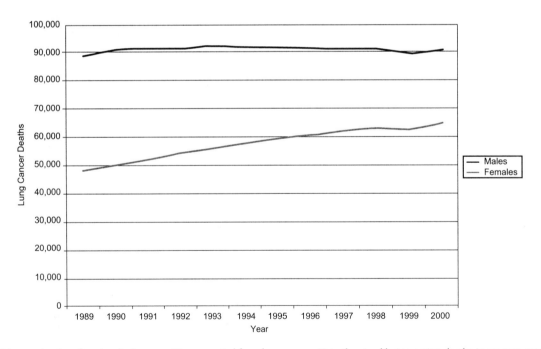

Figure 1. More males than females died over an 11 year period from lung cancer. Note the steadily increasing deaths in women over the same time period.

Source: Landis, S. H., Murray, T., Bolden, A, et al. Cancer Statistics. *CA Cancer J Clin*. 1999, *49*, 8–31.

with a higher risk of lung cancer in nonsmokers, mainly in studies of women. Among these diseases, chronic obstructive pulmonary disease affects more nonsmoking women than men and increases their lung cancer risk; therefore, speculation as to estrogen involvement in this predisposition and further research behind this higher female susceptibility to lung disease may provide valuable insight as to the onset of lung cancer in women and more effective treatment.

Determination of the mechanisms behind various forms of nonsmoking- and smoking-related lung cancer in women will enable more effective treatment options. Since about 80% of lung cancer cases are attributable to smoking, it is clear that smoking rates must be reduced to zero to halt the lung cancer epidemic for both men and women. Lung cancer cases that cannot be prevented must be diagnosed at as early a stage as possible since survival rates are highest for patients who present with early-stage disease. Staging of lung cancer (see Table 2) takes into account location of the tumor, histology, lymph node involvement, and metastasis (spread to various organs). Chest radiograph screening to detect early forms of lung cancer may provide a useful method, but gender differences must be considered when examining for lung cancer risk. Women were only included in 2 of the 11 prospective studies of lung cancer screening to date, and therefore further investigation is warranted to adequately study the role of lung cancer screening for women. In addition, preclinical and clinical trials should address gender as a specific research variable to improve and focus lung cancer therapy. The suggested role of estrogens in lung adenocarcinoma development in many female nonsmokers and the increased susceptibility in women to the carcinogenic effects of cigarette smoke warrant further study to hopefully better target screening studies and develop more effective therapy against lung cancer in women.

Table 2. Staging lung cancer: TNM subsets by stage

Stage 0	Carcinoma in situ	
Stage 1A	T1 N0 M0	T1 = tumor ≤ 3.0 cm, surrounded by lung tissue; no lymph node involvement; no evidence of invasion
Stage 1B	T2 N0 M0	T2 = tumor ≥ 3.0 cm, or tumor of any size that invades visceral pleura or associated atelectasis (collapse of lung alveoli)
Stage IIA	T1 N1 M0	T1 tumor with lymph node involvement in peribronchial or ipsilateral hilar region, or both
Stage IIB	T2 N1 M0	T2 tumor with lymph node involvement
	T3 N0 M0	T3 = tumor of any size with direct extension into the chest wall, diaphragm, etc. without involving the heart, great vessels, trachea, esophagus, etc.; N0 = no lymph node involvement
Stage IIIA	T3 N1 M0	T3 tumor with lymph node involvement
	T1 N2 M0, T2 N2 M0 T3 N2 M0	T1 or T2 tumor; N2 = metastasis to ipsilateral mediastinal lymph nodes and subcarinal lymph nodes
Stage IV	Any T, Any N, M1	M1 = distant metastasis present

Note: T = primary tumor; N = lymph node involvement; M = distant metastasis. Adapted from Mountain, Libshitz, and Hermes (1999).

See Also: Cancer, Hormone replacement therapy, Lung disease, Smoking.

Suggested Reading

Healey Baldini, E., & Strauss, G. M. (1997). Women and lung cancer: Waiting to exhale. *Chest, 112* (Suppl.), 229S–234S.

Mountain, C. F., Libshitz, H. I., & Hermes, K. E. (1999). *Lung cancer: A handbook for staging, imaging, and lymph node classification.* Houston, TX: Charles P. Young Company.

Siegfried, J. M. (2001). Women and lung cancer: Does oestrogen play a role? *The Lancet Oncology, 2,* 506–513.

S. Franco
Marilyn Glassberg

Lung Disease

This entry focuses on lung disease during pregnancy.

PHYSIOLOGY

Hyperventilation is a characteristic feature of pregnancy. During pregnancy, the enlarging uterus causes a progressive upward displacement of the diaphragm, to a maximum of 4 cm. This displacement, however, does not impair diaphragmatic function. The diameter of the chest increases by approximately 2 cm; flaring of the ribs and widening of the rib cage with a subsequent increased angle below the ribs—subcostal angle (up to 50%). Despite these changes, respiratory muscle function appears unchanged. The pregnant woman's ability to move air in and out of the lung remains unrestrained.

The levels of the hormone progesterone increase throughout pregnancy. Placental progesterone stimulates the brain's respiratory centers to increase minute ventilation. The increase in minute ventilation increases the amount of oxygen available to the fetus. Minute ventilation increases by 20–50% before the end of the first trimester and remains the same throughout the duration of the pregnancy. This increased minute ventilation is the result of a marked increase in tidal volume; the respiratory rate remains unchanged throughout pregnancy. Thus, hyperventilation is due to deeper, not more frequent breathing.

Anxiety and uterine contractions associated with labor and delivery further increase the physiologic hyperventilation of pregnancy. Oxygen consumption can double during pregnancy and triples during uterine contractions. Pain relief via intravenous sedation and epidural analgesia can minimize this labor- and delivery-induced hyperventilation.

Shortness of breath or dyspnea is a common feature among 60–70% of normal, healthy pregnant women and is a normal physiologic response in gravid (women in their first pregnancy) patients. The exact cause of dyspnea is not well understood. It occurs in the 1st and 2nd trimesters and plateaus or improves as term approaches. Dyspnea occurs before the upward displacement of the diaphragm. Thus, it is unlikely that the growing uterus plays a significant role in the development of dyspnea. Physiologic dyspnea has been attributed to progesterone's stimulatory effects on the inspiratory neural drive. Others suggest it is due to an increased awareness of the physiologic hyperventilation. Furthermore, increase chemosensitivity may also contribute to dyspnea of pregnancy. Regardless of the exact cause, it remains unlikely that dyspnea of pregnancy is caused by the mechanical burden of the enlarging fetus.

PNEUMONIA

Pneumonia is the most common nonobstetric infectious cause of death during pregnancy and the puerperium. The pathogens involved in pneumonias of pregnant women are similar to those identified in nonpregnant women. Most cases of pneumonia during pregnancy are due to bacteria. The most common bacterial pathogen in community acquired pneumonia in pregnant women is the gram-positive diplococcus, *Streptococcus pneumoniae*. Onset is abrupt and dramatic. Symptoms include fever, chills, pleuritic chest pain, and productive cough with purulent sputum.

Viral pneumonias are also common in pregnant women. Influenza is the most common viral pathogen of pneumonia in pregnancy. Of the three major antigenic types, Type A is most often associated with human illness and epidemics. After a short incubation period, symptoms develop and include general malaise, headache, fever, chills, and upper respiratory symptoms. While initially the respiratory examination may not be remarkable, pregnant women can rapidly develop respiratory failure.

During the course of pneumonia, adverse maternal and fetal effects can occur. Maternal complications can be severe. The most serious complications include bacterial superinfection, respiratory failure, and adult respiratory distress syndrome. Premature labor and delivery is another obstetric problem that can occur including the possible transmission of viral agents to the fetus and newborn. Premature labor may develop during pneumonia as a result of prostaglandin production or from the woman's inflammatory response to the underlying infection. While the transplacental passage of the influenza virus has been documented, it has not been identified as a teratogen (cause of birth defects).

ASTHMA

Asthma occurs in 4% of gravid women, and complicates up to 1.5% of pregnancies, representing the most common obstructive pulmonary disease seen in pregnancy. Asthma is a chronic disease with acute exacerbations; it is characterized by reversible airway obstruction, airway inflammation, and airway hyperresponsiveness to stimuli such as allergens, viruses, exercise, and cold air. Hyperreactive airways result in bronchospasm, mucosal edema, and mucus plugging, producing symptoms of cough, wheezing, dyspnea, and chest tightness.

Poorly controlled asthma is associated with maternal and fetal complications, while well-controlled asthma poses little threat. Maternal decrease in blood oxygen (hypoxemia) is associated with increased incidence of intrauterine growth retardation, prematurity, low birthweight, perinatal mortality, and maternal hypertension. The primary goal in managing the pregnant patient with asthma is to prevent hypoxemia while minimizing the risk to the mother and fetus of adverse effects from medications. Controlling asthma in a pregnant patient should be addressed as in a nonpregnant individual. One of the first steps is to identify triggers that initiate or worsen asthma for a particular person. Triggers may include allergens, exercise, cold air, infections, emotional stress, irritants, gastroesophageal reflux, and drugs such as aspirin.

AMNIOTIC FLUID EMBOLISMS IN PREGNANCY

Amniotic fluid obstruction by clot or debris (embolism) is an uncommon obstetric complication, present in 1/8,000 to 1/80,000 pregnancies. However, it is frequently a fatal event, with a mortality rate in mothers of 50–60% within 1 hour after the onset of symptoms. Permanent neurological damage is suffered by 70% of survivors. This process is triggered by the sudden obstruction (embolization) of amniotic fluid or fetal debris into the maternal blood flow system (venous circulation). Initial alterations in blood flow and pressure (hemodynamics) and oxygenation can be seen and are then followed by abnormalities in blood clotting (coagulopathy). The most common presentation is sudden breathlessness (dyspnea) and hypotension (low blood pressure) followed by cardiorespiratory arrest. The diagnosis does not depend on the detection of fetal debris in the blood vessels (vasculature), but rather on the basis of clinical presentation, since not all patients will have these objective findings.

The neonatal outcome is usually greater than maternal outcome, with 80% of neonates surviving delivery if they are alive at the onset of the event. However, 50% of these neonates suffer permanent neurological damage. In patients who survive amniotic fluid embolism, no recurrence in subsequent deliveries has been reported.

For a pregnant woman with any breathing (pulmonary) complication, the primary goal is to prevent reduced blood oxygen (hypoxemia) and maintain adequate oxygenation for both mother and fetus. Pregnancy may exacerbate or ameliorate other pulmonary diseases. For care providers, it is important to be familiar with the various respiratory infections that may be found among this population. Is it essential to know which antibiotics are contraindicated (not recommended) during pregnancy and to monitor patients on medications to minimize adverse effects. This information is critical in order to provide accurate counseling and education to patients. Finally, it is important to understand that any dyspnea the woman is experiencing will resolve postpartum. As the level of progesterone returns to normal, the increased minute ventilation will also return to baseline.

SEE ALSO: Asthma, Pregnancy

Suggested Reading

Clark, S., Hankins, G., Dudley, D., et al. (1995). Amniotic fluid embolism: Analysis of the national registry. *American Journal of Obstetrics and Gynecology, 172,* 1158.

Contreras, G., Guttierrez, M., & Beroiza, T. (1991). Ventilatory drive and respiratory muscle function in pregnancy. *American Review of Respiratory Diseases, 144,* 837–841.

Oberstein, E. M., Marder, A., Pitts, S., & Glassberg, M. K. (2002). Pulmonary complications in pregnancy, part 1: Infections and asthma. *Journal of Respiratory Diseases, 23,* 41–53.

Oberstein, E. M., Marder, A., Pitts, S., & Glassberg, M. K. (2002). Pulmonary complications in pregnancy, part 2: Emboli and other diseases. *Journal of Respiratory Diseases, 23,* 175–181.

Rigby, F. B., & Pastorek, J. G., II. (1996). Pneumonia during pregnancy. *Clinical Obstetrics and Gynecology, 39,* 107–119.

Venkataraman, M. T., & Shanies, H. M. (1997). Pregnancy and asthma. *Journal of Asthma, 34,* 265–271.

MARILYN GLASSBERG
GEOFFREY HARRIS

Lung Transplantation

The field of lung transplantation has seen steady progress over the past two decades and is now widely accepted as a treatment option for end-stage lung disease. According to the Organ Procurement and Transplantation Network (OPTN), there have been approximately 10,000 lung transplants performed in the United States. Although the list of candidates for lung transplantation is steadily growing, as is the number of transplantation centers, the annual transplant rate is leveling off due to a limited number of donors. As a result, the waiting time for lung transplant can be up to 2 years.

Chronic obstructive pulmonary disease or emphysema (including alpha-1-antitrypsin deficiency) has been the underlying disease process in nearly half of all lung transplants. Cystic fibrosis, idiopathic pulmonary fibrosis, and primary pulmonary hypertension are all disease states that primarily affect the lungs, and are also common reasons for lung transplant. Other causes include sarcoidosis (a disease in which lung tissue develops a granulomatosis or scar-like consistency), bronchiectasis (destruction of the bronchial tubes in the lungs from severe infection), occupational lung disease, Eisenmenger's syndrome (a congenital heart condition which leads to low oxygen levels in blood and elevated red blood cell counts), and rejection of a prior lung transplant.

Lung transplant has been shown to improve lung function and quality of life in all of these diseases, but the procedure does carry significant risk of mortality. Therefore, there are strict guidelines for referring a patient for lung transplant. Specific diseases have their own prognostic criteria used in deciding whether a transplant is appropriate, but general indications for transplant include advanced disease with life expectancy of 2–3 years, unsuccessful medical therapy, severe functional limitation, and poor quality of life. Absolute contraindications to transplant include current smoking, active malignancy, HIV infection, and severe impairment of other organs.

There are four major types of lung transplantation: heart–lung transplantation, single-lung transplant, bilateral lung transplant, and living donor lobe transplant. Heart–lung transplant was the first procedure to have long-term success, and it is now primarily used in patients with Eisenmenger's syndrome or with concurrent severe cardiac dysfunction. Single-lung transplant is the most commonly used technique and has been successful for most types of lung disease except cystic fibrosis. Bilateral transplantation is the preferred method for cystic fibrosis and bronchiectasis, in which both lungs must be removed due to infection. Finally, one technique that is gaining support due to the limited supply of donor lungs is the transplantation of lower lobes from living donors. Cystic fibrosis is the most common disease for which this procedure has been used.

Despite advances in surgical techniques, immunosuppressive therapies, and infection prophylaxis, survival rates after lung transplantation are significantly lower than for other solid organ transplants. Data reported from OPTN for lung transplants performed between 1995 and 2000 show a 1-year survival of 75.4% for men and 76.4% for women and a 3-year survival of 57% for both sexes. Complications from lung transplant include airway complications, rejection, infection, and malignancy. The most important causes of mortality following the time period just after surgery (perioperative period) are acute rejection and infections. The greatest threat to long-term survival is bronchiolitis obliterans, a form of chronic tissue rejection found in up to 60–70% of patients who survive 5 years. The cause of bronchiolitis obliterans is not entirely known, but proposed mechanisms include HLA mismatching (incomplete or imperfect genetic match of the graft tissue to the patient tissue), viral infection (cytomegalovirus), decreased oxygen to the airway (airway ischemia), and problems related to the immune system. Currently, the only definitive treatment for chronic rejection is retransplantation.

SEE ALSO: Acquired immunodeficiency syndrome, Chronic obstructive pulmonary disease, Lung disease

Suggested Reading

Barr, M., Baker, F., Schenkel, F., et al. (2001). Living donor lung transplantation: Selection, technique, and outcome. *Transplantation Proceedings, 33*, 3527–3532.

DeMeo, D., & Ginns, L. (2001). Lung transplantation at the turn of the century. *Annual Reviews of Medicine, 52*, 185–201.

Estenne, M., & Hertz, M. (2002). Bronchiolitis obliterans after human lung transplantation. *American Journal of Respiratory Critical Care Medicine, 166*, 440–444.

Meyers, B., & Patterson, A. (1999). Lung transplantation: Current status and future prospects. *World Journal of Surgery, 23*, 1156–1162.

Speich, R., & van der Bij, W. (2001). Epidemiology and management of infections after lung transplantation. *Clinical Infectious Diseases, 33* (Suppl. 1), S58–S65.

RACHEL LANGE
MARILYN GLASSBERG

Lyme Disease

Lyme disease is an infection caused by a bacterium, *Borrelia burgdorferi*, which is carried around in the adult deer tick, *Ixodes dammini*. It begins as a slowly expanding skin rash and is associated with a tick bite or potential exposure to ticks. The Centers for Disease Control and Prevention (CDC) began surveillance for Lyme disease in 1982 and the Council of State and Territorial Epidemiologists (CSTE) designated Lyme disease as a nationally notable disease in January 1991. Currently all 50 states and the District of Columbia have reporting requirements.

THE VECTOR

Lyme disease is transmitted to humans through the bite of infected *Ixodes* ticks. Ticks feed by inserting their mouths into the skin of unsuspecting prey, and slowly ingesting host blood. The preferred host of nymphal *Ixodes* tick is the white-footed mouse. The preferred habitat for the adult tick is the white-tailed deer. These ticks do not look like the common dog or wood tick, they are much smaller, about 0.2 mm.

Even in endemic regions only 15% of ticks are infected with *B. burgdorferi* (the causative agent of Lyme disease). The vast majority of infection and disease onset occur between May and November, peaking in June and July, when the nymphal stage tick is prepared to feed. For infection to occur, an *infected* tick needs to remain attached for 36–48 hours. Identification of the tick bite and recognition of symptoms are key to early diagnosis. There is no evidence of any person-to-person transmission (respiratory or via body fluids), or of any other vectors (flies, fleas, mosquitoes) transmitting the disease.

THE DISEASE

Lyme disease is a zoonotic (coming from animals), multisystem, multistage disease with the typical sign of an early expanding skin lesion *erythema migrans* (EM) present in 90% or more of patients. If unrecognized or untreated, a patient may present weeks to months later with neurologic, cardiac, and/or joint abnormalities. Tissue damage occurs not as a direct result of spirochetal infection, but rather from a nonspecific immune *response* to infection.

Early Symptoms—Localized Disease

Within 3 days to about 1 month after being infected, 90% of patients experience EM. Erythema begins as a small red macular or papular lesion at the site of the tick bite. As the bacteria migrate outward, the area enlarges and eventually a "clearing" of the central aspect of the lesion occurs (the "bull's-eye" lesion). The leading edge, though infected, remains flat and without scaling. It may be warm, but is not usually painful, thus often missed. As borrelia infection continues, it will enter the bloodstream and disseminate.

Early Symptoms—Disseminated Disease

When the bacteria disseminate, one quarter of patients experience multiple secondary annular skin lesions. Both EM and the secondary skin lesions may fade, but often reoccur. Systemic flu-like symptoms including headache, fatigue, fever, chills, myalgia (muscle pain), and/or arthralgia (joint pains) may present as well, or alone. Few patients may also present with excruciating headache, neck pain, and/or stiffness that resolves in hours, without neurological deficit, and normal cerebrol spinal fluid (CSF) assessment.

Late Disease (Weeks to Months)

Sixty percent of untreated patients experience arthritis, which is classically intermittent, asymmetric with pain, and swelling in large joints, often the knee. Arthritic episodes may last weeks to months, subside, and reoccur with decreasing frequency over several years. Fatigue is common but fever is rare. Ten percent of patients become chronic through the stimulation of an immune response against cartilage and bone similar to that found in rheumatoid arthritis. Fifteen percent of patients experience neurologic symptoms including meningitis, encephalitis, radiculoneuropathy (spinal nerve/nerve root manifestations), and/or facial nerve palsies. These central nervous system symptoms present with abnormal CSF, but patients *do not* have classic meningitis. Symptoms last for months but usually resolve. Eight percent of patients with late symptoms will develop cardiac involvement: A-V block, mild left ventricular dysfunction, or rarely cardiomegaly (enlarged heart). No murmurs are associated and symptoms are brief (days to weeks), but may also reoccur.

Very late sequelae may include the chronic skin lesions, *acrodermatitis chronica atrophicans*, which are firm red patches that atrophy, often on the hands, elbows, or knees. Neuropsychological effects, although rare, may include mild memory dysfunction, subtle mood changes, chronic fatigue, spinal cord inflammation, and sensory neuropathy.

DIAGNOSIS

Clinical symptoms with history of tick bite are sufficient for the diagnosis and treatment of Lyme disease. Early Lyme disease is based on the clinical presentation and there is no need for laboratory testing. Culture is definitive but very difficult, thus not used. Antibody titers (a measurement of antibodies the body produces in response to a specific infection) can prove helpful in diagnosis of patients with nonspecific symptoms. Caution in indiscriminant testing may result in false positives and confusion. Testing is best done to confirm the clinical suspicion, not just to search for a diagnosis.

LYME DISEASE AND PREGNANCY

Though an early report linked Lyme disease with adverse outcomes, a later prospective study of about 2,000 pregnant women refuted the evidence, and concluded that maternal infection of Lyme disease was *not* associated with fetal mortality, decreased birthweight, premature delivery, or congenital malformations. If a pregnant woman, however, becomes infected, it is recommended that she receive prompt treatment to eliminate disease and prevent future manifestations. There have been no known cases of fetal infection from mothers who contracted the disease and were treated.

TREATMENT

Early, nonspecific symptoms in an endemic area are an indication to treat. Successful treatment can occur even with late symptoms, but will be most rapid when identified early. As some symptoms may not clear for 3 months after completion of antibiotics and it is difficult to prove successful elimination of *B. burgdorferi* from the system, the determination of end point for treatment may be difficult! Current guidelines should guide all treatments. Doxycycline, amoxicillin, and cefuroxime axetil are currently the preferred drugs. With late symptoms, intravenous antibiotics are advised. Approximately 10% of patients experience a Jarisch–Herxheimer reaction (temporary worsening of symptoms with the initiation of treatment), headache, musculoskeletal pain, and/or fatigue depending on the severity of their disease.

PROPHYLAXIS AND PREVENTION

Prevention is the key step in avoiding infection.

1. When possible, avoid tick habitats, especially during spring and summer. *Ixodes* prefers a moist shaded environment: areas of leaf litter and forests or areas of low-growing vegetation.
2. Minimize exposed skin when venturing into infested areas: Wear light-colored clothes (to see ticks better), tuck pants into socks, and wear long sleeved shirts.
3. Insect repellants containing DEET are very effective when applied to clothing and exposed skin. DEET can be used safely on children but follow product directions.
4. Perform tick checks regularly and remove attached ticks. If embedded ticks are found, remove them using fine-tipped tweezers. Grab the tick as close to the skin as possible and with a firm steady motion pull the animal away. Do not worry if mouthparts are left behind, they do not transmit disease and human immunity can usually handle the remnants. Next, clean the area thoroughly with an antiseptic, and report any signs of EM or Lyme disease.

There is no indication for prophylactic treatment of asymptomatic patients after tick bite, but if symptoms arise (EM or nonspecific), medical attention and treatment are indicated. As of February 2002, the LYMErix™ Lyme disease vaccine was no longer manufactured, primarily due to concerns that the vaccine itself induced chronic arthritis in certain patients. There is ongoing research into new vaccines.

SEE ALSO: Arthritis, Rheumatoid arthritis

Suggested Reading

Malawista, S. E. (2000). Lyme disease. *Cecil textbook of medicine* (pp. 1757–1761). Philadelphia: W.B. Saunders.
Strobino, B. A., Williams, C. L., Abid, S., Chalson, R., & Spierling, P. (1993). Lyme disease and pregnancy outcome: A prospective study of two thousand prenatal patients. *American Journal of Obstetrics and Gynecology, 169*, 367–374.

Suggested Resources

CDC Lyme Disease Home Page: http://www.cdc.gov/ncidod/dvbid/Lyme/index.htm

September 19, 2001. CDC Division of Vector-Borne Infectious Diseases (DVBID).
September 19, 2001. Lyme disease: Epidemiology.
September 19, 2001. Lyme disease: Prevention and control.
September 19, 2001. Lyme disease: Vector ecology.
September 21, 2001. Lyme disease: Questions and answers.
October 3, 2001. Lyme disease: Diagnosis.
September 17, 2002. Lyme disease: Vaccine recommendations.
November 27, 2002. Lyme disease: The Bacterium.

ROBERT W. SANDERS
LORI B. SIEGEL

Mammary Glands The mammary glands, or breasts, are actually modified sebaceous glands (sweat) that are designed to secrete milk. On average, each breast weighs 200–300 g. They are composed of glandular tissue, fat, and supporting or stromal tissue. Each breast is organized into 12–25 triangular shaped lobes. Each lobe is composed of several smaller lobules. The breast lobules are linked by a collecting duct system which is responsible for the passage of milk. The spaces between the lobules are filled with fatty tissue. This intricate duct system terminates in the central portion of the breast, the areola or nipple area.

Pathologic (disease) changes may occur in any of the breast tissue. For example, the fat tissue in the breasts may actually necrose, or die, in response to trauma. Additionally, the stromal or support tissue of the breasts may give rise to fibrocystic changes, or benign solid tumors, called fibroadenomas. Breast cancer may also develop in any part of the breast.

Breast tissue responds to hormonal changes. Pain and swelling may occur prior to menstruation. Additionally, certain medications, particularly hormonal medications such as oral contraceptives, may also cause changes in the breasts. Early in pregnancy, the breasts prepare for lactation and may become tender and enlarged. After delivery, the breast tissue engorges to prepare for breast-feeding. When a woman chooses not to breast-feed or when she weans her infant, engorgement (swelling due to milk accumulation) may cause pain, and even a low-grade fever. The pain usually responds well to mild pain medications and cold compresses, and will usually resolve in approximately 2 weeks.

As women age, breast pain often diminishes. Hormone replacement therapy, however, may trigger pain in postmenopausal women.

See Also: Breast-feeding, Mammography, Mastectomy, Mastitis, Pregnancy

KAREN L. ASHBY

Mammography Breasts share the same basic structure. The mammary glands produce milk and are found in clusters throughout the breast. Ducts take the milk from the glands to the nipple during breast-feeding. Lymph nodes are present under the arm. The lymph nodes are small, normally bean-sized structures that help to fight infection and enlarge in the presence of infection or cancer in the breast tissue. There are reservoirs within the breast that store the milk. The areola is the part of the nipple that lubricates the nipple with oil. Fat in fibrous tissue surrounds the glands and ducts and gives the breast its smooth shape. Women who have more fat tissue in the breast have a softer breast, while having more fibrous tissue in the breast makes the breast feel firmer. Normally, a lump is easier to locate in a softer or more fatty breast, as compared to a firmer, dense breast.

At the time of each menstrual cycle, the drop in hormones results in a sloughing (breakdown) of the ductal lining. This lining regrows again in a cyclic fashion. The blood vessels around the ducts in other cells also undergo changes during the menstrual cycle. This causes the breasts, in some women, to become swollen, tender, denser, or lumpier in the week before menstruation. During pregnancy, the milk glands, ducts, areolae, and nipples enlarge. The breasts feel heavy, lumpy, and tender when nursing stops. Breasts usually return to their former size; however, they may be less firm. In many parts of the breast, the glandular growth remains until it reduces at the time of menopause. At the onset of menopause, there is a loss of breast tissue, structural components, and an increase in the fat. The milk glands and ducts shrink and the breasts become smaller and softer. The supporting ligaments lose some of their strength. It is important to note that the changes associated with the hormonal changes during a menstrual cycle are not uniform throughout the breast. This can cause some asymmetric findings on physical examination of the normal breast.

EPIDEMIOLOGY

As a result of widespread screening, breast cancer is the most commonly diagnosed cancer and the second leading cause of cancer deaths in women. The most common cause of death from cancer is lung cancer. Breast cancer in women under the age of 55 is an important cause of cancer death; however, half of all new cases and over half of the deaths occur in women over the age of 65 years. The estimated lifetime risk of developing breast cancer is now one out of every eight women.

RISK FACTORS FOR BREAST CANCER

The National Cancer Institute has developed a computer program that uses information to calculate a woman's estimated risk of breast cancer. This program can be found on the institute's website (http://cancertrials.nci.nih.gov).

Factors in the development of breast cancer include increased risk with increased age. The risk of breast cancer is greater with earlier onset of menarche (first menstrual period), which is the age that menstrual cycles begin. The age of the first live birth is important as the risk increases with later age of first pregnancy. Risk increases with the number of first-degree relatives with breast cancer. Prior breast biopsies, especially those showing atypical hyperplasia (abnormal cells on

microscopic exam), help to predict an increased risk of breast cancer. Race is important as the risk is greater in white females. African American women have a lesser risk of breast cancer followed by Hispanic American women. Japanese American women have the lowest risk of breast cancer. It is important for all women to understand that all are at risk for breast cancer and that the majority of women with breast cancer have no identifiable risk factors. Other established risk factors include rare genetic problems that account for 5–10% of breast cancers. These are called *BRCA-1* and *BRCA-2* gene mutations. Risk factors for women with a personal history of breast cancer include a history of some specific breast cancers (ductal or lobular carcinoma in situ), or a history of receiving high-dose radiation therapy at an age of younger than 40. Late age at menopause is another risk factor.

WHAT IS A MAMMOGRAM?

A mammogram is an x-ray of the breast tissue. The mammogram is reviewed by a radiologist, and if he/she finds an abnormality, may recommend other examinations. The mammogram should be scheduled during the time that the breasts are less likely to be tender. This will help to ensure that it is a more comfortable experience. It is important not to use deodorant, powder, lotion, or perfumes on the breasts or under the arms. Mammography is a simple procedure. The woman undergoing the exam undresses from the waist up and the breast is positioned on the x-ray machine and placed between two flat pieces of plastic. The breast is pressed between the plates for a few seconds while the x-ray picture is taken. The pressure is slightly uncomfortable to many women; however, it does not harm the breasts. It is x-rayed from the side and from above. The complete examination takes about 15 minutes.

An ultrasound examination utilizes sound waves to produce an image of the breast tissue. It is used to evaluate whether a lump is a fluid-filled cyst or a solid lump. Fluid-filled cysts are not cancerous. Solid lumps may or may not be a cancer. The next step for a solid lump is usually a biopsy, where a small amount of the tissue or the entire lump is removed and analyzed. It is important to note that most lumps are not cancer.

The average mammogram delivers between 0.7 and 1 rad (x-ray units of measure), which is a minimal amount of radiation. This is about 10% of the exposure delivered 20 years ago. While there is a miniscule increased risk of cancer due to the radiation, the far greater risk is in missing a curable cancer at an early stage.

As in many fields of medicine, there is ongoing reassessment of the way that we look for early cancers, and breast cancer is no exception. The National Guideline Clearinghouse provides a guideline synthesis compiling all the major guidelines for breast cancer screening. The American Cancer Society, the American College of Radiology, and the U.S. Preventive Services Task Force recommend routine mammographic screening for women between the ages of 50 and 69 years. The U.S. Preventive Services Task Force recommends annual or biannual screening, while the American Cancer Society recommends annual screening. The screening should begin earlier in women with high risk for breast cancer (including those having relatives with breast cancer). The organizations that evaluate screening agree that there is no clear age at which mammography should be no longer offered to patients. However, this decision should be made on an individual basis, based on the person's preference and her potential risks and benefits of the procedure. The main area of controversy is the mammographic screening of women between the ages of 40 and 49, who are at average risk for breast cancer. The American Cancer Society, the American College of Radiology, and the U.S. Preventive Services Task Force recommend routine screening in this age group. All three guideline groups acknowledged that the benefit of screening in women younger than 50 is weaker than the evidence for older women; however, they do support the screening. The recommended frequency of mammography in a woman in her 40s is every 1–2 years. This should be decided with her health care provider.

AT WHAT AGE SHOULD WE STOP GETTING MAMMOGRAMS?

Beyond the age of 70, the patient and her physician should make the decision. Frail elderly women with other life-limiting conditions may choose not to have this test performed.

Even though breast self-examination is not a proven way to screen for breast cancer, it is important to emphasize that women should be advised to report any breast changes that they may detect themselves to their physicians. It is important for the patient to look and feel for breast changes on her own.

BRCA-1 TESTING

In recent years, a breast cancer gene called *BRCA-1* has been identified and it carries an 85% lifetime risk of breast cancer and a 60% risk of ovarian cancer. These familial breast cancer syndromes account for less than 1 in 10 breast cancers. Even in women with several family members with breast cancer, routine screening for *BRCA-1* is negative more than 90% of the time. *BRCA-1* gene testing is not indicated in everyday practice, as there are no long-term data to support its use.

SEE ALSO: Breast cancer, Breast examination, Breast-feeding, Breast lumps, Lactation, Mastectomy

Suggested Resources

The American Cancer Society: www.cancer.org and National Comprehensive Cancer Network (NCCN): www.nccn.org
The National Cancer Institute: http://cancertrials.nci.nih.gov

KATHLEEN WOLNER

Manic Depressive Disorder *see* Bipolar Disorder

Marianismo   As projected, the most recent census data have confirmed that the Latino population has become the largest ethnic minority population in the United States. The increase in population reinforces the need for a greater understanding of cultural variables that impact the provision of culturally competent services. One of these variables is the concept of marianismo. The term *marianismo* originated in the anthropological literature and was used to describe the observed behavior of Latina women in Latino society. It implies that women are spiritually superior to men and subsequently able to withstand extreme sacrifices and suffering for the sake of the family. The self-sacrifice involved in this marianista identity, likened to martyrdom, enables the Latina woman in traditional Latino culture to gain respect and admiration from others. This is where she extracts her identity and power. In return for her suffering, she expects to be highly reinforced through others' esteem of her. The reinforcing

Marianismo

components of marianismo send strong messages about what is expected of the Latina woman.

In the mental health literature, Latino professionals discuss marianismo as a framework to help clinicians understand what Latina women are experiencing in mainstream American society. Practitioners found Latinas in treatment often presented with struggles involving cultural conflicts or differing sex role expectations. In treatment, marianismo is a cultural component that can guide understanding and therapeutic intervention with Latinas faced with negotiating these struggles.

Marianismo encompasses traditional cultural dictates related to sexuality, gender roles, family, motherhood, relationships, and behavior. Marianismo defines the Latina "role model" as the Virgin Mary, emphasizing virginity and nonsexuality for the "good" woman. The sexual messages Latinas receive within their cultural contexts tend to be intermixed with issues of duty, honor, security, self-worth, and control, but never with satisfaction or pleasure. The high value placed on sexual morality has great implications for Latinas being raised in the United States. For example, Latina adolescents may face conflict over the dominant society's dating norms and family's restrictions. In addition, traditional sexual mores may put the Latina at risk of sexually transmitted diseases by not questioning her partner's sexual behavior or securing her own sexual protection. It may also place them at risk of becoming victims of domestic violence. The risks identified above are due to: (a) males having the sexual and decision-making rights; (b) acceptance of male infidelity; (c) the denial of bisexuality in the Latino community; and (d) the submissiveness of Latinas.

The Latina is expected to sacrifice her needs for those of her family, especially her children. In traditional Latino culture, the Latina's value is increased when she becomes a mother. The Latina also gains power through subscribing to marianismo and exerting indirect manipulation through her children. It is not surprising then that, when there is a conflict over roles, the Latina will more likely choose the role of mother. These findings have implications for the attainment of both educational and professional goals. Researchers have found that Latinas who delayed marriage and family pursued a college career more often and tended to persist in college longer than women following traditional sex roles. Thus, the conflict between traditional roles of wife and mother and having a career may be particularly significant for Latina women.

Cultural conflicts arising from marianista values versus American values can cause psychological distress. Thus, Latina women must learn to reshape traditional role expectations in response to the majority's structural demands. The Latina must learn to negotiate conflicting values and begin identifying areas of change. The focus of this negotiation process is that of a person–environment fit. It does not place judgment or blame on the Latina. In practice, the clinician needs to be aware of this adjustment and role identification process, while continuing to recognize variability of marianismo values and conflicts within each Latina. The Latina must be able to envision herself as an agent of change in order to accept herself as a competent, successful, worthy Latina, capable of self-love. The Latina woman in the United States must learn to negotiate the components of her marianismo and decide on what she wants to retain, modify, or dismiss and in what environments she chooses to do any or all of the above.

The concept of marianismo is not without critics. Many believe that the term places a negative stereotype on Latina women and believe a more accurate description of marianismo is the concept of a traditional cultural value set. Whether one uses the term marianismo or the concept of values, like any descriptor of a group, both individual and group differences must be accounted for. Thus, it is not assumed that every Latina will have internalized every or any aspect of marianismo nor is it assumed that an "acculturated" or "assimilated" Latina does not struggle with cultural conflicts related to marianismo and American culture. In sum, while marianismo can aid understanding and boost culturally competent services, it is not to be used as a definitive label of the Latina.

SEE ALSO: Acculturation, Gender role, Latinos

Suggested Reading

Comas-Diaz, L. (1988). Mainland Puerto Rican women: A sociocultural approach. *Journal of Community Psychology, 16,* 21–31.

Gil, R. M., & Vazquez, C. I. (1996). *The Maria paradox.* New York: G. P. Putnam's Sons.

Martinez, R. O., & Dukes, R. L. (1997). The effects of ethnic identity, ethnicity, and gender on adolescent well-being. *Journal of Youth and Adolescence, 26,* 503–516.

Stevens, E. (1973). Machismo and marianismo. *Transaction-Society, 10,* 57–63.

Williams, N. (1988). Role making among married Mexican-American women: Issues of class and ethnicity. *The Journal of Applied and Behavioral Science, 24,* 203–217.

MELISSA RIVERA MARANO

Marijuana

Marijuana or hemp (*Cannabis sativa*) is a plant that has been cultivated for thousands of years in various parts of the world for its fiber, seeds, medicinal, and psychoactive properties. The chemical compounds responsible for the intoxicating and therapeutic effects are found in the sticky resin released from the flowers of female plants. The marijuana plant contains more than 400 known compounds of which about 60 have a structure similar to cannabinoids. The main psychoactive substance is generally believed to be delta-9-tetrahydrocannabinol (THC). Cannabinoids act on a specific receptor that is widely distributed in the brain regions involved in cognition, memory, pain perception, and motor coordination.

Marijuana ("grass," "weed," "pot") is prepared by drying the leaves and the flowering tops of the plant, and may be smoked in a rolled cigarette ("joint"), in a pipe, or, more recently, in a cigar ("blunt"). Hashish consists of dried cannabis resin and generally contains higher levels of THC. Cannabis preparations may also be eaten or drunk as a tea, but smoking is the easiest way to achieve the desired psychoactive effects.

In the United States and most of the developed world, cannabis is an illegal substance and is primarily used for its psychoactive properties. However, for centuries marijuana has been used in various parts of the world not only as an intoxicating agent but also as a medicinal substance.

From 1850 until 1937, cannabis was used in American medical practice for a wide range of conditions. The Marijuana Tax Act of 1937 introduced the first federal restrictions on marijuana and outlawed the nonmedicinal, untaxed possession or sale of the drug. The Comprehensive Drug Abuse Prevention and Control Act of 1970 classified marijuana as a Schedule I controlled substance. Since then, there have been several attempts to legalize its medical use. In 1987, the Food and Drug Administration approved dronabinol, a compound containing synthetic THC, as a Schedule II controlled substance for treatment of chemotherapy-induced nausea and vomiting.

In the United States, cannabis became a major drug of abuse in the late 1960s, with peak usage occurring in the late 1970s and early 1980s. According to the Monitoring the Future Survey, in 1979, about 51% of high school seniors reported having used marijuana at least once in the past 12 months. The lowest levels of use occurred in 1992 with about 22% reporting annual use. The 1990s saw the resurgence of use, and annual prevalence rates peaked in 1997 reaching almost 40% among twelfth-grade students. Currently, marijuana is the most commonly used illicit drug in the United States according to the 2001 edition of the National Household Survey on Drug Abuse.

Despite the fact that cannabis is one of the most widely used psychoactive substances in the world, its health and psychological effects are still not well understood and remain the subject of much debate. Due to its legal status, clinical studies of marijuana are difficult to conduct. As a result, data on the adverse effects of the drug are more extensive than data on its therapeutic effectiveness.

Cannabinoids produce a variety of acute psychological effects in humans. THC is rapidly absorbed into the bloodstream after smoking, and acute peak effects appear between 10 and 60 min, diminishing substantially over the next 2–4 hr. Oral administration is slower to take effect and lasts longer. Psychological effects (being "high" or "stoned") are usually characterized by euphoria and relaxation coupled with the intensification of ordinary sensory experiences, including sexual activity. Short-term memory and attention, motor skills, and reaction time are also impaired while a person is intoxicated. High doses of the drug can facilitate anxiety, paranoia, and panic in both experienced and naive users.

For a long time it was thought that marijuana dependence was not possible. Recent research suggests tolerance and withdrawal, and therefore dependence, may occur in long-term, high-dose (daily) users; however, it is not seen in casual or moderate users. The symptoms of withdrawal may include irritability, insomnia, restlessness, loss of appetite, and more, but none are life threatening.

Physiological effects are many and varied but particularly noteworthy for individuals with cardiovascular problems, since the fluctuations in blood pressure and increases in heart rate exacerbate those problems. There are no reports of deaths that are directly linked to cannabis overdose from its acute effects in healthy adults. A number of in vitro and in vivo studies suggested that the immune system may be impaired after exposure to cannabis. However, the clinical significance of these changes is not well understood, and there is no conclusive evidence that consumption of cannabis impairs human immune function. Studies conducted with HIV-positive homosexual men have shown that cannabis use was not associated with an increased risk of development of AIDS among HIV-infected individuals.

Although there is a paucity of information on gender-specific marijuana effects, some evidence suggests that cannabis affects sex hormones. In animal studies, chronic administration of high doses of THC lowers testosterone secretion, impairs sperm production in males, and disrupts the ovulation cycle in females. However, evidence of the effects of cannabis on human fertility is inconclusive. Suffice it to say, individuals experiencing fertility problems would benefit from remaining abstinent from cannabis.

In some parts of the world, cannabis preparations were thought to have therapeutic value in childbirth and pregnancy. In modern medical practice, cannabis is considered to have damaging effects on the fetus. Numerous studies have explored cannabis as a perinatal risk factor, but the results of these studies have been contradictory, and it was difficult to isolate the effects of cannabis from many other variables that could influence the outcomes of pregnancy. Nevertheless, new clinical studies suggest that prenatal exposure to cannabinoids does result in adverse consequences for the offspring. However, these defects are subtle and are not apparent immediately after birth. Again, for pregnant or breast-feeding women, abstinence from cannabis should be the norm.

Advocates of the medical marijuana movement argue that cannabis has numerous therapeutic properties and is less toxic and more effective than some conventional therapies. Considerable debate exists in this area and will not be resolved soon, in large part because there is a lack of clinical studies to evaluate potential benefits and adverse effects in comparison to other existing therapies.

SEE ALSO: Addiction, Substance use

Suggested Reading

Adams, I. B., & Martin, B. R. (1996). Cannabis: Pharmacology and toxicology in animals and humans. *Addiction, 91,* 1585–1614.

Grinspoon, L., & Bakalar, J. (1997). *Marijuana, the forbidden medicine.* New Haven, CT: Yale University Press.

Hollister, L. E. (1998). Health aspects of cannabis: Revisited. *International Journal of Neuropsychopharmacology, 1,* 71–90.

Joy, J. E., Watson, S. J., & Benson, J. A. (Eds.). (1999). *Marijuana and medicine: Assessing the science base.* Washington, DC: National Academy Press.

Mathre, M. L. (Ed.). (1997). *Cannabis in medical practice: A legal, historical and pharmacological overview of the therapeutic use of marijuana.* Jefferson, NC: McFarland.

Onaivi, E. S. (Ed.). (2002). *Biology of marijuana: From gene to behavior.* London: Taylor & Francis.

RAMINTA DANIULAITYTE

Marital Status   Sociologists refer to marital status as an achieved characteristic, in the sense that marital behavior is socially defined and influenced, rather than having any biological properties. Children are typically assumed to be single (never married), whereas adults are generally classified as being single, married, separated, divorced, or widowed, although of course people may change categories at various times in their lives. Virtually every human society assumes that most people will marry when they become adults, and social and biological reproduction tend to take place in the family unit formed by married people.

Data from the 2000 Census in the United States show that 24% of females aged 15 and older had never been married, a slight increase from 23% in the 1990 census. Almost half of women (49%) were currently married with a spouse present in 2000, while 16% were separated or divorced, and 10% were widowed. These figures vary by age, of course, with divorce and especially widowhood increasing with age. Globally, the average age at marriage for women is a key determinant of their social status, and even in the United States, the Current Population Survey in 2000 found that women were marrying 4 years later in life than they had in 1970. In 2000, the median age at first marriage was 25.1 years for women and 26.8 years for men, while in 1970, the corresponding figures were 20.8 and 23.2.

The postponement of marriage has led to a substantial increase in the proportion of young, never-married adults. For example, between 1970 and 2000, the proportion of those who had never married doubled for women ages 20–24, from 36% to 73%, and more than tripled for women ages 30–34, from 6% to 22%. Among existing marriages, the divorce rate has stabilized since the 1980s, with about 40% of marriages likely to end in divorce in the United States.

Marital status is an important factor (along with education, race, and age) influencing labor force participation and differences in economic well-being of households. Single women without children spend a far larger proportion of time over their life cycle in labor market activity, increasing economic inequality among women. However, families headed by females, especially those with children, are among the poorest households in the United States. The obvious disadvantage is that a household with only one earner (e.g., a single mother) will have fewer resources than a household with two or more earners. However, the impact may go beyond that. Research has also demonstrated that family and other social networks can help people find employment and meet basic needs. Many types of resources flow to individuals who have strong network attachments, including childcare, help in emergencies, and resources that allow people to undertake new endeavors such as school enrollment or the purchase of a new home. Married people, who have greater material resources, also have larger support networks, both in the number and the variety of sources of support. Those who have never married and have lower human capital are most likely to reside with relatives or friends. Resources from family and others outside the household are an important income source for low-income single mothers.

The relationship between marital status and health has been a topic of interest for some time. It has been shown in the United States as well as in several other countries that married persons have lower rates of mortality, morbidity, and mental disorders than the unmarried. Among the unmarried, there are several patterns of health differentials. When self-reported health status and health conditions are used, the divorced and separated have the highest rates of poor health, followed by the widowed. Rates of mental illness are lowest for the married and never married, followed by the divorced, widowed, and, finally, the separated.

There are two widely accepted explanations about the relationship between marital status and health: (a) marriage selection and (b) marriage protection. Marriage selection refers to the differential selection into and out of marriage. Generally, spouses may be selected into marriage based on the absence of physical and mental disability, as well as on a range of health-related characteristics such as emotional stability, risk-taking personality, income, and physical appearance. On the other hand, marriage may protect against poor health in several ways. Marriage may strengthen social integration; provide a source of instrumental support for tasks like household work; increase economic resources; contribute to the pool of knowledge and important information processing; and may provide practical assistance and care, especially when a member of the family gets sick. The presence of a spouse may also discourage risky behaviors such as heavy drinking and substance abuse and encourage healthy behaviors like adherence to medical regimens. It is often found that smoking and alcohol abuse are more common among the unmarried, and in particular, the divorced.

Married people may also benefit from emotional rewards from family relationships. However, changes in marital status, such as the death of a spouse, may also be harmful. Such psychological factors may well influence various important lifestyle factors, and thus contribute to a weakening of the patient's physical health. Marital disruption, a particularly stressful life event, elevates the risk of psychological distress thereby contributing over the longer run to poor physical health outcomes. In that case, widowhood, divorce, and separation elevate the risk of poor health compared with marriage (and being never married).

Some researchers have found that marriage tends to be more beneficial to the health of men than of women, whereas others conclude that both sexes benefit equally from marriage, but perhaps for different reasons. Women's marital status is an important predictor of some categories of health problems; however, their influences vary for women of different age. It is observed that divorce and poor female health status are highly correlated in those societies where divorce is uncommon and discouraged, because the divorce decision is usually taken after many difficult years, which can be damaging to health. It has also been suggested by several studies that differences in economic well-being account for much of the difference in marital status and health for women, because with high economic status, women can afford to buy health insurance, housing, and nutrition.

Unmarried men engage in well-established risky health behaviors, including heavy drinking, drinking and driving, substance abuse, and marijuana use, and consequently are more likely to have physiological markers of cardiovascular disease, such as high blood pressure and worse cholesterol levels, than married men. However, the association between marital status and these risk factors is weaker and less consistent for women. The health advantages of marital status probably vary by race and ethnicity. Several researchers suggest, for example, that divorce impacts the mental health of black women less than for white women because divorced black women experience less stigmatization and more support from family and friends than divorced white women.

SEE ALSO: Ethnicity, Morbidity, Mortality, Socioeconomic status

Suggested Reading

Beckett, M. K., & Elliott, M. N. (2002). *Does the association between marital status and health vary by sex, race, and ethnicity?* http://www.rand.org/labor/DRU/DRU2869.pdf

Masculinity

Hibbard, J. H., & Pope, C. R. (1993). Health effects of discontinuities in female employment and marital status. *Social Science and Medicine, 36,* 1099–1104.

Jacobsen, J. P., & Levin, L. M. (2000). The effects of internal migration on the relative economic status of women and men. *Journal of Socio-Economics, 29,* 291–304.

U.S. Department of Health and Human Services, Health Resources and Services Administration (HRSA), Maternal and Child Health Bureau, Women's Health 2002 USA. http://www.mchb.hrsa.gov/whusa02/

Zandvakili, S. (2000). Dynamics of earnings inequality among female-headed households in the United States. *Journal of Socio-Economics, 29,* 73–89.

YUYING LI
JOHN R. WEEKS

Marriage Counseling *see* Couples Therapy, Divorce Mediation, Psychotherapy

---

Masculinity Masculinity defies a simple definition. It is typically represented as a set of stereotypical characteristics that constitutes an energy, an essence, or a state of being. But in this case, the whole would appear to be greater than the sum of its parts. We recognize masculinity when it is encountered, but it is difficult to distill the interacting components into a single, unifying definition that can be applied uniformly.

The most commonly encountered representation of masculinity is best described by sex-role theory, which proposes that humans unconsciously integrate archetypical ways of behaving that are appropriate to their assigned sex from society's institutions (see Femininity). Sex-role theory characterizes masculinity as aggressive, rational, dominant, and objective, and organizes it as the polar opposite of femininity. However, life is not so simple. Instead, a majority of men and women in a given society at a particular point in time will endorse a hegemonic masculinity. This means that social processes are organized in cultures to maintain masculine power by ensuring that subordinate groups view male dominance as fair, reasonable, and in the best interests of society.

Despite varying standards of masculinity throughout history, it has always tended to define itself as different from and superior to femininity. In contemporary U.S. culture, hegemonic masculinity is exemplified by physical strength and bravado, suppression of vulnerability, economic independence, authority over women and other men, and exclusive heterosexuality with associated objectification of women. The fact that few men actually embody all of these qualities is of no consequence. U.S. society supports hegemonic masculinity in its institutions.

Societies tend to value masculinity over femininity. This is exemplified by the extraordinary efforts in which couples engage throughout the world to ensure that they produce at least one son. Furthermore, societies expend tremendous amounts of energy to guarantee that most males do not stray into the feminine realm and will idolize hegemonic masculinity. Additionally, the stereotypical traits embodied within hegemonic masculinity also are not valued equally. For example, gay men may exemplify all of the qualities of hegemonic masculinity, but because they fail on the most valued trait—exclusive heterosexuality—they are not considered *real men.*

Hegemonic masculinity reinforces the division of labor between males and females. Perhaps the most graphic example of this is that when men enter occupations dominated by women, such as nursing and elementary school teaching, they receive better salaries, are promoted faster, and are afforded more respect than their female colleagues. Therefore, despite all of the advances achieved through the hard work and dedication of feminists, power is still solidly within the realm of masculinity. How is this possible? Men have adjusted their relationship to women by accommodating superficial changes but they have not allowed genuine reform. Thus, within the paradoxical context of real progress, hegemonic masculinity has managed to hold and consolidate its privileges.

New movements have recently emerged that attempt to reject hegemonic masculinity in lieu of moving toward a more inclusive social framework. A notable example is the Mankind Project Network. This framework defines a mature masculinity as one that integrates archetypical representations of king, warrior, magician, and lover, and seeks to confront the destructive shadow side of each. For example, the warrior archetype consists of two opposite and equally destructive poles—the sadist and the masochist. A mature masculinity seeks to integrate the opposite poles for each of the four archetypes and find a center between them. The Mankind Project Network relies on the use of ritual and rites of passage as a means of connecting men to their growth process and the expression of moral and ethical behavior within society.

It remains to be seen if these new masculine movements represent a true reform of hegemonic masculinity or if they merely are a new form of accommodation to women that will result in consolidating male dominance.

SEE ALSO: Femininity, Feminism, Gender, Gender role, Homosexuality

Suggested Reading

Connell, R. W. (1999). *Masculinities.* Berkeley: University of California Press.

Moore, R. L., & Gillette, D. (1991). *King, warrior, magician, lover: Rediscovering the archetypes of the mature masculine.* San Francisco: Harper.

Pattatucci, A. M. (1998). *Women in science: Meeting career challenges.* Thousand Oaks, CA: Sage.

ANGELA PATTATUCCI ARAGON

Massage
Massage is derived from the Arabic word *mass* meaning *to press* and has been defined by Westland (1993) as *the aware and conscience manipulation of soft tissues of the body for therapeutic purposes.* Many ancient cultures developed various systems of massage to promote health and healing. Contemporary approaches of massage have included bodywork techniques such as strain–counterstrain, myofascial release, craniosacral therapy, shiatsu, acupressure, Rolfing, and applied kinesiology.

Some women may consider massage to be a luxury; a form of self-indulgence to deal with tension and feel more relaxed. Others may think about massage as a way to manage more specific conditions such as pain, swelling, scar tissue adherence, and muscle or tendon tightness. Knowing and distinguishing between the different benefits that can be derived from various massage approaches can help women determine the best intervention for their given condition or goal. Women will also find it helpful to be familiar with the wide range of practitioners who are skillful in applying massage for a variety of purposes and conditions. Examples of such practitioners include physical therapists, nurses, chiropractors, osteopaths, athletic trainers, and massage therapists.

For the purposes of this entry, massage will be limited to classical Western massage, which includes techniques that have ancient roots, but have been used traditionally in Europe and the United States since the 19th century. The application of massage may produce multiple and/or simultaneous effects. The benefits of massage and the effects of massage have been well described in the scientific literature, and are summarized in Table 1.

Women should be aware that the effects depicted in Table 1 do not necessarily occur with every massage session and individual results may vary based on age,

Table 1. Benefits and effects of massage

Effect	Description	Benefits/outcomes
Mechanical	Movement of body fluids, such as blood and lymph Movement of soft tissue, such as muscle, scar, tendons	↓ Edema (fluid accumulation) ↓ Swelling ↓ Pain ↑ Flexibility of tissues ↑ Mobility
Physiological	At the cellular level, increase flow of nutrients and removal of waste products	↑ Mobility ↓ Edema ↓ Swelling ↓ Pain ↓ Muscle spasm
Psychological/emotional	Promotion of relaxation, decreased anxiety, decreased depression	Relief of pain Relief of stress Release of tension Increased body awareness
Immunological	Enhance immune function and improved cell function	↑ Relaxation ↓ Anxiety ↓ Pain ↓ Cortisol

health status, and receptivity. Women, therefore, should be clear about the benefits they are hoping to achieve through massage. It is recommended that a woman choose a practitioner who not only can examine a client's status, and is skillful in applying massage techniques, but is also able to determine if massage will help the client achieve her goals.

Massage has been used as an intervention or approach to address a wide range of health issues prevalent in women. Some of these health concerns include stress, anxiety, depression, and headaches; gynecological issues such as fibroids and pregnancy/labor and delivery; and premature or low-birthweight infants.

The most compelling benefit of massage is in the area of stress reduction and health promotion. Stress can be defined as a general feeling of fatigue and tension. Psychological consequences of stress can include decreased coping behaviors and alteration of mood patterns. Physiological changes associated with stress include hypertension (high blood pressure); increased respiratory rate and heart rate; changes in levels of glucose, cortisol, adrenaline/noadrenaline; and alterations in blood flow rates to muscle.

In addition to cognitive and behavioral therapies, effective stress management often includes massage as a strategy that can promote relaxation by heightening body awareness and increasing sensory feedback. In several studies, massage has been demonstrated to be effective in reducing both hypertension and rapid respiration. Anxiety and depression are conditions that are distinct from stress, but frequently accompany stressful situations. Symptoms common to anxiety are muscle tension, heart palpitation, sweating, and insomnia. Symptoms common to depression include decreased concentration, irritability, and insomnia. Often a combination of symptoms is presented. As anxiety, depression, or stress become chronic, women are likely to respond to muscle tension, pain, and fatigue with abnormal sitting and standing postures as well as changes in movement patterns. Massage would then be used as a tool to produce the additional changes needed for proper body alignment as well as the necessary physiological and psychological changes.

Researchers have investigated massage as an intervention for depression in subjects with a history of sexual abuse, eating disorders, and postpartum depression. In these studies, massage appears to be helpful in reducing depression and anxiety associated with the given disorder. In some instances, positive changes in

body awareness and body image, and a reduction of stress hormone levels have been noted.

Many women suffer from recurring tension and migraine headaches, which may or may not be associated with stress. Several researchers have demonstrated that massage, when administered as part of a pain management regimen, is beneficial for reducing the severity and duration of headaches. Although the mechanism as to how massage can affect headaches requires additional investigation, researchers suggest that massage can directly affect the soft tissue impairments that lead to abnormal muscular tension and irregular blood flow patterns commonly found with headaches and migraines.

Pregnancy, along with labor and delivery can be responsible for trauma and disorders of the female musculoskeletal and urogenital systems. Back pain during pregnancy, which is often due to postural changes and joint laxity, can frequently be improved with a combination of massage, exercise, posture training, and proper positioning. Historically, massage during labor was used to assist in uterine contractions and movement of the baby's position. Today, the purpose of massage during labor and delivery is to promote relaxation and pain reduction. Researchers have demonstrated that women receiving 20-minute massages every hour during labor report fewer depressed moods, less stress, and less pain compared to women not receiving massages.

Perineal massage is a specific type of massage performed directly to the perineum, the area between the vulva and the anus. Many obstetrician/gynecologists advocate the use of perineal massage to reduce the risk of tearing the perineum during delivery as well as to reduce the need for an episiotomy, a procedure in which the obstetrician surgically cuts the vulva to prevent it from tearing. During pregnancy, women are taught perineal massage and are encouraged to practice it on a regular basis. At the time of delivery, her obstetrician further performs the massage. At present, there are conflicting findings regarding the benefit of perineal massage, although women often report satisfaction with the technique in preparing both physically and psychologically for birth.

For new mothers of premature infants, massage has been demonstrated to facilitate the infant's growth and development. In several studies, premature infants who receive massage have shown improvement in motor function, greater weight gain, and better sleep cycles. The positive effects of massage frequently found in adults, such as a lower heart rate, decreased respirations, and a reduction of stress hormones, are also found in the infants who receive massage. Often the newborn's mother is trained to perform massage with her baby both in the hospital and at home.

There are additional gynecological disorders for which massage may be clinically applied. The effectiveness of massage application for scar management of fibroids, infertility due to scar adhesions, and cosmetic breast scars has yet to be expanded and explored. Further research is needed in these areas. It should be mentioned that massage does not produce changes in subcutaneous fat distribution, cellulite, or change in body contours.

The benefits of massage have been well documented in the scientific literature. To reduce stress and improve overall health, women should consider working with a practitioner who can administer therapeutic massage as part of a health and wellness program. Women who are pregnant should explore massage for its physiological and psychological benefits. Regardless of one's condition, however, it is important to find a practitioner who can examine your condition and assist you in determining if massage will help you reach your desired outcome or goal.

See Also: Anxiety disorders, Depression, Headache, Migraine, Pregnancy, Stress

Suggested Reading

Andrade, C., & Clifford, P. (2001). *Outcome based massage.* New York: Lippincott, Williams & Wilkins.

Freeman, L. W., & Lawlis, G. F. (2001). *Mosby's complementary & alternative medicine: A research-based approach.* St. Louis, MO: Mosby.

Giovanni, D. D., & Wood, E. (1997). *Beard's massage.* Philadelphia: W. B. Saunders.

Holey, E., & Cook, E. (1997). *Therapeutic massage.* Great Britain: The Bath Press.

Westland, G. (1993). Massage as a therapeutic tool: Part 1, *British Journal of Occupational Therapy, 56*(1), 129–180.

Susan Paparella-Pitzel
Ellen Zambo-Anderson

Mastectomy
Mastectomy is a surgical procedure which involves the removal of either the entire breast or a segment of the breast. Usually performed for cancer of the breast, it can also be used for prophylactic removal of the breast for women who are at high risk of developing breast cancer.

Breast cancer begins as a local disease in the breast and if not treated spreads (metastasizes) to other parts of the body. The idea of removing the breast or a part of it goes as far back as Vesalius in the 16th century. Currently the type of surgery performed is determined by the extent or "stage" of the cancer.

STAGES OF BREAST CANCER

Stage 0 (in situ). This includes ductal or lobular carcinoma in situ (CIS), which is noninvasive cancer, and Paget's disease, which is a local cancer of the nipple. There are two types of in situ: (a) intraductal (DCIS) which is noninvasive ductal carcinoma and (b) lobular CIS which is precancerous, more often multicentric (found throughout the breast), more often in both breasts.

Stage I. Early cancer, the tumor is 2 cm (3/4 of an inch) or smaller with no evidence of tumor in the axillary lymph nodes (under the arm) and no distant metastasis.

Stage II. Tumor size is 2–5 cm (3/4–2 in.), lymph nodes may be positive or not; but if the nodes are positive in a tumor less than 2 cm in size, this would qualify as Stage II.

Stage III. III A: The tumor is smaller than 5 cm (2 in.); axillary nodes are positive and it has spread to other lymph nodes; or the tumor is larger than 5 cm and has spread to the lymph nodes under the arm. III B: The cancer has spread outside the breast to the chest wall, muscles, and skin, or the cancer has spread to lymph nodes inside the chest wall near the breast.

Stage IV. There is evidence of distant metastasis to other organs usually the bones, lungs, liver, or brain regardless of size.

TYPES OF SURGICAL PROCEDURES

The surgical technique that was used for the greater part of the 20th century was the radical mastectomy described by Dr. William Halstead in 1894 in the Johns Hopkins Hospital Report. This surgery involved removing the entire breast, skin and chest wall (pectoralis major) muscles, the contents of the axilla (under the arm), and skin, and required an extensive skin graft. Results with this form of surgery resulted in an immediate and drastic decrease in chest wall recurrences. Research in the 1970s and 1980s showed that there was no advantage to removing the chest wall muscles and a new surgical technique, the "modified radical mastectomy," virtually replaced the radical mastectomy. By 1990, only 0.4% of all surgeries for breast cancer were of the radical mastectomy type. Modified radical mastectomy involves a total mastectomy, removing the breast, nipple, and areola with removal of 10–20 lymph nodes under the arm, called an axillary lymph node dissection, without removing the major chest wall muscles. The surgery takes approximately 2–3 hr and breast reconstruction can be performed immediately. It became the most popular surgery for early stage cancers, if the tumor is 5 cm or greater, if the skin or muscle is involved, or four or more axillary lymph nodes are positive for cancer cells.

Total mastectomy without removing the axillary lymph nodes is used for extensive ductal CIS or in invasive cancer when the sentinel lymph node (see below) is negative.

BREAST CONSERVATION THERAPY

More recently, breast conservation therapy (BCT) is being used. This involves combining two modalities: breast conserving surgery, also known as lumpectomy, with 5–7 weeks of postoperative irradiation.

The goal of BCT is local control of the cancer and maintenance of a cosmetically normal appearance of the breast. It was demonstrated in the 1980s to have equal risks of recurrence compared to mastectomy. In 1990, a Consensus Development Statement by the National Institutes of Health recommended lumpectomy for as many as 50–75% of women with early breast cancer.

Breast conserving surgery, the first phase of BCT, also called wide local excision or lumpectomy, leaves a safety margin of healthy breast tissue. It can be done under local or general anesthesia in a standard operating room or an outpatient surgery center and takes approximately 1 hr. The specimen is sent to pathology to assess that the margins of the specimen are without tumor ("clear").

Contraindications to lumpectomy are: (a) the presence of more than one tumor, or if there are suspicious areas of calcifications, small specks of calcium demonstrated on mammography, elsewhere in the breast, (b) if the tumor is so large or the breast so small that cosmetic results following surgery would not be satisfactory, (c) if the tumor is found to extend beyond the margins of the tissue that was removed, (d) if the woman is not willing to have radiation therapy after surgery or has had prior irradiation to the breast or chest wall, or if there is no access to radiation treatment in the community. Collagen vascular disease such as scleroderma poses a risk to irradiation. It cannot be performed for women if they are pregnant. However, if a woman is pregnant in the 2nd or 3rd trimester, she may have surgery and chemotherapy and postpone irradiation until after delivery. Finally, if a woman would prefer to have a mastectomy rather than BCT, she should be given that choice.

SENTINEL LYMPH NODE BIOPSY

This procedure, which has been added to the armamentarium of breast cancer treatment within the past decade, involves obtaining a tissue sample from the sentinel node, the "first lymph node," which drains lymphatic fluid from the breast. It is performed only if there is a single tumor less than 5 cm, the woman has not had prior chemotherapy or hormone therapy, and the lymph nodes feel normal. The surgeon injects either a blue dye or a radioactive substance into the area around the tumor. The lymphatic vessels carry the dye to the first lymph node which is then examined microscopically for the presence of cancer cells. If the node is positive for malignant cells, the surgeon will then proceed with an axillary lymph node dissection.

Potential side effects of axillary lymph node dissection include lymphedema, which is a painful swelling of the involved arm caused by scarring around the lymph duct with resulting limitation of movement and function. The advantage of performing a sentinel node biopsy is that if it is free of cancer there is no need for further axillary lymph node removal.

PSYCHOLOGICAL EFFECTS OF MASTECTOMY

All women diagnosed with breast cancer will experience some degree of emotional distress. It was previously thought that the emotional trauma from breast cancer was the result of the physical disfigurement of amputating the breast. However, with the advent of BCT, it has been shown that despite a better body image, the psychological trauma comes from having a potentially fatal disease.

Women faced with the decision of whether to choose breast conserving surgery versus a mastectomy also carry the psychological burden of having to make the "right choice." The fear of leaving behind cancer cells in a breast or the fear of undergoing irradiation therapy with its side effects of fatigue and vulnerability to depression may prompt a woman to choose a mastectomy. Availability of support groups and individual counseling can help a woman through this very difficult time.

Sexual difficulties may be anticipated in women regardless of whether they have had breast conserving surgery with irradiation or mastectomy with reconstruction. Pain or numbness in the breast or chest wall after surgery with reconstruction will decrease sexual interest. Some women who choose mastectomy without reconstruction may be embarrassed for their partners to see their scar and avoid intimacy. Women should be encouraged to discuss these issues with their partner and health care providers so that referrals to specialty consultants can be made.

A woman's style of coping, which includes attitudes of optimism or pessimism, the availability of social and family support, a woman's ability to discuss emotional issues with her physician, and the way she felt about her body prior to the diagnosis of cancer, all determine her psychological response to breast cancer regardless of whether she has conservative surgery or mastectomy.

SEE ALSO: Body image, Breast examination, Breast-feeding, Breast lumps, Mammography

Suggested Reading

American Cancer Society. (2002, September). *National Comprehensive Cancer Network, Breast Cancer Treatment Guidelines for Patients*, Version IV.

Cody, H. S. (2002). Current surgical management of breast cancer. *Current Opinion in Obstetrics and Gynecology, 14*, 45–52.

Donega, W. L., & Spratt, J. S. (2002). *Cancer of the breast* (5th ed.). Philadelphia: W. B. Saunders.

LaTour, K. (1993). *The breast cancer companion*. New York: Morrow.

Rabinowitz, B. (2002). Understanding and intervening in breast cancer's emotional and sexual side effects. *Current Women's Health Reports, 2*, 140–147.

Rowland, J., & Massie, M. J. (1998). Breast cancer. In J. D. Holland (Ed.), *Psycho-oncology* (pp. 380–401). New York: Oxford University Press.

Sakorafas, G. H. (2001). Breast cancer surgery. *Acta Oncologica, 40*(1), 5–18.

M. MacDougall

Mastitis Mastitis, by definition, is inflammation of the mammary gland. It can occur in any woman; however, it is most common in first-time lactating mothers. This condition is a result of bacterial invasion of breast tissue. Mastitis rarely occurs in the antepartum period (before birth of the baby). Its incidence includes 1–2% of primiparas (first-time mothers) who are postpartum and lactating. It usually occurs 2–4 weeks after delivery.

The presenting symptoms of mastitis include malaise (general sick feeling), fatigue, chills, muscle aches, or localized breast tenderness. The condition progresses to symptoms like fever of greater than 102°F, tachycardia (rapid heartbeat), and a firm, reddened area of breast tenderness. Mastitis is usually preceded by marked engorgement of the affected breast, and is almost always unilateral (one-sided). The most common area of the breast that is affected is the outer quadrant.

Common causes of mastitis include bacteria from the baby's mouth, bacteria entering via breast injuries (bruising, fissures, cracks in the nipple), milk stasis (milk pooling in the breast), and bacteria from the hands of the mother or health care provider. The most common organisms associated with mastitis are the bacterial organisms *Staphylococcus aureus* and beta-hemolytic streptococci. Concurrent infection with mumps is also found to be a cause of mastitis.

Some contributing factors associated with mastitis are: fatigue, stress, lack of sleep, plugged ducts, engorgement, a decrease in number of feedings, inadequate nutrition, breast trauma, and breast constriction by a tight brassiere. Thus, teaching about preventive measures is the most important treatment. Preventive measures include resting when the infant rests, as well as teaching the importance of maternal nutrition, increased fluid intake, and vitamin supplementation. Lactating women require large caloric requirements as a result of milk production and tissue healing from delivery. Proper hand washing, perhaps with an antibacterial soap, should be encouraged. One of the most important preventive measures to emphasize is good breast-feeding habits. For example, early and frequent feedings with complete emptying of breasts will decrease the likelihood of blocked ducts and milk stasis. Proper positioning of the baby on the breast, along with good latch on, could prevent nipple trauma. Lastly, breast care measures include: cleansing with water only and drying adequately, and wearing a nonconstricting, well-ventilated bra.

Treatment for mastitis includes Tylenol for reduction of fever, inflammation, and pain along with antibiotic therapy with penicillin or a cephalosporin. The mother should be instructed to complete the entire antibiotic prescription, even if symptoms subside quickly. She should be assured that breast-feeding can and should be continued in both breasts. Breast-feeding with an infection will not harm the newborn, nor will the antibiotics used for treatment. Both the use of warm compresses and massaging the affected area may help encourage milk drainage toward the nipple. Supportive care, rest, and decreasing stress will also help hasten recovery. The importance of prompt treatment should be stressed. If left untreated, a more serious complication, such as breast abscess, can occur.

SEE ALSO: Breast-feeding, Lactation

Suggested Reading

Auerbach, K. G., & Riordan, J. (1993). *Breastfeeding and human lactation* (pp. 382–384). Sudbury, MA: Jones & Bartlett.

Clark, Cunningham, Gant, Gilstrap, Hankins, Leveno, MacDonald. (1997). *Williams obstetrics* (20th ed., pp. 564–565). Stamford, CT: Appleton & Lange.

Smith, A. BA, IBCLC. (2001). *Breast infections and plugged ducts.* http://www.obgyn.net/pb/articles/bf_smith_1201.htm

Varney, H. (1997). *Varney's midwifery* (3rd ed., pp. 677–678). Sudbury, MA: Jones & Bartlett.

MARYANNE E. MARKOWSKI

Masturbation   Masturbation is self-stimulation of the genitals, energized by fantasy that leads to sexual arousal and orgasm. In addition to generating sexual desire leading to masturbation, sexual fantasies are created, refined, lustily sanctioned, and at a woman's caprice, discarded or retained for future use. Masturbation and fantasy influence one another and are inextricably linked. Historically, masturbation has been labeled as sexually deviant behavior and a social taboo despite its common practice. But as social and moral codes have modernized, masturbation's positive role and importance in sexual health has been endorsed. We now believe it is a normal behavior that most people have practiced at various frequencies throughout the life span.

The mental processes and fantasies determining masturbatory behavior illuminate intimate aspects of a woman's sexual desire. As an infant, localized genital sensations are noted to be pleasurable, help soothe distressing mental states, and are believed to foster development of positive self-regard and bodily image (Levine, 1992). As the young girl learns more control over bodily processes and experiences more complex life situations with sexual themes, she consciously and unconsciously links her mental (fantasy) life with bodily sensations and pleasure. During adolescence and early adulthood, continued exploration of her sexual interests, frequently with an increased role of masturbation, results in the assembly of sexual self-knowledge and facilitates the consolidation of her sexual identity. As an adult, masturbation becomes a conscious means of autonomous self-regulation of bodily sensations and emotional states. Sensual pleasure becomes familiar.

The knowledge she has acquired about masturbation, and sex in general, allows her to make more choices about partner sex. She recognizes that she can be responsible for her own sexual pleasure but may choose to allow her partner to pleasure her. If the goal is orgasm, many women find that masturbatory clitoral stimulation heightens arousal, facilitates orgasm, and can easily be taught to their partners. For a large subset of women, it is the sole means of reaching an orgasm, with or without intercourse. Since masturbation and sexual fantasies are extremely private sexual information, sharing and teaching her partner what pleases her fosters greater mutuality and intimacy for the couple. As the adult woman matures, her sexual creativity evolves and the content of her masturbatory fantasy life changes, altering her behavioral patterns of pleasure. Communication of these changes to her partner helps ward off sexual boredom, fosters continued interest, and deepens intimacy. Men tend to have a more fixed sexual fantasy life over the life span, adding increased importance to the woman's sexual creativity for herself and the couple. Throughout the life span, masturbation can function as a substitute for partner sex.

There is no correct way to masturbate. What stimulates one woman may not work for another: it is individually determined. Physical stimuli such as fingers or vibrators guided to provide a particular type of touch seem to be the most effective and common practice. Most young men do not routinely think about different types of touch associated with masturbation and sexuality, they "just do it." With instruction and patience, they learn to enjoy and include it thoughtfully in their more mature sexual practices. Teaching a partner also helps refine the woman's self-knowledge to new heights.

Not all masturbation is healthy. In 2003, sexually explicit websites on the Internet have become primary sources for adult fantasy and masturbation. Although Internet sexual addiction is male dominated, women are not immune to its addictive qualities. Questions about sexual compulsivity, addiction, or other sexual aberrations should be raised when: (a) the number of times per week that someone has an orgasm by masturbation or any means is greater than seven, (b) sex preoccupies one's consciousness, and (c) interferes with daily life activities. As masturbation (or other sexual activity) becomes increasingly compulsive, relationships are negatively affected and quality of life deteriorates. Personal and professional disasters are common results.

The politics and morality of mainstream America surrounding masturbation has shifted from condemnation to acceptance for both women and men. Primarily negative lies and myths about masturbation are slowly dying and reality is prevailing. When used thoughtfully, it is not only sensually pleasurable, but a fascinating study of the mental and physical components of one's sexuality.

SEE ALSO: Libido and desire

Suggested Reading

Carnes, P. J. (1991). *Don't call it love: Recovery from sexual addiction.* New York: Bantam Books.
Levine, S. B. (1992). *Sexual life: A clinician's guide.* New York: Plenum Press.

Suggested Resources

Betty Dodson Online: http://www.bettydodson.com (1998–2002). Betty Dodson, Ph.D., New York.

GARY MARTZ

Maternal Mortality
Deaths to women that are associated with pregnancy and childbirth fall under the category of maternal mortality. There are more than 500,000 maternal deaths each year in the world, of which almost all (98%) occur in developing nations, but even in the United States two or three women die each day of pregnancy-related causes. Regionally, the lifetime risk of maternal death is highest in Africa, where 1 in every 16 women is likely to be a victim. The risk of maternal death is 1 in 65 in Asia, 1 in 130 in Latin America, but is dramatically lower—1 in 1,800 women—in high-income nations. It is also estimated that for each woman who dies of complications of labor and delivery, at least 30 and possibly as many as 100 women survive childbirth but suffer from disease, disability, or other physical damage as a result of the complications of pregnancy.

An accurate assessment of maternal mortality rates is difficult to obtain, since the areas with the highest rates are often the same places that have the least accurate recordkeeping systems. In developing nations, people often die outside the health care system, and the cause of death is often not recorded even if a death occurs in a hospital. Furthermore, the number of deaths from unsafe (typically illegal) abortion is often underestimated, because the procedure may have been performed in secrecy. In both developing and developed countries, the recorded cause of death may be misclassified if the link to a pregnancy is not recognized.

There are numerous causes of maternal mortality, but 80% of deaths in the world are due to five primary complications. These include hemorrhage (25% of maternal deaths), sepsis (15%), toxemia (12%), unsafe abortion (13%), and obstructed labor (8%). The remaining 20% are often due to associated conditions, such as malaria, anemia, and HIV/AIDS. One in four maternal deaths occurs during childbirth, half occur within the first 24 hours after birth, and the remaining 25% occur in the days and weeks immediately following delivery. Complications that do not result in death can create lifelong conditions such as infertility, impaired mobility, severe anemia, chronic weakness, pelvic pain, uterine rupture, and fistula.

Worldwide, the availability of women's health services makes a significant impact on levels of maternal mortality and morbidity. According to data from the United Nations Population Fund (UNFPA), approximately 15% of pregnant women experience some kind of complication, and about 5% of pregnant women *require* surgery, usually a cesarean section. Note that in the United States nearly one in four deliveries is by cesarean section, but that is a far higher percentage than would be required if it were used solely to save the life of the mother or baby. The World Health

Organization estimates that no population requires more than 15% of births to be by cesarean section. It is estimated that about two thirds of infant deaths each year in the world are a result of poor maternal health and inadequate care during delivery. The UNFPA has recognized three keys to reducing maternal death and disability: (a) family planning to help ensure that every pregnancy is wanted; (b) each birth assisted by a skilled attendant; and (c) access to essential obstetric care so that in the case of complications a woman can reach a functioning health care facility in a timely manner.

Although the proximate cause of maternal death is typically an identifiable medical condition or complication, maternal deaths often represent the culmination of other factors in a woman's situation. Maternal mortality and morbidity are a reflection, in particular, of the status of women in society. When women experience conditions of poverty, lack of education, early and too frequent childbearing, low status, and restricted choices, the likelihood of maternal mortality or morbidity is much higher. Social, cultural, and economic changes that improve the condition and status of women are a necessity to lower the risks of maternal mortality and morbidity throughout the world.

Although the risk of maternal death is considerably lower in industrialized nations than in other parts of the world, with an average of only 12 deaths out of every 100,000 live births, 2–3 women in the United States nonetheless die each day of pregnancy-related causes. Within the United States, the risk of maternal death varies greatly by race/ethnicity. In particular, black women are four times as likely as non-Hispanic whites to die of pregnancy-related complications, and Hispanic women are nearly twice as likely to die of these complications as are non-Hispanic whites. The risk has declined for all racial/ethnic groups over the past 50 years, but most of the improvements were prior to the 1980s. Since then there has been relatively little change in maternal mortality rates. Even so, it is estimated that over half of all maternal deaths could still be avoided through improved health care access, higher quality of care, and altering health and lifestyle habits.

In the United States, the leading causes of pregnancy-related deaths are hemorrhage, embolism, pregnancy-induced hypertension, infection, complications with anesthesia, and heart muscle disease. Although the risk of death is low in the United States, approximately 30% of pregnancies involve some kind of complication before, during, or even after delivery. The most common complications include miscarriage, ectopic pregnancy, excessive vomiting, diabetes, hemorrhage, infection, pregnancy-induced hypertension, premature labor, or the need for a cesarean delivery. Overall, childbirth is the most common reason for hospitalization of women in the United States, both for delivery and for treatment of complications.

In all cases, the repercussions of maternal mortality include children who must now survive without a mother, and the loss of an important member of a family and society.

SEE ALSO: Abortion, Access to health care, Morbidity, Mortality, Pregnancy

Suggested Reading

Sionke, J., & Donnay, F. (2001). *Maternal mortality update 1998–1999: A report on UNFPA support for maternal mortality prevention.* New York: United Nations Population Fund. http://www.unfpa.org/rh/mothers/documents/cmmupdate99.pdf

U.S. Centers for Disease Control. (2000). *Safe motherhood: Preventing pregnancy-related illnesses and death.* http://www.cdc.gov/nccdphp/bb_motherhood/index.htm

World Health Organization. (2001). *Maternal mortality in 1995: Estimates developed by WHO, UNICEF, and UNFPA.* Geneva: Author. http://www.unfpa.org/mothers/pdf/mmin1995.pdf

ELIZABETH CHRISTENSEN
JOHN R. WEEKS

Maternal Separation

Close proximity of a mother to her infant or child is necessary for survival in humans and other mammals. The close contact promotes emotional attachment and helps to provide food, comfort, and safety. Maternal separation is just as important as close contact for the development of individuality and continued growth of the mother–child relationship. Separations that are relatively brief and consistent lead to healthy development of the mother–child relationship. A total lack of separation between the mother and child does not allow for growth and may lead to problems with separation in the future. Separations that are prolonged and/or inconsistent, without other means of comfort, may contribute to relationship problems, distress, illness, anxiety disorders, and/or attachment disorders.

Maternal separation from the neonate, infant, or child may produce stress and anxiety for both individuals. Timing, frequency, and duration of separation all contribute to the degree of stress experienced by the mother–child dyad. There is evidence that immediately after birth infants respond to and prefer the sound of their mothers' voice over that of others. This indicates that infants listen and respond to the sound of their mothers' voice before birth. Newborns also prefer the scent of their own mothers' breast milk. This evidence suggests that newborns know their mothers at birth, therefore, separation from the familiarity of their mothers may be quite stressful. In fact, animal research examining behavioral and physiological reactivity to stress often involves separation of the mother and infant to induce a stressful situation.

It is ideal for a mother and infant to attain close physical contact immediately after birth to enhance and strengthen their relationship. However, it is not critical, as was once thought, that the "bonding" between mother and child happen within a given time frame. Emotional attachment is a process that occurs over time. Women who have complications after delivery, or have newborns who are too ill for interaction, have been able to develop an emotional attachment with their infants similar to mothers who held and interacted with their infants within the first hours after birth. In most circumstances, separation from the newborn can lead to maternal anxiety even if the mother has not yet seen her infant.

Maternal separation anxiety may occur in the natural process of physical separation. It can be evident during the first separation or during significant changes in the relationship that involve separation. The anxiety may be transient and an expected reaction to the separation or it can lead to significant distress, indicating that an anxiety disorder may be present.

Anxiety and stress for the infant increases with age during the first year of life. Between 9 and 12 months of age, infants become more aware that they are separate individuals from their mothers. This can lead to separation anxiety in varying degrees. Consistent return of mother after separation enhances the attachment relationship and contributes to further growth. A mother and her child are continually presented with challenges during separations at each developmental milestone: a toddler spending the first day in preschool, a 5-year-old going to kindergarten, an 8-year-old spending the first night away from home, or even an 18-year-old headed off to college. Separation at any developmental age contributes to feelings of anxiety initially; however, successful separation leads to a sense of accomplishment for both the child and the mother.

SEE ALSO: Anxiety disorders, Child care

Suggested Reading

Feldman, R., Weller, A., et al. (1999). The nature of the mother's tie to her infant: Maternal bonding under conditions of proximity, separation, and potential loss. *Journal of Child Psychology and Psychiatry, 40*(6), 929–939.

Hock, E., & Schirtzinger, M. B. (1992). Maternal separation anxiety: Its developmental course and relation to maternal mental health. *Child Development, 63*(1), 93–102.

Lamb, M. E. (1982). Early contact and maternal–infant bonding: One decade later. *Pediatrics, 70*(5), 763–768.

Mertin, P. G. (1986). Maternal–infant attachment: A developmental perspective. *Australia and New Zealand Journal of Obstetrics and Gynaecology, 26*(4), 280–283.

Stanton, M. E., & Levine, S. (1985). Brief separation elevates cortisol in mother and infant squirrel monkeys. *Physiology and Behavior, 34*(6), 1007–1008.

AMY L. SALISBURY

Medicaid

Medicaid Medicaid was established in 1965 through the Title XIX of the Social Security Act. This federal–state program was developed to finance health care for low-income persons, specifically *the categorically needy and the medically needy*. Categorically needy are those receiving Aid to Families with Dependent Children (AFDC) (now Temporary Assistance for Needy Families) and those who receive Supplemental Security Income (SSI) because they are aged, blind, or disabled. All states must cover the categorically needy. The medically needy are those who have enough money to live on, but not enough to pay for medical care. In 1972, an amendment to the Social Security Act added family planning services to the list of essential services. One purpose of the federal government was to ensure medical care for those on welfare, predominantly single, poor women, and their children. The link to cash assistance is a defining characteristic of the program and makes this an entitlement program.

The Medicaid program, financed by general tax revenues, is a cost sharing program between the states and the federal government. The federal government contributes roughly 57% of the cost and the states pay the balance. The eligibility and benefit structures are determined by each state. In particular, the state defines the scope, amount, and duration of services. Each state defines the eligibility for classification as medically needy, for example. A state Medicaid program must provide the minimum services: (a) inpatient and outpatient hospital services; (b) skilled nursing facilities; (c) physician services; (d) home health care; and (e) early and periodic screening, diagnosis, and treatment (EPSDT) of children under 21 who are eligible. Dental services, prescribed drugs, eyeglasses, intermediate care facilities, and other services are optional services and states may offer any or all of these. Services must be provided to children and pregnant women at no cost. Deductibles (a set amount the patient must pay before Medicaid pays) are not permitted and co-pays (a percentage of charges paid by the patient) generally do not apply. Eligibility for cash assistance is also defined by the state and determines which parents in families can enroll in Medicaid. Many low-income families are not eligible for their state programs. All poor children under 19 years, all children under age 6 years, and pregnant women with incomes up to 133% of the federal poverty level are considered eligible for Medicaid under recent federal requirements.

Medicaid provides coverage to many of the sick and disadvantaged in the society. Children and their parents constitute the majority of the program's beneficiaries (73%) but account for only a quarter of the spending. Individuals with disabilities and older people who are poor (or the dually Medicare–Medicaid eligibles) also receive services through Medicaid. This group of beneficiaries incur the highest per capita expenditures, and consume disproportionate amounts of Medicaid dollars. In 1999, Medicaid covered 5% of nonelderly adults and 15% of those with incomes below 200% of poverty. Medicaid's role as a primary source of long-term care, gap coverage for Medicare, and major source of coverage for the disabled is likely to continue with the increasing growth of the elderly population.

Medicaid costs have risen through a combination of increased enrollment (from 4 million in 1966 to 47 million in 2002) and medical inflation. Total health care expenditures have had the fastest growth since 1991 and have created significant challenges for the federal and state governments in delivering Medicaid services. State-funded Medicaid spending increased by 11% from fiscal year (FY) 2000 to 2001 and is expected to increase by another 13.4% in FY 2002. State Medicaid expenditure increases are most notably due to prescription drugs, enrollment increases, increased cost and use of medical services, and long-term care expenses. In most states, Medicaid costs outstrip state revenue. Selected actions by government intended to address these concerns have influenced the benefits available to Medicaid beneficiaries. In the early 1990s, states concerned about the growing uninsured in their states, submitted applications for waivers under section 1115 of the Social Security Act. This allowed states flexibility in modifying eligibility, payment methods, and other program characteristics, including enrollment of beneficiaries in managed care plans, as an attempt to reduce costs and accommodate increasing enrollment. Another outcome was the extension of health coverage to the working poor and their families who were not previously eligible for Medicaid. Efforts to provide services for poor children prompted the development of State Child Health Insurance Programs, a program to provide coverage for children whose family income was too high for Medicaid. In addition, the 1996 Personal Responsibility and Work Opportunity Act redefined the eligibility, scope, and duration of welfare benefits and set the stage for the work requirements linked to these benefits.

The Medicaid program has achieved access to health care comparable to private insurance for low-income populations. Notable successes are in the provision of care for pregnant women and children and the development of enhanced or special services as part of the benefit package. Further, Medicaid has been a "gap" insurance, and a safety net program for the sickest and the frailest in the society. Medicaid provides coverage for mental health and substance abuse services, expensive drugs for treatment of AIDS, and rehabilitation services not covered by private insurance. In long-term care, Medicaid pays for 44% of nursing home expenditures. Despite this progress, Medicaid is reliant upon the state and federal economy. In more prosperous times, benefits across states may vary less and individual programs may begin to address the needs of beneficiaries. In times of economic distress, however, benefits may be restricted through eligibility, cash assistance, and scope of services or duration of benefits. Reform of Medicaid and the state-to-state variability of services have been a focus of public policy debate for the last decade and will be on the health care agenda for the foreseeable future.

The Medicaid program is of particular relevance to women. Women as single heads of household may rely on Medicaid for themselves and their children, especially during pregnancy. Women who are elderly, disabled, and draw low income count on Medicaid for access to specialized medical care. The overrepresentation of women in the poor and the elderly population, especially those residing in nursing homes, suggests that women have a critical investment in the eligibility and benefits of the Medicaid program.

SEE ALSO: Access to health care, Health insurance, Health maintenance organizations, Medicare

Suggested Reading

(2003). Medicaid comes of age. *Health Affairs, 22*(1), 7–277.

Kovner, A. R. (1990). *Health care delivery in the United States.* New York: Springer.

Novick, L. F., & Mays, G. P. (2001). *Public health administration: Principles for population-based management.* Gaithersburg, MD: Aspen.

Raffel, M. W., & Raffel, N. K. (1994). *The U.S. health care system: Origins and functions.* Albany, NY: Delmar.

BETH E. QUILL

Medical Malpractice

There are many forms of legal regulation of medical practice and its practitioners. Among other legal mechanisms, there are state professional licensing and disciplinary statutes and regulations, mandatory oversight by peer review organizations, federal and state parameters on drug and device prescribing, and financial and quality of care audits by public and private third-party payers. Statutory and regulatory requirements for hospitals and other health care provider institutions and agencies also exert a direct impact on medical practice. One of the most significant mechanisms for regulating physician behavior in the United States is the private civil tort system that encompasses individual professional liability/medical malpractice lawsuits brought by, or on behalf of, patients against their professional caregivers.

A relatively small number of medical malpractice claims are predicated on a theory of violation of contract. In such litigation, the patient/plaintiff claims that an express promise made by the physician about the outcome (for instance, "After this plastic surgery, I guarantee that you will look twenty years younger than before") has not been fulfilled.

The overwhelming majority of malpractice actions, though, are based instead on a theory of tort, which means a civil wrong (as contrasted with a crime) caused by the violation of a duty stemming from something other than a contract. Within the relationship between a patient and physician, a tort is committed by a violation of the physician's fiduciary or trust obligation to act always in the patient's best interests.

A small percentage of the tort actions brought against physicians allege intentional wrongdoing, such as battery, for physically invading the patient's bodily integrity by doing some procedure without appropriate permission. However, the majority of malpractice cases are founded on a theory of negligence, or unintentional (albeit blameworthy) deviation from accepted professional standards. Medical negligence may occur through the failure to supply the individual (or the proxy decision-maker for a decisionally incapable person) with the information necessary to give a truly informed, voluntary consent to a particular intervention. Negligence also may take place through poor-quality, professionally unacceptable rendition of patient care. Many plaintiffs' complaints in professional liability cases allege both lack of adequate informed consent and the substandard performance of medical services.

In any negligence action, the plaintiff who initiates the claim must prove the presence of four elements in order to establish a prima facie case and succeed. The plaintiff's inability to meet the burden of proof—convincing the jury by a preponderance of the evidence—regarding any of these elements warrants dismissal of the case.

First, the plaintiff must show that the professional owed the plaintiff a duty of due care; this responsibility is established by virtue of the existence of a professional/patient relationship. The duty or standard of care owed is that degree of knowledge or skill that would be possessed and practiced by competent, prudent professional peers under similar circumstances. Second, because the present American malpractice system is based on the concept of fault, the plaintiff must show that the physician violated or breached the acceptable standard of care. The law does not require absolute perfection in medical diagnosis and treatment. By the same token, it is not enough for physicians to "do their best" if their conduct does not rise to the applicable level of care under the circumstances.

The third thing that a successful malpractice plaintiff must establish is that physical, financial, and/or emotional injury or damage was suffered. One main purpose of awarding monetary damages in a tort action is to attempt to make the injured victim "whole" again, or returned to the position or condition that existed prior to the negligence, even while recognizing that the ability of money to accomplish that objective very often is a legal fiction.

Finally, proving the element of causation is essential. Specifically, the plaintiff must convince the jury, to a reasonable degree of medical certainty, that the injury incurred was directly or proximately brought about by the defendant's violation of duty, that is, that "but for" (sine qua non) the defendant's negligence, the injury would not have happened and, furthermore, that there were no other intervening, superceding, unforeseeable factors that would explain the injury.

In many medical malpractice cases, the physician is not the only party named by the patient/plaintiff as a defendant. Depending on the specific facts, the health care institution or agency that employs the physician, or with whom the physician is affiliated, may be subject to lawsuit in addition to or in place of the physician. Health care institutions and agencies might be held liable, solely or jointly, for malpractice under theories of vicarious liability for employing (*respondeat superior*) the physician or negligently supervising her, or direct liability for the failure to adequately fulfill their own independent fiduciary responsibilities toward the patient.

SEE ALSO: Informed consent, Physicians

Suggested Reading

Bell, P. A., & O'Connell, J. (1997). *Accidental justice: The dilemmas of tort law*. New Haven, CT: Yale University Press.

Boumil, M. M., & Elias, C. E. (1995). *The law of medical liability in a nutshell*. St. Paul, MN: West.

Danzon, P. M. (1985). *Medical malpractice: Theory, evidence, and public policy*. Cambridge, MA: Harvard University Press.

Kapp, M. B. (1990). The American medical malpractice system: Impediments to effective change. *International Journal of Risk and Safety in Medicine, 1*, 239–254.

Law, S. A., & Polan, S. (1978). *Pain and profit: The politics of malpractice*. New York: Harper & Row.

McClellan, F. (1994). *Medical malpractice: Law, tactics, and ethics*. Philadelphia: Temple University Press.

MARSHALL B. KAPP

Medicare
Medicare (Title XVIII) of the Social Security Act is a federal health insurance program inaugurated on July 1, 1966. The program is the major health insurance for those over the age of 65 years of age, who are covered by the Social Security system, regardless of income. Amendments to the Social Security Act in 1972 extended the benefits to those who do not meet the criteria for the regular Social Security program, but who are willing to pay a premium for coverage. Further amendments in 1973 extended benefits to those entitled to Social Security disability benefits or those who suffer from chronic renal disease requiring a kidney transplant or routine dialysis. Since 1966, the number of enrollees has expanded, and the medical expenditures increased, making Medicare a major budget item for the federal government. Currently, the Medicaid program spends more than $200 billion a year.

Medicare is comprised of two parts: Part A and Part B. Part A of Medicare is the hospital insurance part, funded by Social Security taxes. Coverage includes hospitalization, care in a skilled nursing facility, home health care, or hospice care. The Medicare program has deductibles (set amount the patient must pay before Medicare begins to pay) and co-pays (a percentage of charges paid by the patient). Benefits may also have limitations on the amount of coverage. Hospital care expenses are not paid by Medicare beyond 150 days, for example, and a skilled nursing facility is limited to 100 days. Medicare pays for 14% of nursing home expenditures and Medicaid, which is another source of payment after Medicare expires, pays 44% of nursing home expenditures (1998).

Part B of Medicare is Supplemental Medical Insurance. While it is optional and must be paid for as a Social Security deduction, most elderly enroll in Part B. This part of Medicare pays for reasonable physician charges, inpatient and outpatient medical and surgical services, supplies, physical and speech therapy, ambulance and diagnostic tests, clinical laboratory tests, blood, home health care, and outpatient diagnosis and treatment. Similar to Part A, limitations on the amount of payments and deductibles apply. Physician services, for example, are covered 80% after the deductible ($100) has been met. Although Medicare greatly expanded access to medical services for the elderly, the gaps in benefits and the particular burden of cost sharing requirements on low-income populations have limited the effectiveness of the program.

Managed care, a planned approach to control health care costs, has been enrolling Medicare beneficiaries since the 1990s. A primary incentive is that the Medicare program allows beneficiaries to opt out of the traditional fee-for-Service program and voluntarily enroll in a Medicare-approved Health Maintenance Organization (HMO), provided that the beneficiaries reside in an area that is served by one or more Medicare-approved HMOs. Medicare HMOs typically offer a broader range of benefits (such as prescription coverage or preventive care). Approximately 18% of the nation's 38 million beneficiaries are enrolled in managed care plans. Recently, however, a number of HMOs have declined to participate in the Medicare program or narrowed their service areas. Access to Medicare providers and facilities continues to be a challenge for elderly citizens: About one in seven Medicare beneficiaries do not have a usual source of care or have not seen a physician when they needed medical care.

By the year 2030, it is estimated there will be 120% more elderly than today (65 million) and people over 65 will comprise 22% population. Individuals 85 years of age and older are the fastest growing segment of the population.

Persons over the age of 65 years use 23% of the ambulatory care visits, 48% of hospital days, and 69% of home health services. With increasing availability of community-based services, nursing home utilization has decreased. A major problem for this growing group of elderly is the lack of coverage for prescription drugs. While most adults indicate they have a health problem that requires medication on a regular basis, only 55% of those 50–64 years of age and 49% of those 65–70 years of age noted that their insurance covered prescription costs. The elderly, in particular, report high out-of-pocket costs that often compete with other expenses of daily living or prescription drugs.

Elderly women frequently live longer than men, have more chronic diseases, and are more likely to live alone (except for those over age 85 years). Therefore, Medicare is the primary medical benefit available for health care. Women's contributed earnings are likely to be less than those of men, placing an increased burden for out-of-pocket medical expenses. For example, compared to a 65-year-old man retiring from work in 1990, the average man retiring at 65 in 2030 will require an additional 25 monthly payments of any promised benefit plan. In contrast, the average woman in the same example would require an additional 39 months. Women comprise the majority of nursing home residents, and will likely be the predominant users of Medicare. Thus, elderly women have vested interest in ensuring that specific measures are taken to close currently existing gender gaps in coverage.

The challenge for program officials is to keep the Medicare program efficient, effective, and equitable in providing coverage for a broad scope of services, while containing costs. Therefore, it is expected that the Medicare program will continue to be at the heart of public policy debates.

See Also: Access to health care, Health insurance, Health maintenance organizations

Suggested Reading

Schoer, C., Simantor, E., Duchan, L., & Davis, K. (2000). *Counting on Medicare: Perspectives and concerns of Americans ages*, pp. 50–70. New York: Commonwealth Fund.

Kovner, A. R. (1990). *Health care delivery in the United States*. New York: Springer.

Novick, L. F., & Mays, G. P. (2001). *Public health administration: Principles for population-based managements*. Gaithersburg, MD: Aspen.

Raffel, M. W., & Raffel, N. K. (1994). *The U.S. health care system: Origins and functions*. Albany, NY: Delmar.

BETH E. QUILL

Medicine *see* entry for specific illness or disorder

Meditation Traditionally meditation was used exclusively for spiritual growth. More recently, it has become a valuable tool for relaxation, stress relief, and as an adjunct to medical healing. Those who meditate on a regular basis report a sense of healing, deeper concentration and insight, a heightened sense of intuition, feeling more peaceful, positive, loving, and centered. Medical studies indicate that meditation confers not only strong psychological benefits, but also important physiological benefits. Long-term meditators experience significantly less heart disease and cancer than nonmeditators. Meditation has a profoundly positive effect on blood pressure, chronic pain, and insomnia. Meditators secrete more DHEA than nonmeditators which helps to decrease stress, heighten memory, preserve sexual function, and control weight.

Meditation has been practiced for thousands of years in the Eastern cultures, but is relatively new to the West. Although spiritual more than religious, meditation is practiced in many religions, and also by those who claim no religious affiliation. There are many types of meditation. They include prayer, visualization, Sufi meditation, guided imagery, mindfulness meditation, the relaxation response, biofeedback, transcendental meditation, Zen Buddhist meditation, Native American meditation, movement meditation such as Yoga, T'ai Chi, qigong, and medical meditation. One can meditate alone, with a master/teacher, or in a group of any size. Whatever the form and regardless of the level of practice, all mediations yield similar results. The three most common "methods" of meditation are the relaxation response, mindfulness meditation, and transcendental meditation.

THE RELAXATION RESPONSE

This method begins with the belief that the "normal" state of mind is not a rested one, that the mind bounces from one thought to another followed by emotional and physical reactions, invoking the flight-or-fight response. This response activates the involuntary nervous system which instantly raises blood pressure and heart rate; stimulates the adrenal glands to release adrenaline, noradrenaline, and cortisol; and decreases or increases the production of important hormones. Prolonged periods of time in this mode can cause chronic high blood pressure, heart disease, stomach ulcers, autoimmune diseases, cancer, anxiety, insomnia, and depression. The opposite of the flight-or-fight response is the relaxation response. This response occurs during meditation and produces opposite physiological effects. To reach this response, the meditator sits quietly, clears her mind, and focuses on a calming phrase, image, or thought. Research has documented many health benefits from this type of meditation including decreased PMS symptoms, decreased migraine headaches, reduced anxiety and depression, fewer missed days of work due to illness, significant improvements in insomnia, reduction of chronic pain, and improved high blood pressure.

MINDFULNESS MEDITATION

This type of meditation begins with the concept of mindfulness. Mindfulness has been described as "learning how to stop all your doing and shift over to a 'being' mode." To be mindful is to live in the present moment, to give up the habit of worry, to let all stress drain from mind and body, to let go of ego and the need to control. In this type of meditation, the meditator focuses on the breath and allows the mind to wander striving for a heightened awareness of each passing thought and image. Studies have shown that mindfulness meditation decreases panic attacks and general anxiety, reduces chronic pain and the incidences of headaches, improves recovery to drug and alcohol addiction, and reduces obesity.

TRANSCENDENTAL MEDITATION

This is the most popular and most studied form of meditation in the Western culture. It begins with the concept of restful alertness. As the body becomes deeply relaxed, the mind settles down to a state of inner calm and wakefulness. This form of meditation has been described as easy to learn, effortless to practice, involving neither concentration nor contemplation. It is recommended that one learn this technique from a transcendental meditation teacher. In addition to the results reported with relaxation response and mindfulness meditation, transcendental meditation has been shown to slow the aging process, and significantly lower rates of hospitalization indicating higher levels of health than nonmeditators. Meditation does not require one to believe in a certain way or adopt a particular lifestyle. It will not conflict with one's religion. Whatever meditation technique is practiced, there are many common principles. These include not to worry about doing it exactly right and not to expect an earth-shattering experience. Most meditative results are quite subtle. Accept whatever occurs. Find a quiet comfortable place in which to meditate where disturbances are minimal. Sit in a comfortable chair, on a bed, or on the floor keeping the spine reasonably straight. If physical reasons dictate, lying on the back works fine. Eliminate as many potential distractions as possible, but do not worry about those things that cannot be controlled. No particular time of day is better than another; however, having a specific time in which to meditate will be helpful in making it a regular practice. Call on a spiritual source for assistance while meditating, if that comports with one's individual beliefs. When beginning a meditation practice, start with just 10–15 minutes once a day, increasing the time gradually, but keeping in mind that more is not always better. Meditation taps into very powerful inner energies which are very healing and uplifting, but it does take time to acclimate and is best done gradually.

SEE ALSO: Complementary and alternative health practices, Headache, Hypertension, Massage, Migraine, Pain, Yoga

Suggested Reading

Chopra, D., & Simon, D. (2001). *Grow younger, live longer.* New York: Harmony Books.

Khalsa, D. S., & Stauth, C. (2001). *Meditation as medicine.* New York: Fireside.

Suggested Resources

Maharishi Vedic Education Development Corporation. (2001). Transcendental Meditation Program (June, 2001). http://www.tm.org/main_pages/tm_descrip.html. Accessed on March 24, 2003.

Meditation General Information, Worldwide Online Meditation Center. (1998–2000). Jim Malloy; *General information.* http://www.meditationcenter.com. Accessed on March 10, 2003.

JUDY TRENTMAN

Melanoma Melanoma is a cancer of the skin that occurs when pigmented skin cells begin to grow out of control. Melanoma is often deadly, unlike basal cell and squamous cell skin cancers, which are usually curable. However, if found at an early stage, melanoma can usually be cured. Melanoma often appears as a brown or black spot on the skin, sometimes developing from a mole that has been present for a long time. Melanoma rarely causes obvious symptoms such as pain.

Melanoma begins in the cells that produce skin color. Dark-skinned people are naturally at much lower risk of melanoma compared to fair-skinned individuals. The frequency of malignant melanoma of the skin is increasing faster than any other cancer in the United States. Melanoma is a disease primarily in whites that increases with age.

People with sun-sensitive skin are at increased risk of melanoma. Sun sensitivity refers to the skin's response to sun exposure and is measured by a variety of markers. These markers include light skin color, light hair color, light eye color, tendency to sunburn, inability to tan, and presence of freckles. Studies have also shown melanoma to be related to an increased number of common moles and, especially, abnormal (dysplastic) moles. Studies of total body mole counts and mole counts on the arms have shown that an increased number of moles is related to a higher risk of developing melanoma. Early sun exposure may cause moles to develop, while other risk factors for melanoma, including adult sun exposure, may help change moles into melanoma.

Ultraviolet (UV) light is the main environmental factor responsible for the development of skin melanoma as well as precursor lesions such as common moles (nevi). UV light is often divided into three regions with UV-A ranging from 320 to 400 nm, UV-B ranging from 290 to 320 nm, and with UV-C ranging from 200 to 290 nm, where visible light spans from 380 to 750 nm.

Sunlight is the major source of UV light. Various types of sun exposure are associated with melanoma, ranging from severe sunburns, occupational activities, vacation sun exposure, beach activities, other recreational activities, cumulative sun exposure, and early migration to sunny places. The most consistent risk factor for melanoma has been sunburns, particularly at young ages. The damage from sunburns can cause an increase in melanoma in the area that was burned, but sunburns also appear to suppress the skin's immune system. This allows melanomas to occur in non-sun-exposed skin. While dark-skinned people are naturally at lower risk for melanoma, recent studies suggest there is a higher risk of melanoma with prolonged sun exposure after developing a tan. Growing up in a sunny location or spending a large amount of time in the sun, particularly during childhood and adolescence, also appear to be important. Studies show that both intermittent sun exposure (sunburns and sunny vacations) and total sun exposure (over many years) are risk factors for melanoma.

A second source of UV light is from artificial exposures including tanning beds, sunlamps, and tanning booths. Tanning units are available for use at tanning salons where the patron pays for timed "tanning sessions." Alternatively, entire units may be purchased for home use. Sunlamps, prior to the 1980s, could irradiate only a localized area and emitted primarily UV-B and some UV-C. More recently, tanning beds or standing booths can irradiate nearly 100% of exposed skin, emitting more UV-A and some UV-B. Overall, there appears to be more than a 50% increase in melanoma risk among sunlamp or tanning bed users, with a greater risk associated with more use.

Sunscreens are thought to protect skin from sunburns and many other harmful effects of the sun. Consequently, some professionals suggest that limiting sun exposure through the use of sunscreen can reduce the risk of developing skin cancers by preventing sunburns. However, recent reports have suggested an increased risk of melanoma among sunscreen users. Some researchers think that the increased melanoma risk with sunscreen use may actually be a result of prolonged sun exposure received by those who use sunscreen. However, skin sensitivity to the sun is likely to distort the association between sunscreen use and melanoma, since sun-sensitive individuals are more likely to use sunscreens. Many studies investigating the potential association between sunscreen and melanoma have not accounted for sun sensitivity. When accounting for sun sensitivity, current evidence suggests no association between sunscreen use and melanoma. The lack of a protective effect of sunscreen use may represent the failure of people who use sunscreen to apply enough sunscreen needed for protection, or may reflect a long period of time between protection from sun exposure and development of melanoma. It may be necessary to wait several decades to see if proper application of high-sun-protection-factor (SPF) sunscreen (SPF >15) is truly protective against melanoma.

The use of sunless chemical tanners has increased dramatically in recent years. The tanning effects of sunless tanning products can last 5–7 days; however, the UV protection is shorter lived than the color change. Some dermatologists suggest that using sunless tanning products prior to sun exposure in conjunction with using sunscreens while outdoors may reduce UV damage to the skin, and thereby reduce incidence of skin melanoma. Many dermatologists recommend use of sunless tanning products over intentional sun exposure or tanning bed use for patients who insist on tanning.

The following are important tips to reduce your risk of melanoma: reduce your sun exposure, particularly between 10 AM and 2 PM during Daylight Savings Time; wear protective clothing while in the sun or use a sunscreen with an SPF of greater than 15; when applying sunscreen, use a palm-full of sunscreen and then reapply it every 2 hours; wear protective clothing or use sunscreen even on hazy days or days with light cloud cover; do not use sunscreen to prolong your time in the sun. When there is a strong desire for a tan, use of sunless tanning products combined with sunscreen while in the sun may help prevent melanoma. Avoidance of sun exposure is the only sure way to reduce melanoma risk and aging of the skin. Seeking medical attention for any suspicious moles is important since melanoma can be a deadly disease with few or no symptoms or pain. However, melanoma is also easily curable if identified early and removed.

SEE ALSO: Cancer, Moles, Skin care, Skin disorders

Suggested Reading

Langley, R. G., & Sober, A. J. (1997). A clinical review of the evidence for the role of ultraviolet radiation in the etiology of cutaneous melanoma. *Cancer Investigation, 15*(6) 561–567.

Levy, S. B. (2000). Tanning preparations. *Dermatologic Clinics, 18*(4), 591–596.

Westerdahl, J., Ingvar, C., Masback, A., Jonsson, N., & Olsson, H. (2000). Risk of cutaneous malignant melanoma in relation to use of sunbeds: Further evidence for UV-A carcinogenicity. *British Journal of Cancer, 82*(9), 1593–1599.

LESLIE K. DENNIS

Menarche The average age of menarche, or first menstruation, in the United States is 12.88 years for Caucasian girls and 12.16 years for African American girls. A popular misconception is that menarche marks the beginning of puberty; in reality, menarche occurs later in puberty. According to the widely used "five Tanner stages" of pubertal development, the onset of puberty is identified as Stage 2 at the first signs of pubic hair and breast bud development. The interval between these first signs of puberty and the completion of sexual maturation in girls (measured by the growth of pubic hair, reproductive organs, and breast development) can be as short as a year and a half to as long as 6 years. Menarche generally occurs when girls are in Stage 3 or 4 of their development, which usually takes place somewhere between age 9 and 15 years old.

There has been some debate whether the age at menarche has changed over the last few decades. Examining the average age of menarche globally, the data indicate that the average age of menarche has decreased significantly in the last 100 years. Earlier menarche is attributed to improved nutrition, and the industrial revolution, which brought on a higher stress level due to the faster pace of life. According to a recent review, the age of menarche has remained stable over the last 50 years for Caucasian girls in the United States. Comparable longitudinal data are not available for African Americans or other minority groups, because few studies have included nonwhite girls until recently. Cross-sectional findings, however, suggest that African American girls reach menarche slightly earlier than Caucasian girls (12.16 years vs. 12.88 years), underscoring the important role of ethnicity in understanding menarche. It is notable that the age of menarche has remained relatively stable, while the age of pubertal onset has decreased over the past 30 years in the United States.

GENETIC AND ENVIRONMENTAL INFLUENCES ON TIMING OF MENARCHE

Genetic factors play an important role in the age of menarche. Early menarche tends to run in families, and studies show good correlation (statistically, an average correlation of 0.30) between mother's and daughter's age at menstruation. Environmental influences also affect the onset of menstruation. Delayed menarche is associated with excessive exercise, malnutrition, and significantly low weight. Sports or other activities that require intense physical activity, such as dancing and gymnastics, are associated with later ages at menarche. Such processes, however, can be reversed. One study indicated that stopping exercise for as little as 2 months initiated pubertal development and menarche. Body fat also predicts the onset of menstruation, with obesity linked to earlier onset and low weight related to later onset. Significant weight gain is seen in the years preceding menarche, with girls gaining approximately 40 lb across 4 years before their first menstruation.

Studies have also identified important psychosocial factors affecting menarche. For example, family structure and family relationships are strongly related to the timing of menstruation. Earlier age at menarche is related to the father's absence before puberty and longer father's absence. Moreover, approval and warmth in families, and absence of family conflict is related to later age of menarche. In fact, the quality of family relationships has been shown to influence age of menstruation over and above the effects of breast development and weight.

TIMING OF MENARCHE AND MENSTRUAL EXPERIENCE

The timing of menarche may have considerable impact on how girls remember their initial menstrual experience. Conformity seeking is high during adolescence with girls striving to be like their friends. Girls who menstruate before their peers perceive the experience more negatively than girls who menstruate at the same time or later than their peers. Narratives of women between the ages of 18 and 61 recounting their first menstrual experience indicated that most women

held negative views of the sex education they received in school and at home. They reported that menstruation was either not discussed or the information provided and time spent talking about it was inadequate. Most women also complained that having to ask their questions in front of their classmates made it harder for them to voice their concerns. Particularly interesting, the narratives revealed similar experiences across the sample despite the wide age range among the women. Thus, in spite of our awareness that accurate and informative sex education fosters healthy adolescent development, schools and community resources do not appear to be meeting the needs of adolescents.

Another study offers a fascinating glimpse of how women's perceptions of menarche vary across cultures underscoring the role of environment. In one study, American and Malaysian women reported a greater range of emotional reactions to first menstruation than women from Lithuania and the Sudan, but the former two groups reported primarily negative emotions. The most common emotions reported by Americans and Malaysians were embarrassment followed by anxiety. American women expressed worrying about whether they could play sports, but they also indicated feeling "cooler" and eager to learn about their sexuality. Malaysian women reported feeling wiser, more respected, and mature. In contrast, the Lithuanians were philosophical and more positive in their explanations by placing this experience in a context larger than their selves; they reported feeling a part of nature, knowing the "secret" of life, and appreciating themselves more. Unfortunately, this study did not describe what cultural mechanisms might explain these differences in perceptions, but the data raise important questions about the impact of culture on perceptions of menstruation.

RECOMMENDATIONS

Menarche marks an important transition to adulthood, and being prepared for the experience plays a critical role in girls' perceptions of themselves and the significance of the event. Opportunities to talk about menarche before it occurs, have a venue for asking questions, and increasing communication about the process will diminish anxiety and enhance their understanding of the experience. Indeed, placing the onset of menarche in a positive light, such as marking it with a celebration, can significantly influence how girls interpret and respond to the event. Families and schools can play a special role in providing support and information for young girls to assist them through the transition.

See Also: Adolescence, Genital development, Puberty

Suggested Reading

Coleman, L., & Coleman, J. (2002). The measurement of puberty: A review. *Journal of Adolescence, 25*(5), 535–550.

Graber, J. A., Brooks-Gunn, J., & Warren, M. P. (1995). The antecedents of menarcheal age: Heredity, family environment and stressful life events. *Child Development, 66,* 346–359.

Rierdan, J., & Koff, E. (1985). Timing of menarche and initial menstrual experience. *Journal of Youth and Adolescence, 14*(3), 237–244.

GERI R. DONENBERG

Menopause The age at which 50% of the population will cease menstruation (menopause) is 51.3 years with about 8% of women ceasing menstruation before the age of 40. While the menopause represents the final menstrual period, the diagnosis is made retrospectively after loss of menstruation for 12 consecutive months.

Menopause occurs as a result of a decline in the total levels of circulating estrogen and progesterone, hormones which are produced by the ovary. The ovary is endowed with a finite number of eggs and the menopause represents the loss of any further eggs within the ovarian tissue.

The entire body may be affected by the altered and declining hormonal levels, particularly estrogen deficiency. Virtually all body tissues have estrogen receptors indicating that they are responsive to this hormone. Thus, the possible changes are listed in Table 1.

The immediate symptoms that may occur relate to the loss of menstruation, the onset of vasomotor symptoms (see entry Perimenopause), and the vaginal thinning which can increase susceptibility to infection, be associated with painful intercourse, or blood-stained vaginal discharge.

Of great importance are the hidden potential effects of loss of ovarian activity. Over time, multiple organ systems may be impacted increasing susceptibility to disease. Specifically, these include the cardiovascular system with an increased susceptibility to heart attack, loss of bone, which is accelerated with decline in estrogen and therefore increases susceptibility to bone fracture, and central nervous changes, with suggestion that there might be a relationship to the development of problems like Alzheimer's disease. It should be emphasized that premature menopause, before the age of 40 years, is associated with an earlier increase in incidence of heart attacks, osteoporotic fractures, and Alzheimer's disease.

With increasing life expectancy, menopause in a healthy 50-year-old woman would occur at less than two thirds into the life cycle. The menopause therefore serves as an ideal time to enter the health system for

Table 1. Potential problems in untreated perimenopause

Target organ	Possible symptom or problem
Vulva	Atrophy, dystrophy, pruritus vulvae (change in tissue structure, itching)
Vagina	Dyspareunia (painful intercourse), blood-stained discharge, vaginitis
Bladder and urethra	Cystourethritis (inflammation), ectropion (turning outward), frequency or urgency, stress incontinence
Uterus and pelvic floor	Uterovaginal prolapse (pelvic organ prolapse), abnormal bleeding
Skin and mucous membranes	Atrophy, dryness, or pruritus; loss of resilience
Vocal cords	Voice changes (reduction in upper register)
Cardiovascular system	Atherosclerosis, angina (pain), coronary heart disease
Skeleton	Osteoporosis with related fractures, backache
Breasts	Reduced size, softer consistency, drooping
Neuroendocrine system	Hot flashes, secondary psychological disturbances
Eyes	Dry eyes

a comprehensive examination, based on screening for presence of risk factors for future disease or early evidence of current disease. Logically, the menopause then is also the ideal opportunity for the introduction of a comprehensive preventive health program.

CONFIRMING MENOPAUSE

Although menopause is defined as 12 months of amenorrhea (absence of a menstrual period), any woman with loss of menstruation of greater than 6 months and who is older than age 50 can be confidently diagnosed as being menopausal. It is extremely unusual for a breakthrough ovulation and potential pregnancy to occur in this instance. The diagnosis is more easily confirmed by the development of hot flashes, vaginal thinning, and night sweats.

Menopause can also be confirmed by administration of progestogenic medications (progesterone-containing medications) in an attempt to induce a period. Failure to respond to progestogen indicates lack of the hormone estrogen. The blood level of follicle-stimulating hormone, the brain-produced hormone that stimulates the ovary, can also be measured, but beyond age 50 need not be undertaken on a routine basis. The greatest value for this test is in younger women.

CLINICAL MANAGEMENT

There is a general consensus that the menopause is a normal physiological event occurring in the life cycle of all women. The concept of medicalization of the menopause has been debated. In view of the known effects of reduced ovarian sex steroids on body systems and potential health, there is a need to recognize the potential impact and possibilities for preventive health care.

It is generally recommended that the woman in peri- or postmenopause should have frequent, at least annual, medical checkups which include a comprehensive history and recommended laboratory testing such as routine blood screens, Pap smear, mammogram, stool guaiac (check for presence of blood) for colon cancer screening, blood lipid levels for cardiovascular screening, thyroid testing for coincidental hypothyroidism (underactive thyroid), and, when indicated, screens for sexually transmitted diseases.

There is a broad range of suggested modern therapies for preventive health beyond menopause. The concept of healthy living is of paramount importance and should be focused on healthy diet, including appropriate supplements as necessary, exercise, smoking cessation, moderation in the use of alcohol, avoidance of habit-forming drugs, seat belts, and safe sexual practices. Beyond that, pharmacologic preparations may be indicated dependent upon specific indications.

Recently, there has been considerable debate about the role of hormonal therapies beyond menopause. The situation is becoming clearer and the following is a summary. The use of estrogen alone in women who have undergone hysterectomy, or estrogen plus progestogen in women with an intact uterus can be considered under the following circumstances. It should be emphasized that there is a difference between utilization of these products for the treatment of specific menopause-related effects as opposed to the utilization of these hormones for potential prevention of future disease such as osteoporosis.

The hormonal products remain an essential component in the management of true menopause-related symptoms, most specifically, the vasomotor symptoms (changes in blood pressure), vaginal atrophy (change in the tissue lining the vagina), and night sweats. An additional indication would also be increased urinary frequency (increased need to urinate frequently). Under these circumstances, current recommendations are for the lowest dose products administered for the shortest period of time, consistent with management of symptoms. If symptoms recur upon drug cessation, restarting may be considered based on the risk-to-benefit profile for each individual woman.

Currently, the only preventive indication for hormonal therapy is reduction of bone loss and resultant osteoporosis and bone fracture. Hormones are highly effective for this problem. Use should be balanced for risk and benefit for each individual, and also take into consideration the use of alternate nonhormonal bone sparing products such as the bisphosphonates and the selective estrogen receptor modulators (SERMs). In general, up to 5 years of hormonal use in the younger peri- and postmenopausal women is quite safe, and longer term use needs a careful risk/benefit evaluation. Risks of hormone usage include a slight increase in the incidence of heart attack, blood clot, and stroke in the first year to 18 months of therapy, with no increase beyond that. There is also a slight increase in the diagnosis of breast cancer, but fortunately, there is currently no evidence to suggest an increase in mortality from breast cancer. Indeed, some studies suggest that women on hormones at the time of diagnosis of breast cancer, have longer life expectancy than women who have never utilized these products.

When the only symptom relates to vaginal thinning or dryness, local use of estrogen is the preferred route of administration.

SEE ALSO: Menstrual cycle disorders, Menstruation

Suggested Reading

North American Menopause Society. (2002). *Menopause core curriculum* (2nd ed.). Cleveland, OH: Author.

Utian, W. H. (1980). *Menopause in modern perspective.* New York: Appleton Century Crofts.

Utian, W. H. (2003). Menopause. In R. E. Rakel & E. T. Bope (Eds.), *Conn's current therapy 2003* (pp. 1146–1149). Philadelphia: W. B. Saunders.

WULF H. UTIAN

Menstrual Cycle Disorders Because of the complex interplay of events, which are necessary to facilitate the occurrence of the normal menstrual cycle in the female, multiple factors can play roles in producing disorders of the menstrual cycle. Menstrual cycle disorders can be classified as disorders of the process in which eggs are released from the ovaries (ovulation), cycle length, and menstruation, including duration and volume of menstrual blood flow.

Ovulation depends on the occurrence of proper sequencing of events involving a part of the brain called the hypothalamus and the pituitary gland. Any disruption in hypothalamic function can alter hormonal secretion that affects the ovaries. Disruption in the rhythmic secretion of specific hormones important in ovarian function (FSH and LH) will result in anovulation or lack of ovulation. Common disruptions in the hypothalamic secretion include excess weight changes, athletic and psychologic stresses, as well as eating disorders. In addition, pituitary gland lesions such as adenomas (a type of tumor) can alter hormonal events necessary for ovulation to occur. Endocrine system disorders such as chronic anovulation or polycystic ovary syndrome and thyroid dysfunction may also impact the hormonal changes which affect ovulation. Thus, these conditions can contribute to menstrual cycle disorders.

The interval between menstruations varies from every 21 to 35 days. Even though menstrual cycles vary within this normal range over the reproductive life cycle of a woman, any deviation from her individual pattern often represents a cause for anxiety, and will likely bring her to seek clinical attention. Common diagnoses in this group are oligomenorrhea (menstrual intervals of greater than 35 days), polymenorrhea (intervals of less than 21 days), and amenorrhea (absence of menstruation for more than three normal cycle periods). Causes of these types of abnormal bleeding include underactive thyroid (hypothyroidism), ovulatory dysfunction, pregnancy, premalignant or malignant conditions (some types of tumors), or structural lesions such as polyps. Treatments include correction of hypothyroidism, hormonal contraception, treatment of insulin resistance, progestin (hormone) therapy, and surgery.

The normal duration of menstruation is 4–6 days. Any variation outside of this range represents an abnormality. Common diagnoses in this group are metrorrhagia (irregular periods) and menometrorrhagia (heavy and irregular periods). Usual causes include anatomic lesions such as fibroids and polyps and infections due to cervicitis and endometritis (inflammation of the cervix or lining of the uterus). Often patients will need to undergo an evaluation for bleeding disorders as these may affect the menstrual cycle duration and amount of flow.

Estimates of normal blood flow during menstruation are approximately 20–80 cm^3. Ninety percent of flow occurs within the first 48 hours of the onset of menstrual flow. Common diagnoses in this category of disorders include menorrhagia and menometrorrhagia and causes include anatomic lesions such as fibroids, polyps, excessive tissue in the uterine wall (endometrial hyperplasia), neoplasia (tumor) or hypothyroidism, bleeding disorders such as von Willebrand's disease, or deficiency of blood factors needed for clotting. In addition, any disease causing bone marrow dysfunction or liver disease can contribute to these manifestations. Correction of the underlying cause is usually the basis for treatment.

There are two conditions which merit attention here. One is the condition of midcycle bleeding associated with ovulation. This is due to the rise in the hormones estrogen and progesterone causing shedding of the endometrium (wall of the uterus). It usually lasts for 1–2 days and may be associated with mild cramping. Even though there is no cause for concern, it may cause anxiety in a patient. Although no treatment is usually needed, some patients may receive a hormonal contraceptive method to suppress ovulation. The second condition is called premenstrual tension, which is the cyclic occurrence of symptoms in a specific (luteal) phase of the menstrual cycle. They include somatic complaints (headaches, bloating, or breast tenderness), emotional complaints (anxiety, depression, or irritability), and behavioral complaints (poor concentration, food cravings, or sleep disturbances). Treatment includes suppression of ovulation with medications, exercise, dietary modification, nonsteroidal anti-inflammatory drugs (NSAIDs), hormonal contraception, and medical therapy with selective serotonin reuptake inhibitors (SSRIs).

SEE ALSO: Menstruation, Pregnancy

Suggested Reading

Speroff, L., Glass, R., & Kase, N. G. (1994). *Regulation of the menstrual cycle. Clinical gynecologic endocrinology and infertility* (5th ed., pp. 183–230). Philadelphia: Williams & Wilkins.

MARGARET L. MCKENZIE

Menstruation The menstrual cycle is a combination of a series of events occurring between a part of the brain called the hypothalamus, the pituitary gland in the brain, the ovaries, and the interior of the uterus (endometrium). Normal cycle lengths vary from 21 to 35 days even though considerable variation in the length occurs in individual women over their life span. The menstrual cycle is divided into four phases: the follicular, ovulatory, luteal, and menstrual phases.

HORMONE PRODUCTION AND REGULATION

At puberty, a compound called gonadotropin-releasing hormone (GnRH) is synthesized in a part of the brain called the hypothalamus and travels to the pituitary gland. Here GnRH stimulates the production of follicle-stimulating hormone (FSH) and luteinizing hormone (LH), two hormones important for the functioning of the ovary. These hormones are all secreted in a pulsatile fashion and pulse frequency varies with the phase of the menstrual cycle. Within the ovary, FSH helps to synthesize the "female hormone" estrogen. As estrogen levels become higher (range of 200–300 pg/ml) and are maintained above this level for more than 24 hr,

positive feedback loops on the pituitary gland then trigger a surge of LH and FSH. This leads to release of the egg from the ovaries. The endocrine system then increases synthesis of another hormone, progesterone, which will act on the uterine wall (endometrium) to facilitate the changes necessary for successful egg implantation to occur. In the absence of fertilization, the portion of the uterus that has prepared for egg implantation and pregnancy disintegrates and menstruation occurs. This sloughing of the endometrium is known as menstruation.

The endometrium responds to these cyclical changes of ovarian hormones. Estrogen stimulates growth by increasing both the number and size of the endometrial cells. Progesterone receptors are induced on the membranes of these cells in response to increasing estrogen levels. Estrogen also increases the blood flow to the endometrium. This phase of the cycle is called the proliferative or follicular phase and occurs immediately following menstruation as FSH and thus estrogen levels start to rise.

As the estrogen levels rise and remain in the critical range for 24–48 hr, the positive feedback loop is activated in the pituitary gland resulting in the LH surge. This surge can be detected using ovulation kits.

The luteal phase of the cycle is characterized by progesterone dominance. This action on the endometrium is manifested by decrease in the cell growth (proliferative) effects of estrogen. Progesterone production causes a rise in basal body temperature and forms the basis of tests used to confirm that ovulation has occurred.

In the absence of fertilization, there is a decline in estrogen and progesterone levels. This decline leads to abrupt loss of hormonal support of the endometrium and subsequent decrease in blood flow, loss of the organized architecture, and resultant menstrual flow. This is called the menstrual phase. Normal blood volume during this menstrual phase varies from 20 to 80 cm^3 over the entire menstrual period.

SEE ALSO: Menstrual cycle disorders, Pregnancy

Suggested Reading

Speroff, L., Glass, R., & Kase, N. G. (1994). *Regulation of the menstrual cycle. Clinical gynecologic endocrinology and infertility* (5th ed., pp. 183–230). Philadelphia: Williams & Wilkins.

MARGARET L. MCKENZIE

Mental Illness

Mental illness can be defined as behavioral, psychological, or biological dysfunction that interferes with an individual's daily life and ability to cope with normal stressors. A "mental disorder" is differentiated from a "physical disorder" in order to categorize types of problematic symptoms and behaviors and to guide decisions regarding the boundary between normality and pathology. It is recognized, however, that the mind and body are inherently connected to and affected by one another, as psychological symptoms affect physical symptoms and vice versa.

Nearly 25% of women will experience mental illness in their lifetime. There are biological and psychosocial factors that affect women's mental health differently than men's mental health. Reproductive health events such as the premenstrual period, pregnancy or postpartum, and the perimenopausal period appear to affect psychological functioning. Gender differences in thyroid function, circadian rhythm patterns (sleep cycles), neurotransmitters (brain chemicals), and hormones may also contribute to higher prevalence rates of some mental disorders in women compared to men. Psychosocial factors such as role identity and conflict (family and work), sexual and physical abuse, discrimination, lack of social support, and poverty also affect women's mental health.

Some mental disorders occur equally commonly in men and women (schizophrenia and bipolar disorder), while other disorders, such as postpartum depression, occur exclusively in women. Depression is much more common in women than in men, likely a result of biological, psychological, and social factors. In the past, it was often believed that women were subject to emotional instability as a "side effect" of their reproductive functioning. "Hysteria" (based on the Greek word for uterus) was a term used in the past to describe overreactive emotional states occurring in women. In some cases, women were deprived of personal rights and freedoms as it was believed they were incapable of making rational decisions when in the grip of these "female," overreactive emotional states. While stigma is still a major factor in the lives of both men and women with mental illness, campaigns to improve public awareness of mental disorders and significant developments in understanding and treatments of mental illness have greatly improved conditions for women who experience emotional illness. "Hysteria" is not a term utilized in modern psychiatry.

While mental illness occurs all over the world and prevalence of disorder is remarkably consistent globally (e.g., approximately 1% of the population worldwide has schizophrenia), how illnesses manifest may differ across gender, age, and culture. For example, in cultures where depression is not an "acceptable" illness, individuals with depression are more likely to present with somatic complaints such as fatigue, headache, and pain.

Outcomes of mental illness may differ by gender and culture as well. For example, in most countries suicide attempts more commonly occur in women, while men are more likely to commit suicide. However, in some countries, such as India and China, the reverse is true, with women being more likely to commit suicide as compared to men. It has been speculated that this may be due to differing social roles between men and women, although much more study is needed to better understand how gender and culture affect the causes, presentation, and outcomes of mental illness.

Mental disorders describe, classify, and categorize symptoms rather than people. They are divided into the categories of mood, anxiety, psychotic, somatoform, factitious, dissociative, sexual and gender identity, eating, sleep, impulse control, adjustment, personality, first diagnosed in infancy, childhood, or adolescence, delirium, dementia, amnestic, and other cognitive disorders, mental disorders due to a general medical condition, and substance-related disorders.

Mood disorders include variations of unipolar and bipolar depression. Major depressive disorder is the presence of a major depressive episode, which is sad mood or loss of interest, along with symptoms such as weight loss, sleep difficulty, fatigue, difficulty concentrating, and thoughts of death or suicide. Dysthymic disorder is a chronic depressive symptom that lasts for at least two years. Women are 2–3 times more likely than men to develop unipolar depression and approximately one out of seven women will develop depression in their lifetime. Sixty to eighty percent of women in the postpartum period experience some combination of depressive and anxiety symptoms, 10–20% of new mothers experience more severe symptoms, resulting in a diagnosis of major depressive disorder with postpartum onset (postpartum depression), and in rare cases (0.1%) women who have just given birth will develop psychotic symptoms. It is estimated that approximately 75% of women experience depressive symptoms in the premenstrual period, and that 3% of women experience symptoms severe enough to be diagnosed with premenstrual dysphoric disorder.

Bipolar disorder is characterized by alternating mood changes between severe lows (depressive episodes) and severe highs (manic episodes). A manic episode is elevated or irritable mood, inflated self-esteem, decreased need for sleep, pressured or rapid speech, racing thoughts, and excessive involvement in pleasurable activities such as spending sprees and sexual indiscretions. Women with bipolar disorder tend to experience a depressive episode first, which can be triggered during the postpartum period. Cyclothymic disorder involves 2 years of alternating periods of manic and depressive symptoms that are not as severe as bipolar disorder.

Anxiety disorders are characterized by irrational fear that is usually accompanied by physiological sensations such as palpitations, sweating, shaking, shortness of breath, chest pain, nausea, dizziness, fear of losing control or going crazy, fear of dying, numbness, and chills or hot flashes. Panic disorder is diagnosed when panic attacks (period of intense fear and physiological symptoms) occur along with fear of additional panic attacks and worry about the consequences of having attacks. Agoraphobia is anxiety about being in places or situations where escape might be difficult or help might not be available if a panic attack occurs. Specific phobias are excessive fears of specific objects or situations and are classified by type: animal, natural environment, blood–injection–injury, or situational. social phobia is overwhelming fear of social situations or performance. Obsessive–compulsive disorder (OCD) is the presence of obsessions (persistent ideas, thoughts, impulses, or images that are inappropriate and intrusive) or compulsions (repetitive behaviors or mental acts that a person engages in to prevent or reduce anxiety). Posttraumatic stress disorder (PTSD) is an anxious response to witnessing or experiencing an extremely traumatic or life-threatening event that includes symptoms such as difficulty sleeping, irritability or anger outbursts, difficulty concentrating, hypervigilance, and exaggerated startle response. Acute stress disorder is exposure to a traumatic event combined with dissociative symptoms such as numbing, detachment, or absence of emotional response. Generalized anxiety disorder (GAD) is characterized by excessive worry and anxiety about numerous events or activities and is associated with symptoms such as restlessness, fatigue, difficulty concentrating, muscle tension, and sleep disturbance. Anxiety disorders such as GAD, social phobia, and panic disorder are diagnosed up to 2–3 times more often in women than men. PTSD is

often diagnosed in women who have been raped, physically or sexually abused, or are victims of domestic violence.

Psychotic disorders are characterized by the presence of psychotic features such as delusions (distorted thoughts or false beliefs) or hallucinations (distortions of perceptions). Schizophrenia includes symptoms such as delusions, hallucinations, disorganized speech, disorganized or catatonic behavior, and affective flattening. Schizophreniform disorder is similar to schizophrenia but is less severe and lasts only 1–6 months. Schizoaffective disorder is characterized by the presence of schizophrenia and either a major depressive or manic episode or both. Delusional disorder involves mistaken beliefs about situations that could occur in real life.

Somatoform disorders are characterized by the presence of physical complaints that cannot be explained by a general medical condition, substance use, or another psychological disorder. Somatization disorder is characterized by numerous physical ailments (pain, gastrointestinal, sexual or reproductive, or pseudoneurological symptoms) that result in medical treatment being sought or significant impairment in daily living. Undifferentiated somatoform disorder is similar to somatization disorder but not as severe. Conversion disorder is characterized by unexplained symptoms or problems with voluntary motor or sensory functioning that suggest a neurological or other general medical condition but is judged to be associated with psychological factors. Pain disorder involves pain as the main focus of clinical attention but psychological factors are judged to be significantly related to the pain. Hypochondriasis is characterized by the preoccupation with having a serious illness or disease based on the misinterpretation of bodily symptoms. Body dysmorphic disorder involves a preoccupation with an exaggerated or imagined defect in the individual's physical appearance. Somatization disorder, conversion disorder, and pain disorder are more common in women than men.

Factitious disorders involve pretending to have physical or psychological symptoms to assume the sick role, without the presence of external incentives for this behavior. Factitious disorder includes subjective complaints, self-inflicted conditions, or exacerbation or exaggeration of an existing general medical condition.

Dissociative disorders are characterized by a change in the usually integrated areas of consciousness, memory, identity, or perception of the environment. Dissociative amnesia is an inability to recall important and traumatic information. Dissociative fugue is sudden travel away from home with an inability to recall the past and confusion about personal identity or the assumption of a new identity. Dissociative identity disorder (previously multiple personality disorder) is two or more distinct identities or personality states that recurrently take control of the individual's behavior. Depersonalization disorder is characterized by a persistent feeling of being detached from one's body or mental processes.

Sexual and gender identity disorders include Sexual Dysfunctions such as sexual desire disorders, sexual arousal disorders, orgasmic disorders, and sexual pain disorders, Paraphilias such as exhibitionism, fetishism, frotteurism, pedophilia, sexual masochism, sexual sadism, transvestic fetishism, and voyeurism, and gender identity disorders, which involve cross-gender identification and discomfort with one's assigned sex.

Eating disorders include severe disturbances in eating behaviors. Anorexia Nervosa is a refusal to maintain a minimally normal body weight, Bulimia Nervosa is repeated episodes of binge eating that are followed by inappropriate compensatory behaviors such as abuse of laxatives, self-induced vomiting, fasting, or excessive exercise, and binge-eating disorder is repeated episodes of eating an excessive amount of food without inappropriate compensatory behaviors. It is estimated that 0.5–5% of women suffer from eating disorders, and social factors such as the pressure for women to be attractive and the association of thinness with attractiveness are thought to contribute to these disorders.

Sleep disorders are organized into categories based on the cause of the sleep dysfunction. Primary sleep disorders include dyssomnias (abnormalities in the amount, quality, or timing of sleep: primary insomnia, primary hypersomnia, narcolepsy, breathing-related sleep disorder, and circadian rhythm sleep disorder) and parasomnias (abnormal behavior in relation to sleep: nightmare disorder, sleep terror disorder, and sleepwalking disorder).

Impulse control disorders are characterized by the failure to resist an impulse or temptation to perform an act that is harmful. Intermittent explosive disorder is the failure to resist aggressive impulses that result in serious assaults or destruction of property. Kleptomania is the failure to resist impulses to steal objects that are not needed. Pyromania is a pattern of setting fires for relief of tension, pleasure, or gratification. Pathological

Gambling is maladaptive gambling behavior that is persistent and recurrent. Trichotillomania is recurrent pulling out of one's hair for relief of tension, pleasure, or gratification and results in noticeable hair loss. Kleptomania and trichotillomania are more common in women than men.

Adjustment disorders are characterized by clinically significant emotional or behavioral symptoms in response to an identifiable stressor and are associated with symptoms such as depressed mood, anxiety, and/or behavior problems.

Personality disorders are patterns of experience and behavior that are inflexible and lead to impairment or distress. Paranoid personality disorder is characterized by excessive suspiciousness and distrust. Schizoid personality disorder is diagnosed in individuals who show a restricted range of emotions and have a history of detachment from social relationships. Schizotypal personality disorder is characterized by acute discomfort in close relationships, eccentricities of behavior, and cognitive or perceptual distortions. Antisocial personality disorder is diagnosed in individuals who show disregard for and violation of the rights of others. Borderline personality disorder is characterized by impulsive behaviors and instability in interpersonal relationships, self-image, and mood. Histrionic personality disorder is characterized by excessive emotionality and attention-seeking behaviors. Avoidant personality disorder is diagnosed in individuals who are socially inhibited, feel inadequate, and are hypersensitive to negative evaluation by others. Dependent personality disorder is characterized by submissive and clinging behavior related to an excessive need to be taken care of. Obsessive–compulsive personality disorder is diagnosed in individuals who are preoccupied with orderliness, perfectionism, and control. Borderline, histrionic, and dependent personality disorders are more common in women than in men.

There are disorders that are usually first diagnosed in infancy, childhood, or adolescence, but there is no clear distinction between childhood and adult disorders. Disorders included in this category are mental retardation, learning disorders, motor skills disorder, communication disorders, pervasive developmental disorders (autistic disorder, Rett's disorder, childhood disintegrative disorder, and Asperger's disorder), attention-deficit and disruptive behavior disorders (attention-deficit/hyperactivity disorder, conduct disorder, and oppositional defiant disorder), Feeding and eating disorders of infancy or early childhood (pica, rumination disorder, and feeding disorder of infancy or early childhood), Tic disorders (Tourette's disorder, chronic motor or vocal tic disorder, and transient Tic disorder), Elimination disorders (Encopresis and enuresis), and other disorders such as separation anxiety disorder, selective mutism, reactive attachment disorder of infancy or early childhood, and stereotypic movement disorder.

Delirium, dementia, amnestic, and other cognitive disorders are characterized by a clinically significant deficit in cognition or memory. Delirium is a disturbance of consciousness that develops over a short period of time, Dementia is multiple cognitive deficits including memory, and an amnestic disorder is memory impairment in the absence of other significant cognitive problems.

Mental disorders due to a general medical condition are psychological symptoms (delirium, dementia, amnestic, psychotic, mood, anxiety, sexual dysfunction, or sleep) that are judged to be the result of a general medical condition.

Substance-related disorders are associated with the taking of a drug of abuse, side effects of medication, and toxin exposure. The two groups of substance-related disorders are substance use disorders (substance dependence and substance abuse) and substance-induced disorders (substance intoxication, substance withdrawal, and substance-induced delirium, dementia, amnestic, psychotic, mood, anxiety, sexual dysfunction, or sleep disorders). The 11 classes of substances include alcohol, amphetamines, caffeine, cannabis, cocaine, hallucinogens, inhalants, nicotine, opioids, phencyclidine (PCP), and sedatives, hypnotics, and anxiolytics.

Most mental disorders can be successfully treated in a variety of ways. Psychoactive medications are used to modify emotions and behavior in the treatment of mental disorders and include antidepressant, antianxiety, antipsychotic, and antimanic medications. Antidepressants are commonly used to treat unipolar depression and anxiety disorders and include tricyclic antidepressants, monoamine oxidase inhibitors (MAOIs), and selective serotonin reuptake inhibitors (SSRIs). Antianxiety medications include benzodiazepines, which relieve anxiety symptoms for a short period of time. Antipsychotic medications cannot cure psychosis, but are very effective in treating psychotic symptoms, and antimanic medications stabilize the mood swings in bipolar disorder. Women who are of childbearing age should discuss and carefully weigh the pros and cons of psychotropic medication treatment

with their doctors because of the potential risks while taking birth control pills, possible birth defects in the developing fetus, and the passing of medication through breast milk. Psychosocial therapy includes individual psychotherapy (cognitive-behavioral or interpersonal therapy is commonly used), family therapy, psychoeducation, group therapy (supportive or self-help), inpatient hospitalization, rehabilitation services, and electroconvulsive treatment (ECT).

The changes in laws and public policy in the United States reflect the ever-evolving feminist movement, and the history of women and mental illness is representative of cultural issues reflected in laws and public policy. One historical example is the story of Elizabeth Packard who, in the mid-1800s, was committed to a state mental hospital simply because her husband asserted that she was insane. When she was released, she won a jury trial, and advocated for laws to be changed. She was responsible for changes to commitment laws in many states and was crucial to raising awareness about the treatment of patients in mental asylums. She also fought for the "Bill for the Protection of Personal Liberty," which granted the right to a jury trial to individuals committed to an asylum. In the United States during the years of Packard's story, public policy regarding mental illness also reflected the views regarding women at that time. Women were not yet allowed to vote and husbands were permitted to send their wives to a mental hospital without evidence of insanity.

The "Anti-Psychiatry Movement" that began in the 1960s is another example of the impact of culture on women and mental illness (although criticisms of psychiatry began decades before the 1960s). Much of this movement derived from criticism regarding inhumane treatment of psychiatric patients including lobotomies, ECT, isolation, and restraint. Some also believed that many individuals are misdiagnosed, overdiagnosed, or mistreated. Many people argue against involuntary commitment, coming from a legal or civil liberties perspective. As with Elizabeth Packard, social reform and public policy changes resulted from this movement. Sylvia Plath's *The Bell Jar* and Ken Kesey's *One Flew Over the Cuckoo's Nest* are examples of literary efforts at social reform regarding psychiatric treatment. Plath's work also addressed social and cultural issues related to women and mental illness, including social class and a patriarchal society. More recently, Susanna Kaysen's *Girl, Interrupted* also questioned the symptoms for diagnosing borderline personality disorder, implying that social class and a male-dominated society had a significant influence in her diagnosis and experiences in inpatient psychiatric treatment.

It is evident that culture plays a significant role in various aspects of mental illness, including prevalence rates of diagnoses, as well as treatment implications and access to treatment. Research has shown that racial and ethnic minorities are less likely than the general public to receive quality mental health care. Culture also affects how patients communicate and manifest their symptoms, coping styles and skills, willingness to seek treatment, and family and community supports. A history of racism and discrimination in this country often causes mistrust and fear that deters minorities from utilizing services and obtaining mental health care.

Research has shown that there is a disproportionate number of African Americans who are homeless, incarcerated, in the child welfare system, and victims of trauma; these populations have an increased risk for mental illness. Approximately 40% of Hispanic Americans report difficulty speaking English, therefore, many Hispanic Americans have limited access to Spanish-speaking mental health providers. The American Indians/Alaskan Natives population has a suicide rate that is 50% higher than the national average. It appears that co-occurring mental illness and substance abuse are also higher in this population. Asian Americans/Pacific Islanders often present with more severe mental illnesses than other ethnic groups, possibly due to stigma and shame preventing individuals from seeking treatment.

SEE ALSO: Anxiety disorders, Bipolar disorder, Dementia, Depression, Discrimination, Eating disorders, Hysteria, Obsessive–compulsive disorder, Panic attack, Schizophrenia, Sleep disorders, Substance use

Suggested Reading

American Psychiatric Association. (1994). *Diagnostic and statistical manual of mental disorders* (4th ed.). Washington, DC: American Psychiatric Association.

Suggested Resources

Lawbuzz, Boz & Glaxier, PLC (2000). www.lawbuzz.com
Manteno State Hospital, Manteno, IL. www.themantenoproject.org
Mayo Clinic (April 19, 2001). www.mayoclinic.com
National Alliance for the Mentally Ill (1996–2003). Arlington, VA, www.nami.org
National Institute of Mental Health (2002, May 14). Bethesda, MD, www.nimh.nih.gov
Postpartum Support International (1997–2003). Woodland Hills, CA (March 15, 2003), www.postpartum.net
Psychiatric Survivor Archives of Toronto. www.psychiatricsurvivorar chives.com
United States Surgeon General (2001). Rockville, MD (June 1, 2003). www.surgeongeneral.gov
Wikipedia: The Free Encyclopedia. www.wikipedia.org

TIRA B. STEBBINS

Midwifery   Midwifery is the second oldest profession for women in the world. The practice of midwifery is documented in the Old Testament. The derivation of the word *midwife* means "with woman," giving credence to the most enduring hallmark of midwifery which connotes a human presence during birth.

Exclusive of the North American continent, midwifery care for women has maintained a congruent path throughout history. Organized schools of midwifery have flourished across Europe through the centuries as far back as the 5th century BC when Hippocrates founded the first formal midwifery program. Countries across the world continue to recognize midwives as the caregivers of women, especially during parturition. Today's midwife is very different from the one who counseled Moses' mother to set him adrift in a basket upon the Nile, but her/his role in counseling women remains undaunted.

Midwifery came to America with the first colonists, although birth attendants existed among the Native Americans long before the continent was "discovered." This *new* midwife initially had been trained in Europe or was indigenously apprenticed in America. It was Mary Breckinridge who, having been educated in England, brought the nurse midwife to the United States in the early 1920s to care for Appalachian women and their families in the state of Kentucky. In 1925, she opened the Frontier Nursing Service with nurse midwives who had also been educated in England. These British-trained nurse midwives were the first to practice in the United States.

In 1931, the first nurse midwifery educational program in the United States opened in New York City. It was called the Lobenstine Midwifery School and continues today as the State University of New York (SUNY) Downstate educational program. Currently there are over 40 nurse midwifery educational programs, and nurse midwives practice in all the 50 states. The number of graduates fluctuates each year, but usually over 400 graduate yearly. Currently, there are over 10,000 Certified Nurse Midwives in the United States, and over 7,000 belong to the American College of Nurse Midwives (ACNM). Ninety-five percent are women, and the majority practice in urban and suburban communities.

The American College of Nurse Midwifery was formed in 1955 and changed its name to ACNM when it merged with the Kentucky Association of Nurse Midwives in 1969. The ACNM sets the Standards for nurse midwifery/midwifery practice in the United States. Through the Division of Accreditation, the ACNM accredits its educational programs to ensure a single standard of education; the Certification Council provides the venue for national certification. Within the last decade, the ACNM has expanded its educational horizon and accredited a nonnurse midwifery educational route to practice. Individuals who select the nonnurse route to midwifery must possess a Bachelor of Science degree to be considered for admission. After acceptance they must successfully complete a bridge option which includes basic fundamentals of health care and the trends and ethics of today's health care delivery system. These students then attend and complete the same accredited midwifery education program as their fellow registered nurse students.

There are different routes to midwifery education and care in the United States today. As a future practitioner, it is important for an individual to choose the educational route consistent with his/her philosophy of practice. As a consumer, it is important for a woman to make an informed decision about the practice of midwifery, before entrusting herself and her baby to the birth attendant.

The Certified Nurse Midwife (CNM) and Certified Midwife (CM) are licensed providers who have been educated in programs accredited by the ACNM Division of Accreditation and nationally certified by the ACNM Certification Council. State regulations and/or legislation are promulgated to set the perimeters of the scope of practice.

Direct entry into midwifery education and practice are prospering in its own venue. Midwives' Alliance of North America (MANA) is the official professional organization. Accreditation standards for educational programs and certification of its graduates have been established through the Midwifery Education Accreditation Council (MEAC) and the North American Registry of Midwives (NARM).

Certified Nurse Midwives/Certified Midwives, referred to hereafter as "midwives," provide primary care to women throughout the life cycle. Today, midwives are not just provider of care during pregnancy and childbirth; they provide care that emphasizes well woman care incorporating health promotion and education through the woman's lifetime. Pregnancy and childbirth, however, remain a focal point of midwifery care, since pregnancy is often a healthy woman's first entry into the health care system. Midwives attend about 9% of births nationally each year.

Midwives focus on pregnancy as a normal event, and they inspire women to have confidence and to trust their bodies. Their basic approach is to empower the woman and her family to take an active role in her health care. Midwives respect technology and use it appropriately; they educate women to make informed decisions about childbirth, and they provide the know-how and environment necessary to achieve a safe and satisfying birthing experience.

Increasingly, today's families are choosing midwives, as evidenced by a 118% increase in births attended by midwives in the last decade. However, many legislative, political, economic, and social challenges confront the profession and women's health care. Among them are:

1. High liability premiums
2. Barriers to home birth and trial of labor after cesarean
3. Increasing use of epidurals and induction of labor
4. Emergence of elective cesarean sections
5. Inequitable reimbursement for nurse midwifery services
6. Decrease in scholarship funds for students

In order to sustain and promote the growth in the practice of midwifery observed in the last decade, midwives must educate the public that they are skilled and knowledgeable practitioners who care for women over their lifetimes, rather than only during pregnancy and childbirth.

SEE ALSO: History of Women's Health (pp. 3–13), Women in the Health Professions (pp. 20–32), Labor and delivery, Nurse practitioner, Nursing, Pregnancy, Prenatal care

Suggested Reading

Rooks, J. P. (1997). *Midwifery and childbirth in America.* Philadelphia: Temple University Press.

Suggested Resources

American College of Nurse Midwives: www.midwife.org

ELAINE K. DIEGMANN

Migraine Migraine is the second most common headache disorder, after tension-type headache. The prevalence of migraine is related to age and sex. Before puberty, boys are more susceptible than girls. After puberty, the prevalence in women increases until age 40–50 and then decreases. At age 40, 26% of women will have at least one migraine over the course of a year, compared with 8% of men.

Migraine is a hereditary illness. First-degree relatives of an affected person are 2–4 times as likely to have migraines. The mode of inheritance for most types of migraine is not known, but one form, familial hemiplegic migraine (a type of migraine that runs in families and causes bodily weakness), is known to be transmitted as an autosomal dominant trait (specific method of genetic transmission). The gene has been mapped to chromosome 19.

Migraine consists of two parts, a transient neurological symptom, called the *aura*, and a headache. They can occur together (*migraine with aura*) or separately (*migraine without aura, migraine aura without headache*). The aura usually precedes the headache but may occur during it or afterwards.

The most common auras are abnormalities of vision, sensation, and language ability. An aura may occur alone, or two or three may appear one after another. Visual auras are usually small and unobtrusive at first but enlarge and spread across the field of vision during a period of 10–15 min. Likewise, sensory auras start in one part of the body, usually the fingers or lips, and spread slowly to other parts. Auras usually last 15–30 min and then disappear. Visual auras often consist of an area of visual loss surrounded by a shimmer or a flickering light (scintillating scotoma), or zigzag lines in the form of a horseshoe (fortification spectrum). Sensory auras may consist of numbness or tingling and "pins and needles." A language aura (aphasia) impairs the subject's ability to express herself in words or to understand spoken or written language. Other less common auras include limb weakness, vertigo (dizziness), double vision, lack of coordination, and a reduced level of consciousness.

The pain of migraine may be on one or both sides of the head. It generally has a pulsating or throbbing quality, is moderate to severe in intensity, and is made worse by routine physical activity, such as climbing stairs. The headache is often associated with nausea, vomiting, and sensitivity to light (photophobia) and sound (phonophobia). Untreated, the pain lasts for 4 hr to 3 days.

Migraine headaches respond better to *abortive treatment* the earlier it is given after the pain starts. The choice of medication depends on the severity of the pain. Mild headaches may respond to over-the-counter pain relievers, such as aspirin and acetaminophen (with or without caffeine), and to nonsteroidal anti-inflammatory drugs (NSAIDs), such as ibuprofen and naproxen. Moderate and severe headaches require a prescription drug. The most effective drugs belong to a family of agents called "triptans." Sumatriptan (Imitrex) was the first one marketed. It is available as a tablet, a nasal spray, and a subcutaneous injection. More intense headaches require the nasal spray or injection. Dihydro-ergotamine, another antimigraine agent, is available as a nasal spray (Migranal) and is at least as effective as sumatriptan nasal spray, although not as effective as the injection. The nausea and vomiting of a migraine will respond to antinausea drugs, such as metoclopramide, domperidone, and prochlorperazine, taken as a tablet or suppository.

Using abortive medications for migraine more than 2 days a week can lead to *medication-overuse headache*, a chronic daily headache that improves with each dose of medicine but recurs in a few hours, creating a vicious cycle of withdrawal headache. In order to avoid this, many patients use *preventive therapy* of migraine. Preventive therapy involves taking a drug regularly, everyday, in order to reduce the frequency, severity, and duration of migraine attacks. Once the migraines have been under good control for 3–6 months, the drugs can be withdrawn. Several classes of drugs may be used: beta-blockers such as propranolol, antidepressants such as amitriptyline and phenelzine, calcium-channel blockers such as verapamil, and antiepileptic drugs such as valproate, topiramate, and gabapentin. Although beta-blockers and calcium-channel blockers are also blood pressure medicines, they are usually tolerated well when taken for migraines.

During the first trimester of pregnancy, the risk of exposing the fetus restricts the use of preventive drugs. Among abortive agents, acetaminophen, caffeine,

NSAIDs, narcotic analgesics, and probably sumatriptan are safe, as are the antiemetic agents (prevent vomiting) prochlorperazine and metoclopramide. Amitriptyline, as a preventive drug, is probably safe in the second and third trimesters. Late in pregnancy, NSAIDs should be avoided because they inhibit closure of the fetal ductus arteriosus, causing circulatory problems in the newborn. Breast-feeding mothers should discuss medication choices with their health care provider, to avoid possible ill-effects on the infant.

Many women have migraine headaches only or mainly with their menstrual periods (*menstrual migraine*). These migraines are often intense, long-lasting, and resist abortive treatment. Use of NSAIDs or standard preventive drugs before and during the period, a short course of oral corticosteroids, or therapy with estrogen can prevent or reduce the headaches.

Hormonal contraceptives, including oral and injectable contraceptives, may cause or worsen migraine. This usually occurs within the first few cycles of their use but may not appear for years. Stopping the drug may not bring immediate relief: there may be a delay of several months or no improvement at all.

Migraine with aura and, to a lesser extent, migraine without aura, as well as the use of estrogen-containing contraceptives are all minor risk factors for ischemic stroke. Controversy continues on whether it really is too risky to use estrogen-containing contraceptives in patients with migraine. It seems reasonable, however, not to use them in migraine patients who have other stroke risk factors, such as smoking, high blood pressure, or age over 40 years. If migraine auras appear or worsen during treatment, then these contraceptives should be discontinued.

People with migraines can also develop other types of headache. Some causes of headache, such as bleeding within the skull or meningitis, are quite dangerous. Talk with your health care provider if your headaches change significantly. Warning signs of a possibly serious condition include headache that comes on suddenly without warning, pain that is different from or much worse than your usual migraine pain, headaches occurring more often or lasting longer, pain that gets worse with each new headache, headache that develops after a head injury, headache with fever or stiff neck, or headache with new neurological symptoms such as trouble walking, talking, or weakness.

SEE ALSO: Headache, Oral contraception, Pain

Suggested Reading

Becker, W. J. (1999). Use of oral contraceptives in patients with migraine. *Neurology, 53*(Suppl. 1), S19–S25.

Silberstein, S. D., Lipton, R. B., & Goadsby, P. J. (1998). *Headache in clinical practice*. Oxford: Isis Medical Media.

Silberstein, S. D., Stiles, A., Young, W. B., & Rozen, T. D. (2002). *An atlas of headache*. New York: Parthenon.

MARC WINKELMAN

Military Service

In 2001, there were 1,385,116 active duty members of the United States military, down from 1,610,490 in 1994. In 2001 there were 207,188 women service members, roughly 15% of the total force, up from 199,688 in 1994. Compared to 1994, the total number of active duty military members fell, while the number of women service members rose by about 2.5%.

Until 1948, women could serve as voluntary members of the military. The Army had the Women's Army Auxiliary Corps (WAACs), the Navy had the Women Accepted for Voluntary Emergency Service (WAVES), and the Marines had "Semper Paratus, Always Ready" (SPAR). Usually these volunteers served as nurses, clerks, and sometimes even performed communications jobs, but were not considered full members of the armed services.

The Women's Armed Services Act of 1948 opened the military forces for women to become full members, however limiting their service to noncombat role. Roughly 50% of all military jobs are now open to women. This number varies by branch of service.

In the recent Gulf War, some 540,000 soldiers participated in Operation Desert Storm; of these soldiers, approximately 35,000 were women. The Persian Gulf War was the first major conflict where women saw front-line action. Women were very much in the media spotlight during this war. Media attention and the exceptional performance of female service members during the Gulf War were largely responsible for the changing attitudes and subsequent opening of many previously prohibited jobs to women. Combat exclusion laws have been repealed, however, there are still a number of military occupations closed to women. Among those closed to women are: infantry, armor, field artillery, and special forces in the Army; submarine, SEAL (special forces units), and mining/antimining positions in the Navy; infantry, artillery, armored units, reconnaissance, and combat engineer units in the Marine Corps; and finally, parachute-rescue and combat controllers in the Air Force.

A few of the reasons that opponents of women in combat roles offer for exclusion are: physical differences, reproductive issues, that men would be unable to fight because they would be too concerned with protecting female members, and the potential rape by enemy forces if captured. As military equipment and jobs become more technical and hand-to-hand combat in war decreases, many of these arguments fall by the wayside.

The year 1994 saw an enormous surge of female firsts for the military. In 1994, 1st Lt. Jeanne Flynn became the first Air Force combat jet pilot; Lt. Shannon Workman became the first female Navy pilot to qualify on an aircraft carrier, and 1st Lt. Sarah Deal became the first Marine Corps combat pilot. Also in 1994, the Navy allowed two female pilots to fly combat missions for the first time.

Another area of military service to be opened to women, during the 1990s, came after the United States Supreme Court ruled, in a seven-to-one decision, that the prestigious Virginia Military Institute (VMI) would have to either accept women or go private. VMI's answer was to create the Virginia Women's Military Institute (VWMI). Shortly thereafter, another military academy, the Citadel, admitted their first woman student, Shannon Faulkner.

The United States military has progressed far in the area of women's equality; while not quite there yet, the military continues to progress toward equality.

SEE ALSO: Women in the Workforce (pp. 32–40), Sexual harassment

Suggested Reading

Feinman, I. R. (2000). *Citizenship rites: Feminist soldiers and feminist antimilitarists.* New York: New York University Press.

Gutmann, S. (2000). *The kinder, gentler military: Can America's gender-neutral fighting force still win wars?* New York: Scribner's.

Mace, N. (2001). *In the company of men: A woman at the Citadel.* New York: Simon & Schuster.

Patterson, M. (2001). *A woman's guide to the Army from a survivor.* Pittsburgh, PA: Dorrance.

Weinstein, L., & White, C. C. (Eds.). (1997). *Wives and warriors: Women in the military in the United States and Canada.* London: Bergin & Garvey.

TAMBRA K. CAIN

Miscarriage A miscarriage is a pregnancy that ends before the fetus reaches a point where it would be able to survive outside the uterus. The medical term for a miscarriage is a "spontaneous abortion." About 80% of miscarriages occur in the first trimester, meaning the first 12 weeks of pregnancy. Approximately 20% of pregnancies end in miscarriage. There are probably another 10% of pregnancies lost before women actually realize they are even pregnant.

When a miscarriage occurs, couples are very anxious to understand why this event, which can be devastating, has happened. Approximately 50% of miscarriages are due to genetic abnormalities of the fetus. Most babies are born perfect, and this is "nature's way" of controlling this wonderful phenomenon. Most abnormal fetuses will not continue to grow and will result in miscarriage. The earlier in a pregnancy a miscarriage occurs, the more likely that it was a result of a genetic abnormality. Miscarriages may also be the result of uterine abnormalities such as fibroids or cervical abnormalities. Women with repeated pregnancy losses may require complex evaluations looking for possible autoimmune or endocrine diseases. Miscarriages are not caused by maternal activity (exercise, heavy lifting, etc.) or intercourse. Often patients are concerned about how they may have contributed to this event. It is important to discuss these concerns with your physician. It is unusual to know why a miscarriage occurred.

There are multiple factors that increase the risk of a miscarriage. The most important of these is maternal age. Between the ages of 20 and 30, the risk of miscarriage is 9–17%. At age 35, the risk is 20%, at age 40, the risk is 40%, and at age 45, the risk is 80%. The risk of miscarriage also increases with the more children a woman has had, this is independent of her age. Having had a previous miscarriage is a risk as well. But this is very much dependent on how many miscarriages have occurred. After a single miscarriage, the risk of a second is about 20%, after two miscarriages, the risk is about 28%, and after three miscarriages, the risk is 43%. Most physicians begin an investigation as to why a miscarriage occurs after two or three miscarriages; this will depend upon the patient's specific situation. Smoking and alcohol consumption also increase the risk. Caffeine increases the risk at a significant level when 4–5 cups or more of coffee are consumed a day. There are also, less commonly, risks from maternal exposure to chemicals, medications, or infections.

There are many ways in which a woman may learn that she has had a miscarriage. The most common way is by vaginal bleeding and/or abdominal cramping. These symptoms may also occur, however, in a normal pregnancy or an ectopic pregnancy (pregnancy outside of the uterus). Because of this, ultrasound is key to the evaluation of a possible miscarriage. If a heartbeat is not seen by approximately 6 weeks gestation (6 weeks from the last menstrual period) on a transvaginal ultrasound (specialized procedure using sound waves to visualize the structure around and in the uterus), concern of miscarriage increases. When the diagnosis is not entirely clear, blood levels of the pregnancy hormone, beta-HCG, may be followed over the course of several days. If vaginal bleeding is heavy and the cervix has already begun to dilate, the miscarriage is considered "inevitable." If bleeding is occurring in the face of a heartbeat on ultrasound and a closed cervix, the miscarriage is considered "threatened"; this can be an extremely stressful time for a woman. Continued surveillance with ultrasound is then indicated. There are times when bleeding has occurred to the point that the fetus is passed as well. In these cases an ultrasound reveals an empty uterus. This is called a "complete abortion" and usually no further medical or surgical treatment is necessary. If a significant amount of tissue remains in the uterus, despite loss of a fetal heartbeat, this is called an "incomplete abortion" and often the patient is offered medical or more commonly surgical therapy to complete the miscarriage and clear the uterine cavity. Because of the frequent use of early ultrasound, often a miscarriage is diagnosed even before the patient has experienced any vaginal bleeding. In this case, a routine ultrasound would reveal that the fetus is either not developing normally or no longer has a heartbeat.

Treatment of a miscarriage is varied. If a pregnancy is before approximately 7–8 weeks, often a woman is encouraged to "let nature take its course." In other words, no intervention would be made by the physician and the woman would simply wait to see whether the pregnancy passes on its own. Usually this occurs within 2 weeks, but may take longer. This can result in heavy bleeding and painful cramping, but can be handled well by most women. If at any time the woman felt the bleeding was too heavy or pain too severe, she would contact her physician. In order to expedite passing the pregnancy, or to attempt this later in the first trimester, medication may be considered. More commonly, however, a woman is offered a dilation and curettage (D&C) to complete the miscarriage. This is a surgical procedure done either in the operating room or in the physician's office. This is a decision made by the woman and her physician. The risks of D&C are small, but include bleeding, infection, and uterine perforation.

After a miscarriage, it is usually advised not to have intercourse until after the next normal menses. If intercourse occurs before then, a condom should be used. It is medically safe to attempt pregnancy again after the first normal menses. Many couples are encouraged to wait 2–3 cycles, however, to give themselves some time to heal psychologically from this emotionally difficult event. If a woman feels she is more depressed than she would expect, or is concerned about her mood in any way, it is very important for her to discuss this with her physician.

SEE ALSO: Autoimmune disorders, Ectopic pregnancy, Genetic counseling, Pelvic organ prolapse, Pregnancy, Uterine fibroids

Suggested Resources

American College of Gynecology: www.acog.org

MERRILL S. LEWEN

Mitral Valve Prolapse

Mitral valve prolapse (MVP) is the most common congenital valvular heart disease in adults and has become the most frequent valvular cause of chronic mitral regurgitation (leakiness) in the United States.

The prevalence of this disease in our country varies according to the sources in the literature due to a lack of strict criteria for diagnosis and differences in study design. This condition has been reported to occur in 5–10% of the general population, with the prevalence being highest in young women. However, this finding was based on studies using old diagnostic criteria for this condition. Dr. Levine and colleagues at the Massachusetts General Hospital showed that the supposed epidemic of MVP was created by misinterpretation of echocardiographic findings. The Framingham Study examined 1,845 women and 1,646 men using the current two-dimensional echocardiographic criteria for the diagnosis of MVP. The findings were: disease prevalence of 2.4%, no gender difference and no age group predominance.

Mitral Valve Prolapse

The mitral valve is a bileaflet structure that separates the left atrium and the left ventricle (the upper and lower left-sided chambers of the heart). It is composed of the anterior and posterior leaflets, the chordae tendineae that are attached to the papillary muscles, and the mitral valve annulus. In MVP disease, there is thickening and redundancy of the leaflets, elongation, thinning and occasional rupture of the chordae tendineae, and dilatation of the annulus. Histologically, there is substitution of the normal fibrous tissue of the valve structure by a myxomatous process that is responsible for the above changes. Both leaflets can be involved, but the posterior leaflet is the most commonly affected one.

MVP, floppy mitral valve, click/murmur syndrome, Barlow's syndrome, and myxomatous mitral valve disease are all different names for this disease. The name prolapse comes from the fact that one or both leaflets are displaced above the mitral valve ring into the left atrium during systole, the contraction phase of the heart. MVP can be inherited as an autosomal dominant condition with incomplete penetrance or, less commonly, as an X-chromosome-linked disorder in which males are affected and females are carriers. It can be associated with connective tissue disorders such as Marfan syndrome, Ehlers–Danlos syndrome, adult polycystic kidney disease, anterior chest deformity, scoliosis, and kyphosis. It can be associated with tricuspid valve prolapse as well.

The diagnosis of MVP is based on physical examination of the heart with confirmatory echocardiographic findings. On auscultation of the heart, the typical finding is the midsystolic click, which may or may not be associated with a late systolic murmur of mitral regurgitation because of lack of complete coaptation of the anterior and posterior leaflets. Echocardiography is the most useful tool that can show in real time the prolapsing mitral leaflets, the thickened leaflets, redundant chordae tendineae, and dilated annulus. It can also reveal the severity of mitral regurgitation, if there is any, as well as determine whether there is dilatation of the heart chambers and deterioration of heart function.

Mitral regurgitation is one of the most common complications of MVP disease. Fortunately, the majority of patients have only mild regurgitation or none at all. However, 2–7% of patients progress to severe regurgitation, requiring surgical treatment. Furthermore, the presence of severe regurgitation is a risk factor for heart failure, sudden death, arrhythmias, and congestive heart failure. Symptoms suggestive of hemodynamically significant mitral regurgitation are shortness of breath, decreased exercise tolerance with easy fatigability, and dizziness. Once the patient develops the above symptoms, it is usually indicative that left ventricular contractility is beginning to decrease and surgical treatment with either valve repair or replacement is indicated. Chordae rupture can complicate MVP and can occur spontaneously or during exercise. Mitral valve repair is the treatment of choice over valve replacement when the anatomy is favorable. This is because the former is related to a better outcome with regard to preservation of ventricular function. Isolated posterior leaflet prolapse has better operative success results with lower reoperation rate than anterior or bileaflet prolapse. Indications for surgery in MVP are: (a) development of symptoms of heart failure; (b) asymptomatic patients with severe regurgitation and evidence of left ventricular systolic dysfunction or left ventricular dilatation; (c) chordae rupture with severe regurgitation. Sudden death in patients with MVP is rare (1–2.5%) in the absence of significant mitral valve degeneration and regurgitation. The risks factors for sudden death are: (a) prolapse involving leaflets, (b) significant mitral regurgitation, (c) history of syncope or near syncope, (d) presence of flail mitral leaflet, (e) reduced left ventricular systolic function, and (f) atrial fibrillation.

Infective endocarditis (infection involving the mitral valve caused by bacteria or fungus) is a possible complication of MVP, mainly when it is associated with mitral regurgitation and significant leaflet thickening. Therefore, patients with these two conditions should be advised to take antibiotics prior to any invasive procedures such as dental cleaning and endoscopy with biopsy.

Based on observational studies, the risk of strokes and transient ischemic cerebral attacks in MVP is very low: estimated to be 1 in 11,000 per year. Many people with MVP present with a constellation of nonspecific symptoms that cannot be attributed to advanced valve dysfunction, such as panic attacks, anxiety, atypical chest pain, and palpitations without arrhythmias. This constellation of symptoms has been called MVP syndrome. Many physicians believe that these symptoms are coincidental and that the link between them and the disease is accidental because of the inaccuracy of original studies suggesting an association. It is possible, however, that the autonomic nervous system and neuroendocrine dysfunction found in some patients with MVP may be responsible for some of these symptoms. Further investigation is warranted to confirm this possibility. Patients with these symptoms benefit from reassurance about the benign nature of this disorder, changes in lifestyle, including aerobic exercise, avoidance of stimulants such as caffeine and alcohol, and reduction of stress.

Asymptomatic patients with MVP may engage in exercise and competitive activities. However, patients with mitral regurgitation should avoid weight lifting. Patients with MVP should be followed with a physical examination every 2–3 years. A new murmur or development of symptoms should prompt further evaluation with an echocardiogram.

SEE ALSO: Anxiety disorders, Chest pain, Exercise

Suggested Reading

Boudolas, H., Kolibash, A. J., Jr., Baker, P., King, D. B., & Wooley, C. F. (1989). Mitral valve prolapse and the mitral valve prolapse syndrome: A diagnostic classification and pathogenesis of symptoms. *American Heart Journal, 118*, 796–818.

Braunwald, E. (2001). Heart disease. In E. Braunwald, D. P. Zipes, & P. Libby (Eds.), *A textbook of cardiovascular medicine* (pp. 1665–1671). Philadelphia: W. B. Saunders.

Freed, L. A., Levy, D., & Levine, R. A. (1999). Prevalence and clinical outcome of mitral valve prolapse. *New England Journal of Medicine, 341*, 1.

ELINA YAMADA
CLAIRE DUVERNOY

Moles

Moles Nevi, commonly referred to as moles, beauty marks, or birthmarks, are one of the many types of benign tumors of the skin. Moles can be present at birth or develop during childhood or adulthood. A normal mole can be flat or raised and is generally an evenly colored brown, tan, or black spot on the skin. It can be round or oval. Moles are generally less than 1/4 in. or 6 mm in diameter. Once a mole has developed, it will usually stay the same size, shape, and color for many years.

Congenital moles or birthmarks are a less common kind of mole. Congenital moles are present at birth and are usually larger (>1.5 cm) than moles that develop after birth. They may be brown or black and sometimes pink. Smaller birthmarks are usually pigmented and often slightly raised. Giant congenital moles may be found anywhere on the skin and can cover large areas of the body. The risk of developing melanoma in these giant moles is high.

The number of moles increases with age, especially during childhood and adolescence. Boys tend to have more moles than girls do. Individuals with a family history of skin cancer tend to have more moles. Both children and adults who are sun sensitive are at increased risk of having or developing moles. Sun sensitivity can be measured as red or blond hair, light or fair skin color, a tendency to burn, a tendency to freckle, and a lack of tanning ability. Both benign moles and melanoma (cancer) occur more often in people with a lighter complexion.

Moles that are irregular in shape, size, or color may be referred to as atypical or dysplastic moles. These moles tend to be large. They form a continuum between the common mole and superficial spreading melanoma. Dysplastic moles may occur as multiple moles distributed over the body, a condition known as dysplastic nevus syndrome. People with multiple moles often have a family history of multiple moles and melanoma, and are at higher risk for developing melanoma themselves. Such people need to be closely monitored by a dermatologist. The association of increasing numbers of moles with melanoma suggests that moles are either markers of some exposure that leads to melanoma, or potential precursors of melanoma or both.

Sun exposure is the major risk factor leading to the development of skin melanoma and precursor lesions such as moles. Childhood sun exposure may promote the development of melanoma by increasing the number of moles that develop. Several studies have found more moles on sun-exposed areas of the body compared to sun-protected areas. After early sun exposure causes moles to develop, other risk factors for melanoma may cause the moles to progress to melanoma. Sunburns are related to both sun exposure and the skin's sensitivity to the sun. Various studies have found an increased risk of moles with increasing number of sunburns, similar to the association seen between sunburns and melanoma.

The contribution of tanning bed use or sunless tanning products to the development of moles has not been well-studied at this time. Similar to sun exposure, ultraviolet light from tanning bed use during adolescence is likely to increase the number of moles. Any changes in a mole seen after tanning bed use should be shown to a dermatologist immediately.

Few moles develop into melanoma. Individuals with many moles have a greater chance that progression will occur. It is important to recognize changes in a mole in both children and adults. Photographs or full body charts of your moles can be used to monitor changes in shape, color, and size over time. The most important warning sign for melanoma is a spot on your skin that is changing in size, shape, or color over a period of 1 month to 1 or 2 years. The ABCD rule may help you remember the four signs of melanoma. If you find one of the following, consult a dermatologist: *asymmetric*—if half of the mole does not match the other half; B—irregular *border*—a mole forms irregular borders or becomes ragged, notched, or blurred; C—change in *color*—a mole changes in color or is not the same color all over; D—large *diameter*—a mole is larger than the width of a pencil eraser (more than 1/4 in. or 6 mm in diameter).

Seeking medical attention for suspicious moles is very important because melanoma can be a deadly disease with few or no symptoms or pain. However, melanoma is also easily curable if identified early and removed. Distinguishing between a mole and a melanoma may be difficult, even for dermatologists. The most dependable method to distinguish a normal mole from melanoma is to remove the mole and have it examined under a microscope to determine whether the lesion is cancerous.

SEE ALSO: Cancer, Melanoma, Skin care

Suggested Reading

Augustsson, A., Stierner, U., Rosdahl, I., & Suurkula, M. (1991). Melanocytic naevi in sun-exposed and protected skin in melanoma patients and controls. *Acta Dermato-Venereologica, 71*(6), 512–517.

Dennis, L. K., & White, E. (1994). Risk factors for the prevalence of nevi: A review. In R. P. Gallagher & J. M. Elwood (Eds.), *Epidemiological aspects of cutaneous malignant melanoma.* Boston: Kluwer.

Elder, D. E. (1989). Human melanocytic neoplasms and their relationship with sunlight. *Journal of Investigative Dermatology, 92*(Suppl. 5), 297S–303S.

Rigel, D. S., & Carucci, J. A. (2000). Malignant melanoma: Prevention, early detection, and treatment in the 21st century. *CA: A Cancer Journal for Clinicians, 50*(4), 215–236.

LESLIE K. DENNIS

Mononucleosis The term *mononucleosis* refers to both a specific infection and a syndrome, with considerable overlap between the two. Acute Epstein–Barr virus (EBV) infection produces an illness characterized by sore throat, swollen lymph glands, fatigue, and fever. The clinical illness produced by acute EBV infection is called mononucleosis; the term is also used when other infectious agents produce a similar illness. EBV is a member of the herpesvirus family, which also includes herpes simplex I and II, cytomegalovirus (CMV), discussed below, and varicella-zoster virus, the cause of chicken pox and shingles. Infection due to this family of viruses is characterized by an acute illness followed by lifelong infection, which is usually clinically silent (although chronic infection, and relapses due to immunosuppression can occur).

Infection with EBV usually occurs during adolescence or early adulthood. The virus is found in saliva, and is spread by kissing, shared beverages, or other close contact. Fever, sore throat, and swollen lymph nodes, particularly in the neck area, are the most typical signs and symptoms. Enlargement of the spleen (splenomegaly) is also common. The clinical presentation can be quite varied and is somewhat dependent on age. Signs and symptoms of acute EBV infection occurring in older individuals (in this case, over 30) are often atypical, and individuals may not have the classic symptoms of sore throat and adenopathy. In children younger than 5, acute EBV infection often produces a mild, nonspecific illness. EBV infects lymphocytes and infection results in the presence of significant numbers of abnormal-appearing white blood cells (referred to as atypical lymphocytes). The absence of atypical lymphocytes makes acute EBV infection highly unlikely, and the presence of significant numbers of atypical lymphocytes strongly suggests the diagnosis. Individuals often have mild elevations in liver function tests (LFTs), but LFTs that are increased by more than five times the normal level are unusual, and should prompt investigation for alternative diagnoses.

Individuals can be quite symptomatic from acute EBV infection, and the symptoms often last 2–3 weeks. Swelling in the lymph nodes and tonsils can be significant, and in rare cases may produce obstruction of the upper airway. The most common complication of acute EBV infection is significant fatigue following the acute illness; it is not unusual for individuals to have fatigue for several months following the initial symptoms. Another complication is splenic rupture; spontaneous splenic rupture is rare but individuals with splenomegaly should refrain from activity that produces trauma to the abdomen such as contact sports. Other complications are rare and include encephalitis (brain swelling), hemolytic anemia (low red blood cells), and myocarditis (swelling of the heart muscle).

Therapy of acute EBV infection is largely supportive and there is no role for antivirals in routine cases. Corticosteroids have been used when marked lymphadenopathy (lymph node swelling) and tonsil swelling threaten the upper airway. The role of EBV in chronic fatigue syndrome (CFS) remains unproven, and most evidence suggests that there is no direct relationship between EBV and CFS. Patients with CFS often have elevated levels of antibodies to EBV, but similar levels occur in many asymptomatic individuals. The existence of "chronic Epstein–Barr," defined by symptoms of fatigue that last more than a year following acute infection, or persistent fatigue without acute infection, remains doubtful. In highly immunosuppressed patients EBV infection is associated with the development of lymphoma, particularly in patients with organ transplants and advanced HIV infection.

About 5% of cases of the mononucleosis syndrome (fever, sore throat, adenopathy, and atypical lymphocytes) are due to causes other than EBV. The most common alternative agent is CMV, which can produce a similar illness, although marked adenopathy (lymph node swelling) is unusual and the percentage of atypical lymphocytes (white blood cells) is much smaller (<5% vs. >20%). Acute infection with CMV can be minimally symptomatic, and can also produce an illness characterized by persistent low-grade fever and fatigue. CMV can produce significant illness in immunosuppressed patients, and is a major cause of morbidity and mortality in AIDS patients and organ transplant patients. Acute infection with the parasite *Toxoplasma gondii* can also produce mononucleosis-like illness.

SEE ALSO: Shingles

Suggested Reading

Cohen, J. I. (2000). Medical progress: Epstein–Barr virus infection. *New England Journal of Medicine, 343,* 481–492.

Schooley, R. T. (2000). Epstein–Barr virus (infectious mononucleosis). In G. L. Mandell, J. E. Bennett, & R. Dolin (Eds.), *Principles and practices of infectious diseases* (5th ed., pp. 1599–1608). New York: Churchill Livingstone.

Suggested Resources

http://www.cdc.gov/ncidod/diseases/ebv.htm

KEITH B. ARMITAGE

Mood Disorders Mood disorders, previously called affective disorders, include a number of psychiatric diagnoses where the major symptom is a disturbance of mood. Most individuals experience a wide range of emotional states from sadness and grief to elation. Even the most extreme mood states do not usually interfere with daily functioning for a prolonged period of time. In contrast, a mood disorder occurs when a persistent state of sad, depressed mood, or elevated, irritable mood interferes with daily life. Depressive disorders and bipolar disorders are the two main categories of mood disorders.

DEPRESSIVE DISORDERS

Major depressive disorder (also known as major depression) and dysthymic disorder (or dysthymia) make up the core depressive disorders. Major depressive disorder is the most common of the depressive mood disorders with a lifetime prevalence of 5–12% in men and 10–25% in women. The prevalence of major depression is twice as high in women as it is in men in nearly every country in which epidemiological studies have been conducted. The exception to this finding is among the Orthodox Jewish community across several countries. Cultural differences and a lack of substance use, particularly alcohol, may account for these findings. One theory about the high rate of depressive illness in women compared to men is that there are significant hormonal changes throughout the life span, particularly just after menarche, childbirth, and menopause. Gender roles may also play a part in the incidence of depression in women, especially for women with very young children trying to balance work and home.

The diagnosis of major depression depends upon the presence of a major depressive episode, which is characterized by an overwhelming low mood and/or a loss of interest or pleasure in most activities. An episode is a distinct period of time, lasting at least 2 weeks, that is marked by a significant decline in one's ability to function in a usual manner. The persistent low mood is accompanied by one or more of the following symptoms: loss of appetite (or increased appetite) usually accompanied by weight loss or gain, difficulty sleeping or excessive sleeping, feelings of restlessness or being slowed down, fatigue, loss of energy, and inappropriate feelings of guilt, poor memory or difficulty concentrating, and thoughts of suicide or death. The presence of a manic or hypomanic episode precludes the diagnosis of a depressive disorder.

The first onset of major depression occurs between the ages of 20 and 50 for 50% of those diagnosed with the disorder; however, the mean age of onset is 40 years of age. Depression also occurs in approximately 2% of children and 4–8% of adolescents. Children may present with primary irritability as well as depressed mood. The distress is commonly identified due to school failure, truancy, drug and alcohol use, persistent irritability, violence, or withdrawal from peers and activities. Major depression occurs in 15% of the elderly (>65 years) population, which is more than 60% female. Onset of major depression at this age is not related to the aging process; rather, it is associated with bereavement due to the loss of a spouse or the stress of a chronic medical condition. Depressive symptoms in the elderly commonly include low mood, low self-esteem, worthlessness, and guilt. Cognitive impairment is not uncommon and must be distinguished from dementia related to aging.

The average duration of an untreated major depressive episode is 6–13 months. When treated, the course may be as short as 3 months, typically resolving by 6 months. Often patients discontinue treatment once they are feeling better. This leads to a return of the symptoms if discontinuation occurs in the first 3 months of treatment. Medication should be tapered gradually to avoid side effects and relapse. Over time, the duration and number of episodes can increase.

Depressive episodes are experienced in several ways. Symptom severity in a depressive episode varies from mild to severe. The number of symptoms experienced in a depressive episode varies from as low as 5 to as many as 10 or more. The depressive episodes may also be recurrent, seasonal (Seasonal Affective Disorder), or occurring within 1–6 months after childbirth (postpartum onset or Postpartum Depression). The depressive episode may be further defined by specific coinciding symptoms, namely, psychotic symptoms (delusions, hallucinations), catatonic (extreme disturbance of mobility), melancholic (mood worse in the morning, low reactivity to pleasurable stimuli, significant slowing or agitation, and inappropriate guilt), or atypical features (mood brightens to positive events, excessive sleeping, increased appetite, or weight gain).

Unlike major depressive disorder, which is characterized by one or more depressive episodes in a distinct period of time, Dysthymia is a chronic, persistent depressed mood for at least 2 years. Individuals with dysthymia often report that they have always been depressed or that they have never been as happy as others in their lives. Feelings of inadequacy and persistent irritability, pessimism, withdrawal from social events, and low activity level are common in Dysthymic Disorder. Symptoms of poor appetite or overeating, fatigue, sleep disturbance, low self-esteem, and poor concentration are common but are not severe enough to impair daily functioning. Children and adolescents with dysthymic disorder are usually irritable and pessimistic, have a low self-esteem, poor social skills, and declining school performance. After the initial 2-year period of depressed mood, major depressive episodes may occur in addition to the chronic low mood and has been called "Double Depression." Dysthymia has a lifetime prevalence of 6%. The disorder typically develops early, with most experiencing the onset by 21 years of age. In children, the number of girls affected is equal to that of boys. However, in adulthood, the incidence in women is 2–3 times that of men.

Other depressive mood disorders have been described in the research and clinical literature. Minor depressive disorder has similar episodic symptoms to major depression but with lower symptom severity. Recurrent Brief Depressive Disorder is characterized by recurring depressive episodes meeting criteria for major depression but for durations of less than 2 weeks at one time. Premenstrual Dysphoric Disorder is a diagnosis currently under research investigation to determine its validity as a distinct disorder. The disorder is distinguished by abnormal mood and behavior in addition to physical symptoms, such as headache, breast tenderness, and swelling during the week between ovulation and the onset of menstruation. The symptoms are severe enough to interfere with daily functioning and remit once menses occurs.

BIPOLAR DISORDERS

Bipolar disorders are chronic, often devastating disorders that are characterized by manic or hypomanic episodes. A manic episode is a distinct period of at least 1 week marked by an abnormal elevation of mood that causes a significant loss of daily functioning. A manic episode may initially be a state of euphoria or a period of persistent irritability and low frustration tolerance, which often leads to loss of control. Other concurrent symptoms generally include: exaggerated self-esteem, talkativeness or pressured speech, racing thoughts, a decreased need for sleep, poor attention, and an overindulgence in pleasurable activities (drinking, spending money, sex). An individual in a manic episode may present with delusions, perceptual disturbances, and gross psychotic symptoms. A hypomanic episode is similar symptomatically to a manic episode except that it does not cause significant impairment in social or occupational functioning. There are no psychotic symptoms during a hypomanic episode. A bipolar mood episode may also be mixed in that both depressive and manic symptoms are present simultaneously.

There are three main classifications of bipolar disorders: Bipolar I disorder, Bipolar II disorder, and Cyclothymic disorder. Bipolar I disorder is characterized by at least one manic episode with or without a current or past major depressive episode. Bipolar II disorder is present when there is a current or past major depressive episode and a current or past history of at least one hypomanic episode with no history of a manic episode. The current functioning of the individual is significantly impaired. Psychotic features may be present in bipolar II disorder. The depressive episodes of both bipolar I and II disorders may occur seasonally. The mood episodes of the disorders may be rapid cycling if at least four episodes are identified in a 12-month period. Similar to the depressive disorders, bipolar disorders are also described in terms of specific features of catatonia, melancholia, atypical, or with postpartum onset.

Bipolar disorders have a lifetime prevalence of 1.3–1.6%. Although the onset is usually between 15 and 24 years of age, there is typically a 5- to 10-year delay in seeking treatment. The onset of bipolar disorder may also occur in childhood with symptoms more consistently presenting as irritability and hyperactivity. Early onset of bipolar illness typically follows an initial depressive episode and is frequently a more severe illness than when onset occurs in adulthood. Women and men are affected equally in most bipolar disorders. However, women have a higher incidence than men of rapid cycling and mixed episodes.

Cyclothymic disorder (cyclothymia) is a mild form of bipolar II disorder. It is a chronic disorder with at least 2 years of recurring episodes of hypomania and mild depression with remissions lasting less than 2 months at one time. Cyclothymic disorder is often comorbid with borderline personality disorder. The onset is usually between the ages of 15 and 25 with a lifetime prevalence of 1%. Cyclothymia affects women more than men.

OTHER MOOD DISORDERS

Schizoaffective disorder is classified as a psychotic disorder rather than a mood disorder. However, a depressive, manic, or mixed episode occurring with two or more of the characteristic symptoms of schizophrenia would be considered schizoaffective disorder. These characteristic symptoms are delusions, hallucinations, disorganized speech, grossly disorganized or catatonic behavior, flat affect, and lack of motivation. These symptoms are not usually as severe as when experienced in schizophrenia.

CAUSES OF MOOD DISORDERS

The causes of mood disorders are not fully understood. However, there are strong indications that mood disorders are influenced by the combination of biological, genetic, and psychosocial factors. The biological factors include altered levels of neurotransmitters in the brain, particularly serotonin, norepinephrine, and dopamine. Other significant biological factors include alterations in neuroendocrine systems (stress system), thyroid hormones, circadian rhythm disturbances, and neuroanatomical changes. Family and twin studies have shown that genetics plays a large role in mood disorders, particularly in bipolar I disorder. The particular alterations in these systems may vary depending on the type or subtype of the mood disorder. Psychosocial factors, such as high life stress, multiple losses, poor social support, and trauma, can influence the development of a mood disorder, particularly the depressive disorders.

COMORBIDITY AND MORTALITY

Mood disorders coexist with a variety of other disorders. Depressive disorders are highly comorbid with anxiety disorders. Alcohol and substance abuse/dependence are common in those afflicted with either a depressive or bipolar mood disorder. Individuals with a medical condition (especially one that is chronic) are more likely to have depressive mood disorders. In some cases, the mood disorder may be caused by substance abuse, prescription and nonprescription medications, or a medical condition. A careful, thorough medical and psychiatric evaluation is needed to rule out the causative agent to ensure proper treatment. Mood disorders brought on by medication or a general medical condition are secondary mood disorders that usually resolve once the causative agent is removed or the condition treated.

The greatest risk with mood disorders is the occurrence of suicide with a depressive episode, especially at the onset or end of an episode. It is estimated that 400 of every 100,000 male patients and 180 of every 100,000 female patients commit suicide. Substance abuse and social isolation increases the risk of suicide in mood disorder patients.

TREATMENT

Treatment of mood disorders depends upon the specific symptoms and severity of the illness. Those with severe symptoms, psychosis, or suicidal thoughts or attempts may require hospitalization to prevent self-harm. For most individuals with mood disorders, outpatient therapy in conjunction with medication is the treatment of choice. Psychotherapies are often very helpful for the psychosocial and cognitive aspects of mood disorders. The type of therapy that is best suited for the disorder depends upon the type of disorder, symptom severity and presentation, and individual preference. The therapies include interpersonal therapy, cognitive–behavioral therapy, psychoanalysis, and family therapy.

Medication treatment is generally indicated for major depressive and manic episodes and can have a therapeutic effect in about 2–6 weeks. The choices for medication treatment for depressive episodes include tricyclic antidepressants, such as amitriptyline (Elavil and others) and clomipramine (Anafranil and others), selective serotonin reuptake inhibitors (SSRIs), such as fluoxetine (Prozac) and sertraline (Zoloft), and other novel depressants. Monoamine oxidase inhibitors (MAOIs) such as phenelzine (Nardil) and tranylcypromine (Parnate) are generally used to treat atypical or refractory depression. There is a reluctance to use the MAOIs due to the potential for a hypertensive crisis if the patient does not eliminate tyrosine from their diet. High tyrosine levels are found in many sharp cheeses, cured meats, and fish. The treatment of major depression or bipolar disorder with psychotic features requires additional treatment with antipsychotic medication. The main treatment for bipolar I disorder is mood stabilization with lithium (Lithobid and others), valproic acid (Depakote and others), or lamotrigine (Lamictal).

Atypical antipsychotic medications such as olanzapine (Zyprexa) and risperidone (Risperdal) are also gaining popularity in the treatment of bipolar illness. Obtaining long-term mood stability with medication is reportedly related to a reduction in suicide rates in individuals with bipolar and schizoaffective disorder. Treatment of bipolar II disorder is more complicated due to the frequent depressive episodes which may require medications that induce a hypomanic episode.

Alternative therapies include light therapy, sleep deprivation, and electroconvulsive therapy (ECT). In circumstances of a depressive episode or manic episode with medication failure, intolerance to medications, or severe psychotic or suicidal symptoms, ECT is the treatment of choice. ECT is a generally safe, fast, and effective method of treatment. ECT involves the induction of a generalized seizure by sending pulses of electrical current through the scalp into the brain. ECT is not contraindicated in pregnancy, and has been used for the same indications without apparent harm to the fetus.

Drug treatment in women requires special attention to the possibility of pregnancy and lactation while being treated with the medication. Physicians are sometimes reluctant to prescribe psychotropic medications during pregnancy due to the potential adverse affects on the fetus. However, recent data support the use of some medications during pregnancy, especially when the risk of suicide or self-harm is high. There is also sufficient evidence to suggest that fetal exposure to maternal mood disorders may also impact fetal behavior and development. Antidepressant medications, particularly the SSRIs and tricyclic medications, have been found to be relatively safe during pregnancy between 9 and 36 weeks gestational age. It is recommended that the dosage be tapered in the last month of pregnancy to decrease the risk of neonatal withdrawal. SSRIs are the current first-line choice of clinicians for treatment during pregnancy due to relatively fewer side effects and low risk to the fetus. The use of mood stabilizers such as lithium during pregnancy is associated with greater risk to the fetus; however, the benefits of the medication may outweigh the risks.

SEE ALSO: Anxiety disorders, Bipolar disorder, Depression, Mental illness

Suggested Reading

Altshuler, L. L., Cohen, L., Szuba, M. P., Burt, V. K., Gitlin, M., & Mintz, J. (1996). Pharmacologic management of psychiatric illness during pregnancy: Dilemmas and guidelines. *American Journal of Psychiatry, 153*(5), 592–606.

Altshuler, L. L., Cohen, L. S., Moline, M. L., Kahn, D. A., Carpenter, D., & Docherty, J. P. (2001). Treatment of depression in women. *Postgraduate Medicine, Special Report* (The Expert Consensus Guideline Series), 1–28.

American Psychiatric Association. (2000). *Diagnostic and statistical manual of mental disorders* (4th ed., Text Revision). Washington, DC: American Psychiatric Association.

Cinnirella, M., & Loewenthal, K. M. (1999). Religious and ethnic group influences on beliefs about mental illness: A qualitative interview study. *British Journal of Medical Psychology, 72*(Pt 4), 505–524.

Desai, H. D., & Jann, M. W. (2000). Major depression in women: A review of the literature. *Journal of the American Pharmacology Association (Washington), 40*(4), 525–537.

Loewenthal, K. M., Goldblatt, V., & Lubitsh, G. (1998). Haredi women, haredi men, stress and distress. *Israel Journal of Psychiatry and Related Sciences, 35*(3), 217–224; discussion, 225–226.

Muller-Oerlinghausen, B., Berghofer, A., & Bauer, M. (2002). Bipolar disorder. *Lancet, 359*(9302), 241–247.

Sadock, B. J., & Sadock, V. A. (2003). *Kaplan and Sadock's synopsis of psychiatry: Behavioral sciences/clinical psychiatry* (9th ed.). Philadelphia: Lippincott, Williams & Wilkins.

Sandman, C. A., Wadhwa, P. D., Dunkel-Schetter, C., Chicz-DeMet, A., Belman, J., Porto, M., et al. (1994). Psychobiological influences of stress and HPA regulation on the human fetus and infant birth outcomes. *Annals of the New York Academy of Sciences, 739*, 198–210.

Wisner, K. L., Zarin, D. A., Holmboe, E. S., Appelbaum, P. S., Gelenberg, A. J., Leonard, H. L., et al. (2000). Risk-benefit decision making for treatment of depression during pregnancy. *American Journal of Psychiatry, 157*(12), 1933–1940.

AMY L. SALISBURY

Morbidity
In general terms, morbidity represents illness—any departure from normal well-being. There is a close relationship between mortality and morbidity, because high levels of morbidity (i.e., an unhealthy population) are associated with high death rates, and vice versa. For example, the life expectancy of women in the United States increased from 49 years at the beginning of the 20th century to 79 years at the beginning of the 21st century. These improvements in longevity are a result of significant changes in the patterns of illness and disease among both women and men, although women have seen a bigger improvement than have men. In fact, in 1900, American women had a life expectancy that was 2 years longer than that of men, and the advantage grew to nearly 8 years by the mid-1970s, before dropping to about 6 years in 2000.

Infectious diseases combined especially with complications of pregnancy have historically been the major sources of morbidity (and, at the extreme, of mortality) among women all over the world. Infectious diseases have been brought under reasonable control by better nutrition that helps people resist disease; clean water and adequate sewage systems that help to prevent the spread of disease; better housing, vaccinations, medical care, and a host of other technological innovations that have spread around the world over the last century. These same changes have also reduced pregnancy-related illness, especially in combination with the dramatic decline in the number of pregnancies and births among women. The rising standard of living and improved status of women have been important motivations for limiting family size, but, of course, the success of this has been heavily dependent upon the availability of a wide range of fertility control measures.

Lower morbidity means that people are healthier into the older ages, at which point degenerative (chronic) diseases tend to become sources of illness, disability, and of course death. Patterns of morbidity vary not only by age and sex, but also regionally across the globe. A useful way of making such comparisons is through the calculation of Disability Adjusted Life Years (DALYs). This concept was introduced by the World Bank in 1990 and has been implemented as the global "burden of disease" studies undertaken by Murray and Lopez at the Harvard School of Public Health, and is now accepted and used widely by the World Health Organization of the United Nations. A DALY is equal to the sum of YLL and YLD, where YLL is equal to the years of life lost due to death at an age earlier than expected, and YLD is the number of years lost to disability as a consequence of injury or illness. If a person could expect to live to age 100 in a perfect world, but dies of a stroke (a type of cardiovascular disease) at age 50, then that person "lost" 50 years of life and the sum of all years of life lost in a society to people dying of stroke would be the YLL for that population in that year. Another person might have had a stroke at age 50, but survived. The severity of the disability with which such a person would have to live would then be given a weight and the number of years of normal functioning lost to the disease would be calculated as the YLD. The total burden of a disease is then the number of years of life that a society loses to a disease through its combined impact on mortality and morbidity.

Among women in the world at the beginning of the 21st century, the greatest number of DALYs lost (i.e., the

Morning Sickness

greatest disease burden) is caused by HIV/AIDS, followed by lower respiratory disease, and unipolar depressive disorders. However, World Bank data show that different diseases are important at different ages among women. At ages 15–44, maternal causes are most important, whereas at ages 45 and older, cerebrovascular diseases cause the greatest morbidity burden.

Regional variations in morbidity are now especially related to HIV/AIDS. In sub-Saharan Africa, there is evidence that migrant labor is a powerful source of the spread of the disease because of the sexual networking that is involved in a subcontinent where the use of the condom has not been as widespread as in other parts of the world. Because HIV/AIDS tends to affect young adults more than other age groups, it places a tremendous burden on a society through the loss of not only family members, but also through dramatically reduced economic productivity. Indeed, in the middle of the 20th century, increases in health care access for workers were pushed by labor unions in Europe and North America on the (correct) grounds that improved health levels of workers would make companies more profitable.

SEE ALSO: Disability, Maternal mortality, Mortality

Suggested Reading

Goldman, M. B., & Hatch, M. C. (Eds.). (2000) *Women and health.* San Diego: Academic Press.

Murray, C. J., & Lopez, A. (Eds.). (1996). *The global burden of disease: A comprehensive assessment of mortality and disability from diseases, injury, and risk factors in 1990 and projected to 2020.* Boston: Harvard University School of Public Health.

World Bank. (1993). *World development report 1993: Investing in health.* New York: Oxford University Press.

JOHN R. WEEKS

Morning Sickness The existence of morning sickness early in pregnancy seems difficult to explain. Maybe it is just a mistake, an accident of nature. We all know that the first few months of fetal development are critical for the baby's health. Why then are so many women so sick early in pregnancy, and what can be done to help them? Finally, is it possible that morning sickness is actually a good thing to have?

ALL-DAY SICKNESS

It would be more accurate to refer to morning sickness as "all-day" sickness because for many pregnant women it is, although it is frequently worse in the mornings. The preferred medical term is *nausea and vomiting of pregnancy* (NVP). Morning sickness can range in severity from none (20% of all pregnant women do not get it at all) to persistent vomiting so severe that hospitalization and treatment with intravenous fluids are necessary. Typically, morning sickness is a near-constant feeling of nausea, intermittent vomiting, and an increased sensitivity/aversion to odors. It usually begins about weeks 5 or 6 of pregnancy and usually is fully resolved by about week 14.

WHY DOES MORNING SICKNESS EXIST AT ALL? TRADITIONAL EXPLANATION

Many articles link morning sickness to the pregnancy hormone human chorionic gonadotropin (HCG), which is unique to pregnancy. For example, morning sickness tends to be worse with multiple gestation (a high-hormone state) and it tends to be minimal in pregnancies that end in miscarriage (a low-hormone state). Many patients understand that the sicker they are, the "better" the pregnancy. This theory does not explain everything, however. Why does morning sickness exist at all? Is there some reason, perhaps something related to human evolution, that explains the existence of morning sickness?

AN EVOLUTIONARY EXPLANATION

A promising theory comes from Margie Profet, an evolutionary biologist (and a recipient of a 1993 MacArthur "genius" prize). In her book *Protecting Your Baby-to-Be*, she states that morning sickness is the result of thousands of generations of evolution, and that its purpose is to improve the survival of the human species!

Her theory is that morning sickness is Mother Nature's way of providing humans with an instinctive toxin (or poison) avoidance mechanism. It is a biological radar, warning us when something potentially hazardous is coming our way. For thousands of years, humans were hunter-gatherers, eating whatever and whenever they could.

Many plants produce toxins designed to enhance their survival by damaging the reproductive potential of the animals that ingest them. Today, we extract many of these "toxins" and use them to our advantage, only we now call them herbs, spices, drugs, and medications!

The evidence supporting this theory is extensive. For example, fetal organ development is usually completed by week 14 of pregnancy. During those first 14 weeks, the fetus is exquisitely sensitive to the damaging effects of toxins. The first trimester is also when nearly all miscarriages occur.

SEVERE MORNING SICKNESS

About 1–3% of pregnant women experience severe morning sickness. It can lead to profound dehydration, mineral and electrolyte abnormalities, and acid–base changes in blood chemistry. Treatment requires intravenous fluids and possibly hospitalization. Contact your doctor right away if you have any of the following symptoms:

1. Throwing up everything, food and liquids, for more than a couple of days
2. Losing more than 5% of your body weight (e.g., a 120-lb woman loses 6 lb) compared to your pre-pregnant weight
3. Feeling constantly dizzy, lightheaded, very weak, and having a dry, pasty mouth

MANAGEMENT OF MILD MORNING SICKNESS

From the evolutionary theory comes some helpful advice for dealing with morning sickness. First, trust your instinctive food aversions. If it does not smell good, look good, or "sound" good to you to eat it, then do not. Below are two lists: The "avoid" list is far more important than the "try this" list. Avoidance serves two purposes. One is to help avoid something that can aggravate the morning sickness. The other, and even more important reason, is to avoid substances potentially toxic to the first-trimester fetus.

THINGS TO AVOID

1. Avoid odors as much as possible. Have your partner use breath mints. No smoking in the house. Use air filters. Use odorless hygiene and laundry products. Avoid odor-filled places (crowded public places, public restrooms, smelly gyms, etc.). Have your home cleaned to try to eliminate any musty or moldy household odors. Get rid of smelly stuff in the fridge and place opened boxes of baking soda inside.

2. Avoid unripe fruits and most vegetables (especially mushrooms), canned fruits and vegetables, greasy and high-fat foods (dairy products are usually okay).

3. Avoid burnt foods, barbecued food, raw fish (sushi), nuts, spices, spicy foods and herbs, food flavorings, and condiments (e.g., ketchup, mustard, steak sauce) Small amounts of salt are okay.

4. If vomiting more than once a day, stop all vitamins (yes, even prenatal vitamins) except folic acid (0.4 mg daily) and B6 (25–50 mg daily).

5. Avoid coffee, tea, chocolate, and any substance that is bitter in its native form (before sugar and fat have been added to it).

THINGS TO TRY

1. Keep saltine crackers on your nightstand. Eat one as soon as you awake, while still lying down if possible. Then wait a few minutes before getting up. The crackers will absorb stomach acid that may have accumulated during the night.

2. Eat things a baby would like (boring, bland stuff), like plain white breads, cereal, noodles, rice, plain yogurt. Eat ripe soft fruits. Drink fresh-squeezed fruit juices ice cold and watered down a bit.

3. Eat white cheese. It digests slowly and lessens stomach acid production. Dry, white meats like turkey breast are usually well tolerated.

4. Drink flat, sweetened, clear soda or ginger ale (pour into a cup, then stir). If vomiting, drink Gatorade-type drinks rather than water to replace minerals. Drink liquids with crushed ice, using a straw.

5. Eat small meals all day long, up to 10 times a day. If you have to cook, try to microwave, steam, or boil foods. This lowers the "burned food" odors.

6. To help nausea, try the following (any medications, including vitamins and herbs, should only be taken after consulting with your doctor): vitamin B6, 50 mg once or twice a day. Try ginger, either tea or candied (helps nausea). Try lemon drops (candy). Wear wristbands, also known as acupressure or "sea" bands.

USING MEDICATION

There are times when the morning sickness is so bad that without medication the patient may have to be hospitalized, or alternatively, medication may be necessary for someone to be able to leave the hospital, or for someone to function well enough not to miss work. In those cases, the benefits of using medication may outweigh the risks to the fetus. However, only a qualified obstetrician/gynecologist practitioner should make these types of decisions.

CONCLUSION

Normal (not severe) morning sickness is not a mistake at all. It is an evolutionary miracle, designed to benefit the survival of the species by reducing the risk of miscarriage and birth defects. Hopefully, the information in this article, and understanding what it means, will make dealing with morning sickness just a little bit easier.

SEE ALSO: Pregnancy, Prenatal care, Vitamins

Suggested Resources

www.acog.org

BRYAN S. JICK

Mortality For most of human history, mortality was very high, with life expectancy between 20 and 40 in most societies. At that life expectancy, nearly half of all children born die before reaching age 5, and fewer than 1 in 10 people survive to age 65, with infectious diseases being the biggest killers of humans over the centuries. Over the past 200 years, and especially since the beginning of the 20th century, humans have made great progress in controlling mortality. A combination of factors, including improved nutrition; advances in science that led to vaccinations to prevent severe illness; antiseptics to prevent the spread of bacterial contamination; drug therapies to cure disease; environmental controls such as clean water supplies, sewerage, draining of swamps, improved housing, improved clothing; and the promotion of personal hygiene, all helped to push life expectancy to higher levels all over the world. This happened first in the now-developed countries, but spread quickly to the rest of the world after the end of World War II.

During the Roman Empire, life expectancy was estimated to be 22 years. In the Middle Ages, with some improvement of nutrition, life expectancy increased in Europe to more than 30 years. In the beginning of the 19th century, as a result of improved nutrition, housing, and sanitation due to increasing income, life expectancy in the United States and Europe reached approximately 40 years. Currently in the United States, the odds that a female baby will survive to age 65 are equal to 86%, based on a life expectancy of nearly 80 years. This means that nearly half of all women born will still be alive at age 85.

The process of declining mortality follows a generally predictable path that has come to be known as the epidemiological transition. The main features of the transition are the change from most deaths occurring early in life largely from infectious diseases, to most deaths occurring later in life largely from chronic diseases. As life expectancy increases, a greater fraction of babies born survive to older ages, and human *longevity* gets closer to the human *life span*.

Life span refers to the oldest age to which human beings can survive, which is approximately 120 years, based on the oldest authenticated age to which any human has ever lived. Longevity refers to the actual experience that people have in terms of survival. While life span is thought be largely determined by biological factors, longevity has both biological and social components. Longevity is usually measured by life expectancy, which is the statistically average length of life (or average age at death), and is greatly influenced by the society in which we live, the genetic characteristics with which we are born, and the lifestyle that we maintain.

Human beings still have little control over biological factors such as the strength of vital organs, predisposition to particular diseases, and metabolism rate. Regarding the social factors impacting longevity, there are three major categories: (a) the overall social and economic infrastructure, (b) a person's place within a given society, and (c) a person's lifestyle, regardless of his or her place in society. In general, the wealthier a country is, the better able it is to provide the kind of infrastructure that helps to maintain a lower risk of death for everyone living there. Within any particular society, those at the top of the socioeconomic scale are more likely to have access especially to health care resources, which increase the probability of survival from year to year. Nonetheless, no matter what your status in society might be, certain kinds of behaviors (such as smoking and abusing alcohol and drugs) increase the risk of death, while other kinds of behaviors (such as regular exercise and a moderate, healthy diet) will lower the risk of death.

The major causes of death are (a) diseases that can be transmitted from one person to another, such as malaria, measles, plague, smallpox, and recently HIV/AIDS; (b) degeneration of a body, including chronic diseases such as heart disease, cancer, cerebrovascular disease, chronic lung disease, diabetes mellitus, and chronic liver disease and cirrhosis; and (c) products of the social and economic environment, such as accidental deaths, murders, and suicides.

The "real" causes of death may not necessarily appear on a person's death certificate. In 1993, two physicians, McGinnis and Foege, estimated the "real" or "actual" causes of death in the United States in 1990. Of the 2,148,000 people who died in the United States that year, they found that 400,000 died as a result of tobacco use, and 300,000 deaths were caused by dietary and physical activity patterns of the United States population. Alcohol misuse was the third real cause of death in the United States, followed by infectious diseases, and then toxic agents such as environmental pollutants, contaminants of food and water supplies, and components of commercial products. Finally, they found that firearms were responsible for 36,000 deaths.

There is, of course, still a considerable amount of variability in mortality in the world, despite the world average life expectancy early in the 21st century of 67 years (65 for males and 69 for women). For example, sub-Saharan African countries have life expectancy between 46 and 50 years. The next lowest life expectancy region is South Asia where it is between 58 and 64. The highest life expectancy is found in Japan, where a female baby can expect to live to age 85. Several European countries, including France and Switzerland, have a female life expectancy of 83.

We can also compare urban and rural differentials in mortality. For example, life expectancy in 1841 was 40 years for native English males and 42 for females, but in London it was 5 years less than that. The early differences regarding urban and rural mortality were due less to favorable conditions in the countryside, than to unfavorable conditions in the cities. Over time, medical advances and environmental improvements have benefited the urban populations more than the rural

ones, leading to the current situation of better mortality conditions in urban areas. Differences in mortality by social status are among the most pervasive inequalities in modern society, and they are most noticeable in cities. So, if one is part of a family of low socioeconomic status, this may put him or her at greater risk of death. Data clearly suggest that the higher one's position in society, the longer he or she is likely to live.

As with income, there is a marked decline in the risk of death as education increases. Race and ethnicity are also sources of differentials in mortality in the United States. Data from National Center for Health Statistics showed that in the United States in 1998, at every age up to 70, African American mortality rates are nearly double the rates for the white population. African Americans have higher risks of death from almost every major cause of death than do whites. Marital status also counts for differentials in mortality. Married people tend to live longer than unmarried people do, not only in the United States, but also in other countries.

Gender is also responsible for differentials in mortality. Women live longer than men do, and the gap has been widening until recently. In 1900, women in the United States could expect to live an average of 2 years longer than men in the United States. By 1975, the difference had peaked at 7.8 years, although since then the difference has dropped to 5.7 years. In general, the difference between male and female life expectancy can be an important clue to the status of women in society. Since the evidence points overwhelmingly to an inherent biological superiority of women over men with respect to mortality, any society in which women die at a higher rate, or close to the same rate, as men, is a society in which social customs and inequalities have trumped the biological tendencies. In many Asian societies, women have historically been the last to eat (even though they do most of the cooking), and are less likely to be cared for if sick. These symptoms of lower status are then reflected in higher than expected death rates.

Throughout history, and still today in many developing countries, high rates of pregnancy in a society not well covered by health care systems can lead to high levels of maternal mortality and infant mortality as well. The infant mortality rate (IMR) is the number of deaths of infants under 1 year of age per 1,000 live births in a given year. Included in the IMR are the neonatal mortality rate (calculated from deaths occurring in the first 4 weeks of life) and postneonatal mortality rate (from deaths in the remainder of the first year). Neonatal deaths are further subdivided into early (first week) and late (second, third, and fourth weeks). In prosperous countries, neonatal deaths account for about two thirds of infant mortalities, the majority being in the first week. The IMR is usually regarded more as a measure of social affluence than a measure of the quality of antenatal and/or obstetric care; the latter is more truly reflected in the perinatal mortality rate (the number of deaths after 24 weeks of gestation, including stillbirths, and during the first week of life per 1,000 total births).

As deaths increasingly are pushed to the later ages, the issue has arisen as to whether life span may increase or whether societies will experience a "rectangularization" of mortality. An increase in life span would mean that humans had discovered ways to keep alive beyond the age that any human has thus far lived. While this seems theoretically possible, science has a long way to go before this is likely to be accomplished. Instead, it seems more likely that deaths will become increasingly compressed into a few years late in life. This will lead to a rectangularization of the age curve, in which almost everybody stays alive until age 100 or beyond and then quickly begins to die.

SEE ALSO: Ethnicity, Life expectancy, Marital status, Maternal mortality, Morbidity, Socioeconomic status

Suggested Reading

Caldwell, J. (1986). Routes to low mortality in poor countries. *Population and Development Review, 12,* 171–220.

Hoyert, D. L., Arias, E., Simth, B. L., Murphy, S. L., & Kochanek, K. D. (2001). Deaths: Final data for 1999. *National Vital Statistics Reports, 49*(9). http://www.cdc.gov/nchs/data/nvsr/nvsr49/nvsr49_08.pdf

Hummer, R. A., Rogers, R. G., Nam, C. B., & LeClere, F. B. (1999). Race/ethnicity, nativity, and U.S. adult mortality. *Social Science Quarterly, 80,* 136–153.

Kannisto, V., Lauritsen, J., Thatcher, A. R., & Vaupel, J. W. (1994). Reductions in mortality at advanced ages: Several decades of evidence from 27 countries. *Population and Development Review, 20,* 793–810.

McGinnis, J. M., & Foege, W. H. (1993). Actual causes of death in the United States. *Journal of the American Medical Association, 270,* 2207–2212.

United Nations Statistics Division. (2000). *The world's women: Trends and statistics.* New York: Author.

Weeks, J. R. (2002). *Population: Introduction to concepts and issues* (8th ed.). Belmont, CA: Wadsworth Thomson Learning.

Wilmott, J. R., & Horiuchi, S. (1999). Rectangularization revisited: Variability of age at death within human populations. *Demography, 36,* 475–495.

JOHN R. WEEKS
MANUEL MIRANDA

Multiple Chemical Sensitivity *see* Idiopathic Environmental Intolerance

Multiple Personality Disorder *see* Dissociative Identity Disorder

Multiple Sclerosis

Multiple sclerosis is the most common inflammatory disease of the central nervous system. The cause stems from faulty regulation of the immune system. Myelin, the insulator of nerves, is attacked by the immune system because of improper recognition. Inflammation surrounding the nerves strips the myelin from the nerve fibers and damages some of the fibers (axons) preventing the normal transmission of nerve impulses.

The prevalence of multiple sclerosis is 70/100,000 in the United States with regional variation. Young women are unfortunately disproportionately affected, outnumbering men nearly 2:1. The disease typically begins from age 20 to 50 although onset at both younger and older ages exists. Familial tendencies are apparent. The children of patients with multiple sclerosis have a sixfold greater risk of developing multiple sclerosis than those children of parents without disease. Crucial genetic markers have not yet been identified.

Various subtypes of multiple sclerosis exist. Each subtype depicts the clinical course of the illness. Onset may be either relapsing–remitting (improving, then relapsing) or continuously progressive (worsens over time). The most common subtype, relapsing–remitting, begins before the progressive subtypes by nearly a decade. The peak incidence of relapsing–remitting multiple sclerosis occurs between the ages of 25 and 29, whereas progressive is most commonly diagnosed between ages 35 and 39. Distinguishing a person's subtype is important because therapy depends upon disease classifications.

The clinical symptoms and physical findings in multiple sclerosis are varied. No region within the central nervous system is spared. Cognitive impairment (loss in memory and concentration) occurs to variable degrees in more than one half of individuals with multiple sclerosis. Cognitive speed, recent memory, attention, and abstraction are commonly impaired. Mood disorders ranging from euphoria through depression are not uncommon.

The optic nerve (primary nerve supply to the eye) is often involved. Optic nerve inflammation causes eye pain worsened with movement and visual blurring. Progression over several days with decrease in color vision is classical for the diagnosis. Central visual loss reflecting swelling within the optic nerve is frequently noted during ophthalmologic testing.

Additional cranial nerves (nerves to the head and neck) also may be involved. Eye movement difficulties caused by disturbances in brainstem pathways result in double vision or feelings of imbalance. Facial pain may occur associated with numbness and tingling. Unexplained facial pain in a young adult may be the first symptom of multiple sclerosis. Slurring of speech (dysarthria) and difficulty swallowing (dysphagia) are frequent.

Disturbances of sensation and strength often occur. Regional inflammation within the brain results in loss of sensation or strength usually on the opposite side of the body. Problems with strength or sensation occurring simultaneously on both sides of the body imply inflammation within the brainstem or spinal cord.

Coordination difficulties often are seen. Clumsiness of the body or legs frequently impairs walking. Speech may be affected resulting in an awkward speaking pattern. Poorly coordinated eye movements may cause imbalance or a sense of movement when none is apparent.

Autonomic nervous system involvement commonly causes urinary incontinence. Persons may lose the ability to inhibit their bladder from emptying when the urge arises. Less frequently, the bladder loses its tone and distends until pressure builds and leakage occurs. Problems with defecation are less common. Erectile dysfunction (difficulty having an erection) in men and absence of orgasms in both men and women are not infrequent.

External factors influence the course of multiple sclerosis. Infectious agents such as viruses and some bacteria often precede worsening of the illness. Trauma has not been shown to convincingly worsen the illness. It has been suggested that vaccination has been implicated to exacerbate disease, although most experts no longer hold this to be true, and recommend vaccination when indicated. Pregnancy seems to inhibit disease activity. However, attacks seem to increase in frequency in the first 3–6 months after delivery.

Diagnosis is based on historical information requiring multiple episodes affecting various regions of the central nervous system at different times. Laboratory tests and radiographic imaging are used for confirmation. Blood and cerebrospinal fluid samples along with magnetic resonance imaging are frequently obtained. Alternative diagnoses including infections, a variety of immune disorders, metabolic and inherited disorders should be excluded.

Pharmacologic therapy (medication management) for multiple sclerosis has evolved during the last decade. Acute treatment with intravenous or oral anti-inflammatory steroids speeds functional recovery following acute worsening. Individuals who do not respond to standard treatment of a severe initial attack may benefit from plasma exchange. Subcutaneous and intramuscular medications (medications injected beneath the skin) decrease the frequency of relapses in patients with either relapsing–remitting or relapsing–progressive subtypes. Various other intravenous and oral immune system inhibitors have met with mixed success.

Scant information exists regarding the social impact of multiple sclerosis and a woman's ability to fulfill the demands of an active lifestyle. Chronic illness often strains relationships resulting in marital or familial discord. Employment may be jeopardized from either physical or cognitive disability. Rehabilitative experts with interest in multiple sclerosis and its associated conditions may be available. Social support thankfully exists through local MS Society chapters. Counseling and pharmacologic management of depression should be sought early to prevent social isolation.

See Also: Autoimmune disorders, Pregnancy

Suggested Reading

Galetta, S. L., Markowitz, C., & Lee, A. G. (2002, October 28). Immuno-modulatory agents for the treatment of relapsing multiple sclerosis: A systematic review. *Archives of Internal Medicine, 162*(19), 2161–2169.

O'Connor, P., & Canadian Multiple Sclerosis Working Group. (2002, September 24). Key issues in the diagnosis and treatment of multiple sclerosis. *Neurology, 59*(6 Suppl. 3), S1–S33.

Stuifbergen, A. K., & Becker, H. (2001, February). Health promotion practices in women with multiple sclerosis: Increasing quality and years of healthy life. *Physical Medicine and Rehabilitation Clinics of North America, 12*(1), 9–22.

Joseph P. Hanna

Myasthenia Gravis

Myasthenia gravis (MG) is an autoimmune disorder of the neuromuscular junction (NMJ) that results in muscle weakness and fatigability. Muscle contractions occur when electrical impulses travel along motor nerve fibers and end at the NMJ. When an electrical impulse reaches the nerve fiber terminal, it causes the release of a molecule called acetylcholine (ACh). ACh diffuses across the gap (NMJ) and activates specialized ACh receptors (AChR) on the muscle fiber. AChR activation causes electrical activation of muscle fibers and contraction. Excess ACh in the NMJ is eliminated by an enzyme called cholin esterase (ChE). In MG, there are circulating antibodies directed against AChR. These attach and cause elimination of AChR. With a paucity of AChR, there is failure of nerve-to-muscle transmission, especially high levels of activity. This presents as fatigability or muscle weakness with repeated contraction. Muscles around the eye and muscles of the face and throat are particularly vulnerable in MG.

The prevalence of MG is about 150 per million. Onset is early in women (late teens and 20s) and late in men (60s and 70s). Prevalence used to be higher in women, but with the aging of the population, may be higher in men now. Ten percent of patients with MG have a tumor of the thymus gland (thymoma) in the chest. In others, there may be enlargement of the thymus (hyperplasia).

MG manifests as waxing and waning drooping of eyelids; double vision or squint; facial weakness and loss of expression; weakness/fatigability of chewing, swallowing, and speech; neck weakness; weakness/fatigability of arm and leg muscles; and weakness of breathing muscles in varying combinations. Prolonged activity worsens symptoms. Examples are double vision while reading or watching television, voice slurring during a long conversation, chewing or swallowing difficulty as the meal progresses, or hands getting weak with repeated activity. Symptoms are commonly worse in the evenings than in the mornings. If weakness is restricted to the muscles around the eyes, the disorder is termed ocular MG. More commonly, it is diffuse and is called generalized MG. Generalized MG can be mild or can be severe. Acute severe worsening of MG (myasthenic crisis) may be precipitated by infection, surgery, or some medications. Weakness of breathing muscles during a myasthenic crisis may necessitate ventilatory support.

Often, MG starts around the eyes and becomes generalized in ensuring months. Infrequently, MG spares the eye and face muscles. MG is usually a life-long problem. Most of the worsening and fluctuation in severity is seen in the first few years of the disease. After several years, the disease tends to stabilize, but there may be some residual fatigability and weakness. Most myasthenics receiving appropriate medical care can remain independent and lead productive lives.

The diagnosis of MG is challenging, and clinical suspicion needs to be high. If MG is suspected, a bedside test (Tensilon® test) which assesses transient improvement after injection of edrophonium may be performed. Often, the physiological change in NMJ transmission can be demonstrated by a decrement in muscle response on repetitive electrical stimulation of nerve. The most sensitive test for MG is an electrical test called single fiber EMG. A blood test for the detection of AChR antibodies is quite sensitive and specific.

Treatment options include ChE inhibitors (such as pyridostigmine and neostigmine, which increase availability of ACh by blocking its destruction), corticosteroids (which reduce the autoimmune response), and azathioprine and other immunosuppressants. Most experts believe that removal of the thymus gland (thymectomy) early in the course of generalized MG improves the long-term course. In periods of acute worsening, removal of antibodies from the blood (plasma exchange) can rapidly improve symptoms. Intravenous immunoglobulin is also an option for acute worsening. Several classes of medications, especially anesthetic agents, some cardiac medications, and some antibiotics can cause worsening of MG and need to be avoided.

Pregnancy has special implications for myasthenics. About one third get worse during pregnancy or after delivery. Weakness of muscles may make vaginal delivery difficult. About 10–20% of infants born to myasthenic mothers may have transient weakness and trouble feeding for the first few weeks after birth (neonatal myasthenia) because of antibodies crossing the placenta.

MG is not a genetic disease. Rarely, disorders closely resembling MG are seen running in families. Such congenital myasthenic syndromes are not autoimmune; rather, they are genetic defects in proteins of the NMJ. Some other disorders of the NMJ of note that have only a passing similarity to MG are Lambert–Eaton myasthenic syndrome and botulism.

SEE ALSO: Autoimmune disorders, Pregnancy

Myasthenia Gravis

Suggested Reading

Engel, A. (Ed.). (1999). *Myasthenia gravis and myasthenic syndromes* (Contemporary neurology series, no. 56). New York: Oxford University Press.

Richman, D. P. (Ed.). (1998). Myasthenia gravis and related diseases: Disorders of the neuromuscular junction. *Annals of the New York Academy of Sciences, 841*, 1–831.

Vincent, A., Palace, J., & Hilton-Jones, D. (2001). Myasthenia gravis. *Lancet, 357*, 2122–2128.

NIMISH THAKORE

Nail Care One of the most common problems in caring for nails is picking and biting. The habit is common across all age groups. Picking and biting nails and cuticles increases the risk of infection by introducing bacteria. In general, the behavior often occurs as a result of anxiety or nervousness.

Filing, even of the cuticles, is often recommended in place of cutting or clipping. This allows the removal of dead skin and reduces the likelihood of injury. Lotions and exfoliants can be used to moisturize the area around the nails; cuticles should be kept moist and pushed back. Nails should be cared for in this manner at least once a month. Individuals with dry skin may wish to do it more frequently. Products containing aloe vera are often recommended, especially for individuals with eczema or other conditions involving dry skin.

Pain, swelling, and redness are signs that may indicate an infection or other problem, such as an in-grown nail. It is important to keep the area clean and to avoid "digging" into it in an attempt to cure the problem. In such situations, the individual may wish to consult a podiatrist (doctor who specializes in the care of feet).

A wide selection of "false" nails is available. If applied properly, acrylic nails are often the best because they adhere to the nail directly, so that the risk of infection is reduced. Other products, such as silk and fiberglass nails, are glue-based and are more likely to lift, increasing the time required to maintain and care for them properly as well as the risk of infection.

A manicurist should be selected based on the cleanliness of the facility and his or her practice, rather than on the basis of price. Consider the following.

1. If the state requires a license to provide manicures to the public, the license should be appropriately displayed and should be current.
2. All instruments used should be sterilized after each use or thrown away. Barbicide can be used to clean the equipment.
3. Cuts on the manicurist's hand(s) should be covered to avoid possible transmission of infection to others.
4. The manicurist should ask, or be informed if she does not, if the client has a particular medical condition that may predispose the client to a greater risk of injury or infection. For instance, individuals on blood thinners (such as Coumadin) may be at greater risk of seriously bleeding if they are cut by accident. Diabetic clients may be more prone to infection.

The provision of nail care provides an important service to many women. A manicure enhances a woman's appearance and the experience is often relaxing.

Women interested in becoming manicurists will find that the profession offers flexibility and independence. The practice can be easily moved and the hours can be tailored to fit any schedule. Manicurists can rent a booth at someone else's salon or can enter an arrangement whereby they are paid minimum wage and a commission for working at a particular salon.

MARA MEZA

SEE ALSO: Diet, Foot care, Hair care, Skin care, Skin disorders

Suggested Reading

Ferri, E., Kenny, L., and Epstein, D. (1998). *Style on hand: Perfect nail and skin care.* New York: Universe Publishing.
Manos, F. (1998). *Beautiful hands and nails naturally.* New York: Avery Penguin Putnam.
Tourles, S. (1998). *Natural foot care: Herbal treatments, massage, and exercises for healthy feet.* North Adams, MA: Storey Books.

Natural Childbirth What is natural childbirth today and what does the word "natural" mean to today's woman in this world of technologic intensive labor? The dictionary definition of the word "natural" means legitimate; a state of nature untouched by influences of civilization and society; freedom from artificiality or constraint. Could not this be a definition of the birth process? But what one lives and breathes, becomes normal and natural to you. We are losing the normalcy of birth: women doing women's work with women's bodies and resources birthing a healthy mother and baby. As professionals, we can never forget that the woman must be at the center of the experience.

It is such a dichotomy in our society that we revere and admire the athlete who pushes to the limit of endurance; handling pain pumped up by the powerful pull of winning and success; pushing the human body to new limits to set new records. Labor is the true contact sport. Women must want to participate to win. Yet professionals attempt to evaluate the forces of labor to levels of distress that equate the natural forces of a normal process to the pain of death and disease.

Women and practitioners must be reeducated that pain is a valuable tool during labor. As the woman handles pain, she can use it as a guide to find the positions and practices that give her comfort and actually facilitate the birth process. Pain is like a catalyst that helps contractions intensify and assists the baby progress through the birth canal. Nature's medication, endorphins, are released in response to pain and may decrease the woman's perception of pain. With support from the practitioner, the family, and a secure environment, the woman can surrender to the experience and give birth. So in the hospital, flat on her back with tubes coming from every orifice, completely devoid of stimulation, is it surprising that the contractions decrease; labor arrests; and almost 30% of women need operative intervention.

Unless something has happened to change her anatomy, today's woman is just as capable if not more so, with her state of health and nutritional stores to give birth. Unfortunately, today's woman has bought the advertising hype that technology guarantees a normal healthy child; that operative birth saves the vagina from trauma; that women have no responsibility for the birth outcome. This is not to say that technology is not an effective tool when the pregnancy is at risk and interventions are necessary to effect a safe outcome. Women and practitioners must never forget that these interventions are simply tools to be utilized as appropriate to give nature a helping hand. Many women are simply not interested in pursuing natural childbirth. This technology seems to be too readily available to them and is championed by care providers and the mass media as the "intelligent" choice.

Natural childbirth simply stated means a spontaneous birth through the vaginal canal utilizing the forces of the uterine contractions under the control of the woman. This author feels that it should be taken a step further to mean that the woman should be educated to understand the forces of labor and how to use these forces in conjunction with her own natural resources to give birth. She should be allowed to ambulate, eat and drink, choose the position of birth, feel the forces of birth, and choose who will support her and who will assist her to birth within a safe environment.

Women, this author intreats you to listen and take control of your birth again. It is a fulfilling natural process, not a disease. It should be celebrated with family with tears of joy, not fear. Only when women truly take control and make informed decisions about their birth, will normal birth become the standard again.

See Also: Cesarean section, Labor and delivery, Pregnancy

Suggested Reading

Lothian, J. A. (2000). Why natural childbirth? *The Journal of Perinatal Education, 9*(4), 44–46.
Lothian, J. A. (2002). Position paper—Lamaze for the 21st century. *The Journal of Perinatal Education, 11*(1), x–xii.

Elaine K. Diegmann

Natural Family Planning Natural family planning is a method of understanding signs and patterns of fertility during the menstrual cycle to achieve or avoid pregnancy. Other terms for this method are fertility awareness method (FAM), the rhythm method, or periodic abstinence. The use of the term natural does not imply that other methods are "unnatural." The expression actually means that the natural signs and symptoms of the menstrual cycle are observed, recorded, and interpreted to ascertain when a woman is fertile. The couple then abstains or uses a barrier method or withdrawal during these times.

There are several methods that are considered to be natural family planning. All of these methods overestimate the time of fertility in order to compensate for the life span of the sperm and ova (egg). The sperm can live for 5 days within the female reproductive tract. The life span of the ova is 24 hr. The calendar method is the recording of the intermenstrual period (the number of days from the onset of one period to the onset of the next) for 6 months in order to ascertain the shortest and longest cycle length. The fertile time can then be determined by subtracting 18 from the shortest cycle length and 11 from the longest cycle. The couple then abstains from intercourse on the days corresponding to the fertile time. This would require periodic abstinence for an average of 16 days a cycle. The effectiveness rate of this method for perfect use is 3.1% for the first year. For imperfect use the failure rate is as high as 86.4%, however.

A second type of natural family planning is the basal body temperature (BBT) method. Fertility is determined by taking the temperature first thing in the morning before getting out of bed with a special thermometer for this purpose. The temperature is recorded. An increase of 0.2–0.4°F that continues for 3 days indicates that ovulation has occurred. The couple abstains or uses another method until after the ovulation temperature spike. Perfect use of this method has a failure of 2% and a typical use failure rate of 20%.

Another method of detecting fertility is observing the cervical mucus beginning the first day after menstruation stops. Just after menses, the vagina may feel moist for a few days. The mucus then becomes thicker and cloudy. As ovulation approaches, the mucus becomes more clear, slippery, stretchy, and abundant. The mucus may be stretched for 2–3 in. between the thumb and index finger during peak times. Ovulation occurs at the peak of this wetter, clearer mucus. The fertile time is the first day of peak mucus until 4 days after the peak day. Some issues that can make this method more difficult to interpret are the use of douching, having unprotected intercourse the day before since semen and arousal fluids can be confused with mucus, vaginal infections, and menstruation. Couples may either have intercourse only during the pre and post peak days or use another method during the peak times. Some choose to avoid having intercourse until after the peak each month. This method typically requires the help of a professional to correctly interpret the mucus findings.

The symptothermal method combines more than one indicator of fertility. Many use the temperature and mucus observations to determine fertile times. Other signs can also be used such as checking the position and consistency of the cervix and noting midcycle pain called mittelschmerz or ovulation pain.

The advantages for using these methods are that the cost is free, the Catholic Church sanctions the methods, and there are no hormones introduced into the body. Often these methods are used to determine the most fertile time of the month when couples are attempting pregnancy. Women become more aware of their bodies as well. The disadvantages are that these methods are very complex and require highly motivated couples willing to abstain from intercourse during fertile times. Conditions that cause the menstrual cycle to be irregular or alter cervical mucus such as breastfeeding or recent childbirth may make these methods more difficult to use.

It is recommended that couples seek professional education and monitoring when learning to use these methods as they often require several cycles of observation to become familiar with the fertility signs and symptoms.

SEE ALSO: Birth control, Menstruation

Suggested Resources

www.plannedparenthood.org

NANCY MYERS-BRADLEY

Nausea Nausea is a common symptom that is associated with a wide variety of conditions. Nausea is an unpleasant sensation in the upper abdomen often referred to as "queasiness," which is usually accompanied by an urge to vomit. Vomiting, usually preceded by nausea, is defined as the forceful ejection of stomach contents up to and out of the mouth. It is important to recognize that nausea and vomiting are not diseases in and of themselves but rather symptoms of an underlying process. Usually nausea and vomiting are due to an illness that improves on its own or is easily treated.

CAUSES

The list of conditions that can cause nausea and vomiting is long and includes disorders affecting the digestive tract, abdominal organs, central nervous system, metabolism, and endocrine system. Examples of digestive tract disorders that may be associated with nausea include gastroparesis (poor stomach emptying in the absence of an anatomical obstruction), gastroesophageal reflux disease, irritable bowel syndrome, peptic ulcer disease, and gastrointestinal obstruction. Nausea may be due to infections involving the digestive tract like viral gastroenteritis and food poisoning. Inflammatory abdominal conditions like gallbladder disease, hepatitis, and pancreatitis frequently cause nausea. Nausea is a common symptom reported by patients with balance and equilibrium problems (such as motion sickness), other intracerebral disorders (such as migraine headaches, tumor, hemorrhage, meningitis), and psychiatric disorders (such as anxiety, depression, anorexia nervosa, bulimia). Endocrine and metabolic causes of nausea and vomiting include pregnancy (nausea occurs in 70% of women during the first trimester), diabetes, kidney failure, and thyroid disorders. Medications are among the most common causes of nausea and vomiting, usually during the first few weeks the medication is used. Examples of medications that frequently cause nausea and vomiting are aspirin, nonsteroidal anti-inflammatory drugs (such as ibuprofen), digoxin, theophylline, oral contraceptives, narcotics, and many cancer chemotherapy agents. Nausea and vomiting may also occur in patients with heart attacks, congestive heart failure, or during the first few days following surgery.

DIAGNOSIS

Although the causes of nausea and vomiting are numerous, careful consideration of each patient's individual circumstances gives clues to the likely cause. This, along with a thorough history and physical examination, can narrow down the diagnosis. Important factors to consider are duration, severity, and frequency of symptoms as well as recent ingestions (e.g., spoiled foods, toxins), new medications, similar illness in family or friends, description of vomit (if any), and any other associated symptoms. Acute nausea and vomiting, lasting on the order of hours to a few days, is typically due to infection (e.g., gastroenteritis, meningitis), medications, acute inflammatory conditions (e.g., gallbladder disease), or toxins (e.g., alcohol). Nausea and vomiting symptoms lasting more than 1 month may be due to a number of chronic medical conditions (e.g., gastroparesis, irritable bowel syndrome, cancer, and diabetes), pregnancy, medications, or psychiatric disorders. Vomiting early in the morning may suggest causes including pregnancy,

kidney failure, alcohol, narcotic withdrawal, and increased intracranial pressure (increased pressure on the brain due to causes like cerebral hemorrhage, tumor, or meningitis). Vomiting occurring 1–3 hr after meals is seen in gastric outlet obstruction and gastroparesis whereas symptoms during or immediately after meals are often associated with psychiatric disorders (e.g., anorexia nervosa and bulimia). Associated symptoms that may aid in the evaluation and diagnosis include fever, abdominal pain, diarrhea, red blood or black "coffee grounds" in the vomit, weight loss, chest pain, headache, stiff neck, ringing in the ears, and vertigo.

A complete physical examination is performed not only to provide diagnostic information but to determine whether any complications of nausea and vomiting have occurred. The patient is specifically assessed for signs of weight loss, dehydration, fever, jaundice, abdominal tenderness and location, abdominal masses, enlarged lymph nodes, neurologic abnormalities, and blood in the stool.

A number of diagnostic tests may be used to evaluate nausea and vomiting, and the choice is dictated by the clinical situation. Laboratory studies may include blood, urine, and stool tests. A pregnancy test should be considered in women of reproductive age. A variety of radiologic studies may also be useful, including abdominal x-rays, abdominal ultrasound, abdominal or head CT scan, and contrast imaging studies (where the patient drinks barium and then x-rays are taken of the stomach and small intestine). At times, endoscopy (insertion of a flexible tube containing a camera into the mouth or rectum) may be required to diagnose the underlying cause of nausea and vomiting.

TREATMENT

Treatment of nausea and vomiting will depend on the severity and cause. Important issues to be addressed are: correction of fluid and electrolyte losses; identification and treatment, or removal, of the underlying cause; and symptom treatment. Minor self-limited symptoms can often be managed with rest and a bland diet consisting of cold or room-temperature clear liquids (e.g., ginger ale, broth) and small frequent meals of nonfatty foods (e.g., crackers, toast). Oral rehydration fluids (e.g., sports drinks) provide important sugar and salt in addition to water when vomiting has persisted for more than 24 hr. However, young children and infants should not be given sports drinks, and should be rehydrated under medical supervision. Medical attention should be sought if nausea lasts more than a week or if pregnancy is suspected. Immediate attention should be sought if there is persistent vomiting, vomiting with diarrhea, severe abdominal pain, severe headache, stiff neck, high fever, red blood or "coffee grounds" in the vomit, lightheadedness, confusion, decreased consciousness, chest pain, rapid heart rate, or shortness of breath.

At times, hospital admission may be necessary for intravenous fluids, testing, and/or treatment. Specific treatments are directed at the underlying cause and can range from simple measures such as over-the-counter medications for motion sickness to invasive treatments such as dialysis for kidney failure or surgery for gallbladder disease. Sometimes the cause of symptoms cannot be identified or treatment is unsuccessful or incomplete. In these cases, antiemetic ("antivomiting") medications may be given. There is a wide variety of antiemetic agents available and the clinician must decide which is most appropriate given the situation and severity of symptoms. Acupuncture and acupressure have been effective in reducing nausea and vomiting in chemotherapy patients and in people with symptoms following surgery. Acupressure may reduce nausea in pregnancy. In cases of chronic nausea and vomiting in which a physical explanation has been ruled out, a psychiatric evaluation may be helpful.

SEE ALSO: Abdominal pain, Acupuncture, Bulimia, nervosa, Migraine

Suggested Reading

Hasler, W. L. (1999). Approach to the patient with nausea and vomiting. In T. Yamada, D. H. Alpers, L. Laine, C. Owyang, & D. W. Powell (Eds.), *Textbook of gastroenterology* (3rd ed., pp. 775–794). Philadelphia: Lippincott.

Koch, K. L., & Frissora, C. L. (2003). Nausea and vomiting during pregnancy. *Gastroenterology Clinics of North America, 32*(1), 201–234.

Quigley, E. M., Hasler, W. L., & Parkman, H. P. (2001). AGA technical review on nausea and vomiting. *Gastroenterology, 120*, 263–286.

Suggested Resources

Medical encyclopedia: Nausea and vomiting. MEDLINEplus health information. U.S. National Library of Medicine and the National Institutes of Health. (2003, April). http://www.nlm.nih.gov/medlineplus/nauseaandvomiting.html

Nutrition tips for managing nausea and vomiting. Mayo Clinic health information/MayoClinic.com. Mayo Foundation for Medical Education and Research. (2002, June). http://www.mayoclinic.com/invoke.cfm?id=HQ01133

MARGARET JAKUBOWICZ
MARGARET F. KINNARD

Neonatal Care Ethics

During the year 2000, there were over 4.5 million births in the United States. Nearly 12% of these births were defined as premature, that is, occurring at less than 37 weeks gestation, and 1% of these births were infants weighing less than 1,500 g. We have developed specialized expertise and technologies in order to take care of the smallest of these very low birth-weight (VLBW) infants, referred to as "micropremies."

Mortality and morbidity, in general, inversely correlate with gestational age and birthweight of infants born prematurely. The neonatal mortality rate drops significantly at 1,000 g, which typically correlates with a gestational age of 27 weeks. Currently the limit of our ability to resuscitate an extremely premature newborn is 22 weeks of gestation or just over half of a normal gestation of 40 weeks. More than half of these infants do not survive despite intensive efforts and the survivors most commonly experience enduring deficits and morbidity. Morbidity associated with extreme prematurity includes: cerebral palsy, which is a nonprogressive neuromuscular disorder involving primarily the extremities often with associated cognitive defects; bleeding in the brain (intraventricular hemorrhage, IVH), bleeding-related swelling of the brain (posthemorrhagic hydrocephalus) and conditions affecting the white matter of the brain (periventricular leukomalacia, PVL); chronic lung disease sometimes necessitating a home ventilator; disorders of the eye (retinopathy) of prematurity, which in some cases can lead to vision difficulties or retinal detachment and blindness; hearing loss; and long-term growth and development delays.

Along with the ability to save some of the smallest babies come many ethical considerations. Four central ethical concerns in the clinical care of premature infants relate to: (1) the process of obtaining informed consent for these interventions; (2) the quality of life we are creating for a population of former extremely low birth-weight infants and their families; (3) optimal approaches to palliative care for these critically ill infants; and (4) the distribution of scarce societal resources and technology for the entire neonatal population.

INFORMED CONSENT

In theory, informed consent occurs in a context of trust and understanding and is predicated on three elements: a substantive process for information sharing; the ability of the appropriate decision-maker to make knowledgeable, reasoned, and meaningful choices; and the ability to make decisions freely and in the absence of coercive pressures. In reality, the existence of true informed consent in the neonatal intensive care unit (NICU) is often under debate. Neonatologists (doctors who care for premature infants) are asked to explain the risks of delivering a premature infant to mothers and families at moments of extreme vulnerability in the mother's life: she is in preterm labor, or ill herself and hearing for the first time that she is having a premature infant; these are also conversations that may be rushed due to clinical circumstances. The detail and significance of these discussions must increase with the decreasing gestational age of the infant. There are a variety of issues that need to be reviewed. These encompass the risks of cardiopulmonary resuscitation in the delivery room, the possible clinical course while in the NICU, including the types of respiratory support available to these infants such as specialized mechanical ventilation (high-frequency ventilation), the possibility of surgery to correct a heart defect (patent ductus arteriosus), the occurrence of IVH and PVL, and the inherent risks of long-term neurodevelopmental disabilities associated with an extremely low birthweight infant.

Inherent in the *ability to* resuscitate an extremely premature infant is the decision of *whether to* do so. This decision comes to intimately involve both parents and physician. Consent discussions are shaped by evidence and standards of care, but personal values, cultural influences, and religious beliefs affect the family's understanding of what is good and right and possible. The values of clinicians and counselors may enter into these discussions, as it is often difficult to be completely "objective" in the face of such uncertainty and risk. In present-day medicine, parents hold ultimate responsibility for the choices made in the care of a premature infant, even if it is the clinician who must present and, at times, guide these choices. It is apparent that this represents an extraordinary and often painful burden for the family to shoulder. Sensitive, supportive efforts on the part of the clinical team can make the process less difficult. Ongoing discussions after the infant is born are also important; it may not be until birth of the infant that the family truly develops an understanding of the type of support that children born prematurely will require.

QUALITY OF LIFE

The eventual quality of life for a premature baby is greatly influenced by gestational age at the time of birth.

Infants born at the limits of viability, that is, 22–25 weeks, tend to be the most profoundly affected in their neurodevelopmental outcomes. Unfortunately we have no way of foretelling which infants may eventually have deficits; the prognostic ability of head ultrasounds demonstrating bleeding in the brain (IVH) is called into question in the extremely low birthweight population. We do know that when surveyed, parents of VLBW infants with developmental delay feel no worse impact than those families with normal term infants. In addition to the ability to "save" extremely premature infants we have also advanced technology with regard to the surgical correction of many previously lethal deformities. We have seen advances in the repair of severe bowel diseases. The diagnosis of abnormal placement of the tissue beneath the lungs (congenital diaphragmatic hernia, CDH) is no longer a death sentence and congenital heart disease including underdevelopment of the heart (hypoplastic left heart syndrome) is readily correctable at large institutions via staged surgery or cardiac transplant. Fetal therapy is available for some surgical interventions including correction for CDH and fetal gene therapy is on the horizon for inheritable diseases such as some types of disorders of immune system functioning (severe combined immune deficiency).

Optimism about the health outcomes of premature infants is often well founded. Moreover, even when deficits persist, the physical difficulties accompanying prematurity are not determinant of one's eventual strengths and capacities, nor are they predictive of one's sense of personal satisfaction, life meaning, individualism, and societal contributions. This said, there are very real concerns about the very devastating health outcomes experienced by many of the littlest or sickest of premature infants. These issues merit our continued attention as technological abilities push back the defining line for infant viability.

PALLIATIVE CARE APPROACHES

It is increasingly acknowledged that integrated palliative care and pain programs are central to optimal care for infants. Dismissed are the thoughts that infants do not experience pain as older children and adults do, and modern training in neonatology includes skills in evaluating and treating the pain of infants just as in the care of patients by other subspecialties. Palliative care consultation services are slowly making their way into the NICU. When the time comes for palliative care in the infant's life we must apply what we have learned from other populations. Easing the passage to death is a gift the physician can give the family and their baby. Palliative care studies in infants demonstrate that fewer medical procedures are performed and more supportive services are provided to families that are involved with palliative care consultation. As the availability of palliative care programs increases we will see a greater number of clinicians skilled in providing pain relief, emotional support, and access to services for these families to ease their burden.

RESOURCE ALLOCATION

One consideration that permeates all of medicine, and especially intensive care medicine, is the challenge of appropriate resource allocation. Costs associated with successful resuscitation of the very littlest of newborns are substantial, and they are overshadowed by the costs of caring for children and adults with the sequelae of prematurity. Creating a health care system where pregnant women have access to the prenatal care that they need may have the biggest impact on the rate of premature birth over the next decade. It is encouraging that the rate of premature birth declined in 2000 for the first time in over a decade from 11.8% to 11.6%. However, lack of access to prenatal care remains a huge contributor to the rate of premature births, especially in rural and poor areas of the country. Without serious attention to this issue, this will become a worsening problem in coming years.

Until premature birth can be prevented there will be challenges surrounding the care of the VLBW infant. There are difficult decisions to be made regarding consent of the family in danger of delivering a very premature infant, resuscitation of that infant, long-term quality of life for the infant and family, and when treatment fails providing a pain-free death with dignity, which also provides emotional support for the family. The best care will be provided by physicians and support staff working closely with families to alleviate some of the inherent emotional distress associated with NICU care.

SEE ALSO: Informed consent, Prenatal care

Suggested Reading

Catlin, A. (Ed.). (2001). Special issue: Neonatal ethics. *Journal of Clinical Ethics, 12.*

Hack, M., Flannery, D. J., Schluchter, M., et al. (2002). Outcomes in young adulthood for very-low-birth-weight infants. *New England Journal of Medicine, 346,* 149–157.

Jonsen, A. R., Siegler, M., & Winslade, W. J. (2002). *Clinical ethics: A practical approach to ethical decisions in clinical medicine* (5th ed.). New York: McGraw-Hill.

Lantos, J. D., Mokalla, M., & Meadow, W. (1997). Resource allocation in neonatal and medical ICUs. *American Journal of Respiratory Critical Care Medicine, 156,* 185–189.

Lee, S., Penner, P. L., & Cox, M. (1991). Impact of very low birth weight infants on the family and its relationship to parental attitudes. *Pediatrics, 88,* 105–109.

Meadow, W., Goldblatt, A. D., & Lantos, J. (2002). Current opinion in pediatrics: Ethics and law 2001. *Current Opinion in Pediatrics, 12,* 170–173.

Philip, A. G. (1995). Neonatal mortality rate: Is further improvement possible? *Journal of Pediatrics, 126,* 427–433.

Pierucci, R. L., Kirby, R. S., Leuthner, S. R., et al. (2001). End-of-life care for neonates and infants: The experience and effects of a palliative care consultation service. *Pediatrics, 108*(3), 653–660.

REBECCA H. MORAN
LAURA WEISS ROBERTS

Neural Tube Defects

Defects of neural tube development are congenital anomalies with an estimated incidence of 1 in 2,000 live births. Formation of the neural tube is completed by 28 days of gestation, before most women are even aware that they are pregnant. Neural tube defects (NTDs) result from the failure of closure of the neural folds at one or more of sites.

The most severe form of NTDs occurs when there is a total failure of neural tube formation. Failure of closure of the anterior portion of the neural tube results in anencephaly, a total or partial absence of the brain and skull. Anencephalocele occurs when there is a limited closure defect of the skull with brain and membrane tissue protruding through the opening. Spina bifida results from failed closure of a portion of the posterior neural tube. Myelomeningocele is a form of spina bifida in which a protruding sac contains nerves, covering membrane tissue, and cerebrospinal fluid. A meningocele is a less frequent type of spina bifida in which the sac protruding through the vertebral defect contains meninges, the membrane tissue enclosing the spinal cord. In another form of spina bifida, intact skin covers the vertebral defect, often concealing the lesion and leading to the term spina bifida occulta. Skin lesions such as hair tufts, sinus tracts, or birthmarks may raise suspicion of an underlying spina bifida occulta, which occurs in approximately 10% of otherwise healthy people. Thus mild forms are considered normal variants. However, some forms of spina bifida occulta are associated with fibrous bands that limit mobility of the lower spinal cord. The tension transmitted to the spinal cord during movement can cause injury and progressive neurological symptoms such as lower back pain, muscle atrophy, and urinary incontinence.

Screening the pregnant population for NTDs is accomplished by measuring maternal serum levels of the major fetal tissue protein, alpha-fetoprotein (AFP). If the fetal skin layer is not intact, greater amounts of AFP leak into the amniotic fluid and then diffuse into the maternal bloodstream. AFP values that are 2–2.5 times above the average identify the pregnancy as high risk and lead to the detection of over 80% of fetuses with NTDs. High-resolution ultrasound is recommended if screening detects an elevated AFP level as it is able to identify nearly 100% of open NTDs. Although AFP screening is noninvasive and does not physically harm the mother or fetus, receiving abnormal results can cause great emotional stress. Awareness of congenital anomalies in the fetus leads to ethically complex decisions about whether to terminate the pregnancy.

Neural tube closure is a complex process, and defects have genetic and environmental etiologies. The incidence of NTDs varies greatly among populations and ethnic groups. In the United States, African and Asian Americans have a lower rate of NTDs than those of Hispanic or European heritage. Risk factors for neural tube defects include diabetes, hyperthermia, and use of the anticonvulsant valproic acid. In addition, alterations in genes involved in the processing of folate, a form of B vitamin, are found in some mothers of affected infants.

Randomized investigations have shown a 60% reduction in the occurrence of NTDs when women received folic acid vitamins. As a result the Public Health Service recommends that women capable of becoming pregnant consume 0.4 mg of folic acid daily and high-risk women take 4 mg of folic acid per day around conception. Estimates of folic acid intake from natural food sources show that only 8% of women consume 0.4 mg daily. Folic acid intake can be increased by consuming foods such as leafy greens, legumes, citrus fruits, liver, and whole wheat. Alternatively, folate fortified processed foods or vitamin supplements can be taken. Since the implementation of grain fortification in 1998, the average woman receives about one quarter of her daily folate requirement from cereal products.

Vitamin supplements were the only form of folate tested in the clinical trials demonstrating decreased incidence of NTDs.

Elective cesarian section and in utero surgery for infants with spina bifida have been advocated to decrease trauma to the spinal cord. Cesarian delivery prior to onset of labor remains controversial because of a lack of planned research studies demonstrating a benefit. Surgery to cover the exposed spinal cord in fetuses with spina bifida during the second trimester of pregnancy is still investigational. Early results show improved neurological outcomes, but the benefit should be weighed against the increased risk of preterm labor and maternal complications.

Anencephalic infants are either stillborn or do not survive beyond a few weeks. In the United States over 90% of infants with spina bifida survive beyond a year, although most experience serious lifelong disability. All have varying degrees of paralysis and decreased sensation, and the majority also have an obstruction to the flow of cerebrospinal fluid. Complications of progressive brainstem dysfunction are the leading early cause of death in infants with spina bifida.

As children with spina bifida mature, the neurological, genitourinary, and musculoskeletal systems require ongoing surveillance. Lack of bladder control may lead to recurrent urinary tract infections and renal damage. Since spina bifida involves the spinal cord, it also inevitably affects sexual functioning. Orthopedic abnormalities include curvature of the spine and imbalanced muscle groups producing joint dislocation. Individuals with spina bifida are also at risk for severe latex allergy from repeated exposures during hospitalizations.

Spinal nerve damage may result in urinary retention, reduced rectal sensation, or an inability to retain stools. Control of urinary and fecal incontinence is essential for achieving personal and social independence. Bladder emptying at routine intervals by insertion of a clean urine catheter is an important management technique, and a range of dietary, pharmacologic, and surgical interventions also exist.

The effects of spina bifida lesions on sexual functioning vary widely between individuals. Puberty may occur earlier in those with spina bifida when compared to their siblings. Altered genital sensation is frequent in both males and females. While women usually have normal fertility, functional problems with erection and ejaculation can lead to decreased fertility in males. The course of pregnancy in women with spina bifida is similar to unaffected women except for an increased risk of urinary tract infections, pressure sores, and lower pelvic pain. Pregnant women with spina bifida are encouraged to deliver vaginally, as cesarian section is associated with higher risk of complication rates. The risk of NTDs in the offspring of individuals with spina bifida is estimated at 1 in 25, which is higher than the risk in the general population. The majority of individuals with spina bifida have never discussed spina bifida-related sexual issues with their physician and providing a supportive environment can greatly improve their quality of life. Assisted reproductive technologies are available to improve male fertility and periconceptual counseling can help in pregnancy planning.

The long-term prognosis for individuals with spina bifida is difficult to estimate as improvements in medical care continue to increase life expectancy. Recent studies show survival to the third decade of life in over 50% of affected persons. Early mortality places NTDs as the fifth leading cause of years of potential life lost. Despite daunting medical problems, most children with spina bifida have normal intelligence and lead a nearly independent life.

SEE ALSO: Activities of daily living, Alpha-fetoprotein screening, Disability, Nutrition, Prenatal care, Quality of life

Suggested Reading

Anon. (2002). Spina bifida: Key primary care issues. *Australian Family Physician, 31,* 66–105.

Botto, L. D., Moore, C. A., Khoury, M. J., & Erickson, J. D. (1999). Neural-tube defects. *New England Journal of Medicine, 341,* 1509–1519.

Locksmith, G. J., & Duff, P. (1998). Preventing neural tube defects: The importance of periconceptual folic acid supplements. *Obstetrics and Gynecology, 91,* 1027–1034.

Northup, H., & Volcik, K. A. (2000). Spina bifida and other neural tube defects. *Current Problems in Pediatrics, 30,* 317–332.

Volpe, J. (1995). Neural tube formation and prosencephalic development. In *Neurology of the newborn* (3rd ed., pp. 3–41). Philadelphia: W. B. Saunders.

N. K. YEANEY

Neuropathy Nerves extend out from the central nervous system (spinal cord or brain) to supply muscle, skin, and other tissues. Nerves are comprised of a large number of microscopic nerve fibers. The core of each nerve fiber is the axon, which is a long, thin extension of a nerve cell located within or near the spinal cord or brain. The axon carries electrical impulses. Nerve fibers can be motor (making muscles contract), sensory, or autonomic (controlling blood vessels, sweat glands, and viscera). Large nerve fibers (which serve motor or fine sensory function) have an insulation of a fatty substance called myelin surrounding the axon. Small nerve fibers (which may be myelinated or unmyelinated) carry the sensation of pain or temperature, or are autonomic.

Neuropathy means a disorder of nerves. More specifically, it is used synonymously with polyneuropathy, implying a disorder affecting the nerves of the body diffusely. Polyneuropathy needs to be distinguished from mononeuropathy (disorder of a single nerve). The most common mononeuropathy is carpal tunnel syndrome, or median nerve entrapment in the hand, which causes fingers to go numb in sleep. Mononeuropathies of nerves arising from the brain are called cranial neuropathies. The most common cranial neuropathy is unexplained facial neuropathy, or Bell's palsy.

Polyneuropathies are usually symmetrical. In general, the longest nerve fibers (which supply the feet) are affected first. As the disease advances, progressively shorter nerve fibers are involved and symptoms ascend up the legs. When the knees get affected, the fingers get affected too. Symptoms of polyneuropathy include numbness, tingling, burning, shooting pains, loss of sensation (leading to unnoticed injuries to feet), loss of muscle bulk in the feet, hammertoes, weakness advancing to foot drop, hand weakness and even thigh weakness, loss of balance, loss of sweating in the feet, and skin changes.

The most common cause of polyneuropathy in the developed world is diabetes. Prevalence of neuropathy in longstanding diabetics may be as high as 50%. Diabetic polyneuropathy can be mild or can be severe and disabling. Good control of diabetes decreases the risk of polyneuropathy. The list of other causes of polyneuropathy is long. A short list includes (a) heredofamilial neuropathies: Charcot–Marie–Tooth disease, others, (b) infectious: HIV, leprosy, diphtheria, (c) toxic: drugs (some drugs used for cancer and HIV, INH, amiodarone, others), metals (lead, gold, arsenic, thallium), industrial toxins, and possibly alcohol, (d) nutritional: deficiencies of thiamine, niacin, vitamin B12, vitamin E, (e) metabolic: renal failure, thyroid deficiency, (f) paraproteinemia (abnormal immunoglobulin-like protein in the blood) and paraneoplastic (distant effect of cancer), and (g) vasculitic: from autoimmune inflammation of blood vessels, either in isolation or in association with disorders like rheumatoid arthritis. Vasculitic neuropathy is often severe and could be diffuse (spread out), asymmetrical, or affect multiple individual nerves (mononeuritis multiplex).

A specific neuropathy called Guillain–Barré syndrome (also called acute inflammatory demyelinating polyradiculoneuropathy) is caused by an autoimmune attack on myelin. It develops over days to weeks and can affect short as well as long nerves. Unlike other neuropathies, weakness of muscles predominates and can be so profound that the patient's breathing has to be supported on a ventilator. The vast majority make an excellent recovery over weeks to months. Recovery is hastened by plasma exchange (removal of antibodies and other offending molecules from blood) or by injecting high doses of immunoglobulin intravenously. A chronic demyelinating neuropathy (CIDP) also occurs. Some forms of Charcot–Marie–Tooth disease are also demyelinating. Most other polyneuropathies, in contrast, are axonal.

In a large minority (if not the majority) of nondiabetic individuals with neuropathic symptoms, a cause of neuropathy is not found. Such cryptogenic neuropathy tends to be relatively mild and indolent.

Evaluation for neuropathy includes a careful neurological and physical examination and blood and urine tests to look for possible causes. Electrodiagnostic examination (or electronography and nerve conduction studies) is invaluable for the objective diagnosis of neuropathy, assessment of severity, and identification of demyelinating neuropathy. In rare cases a nerve biopsy is indicated.

Treatment involves reversing the cause (if identified), pain control (medications known as tricyclic antidepressants and some antiepileptic drugs are commonly used), foot care, orthotic devices (if there is foot drop), and aids for walking and hand use. Some mononeuropathies are amenable to surgery.

SEE ALSO: Chronic pain, Pain

Suggested Reading

Dyck, P. J., & Thomas, P. K. (Eds.). (1999). *Diabetic neuropathy.* Philadelphia: W. B. Saunders.

Dyck, P. J., Thomas, P. K., Griffin, J. W., et al. (Eds.). (1993). *Peripheral neuropathy.* Philadelphia: W. B. Saunders.

Mendell, J. R., Kissel, J. T., & Cornblath, D. R. (Eds.). (2001). *Diagnosis and management of peripheral nerve disorders* (Contemporary Neurology Series, 59). New York: Oxford University Press.

Stewart, J. D. (2000). *Focal peripheral neuropathies.* Philadelphia: Lippincott, Williams & Wilkins.

NIMISH J. THAKORE

New England Female Medical College

The world's first medical college for women was established in the United States in 1848. Originally the school was called the Boston Female Medical College, but later the name was changed to the New England Female Medical College. The school first opened its doors in 1848 and immediately enrolled 12 women in its first class. By 1850 all 12 women graduated with medical degrees and began practicing medicine. Among the graduating 12 was Rebecca Lee, the first African American woman to become a physician in the United States. The New England Female Medical College was founded with the ultimate goal of educating women in obstetrics and gynecology.

The establishment of a medical school for women stirred up an enormous amount of controversy. At the time there was a common misbelief that women could never become doctors because all women had certain characteristics that made them ill-suited for the role of a physician. Male leaders in medicine attributed these characteristics to a woman's inability to make decisions, lack of rational judgment, emotional instability, lack of stamina, and biological inferiority.

Nonetheless, social reform helped women in their struggle to become doctors, since there was a need in society for women to care for the poor, children, and other women. In addition, society became more accepting of women taking on significant roles in the areas of sanitation, personal hygiene, and diet. Furthermore, the women's suffrage movement had just begun and it fueled the momentum for women's physicians.

Although the New England Female Medical College allowed women to study medicine, the curriculum still oppressed women. The basic medical curriculum was limited in its focus, which was only on obstetrics and gynecology. Samuel Gregory, the school's founder, was the leader of a crusade against men delivering babies because he believed it was immoral for men to be involved in the birth process. His intention for creating the school was to train women only as midwife physicians rather than true physicians.

The next obstacle a woman with medical degrees had to overcome was a lack of adequate clinical training. Many hospitals denied female medical students the opportunity to obtain clinical experience. Further, even if a hospital did permit female students to do a clinical rotation, the students were still limited to obstetrics and gynecology. This forced many women to go overseas for clinical training. The expense of such an endeavor discouraged many women from pursuing medicine. Furthermore, medical societies refused to give women physicians a medical license. In an effort to discourage the training of women, any male physician who taught or consulted with women physicians was threatened with loss of his medical license.

To enroll in the New England Female Medical College, a woman had to have an English education and submit a medical thesis. The 3-year medical program required 30 hours of instruction per week over a period of 17 weeks. During the last 2 years the student was required to do a preceptorship under a supervising physician.

In 1874, the New England Female Medical College made an offer to merge the school with Harvard Medical School. However, Harvard rejected the offer because its board believed women should not be doctors. After 26 years of training women physicians to deliver babies, in 1873 the school merged with the Boston University School of Medicine, creating one of the first coeducational medical schools in the world.

Although there has been progress for women in medicine in the last century, women are still underrepresented in medicine. By 1979 only 10% of the physicians in the United States were women. This disparity led to the American Medical Association's Outreach Program for Women Physicians, which focused on the recruitment of women physicians to medical leadership positions. Today, this program has been expanded and now includes the Women Physicians Congress. As a result, medical student enrollment among females is quickly rising. In 2002, 45.7% of enrolled medical students were women. Despite the increased enrollment, only 24.6% of physicians in the United States today are women. Another disparity is that women physicians, on average, make $45,000 less than their male counterparts.

Women are also underrepresented in academic medicine. For instance, in academic medicine, when comparing the makeup of medical school faculties, on average there are only 21 women per 161 men. In addition, only 7.5% of medical school department chairs are held by women and only 4 of the 125 U.S. medical schools have women as deans.

The creation of the New England Female Medical College was a landmark event for women in medicine. The school not only allowed women to obtain their medical degrees but was also key in the creation of one of the first coeducation medical schools in the world. Undoubtedly, there has been much progress for women in medicine since the mid-1800s. However, much more

work remains. Women are still significantly underrepresented in the practice of medicine, academic medicine, and other medical leadership positions. Even as we have entered the new millennium efforts to advance women in medicine are still needed.

SEE ALSO: Discrimination, Education, Midwifery, Pregnancy, Woman's Medical College of Pennsylvania

Suggested Resources

American Medical Association. (2003). Celebrating women in medicine: 20 years of progress (1999, September 20 editorial). http://ama-assn.org/scipubs/amnews/amn_99/edit0920.html

American Medical Association. (2003). Table 1—Physicians by gender (excludes students). Retrieved January 23, 2003, from http://www.ama-assn.org/ama/pub/article/171-195.html

American Medical Association. (2003). Table 3—Women in US medical schools over a 20 year period. Retrieved January 23, 2003, from http://www.ama-assn.org/ama/pub/article/171-197.html

American Medical Association. (2003). Table 11—Income/total by year. Retrieved April 10, 2003, from http://www.ama-assn.org/ama/pub/article/171-206.html

The Joint Committee on the Status of Women. (2003). The matriculation of women at Harvard Medical School 1847–1870. Retrieved February 10, 2003, from http://www.hms.harvard.edu/jcsw/matriculation/matriculation1.html

Justin, M. S. (2002–2003). *The entry of women into medicine in America: Education and obstacles 1847–1910.* Hobart and William Smith Colleges. http://campus.hws.edu/his/blackwell/articles/womenmedicine.html

ELIZABETH M. VALENCIA

Nicotine Nicotine was first identified in the early 1800s. It is a stimulant from the same family as cocaine. Nicotine is a naturally occurring colorless liquid that turns brown when burned and acquires the odor of tobacco when exposed to air. Most nicotine is obtained through tobacco use.

THE EFFECTS OF NICOTINE

Most cigarettes in the U.S. market contain 10 mg or more of nicotine. The effects of nicotine in people are influenced by: (a) the rate and route of dosing, (b) the development of tolerance, and (c) the metabolism of nicotine.

The average smoker smokes about $1\frac{1}{2}$ packs of cigarettes a day and takes between 10 and 20 puffs per cigarette. According to the National Institute on Drug Abuse, this average smoker gets 300 "hits" of nicotine to the brain each day. The average smoker takes in 1–2 mg of nicotine per cigarette. It takes only a few seconds for nicotine to enter the bloodstream after inhalation and less than 10 s to reach the brain. It is likely that the targets of nicotine in the central nervous system (CNS) are receptors found throughout the brain called nicotinic acetylcholine receptors (nAChRs). Cigar and pipe smokers typically do not inhale the smoke, so nicotine is absorbed more slowly through the mucosal membranes of their mouths.

Unlike most abused drugs, a smoker does not become intoxicated on cigarettes. In fact, the immediate effects of smoking are positive effects on mood, alertness, and ability to concentrate. This is because nicotine is activating the brain circuitry that regulates feelings of pleasure. The acute effects of nicotine dissipate in a few minutes, causing many smokers to continue dosing frequently throughout the day to maintain the drug's pleasurable effects. These effects are the primary reasons why so many smokers continue to smoke.

Eventually, the body develops a tolerance to nicotine's effects and physical dependence develops. When someone who is nicotine dependent tries to quit smoking, they experience a nicotine withdrawal syndrome. Symptoms of nicotine withdrawal include irritability, insomnia, anxiety, difficulty concentrating, depressed mood, decreased heart rate, and increased appetite. The withdrawal symptoms may peak within 1–4 days and persist for 3–4 weeks. Their persistence makes cessation difficult; most smokers who try to quit on their own relapse within a few days.

Nicotine has a rapid onset and short duration of action. Nicotine disappears from the body in a few hours. Under natural conditions, persons may have some cigarettes as often as every 20–30 min to keep a steady dose of nicotine in their body. Recent studies are looking at genetic variations in the enzymes that metabolize nicotine. According to Walton and colleagues "it should soon be possible to identify fast metabolizers (of nicotine) by DNA analysis."

Nicotine has different effects on mood. At first, it acts as an "upper" and, after a while, it acts as a "downer." Recent studies are examining the relationship between nicotine and depression.

Niaura et al. (2001) review the literature on maternal influences of smoking behaviors on their offspring. In particular, several studies have examined the effects of in utero exposure to smoking and the neuropsychiatric effects on the offspring. In women who smoke, neuropsychiatric deficits may be transmitted from mother to child.

NICOTINE ADDICTION

The addictive power of nicotine is shown in animal studies in which rats will self-administer intravenous nicotine. Despite knowing the negative health consequences, many adult smokers are addicted to nicotine. They crave for the cigarette within 15 min of awakening; they compulsively seek out nicotine throughout the day; and they find it difficult to refrain from smoking in areas where it is prohibited. Recent research studies are examining whether smoking, nicotine dependence, and nicotine addiction runs in families and whether genetic variations in brain neurotransmitter receptors may predispose someone to nicotine addiction.

TREATING NICOTINE ADDICTION

According to the Tobacco Advisory Group of the Royal College of Physicians in London, nicotine addiction is "a life-threatening, but treatable disorder." In fact, nicotine has been developed as a medication to assist smoking cessation. Nicotine replacement therapy (NRT) is a safe, approved method that helps take care of the nicotine addiction, while the smoker works on breaking the smoking habit. Often, NRT in the form of nicotine patch, gum, or inhalant is combined with some form of behavioral treatment program. Another medication used for nicotine addiction is the Bupropion slow-release (SR). NRT and Bupropion SR are Food and Drug Administration (FDA) approved and are prescribed to alleviate withdrawal symptoms, depressive symptoms, or to delay weight gain following smoking cessation.

See Also: Cardiovascular disease, Coronary risk factors, Lung disease, Smoking, Tobacco

Suggested Reading

Coleman, T., & West, R. (2001). Newly available treatment for nicotine addiction. *British Medical Journal, 322*, 1076–1077.

Manuda, M., Johnstone, E., Murphy, M., & Walton, R. (2001). New directions in the genetic mechanism underlying nicotine addiction. *Addiction Biology, 6*, 109–117.

National Institute on Drug Abuse Report Series: *Nicotine addiction.* www.nida.gov/researchreports/nicotine/nicotine2.html

Niaura, R., Bock, B., Lloyd, E. E., Brown, R., Lipsitt, L. P., & Buka, S. (2001). Maternal transmission of nicotine dependence: Psychiatric, neurocognitive and prenatal factors. *American Journal of Addiction, 10*, 16–29.

Tobacco Advisory Group of the Royal College of Physicians. (2000). *Nicotine addiction in Britain.* London: Author.

Walton, R., Johnstone, E., Nunafo, M., Neville, M., & Griffiths, S. (2001). Genetic clues to the molecular basis of tobacco addiction and progress towards personalized therapy. *Trends in Molecular Medicine, 7*, 70–76.

Watkins, S. S., Koob, G. F., & Markou, A. (2000). Neural mechanisms underlying nicotine addiction: Acute positive reinforcement and withdrawal. *Nicotine Tobacco Research, 2*, 19–37.

MARILYN DAVIES

Nightingale, Florence

During her parents' 3-year honeymoon in Europe, Florence Nightingale was born on May 12, 1820, in Florence, Italy. She was named after her birthplace. Her only sister, Frances Parthenope, or Parthe, had been born a year before, also named after her birthplace (Parthenope is the Greek name for Naples). Florence's parents were socially and politically connected, due to their wealth and membership in England's upper class. The family had two homes, although they spent the majority of the year at Embley Park in southern England. Their summer home in Derbyshire, Lea Hurst, was Florence's favorite of the two. Religion and education were integral parts of the Nightingale home; both would have a monumental impact on Florence's later life.

There was little opportunity for formal education during this time since universities were generally closed to women. Fortunately, Florence's father, William Edward Nightingale, was an educated man and desired to share this education with his daughters. Florence studied history, philosophy, ethics, grammar, writing, and mathematics. She learned to speak Latin, Greek, French, German, and Italian. These teachings would prepare Florence for her later role in life.

In 1837, while at Embley Park, Florence received her first "call from God." At that time, she did not fully understand what it meant, but the call drove her to become more active in helping the local poor. In 1849, while traveling in Egypt with friends, Florence received her second call from God. The following year she vowed chastity and obedience to God. After this time in her life, nursing took a priority for Florence. Although she received two marriage proposals, Florence never married; instead she chose to remain true to her calling.

Florence knew her calling was to serve the poor and sick. Her parents refused to allow her to become a nurse as nursing was not considered to be a suitable profession for a well-educated woman. However, during her trip to Europe and Egypt with friends, Florence visited Pastor Theodor Fliedner's hospital and school for deaconesses at Kaiserswerth, near Dusseldorf. In 1851, the following year, she returned to Kaiserswerth and spent 3 months training as a nurse. This training and her experience working with the sick and poor led her to Harley Street, London, where in 1853 she was offered an unpaid position as the Superintendent of the Establishment for Gentlewomen during Illness.

Florence Nightingale, the founder of modern nursing, thus began her career in nursing and hospital reform. She was able to utilize not only her fine education, but also her natural organizational skills to revamp the administration of the Establishment. In 1854, Sidney Herbert, the Minister at War, appointed Florence to oversee the introduction of female nurses into military hospitals during the Crimean War; Herbert selected Florence since he knew her both socially and professionally through her work at Harley Street. In November 1854, Florence Nightingale arrived at the Barrack Hospital in Scutari, Turkey, with 38 nurses. Although the doctors did not want the nurses there, within 10 days the medical and nursing staff were stretched to their limits due to the arrival of fresh casualties.

The British hospital at Scutari was in shambles; there were no beds, no kitchen, little water, and few doctors. Florence was not only a caretaker, but also an administrator, organizing nursing support for the doctors and provisions and facilities for the hospital. During this time, Florence came to be known by the soldiers as a caring and dedicated woman; one who cared no matter what the social status of the person was. It was during this time that Florence Nightingale became known as "the Lady with the Lamp." After the Crimean War, Nightingale quietly returned home. During the next few years, Florence made Army nursing reform the focal point of her career.

In 1860, at the St. Thomas's Hospital, the Nightingale School of Nursing opened in London. During this time, Florence was also consulted by U.S. President Abraham Lincoln for advice on Civil War nursing. In 1861, Florence developed severe spinal pain, which would limit some of her later endeavors. However, she did not let poor health keep her from implementing sanitation reform in India, which became the focus of her attentions for the next several years. After India, Florence turned to reform of another kind: nursing reform and women's progress. In 1893, at the Chicago World's Fair, Florence's last paper was read to the Nurse's Congress. On August 13, 1910, she died in her sleep at age 90. Today, Florence Nightingale is remembered for her pioneering work in public health, hospital administration, sanitary reform, and the use of statistical data for decision-making processes.

SEE ALSO: Blackwell, Elizabeth; Healers, Nurse practitioner, Nursing, Women in the Health Professions (pp. 20–32), Women in Health: Advocates, Reformers, and Pioneers (pp. 40–48)

Suggested Reading

Dossey, B. M. (2000). *Florence Nightingale: Mystic, visionary, healer.* Springhouse, PA: Springhouse.
Goldie, S. (Ed.). (1997). *Letters from the Crimea, 1854–1856/Florence Nightingale.* New York: Mandolin.
Hobbs, C. A. (1997). *Florence Nightingale.* New York: Twayne.
Webb, V. (2002). *Florence Nightingale: The making of a radical theologian.* St. Louis, MO: Chalice Press.
Woodham-Smith, C. (1983). *Florence Nightingale, 1820–1910.* New York: Atheneum.

Suggested Resources

Florence Nightingale Museum. (2003). London. Retrieved July 2003, from http://www.florence-nightingale.co.uk

TAMBRA K. CAIN

Novello, Antonia Born in 1944 in a small town in Puerto Rico, Antonia Novello experienced the hardships of pain and disease early in life. Like many who go on to do great works, rather than breaking her, the challenges she faced shaped her character. Her father died when she was 8 and her childhood was overshadowed by illness. She had an abnormality of the colon that was not fully corrected until she was 20 years old. Overlooked by the public health system in Puerto Rico and hospitalized every summer, she learned firsthand what it is like to be a helpless patient. Through these experiences came the desire to be a doctor. Not only did she become a physician, she specialized in health problems of children and adolescents and has dedicated her life to the service of public health.

Dr. Novello finished high school at age 15, entered medical school at age 20, and graduated in 1970. She began her career in medicine, excelling immediately. She was named "Intern of the Year" by the University of Michigan for her work in pediatric nephrology, the first woman to receive that honor. She did a fellowship in pediatrics at Georgetown University Hospital in Washington, DC, and then spent a few years in private practice.

In 1978, she began her career in public health. She joined the Commissioned Corps of the U.S. Public Health Service, headed by the U.S. Surgeon General. The Commissioned Corps works in poor areas, on Indian Reservations, or wherever there is a scarcity of medical personnel. In 1982 she received a master's degree in public health (MPH). She became deputy director of the National Institute of Child Health and Human Development, where she was an influential spokesperson for children with AIDS. She was a major contributor to the drafting of the Organ Transplant Procurement Act of 1984, and she was integral in lobbying for mandatory warning labels on cigarette packaging.

In 1989, when AIDS had become fully recognized as a national and worldwide health crisis, Dr. Novello was nominated as Surgeon General of the United States by the then president, George H. Bush. She served in that capacity from 1990 to 1993, having the special distinction of being the first woman and the first Hispanic to be the Surgeon General. As the country's lead physician she continued to work on issues surrounding children, women, and minorities. She brought attention to the problems of underage drinking and smoking; she worked to raise awareness about the AIDS virus, especially the plight of children with AIDS. She was the first Surgeon General to bring the issue of domestic violence as a public health concern into the national spotlight. Because of her efforts, the medical community is more aligned with legal and social support services in the effort to end abuse against women. She acknowledged violence among young people as a public health issue, recognizing that those at highest risk are largely the poor and minorities.

After her tenure as Surgeon General, Dr. Novello served as a Special Representative for Health and Nutrition for the United Nations International Children's Emergency Fund (UNICEF), and in 1996 was a visiting professor of Health Policy and Management at Johns Hopkins University. She has received numerous awards, including the U.S. Public Health Service Achievement Award and the Congressional Hispanic Caucus Medal. She has edited a book on Hispanic/Latino health and is the author of the foreword to

Nurse Practitioner

Salud!: A Latina's Guide to Total Health—Body, Mind, and Spirit. In 1999, she became the Health Commissioner of the State of New York, the first Hispanic to hold that position. There she continues to advocate for children, adolescents, and families. She has worked toward solutions for the medically uninsured, teen pregnancy, underage smoking, substance abuse, AIDS, and vaccination shortages. She continues to spend energy on reducing domestic violence, increasing organ donation, and pushing for clean air legislation.

In a commencement speech given by Dr. Novello in 1992 at Providence College, she encouraged graduates to set their goals high but to plan realistically and thoughtfully, and to remember that while "getting there" is important, how you get there is what matters most. She endorsed that failure can be a useful experience, because what is learned along the way is what will shape your life; that each person, in spite of the odds, has the most wonderful opportunity to make a difference. Dr. Novello has certainly made a difference with her life.

SEE ALSO: Acquired immunodeficiency syndrome, Adolescence, Domestic violence, Latinos

Suggested Resources

Academy of Achievement, The Hall of Public Service, Interview (June 18, 1994). *Antonia Novello, M.D. Former Surgeon General of the United States* (December 5, 1996). Retrieved March 10, 2003, from http://www.achievement.org

Anders, G. (2002). Dr. Antonia Novello: Crusading for health care. *Hispanic Magazine.* Retrieved March 10, 2003, from http://www.hispaniconline.com

Novello, A. (1992). *Gifts of speech. To the graduating class of Providence College* (May 17, 1992). http://www.gos.sbc.edu

JUDITH TRENTMAN

Nurse Practitioner In the year 2000, the U.S. Department of Health and Human Services reported that 2,694,540 of the workforce were licensed registered nurses, representing the largest segment of health care personnel. Of this number, 102,829 were nurse practitioners (NPs). The most recent Advanced Practice Nursing Survey indicates that women represent 81% of this population with approximately 80% being women over 40 years of age.

Broadly defined, an NP is an advanced practice registered nurse who has attained a formal NP education, primarily at the master's degree level. The NP's scope of practice is delineated by The Nurse Practice Act in each state, with specialization in one of seven patient populations, including acute care (ACNP), adult (ANP), family (FNP), gerontology, pediatrics, women's health care, and adult or family psychiatric and mental health. Other advanced practice nursing specialties that are not considered to be part of the NP discipline, include the nurse anesthetist (CRNA), clinical nurse specialist (CNS), and midwife. Formal educational programs for NPs and all advanced practice nurses must meet accreditation standards and graduates must pass a certification exam administered by one of five certifying bodies: The American Academy of Nurse Practitioners (AANP), American Nurses Credentialing Center (ANCC), the National Certification Board of Pediatric Nurse Practitioners (NCBPNP/N), the Council on Certification of Nurse Anesthetists, and The National Certification Corporation for the Gynecological/Obstetrics and Neonatal Nursing Specialties. Currently, a minimum of a master's level education is required by some of the organizations listed, but will be required by all by the year 2007.

The NP's scope of practice is continually evolving, but in general is characterized by education and health promotion, diagnosis, and the provision of services necessary for the treatment of acute and chronic illnesses. In all 50 states, NPs are granted at least some prescriptive privilege, with state formularies that include controlled substances, to states that require physician supervision and impose formulary limits.

Advanced practice in nursing dates back to 1877 when Sister Mary Bernard administered anesthesia at St. Vincent's Hospital in Erie, Pennsylvania. Schools for nurse anesthesia were established from 1909 to 1914. The American Association of Nurse Anesthetists was founded in 1931. Midwifery, the second oldest advanced nursing specialty, began when Clara D. Noyes proposed the training of nurses as midwives and Mary Breckinridge established the Frontier Nursing Service in eastern Kentucky. A long-established discipline in Europe, Mary Breckinridge traveled throughout England and France observing the nurse midwives' contributions to health care. In 1929, she brought British nurse midwives to the United States to join with public health nurses to serve in rural and remote areas. Neither anesthesia nor midwifery advance practice required an advanced education until the late 1950s and early

1960s. The first advanced practice program to require a master's degree was the Clinical Nurse Specialist track developed by Hildegard Peplau at Rutgers University in 1963.

Responding to a physician trend toward medical specialization and a subsequent shortage of primary care providers, the first NP program was established at the University of Colorado in 1965. Loretta Ford, collaborating with a physician, Henry Silver, developed a collaborative practice certificate program, with an emphasis on health and wellness. Diagnosing and treating health problems in children, particularly in rural areas, signaled a trend toward broadening the NP's responsibilities and increased autonomy. Federal funding increased to support the NP's professional development and set the stage for nurses to be designated as primary care providers. In 1971, additional support for NPs assuming primary care for patients came when the secretary of Health, Education, and Welfare issued the recommendation that NPs and physicians could share the responsibility of providing primary care for all populations. By the mid-1970s there were more than 500 NP certificate programs across the United States. The emphasis shifted to advanced education in nursing and by the beginning of the 1980s several master's programs were developed, outnumbering certificate programs. Currently, 70% of nurse-midwives graduate from Master's of Science in Nursing (MSN) programs accredited by the American College of Nurse Midwives. There are over 7,000 certified nurse-midwives in the United States and abroad in developing countries. In the year 1995 there were more than 200 university or college programs offering a master's level preparation. This rapid increase in advanced practice necessitated The American Nurses Association (ANA) to establish standard curriculum guidelines for the burgeoning number of preparatory programs and initiate credentialing requirements to ensure a level of competence.

Presently, the NP works in a number of settings, including the community or public agencies, private practice with their collaborating physician, or in the ambulatory, inpatient, or emergency and operating room settings of hospitals. Nurse-midwives attend approximately 300,000 deliveries per year. However, despite continued rural health care shortages, and the role these shortages played in the development of the NP role, less than 15% of all NPs practice in rural areas. Additionally, rural areas continue to lose primary care physicians as managed care recruits MDs out of these rural settings. Telemedicine may potentially present a solution by making it possible for NPs to communicate and collaborate with urban-based physicians, and thereby to work independently in remote areas.

Since the inception of the NP role, there have been several studies supporting the NP's effectiveness and safety in providing independent care comparable to that of a primary care physician. The most recent findings of a Columbia University study were published in the *Journal of the American Medical Association*, which concluded that in an ambulatory care site, with no disparity in assigned responsibilities, there were no significant differences between the primary care outcomes of a physician and those of an NP.

Traditional registered nurses, drawn to advanced practice role, with its greater professional autonomy and more flexible work scheduling, is likely a factor in today's nursing shortage. However, as the largest group of nonphysician, primary care providers, NPs occupy an important place among the health care workforce, and offer health care consumers an additional choice, while permanently altering health care delivery in this country.

SEE ALSO: Midwifery, Nursing, Physicians, Rural health

Suggested Reading

Brown, S. A., & Grimes, D. E. (1995). A meta-analysis of nurse practitioners and nurse midwives in primary care. *Nursing Research, 44,* 332–339.

Catalano, J. T. (1996). *Contemporary professional nursing* (pp. 1–18, 171–187). Philadelphia: F. A. Davis.

Mundinger, M. O., Kane, R. L., Lenz, E. R., Totten, A. M., Teal, W. Y., Cleary, P. D., et al. (2000). Primary care outcomes in patients treated by nurse practitioners or physicians: A randomized trial. *Journal of the American Medical Association, 283*(1), 59–68.

Sherwood, G. D., Brown, M., Fay, V., & Wardell, D. (1997). Defining nurse practitioner scope of practice: Expanding primary care services. *The Internet Journal of Advanced Nursing Practice, 1*(2).

Spratley, E., Johnson, A., Sochalski, J., & Spencer, W. (2000). The registered nurse population: Findings from the national sample survey of registered nurses. Washington: Health Resources and Services Administration, Bureau of Health Professions, Division of Nursing.

DOROTHY M. MEYER

Nursing Nursing is the profession of caring for the health of others; it is as much an art as it is a science. Nursing care was given by family members for many centuries and soldiers took care of wounded comrades in battles. However, nursing education did not begin until the 1800s when a hospital in Kaiserswerth, Germany, opened a training school for deaconesses in 1836. Doctors began educating women about childcare and nursing. Florence Nightingale, the forerunner of modern nursing, spent a short time there gaining a limited amount of formal training.

The modern-day profession of nursing is defined thanks to the contributions of Florence Nightingale, a British woman who led 38 women to care for the wounded and dying soldiers in 1854 in the Crimea. While dealing with the tragedies of war, Nightingale made sweeping social changes that have influenced how care is given for sick and wounded people today. After the war, Nightingale wrote extensively about nursing and developed London's first training school for nurses in 1860. She believed there was a need for education in both the classroom and the health care setting. Students worked in the hospitals and acquired skills and applied their knowledge while caring for their patients.

In the United States, within a few years, two female physicians began The New England Hospital for Women and Children and started the first general training school for nurses. Linda Richards completed the training in 1867 and is noted as America's first "trained" nurse. Training schools soon opened in New York (Bellevue Hospital), New Haven, and Boston. The educational programs proliferated across the country and by the 1920s many hospitals were staffing their units with inexpensive student labor. The older design of the large wards for patients evolved due to the need for one supervisor to oversee a larger number of students.

Education for nurses has changed dramatically since then. Today there are different programs for the entry-level education offered at colleges and universities, while some hospital-based diploma programs still survive. Diploma programs, an outgrowth of the original hospital-based training education, take about 3 years to complete. Due to declining hospital funding, rising education costs, and the increasing need for degreed professionals, only a small number of programs still exist. Associate degrees in nursing (ADN) are offered at community and junior colleges and take 2–3 years to complete. In 2000, approximately 40% of registered nurses (RNs) received their basic education in associate degree programs while only 6% of RNs graduated with a "Diploma in Nursing."

The Bachelor of Science in Nursing (BSN) degree programs are offered by colleges and universities and take 4 or 5 years to complete. The American Nurses Association (ANA), the national professional organization for nurses, has designated the BSN as the entry level for professional nursing. This preparation allows for greater advancement and opportunity and is often required for administrative positions. By 2000 about 38% of RNs had graduated from baccalaureate programs with another 16% (ADN and Diploma RNs) returning to school to advance their education to a bachelor's degree. All three levels of education permit the nurse to be a candidate for the licensing exam, which, when successfully passed, results in licensure as an RN in the state the exam was taken. State laws provide for the election or appointment of members who form a Board of Nursing. The Board of Nursing for each state regulates the practice and standards of nursing in that state.

Advanced degrees in nursing have also developed, and as of 2000, more than 196,279 RNs have the education to work as advanced practice nurses (APNs). Advanced practice nurses complete a BSN, and most pursue a graduate program in nursing (MSN) and take a nationally recognized certifying exam. The four categories of advanced practice are nurse anesthetists, nurse-midwives, nurse practitioners, and clinical nurse specialists. Advanced practice nurses receive advanced education and specialization, which prepares them for more complex tasks in their chosen clinical area. Advanced practice nurses may specialize in the primary care of children, adults, or geriatrics, or focus on anesthesia, cardiac care, mental health, community health, or obstetrics. Depending on state laws they may perform history and physicals, prescribe medications or treatments, offer education and consultation, and even attend or assist in childbirth.

Registered nurses today are offered a variety of fields and settings in which to work. Nurses work to promote health and prevent disease as well as educate and advocate for vulnerable populations. They work in collaboration with physicians to perform complex procedures and staff various inpatient and outpatient areas that provide comprehensive care to a wide variety of patients. They also supervise licensed practical nurses and other unlicensed personnel in administering direct care to patients. Usually, nurses choose a specialty area and become experts in providing care in a particular setting and/or for a specific subgroup of patients, such as geriatrics, orthopedics, school nursing, occupational or forensics, psychiatry, medicine, surgery, oncology, maternity, pediatrics, or one of the acute or critical care areas, like emergency rooms or cardiac care. Some nurses become managers within the hospital and direct nursing activities and are administratively responsible for a specific section of the hospital or at higher levels often designated as a vice president of patient care.

Apart from hospital settings, nurses work in nursing homes, within the military, in doctors' offices, home health care, and rehabilitation; occupational nurses work in manufacturing plants and industry providing both emergency care and preventive wellness and while maintaining safety, nurses are recruited today to work for health maintenance organizations and insurers as case managers.

DEMOGRAPHICS OF NURSES

Generally, women predominate in the nursing profession. Gradual changes have helped the number of men in nursing increase. The military excluded men from serving as nurses from 1901 until after the Korean War and the ANA did not permit males to join the organization until 1930. The proportion of men in the profession of nursing increased from 1% in 1966 to 6% in contemporary times. This increase may have resulted from greater employment opportunities in nursing, the growing acceptance of men in the profession, as well as the improved gender balance elsewhere—in areas that were dominated by one gender versus another.

In 2000, 59% of employed nurses were working in hospitals; 71.5% were married and 17.9% were widowed, divorced, or separated. People of Caucasian origin represent 88% of the RN population, while roughly 12% of the employed nurses come from non-Caucasian backgrounds. In 2000 only 9.1% of RNs were under the age of 30.

The "typical" RN is now a 46-year-old married woman from the baby boom generation. Since population growth has declined, the number of people entering the workforce will be less and a decreasing number of nurses will be available to take care of a growing number of aging Americans. Currently, nurses have reported working longer hours in highly stressful environments and a significant proportion of nurses are leaving the profession in search of working opportunities that are more flexible and less stressful. A long-term shortage of nursing is projected due to the increasing demand for nurses, the aging of the current workforce, and the decline in the number of people seeking to enter the profession. The shortage of nursing as well as the heightened level of stress and job dissatisfaction have raised important concerns over quality of care. California is the first state to attempt to regulate the nurse–patient ratios, by limiting the number of patients per RN. The outcome of this regulation remains to be seen.

Research has shown that women who graduated from high school in the 1990s were 30–40% less likely to enter nursing than those who graduated in the 1970s. Changing the image of the profession may improve recruitment, but there is a need to raise relative wages, improve working conditions and other benefits, and lower education costs, so nursing can retain its workforce rather than lose people to other occupations that may offer greater opportunity or prestige. Despite the stress and demands of health care, nurses continue to find great personal rewards when able to practice the art and science of the profession.

SEE ALSO: Women in the Health Professions (pp. 20–32), Women in the Workforce (pp. 32–40), Midwifery, Nurse practitioner

Suggested Reading

Baer, E., D'Antonio, P., Rinker, S., & Lynaugh, J. (Eds.). (2000). *Enduring issues in American nursing.* New York: Springer.

Buerhaus, P. I., Staiger, D. O., & Auerbach, D. I. (2000). Implications of an aging registered nurse workforce. *Journal of the American Medical Association, 283*(22), 2948–2954.

Griffin, G. J., & Griffin, J. K. (1973). *History and trends of professional nursing* (7th ed.). St. Louis, MO: C.V. Mosby.

Group, T. M., & Roberts, J. I. (2001). *Nursing, physician control and the medical monopoly: Historical perspectives on gender inequality in roles, rights, and range of practice.* Bloomington: Indiana University Press.

Schrefer, S. (Ed.). (2000). *Nursing reflections: A century of caring.* St. Louis, MO: C.V. Mosby.

United States Department of Labor Bureau of Labor Statistics (n.d.). *Registered nurse.* Retrieved February 13, 2003, from http://www.bls.gov/oco/ocos083.htm

MELISSA ZUPANCIC

Nursing Home Nursing homes serve as residence for individuals who are too frail, too sick, or too disabled to live in their homes. It is estimated that nearly 12 million individuals are disabled enough to require long-term care. As of 1999, 1.5 million resided in nursing homes and over one third of nursing home residents were 85 years of age or older. Residence in a nursing home can be temporary, during a recovery period in which the patient requires skilled nursing care, or permanent, in the presence of severe and irreversible decline of functional and cognitive abilities. Most individuals prefer to reside in their homes, especially when a network of friends, family members, and professional individuals is available to provide help. The decision to reside in a nursing home is postponed both for financial and psychological reasons. Psychologically, the impact of placement in a nursing home suggests this is the final move and represents a loss of function and familiarity. Placement is postponed while the caregiver tries to provide as much care as possible for as long as possible; it is materialized when the caregiver is physically and psychologically exhausted because care for physical and/or behavioral problems is required 24 hours a day. Also, when resources in the community are not predictably and promptly accessible, the individual may be no longer safe in the community and a move to a nursing home becomes warranted. Despite the number of services available to support long-term care to community-dwelling residents, long-term care has remained fragmented and care management or care coordination among various agencies to promote individual choice and control has been less than optimal.

Nursing home care is very costly, amounting to $90 billion in 1998. Out-of-pocket expenditures by consumers have accounted for nearly one third of the total costs. Nearly 50% of all nursing home residents pay for their care out of their own savings. Medicare provides coverage for such services only on a temporary basis. Individuals with low incomes/resources can qualify for Medicaid to obtain coverage for care in nursing homes. Most individuals "spend down" to levels of income/resource that are low enough to qualify for Medicaid, a mechanism that often leads to spousal impoverishment. It is important to note that Medicare and Medicaid programs will reimburse only to nursing homes that are certified by the government to provide service to Medicare and Medicaid beneficiaries.

Nursing home residents have certain protections under the law, and, similar to all patients, they have the right to be treated with respect and dignity; to be informed about their medical condition and medications, to see their own doctor; to be informed in writing about the services and associated fees before being admitted to the nursing home; and to manage their own resources or choose an individual whom they trust to do so. On the other hand, nursing homes are not required to admit a patient if he or she cannot show how they will pay for services and may legally discharge a resident for nonpayment. Although a patient's family is not liable to reimburse for services received in a nursing home, the patient's estate is. Families get pursued by nursing homes for debt collection after the patient's death. Some are able to pay, and others not, especially in the event that they are financially devastated by the lengthy episode of illness. Families can seek financial advice through the legal services of the Area Agency on Aging.

There have been concerns about the quality of care rendered in nursing homes, following a report by the United States General Accounting Office in 1997 noting the presence of "serious or potentially life-threatening problems associated with nursing home care." Issues such as the qualification and level of staffing have been central to such concerns. Several indicators of quality of care have improved over time, including the lower use of antipsychotic drugs and a decrease in the inappropriate use of each of physical restraint, indwelling urinary catheters, and the increase in the number of nursing home residents receiving hearing aids. Many areas still need improvement, however. For example, a number of patients continue to suffer unnecessarily from pressure ulcer, malnutrition, and dehydration. Furthermore, many elderly continue to experience verbal abuse and neglect.

The Center for Medicare and Medicaid Services proposes a checklist of items to inquire about when selecting a nursing home. This checklist is available through their website, cited below. Briefly, the person inquiring about a nursing home must check that the institution is Medicare and Medicaid certified; can provide the level of care and special services needed for the patient, if the patient has dementia, is on a ventilator, or needs rehabilitative services; the residents are dressed appropriately for the season of the year and time of the day; the facilities are clean and odor-free; the temperature and the lighting are adequate; the noise level is comfortable; the furnishings are sturdy; and the facility is located at a reasonable distance from family and friends. With respect to the staff, the person inquiring about the nursing home must ensure that staff members are warm, polite, and respectful to patients; there is a full-time RN in the nursing home at all times, in addition to the Director of Nursing; the same team of nurses and Certified Nursing Assistants (CNAs) work with the same resident 4–5 days a week; that the ratio of CNAs to residents is reasonable; that there is a full-time social worker; and that a licensed physician affiliated with the facility can be easily accessible. Serious quality problems can be reported to the Ombudsman of the Area Agency of Aging if matters are not resolved through discussions with the nursing home staff.

Parallel to the increase in life expectancy, the size of the elderly population is projected to grow substantially in the next decades. For example, the population 85 years of age or older, the frailest group of the elderly, and comprised of 4.2 million individuals in 1999, is expected to double in 2030, and more than quadruple by 2050. Such changes in population demographics are bound to strain the existing system for providing long-term care to elderly Americans. Given the disproportionate representation of women among nursing home residents, women are encouraged to be active participants in debates shaping relevant public policies.

SEE ALSO: Activities of daily living, Long-term care, Medicaid, Medicare, Patients' rights

Suggested Resources

American Association of Retired People: www.aarp.org
Center for Medicare and Medicaid Services: www.cms.gov
Legal Counsel for the Elderly: www.uaelderlaw.org

SIRAN M. KOROUKIAN
EVANNE JURATOVAC

Nutrition Nutrition is the sum of the processes involved in consuming food and assimilating and utilizing it. Nutrition is concerned with all the nutrients that are needed to build sound bodies and promote health such as proteins, fats, carbohydrates, vitamins, minerals, water, and fiber. Good nutrition provides the essential nutrients that the body needs to function normally and to have an optimum nutritional status.

Malnutrition is poor nutritional status resulting from dietary intakes either above or below the required range. Thus a person may be obese, but still be malnourished if he or she has poor stores of protein, iron, or vitamins. Malnutrition can result from poor food choices, fasting, starvation, poor absorption from the

gastrointestinal tract, or interference with nutrient utilization by drugs, alcohol, or metabolic diseases.

Protein–energy malnutrition is the result of deficiencies of protein and energy. Fasting and starvation can lead to severe protein–energy malnutrition. This kind of malnutrition causes rapid weight loss and decreased resistance to infection. Anorexia nervosa, a self-induced aversion to food, is a unique type of malnutrition. People with anorexia nervosa take extreme measures to maintain a low body weight, including constant exercise. This disease can be fatal if not treated early.

Marasmus and kwashiorkor are diseases due to protein–energy malnutrition among children. These are widespread nutritional disorders in developing countries especially in children under 5. Marasmus is derived from the Greek word *marasmós*, meaning wasting or withering. Marasmus is due to the deficiency of protein and calories, while kwashiorkor is due to a deficiency of protein only. When children are weaned from mother's milk and fed on a starchy low-protein diet, they develop kwashiorkor.

NUTRITIONAL NEEDS THROUGH THE LIFE CYCLE

Nutritional needs vary, depending on the body's requirements at different stages of life. Growth is most rapid before birth, and therefore maternal nutrition is extremely important. Each stage of life has its own special requirements and meeting these needs is vital for a healthy life.

Nutrition in Infancy

Nutrition during the first year of life lays the foundation for future health, growth, and development. Growth during the first year of life is more rapid than at any other period of life beyond intrauterine life. Without adequate nutrients, signs of nutritional deficiency appear in infants much sooner than in any other age group. The consequences of malnutrition in infancy are more severe, delaying physical and mental development and resulting in learning disabilities.

During infancy, caloric needs per unit body weight exceed those of all other age groups. Infants require more calories because they are very active and have a greater surface area in proportion to their

Nutrition

weight, resulting in greater heat loss. By the end of first year of age the birthweight has usually tripled. An intake of about 100 cal/kg is optimal. Intake of less than 80 cal/kg is usually inadequate and intake of more than 120 cal/kg leads to obesity.

Breast-feeding is the optimal way of providing food for infants. Human milk provides important immunologic protection. Breast-fed infants have a slower rate of weight gain than formula-fed infants and lower rates of obesity. Breast-fed infants do not require solid foods during the first 6 months of life. Cow's milk should not be given until after the first birthday because it can cause intestinal bleeding. For optimal brain development, only whole milk should be used between the ages of 1 and 2.

Nutrition in Childhood and Adolescence

After the first year, the rate of growth slows and changes in body structure begin to occur. Much of the fat present during infancy is lost. Muscles become stronger and bones lengthen and increase in density. Children should participate in vigorous physical activity and establish healthy nutritional habits that will last into adulthood. Children should eat a variety of foods in three meals each day with healthy snacks between meals. Serving milk with all meals increases the protein intake. The nutrients most commonly deficient in childhood are calcium, vitamin C, thiamine, and riboflavin. Instead of soft drinks, candy, and other less nutritional snacks, offer cheese, yogurt, fruits, and raisins, which will supply these essential nutrients.

During adolescence, growth occurs in spurts. Calcium is very important because bone density increases. Adolescents require adequate calories to support their activity level and growth needs. A nutritious breakfast improves mental alertness and provides energy for physical activity until lunchtime.

Nutrition in Pregnancy and Breast-Feeding

A woman's nutritional status prior to her pregnancy and during pregnancy influences the pregnancy outcome. Adequate weight gain is an important factor in ensuring a healthy pregnancy. Mothers with a weight gain of less than 15 lb are at a greater risk for delivering low-birthweight babies. Babies who weigh less than 5.5 lb have a higher rate of infant mortality and decreased resistance to infection. A normal weight gain for most women is 25–30 lb. Generally a woman should gain 2–4 lb during the first trimester and about 1 lb per week during the second and third trimesters.

The nutritional needs of pregnant women and nursing mothers are greater than in nonpregnant women. During the second and third trimesters, an extra 300 cal/day is required. Women use up an extra 500 cal/day during lactation, which can help breast-feeding mothers return to their prepregnancy weight. The growing baby needs a considerable amount of calcium to develop. If the mother does not take in enough calcium-rich foods, calcium from her bones is used instead. However, the mother's bones are replenished after breast-feeding stops, and breast-feeding does not seem to increase the risk of osteoporosis. The need for folic acid doubles during pregnancy. Eating adequate amount of folic acid-rich foods during pregnancy and throughout the childbearing years reduces the chance of having a baby with birth defects of the brain and spinal cord known as neural tube defects (anencephaly and spina bifida). Excess vitamin or mineral intake during pregnancy can harm the fetus. Consult a physician before taking any supplements. Alcohol and cigarette smoking are known to cause low birthweight. Excessive caffeine may also impair the growth of the fetus. To maintain fluid balance and increase blood volume, salt intake should not be restricted during pregnancy unless there is a medical reason. Drugs taken by the nursing mother appear in the breast milk. Nursing mothers should exercise caution while nursing and consult with the physician before taking any medication.

Geriatric Nutrition

Physical, mental, and social factors affect the food habits of the elderly. Aging is characterized by a decline in the basal metabolic rate, which decreases by 2% per decade. The elderly are often less active, and as a result have reduced caloric requirements. Older people also need more calcium to prevent bone loss. When planning meals to meet the nutritional needs of elderly people, special attention should be paid to factors that affect their food intake. Since the sense of taste declines with age, plan for colorful and nutritionally dense foods.

See Also: Diet, Vitamins

Suggested Reading

American Council on Science and Health. (1982). Alcohol use during pregnancy: A report. *Nutrition Today, 17,* 29.

Bendich, A., & Deckelbaum, R. J. (Eds.). (2001). *Preventive nutrition: The comprehensive guide for health professionals* (2nd ed.). Totowa, NJ: Humana Press.

Elwood, T. W. (1975). Nutritional concerns of the elderly. *Journal of Nutrition Education, 7,* 50.

McWilliams, M. (1980). *Nutrition for the growing years* (3rd ed.). New York: Wiley.

Mitchell, M. K. (2003). *Nutrition across the life span* (2nd ed.). Philadelphia: W. B. Saunders.

Westcott, P. (2000). *Diet and nutrition.* Austin, TX: Raintree Steck-Vaughn.

RAJKUMARI RICHMONDS

O

Obesity

Obesity is a rapidly growing problem in the United States today, reaching epidemic proportions. According to the Centers for Disease Control and Prevention, during 1999–2000, 64% of Americans were overweight or obese, with 23% actually defined as being obese (see definitions below). Thirty percent of children and adolescents during the same time period were found to be overweight. The prevalence of obesity has escalated over the years: between 1971 and 1974, only 24.7% of the adult population was affected. Obesity is more common in women, affecting 34.8 million women compared with 26.4 million men. Obesity affects all socioeconomic and ethnic groups, particularly the less privileged and minorities. Nationally, this problem needs to be addressed promptly because obesity leads to multiple medical problems that substantially affect the quality of life, longevity, and health care costs.

Table 1. Classification of overweight and obesity

	Body mass index (kg/m^2)
Underweight	< 18.5
Normal	18.5–24.9
Overweight	25.0–29.9
Obese	
Class I	30–34.9
Class II	35.0–39.9
Class III	≥ 40 (extreme obesity)

is associated with insulin resistance, high cholesterol, and coronary artery disease. Obesity can be described as android (abdominal fat accumulation, or "apple-shaped") or gynecoid (mostly peripheral fat distribution, favoring the hips and lower extremities, or "pear-shaped").

DEFINITION

Overweight refers to increased weight for given height. Obesity refers to excessive amounts of body fat relative to lean body mass. Weight is proportionate to height and is adjusted using the body mass index (BMI). BMI is calculated as a ratio of an individual's weight in kilograms, divided by the square of height measured in meters. A BMI greater than 30 defines obesity (Table 1).

Other measures of obesity include measurement of the waist circumference. Waist circumference greater than 88 cm (35 in.) in women or greater than 102 cm (40 in.) in men indicates increased abdominal fat, which

CAUSES OF OBESITY

Why is obesity such a growing problem? Nationally, the main problem appears to be that calorie-dense foods are easily available, which increases caloric intake, along with *lifestyle changes,* including reduced physical activity. There are complex interactions between hormones that control feeding, fat breakdown, and fat storage. These include insulin, leptin, neuropeptide Y, and others. There are also rare genetic syndromes that affect a small minority of people. The number of overweight and obese children has been rising, which contributes to the growing pool of obese adults.

COMPLICATIONS OF OBESITY

Obesity leads to complications that involve many organ systems (Table 2). Obesity is a leading cause of type 2 diabetes. In android (apple-shaped) obesity, fat is deposited in the abdomen in the form of triglycerides, or storage fat. Triglycerides in the abdomen are broken down into free fatty acids, which oppose the action of insulin and prevent tissues and organs from using glucose in the blood. High blood sugars result, and this eventually progresses to diabetes. Problems with insulin secretion may also occur as a result of this process. Triglyceride deposits also provide a source of fatty acids for lipid and cholesterol production, leading to clogged arteries. Blocked arteries can lead to heart attacks, strokes, kidney failure, impotence, abdominal pain, leg pain, and even gangrene.

Restrictive lung disease can result if obesity interferes with the ability to deeply inhale and adequately

Table 2. Complications of obesity

Cardiovascular
  High blood pressure
  Heart failure
  Angina, heart attack
  Stroke
  Blood clots in leg veins and lungs
  Lower leg swelling
Respiratory
  Sleep apnea
  Restrictive lung disease
Female reproductive and urinary problems
  Irregular menstrual cycles
  Infertility
  Increased risk of cancer of the breast, uterus, colon
  Urinary incontinence
Infectious
  Superficial fungal skin-fold infections
  Leg ulcers
Gastrointestinal
  Gallstones, inflamed gallbladder
Metabolic
  High cholesterol, high triglycerides
  Diabetes
  High uric acid, causing gout and kidney stones
Musculoskeletal
  Low back pain
  Degenerative arthritis, particularly knees and spine
Psychological/social
  Depression
  Social isolation
  Impaired activities of daily living
  Limited physical activity choices

exhale, resulting in low blood oxygen levels and occasionally high carbon dioxide levels. Such patients may require long-term, low-dose oxygen therapy. Sleep apnea due to excess amounts of tissue in the neck can lead to loud snoring and blockage of airway at the level of the pharynx. This leads to a drop in oxygen levels, which produces strain on the right side of the heart, resulting in heart failure and widespread swelling (edema). Sleep apnea with loud snoring has been known to result in marital discord as well. Finally, sleep apnea is associated with abnormal heart rhythms and high blood pressure.

Obese persons who are sedentary are at risk of forming clots in the deep veins of their legs. Clots in the veins can occasionally fragment and travel upward to the heart and lungs, which can be fatal.

Women with obesity are prone to developing menstrual irregularities. Abdominal fat deposition leads to insulin resistance, which can lead to hormonal imbalances in the ovary, which prevent ovulation. Infertility may result and some women may need assistance with ovulation and expert fertility evaluation. Also, higher levels of testosterone and other ovarian hormones can lead to acne and excess facial, abdominal, and chest hair. This is a difficult cosmetic problem and is a source of low self-esteem. Missed menstrual cycles can lead to an abnormal buildup of the inner lining of the uterus (endometrium), which can lead to uterine cancer. Finally, obesity is associated with an increased risk of breast cancer.

Low back and knee pain are frequent consequences of excess weight. Joint degeneration occurs faster in obese individuals. Joint replacement surgery is often difficult in these patients. Chronic pain often occurs even in spite of surgery. Many individuals require canes, walkers, wheelchairs, or motorized vehicles to assist with mobility for activities of daily living.

Superficial skin fungus infections may occur beneath the breasts, in the neck folds, armpits, and groin as a result of moisture from sweating between adjacent folds of skin. These can be a chronic problem and may predispose to bacterial infection, as well as causing social embarrassment.

Many obese patients are depressed. It can be difficult to tell whether depression causes altered feeding behavior leading to obesity, or whether obesity leads to depression. In some patients, a vicious cycle of obesity and depression may occur. Body-image consciousness in society leads to great difficulties for obese persons, who are often viewed in a negative light by their nonobese peers. This may lead to social isolation, difficulties obtaining employment, and in forming meaningful relationships.

TREATMENT

Obesity is typically a chronic disease that is difficult to treat and requires ongoing management. Many patients will require lifelong attention to control weight with diet and regular exercise. Patients need to be informed that obesity-related illness and death can be significantly reduced with a weight loss of only 5–10% of their body weight. The physician and patient need to openly discuss realistic weight loss goals and assess the patient's readiness to participate in a weight loss program. Gradual changes should be encouraged, potential adverse outcomes discussed, and ongoing positive reinforcement provided.

DIET

There are a variety of recommended diets to promote weight loss. Regardless of the type of diet, a net reduction in caloric intake is required to lose weight. Popular low-carbohydrate diets go *against this rule (not really as even they produce a net caloric deficit, but with a skewed nutrient intake)* but need further study to see if they are safe and effective in the long term. Obese patients on low-calorie diets (LCD) of 1,000–1,500 kCal per day can lose about 8% of their weight. Very low-calorie diets (VLCD) of 400–800 kCal per day understandably lead to greater weight loss, up to 13–23 kg. However, this weight loss is hard to maintain. Evidence shows that at the end of 1 year, those who followed either a VLCD or a LCD approached similar weights. VLCD should therefore be recommended only if immediate weight loss is required for health reasons or surgery. Patients should be encouraged to eat a variety of nutrient-rich foods incorporating fruits, vegetables, fiber, and vitamins. Carbohydrates should be derived from whole foods; processed foods should be avoided. Low-fat diets can be effective in cutting back calories.

The primary care provider should evaluate the obese patient for obesity-related diseases. Consultation with a nutritionist is essential to calculate caloric needs according to the estimated ideal body weight and level of physical activity. Special diets may be needed for the patient with diabetes, high blood pressure, cholesterol or triglyceride disorders, kidney stones, and heart failure.

EXERCISE

Thirty-eight percent of adult Americans reported no leisure-time physical activity in 1997–1998. Physical inactivity increases the risk for heart disease and for high blood pressure. Women were found to be less physically active than men. More African Americans and Hispanics than whites were found to be sedentary, as were the elderly and the less affluent. Girls with a higher BMI exercised even less. Introducing physical activity in an obese patient should be a gradual process and slowly increased as tolerated. Regular aerobic exercise (brisk walking, aerobic dancing, jogging/running, swimming, exercise bike) will produce modest weight loss in overweight and obese adults, even without dietary calorie reduction. Finally, a combination of LCD and exercise produces more weight reduction than either one alone.

BEHAVIOR THERAPY

Behavior modification is important in achieving successful weight loss. This can be done either with a therapist (individually or in a group) or with a physician. Weight loss of about 10% of body weight can be expected with behavior modification alone. Attention to self-monitoring of eating behavior is important, by keeping a food diary of calories, portion sizes, emotions leading to eating, and location of eating. A similar exercise log is also useful. Patients need to work on controlling their impulses when shopping for food or making menu selections. Positive changes lead to reinforcement, such as monitoring weight loss. Involvement in a support group *may* avoid relapses.

MEDICATION

Medications are not routinely recommended because of side effects, limited effectiveness, and the need for more healthful interventions in the form of diet and exercise. Medications are recommended only in patients with a BMI > 30 who do not have obesity-associated risk factors or diseases, or in those with a BMI > 27 who do have obesity-related risk factors or diseases. Medication should be used along with, rather than as a substitute for, diet and exercise. The two medications that are currently approved for long-term treatment of obesity are orlistat and sibutramine. Orlistat inhibits 30% of fat absorption from the intestines and can also lower cholesterol somewhat. In studies, orlistat produces a 5–10% reduction in body fat. Side effects are excess gas, abdominal pain, oily rectal spotting, and incontinence of stool. The symptoms improve with time and fiber may help. Fat-soluble vitamins can be lost in the stool and supplements are recommended.

Sibutramine acts in the brain by suppressing reuptake of the transmitters norepinephrine and serotonin. This reduces appetite and therefore caloric intake. Patients may lose 5% or more of their body weight with this medication. Blood pressure elevation can occur and needs to be monitored closely. Other side effects, including dry mouth, insomnia, headache, and constipation, are mild and diminish with time.

SURGERY

Bariatric surgery is the most effective treatment for severe obesity. Bariatric surgery can be considered in patients who are 18 years or older with BMI $\geq$ 40, or BMI between 35 and 40 if there are major weight-related complications. Patients must have failed nonsurgical methods of weight loss and/or failed treatment in obesity clinics and must be committed to long-term follow-up. They must not have medical or psychological conditions that prevent the use of anesthesia or surgery. The goal of bariatric surgery is to reduce the size of the stomach (as in vertical banded gastroplasty) or to create malabsorption of nutrients (as with the Roux-en-Y gastric bypass).

Vertical banded gastroplasty ("stomach stapling") allows for weight loss of 20% of body weight during up to 5 years of follow-up. However, weight gain can occur in patients who consume high-calorie foods in the form of soft foods or liquids (ice cream or sugary drinks). Gastric bypass is the most effective surgery for extreme obesity, but leads to diversion of the stomach into the small intestine, and results in malabsorption of nutrients. Weight loss after gastric bypass ranges from 50 kg to as much as 100 kg, but this procedure carries a higher risk of complications and patients need to be followed closely for nutrient supplementation.

SEE ALSO: Body mass index, Diabetes, Nutrition, Weight control

Suggested Reading

Centers for Disease Control and Prevention, National Center for Chronic Disease Prevention and Health Promotion. *Overweight and obesity.* www.cdc.gov/nccdphp/dnpa/obesity/index.htm

Nambi, V., Hoogwerf, R., & Sprecher, D. (2002). A truly deadly quartet: Obesity, hypertension, hypertriglyceridemia, and hyperinsulinemia. *Cleveland Clinic Journal of Medicine, 69,* 985–989.

NHLBI Obesity Education Initiative Expert Panel on the Identification, Evaluation, and Treatment of Overweight and Obesity in Adults. (1998).

Prystowsky, J. (2002). Surgical management of obesity. *Seminars in Gastrointestinal Disease, 13,* 133–142.

Yanovski S. Z., & Yanovski J. A. (2002). Drug therapy: Obesity. *New England Journal of Medicine, 346,* 591–602.

ASRA KERMANI

Obsessive–Compulsive Disorder Obsessions and compulsions are fairly common mental phenomena that most people have experienced, but they can become severe enough to interfere with one's functioning. At this point they are known as a disorder. Obsessions are repeated intrusive thoughts, usually unwelcome to the thinker, and may include ideas of a harmful, violent, sexual, or religious nature. Frequently the ideas are not those the individual can accept and they cause anxiety or tension. They may relate to contamination or the fear that something terrible will happen if the person does not perform perfectly some act that will take away the idea. These acts are called rituals. Compulsions are behaviors or thoughts that must be done in order to undo the terrible ideas. They may include frequent hand washing, saying certain numbers, checking the stove or windows and doors, arranging furniture or objects in a certain way, cleaning, hoarding, or other acts. Individuals who suffer from these conditions know that the obsessions and compulsions are not real, but they cannot refrain from experiencing them and they can consume a considerable amount of time taken from ordinary life.

Obsessions and compulsions must be distinguished from excessive worrying about real-life events and often there is a fine line between them. Adults usually have some insight into the realization that the ideas and behaviors are excessive, while children may not. Often these disorders occur along with other psychiatric problems such as major depressive illnesses, anxiety disorders such as phobias or posttraumatic stress disorders, and drug and alcohol abuse. Often people experiencing these disorders have obsessive–compulsive personalities

Obsessive–Compulsive Disorder

that have been very helpful in organizing their lives and have contributed to their successful management of difficult situations, but the disorder becomes sufficient to meet the criteria outlined in the *Diagnostic and Statistical Manual of Mental Disorders*, fourth edition of the American Psychiatric Association. The definition in this book requires that for the diagnosis, the person must experience the obsessions and compulsions for at least over 1 hour a day and that they interfere with functioning such as work, school, social relationships, and self-care. It is important to find out that they are not due to the use of drugs or alcohol, or due to another medical condition. It is also important to distinguish them from the delusions of a psychotic condition such as is noted in schizophrenia, the manic thoughts in bipolar disease, or the excessive preoccupation with food and body image in eating disorders. Certain other preoccupations with body image are also distinguished from this. Sometimes it is hard to tell the difference between delusions and obsessions and compulsions or specific phobias, but careful discussion with a trained mental health professional can clarify this, which is important because of treatment considerations.

CAUSES

The exact causes of obsessive–compulsive disorders (OCDs) are not known at this time, although extensive research is being done. Special interest has been in the genetics of the disease. In some cases a family history can be found and studies show an autosomal dominant mode of inheritance with incomplete penetrance. In some cases there is an association with Tourette's syndrome (a disorder in which individuals experience involuntary tics among other symptoms). Certain brain pathways and structures are affected including the orbitofrontal cortex, the caudate nucleus, and the cingulate cortex. There is a disturbance in the function of serotonin transmission in the orbital cortex and caudate nucleus. Recent research has suggested some cases may be due to autoimmune problems such as infection with betahemolytic streptococcal infection in children. Brain imaging techniques have helped greatly in clarifying more of these causes.

COURSE

While the mean onset of this disorder is usually between ages 20 and 24, many cases occur in childhood or adolescence and some later in life, though usually before age 35. Men and women have similar prevalence rates of OCD, although men seem to have an earlier age of onset. The disorder starts often after a very stressful life event, but for women it may very well begin or be exacerbated during or after a pregnancy. Women are often very loathe to tell their doctors or midwives about their condition because it may include ideas about harming their babies. They know that they would not hurt them but their fears are major. They are usually relieved when a knowledgeable trained person can help. They are to be distinguished from women who are psychotic with delusional ideas about harming themselves or their fetuses and babies. Women tend to have depression associated with OCD more than men and the depression may resolve while the OCD persists. Gender differences in the expression of the disorder include the finding that women tend to have more hand washing rituals while men tend to have more checking rituals. Men seem to be more treatment resistant. Many individuals may keep their symptoms secret so there is often a long lag between onset and presentation of the troublesome symptoms to the attention of any professional person. Onset often happens after a very stressful life event or frequently during or after a pregnancy in women.

Treatment usually requires the integration of a few different types of therapies. These include behavioral therapy, use of serotonin reuptake inhibitor drugs such as fluoxetine (Prozac) or sertraline (Zoloft), other antidepressant or antianxiety medications, and making sure that all helpful approaches are used. Behavioral therapies include exposing the person to the feared objects or situation and trying to help the person resist the ritual. This is often called exposure therapy. In the most difficult cases neurosurgery has occasionally been used. There have been tremendous advances in this area in the past 30 years. Treatment has improved, as we understand more of the underlying neurobiological and psychosocial causes.

SEE ALSO: Anxiety disorders, Depression

Suggested Reading

Sadock, J. B., & Sadock, V. S. (2000). *Comprehensive textbook of psychiatry* (7th ed.). Philadelphia: Lippincott, Williams & Wilkins.

MIRIAM B. ROSENTHAL

Occupational Therapist

Occupational therapy is the holistic health profession that works with individuals to attain, restore, and maintain function in daily life activities and meaningful life roles such as student, homemaker, hobbyist, and worker. The word "occupation" in the context of occupational therapy refers to activities that are valued by that individual in his or her culture. Areas of occupation include activities of daily living (grooming, dressing, eating); instrumental activities of daily living (financial, household, and health management); work (job performance, volunteering); social participation (family, friends, community); education; play; and leisure.

As a profession established in 1915, the first occupational therapists were women, a trend that continues today with 90% of women in the workforce. As of December 31, 2002, there were 104,741 registered occupational therapists (OTRs) and 43,019 certified occupational therapy assistants (COTAs). Ninety percent of OTRs and 89% of COTAs are women. Occupational therapists treat a variety of human conditions and are found in diverse practice areas such as mental health, rehabilitation, schools, home health care, nursing homes, pediatrics, outpatient, community/day treatment, hospice, teaching, management, and research. Therapists can be self-employed contracting their services and/or providing staff to facilities needing occupational therapy. Those with entrepreneurial aspirations can find new niches for occupational therapy to benefit populations either underserved or not yet identified. Work in these settings can provide flexibility in work hours beneficial to women with other responsibilities and roles.

The profession of occupational therapy has two classifications of therapists: OTRs and COTAs. OTRs must graduate from an accredited master's or doctoral program in occupational therapy, successfully complete a minimum of 24 weeks of supervised fieldwork experience, and pass the national certification exam. COTAs work under the supervision of the occupational therapist, must graduate from an accredited associate's degree or certificate program in occupational therapy, successfully complete 16 weeks of supervised fieldwork experience, and pass the national certification exam.

Educational programs for both the occupational therapist and occupational therapist assistant include the following: biological, behavioral, and health sciences, human development, anatomy, pathology, activity analysis, health policy, reimbursement, and ethics. Occupational therapist programs emphasize physiology, kinesiology, the neurosciences, occupational therapy theory, evaluation, and research. Assistant programs emphasize occupational therapy skills and treatment. Occupational therapists evaluate, establish, and implement treatment programs. The occupational therapy assistant focuses on the implementation of the treatment.

The fieldwork experience is designed to blend theory and practice. These integrated experiences promote clinical reasoning and the development of a repertoire of clinical skills.

Upon passing the national certification exam, occupational therapists are registered and assistants are certified. If working in the United States, they must adhere to licensure laws regulating the practice of occupational therapy, which vary from state to state.

In most instances the process of occupational therapy begins with a referral from a physician. The referred individual is first interviewed and evaluated. The evaluation gives the therapist an understanding of the individual's experience, builds a therapeutic relationship, identifies strengths and limitations, defines what the individual feels is important regarding goals, and establishes treatment priorities. Evaluations assess areas of occupation and performance components (motor, process, and psychosocial skills needed to do daily activities). Motor skills include muscle strength, joint range of motion, sensation, balance, mobility, and coordination. Process skills include concentration, problem solving, judgment, and memory. Psychosocial skills include reality testing, orientation, coping skills, and self-esteem.

After the initial occupational therapy evaluation, goals are established collaboratively with the individual and their significant others. Treatment interventions are identified and implemented. Clients can be seen individually or in group treatment sessions. Examples of diagnoses and treatment include the following:

Diagnosis	Treatment
Stroke	Increase coordination and balance for grooming
Hip replacement	Adaptive equipment training to simplify self-care
Hand injury	Purposeful activities to improve range of motion
Chemical dependency	Explore healthy leisure pursuits to structure time
Mental retardation	Practice and simulation of job performance activities
Chronic pain	Biofeedback techniques to better manage pain
Depression	Coping, stress management, and assertiveness training
Dementia	Adapt the environment to help orient the individual

Oophorectomy

Diagnosis	Treatment
Pediatric	Play activities that promote balance and coordination
Learning disabilities	Adaptive techniques to enhance the educational process

The occupational therapy treatment plan may warrant more extensive testing. Occupational therapy assessments can help clarify diagnoses and aid in determining legal issues such as competency, guardianship, and placement. The data and recommendations of an occupational therapist can more clearly identify functional abilities and illuminate appropriate options to pursue.

Throughout treatment the occupational therapist monitors and reassesses the individual's response to treatment and documents progress in accordance with regulatory agencies to ensure reimbursement by third-party payers. Communication with team members (physician, nurse, social worker, physical therapist), the patient, family, or caregivers is important in developing appropriate discharge plans to maintain and promote wellness.

Helping individuals achieve optimal function and satisfaction in their life roles is the unique ability of occupational therapists.

SEE ALSO: Activities of daily living, Alzheimer's disease, Dementia, Disability

Suggested Reading

American Occupational Therapy Association. (1999). Standards for an accredited educational program for the occupational therapist. *American Journal of Occupational Therapy, 53,* 575–582.

American Occupational Therapy Association. (1999). Standards for an accredited educational program for the occupational therapy assistant. *American Journal of Occupational Therapy, 53,* 583–589.

American Occupational Therapy Association. (2002). Occupational therapy practice framework: Domain and process. *American Journal of Occupational Therapy, 56,* 609–639.

Crepeau, E. B., & Neistadt, M. E. (1998). *Willard and Spackman's occupational therapy* (9th ed.). Philadelphia: Lippincott.

NBCOT certifies 6,727 during 2002. (2003, Spring). *Report to the Profession,* p. 6.

CYNTHIA OLSCHEWSKY

Oligomenorrhea

Oligomenorrhea is infrequent menstrual bleeding that occurs at intervals greater than 5 weeks or 35 days. Normal menstrual bleeding occurs every 28 days with a normal range of 21–35 days. The duration of flow is 4.5 days with a range of 2–7 days. Normal blood loss at menses is 35 ml with a range of 20–80 ml.

Causes of oligomenorrhea include any condition that may disrupt key components of the body endocrine system (the hypothalamic–pituitary axis). Common groups in which this may be seen include patients with eating disorders, ballet dancers, and competitive athletes such as runners, gymnasts, and ice skaters, especially if training started in the prepubertal years. This condition can also be found in patients with polycystic ovarian syndrome, conditions of abnormal metabolism (dysmetabolic syndromes), and in patients with fluctuating weight patterns.

Treatment includes cyclic progestin therapy or oral contraceptives to induce periods and protect the lining of the uterus (endometrium) long term from the development of abnormal, excessive cell growth (hyperplasia).

SEE ALSO: Menstrual cycle disorders

Suggested Reading

Emans, S. J. H., & Goldstein, D. P. (1990). *Pediatric and adolescent gynecology.* Boston: Little, Brown.

Herbst, A., Mishell, D., Stenchever, M., & Droegemueller, W. (1992). *Comprehensive gynecology.* St. Louis, MO: Mosby-Year Book.

Stenchever, M. (1991). *Office gynecology.* St. Louis, MO: Mosby-Year Book.

DIANE YOUNG

Oophorectomy

Oophorectomy, also called ovariectomy, is the surgical removal of one or both ovaries. According to the Centers for Disease Control and Prevention (CDC), 491,000 oophorectomies and salpingo-oophorectomies (surgical removal of the fallopian tubes along with the ovaries) were performed in the United States in the year 1998. Removal of the ovaries is often done along with a hysterectomy (removal of the uterus). The ovaries produce ova (reproductive egg cells) and the sex hormones androgens, estrogens, and progesterones. Excision of both ovaries (bilateral oophorectomy) causes a surgical menopause, with the cessation of menses and fertility.

Between the years 1988 and 1993, approximately 50% of women in the United States undergoing hysterectomy also had both ovaries removed. During these years, the proportion of women having oophorectomy along with hysterectomy increased. Oophorectomy was done more frequently when the surgical approach was abdominal—63% for abdominal hysterectomy versus 18% for vaginal hysterectomy. Approximately two thirds of women with a diagnosis of cancer or endometrial hyperplasia had an oophorectomy along with their hysterectomy. Younger women are less likely to have oophorectomy accompanying hysterectomy—the incidence is 18% in the 18- to 24-year-old age group, 76% in those 45–54 years old, and 62% in women 55 years or older.

Oophorectomies are performed for a variety of reasons. With cancer of the ovary or ovaries, both ovaries are removed. In the past, prophylactic oophorectomy was often performed in women who were nearing menopause and undergoing hysterectomy in order to prevent future ovarian cancer. Since ovarian tissue can also grow elsewhere in the abdomen, oophorectomy does not always protect against the future development of ovarian cancer. Ovarian cancer, when caught early, has excellent 5-year cure rates. However, early detection is not common due to the lack of early signs and symptoms. Some high-risk women choose prophylactic oophorectomy to prevent ovarian and even breast cancer. Studies have shown significant risk reduction of both of these cancer types with the surgery, but the procedure is still somewhat controversial and the optimal timing for such intervention is not clear.

Prophylactic oophorectomy may also be performed in young women who have already developed breast cancer. Since some breast cancers grow larger in response to estrogen or progesterone, the removal of the ovaries can cut the supply of these hormones to the tumor. Other indications for oophorectomy are the excision of large ovarian cysts, removal of ovarian abscess, and treatment of endometriosis.

Obstetrician/gynecologists are the surgical specialists who perform oophorectomies. Oophorectomy may be carried out through an abdominal surgical incision—either horizontal or vertical. The surgery can also be done through the vagina, which speeds recovery. Another option with a relatively quick recovery time is laparoscopic surgery. With an abdominal incision, recovery typically takes up to 8 weeks while women who have vaginal and laparoscopic surgeries usually recover within 2–4 weeks. Surgery to remove ovarian cancer requires an abdominal incision.

Following bilateral oophorectomy, a woman usually receives treatment with female hormones, such as estrogen (if the uterus is also removed) or combination therapy of estrogen and progesterone if the uterus is left intact. Use of selective estrogen receptor modulators (SERMs) and testosterone replacement are two other options. If only one ovary is resected, the remaining ovary typically makes enough estrogen to negate the need for hormone replacement therapy postsurgically.

Women who have undergone bilateral oophorectomy and who do not take hormones may experience the usual signs and symptoms of menopause including hot flashes, sleep disturbance, vaginal atrophy, and decreased vaginal lubrication. A surgical menopause such as this causes an abrupt loss of ovarian secretion of androgens, estrogens, and progesterone. Potential psychological reactions include grief over the loss of the ability to become pregnant and/or depressive symptoms. Women who have experienced depression during times of significant hormonal shifts, such as during pregnancy or in the postpartum period, are more likely to experience depression following oophorectomy. Overall, the abrupt change in hormonal levels tends to produce more severe and pronounced symptoms than a natural menopause with its more gradual decrease in hormone production.

SEE ALSO: Hormone replacement therapy, Hysterectomy, Menopause

Suggested Reading

Kornstein, S. G., & Clayton, A. H. (Eds.). (2002). *Women's mental health: A comprehensive textbook.* New York: Guilford Press.

Krasnoff, R. D. (1994). In P. B. Doress-Worters & D. Laskin Siegal (Eds.), *The new ourselves, growing older: Women aging with knowledge and power* (pp. 315–332). New York: Simon & Schuster.

Suggested Resources

Centers for Disease Control and Prevention website: www.cdc.gov

PAULA L. HENSLEY

Oral Contraception

Oral contraceptives (birth control pills) are either combined estrogen and progestin or progestin-only formulations that prevent conception. Estrogen is the female hormone secreted by

Oral Contraception

the ovary in the first half of the menstrual cycle. Progesterone is the hormone produced by the ovary in the second half of the cycle. The pill's estrogens and progestins (substances that behave like progesterone in the body) are synthetic imitators of the body's natural hormones.

The most commonly used type of birth control pill is the combined oral contraceptive. These are formulations containing combinations of various types and dosages of estrogens and progestins. The combined pills are cycles of 3 weeks of active, hormone-containing pills and 1 week of inactive placebo pills. Combined oral contraceptives may be monophasic (contain the same dose of hormone for 3 weeks of active pills) or multiphasic (containing various doses of hormones in the active pills). Monophasic pills are one color for the three weeks of active pills and a different color on the inactive week. Multiphasic oral contraceptives are multicolored pills during the active pills specifying different dosages throughout the cycle as well as a separate color for the inactive week. There is no real advantage to either type of pill. Pills are taken daily at about the same time. Menses begins during the week of inactive pills. The primary action of combined oral contraceptives is suppression of ovulation, thus preventing conception. In addition, they also thicken the cervical mucus preventing sperm from ascending into the uterus and fallopian tubes and change the lining of the uterus making implantation less likely.

Birth control pills are sometimes prescribed "continuously." In this case the patient does not take the placebo pills and rather goes directly to the next pack of active pills. This method is used to eliminate some or all menstrual periods.

A second type of oral contraceptive pill is the progestin-only or "minipill." These formulations contain only a progestin. The pill pack contains 28 active hormonal pills that are the same color throughout. There is no week of inactive/placebo pills. The progestin-only oral contraceptives prevent ovulation in some women; however, the primary method of contraceptive action is to thicken cervical mucus, preventing sperm from ascending into the upper reproductive tract, thus inhibiting conception. The cervical mucus begins to thin within 23 hr so these pills must be taken very consistently every 24 hr. Because the progestin-only pills contain no estrogen, they can be used by women who may have conditions that preclude the use of combined oral contraceptives such as history of blood clotting disorders; smokers who are over 35; women who are lactating; those who experience severe nausea with estrogen intake; those who experience breast tenderness, severe headaches, or hypertension while taking combined pills.

BENEFITS OF ORAL CONTRACEPTIVES

The benefits of both types of pills include:

1. *Excellent contraception.* Combined oral contraceptives have a perfect use failure rate of 0.1% (number of pregnancies per 100 couples using it for 1 year of use). Progestin-only pills have a perfect use failure rate of 0.5%. Typical use pregnancy rate for both types of oral contraceptives is 5%. Because of the effectiveness of the pill, it is estimated that for every 100,000 users, 117 ectopic pregnancies, 10,500 spontaneous abortions (miscarriages), and 10,407 term pregnancies requiring cesarean sections are prevented (Dickey, 2000).

2. *Reversibility.* Fertility returns rapidly after stopping oral contraceptives. Pills have absolutely no effect on future fertility although it can take somewhat longer to become pregnant after stopping pill use. The median time from discontinuation to conception is 3 months for combined pills and less than 3 months for minipills.

3. *Not coitally related.* Pills are taken daily, not just used at the time of intercourse. Therefore, women are protected consistently from unintended pregnancy. It is not necessary to interrupt the spontaneity of sexual activity to use this method.

4. *Safety.* Pills are a very safe method of contraception throughout the reproductive years. No studies have demonstrated adverse effects of long-term use. Oral contraceptives are safe for use during the full span of reproductive years in healthy, nonsmoking women. It has been well demonstrated that hospitalizations for adverse health events prevented by oral contraceptives (unintended pregnancy, ovarian cysts, and invasive cancers of the ovary and endometrium) vastly outweigh hospitalizations for conditions related to pill use. There is also no reason to take a rest or holiday from taking the pill. This increases the risk of pregnancy and has no benefit whatsoever.

5. *May be used for emergency contraception.* Within 72 hr of unprotected intercourse, larger doses of certain birth control pills may be used to prevent an unintended pregnancy. The failure rate with this method is between 1 and 3% depending on what

method is used. Telephone hotline: 1-888-NOT-2-LATE (1-888-668-2528).

6. *Noncontraceptive benefits.* Combined pills provide protection against osteoporosis, functional ovarian cysts, and benign breast disease. They also decrease the risk for ovarian cancer and endometrial cancer (cancer of the lining of the uterus) significantly. Longer use conveys greater protection. The pills improve acne and decrease hirsutism (unwanted facial and body hair resulting from excessive male hormones). Both combined and progestin-only pills decrease menstrual cramps and menstrual flow, reduce symptoms of endometriosis, decrease premenstrual syndrome, diminish anemia related to heavy periods, decrease the midcycle pain of ovulation, and lower the risk for pelvic inflammatory disease (infection of the uterus, tubes, and pelvic cavity that can be life threatening).

DISADVANTAGES

Disadvantages of oral contraceptives include:

1. *Risk of cardiovascular diseases.* Although the risk is very small, use of the pill can predispose women to the most serious risk attributable to combined oral contraceptives, diseases of the heart and circulatory system. Cardiovascular problems such as heart attack, stroke, and blood clots are due to: (1) an increase in coagulability (blood clotting) due to estrogen; (2) an unfavorable change in cholesterol and other fats in the blood due to male hormone activity of progestins; and/or (3) increased blood pressure in susceptible patients due to the estrogen and/or progestin components of the pill. The risk increases with age. Concomitant smoking is a major cause of these complications.

2. *Cost of method.* Oral contraceptives can be expensive if they are not covered by insurance. Unfortunately, many insurance companies do not cover oral contraceptives for birth control purposes only. If they are used to treat a medical condition such as severe cramps or irregular periods, the cost may be covered. The cost of pills depends on the type and pharmacy, but they average between $30 and $35 a cycle. They can be obtained at health departments, birth control clinics, or, in some instances, pharmaceutical company programs at reduced cost.

3. *No protection against sexually transmitted diseases.* While birth control pills thicken cervical mucus and may decrease the likelihood of pelvic inflammatory disease, they do not prevent gonorrhea, chlamydia, trichomoniasis, HIV, or genital warts and human papillomavirus (HPV) that can cause cervical dysplasia and cancer. Because of changes in the cervix called ectopy, a condition that causes vulnerable cells to be more exposed in the cervical opening, chlamydial infections may be acquired more easily on oral contraceptives. For this reason, it is recommended that latex condoms be used in addition to oral contraceptives for those who are at risk for sexually transmitted infections.

4. The need to remember to take a pill each day is difficult for many patients. The vaginal ring method of hormonal contraception and the birth control patch may be excellent options for these patients.

5. *Adverse effects directly related to pill use.* These include nausea and vomiting, menstrual changes including spotting, headaches (may increase or decrease on the pill), depression (may increase or decrease), decreased libido due to decreased levels of circulating free male hormone, and increased risk of gallstones. These effects can generally be ameliorated by adjustment of dosage or formulation of pills.

6. *Adverse effects that may be related to pill use.* Certain types of benign liver tumors have also been associated. Since cervical cancer is related to HPV, pill users may be more susceptible, because they have more sexual partners. Studies that have attempted to control for confounding risk factors have found that the risk of cervical cancer still seems to be slightly higher in patients using the pill.

Birth control pills are safe, effective, and generally very well tolerated. The decision to use an oral contraceptive should be based on personal preference, medical history including conditions that may be exacerbated or improved by pills, the ability to take a pill each day, and economics. They require a prescription by a medical provider who should monitor the patient's response to the pills and provide preventive screening for breast and cervical cancer as well as sexually transmitted diseases where the risk is great.

SEE ALSO: Acquired immunodeficiency syndrome, Birth control, Chlamydia, Condoms, Ovarian cancer, Ovarian cyst, Pelvic pain, Sexual organs, Uterine cancer

Suggested Reading

Dickey, R. (2000). *Managing contraceptive pill patients* (pp. 10–11). Dallas, TX: EMIS.

Hatcher, R., Trussel, J., Stewart, F., Cates, W., Stewart, G., Guest, F., et al. (1999). *Contraceptive technology* (pp. 405–509). New York: Ardent Media.

Suggested Resources

Planned Parenthood Federation of America. (2000, April). *You and the pill.* http://www.plannedparenthood.org/bc/you_and_pill.htm

NANCY MYERS-BRADLEY

Oral Health   This entry focuses on oral health during pregnancy. The imbalance of female sex hormones during pregnancy has been implicated in changes in the oral cavity. Many of the changes can be minimized or prevented with good oral hygiene and regular oral health care.

PREGNANCY GINGIVITIS

Gingival (gum) changes become noticeable from the second month of gestation and reach a maximum level in the eighth month. Hormonal changes may cause the gingiva to become inflamed and edematous (swollen). "Pregnancy gingivitis" is characterized by a tendency to bleed easily.

PREGNANCY TUMORS

Single, tumor-like growths may develop on the tissue between the teeth. The "pregnancy tumors" may grow rapidly reaching 2 cm during the second trimester of gestation. Most of these lesions regress spontaneously several months after the termination of pregnancy.

TOOTH MOBILITY

Tooth mobility may be related to the degree of gingival disease and disturbance of the attachment apparatus (tissue attaching teeth to bone). Mineral changes in the bone may also contribute to tooth mobility. Tooth mobility due to hormonal changes during pregnancy usually reverses after delivery.

TOOTH DECAY

Pregnancy does not directly contribute to tooth decay. However, the frequent vomiting associated with morning sickness can cause acid erosion of the teeth. Snacking on starches and sugar-rich foods between meals increases acid production in the mouth. It can damage tooth enamel. The pregnant woman should try to limit sugary and starchy foods to mealtime.

ORAL HYGIENE CARE DURING PREGNANCY

The most important objectives in planning dental treatment are establishing a healthy oral cavity and optimum oral hygiene practices. Conscientious oral hygiene care during office visits as well as at home can help control bacterial plaque formation. Gingival conditions occur most frequently among pregnant women whose oral hygiene is inadequate and promotes plaque buildup. The hormonal and vascular changes that accompany pregnancy often exaggerate the inflammatory response to plaque. The dentist is charged with monitoring the pregnant patient's oral hygiene to obtain good plaque control throughout pregnancy. Scaling, polishing, and root planing visits may be scheduled more frequently than for nonpregnant patients. Pregnant women should brush after each meal with a fluoride-containing toothpaste and floss thoroughly daily. Research has shown that women who have low-birthweight infants as a consequence of either preterm labor or premature rupture of membranes tend to have more severe periodontal (gum) disease than mothers with normal-birthweight babies. However, it remains unknown whether there is a causal relationship.

THE ROLE OF DIET

Diet plays an important role in the developing dentition of the fetus. Vitamins, minerals, and proteins are transferred through the mother's blood to the fetus. Vitamin C maintains the structure of bone and teeth. Proteins build teeth and bones. Calcium builds and strengthens healthy bones and teeth. If the mother is receiving an insufficient supply of calcium, it will be extracted from the mother's bones to meet the fetus's needs. The mother could experience skeletal problems later as a result.

DENTAL CARE

Elective dental care is not advised during the first trimester or last half of the third trimester. Organogenesis (development of the organs of the fetus) takes place during the first trimester and therefore, the fetus is very sensitive to environmental influences. During the last half of the third trimester, the uterus is very sensitive to external stimuli. Dental care during this time involves the risk of premature delivery. Moreover, third-trimester pregnant patients should not be subjected to prolonged chair time in a supine or semireclining position. The safest period during which a pregnant woman can obtain dental care is the second trimester. The focus should be on simple and short procedures. Any proposed emergency treatment should be discussed with the patient's physician first.

RADIOGRAPHS

Whether or not pregnant women should be exposed to dental radiographs (x-rays) is a controversial area. Exposure to radiographs should be minimized. Radiographs should only be taken when absolutely necessary and high-speed film should be used to minimize exposure. As with any patients, the pregnant woman should wear a protective lead apron with a thyroid collar.

POSTPARTUM TRANSMISSION OF MUTANS STREPTOCOCCI

Research has shown that dental caries is an infectious and transmissible disease. Studies have shown that babies can acquire mutans streptococci, bacteria most strongly associated with dental caries, from their mothers. Mothers with untreated dental caries possess reservoirs of mutans streptococci.

SEE ALSO: Pregnancy

Suggested Reading

Berkowitz, R. (2003). Acquisition and transmission of mutans streptococci. *California Dental Association Journal, 31,* 135–138.

Offenbacher, S., & Beck, J. (1999). Periodontitis: A potential risk factor for spontaneous preterm birth. *Compendium of Continuing Education in Dentistry,* Fall, 32–39.

Rose, L., & Kaye, D. (1983). *Internal medicine for dentistry.* St. Louis, MO: C.V. Mosby.

PAMELA ARBUCKLE
JOY A. JORDAN

Osteoarthritis

Osteoarthritis, or degenerative joint disease, is the most common form of arthritis in the United States, affecting 15.8 million Americans. More than 15% of women over the age of 80 have symptomatic osteoarthritis of the knee. Osteoarthritis is a leading cause of disability and thus has a significant economic impact. Although there is no cure for osteoarthritis, individualized treatment programs can limit loss of function, reduce pain, and maintain joint mobility.

Osteoarthritis results from degeneration of cartilage within joints. This cartilage provides a cushion between the two bones and forms the smooth gliding surface needed for normal joint function. Cartilage is composed of water, cells, and matrix. Seventy percent of cartilage is water. The cells make the stiff matrix that is composed of proteoglycans, collagen, and glycoproteins. Damage to cartilage is caused by multiple factors including biomechanical, metabolic, biochemical, and genetic factors that combine to produce inflammation. The main cause of osteoarthritis is repeated exposure to physical forces that injure cells within the cartilage, leading to the release of enzymes that degrade cartilage. Less commonly, defective cartilage can fail under normal joint loading. Multiple risk factors have been associated with the development of osteoarthritis, including age (over 50), gender, obesity, occupation, injuries, genetics, and others. Secondary osteoarthritis can also result from other conditions such as trauma, calcium deposition diseases, and other bone and joint disorders such as rheumatoid arthritis.

The main symptom of osteoarthritis is joint pain. Stiffness is also a common complaint and is usually worse in the morning or after periods of inactivity, but generally resolves in less than 30 min. The diagnosis is made by noting a characteristic pattern of joint involvement, characteristic appearance on x-rays, and the absence of clinical and laboratory evidence for other types of arthritis. The most commonly affected joints are the small joints of the fingers and the weight-bearing joints such as the knees, hips, and spine. On x-rays, osteoarthritis appears as joint space narrowing with formation of bone spurs near joints.

Osteoarthritis

Osteoarthritis of the knee is common in patients over the age of 50 and in obese patients, and is diagnosed based on the presence of knee pain with bony tenderness and enlargement, and less than 30 min of morning stiffness. Osteoarthritis of the hands causes bony enlargement of the small finger joints as well as the joint at the base of the thumb. This form of osteoarthritis is often seen in mothers and grandmothers and is inherited as an autosomal dominant trait. When the feet are involved with osteoarthritis the joint at the base of the first toe is often affected and results in a bunion. Osteoarthritis of the hip usually produces pain in the groin area. Osteoarthritis of the spine is common in the neck and lower back. When the joints between the vertebrae are affected, nerve roots can be compressed as they exit the spine, causing nerve-related pain and weakness. Osteoarthritis of the spine can also lead to slippage of the vertebral bodies on each other and compression of the spinal cord itself.

Treatment for osteoarthritis includes medication, nondrug treatment, and surgery. Nondrug treatment includes weight loss, rest, physical therapy, bracing, and exercise. Obesity is strongly associated with the development of osteoarthritis; being obese more than doubles the risk for osteoarthritis of the knee. In one study, losing just 10 lb reduced the risk of osteoarthritis of the knee by 50%. Rest relieves pain but prolonged rest can lead to muscle weakness, so rest is recommended for only short periods of time. Physical therapy can improve flexibility and muscle strength, which is important for supporting the affected joints. By supporting more weight, strong muscles unload the joint and cartilage. Braces (e.g., to correct deformity in the knee) and knee sleeves that correct abnormal tracking of the kneecap may help pain. Exercise is important to maintain flexibility and strengthen muscles.

Pain relief is an important goal of therapy in osteoarthritis, and pain-relieving drugs are a mainstay of treatment. Acetaminophen (Tylenol) in doses of up to 4 g per day is recommended as the first treatment and has few side effects. Liver damage may occur with large doses of acetaminophen in people who also drink alcohol. Nonsteroidal anti-inflammatory drugs (NSAIDs) are useful in patients who do not respond to acetaminophen. NSAIDs such as ibuprofen, naproxen, and ketoprofen are available over the counter or by prescription. Side effects of these medications include gastrointestinal (GI) problems such as gastritis and ulcers, which occasionally can be serious. Rash and impairment of kidney, liver, and bone marrow function are rare but do occur. Newer NSAIDs called COX-2 inhibitors (celecoxib, rofecoxib, and valdecoxib) have slightly fewer GI side effects compared to other NSAIDS. Other medications such as codeine, Tramadol, and propoxyphene should be limited to short-term use only. However, these medications may be useful for some patients who are at high risk for side effects with NSAIDs (such as people with a history of stomach ulcers or allergic reactions).

When oral medications are not enough, injection of corticosteroids into the joint is usually quite effective for short periods of time (weeks to months). These injections should be limited to 3–4 times per year in the same joint. Newer hyaluronic acid derivatives (another class of medications; Synvisc and Hyalgan) may be effective in osteoarthritis of the knee in selected patients. These medications are given in a series of 3–5 weekly injections and can be repeated twice per year.

Surgery is helpful in patients with significant limitations of joint function who are not helped by other treatments. Joint replacements of the knee and hip provide marked pain relief and improve function in most patients.

See Also: Arthritis, Obesity, Rheumatoid arthritis

Suggested Reading

Bradley, J. D., Brandt, K. D., Katz, B. P., Kalasinski, L. A., & Ryan, S. I. (1991). Comparison of an anti-inflammatory dose of ibuprofen, an analgesic dose of ibuprofen, and acetaminophen in the treatment of patients with osteoarthritis of the knee. *New England Journal of Medicine, 325*(2), 87–91.

Buckwalter, J. A., & Lohmander, S. (1994). Operative treatment of osteoarthrosis: Current practice and future development. *Journal of Bone and Joint Surgery—American Volume, 76*(9), 1405–1418.

Hochberg, M. C. (1996). Prognosis of osteoarthritis. *Annals of the Rheumatic Diseases, 55*(9), 685–688.

Hochberg, M. C., Altman, R. D., Brandt, K. D., Clark, B. M., Dieppe, P. A., Griffin, M. R., et al. (1995). Guidelines for the medical management of osteoarthritis. Part I and II. *Arthritis and Rheumatitis, 38*(11), 1535–1540, 1541–1546.

Holderbaum, D., Haqqi, T. M., & Moskowitz, R. W. (1999). Genetics and osteoarthritis: Exposing the iceberg. *Arthritis and Rheumatitis, 42*(3), 397–405.

Recommendations for the medical management of osteoarthritis of the hip and knee: 2000 update. (2000). American College of Rheumatology Subcommittee on Osteoarthritis Guidelines. *Arthritis and Rheumatitis, 43*, 1905–1915.

Chad Deal

Osteoporosis and Osteopenia

Osteoporosis, or porous bone, is a disease characterized by low bone mass and reduced bone strength, with increased risk of fractures. The term *osteopenia* means low bone mass, which is one aspect of osteoporosis. Osteopenia is often used to describe a mild form of osteoporosis because osteoporosis is diagnosed primarily by low bone density. Several diseases produce low bone density and osteoporosis is the most common of these.

Osteoporosis is often called the "silent disease." It can go undetected until a fracture suddenly occurs. Any bone can be affected, but osteoporotic fractures most often involve the hip and spine. The wrist is also a common fracture site. Spinal (vertebral) fractures can be very painful or they can occur silently over many years, without pain, causing a gradual loss of height or a bent upper back (dowager's hump).

RISK FACTORS

In general, older women are at greater risk of developing osteoporosis than men, because the decline in estrogen production at menopause speeds the loss of bone. Half of all women who live to 85 will have an osteoporosis-related fracture at some point. Although older women are at highest risk, osteoporosis can also develop in older men, and occasionally even in younger women and men. Risk factors for osteoporosis include: a personal history of fracture, family history of fracture in a first-degree (closely related) relative, a family history of osteoporosis, being female, lower body weight (weighing <154 lb or <70 kg after age 60) or having a small frame, advanced age, estrogen deficiency (because of menopause or due to surgical removal of the ovaries), abnormal absence of menstrual periods (amenorrhea), low dietary calcium intake, inactive lifestyle, excessive drinking of alcohol, and cigarette smoking. People of European and Asian descent are at more risk than African Americans or Hispanic Americans. Because certain medications such as corticosteroids or excessive thyroid hormone can cause osteoporosis, a woman should ask her physician to review her medications with this in mind.

DIAGNOSIS AND SCREENING

Regular x-rays are not accurate for measuring bone density. Osteoporosis is best diagnosed by measuring bone density at the hip, spine, and/or forearm using a special x-ray known as DEXA. Ultrasound (of the heel for instance) is sometimes used to diagnose osteoporosis, but is less accurate. When a patient's bone mineral density (BMD) is measured, it is compared against the average bone density for a young healthy person of the same gender. DEXA results include the "*T* score," which is the number of standard deviations above or below the bone density for young healthy people. Osteoporosis is diagnosed when the bone density is more than 2.5 standard deviations below this average (*T* score less than −2.5). Bone density between 1 and 2.5 standard deviations below the average (*T* score between −1 and −2.5) is called osteopenia.

Because osteoporosis develops silently, screening with DEXA is recommended for women age 65 and older, according to the U.S. Preventive Services Task Force (USPSTF). Between age 60 and 65, women at higher risk (body weight <154 lb or <70 kg, not using estrogen) should be screened.

PREVENTION

Bone mass peaks before age 30. Osteoporosis can be postponed by building up a healthy bone mass in childhood and young adulthood. By starting adult life with a higher bone mass, more time will pass before the bone mass becomes dangerously low. Bone mass can be maximized and maintained by including enough calcium in the diet, regular weight-bearing exercise, avoidance of smoking, and avoidance of more than moderate alcohol intake.

Calcium in the diet is very important. A daily total of 1,000 mg of calcium is recommended for most adults, but 1,500 mg is suggested for postmenopausal women. Teens, women in their early 20s, and breast-feeding women should get 1,200–1,500 mg per day. Foods high in calcium include milk, cheese, yogurt, sardines, broccoli, eggs, salmon, peanuts, soybeans, tofu, and spinach. One cup of 1% milk contains about 250 mg of calcium, one cup of broccoli has about 178 mg, and 1 cup of kidney beans has about 115 mg. Orange juice, soy milk, and other nondairy "milk" with added calcium are available. However, some women have difficulty obtaining enough calcium from foods alone, especially if they avoid dairy products.

Calcium supplements are recommended if the diet does not supply enough calcium. There are several kinds of calcium supplement (such as calcium carbonate or calcium citrate), some containing vitamin D as well.

When reading the label on calcium supplements, look for the amount of "elemental calcium." The body will not absorb more than about 500 mg of elemental calcium at a time, so if more is needed, the doses should be spread out through the day. Postmenopausal women should consider taking vitamin D as well, especially in winter in the northern latitudes. Calcium can interfere with the absorption of some medications, and people with a history of kidney stones should check with their doctor before taking calcium supplements.

Weight-bearing exercise can help prevent the development of osteoporosis, and of course is beneficial for other health reasons. Weight-bearing exercise is activity that exerts a force or stress on bones, such as walking. Bone responds to even mild forces or pressure by becoming more dense. The key is to include moderate weight-bearing exercise in your daily routine. Vigorous exercise is not needed for maintenance of bone density, and can increase the risk of fracture in a person who has osteoporotic bones. Very vigorous exercise, as may be performed by an elite athlete, can actually cause a decrease in bone mass in young women by decreasing the body's production of estrogen. For many older women, a daily walk with good supportive shoes or sneakers is effective. Walking provides good gentle stress to the bones in the spine and legs. For women who can safely exercise more vigorously, jogging and climbing stairs are good. Exercises to strengthen the muscles that hold the back erect are beneficial. These include exercises that gently arch the back. Resistance training is also helpful. This involves exercise against a resistance, by using an elastic exercise band (one brand name is Theraband), or walking in water (water exercises), or lifting weights. Your physician or physical therapist can help you design an exercise program that is appropriate for you.

Smoking and excessive alcohol intake are both known to increase the risk of osteoporosis, so efforts to stop smoking and limit alcohol intake are important.

TREATMENT

If you have osteoporosis, it is important to follow your physician's recommendations. Your physician may consider laboratory tests to rule out various secondary causes of osteoporosis. Treatment of osteoporosis includes continuing the above preventive measures, and usually adding medications, with the goal of slowing the progression of the disease and reducing the chance of fractures. Currently there are several effective medications that have been approved by the Food and Drug Administration for the treatment (and prevention) of osteoporosis. These include hormones such as estrogen, raloxifene, and calcitonin, as well as bisphosphonate medications such as alendronate. Women who take calcium supplements regularly should also take vitamin D, to help the calcium be absorbed into the bones.

Once osteoporosis has developed, the risk of fractures can be reduced by minimizing the chance of falls. This may involve such measures as wearing sensible low shoes, using a cane or a walker if needed, avoiding clutter or throw rugs on the floor in the home, installing helpful wall rails in the bathroom, and avoiding medications that can cause grogginess or dizziness. Other precautionary antifall measures may be needed, depending upon your level of ability or disability.

SEE ALSO: Falls Prevention, Hormone replacement therapy, Menopause, Vitamins

Suggested Resources

National Institutes of Health (NIH). *Osteoporosis and related bone diseases, National Resource Center.* http://www.osteo.org

National Osteoporosis Foundation, Washington, DC: http://www.nof.org/osteoporosis

National Women's Health Resource Center, U.S. Department of Health and Human Services: http://www.4woman.gov/

Screening for osteoporosis in postmenopausal women. What's new from the USPSTF? (2002, September). AHRQ Publication No. APPIP02-0025. Rockville, MD: Agency for Healthcare Research and Quality. http://www.ahrq.gov/clinic/3rduspstf/osteoporosis/osteowh.htm

JUDITH M. FRANK
ALICIA M. WEISSMAN

Ovarian Cancer Ovarian cancer refers to a heterogeneous (diverse) group of diseases. The most common form of ovarian cancer, the epithelial ovarian cancers, tends to occur in women after the age of 50. This type of ovarian cancer was highly publicized with the diagnosis and death of actress and comedienne, Gilda Radner. It is this form of cancer that most individuals think of when they hear the term "ovarian cancer." There are, however, two other forms of ovarian cancer: the germ-cell tumors and the stromal tumors.

The germ-cell tumors that are responsible for only 2–3% of ovarian cancers are identical to the tumors that cause testicular cancer in young men. Germ-cell tumors arise from the portion of the ovary that gives rise to the oocyte or "egg." They tend to be diagnosed in the late teens and early 20s, they tend to involve only one gonad (sex gland) thus removal of the gonad (castration) is not required, and they are highly curable with chemotherapy. The stromal tumors that account for only 7% of all ovarian cancers arise from the portion of the ovary that produces hormones. These tumors can occur at any point of the life cycle. Because of their tendency for hormone production, these tumors can cause early puberty as well as masculinization. Like germ-cell tumors, ovarian stromal cancers tend to be diagnosed before they have spread and are associated with a favorable prognosis.

Epithelial ovarian cancer, which is by far the most common form of ovarian cancer, arises from either the surface of the ovary or from embryologic tissue (rests) within the ovary. There is no analogous (similar) tumor seen in men. The remainder of this section will focus on epithelial ovarian cancer.

While epithelial ovarian cancer is not the most common of the gynecologic cancers, it is responsible for more deaths than uterine and cervical cancer combined. For this reason, ovarian cancer is one of the most dreaded of the female cancers. The primary reason for the high mortality rates seen with epithelial ovarian cancer is the fact that this disease is usually discovered only after it has spread well beyond the ovary (only 25% of cases have not spread beyond the ovary at the time of diagnosis). When epithelial ovarian cancer is diagnosed in the early stage (i.e., still limited to the ovary), the likelihood of cure is actually quite high (approximately 70–90% cure rate). Unfortunately, once the disease has spread outside of the pelvis, the cure rates are low (less than 20% likelihood of cure).

The reason for later diagnosis of epithelial ovarian cancer is that this disease tends not to cause symptoms in its early stages. The female pelvis is built to carry a pregnancy, thus there is an ingrained tolerance for the presence of a "mass" in the pelvis. The early symptoms are often nondescript. A vague sense of bloating or abdominal discomfort and indigestion are the more commonly reported symptoms of ovarian cancer. These symptoms are common in the general population and usually do not represent the presence of a malignancy. However, if any such symptom is progressively worsening or significant enough that the physician feels a diagnostic evaluation should be undertaken, it is wise to include a pelvic ultrasound in the evaluation, even if the symptoms are more in the abdomen than the pelvis. It is not at all infrequent for a patient, who ultimately

turned out to have ovarian cancer, to have undergone an extensive gastrointestinal evaluation with specialized evaluation of the colon (colonoscopy) and stomach (gastroscopy)—both of which tend to be negative in women with ovarian cancer. Often neither specialized imaging techniques (computed tomography [CT] scan) of the abdomen and pelvis nor pelvic ultrasound (both of which would likely have made the diagnosis) are performed until a much later date, when symptoms are extreme.

SCREENING

Because of high cure rates when discovered early and because at present most cases are diagnosed late, ovarian cancer is an excellent candidate for using a screening test. Unfortunately, development of a highly effective screening methodology has been difficult. There is a general misconception that measurement of a specific compound found to be abnormal in ovarian cancer (serum CA-125) should be performed on all women to screen for ovarian cancer. While a rise in CA-125 is associated with ovarian cancer, a large body of data has shown that in most cases, elevation of CA-125 is due to a cause *other* than ovarian cancer in the general population. For this reason, CA-125 measurement alone is not an effective screening tool, as most abnormal readings will not be due to ovarian cancer and will thus lead to unnecessary anxiety and the performance of unnecessary diagnostic evaluations and surgical treatments.

Pelvic ultrasound performed with a vaginal probe has also been investigated as a screening tool. While it has been shown to detect the presence of asymptomatic ovarian cancers, its usefulness is limited by the fact that the "false positive rate" (the percentage of women who have an abnormal ultrasound who turn out not to have ovarian cancer) is high, perhaps as high as 80%. Many of the cancers detected by ultrasound screening are of the better prognostic variety (and would have likely remained localized to the ovary even if the diagnosis had been made without screening). Some cancers, mostly those that carry a poor prognosis, are missed by ultrasound screening. The British have conducted a study on approximately 20,000 women using pelvic ultrasound in conjunction with CA-125. They found that women diagnosed with ovarian cancer while undergoing screening lived longer than women with ovarian cancer who were not screened. However, a significant difference in long-term survival was not detected, though there appeared to be a trend toward lower mortality in the screened group. A much larger study is presently under way, which will hopefully definitively answer the question regarding the use of a combined serum CA-125 and ultrasound as a valuable screening tool. It is important to note that these studies are generally performed on postmenopausal women because they are far less likely than premenopausal women to have false-positive CA-125 or ultrasound readings.

At present, screening is offered to women at markedly increased risk of ovarian cancer because they carry a genetic mutation associated with a high likelihood of development of ovarian cancer. For the general population, ovarian cancer screening has not so far been proven to be beneficial in reducing the mortality from this disease. Modalities other than CA-125 and ultrasound, such as serum proteomics (a technique whereby serum is "fingerprinted" to identify its protein signature to look for patterns highly suggestive of ovarian cancer), are under investigation and show promise.

TREATMENT

If a woman is suspected to have ovarian cancer on the basis of her diagnostic evaluation, referral to a gynecologic oncologist is necessary. This specialist who is highly trained in the management of ovarian cancer will optimize both the surgical and chemotherapeutic management of the patient. It is extremely important that the initial surgery be performed in a fashion that can optimize chances for survival. In women with apparently early tumors, it is key that a complete "staging" procedure be done to look for hidden sites of disease that are not obvious to the naked eye. This involves biopsies at multiple sites of the intra-abdominal lining and of strategic lymph nodes. Microscopic metastases (clusters of tumor cells that have spread to other parts of the body) to these structures have been reported to occur in up to 30% of individuals whose disease appears limited to the ovary. Detection of such metastases would lead to a different, more aggressive, treatment plan. For women with disease that has already metastasized, the goal of the initial surgery is to remove as much of the disease as possible, because the amount of disease remaining at the end of surgery has consistently been shown to affect outcome. This surgery can be extremely challenging and requires both the technical skill and judgment that come with experience from

treating ovarian cancer. It has been shown that the outcome of the initial surgery is clearly improved when a gynecologic oncologist is involved, as compared to a general gynecologist or a general surgeon. In some cases, it may be advisable to delay the surgery and use chemotherapy first to contain the disease because the patient is so weakened by the cancer that a large surgery is too risky.

Once a diagnosis has been made, chemotherapy is usually, but not always, necessary. The initial chemotherapeutic approach involves the use of two agents, called carboplatin and paclitaxel. These agents are usually given in an outpatient setting over approximately 5–6 hr. Generally 3–6 courses of chemotherapy are given (depending on how advanced the initial disease was), 3 weeks apart. After chemotherapy is complete, some women who had advanced disease may benefit from a second operation referred to as second-look, to try to ascertain whether the disease is no longer evident. Frequently, after the initial six cycles of chemotherapy, consolidation chemotherapy with paclitaxel alone is recommended for women who initially had advanced disease, to try to optimize outcome. While the majority of women respond well to chemotherapy eventual relapses are common. There are a variety of agents available to treat women with recurrent ovarian cancer, but cure after recurrence is extremely rare. The goal of treatment in the recurrent situation is to lengthen life (and hopefully preserve quality of life) for as long as possible.

SEE ALSO: Cancer, Hysterectomy

Suggested Resources

www.lynnecohenfoundation.org

LYNDA D. ROMAN

Ovarian Cyst An ovarian cyst is a fluid-filled sac that can occur within or on the surface of the ovary. Many women will develop an ovarian cyst at some time during their lives. Most cysts are benign (not cancerous), not dangerous, resolve on their own, and require no treatment. Ovarian cysts are generally painless, causing discomfort only if they twist, rupture, or bleed.

Most ovarian cysts result from hormonal changes that occur during the menstrual cycle. A follicular cyst results when a follicle that is produced in the ovary each month, does not release its egg and continues to grow until it forms a cyst. These cysts usually do not cause pain, and usually disappear without treatment after several months. A corpus luteum cyst occurs in the ovary after an egg is released. The small cyst that contained the egg seals off and tissue and fluid collect inside. This cyst usually disappears on its own, but can become large, may bleed into itself, and can cause pelvic pain. It may also rupture causing severe pain and internal bleeding.

An ovarian cyst may be detected on pelvic examination or during a pelvic ultrasound. A pelvic ultrasound uses sound waves to image the internal organs. A cyst that only contains fluid tends to be benign and unless it is very large requires no treatment. A cyst that contains more solid components usually requires further evaluation.

There are several other common types of ovarian cysts. A dermoid cyst may contain different tissues, such as hair, fat, and even teeth. They are almost always benign, but they can become very large, and can actually twist or torse causing pain. These cysts usually require surgical removal. Another common cyst is an endometrioma that usually occurs in women who have the condition "endometriosis," where uterine lining cells grow outside the uterus. Endometriomas may become large and painful, requiring surgical treatment. Cystadenomas come from the ovarian tissue itself, and may be filled with fluid or mucus-like material. They may also become very large.

The majority of ovarian cysts are benign. There are several factors that can help predict whether or not a cyst is cancerous. The first is the size of the cyst. Very large cysts, usually greater than 9 or 10 cm, are less likely than small cysts to resolve spontaneously. If a cyst has a large number of solid components, or separations or septations, this may also be a sign of malignancy. A postmenopausal woman who develops an ovarian cyst is less likely to have a benign cyst than is a reproductive-age woman.

The treatment of an ovarian cyst depends upon the type and size of the cyst, and the woman's age. Small cysts that are purely fluid-filled and less than 4 or 5 cm may be observed for 1–3 months and will usually resolve without treatment. Women who have a tendency to develop functional cysts are sometimes placed on oral contraceptives, which can prevent new cyst formation. In older women a cyst usually requires surgical evaluation. Surgery may also be required if a cyst is large, has solid components, is growing, or is causing pain. When ovarian cysts do require further assessment, they can usually be evaluated and treated with laparoscopic surgery, in which a narrow, telescope-like instrument is used to visualize the pelvic organs. Additional surgical instruments are placed through small incisions to perform the surgery. This is usually done under general anesthesia. Very large cysts or cysts that are more suspicious for cancer may require more extensive surgery.

SEE ALSO: Endometriosis, Laparoscopy

KAREN L. ASHBY

Pacemaker Therapy The heart is a unique structure in the human body in that it combines both mechanical and electrical properties in the same cell. Normal electrical function in the heart includes the firing of a dominant pacemaker, an area of heart tissue that initiates heartbeat. The dominant pacemaker is usually in the area of the heart called the sinus node, which is located in the right atrium (one of four chambers of the heart: two atria and two ventricles). The pacemaker generates a resting heart rate between 60 and 100 beats per minute. This dominant impulse is then transmitted throughout the heart by a wiring system called the auriculoventricular (AV) node and His–Purkinje fibers, which carries the impulse down into the ventricles, resulting in synchronized contraction of the cardiac chambers for optimal performance. When problems occur in this system, it is possible to implant a man-made pacemaker to replace the heart's own intrinsic pacemaker function.

Pacemakers have undergone a remarkable evolution since their initial implantation in 1958. The first pacemaker was a primitive device by today's standards, a ventricular pacemaker used for patients with Stokes–Adams attacks (passing out or syncopal spells due to complete heart block with slow or absent pulse). Since then, pacemakers have evolved into devices of great technical sophistication. As of 2001, more than 500,000 patients have received pacemakers, and up to 115,000 new devices are implanted each year in the United States alone. Today's permanent pacemakers can be programmed to perform complex functions, allowing clinicians to meet patients' specific clinical needs and also to optimize hemodynamic (blood flow

and blood pressure) support. Depending on the patient's specific diagnosis, the cardiologist may elect to place a single- or dual-chamber pacemaker either in the right atrium, right ventricle, or both. It is even possible now to place a so-called biventricular pacemaker, which can stimulate both the right and the left ventricles and can improve cardiac performance in patients with heart failure under certain circumstances.

TEMPORARY AND PERMANENT PACEMAKERS

Temporary pacemakers are used only in the hospital to support patients who require temporary and intermittent support due to various degrees of heart block. The goal for the use of temporary pacemakers is the resolution of the indication (heart block) or the implantation of a permanent pacemaker. Permanent pacemakers, as the name indicates, are placed for permanent cardiac rhythm dysfunction and various degrees of heart block.

Indication

The indications for permanent pacemaker can be summarized according to the American College of Cardiology/American Heart Association published guidelines.

Complete Heart Block

Where there is no electrical communication between atria (upper chambers) and ventricles (lower chambers). Patients will require a pacemaker in this situation regardless of whether or not they have symptoms.

Second-Degree Heart Block

Where there is some synchrony (timing compatibility) between atria and ventricles, but it is not constant (or 1:1) like the normal heart. If patients have symptoms due to this conduction disturbance, they will require a pacemaker. For asymptomatic patients, a pacemaker may be required after further evaluation by a cardiologist.

Sinus Pause

When the heart's sinus node fails to fire at a regular and expected interval and the pause is longer than 3.0 s or the heart rate is less than 40 beats/min.

Syncope ("Passing Out")

If patients "pass out" due to carotid sinus hypersensitivity (excessive excitability of heartbeat-generating tissue in the carotid artery) or due to recurrent cardiogenic (from the heart tissue) syncope despite optimal medical therapy, a pacemaker is indicated.

PACEMAKER IMPLANTATION AND FOLLOW-UP INSTRUCTIONS

Pacemaker implantation is done in a designated aseptic radiation theater (procedure room) by an experienced cardiac electrophysiologist (heart conduction specialist) or, in some cases, by a cardiac surgeon. The majority of pacemaker generators are placed in a subcutaneous "pocket" underneath the skin in the right or the left (depending on whether the patient is left or right handed) pectoral region. The leads are inserted via the cephalic or the subclavian veins (veins located in the chest/neck area) and are advanced under fluoroscopic (x-ray) guidance into the right atrium and/or right ventricle, depending on the pacemaker mode. The patient is treated with broad-spectrum antibiotics periprocedurally (before the procedure). The patient is subsequently monitored for 24 hr in the hospital. A chest x-ray and 12-lead electrocardiogram (EKG) are obtained postprocedure. The patient is then discharged home with restrictions on activity and follow-up appointments to check the wound site and pacemaker function.

Patients in general are recommended to stay away from electromagnetic fields, arc welding, large stereos, and chain saws. When passing through security checkpoints at airports, patients are instructed to inform the security personnel about the pacemaker, in order to limit the time spent in antitheft entrances. Scanning wands and cell phones must be kept at a distance of more than 6 in. away from the pacemaker. Patients cannot undergo magnetic resonance imaging (MRI) scans with a pacemaker, and therefore alternative imaging is required, depending on the clinical condition. Device-specific questions for home and work are made available to the patient via manufacturers' booklets. Moreover, patients are instructed to carry a pacemaker identification card at all times.

Placing a magnet over the pacemaker resets the device. The magnet can be left in place over the pacemaker in order to provide continuous pacing without sensed input under specific circumstances, such as when the patient is undergoing surgery and a cautery device is being used.

COMPLICATIONS OF PACEMAKER IMPLANTATION

Potential complications include pneumothorax (air in the chest), hemothorax (blood in the chest), ventricular puncture leading to hemorrhage, lead displacement or fracture, infection, and problems with pacing and sensing inappropriately. Many problems due to inappropriate sensing and pacing (both under- and oversensing and pacing) can be corrected by placing the pacemaker programming device over the pacemaker and changing the settings as appropriate. Excision of the pacemaker is required only for physical problems with the leads (such as displacement or fracture) and battery change at the pacemaker's end of life. Pacemaker batteries are now extremely energy efficient and can last 10 years or more without requiring replacement.

WOMEN AND PACEMAKERS

The indications and management of pacemakers are generally the same for female patients as compared to the general population. No extra follow-up is needed during pregnancy, as long as the patient is not on any antiarrhythmic medications (medications used to treat abnormal heart rate/rhythm). Routine pacemaker checkup is strongly recommended even for asymptomatic and uneventful pregnancies.

SEE ALSO: Cardiovascular disease, Pregnancy

Suggested Reading

Braunwald, E., Zipes, D. P., & Libby, P. (Eds.). (2001). *Heart disease. A textbook of cardiovascular medicine* (6th ed., Chapter 24). Philadelphia: W.B. Saunders.

Gregoratos, G., Cheitlin, M., Conill, A., et al. (1998). ACC/AHA guidelines of cardiac pacemakers and anti-arrhythmia devices: A report of the ACC/AHA task force on practice guidelines (Committee on Pacemaker Implantation). *Circulation, 97,* 1325–1335.

Suggested Resources

General pacemaker information for patients and physicians is available on the Internet at www.medtronic.com

KAMALA TAMIRISA
CLAIRE DUVERNOY

Pain Persons perceive pain when their internal environment is threatened. Threats may occur from a variety of sources. Pain receptors are present in the skin, connective tissue, blood vessels, bony surface, and most organs. A major exception is the brain where pain is sensed rather than originated.

Stimuli exiting these pain receptors travel from distant surfaces and tissues by nerves first to the spinal cord and up to the brain. Once signals enter the brain, they stop in a central relay station, the thalamus. Here, the quality and severity of the pain is realized. Within the thalamus, pain is recognized but not located. Localizing pain requires transmission from the thalamus to the map of the body surface located in the cerebral cortex. Surface pain is referred to the region or its origin. Organ pain is referred to various areas on the body surface sometimes creating confusion in finding the source of the pain. Some examples of referred organ pain include left arm and jaw pain with heart attack and right shoulder pain from gallbladder disease.

Pain also occurs when the brain loses some or all sensation to portions of the body. Injury to peripheral nerves from trauma, infection, or toxins often results in permanent sensory loss and pain. A common example occurs in diabetes where nerve injury in the feet results in incessant pain. Even after removal of an arm or leg, phantom limb pain may persist.

Pain resulting from nerve injury, neuropathic pain, may assume several qualities. Descriptions of incessant burning and tingling, parathesias, commonly are associated with nerve injury or removal. Intermittent stabbing pains, neuralgias, may occur in the face, trigeminal neuralgia, or back of head, greater occipital neuralgia. Nerve compression in the back commonly caused by degeneration of the spine causes intermittent stabbing pain that radiates from the thigh to foot, sciatica.

Injury to nerves in the arms and legs may result in persistent pain syndromes that clearly are in excess of the degree of nerve involvement. Heightened sensitivity of the sympathetic pathways (a part of the nervous system called the autonomic nervous system) results in a regional pain syndrome. Multiple classifications of these pain disorders exist.

Complex regional pain syndromes commonly involve the hand more than the foot. Burning, overly sensitive, and spreading pain throughout the limb are common characteristics. The dysfunctional sympathetic nervous system also causes swelling in the affected limb, skin changes with loss of hair and nail changes, overactive sweating, thinning of the underlying bone, coolness to touch, and bluish discoloration.

Pain that does not result from either an environmental threat or disruption of nerve pathways is currently designated idiopathic, cause unknown. Migraine headaches until recently dwelled within this group. Painful diagnoses still classified as idiopathic include tension headache and fibromyalgia. Depression is uncommonly the solitary cause for regional pain. Alternative diagnoses must be excluded prior to assigning a diagnosis of psychogenic pain. Even when a strong psychogenic component is evident, an exhaustive search for the root cause of the pain must be completed.

Understanding the cause of a person's pain should be the first step in care. An attempt to find and eliminate or lessen the pain's origin is essential. Patients with pain often have associated depression. This component must be addressed separately from the root source of the pain. Lack of clear separation of the emotional from the physical component may interfere in both communication and treatment.

Treatment of pain can be divided into several arenas: (a) medical, (b) surgical, and (c) behavioral. Medical management stresses pharmacologic intervention.

Surgical therapy includes both peripheral and central nervous system procedures along with implantation of analgesic pumps. Behavioral therapies include modalities such as biofeedback, exercise, and meditation.

Pain-reducing medications abound including both prescription and over-the-counter analgesics. Acetaminophen, aspirin, and nonsteroidal anti-inflammatory drugs (NSAIDs) are the most commonly used pain relievers. These over-the-counter (available without prescription) remedies are appropriate for pain caused by irritations from the environment. These medications interfere in the inflammatory cascade that is commonly engaged at sites of tissue injury.

Analgesic medications unfortunately can cause toxicity. Acetaminophen, the active ingredient in Tylenol, is the commonest cause of accidental liver failure. Daily doses of 3–4 g and solitary doses of more than 200 mg/kg can proceed to death from liver injury. Aspirin predisposes to hearing loss, kidney failure, and significant upper intestinal irritation and ulceration. NSAIDs, similar to aspirin, inhibit the normal protective coating of the stomach and upper small intestine. The stomach's acid irritates and destroys the lining predisposing to ulcer formation. Kidney failure from NSAIDs is also a concern.

Opiates, one type of prescription analgesics, have been used for both recreational and medicinal purposes for several milleniums. These medications produce a sense of euphoria relieving pain of all types. Morphine, codeine, oxycodone, meperidine, fentanyl, and hydromorphone are some of the commonly available forms. Administration can occur by most methods imaginable including by mouth (oral), across skin (transdermal), through injection into veins (intravenous) or muscle (intramuscular), by inhalation, or through placement in the rectum by suppository. Electronic pumps are available that can be implanted under the skin for direct administration into the fluid surrounding (intrathecal) or space directly surrounding (epidural) the central nervous system.

Adverse effects abound with opioid use. Common side effects include nausea, constipation, and a feeling of uneasiness, dysphoria. Escalating doses lead to confusion, sleepiness, and depressed breathing. Tachyphylaxis, failing effectiveness over time, and dependence commonly develop with use in excess of several weeks. These effects are caused by changes within the central nervous system with increasing number of pain receptors being produced in response to chronic stimulation. If a person is thought to be dependent on narcotic analgesics, the patient's pain management program should be reviewed.

Additional agents may complement opiates, acetaminophen, and NSAIDs. Anticonvulsants including carbamazepine, oxcarbazepine, and gabapentin may be used predominately when pain stems from a nerve injury. Conditions with predominant neuropathic pain (pain related to nerve damage) include trigeminal neuralgia (a disease of a facial nerve), reflex sympathetic dystrophy (disease of the autonomic nervous system), painful polyneuropathies (damage to multiple nerves), and all forms of nerve root irritation including postherpetic pain from shingles (nerve damage that sometime occurs after herpesvirus infection).

Tricyclic antidepressant medications including amitriptyline and nortriptyline act as enhancers or adjuvants to opiates for pain relief. These antidepressant compounds act by blocking the reuptake after release of the neurotransmitters serotonin and norepinephrine in the brain. Newer antidepressants classified as selective serotonin reuptake inhibitors (SSRIs) do not seem as effective as their predecessors. The older agents also cause drowsiness that may be desirable when sleep is disturbed by pain.

Corticosteroids such as prednisone affect pain related to local tissue injury similar to the NSAIDs. Additional benefits include increased energy and euphoria. However, significant side effects exist especially with prolonged use. Diabetes mellitus, thinning of bone (osteoporosis), central obesity, high blood pressure, and gastrointestinal irritation are among the most common and serious treatment-related complications. Careful surveillance for ill effects related to corticosteroid use is essential when prolonged use is necessary.

Several ointments also relieve pain. Liniments have been used for generations to alleviate joint and muscular pain. Topical capsaicin ointment was developed to relieve superficial burning pain. This ointment derived from hot peppers releases and eventually depletes the stores of the pain-producing neurotransmitter, substance P, from nerve terminals. Initial use, unfortunately, temporarily increases pain. Premature abandonment of this effective therapy is common. Lidocaine ointment and sprays are available providing local relief of painful skin and mucosal surfaces.

Surgical procedures to alleviate pain are available. Regional blockade through injection of local anesthetics along with corticosteroids into joints and the epidural space can reduce pain significantly. Cutting peripheral nerves or the sensory root involved in pain may be used in refractory cases. However, the pain that is relieved may be replaced by additional regional pain after normal sensation from that region is reduced or eliminated. Central nervous system operations for pain are usually reserved until all other mechanisms for pain relief have been eliminated. Cutting specific pain tracts within the spinal cord or destroying pain regions in the thalamus have been used successfully.

Other pain-modifying procedures also may be used. Electrical impulses applied to the skin surface may alleviate regional pain. The mechanism of action is believed to be mediated through pain gates that are blocked when the impulses occur. Acupuncture, cool and warm compresses, massage, and vibration are thought to act by a similar mechanism.

Vigorous exercise relieves pain through central mechanisms. Internal neurotransmitters, encephalins and endorphins, released by exercise are believed to lessen pain by binding to opiate receptors. Psychic distraction in the form of meditation, biorhythm training, or prayer may also lessen pain both during and following the activity.

SEE ALSO: Arthritis, Cancer, Depression, Headache, Pregnancy

Suggested Reading

Battista, E. M. (2002). The assessment and management of chronic pain in the elderly. A guide for practice. *Advance Nurse Practitioner, 10*(11), 28–32.

Bernstein, R. M. (2001). Injections and surgical therapy in chronic pain. *Clinical Journal of Pain, 17*(S4), S94–S104.

Frank, A. O., & DeSouza, L. H. (2001). Conservative management of low back pain. *International Journal of Clinical Practice, 55*(1), 21–31.

Hoffert, M. J. (1989). The neurophysiology of pain. *Neurology Clinics, 7*(2),183–203.

Leland, J. Y. (1999). Chronic pain: Primary care treatment of the older patient. *Geriatrics, 54*(1), 23–28, 33–34, 37.

Reid, M. C., Engles-Horton, L. L., Weber, M. B., Kerns, R. D., & Rogers, E. L. (2002). Use of opioid medications for chronic non-cancer pain syndromes in primary care. *Journal of General Internal Medicine, 17*(3), 173–179.

Salerno, S. M., Browning, R., & Jackson, J. L. (2002). The effect of antidepressant treatment on chronic back pain: A meta-analysis. *Archives of Internal Medicine, 162*(1), 19–24.

JOSEPH P. HANNA

Panic Attack   A panic attack is intense fear in the absence of real danger, which lasts for a period of time (usually 10–30 minutes) and then stops. The fear is accompanied by at least four of the following symptoms: (a) heart racing, pounding, or skipping beats, (b) sweating, (c) trembling or shaking, (d) difficulty breathing, (e) feeling of choking, (f) chest pain, (g) nausea or upset stomach, (h) dizziness, (i) a sense that the external world is strange or unreal (derealization), or a sensation of detachment from one's own body or experience (depersonalization), (j) fear of losing control or "going crazy," (k) fear of dying, (l) odd sensations (pins and needles, tingling, or numbness in parts of the body), or (m) chills or hot flushes. Panic attacks come on suddenly and rise to a peak within about 10 minutes.

Panic attacks are the main feature of panic disorder, but they can also occur in other conditions such as posttraumatic stress disorder. Attacks can come daily, weekly, or at longer intervals, and may come in bursts of more frequent attacks with attack-free periods in between. Some people become afraid of having a panic attack in public or somewhere that may be difficult or embarrassing to escape from. This can develop into agoraphobia, in which public places are avoided or endured only with extreme anxiety.

Panic attacks are real. Panic attacks happen when the body's "fight or flight" response is activated even when there is no real danger. Adrenalin is released into the bloodstream, so an attack feels real—and biochemically, it *is* real. Someone having a panic attack feels that something terrible is happening or that she is going to die. A natural response is to try to figure out why she feels this way. A person suffering from panic attacks may believe that the attacks indicate an undetected life-threatening illness, and may not be reassured by repeated medical evaluation. She may change her behavior to avoid places and situations that trigger the attacks. She may fear that panic attacks mean that she is "going crazy." Panic attacks are not caused by weak character. While one part of the brain may understand that "this is only a panic attack," another part of the brain is convinced that there is imminent danger.

Panic disorder consists of recurrent unexpected panic attacks followed by at least 1 month of persistent concern about having another panic attack, worry about what the attack means, or behavioral change as a result of the attacks. To diagnose panic disorder, the panic attacks cannot be caused by another condition such as hyperthyroidism, excessive caffeine intake, drug use (cocaine or amphetamines), alcohol withdrawal, or another mental disorder. Symptoms like loss of consciousness, loss of bladder or bowel control, slurred speech, loss of memory are not typical of panic disorder and suggest there must be another underlying condition.

A person who only has panic attacks in one or a few specific situations probably has a different disorder. For example, social phobia is a disorder in which panic attacks are caused by social situations such as attending a party. Posttraumatic stress disorder involves panic attacks that are triggered by events that bring a previous traumatic experience to mind. Panic attacks can also be caused by medical conditions such as asthma, hyperthyroidism, and others. There are no laboratory tests that diagnose panic attacks or panic disorder, but laboratory tests can help rule out underlying causes of panic attacks.

Between 0.5% and 1.5% of the population has panic disorder in any given year. It usually begins between the late teens and mid-30s. Panic disorder is twice as common in women than men. It affects all ethnic groups. Having a close relative with panic disorder raises the chance of developing panic disorder, but most people with panic disorder do not actually have affected family members. Compared to the general population, people with panic disorder have higher rates of depression and other anxiety disorders at some time in their life. A person with panic attacks may self-treat the intense anxiety with alcohol or other drugs, and can develop a substance-abuse problem as a result.

Untreated, panic disorder can continue for years. Fortunately, treatment is available that can help almost everyone with panic attacks. Antidepressant medications (either tricyclics or selective serotonin reuptake inhibitors) reduce or eradicate symptoms but may take a few weeks to work. Valium-type medications (benzodiazepines) work immediately, but have more side effects and can be addicting. Sometimes a benzodiazepine will be used for a few days or weeks along with an antidepressant until the antidepressant takes effect. Talking therapies are also effective, but may take longer to work. Cognitive–behavioral therapy for panic disorder is the best studied, but other kinds of therapy may work too. Treatment of agoraphobia (fear of open or public places) may involve careful exposure to anxiety-provoking situations as part of the treatment. After the panic attacks are eliminated, medication is usually continued for a year or so to prevent relapses.

SEE ALSO: Anxiety disorders, Mood disorders, Phobia, Posttraumatic stress disorder, Substance use

Suggested Reading

Bemis, J., & Barrada, A. (1994). *Embracing the fear: Learning to manage anxiety and panic attacks.* Hazelden Information Education.

ALICIA M. WEISSMAN

Pap Smear *see* Pap Test

Pap Test

The Pap test, also called "Pap smear," was developed over fifty years ago. This test, in which cells are removed from the cervix and evaluated through a microscope, has dramatically decreased the number of cervical cancer deaths in this country. The Pap test can detect precancerous and cancerous changes of the cervix, allowing early detection and prevention of cervical cancer. How often women should be screened depends on age, history, and risk factors. Screening should start no later than age 21 years, and no later than 3 years after starting sexual activity. Cervical cancer is rare under age 25. Women who have had a total hysterectomy (removal of uterus and the cervix) may not require Pap smear screening if the surgery was for a benign condition. The Pap smear is currently our best screening test for cervical cancer.

The actual test itself can be performed during any part of the menstrual cycle, except during active (heavy) menses. A small brush and spatula are used to scrape cells from the inside and outside of the cervix. Usually this is not painful. The sample is then either placed in a glass slide or in a small jar. The cells are then looked at under a microscope (or by a computer). There are several new technologies that help improve the accuracy of the Pap test. One is the liquid-based, thin-layer slide preparation in which the cells are placed into a vial and the Pap smear is read from the slides that are prepared from this medium. This helps eliminate some of the air-drying artifact that can occur with a traditional slide preparation. There are also automated readers that utilize a microscope that sends images to a computer, which analyzes the slide for abnormal cells, eliminating some of the human error.

Pap smear results may be reported as normal, "ASCUS" (atypical squamous cells of undetermined significance), "AGUS" (atypical glandular cells of undetermined significance), low-grade SIL (squamous intraepithelial lesion), high-grade SIL, or cancer. Sometimes vaginal infections such as yeast, trichomonas, and bacterial vaginosis can be identified by Pap test.

Of all the Pap tests performed in this country, approximately 6% will be abnormal and require further evaluation. Significant abnormal results require evaluation with colposcopy. A colposcope is a tool that helps magnify the cervix and will usually demonstrate the area of the cervix where the abnormal cells are coming from. After visualization with a colposcope, abnormal areas are biopsied, which involves removing a small pinch of tissue from the cervix. This procedure can usually be done in the office, with minimal discomfort. An ECC (endocervical curettage), or scraping from the cervical canal, is often performed at this time. Mild abnormalities on Pap (including some cases of ASCUS) can be followed with frequent Pap testing, rather than immediate colposcopy. Recurrent abnormal findings should be evaluated with colposcopy.

The treatment depends on the biopsy results. Sometimes after the biopsy is performed, more frequent Pap smears are the only necessary follow-up. More serious abnormalities may require a minor surgical procedure to remove the abnormal cells. There are several ways in which this can be achieved. One method of treatment is a LEEP, or loop electrosurgical excision procedure, where a wire loop acts as a scalpel and removes the abnormal cells from the cervix. Another method called "cryotherapy" involves freezing the abnormal tissue and laser therapy involves using light beams to destroy the abnormal cells. Sometimes a procedure called a "conization," or cone biopsy, is required to remove a larger cone-shaped wedge of abnormal tissue with a scalpel or laser.

Many Pap smear abnormalities, particularly SIL or dysplasia, are related to a virus called human papillomavirus (HPV). HPVs are a family of hundreds of viruses that may also cause genital warts or warts on the hands and feet. There are hundreds of serotypes of HPV, but only a few are associated with cervical cancer. Most cervical cancers are preventable with regular screening.

Because the Pap smear is a screening test, it is not 100% accurate. Both "false-positive" and "false-negative" results may occur. A false-positive Pap smear means that a Pap test appears abnormal, but there is actually no underlying abnormality. A false-negative Pap test occurs when there is actually an abnormality and the Pap smear is reported as normal. One of the benefits of regular screening with Pap tests is that an abnormality that may initially not be detected can be identified with a subsequent test.

SEE ALSO: Cervical cancer, Colposcopy, Human papillomavirus, Pelvic examination, Trichomoniasis, Yeast infection

KAREN L. ASHBY

Parenting Parenting is a relatively new word about a very old topic—raising children. Parenting can be done by one or both biological parents, by adoptive parents, or by any other person who informally takes the place of a parent. The goal of parenting is to raise children to be happy, healthy adults who can think for themselves and make good choices in their lives. Good parenting requires self-control, consistency, and persistence. Most parents find that parenting is the most difficult and most rewarding job they ever do. A full description of effective parenting is beyond the scope of this book but many helpful guides are available at any library or bookstore.

Custody is a part of parenting that refers to the legal responsibility for a child. When parents separate from each other or divorce, or when parents live separately from their child, a judge usually decides who will have custody of the child. Judges who make decisions about custody often look closely at parenting issues. A judge will consider whom the child turns to when the child has problems and how the parent makes decisions about the child.

Parenting can also play a role in determination of parental fitness or termination of parental rights. Courts often become involved in families where there is abuse or neglect of a child. If the situation cannot be made safe for the child, the state takes custody of the child at least temporarily. If the parents cannot or will not work toward creating a healthy environment for their child, then the state could ultimately end the parents' legal connections with the child and allow the child to be adopted.

SEE ALSO: Adoption, Child care, Cohabitation, Day care, Divorce, Domestic partnership, Marital status

Suggested Reading

Brazelton, T. B., & Greenspan, S. (2000). *The irreducible needs of children: What every child must have to grow, learn, and flourish.* Cambridge, MA: Perseus.

Lyster, M. (1996). *Building parenting agreements that work.* Berkeley, CA: Nolo Press.

Peters, D., & Strom, R. (1997). *Divorce and child custody: Your options and legal rights.* Philadelphia: Chelsea House.

Watnik, W. (1997). *Child custody made simple.* Claremont, CA: Single Parent Press.

SHEILA SIMON

Parkinson's Disease

Parkinson's disease (PD) is a chronic neurodegenerative disorder of unknown cause, which typically affects people in middle to late life. Named for Dr. James Parkinson, who first described the disease over 180 years ago, PD needs to be distinguished from Parkinsonism, a descriptive term applied to various features of the disease. *Parkinsonism* applies to the syndrome of hand tremor, muscle stiffness, slowed body movements, and unsteady posture and gait. Parkinsonism can be caused by certain medications or illicit drugs, as a result of viral infection, secondary to a number of environmental exposures (insecticides, contaminated water supplies), or by PD. A diagnosis of PD implies that the Parkinsonism is of unknown cause, chronic and progressive in nature, and other prominent neurological dysfunctions are absent.

PD is newly diagnosed in approximately 5,000 Americans each year. It is believed to affect 1 million Americans and 1–2 per 1,000 people will likely develop the disease. The incidence of PD is expected to rise as the population continues to age. Two in 100 seniors over the age of 65 have the disease and perhaps up to 50% of those 85 and older meet criteria for the diagnosis. Disease onset is often between the ages of 55 and 65, and men are affected roughly 1.5 times as often as women. Less than 5% of all cases are in people under 40, with many such cases having a genetic link.

Nerve cells in the midbrain, which produce the neurotransmitters dopamine and norepinephrine, are known to degenerate in PD, although the reason for this is unclear. The decrement in these neurotransmitters yields decreased stimulation of the brain's motor cortex, and the resulting core symptoms of the disease.

Cardinal features of PD can be recalled using the mnemonic "TRAP"—tremor, rigidity, akinesia, and postural abnormalities. Patients typically exhibit a hand tremor at rest, often more pronounced unilaterally. Rigidity or stiffness of the arms, legs, and/or neck is quite common. Akinesia, the absence of spontaneous motor movements, or bradykinesia, a slowing of the body's overall motor activity, can be the most striking feature of the illness. Patients with PD may appear statue-like with expressionless faces, in the extreme. They frequently have postural abnormalities as well, such as impaired balance and unsteady gait. The presence of two or more such signs or symptoms make the diagnosis quite likely.

A number of other symptoms are common, including constipation, urinary incontinence, sexual dysfunction, difficulty swallowing, weakened speech, sleep disorders, and visual disturbances. Psychiatric illness is common as well, with depression and dementia each seen in approximately 40% of patients and psychosis in up to 10%. Half of all patients may experience pain as a result of their disease. Muscle or joint pains from abnormal posturing, headaches, gastrointestinal discomfort, and sleep-related discomfort are fairly common.

Treatment includes both lifestyle modification and medications. Patient and family education is essential. Routine exercise, dietary advice, a review of optimal sleep hygiene, and referral for physical, speech, or occupational therapy as indicated are also vital. Pharmacological treatments are focused on decreasing symptoms, enhancing mobility, slowing the progression of illness, and minimizing frequently encountered side effects. Commonly used medications aim to enhance the amount of dopamine receptor stimulation in the brain. This can be accomplished by (a) direct dopamine replacement (carbidopa/levodopa), (b) synthetic dopamine agents (bromocriptine, pergolide, ropinarole, and others), and (c) blocking the clearance of available dopamine (amantadine).

Potential side effects from such treatments include motor tics, delusional thinking, hallucinations (commonly visual), anxiety, restlessness and agitation, nausea, confusion, sedation, decreased blood pressure with an increased risk of falls, and other cardiac side effects. In treatment-refractory cases, neurosurgical procedures may be considered. Options include resection, or more recently, implantable electrode stimulation of different deep brain regions collectively known as the basal ganglia. A partial response or better is reported in up to 90% of patients with such procedures. However, potential complications include infection, hemorrhage, or stroke.

Limited evidence exists to support the role of medicines such as selegiline or vitamin E in prevention of PD. Estrogen replacement, which is known to modulate neurotransmission, may have an undefined role in preventing PD.

Parks, Rosa

SEE ALSO: Dementia, Depression

Suggested Reading

Aminoff, M. J. (2001). *Parkinson's disease and other extrapyramidal disorders.* (Harrison's Online, Pt. 14, sec. 2, chap. 363).

Hermanowicz, N. (2001). *Management of Parkinson's disease* (Postgraduate Medicine Online). New York: McGraw-Hill.

Kaufman, D. M. (2001). *Clinical neurology for psychiatrists.* Philadelphia: W.B. Saunders.

JOHN SANITATO

Parks, Rosa On December 1, 1955, when Rosa Parks climbed on board the bus in Montgomery, Alabama, she had no way of knowing that her actions that day would change a world, and later result in her being considered one of the founders of the civil rights movement.

Rosa Parks was born Rosa Louise McCauley on February 4, 1913, in Tuskegee, Alabama. At the time of her birth, Rosa's mother, Leona Edwards, was a school teacher dedicated to learning, from Pine Level and Rosa's father, James McCauley, was a carpenter and stonemason from Abbeville. After their marriage, the young couple moved to Tuskegee, the cultural center for blacks in the South. Tuskegee claims ties with many famous southern blacks; most notable are Booker T. Washington and George Washington Carver. Washington founded The Tuskegee Normal Industrial Institute, or simply the Tuskegee Institute. It was this cultural and social environment that Rosa Parks was born into, but she was not to live in Tuskegee for long. The McCauleys had to leave Tuskegee for economic reasons and moved back to Abbeville to live with James' parents. This caused the permanent separation of Rosa's parents when she was just 2 years old. Leona McCauley and Rosa moved back to Pine Level with Rosa's younger brother, Sylvester, to live with Leona's parents. Rosa spent her childhood in Pine Level, before moving to Montgomery in 1923 at the age of 10. In 1932, Rosa married Ray Parks, a barber by profession and an active civil rights activist. Two years later, Rosa Parks earned her high school diploma.

The bus incident was not Rosa's first introduction to activism. Rosa and Ray had long been active members of the National Association for the Advancement of Colored People (NAACP) and the St. Paul AME (African Methodist Episcopal) Church. Rosa had attended at least one lecture by Dr. Martin Luther King, Jr. Perhaps Rosa's introduction early in life to the cultural environment of Tuskegee or her later exposure to some of the finest activists of her time prepared her for her stand that December day on a Montgomery, Alabama bus. Rosa did not intend to become the catalyst who would change history that day; she was just a tired woman who was tired of being pushed around. Rosa did not sit in the all-white section, rather she sat in the neutral middle, where blacks could sit if there was no need for more white seats. When the bus driver asked the blacks seated in the middle section to move to the back of the bus to accommodate the whites who had just gotten on the bus, she refused. Rosa Parks was arrested and fined for violating a city ordinance.

Rosa's arrest and subsequent conviction charged the black civil rights movement. The weekend of Rosa's arrest, a meeting was called with leaders of the black community and the bus boycott was planned. On Monday, December 5, 1955, the 381-day Montgomery Bus Boycott started and the Montgomery Improvement Association was formed, with Dr. Martin Luther King, Jr., a newcomer to Montgomery, placed in charge. One week later, some 7,000 blacks rallied in protest of her conviction. In 1956, the United States District Court held that segregated buses were unconstitutional, a decision that the United States Supreme Court upheld. Rosa Parks remained active in civil rights. In 1980, Rosa became the first woman to receive the Martin Luther King Jr. Nonviolent Peace Prize. She also received the Presidential Medal of Freedom in 1996 and a Congressional Gold Medal in 1999.

SEE ALSO: Affirmative action, African American, Discrimination, United States Civil Rights Acts of 1964

Suggested Reading

Brandt, K. (1993). *Rosa Parks: Fight for freedom.* Mahwah, NJ: Troll Associates.

Brinkley, D. (2002). *Rosa Parks.* New York: Viking Penguin.

Felder, D. G. (1996). *The 100 most influential women of all time.* New York: Carol Publishing Group.

Nelson, G. (1993). *Rosa Parks: Hero of our time.* Cleveland, OH: Modern Curriculum Press.

Scholastic, Inc. (2003). *Rosa Parks: My story.* New York (July, 2003). http://teacher.scholastic.com/rosa

Siegel, B. (1992). *The year they walked: Rosa Parks and the Montgomery Bus Boycott.* New York: Four Winds Press.

Time Online Edition. (2003). *The 100 most influential people of the 20th century.* The Torchbearer: Rosa Parks (July, 2003). http://www.time.com/time/time100/heroes/profile/parks01.html

TAMBRA K. CAIN

Patients' Rights The mystique of medicine and technology combined with an innate desire to maintain the well-being of our bodies has led us to grant a tremendous amount of power to both health care providers and the insurance industry. Health care providers carry an acquired knowledge of corporeal mechanics and the insurance industry holds the purse strings for health care spending. The patients who were the recipients of health care were left with little or no power to negotiate on their own behalf.

In 1972, I was witness to an example of this type of discrepancy in power. My position was that of a nurse's aide on the maternity ward of a small hospital. One evening I was in the room of a patient who had been admitted for a cesarean section that had been scheduled for the following morning. While I was present, the obstetrician entered the room, greeted the patient, and began a discussion that led me to believe that she had been following the patient throughout the pregnancy. The physician then directed me to expose the woman's abdomen in preparation for an examination. Once exposed, the very pregnant abdomen displayed two well-healed scars from previous surgical procedures. While looking at the scars, the physician said to the patient in a chastising tone, "what do you expect me to do with this?" as if to infer the surgical scars were an imposition. Without further comment, she (the physician) left the room. The patient was left lying in bed with a look that displayed some combination of horror, fear, embarrassment, and demoralization. I spent the remainder of the evening pondering over the patient's situation and was much relieved the next day when I saw her with her newborn child.

This and other stories with similar themes reflect a violation of patients' individual "rights." But what is a "right"? According to *Webster's New Universal Unabridged Dictionary*, a "right" can be defined as "… a just claim or title, whether legal, prescription or moral." The American Civil Liberties Union (ACLU) states that "rights give us dignity and protection; if we have a right to something we can insist on it without embarrassment." That patients have rights is surprising to some. The demanding force of the "baby boomer generation" has been instrumental in the establishment of rights to protect vulnerable citizens, including patients. Some patients have crossed an emotional line from being self-confident, independent persons to becoming dependent individuals who are at the mercy of the health care system. Patients have had little input into the framework and structure of the system they are now dependent on for delivering the remedies needed to reclaim their desired state of being.

In 1990, The Patient Self Determination Act was enacted as part of the Omnibus Budget Reconciliation Act of 1987. This law applies to all institutional providers that receive Medicare or Medicaid funding. The law is described in the text, *Health Law*: "The statute requires that each of those covered by the Act provide every patient with written information describing that person's rights under state law 'to make an informed decision concerning medical care, including the right to accept or refuse medical treatment or surgical treatment and the right to formulate advance directives'."

The Patient Self Determination Act has placed the health care provider and the health care recipient in a face-to-face position to address issues that deal with the mandates of the patient. Patients have the opportunity to define their values (as they relate to medical care), their quality of life preferences, and to whom the patient will entrust the position of surrogate for health care decision-making.

To make well-informed decisions regarding one's own health care, one must be knowledgeable about their own health issues. The major source of knowledge for a patient is the health care provider. The information that the health care provider has must be shared with the patient in language and at a level that the patient understands. This concept is the embodiment of the doctrine of informed consent. The importance and significance of this concept was stressed by The President's Commission for the Study of Ethical Problems in Medicine and Biomedical and Behavioral Research: Making Health Care Decisions, "ethically valid consent is a process of shared decision making based upon mutual respect and participation, not a ritual to be equated with reciting the contents of a form that details the risks of particular treatments. Its foundation is the fundamental recognition that adults are entitled to accept or reject health care interventions on the basis of their own personal values and in furtherance of their own personal goals." The American Hospital Association has developed a list of guidelines in support of patients' rights. Many hospitals throughout the United States have implemented these guidelines as part of their standard of care. This document was recently revised and renamed "The Patient Care Partnership" (see Exhibit 1).

Patients' rights are extensive and announced, acknowledged, and explained in several laws, including: The Rights of Minors; The Americans with Disabilities

Exhibit 1.

THE PATIENT CARE PARTNERSHIP: UNDERSTANDING EXPECTATIONS, RIGHTS, AND RESPONSIBILITIES

When you need hospital care, your doctor and the nurses and other professionals at our hospital are committed to working with you and your family to meet your health care needs. Our dedicated doctors and staff serve the community in all its ethnic, religious, and economic diversity. Our goal is for you and your family to have the same care and attention we would want for our families and ourselves.

The sections below explain some of the basics about how you can expect to be treated during your hospital stay. They also cover what we will need from you to care for you better. If you have questions at any time, please ask them. Unasked or unanswered questions can add to the stress of being in the hospital. Your comfort and confidence in your care are very important to us.

WHAT TO EXPECT DURING YOUR HOSPITAL STAY

- **High-quality hospital care.** Our first priority is to provide you the care you need, when you need it, with skill, compassion, and respect. Tell your caregivers if you have concerns about your care or if you have pain. You have the right to know the identity of doctors, nurses, and others involved in your care, as well as when they are students, residents, or other trainees.
- **A clean and safe environment.** Our hospital works hard to keep you safe. We use special policies and procedures to avoid mistakes in your care and keep you free from abuse or neglect. If anything unexpected and significant happens during your hospital stay, you will be told what happened and any resulting changes in your care will be discussed with you.
- **Involvement in your care.** You and your doctor often make decisions about your care before you go to the hospital. Other times, especially in emergencies, those decisions are made during your hospital stay. When they take place, making decisions should include:
  - *Discussing your medical condition and information about medically appropriate treatment choices.* To make informed decisions with your doctor, you need to understand several things:
    - The benefits and risks of each treatment.
    - Whether it is experimental or part of a research study.
    - What you can reasonably expect from your treatment and any long-term effects it might have on your quality of life.
    - What you and your family will need to do after you leave the hospital.
    - The financial consequences of using uncovered services or out-of-network providers.
  - Please tell your caregivers if you need more information about treatment choices.
  - *Discussing your treatment plan.* When you enter the hospital, you sign a general consent to treatment. In some cases, such as surgery or experimental treatment, you may be asked to confirm in writing that you understand what is planned and agree to it. This process protects your right to consent to or refuse a treatment. Your doctor will explain the medical consequences of refusing recommended treatment. It also protects your right to decide if you want to participate in a research study.
  - *Getting information from you.* Your caregivers need complete and correct information about your health and coverage so that they can make good decisions about your care. That includes:
    - Past illnesses, surgeries, or hospital stays.
    - Past allergic reactions.

○ Any medicines or diet supplements (such as vitamins and herbs) that you are taking.

○ Any network or admission requirements under your health plan.

— *Understanding your health care goals and values.* You may have health care goals and values or spiritual beliefs that are important to your well-being. They will be taken into account as much as possible throughout your hospital stay. Make sure your doctor, your family, and your care team know your wishes.

— *Understanding who should make decisions when you cannot.* If you have signed a health care power of attorney stating who should speak for you if you become unable to make health care decisions for yourself, or a "living will" or "advance directive" that states your wishes about end-of-life care, give copies to your doctor, your family, and your care team. If you or your family need help making difficult decisions, counselors, chaplains and others are available to help.

- **Protection of your privacy**. We respect the confidentiality of your relationship with your doctor and other caregivers, and the sensitive information about your health and health care that are part of that relationship. State and federal laws and hospital operating policies protect the privacy of your medical information. You will receive a Notice of Privacy Practices that describes the ways that we use, disclose, and safeguard patient information and that explains how you can obtain a copy of information from our records about your care.

- **Help preparing you and your family for when you leave the hospital**. Your doctor works with hospital staff and professionals in your community. You and your family also play an important role. The success of your treatment often depends on your efforts to follow medication, diet, and therapy plans. Your family may need to help care for you at home.

  You can expect us to help you identify sources of follow-up care and to let you know if our hospital has a financial interest in any referrals. As long as you agree we can share information about your care with them, we will coordinate our activities with your caregivers outside the hospital. You can also expect to receive information and, where possible, training about the self-care you will need when you go home.

- **Help with your bill and filing insurance claims**. Our staff will file claims for you with health care insurers or other programs such as Medicare and Medicaid. They will also help your doctor with needed documentation. Hospital bills and insurance coverage are often confusing. If you have questions about your bill, contact our business office. If you need help understanding your insurance coverage or health plan, start with your insurance company or health benefits manager. If you do not have health coverage, we will try to help you and your family find financial help or make other arrangements. We need your help with collecting needed information and other requirements to obtain coverage or assistance.

While you are here, you will receive more detailed notices about some of the rights you have as a hospital patient and how to exercise them. We are always interested in improving. If you have questions, comments, or concerns, please contact ———.

Note: Reprinted with permission of the American Hospital Association, copyright 2003.

Act; Title VII of the Civil Rights Act of 1964; The Rehabilitation Act of 1973; The Child Abuse Prevention and Treatment Act of 1974; The Public Health Service Act; The Uniform Determination of Death Act; and The Uniform Anatomical Gift Act. Under the Omnibus Budget Reconciliation Act of 1987, residents of long-term care facilities have listed among their rights the right to be free of physical and chemical restraints. This further reflects the multitude of rights that are in place to protect us as patients. An act that is currently being implemented is the Health Insurance Portability and Accountability Act, also known as the HIPAA privacy rule. This rule defines how to use and disclose the personal health information of the patient. In addition, the rule contains regulations that all health care providers must follow in order to comply with the protection of patient privacy.

SEE ALSO: Confidentiality, Durable power of attorney for health care, Informed consent, Living wills, Medical malpractice, Quality of life

Pedophilia

Suggested Reading

Annas, G. J. (1989). *The rights of patients. The basic ACLU guide to patients rights.* Carbondale: Southern Illinois University Press.

Fremgen, B. F. (2002). *Medical law and ethics.* Upper Saddle River, NJ: Prentice–Hall.

Furrow, B. R., et al. (Eds.). (2000). *Health law* (2nd ed.). Florence, KY: West.

Medicare and Medicaid programs: Survey certification and enforcement of skilled nursing facilities and nursing facilities—final rule. *Federal Register*, Vol. 59, November 10, 1994.

ANNE SIMPSON

Pedophilia The sexual molestation of a child is considered by many to be the most morally reprehensible act imaginable. The terms pedophile, child molester, perpetrator, and sex offender are often used interchangeably; they overlap and yet refer to distinct aspects of the behavior and the people who commit sexual acts with children. "Perpetrator" and "sex offender" are legal terms that refer to people who have been convicted of a sexual crime against a minor. "Child molester" is a social term that describes anyone who has sexually molested a child, regardless of legal status. Neither the legal nor the social definitions consider the eroticism of the person committing the behavior, that is, whether or not they are sexually attracted to children. Indeed, many sexual acts against children are committed by people who do not evidence a sexual attraction to children but who are motivated by other factors such as immaturity, opportunity, mental retardation, mental illness, or psychopathy. Most child molesters are male although female child molesters are reported in legal records. A significant number of the reported female molesters are accompanied and often directed by an adult male companion when they engage in the behavior in contrast to male child molesters who most frequently act alone.

The term "pedophilia" is a psychiatric diagnosis classified in the *Diagnostic and Statistical Manual of Mental Disorders* (DSM-IV-TR) as a sexual disorder or paraphilia. It is characterized by the following: (a) recurrent, intense sexually arousing fantasies, sexual urges, or behaviors involving sexual activity with a prepubescent child or children (generally age 13 years or younger) over a period of at least 6 months; (b) the person has acted on these sexual urges, or the sexual urges or fantasies cause marked distress or interpersonal difficulty; and (c) the person is at least age 16 years and at least 5 years older than the child or children. It does not include an individual in late adolescence involved in an ongoing sexual relationship with a 12- or 13- year old. While the DSM-IV-TR diagnosis specifies that the person has either acted on these urges or is distressed by them, many believe that actual touch or distress are not necessary components; that is, someone who has the recurrent intense urges but never acted on them nor been distressed by them, should still be considered a pedophile. Most pedophiles are male; as stated above, there are relatively few female child molesters and a very small percentage of those actually evidence a sexual attraction to children. However, all prevalence data are suspect because of the secrecy surrounding these behaviors.

Pedophiles typically report an attraction to children of a specific gender and age range. Those attracted to females usually prefer 8- to 10-year-old girls while those who prefer males usually seek out 11- to 13-year-old boys. A sexual attraction to young girls is more often reported than to young boys but this may reflect a greater reluctance to admit same-sex attraction. Some pedophiles are exclusively attracted to children while others profess a sexual attraction to adults as well. The stereotypic pedophile—single, shy, interpersonally awkward with adults, preferring to be in the company of children—certainly exists but is, by no means, the only presentation. Many pedophiles, particularly the nonexclusive type, marry, raise families, and function acceptably in an adult world. Incest offenders, those who engage in sexual behaviors with their own children, stepchildren, or other children with whom they function as a parental figure, may or not meet criteria for pedophilia. Those who do are most likely to have sexually transgressed with nonrelated children as well.

Once established, the sexual attraction to children is ever present although the frequency and strength of the urges and behavior may fluctuate with stress and opportunity. Opportunity may randomly present itself, such as a family with two children moving in next door, or it may be carefully orchestrated, such as the deliberate courtship of a woman with young children or the participation in a specifically youth-oriented event or activity.

Pedophiles may or may not be distressed by their sexual attraction to children. On one end of the continuum are those who seek each other out on the Internet, forming large networks to chat, trade child pornography, or hook up with children, and join societies

490

such as NAMBLA (North American Man–Boy Love Association) that promote sexual behaviors between adults and children. They profess the belief that it is a repressive society, not sexual contact, that harms children. On the other end are those who experience their urges as intrusive, unwanted, and "sick." They feel compelled to act upon these urges despite efforts to refrain and attempt to rationalize their behavior in order to reduce the internal conflict.

While cases of assault, rape, abduction, and murder of a child receive the most media attention, they represent a tiny fraction of the spectrum. Pedophiles are more likely to use psychological seduction rather than physical coercion to engage a child. This is often referred to as "grooming" and consists of a number of discussions and gentle touch designed to win over the child's trust and complicity in suggested sexual behaviors such as fondling, genital exposure, oral–genital contact, and viewing of pornography and posing naked for photos. Anal or vaginal penetration are less frequent behaviors. They are more difficult to accomplish and are less likely to be agreed upon by a child. When the sexual interaction falls short of penetration, pedophiles often rationalize that they are not harming the child because, in their eyes, the child has agreed to participate and may even experience emotional and physical pleasure from the contact.

For all of us, the awareness of sexual attraction begins in childhood and evolves over time. Boys and girls interact in a number of settings and discover an excitement and interest in the opposite or same sex as they enter puberty. Most of the time, their sexual interest is directed toward peers within a narrow age range (1 or 2 years on either side). Pedophiles also trace their urges back to adolescence when they first became aware that they were attracted to a much younger age group than were their peers. Some explored this with younger siblings or children in the neighborhood; others confined their longings to fantasy and masturbation. Many felt guilty and ashamed and prayed to have their urges taken from them. All knew that what they were feeling was wrong and went to great lengths to hide or disguise any outward demonstration of their feelings.

Fear of condemnation and punitive consequences keep even those desperate for help from seeking it. By the time most pedophiles are caught, they have been acting out with children for years. Reports concerning number of victims and acts vary from study to study. Meaningful statistics are difficult to ascertain. It appears, however, that the largest number of victims and acts per offender occurs with those who molest nonrelated males (median of 10.1 acts) as compared with those who molest nonrelated females (median of 1.4 acts).

The etiology of pedophilia is unclear. Theories range from regarding pedophilia as a normal variant of sexual development to seeing it as a deviant pathway of sexual attraction occurring at some critical juncture of sexual development. Efforts have been made to examine underlying neurobiological, neuropsychiatric, and hormonal abnormalities. Many investigators have focused on the presence of childhood sexual abuse in the histories of abusers as the central cause. While data do suggest a significant number (43–57%) of pedophiles were sexually abused as children, an equal number were not. Moreover, it is important to recognize that childhood molestation per se will not automatically lead any child victim to an adult life of offending behavior against children. The impact of childhood sexual abuse is multidetermined and includes factors such as the personality of the child victim, the environment in which he or she lives, the nature and type of abuse, the relationship to the abuser, and the reaction and care given to the victim.

Pedophilia is considered a chronic disorder and, as such, is not curable. Treatment efforts to eradicate the unwanted sexual attraction to children and substitute a socially acceptable interest in adults have not been successful. However, the intensity or strength of the urges can often be significantly reduced by use of medications. For a long time, testosterone-lowering medications such as Depo-Provera and Depo-Lupron have been used to suppress sexual drive. More recently the class of antidepressants that are selective serotonin reuptake inhibitors have been successfully used to lower sexual drive by increasing the levels of serotonin. By lessening the intensity of the drive or urge, these medications increase the pedophile's capacity to exercise self-control and to make use of therapeutic interventions. Cognitive–behavioral techniques done in group therapy settings have proven to be the most helpful in altering thinking patterns and preventing relapse. While ideally professionals treating pedophiles would like to develop a drug or a treatment intervention that would do away with the attraction to children altogether, ultimately it is the victimization of children, not the attraction to children, that must be addressed.

SEE ALSO: Incest, Sexual abuse

Suggested Reading

Abel, G., & Osborne, C. (1992). The paraphilias: The extent and nature of sexually deviant and criminal behavior. *Clinical Forensic Psychiatry, 15*, 675–687.

Cohen, L., & Galynker, I. (2002). Clinical features of pedophilia and implications for treatment. *Journal of Psychiatric Practice, 8*(5).

Fagan, P., Wise, T., Schmidt, C., & Berlin, F. (2002). Pedophilia. *Journal of the American Medical Association, 288*(19).

Zucker, K. (2002). Introduction to the special section on pedophilia: Concepts and controversy. *Archives of Sexual Behavior, 31*(6), 465–477.

CANDACE B. RISEN

Peer Relationships Peer relationships are among the most influential means of support for people of all ages and have critical implications for social behavior and development. Among the most commonly referenced peer relationships are friendships. Friendships are voluntary relationships that are rooted in common interests and experiences. In childhood, friendships contribute to the acquisition of social competencies and skills such as cooperation, negotiation, and compromise. Peer relationships often cultivate salient bonds among children and these are strengthened as children learn to communicate effectively with each other, share feelings, become sensitive to others' needs and concerns, and gain perspective on different points of view. Thus, peer relationships are not only critical to social development but also have significant implications across the life span.

Healthy peer relationships in childhood are believed to be the foundation of future success and positive adjustment in adolescence and adulthood. In fact, friendships and general popularity among peers allow children to develop intimate relationships with others. This intimacy often enables youth to cope more effectively with life's challenges, manage stress through supportive relationships, and acquire knowledge about close bonds with others. According to research, having approving and encouraging friendships during childhood is associated with increased life satisfaction, good academic adjustment, decreased depression, and increased self-worth. Further, individuals who reported having supportive friendships as children were less victimized by bullies in later youth. Thus, early peer relationships have significant implications for young people's social and behavioral outcomes.

Changes in peer relationships can also change individual behavior. Shifts may occur through a variety of mechanisms. For example, through imitation and modeling, peers may train each other to abide by or reject social conventions. Research suggests that youth associate with like-minded peers, but it is not clear if children choose peers who are already like themselves, or if they alter their behavior to be more consistent with their peers. Indeed, youth may conform to each other's belief systems to win acceptance and approval or they may seek out peers with similar values and beliefs. For example, children with high-achieving, studious friends may be influenced to become more invested in their schoolwork, or youth who use illegal substances may seek out peers who also engage in drug and alcohol use. Peer influence increases with child age, but evidence indicates that parents remain important confidants during adolescence. Peer influences can be short lived or may persist throughout development depending on the amount of time peers spend together and the extent to which they are involved in each other's lives. Peers who spend little time together have less impact on each other.

Poor outcomes have been found among youth whose early peer relationships were problematic. Superficial peer affiliations among children diminish attachment to others and fuel loneliness, which may have deleterious effects on children's self-worth and self-perception. Children who experience social isolation and detachment tend to be rejected by their peers because they are coy, withdrawn, or even aggressive. These behaviors interfere with acquiring the necessary social skills to establish successful and meaningful relationships. A cyclical pattern emerges whereby children's socially inappropriate behavior interferes with establishing meaningful friendships, and then the absence of meaningful friendships diminishes these children's opportunities to interact with others in order to develop more effective social skills. Research indicates that as these children mature, they continue to show important skill deficits and have difficulty fitting into mainstream peer cultures. Furthermore, these children have significant adjustment problems in adolescence and adulthood.

Despite the absence of meaningful positive social interactions with peers, these youth seek out friends and as a result often affiliate with other rejected youth who have similar social deficits. These affiliations pose a significant problem, because they are based on similar experiences of social rejection, marginalization, and alienation. Youth who come together as a function of social rejection and alienation from mainstream culture are at elevated risk for poor outcomes (e.g., delinquency, substance use). For example, children who bully and fight with peers are typically rejected and turn to youth with similar behavior patterns. As these children mature, they may engage in more serious problem behaviors (e.g., fighting with weapons, selling drugs). Thus, the peer group that was founded on a common experience of marginalization may transform into a group of delinquent adolescents (e.g., gang). These networks then reinforce each other through deviant social skills that further contribute to their maladjustment. Indeed, delinquent peer influences are among the most significant predictors of antisocial behavior among adolescents.

In sum, peer relationships contribute in significant ways to the development of social competencies, individual functioning, the capacity for intimacy, and the formation of healthy adult relationships. Youth who experience social rejection and problematic relationships are at elevated risk for behavioral and emotional maladjustment.

SEE ALSO: Adolescence, Youth

Suggested Reading

Asher, S. R., & Coie, J. D. (Eds.). (1990). *Peer rejection in childhood.* Cambridge, UK: Cambridge University Press.

Bukowski, W. M., Newcomb, A. F., & Hartup, W. W. (1996). *The company they keep: Friendship in childhood and adolescence.* Cambridge, UK: Cambridge University Press.

Dishion, T. J., McCord, J., & Poulin, F. (1999). When interventions harm: Peer groups and problem behavior. *American Psychologist, 54,* 755–764.

Erwin, P. (1993). *Friendship and peer relations in children.* New York: John Wiley & Sons.

Schneider, B. (2000). *Friends and enemies.* London: Arnold.

Weisfeld, G. E. (1999). *Evolutionary principles of human adolescence.* New York: Basic Books.

KRISTI JORDAN
GERI R. DONENBERG

Pelvic Examination The pelvic examination is the most important part of the overall gynecologic exam. While the examiner must think about the whole patient, the purpose of the pelvic exam is to screen for abnormalities of the cervix, pelvic masses, including abnormalities of the patient's uterus, fallopian tubes, and ovaries as well as observing any abnormalities in pelvic support structures. At its best, the pelvic exam should be performed in a thoughtful, compassionate manner, instilling in the patient a sense of trust, which should never be violated. At its worst, the thoughtless, hurried examiner can traumatize the patient and cause anxiety about the examination that will never be overcome. This trust should weigh heavy on the examiner's thoughts while performing this important aspect of the gynecologic exam.

With the woman fully clothed, the examiner should first describe what will happen during the examination, since people tend to retain more information in this setting. Once the patient has been examined in the sitting and lying position from the head to the abdomen, the patient places her feet in the exam table's stirrups, which are ideally covered with stirrup warmers (this is termed the lithotomy position). The examiner now sits in front of the patient with a suitable flexible light source and appropriately drapes the patient, covering her except for her vaginal area. Prior to introducing the previously warmed speculum (which comes in a variety of sizes, see Figure 1), the examiner should inspect the external anatomy for any abnormality, including the lower abdomen, the external genitalia including the folds of the vaginal opening, the hymen, and the pubic hair area. The examiner should explain to the patient during and prior to each step what he or she is doing and why. Separating the opening of the vagina, the examiner should continue to inspect the anatomy including the urethral opening, the area between the

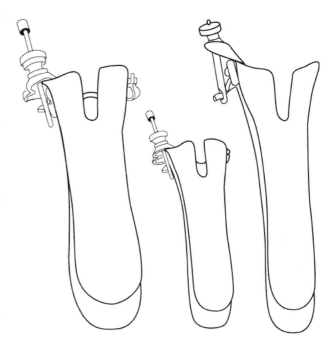

Figure 1. Various sizes of the speculum. (Courtesy: Illustration drawn by Ginny Canady, Director of Audio/Video Resources, Department of Obstetrics/Gynecology, Medical University of South Carolina.)

Pelvic Examination

bottom of the vagina and anus (the perineal body) for abnormal hair distribution, skin color changes, skin lesions or any generalized abnormalities (irritation, ulcers, dryness, etc.), abnormal positions of anatomy, and/or pelvic relaxation. The patient should be asked to cough to inspect for any evidence of pelvic relaxation (lack of muscular support), cystocele (bulging of the bladder into the vagina), or urinary leaking. While separating the opening of the vagina and depressing the perineal body, the speculum should be inserted into the vagina, usually in a vertical fashion keeping continuous pressure on the bottom part of the vagina so as to avoid the more sensitive structures above (urethra, bladder). The speculum should be carefully turned as it is introduced, always mindful of the patient's labia (opening of the vagina) to avoid inadvertent discomfort. This is accomplished best with the insertion at the proper angle, downward pressure on the vagina, and the slightly rotating technique (Figure 2). Once the speculum is inserted to its full length, the speculum blades are then opened exposing the cervix at the top (apex) of the vagina. One should open the blades only enough to clearly visualize the cervix without undue discomfort to the patient (Figure 3). The Pap smear may then be performed with the thin prep technique (using a small brush and placing the cells in a small container of liquid for computer evaluation) or using the time-honored microscopic slides. A cotton swab may be used to help further expose the cervix if needed. Cultures for gonorrhea and chlamydia may be obtained with small swabs placed in the opening of the cervix. The inspection of the vaginal side walls may be accomplished at this time. Any abnormalities of the cervix should be biopsied, as the Pap smear is only a screening test for use when the cervix appears normal. Any discharge may then be examined for evidence of vaginitis (discharge with inflammation), vaginosis (discharge without inflammation), or other abnormalities. As the speculum is withdrawn (repeating the careful rotation), the anterior and posterior fornix (the area of the vagina around the top and bottom of the cervix) may be inspected.

Attention should be turned to the bimanual aspect of the pelvic exam. This is accomplished by placing one or two fingers of the physician's dominant hand (which should feel most comfortable and proficient in examining any body part) into the hymenal/vaginal opening while using the opposite hand on the external lower abdomen (Figure 4). The fingers should be inserted at the proper angle (similar to the speculum)

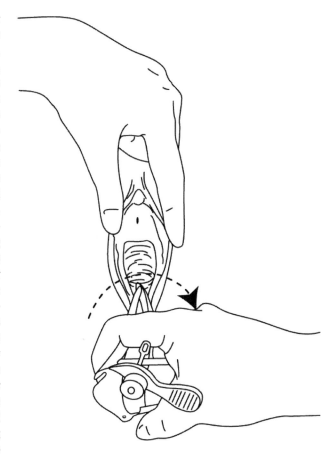

Figure 2. The slightly rotating technique followed during the insertion of the speculum into the vagina. (Courtesy: Illustration drawn by Ginny Canady, Director of Audio/Video Resources, Department of Obstetrics/Gynecology, Medical University of South Carolina.)

while depressing the perineum, which will further expose any weakness in the pelvic muscle support (pubococcygeal muscles) or confirm the muscles' strength. The physician should now be examining the length of the vagina, the vaginal wall, and external aspect of the cervix at the top of the vagina. The cervix is gently examined and lifted while the external hand gently examines the top of the uterus as it is lifted up by the internal exam. The examiner should then begin to outline the size, firmness, mobility, shape, and position of the uterus, ovaries, and any palpable pelvic masses. The vaginal canal, ovaries, and fallopian tubes are then examined in a similar fashion. The vaginal fingers are then turned laterally to feel the pelvic walls (Figure 5). It should be noted that normal adnexa (ovaries and fallopian tubes) are frequently not detectable even under the best of conditions because

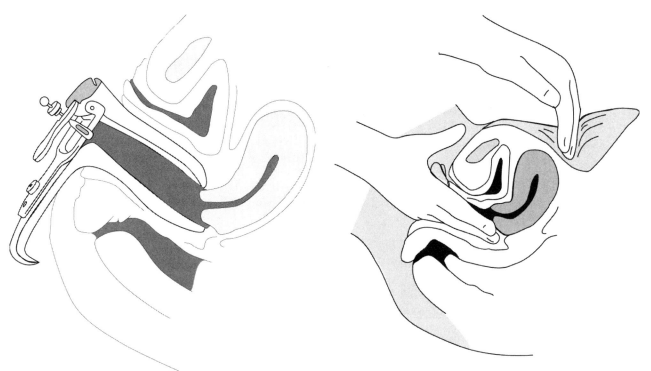

Figure 3. Opening the blades of the speculum to clearly visualize the cervix. (Courtesy: Illustration drawn by Ginny Canady, Director of Audio/Video Resources, Department of Obstetrics/Gynecology, Medical University of South Carolina.)

Figure 4. Bimanual pelvic exam. (Courtesy: Illustration drawn by Ginny Canady, Director of Audio/Video Resources, Department of Obstetrics/Gynecology, Medical University of South Carolina.)

normal ovaries and tubes are so small. In the obese patient even enlarged adnexa may be missed (thus vaginal ultrasound is frequently used). Normal-sized ovaries (approximately 3 × 2 × 2 cm or 1.3 × 0.8 × 0.8 in.) may be felt in the premenopausal woman with active ovarian function. However, if the ovaries are felt in the postmenopausal woman, this may be abnormal, as the ovaries should be too small to be felt when they are not ovulating (making eggs). In this case, further investigation is required.

Finally, the rectal–abdominal bimanual exam is performed. This portion of the exam is to look for external and internal hemorrhoids, fissures (cracks in the skin), fistulas (small connections between the vagina and rectum, which are not normal), polyps in the rectum near the anal opening, or tumors. The uterus is palpated bimanually with the index finger in the vaginal opening and the middle finger in the rectum. With a posterior uterus (a uterus that is tipped backward, which is completely normal), only now will the top of the uterus be felt. The ovaries and particularly the space behind the uterus and uterine support structures (the uterosacral

ligaments) and the internal areas alongside the vagina and cervix are palpated. These areas are best examined rectally and here the diagnostic findings of endometriosis or the spread of cervical cancer may be found. With one finger in the vagina and another in the rectum the rectovaginal septum (the structure separating the vagina from the rectum) can be examined. Having the patient strain may further discover any pelvic support weaknesses including the presence of an enterocele (bulging of small bowel into the vagina) or rectocele (bulging of rectum or large bowel into the vagina). When the bimanual exam is completed the examiner may use his or her rectal finger to place a stool specimen on a hemoccult card to check for blood, which screens for colon cancer in the older patient. The examiner should not perform this blood test if the patient is menstruating or if the cervix had some blood on it without changing gloves. The physician can also give the patient a set of three stool cards to take home with instructions to bring them back to be tested for blood.

Once the pelvic examination has been completed, the examiner should assist the patient to return to the

495

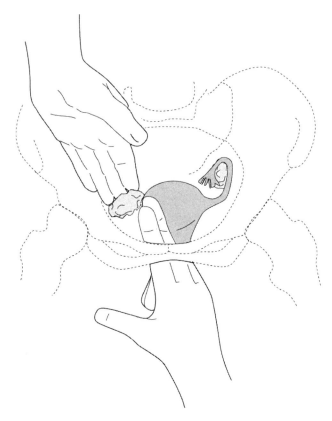

Figure 5. Examining the ovary and the pelvic wall with the examiner's fingers. (Courtesy: Illustration drawn by Ginny Canady, Director of Audio/Video Resources, Department of Obstetrics/Gynecology, Medical University of South Carolina.)

sitting position. The examiner should then talk with the fully clothed patient to discuss the findings of the examination and answer any questions that she may have. Thus the pelvic examination, which screens for cervical cancer and pelvic disease, has been completed. Giving the patient some time to collect her thoughts and to discuss the findings, we think, is the optimal way to complete this very important medical exam.

SEE ALSO: Pap test, Pelvic examination, Pelvic pain

Suggested Resources

The American College of Ob/Gyn. *Patient education.* www.acog.org
Having a pelvic exam and pap test. www.cancer.gov/cancerinfo/having-a-pelvic-exam

JAMES F. CARTER

Pelvic Inflammatory Disease *see* Pelvic Pain

Pelvic Organ Prolapse Pelvic organ prolapse is a condition denoting the descent of pelvic organs toward or through the vaginal opening. References to prolapse of the womb have first been made in ancient Egypt dating back to 1550 BC. Vaginal vault prolapse refers to significant descent of the vaginal apex ("the top of the vagina") following a hysterectomy. Although obviously not a new condition, prolapse is becoming increasingly common due to increased life expectancy.

Prolapse of the top of the vagina or uterus is rarely an isolated finding. The anterior vagina (front side or the bladder side of the vagina) and the posterior vagina (back or rectal side of the vagina) can and often do protrude independent of the uterus or the apex. Protrusion of the anterior vagina is also called a cystocele, while posterior vaginal prolapse is called a rectocele, named after the organs which are thought to descend along with the vagina, the bladder, and rectum. Prolapse of the vaginal apex can, but need not necessarily, be accompanied by an enterocele. Enterocele is defined as the presence of abdominal contents (such as small bowel or omentum) dissecting between the vagina and the adjacent rectum.

SYMPTOMS

Patients may present with an obvious vaginal bulge that is seen or felt by the woman. Conversely, she may complain of a vague sense of pelvic heaviness or a sensation as if "something is about to fall out." Bulging is often noted to be worse toward the end of the day when compared to when she first awakes. When the vaginal lining remains exteriorized for a prolonged period of time, it undergoes thickening from the constant rubbing on undergarments. The vaginal tissue may develop sores (ulcers) and become infected. Urinary incontinence as well as difficulty voiding is common with pelvic organ prolapse and in severe cases complete urinary retention may be seen. Voiding difficulties may result in frequent urinary tract infections and, occasionally, overflow incontinence. Due to kinking of the urethra, urinary incontinence may be masked, in which case the woman does not think she has incontinence, but if the prolapse is fixed surgically or otherwise without further attention to the problem, severe incontinence may surface. Especially concerning the presence of occult stress incontinence, is a history of stress incontinence that spontaneously improved and/or resolved as the prolapse progressively worsened. Although rare, severe pelvic prolapse may result in kinking of the ureters with the potential for kidney damage.

Difficulties may be encountered during sexual intercourse. Defecation may be difficult with associated constipation being very common.

FREQUENCY AND ETIOLOGY

In a routine gynecologic clinic population, most women had mild to moderate prolapse (43.3% and 47.7%, respectively) and few had no or severe prolapse (6.4% and 2.6%, respectively). Complete eversion of the vagina is even more rare. If one imagines the vaginal tube analogous to a sock, complete eversion is similar to completely turning the sock inside-out.

Significant trends for increasing prolapse were found with advancing age, number of children, postmenopausal status, hysterectomy, and prior surgery for prolapse. A Swedish study of the general population reported a prevalence of 30% of any prolapse. Statistical associations with age, number of children, maximal birthweight, and pelvic floor muscle strength were found. Such associations were not found regarding the woman's weight or history of hysterectomy. Indeed, vaginal vault prolapse is thought to occur in less than 0.5% of patients who have had hysterectomies, whether done vaginally or abdominally.

PATHOPHYSIOLOGY

The anatomy of pelvic organ prolapse can be understood in terms of three levels of support. Level I represents the support of the top part of the vagina in terms of the cervix (with no prior hysterectomy) or the vaginal cuff (in a woman who has undergone total hysterectomy) by the cardinal–uterosacral ligament complex. This is analogous to the toe of the sock being suspended by two ropes, one on either side. The cardinal–uterosacral ligament complex serves to keep the upper vagina and uterus resting on the levator ani muscles, which comprise the majority of the pelvic diaphragm that rests in a near-horizontal plane in a

woman standing erect. Level II denotes the lateral support of the midvagina to the pelvic sidewall. Level III is represented by the fusion of the distal vagina (the opening of the sock) to tissue of the perineum.

The U-shaped levator ani muscles, as long as they are functioning properly, essentially support the pelvic organs by preventing their descent through the hiatus (the opening of the "U"). Once the muscles cease to function properly the structures described earlier come under increasing tension and are apt to fail. The conditions of enterocele and apical prolapse represent failures of level I support. Apical prolapse occurs due to tearing or attenuation of the cardinal–uterosacral ligaments (the ropes). This results in failure to support the top part of the vagina and uterus over the pelvic diaphragm. Enterocele following a hysterectomy is analogous to opening of the stitch along the toe of the sock. Level I support is considered the most important in maintaining adequate overall pelvic support, because once that fails, usually the pressures exerted will result in further failure of the support systems. Failure of level II support results in a cystocele and/or rectocele. Failures of level III are very rare and limited to women who have undergone radical vulvar surgery.

A cystocele, named after the organ that descends with the anterior vagina—the bladder, occurs due to the fact that the bladder sits passively atop the anterior vaginal wall. If the support of the anterior vagina is compromised, the bladder will follow the vagina down its descent toward the vaginal opening. This support may be compromised in several ways. One way it can be compromised is if one or both of its sidewalls break away from the pelvic sidewall. If one imagines the anterior vagina as a trampoline, this is analogous to the breakage of the springs on opposite sides. Another way is by breakage of the strong layer of tissue in its midportion, which is analogous to ripping the tarmac that represents the trampoline's surface. A final method is due to general attenuation of the vagina, which is analogous to having the fabric of the tarmac fray and get worn with repeated use in a particular spot on the trampoline.

MANAGEMENT

It has been suggested that early, persistent, and well-performed pelvic floor muscle exercises (Kegel exercises) may be helpful in preventing pelvic organ prolapse and may slow the progression of early signs of prolapse. Success depends upon early intervention and exercising the correct muscle group, which is best verified during a pelvic examination. The levator ani muscles are the target of such exercises and are comprised of two types of muscle fibers: slow twitch and fast twitch. Proper exercising involves utilizing and strengthening these two types of muscle fibers. One component of exercise is maximal contraction of the muscle over a period of time, the other is rapid maximal contraction followed by relaxation done in sequence. The difficulty of the exercise routine is gradually increased by increasing the amount of time on the continuous contraction exercises while increasing the number of consecutive quick contractions. It is now possible to find physical therapists able to work with patients on this problem.

A pessary is a medical device that is worn in the vagina to help prevent protrusion of the prolapse. Most pessaries are made of silicon and they come in various shapes and different sizes. Some remain in the vagina for months at a time, while others can be removed and reinserted by the patient. Some allow sexual intercourse, while others do not. Although pessaries do not cure the problem, they are appropriate as an option to avoid the need for surgery in motivated patients. Pessaries must be properly fitted by an experienced clinician and removed for vaginal inspection on a routine basis because the biggest risks of pessary use result from their neglect for a prolonged period of time.

Surgery is reserved for patients who have significant symptoms related to their pelvic organ prolapse. Multiple procedures are available, which can be done through a vaginal or abdominal route. The key to the decision-making process, however, is careful evaluation of all pelvic floor defects both in the office and during the surgery and addressing each of them at the time of surgery. Careful consideration for the potential risks and benefits of surgery should be done prior to any such undertaking.

SEE ALSO: Hysterectomy, Kegel exercises, Urinary incontinence and voiding dysfunction

Suggested Reading

Adam, R. A., & Preston, M. R. (2002). Urinary incontinence: Diagnosis and treatment. *Women Health Gynecology Edition, 2*(4), 218–229.

Agency for Healthcare Policy and Research. (1992). *Urinary incontinence in adults* (Publication 93–0552). Rockville, MD: United States Department of Health and Human Services.

Bent, A. E., Ostergard, D. R., Cundiff, G. W., & Swift, S. (Eds.). (2002). *Ostergard's urogynecology and urodynamics.* Philadelphia: Lippincott.

Walters, M. D., & Karram, M. M. (Eds.). (1999). *Urogynecology and reconstructive pelvic surgery.* St. Louis, MO: C. V. Mosby.

RONY ADAM

Pelvic Pain Pelvic pain is one of the most commonly reported symptoms in gynecology practice. Pelvic pain can be acute (of short and limited duration) or chronic (of longer duration).

ACUTE PELVIC PAIN

Acute pelvic pain is pelvic pain lasting no more than one month. Acute pain of the pelvis can originate from the gastrointestinal organs (bowel or stomach), genitourinary system (gynecologic organs—uterus, fallopian tubes, or ovaries or urinary system—bladder, kidneys, ureters, or urethra), or can be musculoskeletal (muscles and bones of the pelvis) in nature.

Pregnancy

The causes of acute pelvic pain with pregnancy include ruptured ectopic pregnancy, threatened or incomplete abortion (miscarriage), and degeneration of fibroids. An ectopic pregnancy occurs when the fetus implants outside the uterine cavity—in a fallopian tube, for example. The pain associated with ectopic pregnancy is due to dilation of the tube or blood in the peritoneal cavity, which causes irritation.

Pelvic Inflammatory Disease (PID)

This is an acute infection involving the uterus, fallopian tubes, and ovaries. Often, PID is caused by a sexually transmitted infection such as chlamydia or gonorrhea. The diagnosis is usually made when lower abdominal pain and tenderness develop in association with fever, vaginal discharge, and an abnormal increase in the white blood cell count. Treatment consists of antibiotic therapy.

Leaking or Ruptured Ovarian Cyst

With either condition, a small amount of blood can leak into the pelvic cavity and cause local irritation and pain. There are many different types of ovarian cysts, most of which are benign (not cancer). Some of these resolve on their own and some require surgical intervention.

Twisted Ovary or Fallopian Tube

The twisting of an ovary or fallopian tube is called "torsion." This can cause blood supply to be compromised to the tube or ovary and intense pain can result. The diagnosis is usually made using ultrasound and physical examination. Treatment consists of surgical intervention.

Fibroid Uterus

Fibroids occasionally cause pelvic pain, especially when they encroach on adjacent structures like the rectum or bladder. Pain can also develop if the fibroid begins to degenerate as it outgrows its blood supply; this is occasionally seen in the pregnant uterus. In rare instances, acute pain is caused by fibroid torsion. If fibroids remain painful it is usually recommended that these be removed. If this is not possible, pain medication will be prescribed.

Appendicitis

This is the most common intestinal source of acute pelvic pain. Symptoms include pain with loss of appetite and nausea, fever, chills, and vomiting. Usually pain begins in the area of the belly button and moves to the lower right area of the pelvis. Diagnostic laparoscopy (surgery where small "stab-wound" incisions are made to look through a laparoscope and then operate if necessary in the pelvis or abdomen) may be useful in ruling out other sources of pelvic pain. Appendicitis often is mistaken for PID.

Diverticulum

A diverticulum is an outpouching of the colonic mucosa through the colon wall. Inflammation and infection of the diverticulum cause diverticulitis. This diverticulum usually affects older women; it rarely occurs in women who are younger than 30–40 years. The diagnosis is usually made using computed tomography (CT) scan and treatment consists of antibiotics.

Intestinal Obstruction

Obstruction is a common cause of pain in women with adhesions (scar tissue) from previous abdominal surgery. Symptoms include colicky abdominal pain and distension, vomiting, and constipation. Abdominal x-ray films determine whether obstruction is partial or complete. Nasogastric suction, intravenous fluid, and surgical intervention may be needed.

Urinary Tract Infection and Stones

The pain can be severe and crampy and may radiate to the groin. The sensation of having to go to the bathroom frequently and urgently, and blood in the urine are common findings. Kidney ultrasound, urine culture, and blood tests are used to make a diagnosis. Antibiotic and surgical management may be necessary.

CHRONIC PELVIC PAIN

One of the most common reasons for a woman to visit her provider is for chronic pelvic pain. A diagnosis is made when the duration of pain is more than one month. Approximately 15% of hysterectomies in the United States are performed due to chronic pelvic pain. Below are some common causes of chronic pelvic pain.

Endometriosis and Pelvic Adhesions

This is the most common gynecologic reason for chronic pelvic pain. Endometriosis is a disease where endometrial tissue, which usually is only present as the uterine lining, implants itself on other areas in the pelvis. This diagnosis must be made surgically, although on occasion a large area of endometriosis on the ovary (an endometrioma) can be identified on ultrasound.

Irritable Bowel Syndrome

The exact cause of this condition is unknown but it is a common cause of lower abdominal pain. Symptoms include excessive flatulence, alternating diarrhea and constipation, and abdominal distension. The diagnosis is usually based on physical examination and history. A multidisciplinary program consisting of medical and psychological approaches is needed. The patient must be evaluated for more serious forms of intestinal disease, such as Crohn's disease, ulcerative colitis, intestinal neoplasms, and hernia.

Interstitial Cystitis

This is an autoimmune disease of the lining of the bladder that leads to pain with urination and lower abdominal pain and discomfort. The pain can be partially relieved by emptying the bladder. The diagnosis is usually made by performing cystoscopy (when a tiny scope is placed into the bladder) looking for pinpoint hemorrhages on the bladder wall. This is considered the hallmark finding. Treatment may consist of anticholinergic, antispasmodic, and anti-inflammatory medications. Distending the bladder with fluid may provide temporary relief.

Myofascial Syndrome

This condition is responsible for chronic pelvic pain in up to 15% of all cases. Trigger points can be observed upon examination and local injection of anesthetic into the painful points can be helpful.

The uterus and ovaries share the same visceral innervation with the ileum, colon, and rectum. Therefore, it is often difficult to differentiate the source of the pain. A multidisciplinary team consisting of psychologists, anesthesiologists, physiotherapists, gastroenterologists, and gynecologists can best help a patient manage chronic pelvic pain.

Patients typically require pain medication, although tricyclic antidepressant and behavioral therapy usually reduce the need for such medication. The approach should be supportive, therapeutic, and sympathetic. Specific skills are taught using cognitive-behavioral approaches. Relaxation techniques, stress management, sexual and marital counseling, and psychotherapy are also useful.

Acupuncture and nerve blocks to pelvic structures (uterosacral—associated with the uterus, hypogastric—associated with the stomach, or epidural—spinal area nerve blocks) can also be used to control the pain. A presacral neurectomy (cutting of specific nerves leading to pelvic structures) or sympathectomy (cutting of specific nerves that are associated with pelvic pain) can help patients whose pain does not respond to standard treatment.

SEE ALSO: Abdominal pain, Endometriosis, Irritable bowel syndrome, Laparoscopy, Ovarian cyst, Ultrasound, Urinary tract infections, Uterine fibroids

Suggested Resources

www.endometriosisassn.org
www.endocenter.org

HABIBEH GITIFOROOZ

Peptic Ulcer Disease

A peptic ulcer is an erosion in the lining of the stomach or of the duodenum, the first portion of the small intestine. Ulcers develop when the normal defense and repair mechanisms of the lining (mucosa) are impaired, making it susceptible to damage by stomach acid and the digestive enzyme, pepsin. The majority of peptic ulcer disease (PUD) is caused by an infection with a bacterium called *Helicobacter pylori* and by nonsteroidal anti-inflammatory drugs (NSAIDs), like ibuprofen and aspirin. Rarely, PUD may be due to Zollinger–Ellison syndrome (a disorder involving tumors in the pancreas and duodenum, which secrete a hormone that stimulates excess acid production leading to ulceration), viral infection, cocaine use, or Crohn's disease. Smoking increases the risk for PUD and also impairs ulcer healing.

PUD is a very common problem. Duodenal ulcers are diagnosed four times more often than gastric (stomach) ulcers. Approximately 10% of men and 5% of women will have a duodenal ulcer at some point during their lifetime. Although gastric ulcers occur in similar frequencies in men and women, there is a female predominance of gastric ulcer disease among people taking NSAIDs. In recent years, there has been a fall in the number of duodenal ulcer diagnoses, which has been attributed to declining *H. pylori* infection in the general population. However, rates of gastric ulcer have been increasing with the rise attributed to greater NSAID use.

In the United States, approximately 30% of the population is infected with *H. pylori*, in contrast to 80–90% of people in developing countries. Although *H. pylori* has been shown to be a strong risk factor for PUD, most infected people never develop ulcers. The factors that make one infected person more likely to get PUD than another are not well understood and are a subject of intense research. Chronic *H. pylori* infection has also been found to increase the risk for gastric cancer.

NSAIDs promote ulceration not only by direct damage to the mucosa through their weak acid properties, but also by blocking normal mucosal defense mechanisms. NSAIDs inhibit the production of the protective prostaglandins that are hormone-like substances important in maintaining the mucosal defense against acid and digestive enzymes. Approximately 2–5% of chronic NSAID users are diagnosed with duodenal ulcers and as many as 10–20% are diagnosed with gastric ulcers. Among chronic NSAID users, 1–2% will develop serious ulcer complications each year. These include gastrointestinal bleeding, perforation (extension of an ulcer through the stomach or duodenal wall), and gastric outlet obstruction (blockage of stomach contents from entering the duodenum). A number of factors have been found to increase the risk for major gastrointestinal complications in NSAID users and these include a history of PUD, older age, corticosteroid (e.g., prednisone) use, clot-preventing medication (e.g., coumadin, heparin) use, high doses of NSAIDs, multiple NSAIDs, and poor overall medical condition. In recent years, a new class of NSAID, "Cox-2 inhibitors," has been introduced, which inhibits the prostaglandins responsible for pain and inflammation but does not affect prostaglandins important for gastroduodenal mucosa protection. They have been shown to cause fewer ulcers and ulcer-related complications.

Pain is the most common symptom of PUD and is typically located in the upper abdomen. However, many people who develop ulcer complications, including bleeding, will have had no prior symptoms. This is especially true in chronic NSAID users. The pain usually comes and goes over a period of days to weeks and is frequently described as "gnawing," "burning," or "hunger-like." Some people will describe a pain that is relieved by meals, particularly those with duodenal ulcers, while others will have pain without any relationship to eating. Sometimes the pain is relieved with antacids. Pain radiating to the back suggests a penetrating duodenal ulcer (extension of the ulcer through the duodenal wall into the pancreas). It is important to recognize that "ulcer-like" symptoms may be seen in many other disorders including gastritis, malignancy, gastroesophageal reflux, vascular disease, gallbladder and bile duct disease, and pancreatic disease.

People with "alarm" symptoms such as vomiting blood, bloody stool, and sharp, sudden, persistent abdominal pain should seek medical attention immediately. Bleeding is the most common ulcer complication, especially in the elderly, and the symptoms include vomiting red blood or "coffee grounds" (dark blood) and passing black, tar-like, or maroon stools. Pain that becomes abruptly worse and/or generalized suggests the possibility of perforation. Nausea and vomiting may indicate the presence of a gastric outlet obstruction. Weight loss suggests the possibility of gastric malignancy.

The diagnosis of PUD can be made either by an upper gastrointestinal (UGI) series (x-rays of the stomach and intestines are taken after the patient drinks barium, a thick white liquid) or by upper endoscopy (insertion of a thin flexible tube containing a camera into the mouth). Endoscopy is superior to UGI series in making the diagnosis, especially with small ulcers. It also has two other advantages, the ability to obtain biopsies and the ability to directly treat bleeding ulcers. Because of the association of gastric ulcers with malignancy, endoscopy allows for direct inspection and biopsies of suspicious-appearing or poorly healing gastric ulcers. During endoscopy, biopsies of the gastric mucosa can also be obtained and tested for the presence of *H. pylori*. However, endoscopy should not be performed solely for detecting *H. pylori* infection (see below). When a bleeding ulcer is suspected, there are a number of endoscopic treatments available, which can decrease blood transfusion requirements and prevent the need for surgery. Factors favoring endoscopy over UGI as the diagnostic test of choice are age over 50, weight loss, gastrointestinal bleeding, and severe symptoms or those which do not respond to treatment. A gastric ulcer found on UGI should be followed by endoscopy at approximately 8 weeks to assess healing and, if suspicious features for gastric cancer are present, to obtain biopsies.

In people with known PUD or who have ulcer symptoms, there are several methods, both invasive and noninvasive, for diagnosing *H. pylori* infection. Noninvasive methods test blood, urine, breath, and stool for evidence of infection whereas invasive methods involve endoscopically (using a small tube inserted into the body) obtained gastric biopsies. If endoscopy is indicated for a reason other than the diagnosis of the bacteria *H. pylori*, then gastric (stomach) biopsies can be obtained for either rapid urease testing or histologic examination. The rapid urease test is a quick and accurate test of stomach fluid with results in less than an hour. Histologic examination involves a pathologist reviewing the biopsy specimens under a microscope for the presence of *H. pylori* organisms and may take several days to a week for results to be reported. However, because rapid urease and breath tests may be falsely negative in patients taking some types of medication (proton [acid] pump inhibitors, PPI), antibiotics, or bismuth, microscopic cell testing (histology) should be performed.

The goals of PUD treatment are to relieve symptoms, promote ulcer healing, prevent ulcer recurrence, and prevent ulcer complications. Acid-suppressing medications, like H_2 blockers and PPI, reduce the amount of gastric acid produced allowing ulcers to heal and reducing pain. PPIs, for example, omeprazole and lansoprazole, are the most effective PUD therapy, healing over 90% of duodenal ulcers within 4 weeks and gastric ulcers within 8 weeks of therapy. After PUD treatment is complete, continued PPI therapy is not generally recommended unless the individual also has gastroesophageal reflux disease or is a chronic NSAID user. The elderly and people in poor general medical condition who have experienced an ulcer complication should also be considered for long-term (maintenance) therapy. Drugs that block specific receptors on the stomach lining, H_2 blockers, like ranitidine and cimetidine, are less expensive alternatives to PPIs and have healing rates of approximately 80% at 4 weeks.

Treatment *of H. pylori* infection should be considered in all patients with gastric or duodenal ulcer or a documented history of PUD. Eradication of the organism is associated with a reduction in ulcer recurrence from 60–70% to less than 10%. The most effective treatment regimens for *H. pylori* include a 10- to 14-day course of a combination of two antibiotics (amoxicillin, clarithromycin, and/or metronidazole) and a PPI or ranitidine bismuth citrate. Acid-suppressing medication is then continued for another 4 weeks in duodenal ulcers and 6 weeks in gastric ulcers.

In NSAID-induced ulcers, the NSAID should be discontinued if possible. If not, once daily PPI has been shown to be the most effective regimen in preventing NSAID-induced ulcers with over 80% healing of gastric and duodenal ulcers at 8 weeks. In high-risk patients on chronic NSAIDs, a newer class of medications, the Cox-2 inhibitors, may be considered. Although effective in preventing ulcers in NSAID users, many people suffer side effects such as cramping and diarrhea. Moreover, since misoprostol causes miscarriages, it absolutely must not be used by women of reproductive age who are not using contraception.

While PUD almost always responds to treatment, there are risk factors for poor ulcer healing. These include persistent *H. pylori* infection, continued NSAID use, and smoking. Rarely, recurrent or poorly healing ulcers may indicate the presence of gastric cancer or Zollinger–Ellison syndrome. Surgery is rarely necessary and typically only required for ulcers that fail to heal or major ulcer complications, like perforation.

SEE ALSO: Abdominal pain, Chronic pain, Nausea, Pelvic pain

Suggested Reading

Del Valle, J., et al. (1999). Acid peptic disorders. In T. Yamada, D. H. Alpers, L. Laine, C. Owyang, & D. W. Powell (Eds.), *Textbook of gastroenterology* (3rd ed., pp. 1370–1444). Philadelphia: Lippincott, Williams & Wilkins.

Suggested Resources

U.S. National Library of Medicine: http://www.nlm.nih.gov/ medline/ency/article/003120.htm

MARGARET F. KINNARD

Perimenopause The term perimenopause is defined as that time about or around menopause. Internationally, the Council of Affiliated Menopause Societies has used the term *climacteric* to describe the phase during the aging of women marking the transition from the reproductive phase to the nonreproductive state. Generally, it is recommended that perimenopause and climacteric be used synonymously and to represent the transition from the reproductive stage to 12 months following the final menstrual period. This term is also often referred to as the menopause transition.

Perimenopause generally starts in a woman's early 40s when increasing symptoms may develop. The most frequent symptoms are menstrual cycle irregularities, vasomotor symptoms (hot flashes), sleep disturbances, and less frequently vaginal thinning and dryness. The response to symptoms is impacted by psychological, social, and cultural influences, but the most significant initiator of symptoms in the perimenopause is related to the declining or changing levels of estrogen and progesterone, produced from the ovary. As the menopause transition is a normal process, there is a disinclination to call the effects "symptoms," but these can be quite severe and need medical intervention. There are potential long-term effects from the hormonal changes (see Menopause).

Our current knowledge about the perimenopause is limited to few studies, but what is known in terms of changes through the perimenopause are listed as follows:

1. *Declining fertility.* The ability to reproduce declines rapidly between the ages of 35–38 and onwards. Fertility beyond age 45 is much less frequent.

2. *Changes in the menstrual cycle.* The menstrual cycle changes are the most frequent symptoms reported by women in the premenopause. These include heavier flow (menorrhagia), reduced flow (oligomenorrhea), more frequent menstruation (polymenorrhea), and ultimately loss of menstruation (amenorrhea).

3. *Vasomotor symptoms.* The most frequent symptom after menstrual cycle changes relate to vasomotor symptoms. The hot flash, which is a feeling of sudden transient warmth that may spread across the face or the entire body, usually followed by a sensation of perspiration and possible shivering, is frequently a problem. The vasomotor symptoms may last a few months or several years, but usually disappear spontaneously. The best therapy remains some form of estrogen or estrogen plus progestin therapy.

4. *Sleep disturbances.* Changing or declining estrogen levels have a negative impact on the quality of Rapid Eye Movement (REM) sleep. REM sleep is an important component of normal sleep. Disrupted sleep patterns can be exacerbated by night sweats (hot flashes during the night). A result of poor sleep is morning fatigue, irritability, complaint of reduction in short-term memory, and minor depression.

5. *Urogenital changes.* Thinning of the vaginal lining with increasing susceptibility to infection or to painful intercourse is not usual prior to cessation of menses and the presence of a low estrogen level.

6. *Urinary complaints.* There is very little evidence to suggest any impact of the perimenopause on urinary stress incontinence (leaking bladder). However, there may be an increase of urgency or the sensation of the need to urinate immediately.

7. *Central nervous system changes.* There is no direct evidence of any major central nervous system change in terms of direct causation of perimenopause with increased depression, loss of cognition, or headache, although indirect evidence has been presented.

8. *Sexuality.* There is evidence that sexual activity decreases with age in both sexes and problems of sexual desire and sexual arousal may be related to declining ovarian estrogen and androgenic hormones.

The perimenopause represents a good opportunity for a complete health evaluation, identification of risk factors for development of future medical problems, screening for early evidence of existing problems, and commencement of a proactive preventive health program.

SEE ALSO: Fecundity, Libido and desire, Menstrual cycle disorders, Menstruation, Oligomenorrhea

Suggested Reading

North American Menopause Society. (2002). *Menopause core curriculum* (2nd ed.). Cleveland, OH: Author.

WULF H. UTIAN

Periodontics The cyclic nature of the female sex hormones is often reflected in gingival tissue changes. Fluctuating levels of progesterone and estrogen may have an adverse effect on gingival response to bacterial plaque. During puberty, the female experiences an increase in the production of estrogen and progesterone resulting in an increase in the prevalence of gingivitis without an increase of plaque. However, in areas where food debris, plaque, and calculus are deposited, clinically there may be a nodular hyperplastic reaction of the gingiva. Milder gingivitis cases respond well to scaling and root planing with frequent oral hygiene instructions. Severe cases may require microbial culturing, antimicrobial mouth rinses, and slow-release subgingival antimicrobial therapy. Whenever possible, involvement of a parental figure with home care procedures is recommended.

EATING DISORDERS

Adolescent girls are susceptible to the eating disorders bulimia nervosa and anorexia nervosa. Signs and symptoms of chronic regurgitation of gastric contents on intraoral hard and soft tissues consist of smooth erosion of the tooth, usually on the tongue surfaces of the upper front teeth. In addition there can be an enlargement of the salivary glands, which can decrease salivary flow resulting in increased oral mucous membrane sensitivity and gingival redness.

MENSTRUATION

Gingival inflammation is often aggravated by an imbalance and/or increase in estrogen and progesterone. In certain individuals they are more inflamed and red preceding the onset of menses. At times during the menstrual period there may be minor increase in tooth mobility. Intraoral apthous ulcers, herpetic lesions, and candida (yeast) infections occur in some women during the phase of the cycle when progesterone is the highest. Frequent supportive periodontal therapy appointments with particular emphasis on oral hygiene are recommended for those women who are clinically symptomatic with their menstrual cycle.

PREGNANCY

The net effect of gestational changes is twofold: increased gingival swelling, redness, and bleeding occurring as a physiologic change during pregnancy; and alterations in host response and tissue physiology serving to increase the gingival inflammatory response to bacterial plaque. Increased signs of gingival inflammation become evident after the first trimester and peak during the latter part of the third trimester, regressing after parturition. The most common site of gingivitis is usually seen in the anterior regions of the mouth, but can be more generalized and may cause false pocketing with increased probing depths but minimal changes in attachment levels. Pyogenic granulomas, "pregnancy tumors," may develop, which generally will regress postpartum. Increased tooth mobility unrelated to attachment loss has also been noted but usually requires no treatment. Expectant mothers should be provided with a comprehensive plaque control program to minimize the exaggerated inflammatory response to the gingival tissues.

ORAL CONTRACEPTIVES

Oral contraceptives may produce the gingival changes seen during pregnancy. Certain brands of oral contraceptives may cause more significant changes than others. In recent years, the quantity of synthetic hormones contained in most oral contraceptive agents has decreased and it appears that current oral contraceptive agents no longer affect the gingiva to the same degree as previously reported. While the increased gingival inflammation associated with pregnancy regresses after parturition, many women take oral contraceptives for extended periods of time, emphasizing the need for long-term periodic office visits to monitor periodontal health. While the effects of progesterone and estrogen on the gingiva cannot be avoided, thorough plaque control reduces the incidence and severity of adverse gingival changes.

MENOPAUSE

Some patients report experiencing burning sensations in the oral cavity and altered taste sensations. For many years menopause-related desquamate gingivitis have been described among postmenopausal women and are thought to be related to the hormonal changes of menopause. Ongoing studies are examining the association of postmenopausal primary osteoporosis with upper and lower jawbone mineral density, tooth loss, bony ridge atrophy, and periodontal attachment loss. Most recent evidence points to a probable cause

between osteoporosis and tooth loss as well as alveolar bone loss.

SEE ALSO: Menarche, Menopause, Oral contraception, Oral health

Suggested Reading

Mahn, L. K., & Escott-Stump, S. (2000). *Krause's food, nutrition, and diet therapy* (10th ed., pp. 516–533). Philadelphia: W. B. Saunders.

Newman, M. G., Takei, H. H., & Carranza, F. A. (2000). *Carranza's clinical periodontology* (9th ed., pp. 513–526). Philadelphia: W. B. Saunders.

Rose, L. F., Genco, R. J., Cohen, D. W., & Mealey, B. (2000). *Periodontal Medicine*, 252–253.

Wilson, W. G., & Kornman, K. S. (1996). *Fundamental of Periodontics*, 151–163. Chicago: Quintessence Publishing Co.

World Workshop in Periodontics. (1996). *Annals of Periodontology*, *1*(1), 290–292.

VALERIE GODFREY

JOY A. JORDAN

Permanent Makeup   *see* Tattoos

Personality Disorders The *Diagnostic and Statistical Manual of Mental Disorders*, fourth edition (DSM-IV), defines a personality disorder as "…an enduring pattern of inner experience and behavior that deviates markedly from the expectations of the individual's culture, is pervasive and inflexible, has an onset in adolescence or early adulthood, is stable over time, and leads to distress or impairment." The DSM-IV defines these disorders categorically, and requires that a certain number of established "criteria" be met before the diagnosis is made. However, many experts argue that personality traits are dimensional and that these disorders represent maladaptive variations of normal traits. In addition, these categories are not objective disease entities, but are instead hypothetical constructs developed for their utility in describing recurrent observations in clinical practice. Individuals who meet the criteria for a diagnosis of a personality disorder also are often diagnosed with other mental disorders, especially mood disorders, anxiety disorders, and substance abuse or dependence. There are 10 recognized personality disorders in all, which the DSM-IV groups into "clusters."

Cluster A includes personality disorders characterized by oddness or eccentricity: paranoid, schizoid, and schizotypal. Those who meet the criteria for a diagnosis of paranoid personality disorder are generally distrustful and habitually suspect that others are trying to harm them. As a result, they have difficulty forming and maintaining relationships. Individuals diagnosed with schizoid personality disorder do not desire or enjoy close relationships with others. They are restricted in emotional expression and thus may appear cold or detached. Similarly, those with a diagnosis of schizotypal personality disorder exhibit social detachment. However, they also exhibit odd beliefs (e.g., clairvoyance and telepathy), odd behaviors, and peculiar perceptual experiences.

The Cluster B personality disorders are characterized by dramatic, emotional, or self-centered behavior: antisocial, borderline, histrionic, and narcissistic. Those who exhibit antisocial personality disorder consistently violate the rights of others and often use aggression, dishonesty, and criminal behavior in order to meet their goals. They tend to be impulsive and tend to lack remorse. There is a high prevalence of this disorder in prison populations. Individuals who meet the criteria for borderline personality disorder (BPD) have lives characterized by a pattern of instability of behaviors, emotions, relationships, and self-image. They tend to be impulsive and may repeatedly engage in self-injurious behavior or attempt suicide. Completed suicide occurs in approximately 10% of this population. Individuals diagnosed with histrionic personality disorder are only comfortable when they are the center of attention. They are often dramatic in their emotional expressions, speech, and gestures. Narcissistic personality disorder is characterized by an inflated sense of self-importance, a need for excessive admiration, an expectation of special treatment from others, and a lack of empathy.

Cluster C includes personality disorders characterized by anxiety and fear: avoidant, dependent, and obsessive–compulsive. Individuals who have a diagnosis of avoidant personality disorder shun interactions with others because they see themselves as socially inadequate and fear they will be rejected or criticized. If they do have an intimate relationship, they are emotionally restrained within that relationship for fear of ridicule. There is much overlap in the diagnostic criteria of avoidant personality disorder and that of social phobia. Individuals who meet the criteria for dependent personality disorder have an excessive need for nurturance and support, which leads to passivity and fears of

separation from others. They believe they need others to take responsibility for major areas of their lives. Individuals who meet the criteria for obsessive–compulsive personality disorder are fearful of being out of control and thus are very rigid in their thinking and activities. They are preoccupied with orderliness, perfectionism, and control of themselves and their environments.

Estimates of the prevalence of personality disorders are based on limited research. The best available data indicate that the personality disorders have prevalence rates between 0.5% and 3% in the general population. BPD is one of the most common personality disorders among individuals seeking mental health treatment, and is seen in approximately 10% of mental health outpatients and 20–40% of mental health inpatients. Prevalence rates according to race, ethnicity, and culture remain largely undetermined.

Three of the personality disorders are diagnosed more commonly in women than in men: dependent, histrionic, and borderline. Antisocial personality disorder is less common in women than in men. These gender differences in prevalence rates may exist for a number of reasons: (a) Real gender differences in the presence of the disorders. For example, invalidating environments, particularly those characterized by abuse, are hypothesized to be important in the etiology of BPD. Girls are more likely to be victims of child abuse than boys are, and therefore, BPD may actually be more common in women than in men. (b) Gender bias in the development of the criteria. In particular, the criteria for dependent and histrionic personality disorders have been criticized by feminists for including personality characteristics that are stereotypically feminine (e.g., difficulty expressing disagreement with others, easily influenced by others), thus increasing the likelihood that normal women who adhere to traditional female gender roles will be diagnosed with one of these personality disorders. (c) Bias in clinicians diagnosing personality disorders. For example, research has indicated that clinicians are more likely to diagnose histrionic personality disorder if the patient is female than if the patient is male, even when given identical information in written case histories.

The most promising theories regarding the etiology of personality disorders are integrative, acknowledging that personality disorders are most likely determined by multiple factors having reciprocal influences over time. One etiological theory that takes this approach is the biosocial theory of BPD. This theory hypothesizes that

Pharmacists

BPD develops because of a lack of "good fit" between the child's biological vulnerabilities and the environment. According to the theory, individuals with BPD have a biological vulnerability to emotion dysregulation that they either were born with or developed very early in life. The "poor fit" environment for these children is an "invalidating environment," in which the child's private experiences (e.g., thoughts, feelings, desires) are chronically and pervasively dismissed as wrong, inappropriate, or otherwise invalid. These factors act in a reciprocal fashion over time, each eliciting and amplifying the other, to create severe emotion dysregulation, which consequently results in dysregulation of behavior, relationships, cognitive processes, and self-image. Continued research in psychology and neurobiology will provide important information about the validity of integrative theories of personality disorders like this one.

The development of effective and proven treatments for personality disorders has lagged behind advances in the treatment of other mental health problems, in part because of a belief that these disorders were untreatable. Currently, pharmacological treatments focus on the management of symptoms that may be associated with a personality disorder, such as cognitive–perceptual disturbances, mood dysregulation, aggression, and impulsivity. However, pharmacological treatments alone are inadequate for the treatment of personality disorders, and therefore psychotherapy is the recommended treatment method. Psychodynamic and cognitive–behavioral psychotherapies are popular treatment approaches, but there is surprisingly little research on their effectiveness. Treatments for BPD are among the most studied. "Dialectical behavior therapy" is the type of outpatient psychotherapy for BPD that currently has the most evidence for its effectiveness. There is also demonstrated efficacy for a psychodynamic treatment of BPD that relies on a partial hospitalization program. Avoidant personality disorder has been shown to respond well to behavioral treatments, including systematic desensitization and social skills training. "Multisystemic therapy" has been demonstrated to be effective for adolescents exhibiting behaviors associated with antisocial personality disorder. A few published studies have suggested that cognitive therapy may be effective in the treatment of several personality disorders, including borderline, antisocial, narcissistic, dependent, and avoidant.

SEE ALSO: Mood disorders, Phobia, Substance use

Suggested Reading

American Psychiatric Association. (1994). *Diagnostic and statistical manual of mental disorders* (4th ed.). Washington, DC: American Psychiatric Association.

Ballou, M., & Brown, L. S. (Eds.). (2002). *Rethinking mental health and disorder: Feminist perspectives.* New York: Guilford Press.

Henggeler, S. W. (1999). Multisystemic therapy: An overview of clinical procedures, outcomes, and policy implications. *Child Psychology and Psychiatry Review, 4,* 2–10.

Linehan, M. M. (1993). *Cognitive behavioral treatment of borderline personality disorder.* New York: Guilford Press.

Millon, T. (1996). *Personality and psychopathology: Building a clinical science.* New York: Wiley-Interscience.

Young, J. E., & Klosko, J. S. (1993). *Reinventing your life: How to break free from negative life patterns.* New York: Dutton.

AMY S. HOUSE
JOSEPHINE ALBRITTON

Pharmacists According to the U.S. Bureau of Labor Statistics, there were approximately 217,000 licensed pharmacists in the United States in the year 2000, representing the third largest health care profession (following nurses and physicians). While pharmacists traditionally are known to dispense medications, many are becoming more involved in drug therapy decision-making and patient counseling. Some specialized pharmacists function as primary care providers. All states require pharmacists to have a license to practice pharmacy. To obtain a license, one must complete an internship under a licensed pharmacist, graduate from an accredited college of pharmacy, and pass a state licensure examination.

In 2000, 82 colleges of pharmacy were accredited to confer degrees. Pharmacy programs grant the degree of Doctor of Pharmacy (Pharm.D.), which requires at least 6 years of postsecondary study as well as passing the state licensure examination. The Pharm.D. degree has replaced the Bachelor of Science (B.S.) degree, which will cease to be awarded after 2005. Approximately 70% of first-year pharmacy students are women and 13% are of minority groups.

The job opportunities available for pharmacists are extensive, ranging from community or retail pharmacy to basic science research in a laboratory. Traditionally, pharmacists either worked in a retail store, whether it be a chain or independent pharmacy, or in a hospital; however, they may also work in industry, academia, or as a primary care provider. Still other graduating pharmacists will go on to do residencies and specialty fellowships.

The primary role of the pharmacist is to provide pharmaceutical care. Modern pharmacists are responsible for the outcomes from the use of medication and are to ensure that the treatment administered improves the quality of life for patients. Pharmacists are well trained in pharmacology and therapeutics, as well as in pharmacokinetics, pharmacodynamics, and drug–drug interactions. The provision of pharmaceutical care involves various functions. One of the vital functions a pharmacist performs is a review of patient profiles by seeking to identify an indication for each medication that a patient may be receiving. Once the indication has been ascertained, the pharmacist determines if each medication is appropriate for the indication, in which case the dose and dosing interval are evaluated. Next, the entire medication profile is assessed to identify potential drug–drug interactions that may hinder the patient from achieving the desired therapeutic effect. One takes into account any gender and ethnic issues that may result in metabolic or pharmacodynamic concerns as well as the patient-specific kidney and liver functions. This is because the liver and kidney are the primary organs that break down and remove most drugs from the body and the prescribed medications may be ineffective or toxic in the event that the liver and kidney exhibit poor function. Taken together, the above steps represent the process of pharmaceutical care.

Pharmacists have other roles as well. For example, they play a critical role in improving patient adherence to their prescribed medications. Nonadherence has long been cited as a major reason for the lack of effect of medications. Since the pharmacist is often the last person to see the patient before they take their medications, especially in the retail setting, they are in an excellent position to advise and aid adherence to prescribed medication regimens and to intervene on the patient's behalf if problems exist. Adherence may be improved by educating patients about medications and the conditions being treated. An assessment of the patients' needs should be made to include the proper use of aids that are appropriate for language, readability, and font size (especially for the elderly).

Within a few years, there will likely be a critical shortage of pharmacists. Employment opportunities for pharmacists are expected to grow faster than the average of all occupations through 2010. This is largely due to the increased pharmaceutical needs of a growing elderly population and greater use of medication. Other factors include scientific advances, new development in genome research and medication distribution systems,

and consumer's desire for more drug information. By 2020, it is estimated that there will be a shortfall of 157,000 pharmacists. This is in part due to the aging population and the increase in health care services for this group but also due to other health care issues including the increased prevalence of chronic diseases, the complexity and number of medications available, the increased emphasis on primary care, home health care, and long-term care, and also concerns regarding cost containment. While new pharmacy schools have opened in recent years it is unclear if they will be able to fill the projected void between supply and demand. The role of the pharmacist will continue to evolve as changes in health care demand.

SEE ALSO: Disability, Morbidity

Suggested Reading

Schumock, G. T., Butler, M. G., Meek, P. D., et al. (2003). Evidence of the economic benefit of clinical pharmacy services: 1996–2000. *Pharmacotherapy, 23*(1), 113–132.

Suggested Resources

Retrieved February 11, 2003, from www.aacp.org/docs/mainnvigation/ for Dean/ 4108_cpspharmtrends.doc
Retrieved May 15, 2003, from www.bls.gov/oco/content/ocos079.stm

MATTHEW A. FULLER

Phobia
Phobias are irrational and excessive fears of specific things or situations. Phobias are categorized as a type of anxiety disorder. In modern psychiatry, phobias may be described as *specific* or simple phobias centered around clearly defined objects or circumstances, or fears around more general circumstances such as agoraphobia (fear of sudden, severe panic attacks) or social phobia (fear of social or performance situations in which extreme embarrassment may occur). There are many subtypes of specific phobias including fears of animals or insects (e.g., fear of spiders or snakes), fears of circumstances in the natural environment (e.g., fear of heights), fear of blood or injury, and fear of a variety of life circumstances (e.g., fear of enclosed spaces).

It is important to distinguish phobias from natural concern regarding potentially dangerous objects or circumstances. For example, a person who is concerned about snakebite if he or she is for some reason required to remove a venomous snake from the snake's hiding place would not generally receive a diagnosis of phobia. If, on the other hand, a person lived in an environment relatively devoid of snakes, was distressed by her fear of snakes, and had some degree of functional incapacitation because of her fear of snakes, then she might qualify for a diagnosis of a phobic disorder. Individuals with phobias have a marked and persistent fear that is cued by the presence of the phobic situation. Exposure to the phobic stimulus nearly invariably provokes an immediate anxiety response; sometimes individuals will experience a panic attack with rapid heartbeat, sweating, shortness of breath, and feeling dizzy. In cases of blood/body injury phobia vasovagal fainting can occur, indeed approximately 75% of individuals with blood/body injury phobia report a history of fainting in situations of blood drawing, injection, or body injury. Traumatic experiences such as being bitten by an animal or being trapped in a closet may predispose to the development of phobias as may informational transmission (e.g., repeated media coverage of airplane crashes may be associated with the development of phobia regarding air travel in some vulnerable individuals).

The content of phobia as well as their frequency of occurrence varies among cultures and ethic groups. For example, fear of magic or ancestral spirits is not uncommon in some cultures, and a diagnosis of phobia is only warranted in situations where the fear is excessive for a given culture and causes significant disability or distress. Phobias are relatively common in the populations with a community sample 1-year prevalence rate of 9% and a 10% lifetime rate. Gender ratios differ among phobia, with women being more likely to experience some specific types of phobias. Approximately 75–90% of individuals with animal- and natural environment-type phobias (e.g., fear of spiders) are women. An exception to this is fear of heights where women make up 55–70% of individuals with fear of heights. Approximately 55–70% of individuals with blood/body injury phobias are women as well. Phobias generally have their onset in childhood or young adulthood, in some cases persisting into adulthood. Treatment may involve a variety of behavioral or cognitive interventions. In one approach, exposure therapy, individuals are exposed to the feared object/situations to varying degrees of intensity and the focus of therapy is on lessening fear and anxiety related to the phobic object or situation. With some types of phobias, such as social phobia and agoraphobia (when individuals are

fearful of leaving their homes), medications may be helpful as well. Medications known to be useful in social phobia include selective serotonin reuptake inhibitors (SSRI), antidepressant medications, and beta-blockers, which reduce biologic anxiety symptoms.

SEE ALSO: Anxiety disorders, Cognitive-behavioral therapy, Depression

Suggested Reading

Heimberg, R. G., & Juster, H. R. (1994). Treatment of social phobia in cognitive behavioral groups. *Journal of Clinical Psychiatry, 55*(Suppl.), 38.

MARTHA SAJATOVIC

Phototherapy *see* Light Therapy

Physical Examination
The concept of the adult physical examination has changed significantly in the past several years. As compared to many years ago when having a "physical" meant an annual hour-long history and physical examination, medical care has changed to consist of a series of visits where a broad array of issues are addressed. The care is tailored to the patient's gender, health history, and family history. Screening for illnesses for which she is at risk, counseling for problems that she is at risk of, and immunizations are addressed during the visits. The extent of the physical examination is based on the clinical situation. The purpose of the physical examination is to allow the patient to express concerns and explain symptoms she is experiencing. It allows the physician to investigate physical complaints further as he or she examines the patient, and in some cases to establish a baseline of normal physical findings. It is an opportunity to obtain not only further history but to share a multitude of information between the patient and the physician.

WHAT IS A COMPREHENSIVE EXAMINATION?

A critical part of every physical examination is an assessment of the vital signs. This includes the pulse, respiratory rate, and blood pressure. Blood pressure is a very important part of any physical examination and if there are symptoms, it is important to check the temperature. An elevated blood pressure of greater than 140 systolic should be repeated with the patient at rest for 5 min. Antihypertensive medication should not be started based on a single high reading. At least three abnormal readings should be obtained before starting the medication. The blood pressure should be repeated to confirm that it is real and not due to anxiety.

Any skin lesions should be assessed and if the patient has any complaints regarding her hair or scalp, a thorough examination of the entire scalp, skull, and face should be done. A comprehensive examination of the eyes is generally done in an ophthalmologist's or optometrist's office. The primary care provider, however, does need to assess the position of the eyes and the health of the eyelids and conjunctiva of each eye.

Examination of the ears allows one to inspect the eardrums, canals, and external ears. The nose and sinuses are examined by palpating the areas above the eyebrows in the midline (frontal sinus) and the maxillary sinuses (below each eye). Palpation may reveal tenderness and provide clues to the presence of infection. Examination of the mouth and throat includes a check of the lips, oral mucosa, gums, teeth, and tongue. Lymph nodes are present in the neck, both in the front and the back of the neck and are referred to as anterior and posterior cervical lymph nodes. The thyroid gland rests in the middle of the neck in the midline and is palpated to check for enlargement or nodules. Examination of the chest is done using visual inspection, palpation of the chest wall, and listening with the stethoscope. The purpose of listening with the stethoscope is to identify any abnormal sounds that might indicate bronchospasm (wheezing) or crackling sounds that would be consistent with fluid in the lungs or infection. Examination of the breasts is done usually with the patient's arms relaxed and then elevated. It is also helpful to bring her hands to her hips and ask her to press down on the hips so that it may make any abnormalities more prominent.

The musculoskeletal system examination includes assessment of the arms, legs, shoulders, neck, and the temporomandibular joint, where the mandible (or jaw) connects with the skull. It is important that any painful joints be palpated and an evaluation of the range of motion of the joint be done.

In order to fully evaluate the heart, it is important to look at and palpate the carotids that are the large arteries in the neck. One may listen for carotid bruits that are

muffled sounds indicating possible obstruction in the vessels. Examination of the heart is done by listening to all areas of the heart that coincide with the four heart valves. When examining the abdomen it is important to first look then listen for the presence of bowel sounds. After bowel sounds are identified, it is appropriate to percuss the abdomen to identify the span of the liver. At this point, the examiner can examine lightly and then more deeply with the fingers. The genital and rectal examination in women is performed with the woman in the stirrups. The external genitalia are examined along with the vagina and cervix. A Pap smear is obtained; palpation of the uterus and the annexa (ovaries) is done.

The examination of the legs includes palpation to check for swelling in the legs, also known as edema. The pulse on the top of the foot is known as the dorsalis pedis and is one way to assess the adequacy of blood flow to the feet.

A neurologic examination assesses the health of the cranial nerves, which are the nerves that supply the face, head, and neck. The cranial nerves can be checked by looking for the patient's sense of smell, strength of the jaw muscles, corneal reflexes that are the reflexes of the eye when touched, facial movements, the gag reflex, and the strength of the muscles in the neck. Muscle strength testing is part of the neurologic examination, as is sensation and the evaluation of balance to further assess the cerebellar system.

WHAT IS THE APPROPRIATE DEPTH OF A PHYSICAL EXAMINATION?

This clearly must be based upon the patient's age, her known health problems, and her complaints. The depth of an examination for a healthy 40-year-old with no symptoms is very different from the depth of an examination given to a 30-year-old with severe illnesses. In general, what has been described above is a very comprehensive examination and not necessarily what is indicated for each patient at each visit.

It is important to realize that a physical examination provides an assessment of the person's physical status at the time of the examination. For example, a normal physical examination is no guarantee of normal health as it simply allows the physician to evaluate that person on that day. Taking a good history and doing a good examination so that appropriate testing may be ordered allows the physician to evaluate any symptoms that the patient may be having. However, unfortunately, it does occur that a person with no symptoms can become ill shortly after having a normal physical examination. This makes the point that a physical examination is no guarantee of sound health, but it is a great opportunity to identify and evaluate symptoms.

The frequency of the examination depends on the health status of each person. A well woman with no physical problems may go for a long period of time between physical examinations.

However, special populations do exist that do require much more compulsive care in order to prevent physical abnormalities in the future. Diabetic women require much closer monitoring of many aspects of their health, in addition to monitoring of their glucose levels. Because diabetics suffer from a certain set of illnesses, very specific examinations need to be done on a regular basis. Diabetes can cause retinal damage and result in blindness. Thus, it is very important for diabetic patients to have routine eye examinations by an ophthalmologist or optometrist. The blood pressure must be monitored and maintained within a very safe level. A foot examination utilizing a sensitive test called a monofilament examination is used to identify decreased sensation. By identifying women with decreased sensation in the feet, they can be targeted for interventions by the podiatrist to maintain healthy feet and reduce the risk of amputation that accompanies sensory loss. With regard to lab work, diabetic patients require routine monitoring of their glycosylated hemoglobin levels. This level indicates the overall control of the diabetes. Other routine monitoring that must be done is measurement of kidney function, evaluation and management of high cholesterol, and checks for protein in the urine.

There are other populations of patients who are disadvantaged, either due to homelessness, mental illness, or being in abusive situations. Many times these patients have difficulty keeping appointments, thus, when they do present for care, as much care should be given to them as possible.

SEE ALSO: Preventive care

Suggested Reading

Barker, L. R., Burton, J. R., & Zieve, P. D. (Eds.). (2003). *Principles of ambulatory medicine* (6th ed.). Philadelphia: J.B. Lippincott.

Bates, B. (1995). *A guide to physical examination and history taking* (6th ed.). Philadelphia: J.B. Lippincott.

Carlson, K. J., Eisenstat, S. A., Frigoletto, F. D., Jr., & Shift, I. (1995). *Primary care of women.* St. Louis, MO: C.V. Mosby.

Suggested Resources

The American College of Physicians, American Society of Internal Medicine, Ambulatory Medicine and Oncology sections, The Medical Knowledge Self Assessment Program 12.

KATHLEEN WOLNER

Physical Therapy

Physical therapy as a profession started in the late 1800s to early 1900s as a way of aiding rehabilitation of patients with poliomyelitis, which first affected children in the United States in 1894. One of the first people to practice physical therapy as a profession was a woman named Mary McMillan, who later served in World War I. She and other physical rehabilitation specialists and reconstruction aides, as they were called then, founded the American Women's Physical Therapeutic Association in 1921. The next year, the name of the organization was changed to the American Physiotherapy Association, and men were admitted. Current practitioners are physical therapists and physical therapist assistants. According to the Bureau of Labor Statistics' most recent data (annual average, 2002), 72% of physical therapists are women. Approximately 200 colleges and universities offer educational programs in physical therapy. The minimum educational requirement is a post-baccalaureate degree earned at an accredited program. Most programs offer a master's degree, but a Doctor of Physical Therapy degree is also available. Following graduation, licensure requires that the trainee pass a state-administered national exam. Other practice requirements vary from state to state. In 38 states, physical therapists may practice independently (without physician or other provider referral or consultation).

Patients are referred to physical therapy for a variety of reasons—some conditions include orthopedic complaints (back, neck pain), orthopedic injuries or surgery, traumatic brain injury, stroke, congenital disorders (in children), and urinary incontinence (especially in women). Physical therapy services typically require prior authorization from insurance companies and services are not covered in all plans. According to the American Physical Therapy Association, physical therapy includes several steps. First, the physical therapist or physical therapy assistant examines and evaluates patients with disabilities, impairments, functional limitations, and health conditions in order to formulate a diagnosis, prognosis, and intervention. *Impairment* refers to the loss of a psychological, physiological, or anatomical structure or function. *Disability* means a loss in the ability to perform activities of daily living (ADLs). The person referred for physical therapy may undergo a specialized physical examination by the physical therapist or assistant to evaluate the functional limitation that is of concern.

Second, the physical therapist or assistant designs, implements, and modifies therapeutic interventions to lessen existing impairments and functional limitations. Examples of interventions include therapeutic heat, therapeutic cold (cryotherapy), therapeutic ultrasound, ultraviolet light or laser light, hydrotherapy (using whirlpools and aquatic pools), traction devices, continuous passive motion, compression, and electrical stimulation. Examples of the use of these interventions are discussed below.

Third, the physical therapy professional helps people prevent injury and disability by promoting the maintenance of fitness, health, and quality of life. An excellent use of physical therapy is preventative, ranging from work with the elite athlete on proper athletic techniques to work with the elderly to prevent falls. Fourth, the professional engages in consultation, education, and research.

Physical therapy often involves exercises to promote a range of motion and improve strength. The physical therapist or assistant typically teaches these exercises to the patient, who performs the exercises with the therapist initially. Homework is usually assigned between sessions to improve the physical outcome. When most people think of physical therapy, this modality is what they envision. As mentioned previously, many other agents and techniques are utilized by the physical therapy professional.

Many people are referred to physical therapy treatment when an injury occurs, often leading to pain. Therapeutic heat is frequently utilized to ease pain, reduce muscle guarding and spasm, and aid tissue elasticity. Heat application may be superficial (e.g., using hot packs, whirlpool, and paraffin) or deep (e.g., using ultrasound or electromagnetic radiation in nonionizing form). Cryotherapy, or cold therapy, helps manage pain, edema, and muscle guarding/spasm. Cold packs, cool whirlpool, and ice massage are three cryotherapy agents. Cold therapy is used for acute injuries, as heat is contraindicated in the acute period because it may increase inflammation.

Ultraviolet light has been useful in the treatment of dermatological conditions including psoriasis; lasers have been helpful in promoting tissue healing and treating pain. Whirlpool therapy has several clinical uses, including pain relief, wound debridement, wound cleansing, and stimulation of circulation. Traction techniques, such as cervical traction and lumbar traction, are useful in conditions that may benefit from an increase in intervertebral space, such as disk herniation, muscle spasm, and arthritis of the spine. Traction works by applying a pulling force via either free weights or a traction machine to the spine.

Continuous passive motion is a type of passive motion which is produced using a mechanical device. It is often used postoperatively for joint injuries and reconstructions and is best started within the first postoperative week. Mechanical compression units are another type of motorized device that is used in physical therapy. Such devices deliver compression intermittently to reduce edema. Typically, patients wear compression garments between treatments to maintain improvement.

Lastly, electrical stimulation is used to help manage pain, strengthen muscle, stimulate denervated muscle, and ease edema. It is also beneficial in encouraging circulation, wound healing, and fracture repair. A device called a TENS (transcutaneous electrical nerve stimulation) unit has been especially helpful in the management of pain.

In summary, physical therapy is useful in the prevention and treatment of disability and physical limitation. Multiple techniques are employed by the physical therapy professional to achieve the goals of therapy.

SEE ALSO: Activities of daily living, Disability, Occupational therapist

Suggested Reading

Behrens, B., & Michlovitz, S. (1996). *Physical agents: Theory and practice for the physical therapy assistant.* Philadelphia: F. A. Davis.

Rothman, J., & Levine, R. (1992). *Prevention practice: Strategies for physical therapy and occupational therapy.* Philadelphia: W. B. Saunders.

Scott, R. (2002). *Foundations of physical therapy: A 21st century-focused view of the profession.* New York: McGraw–Hill.

Suggested Resources

American Physical Therapy Association website: www.apta.org

PAULA L. HENSLEY

Physicians The first woman who was formally academically trained as a physician in the United States was Elizabeth Blackwell, who graduated at the top of her class in 1849. In 2000, women represented 22.8% of U.S. physicians, and this is increasing, as women now enroll in medical schools at the same rate as men. Currently, during college, biology, chemistry, and physics classes are required as part of a "premed" curriculum. Medical school is 4 years long at present. Medical school combines classroom learning (including learning about normal physiology, anatomy, and abnormal pathology) and "rotations." Rotations occur in health care settings, such as hospitals and clinics, so that students can both observe physicians and learn experientially. More than 40% of medical students in the United States are currently women, which has been consistent with increases in female applicants. Some medical schools offer MD/PhD programs, which confer a dual degree on their graduates, preparing them to be both clinicians and researchers. Other medical schools offer DO (Doctor of Osteopathy) programs, with a holistic approach to medicine. During and after medical school, national standardized examinations, called USMLE (United States Medical Licensing Exams), are taken in addition to any exams in the medical school itself, to establish a standard for practicing doctors.

"Residency" is the physician training that occurs after medical school graduation, in the new doctor's choice of a generalist (primary care) or specialty field. Primary care physicians include pediatricians, family doctors, and general internists. Specialties include such diverse fields as psychiatry, ophthalmology, and surgery, among others. Based upon the chosen specialty, residencies are of different lengths, usually ranging from 3 to 5 years. The highest percentages of women residents can be found in OB/GYN (67%) and pediatrics (65%), caring for other women and children. Fields such as cardiology and surgery are still dominated by men. During medical school and training, doctors-in-training often work long hours, though this is currently undergoing change on a national level. Different medical specialties have various certification national procedures, including a written examination in that specialty and possibly an oral examination. "Chief residency" is a coveted position of authority at the senior resident level, which is an honor, as well as being a significant additional commitment. After residency, the physician may pursue a fellowship.

Fellowships are additional training in "subspecialties," such as colorectal surgery or forensic psychiatry, to gain additional expertise.

Physicians evaluate, diagnose, and treat patients, usually as part of a "treatment team" in which members of various professions collaborate (e.g., nurses, social workers, and physical therapists). Physicians may focus on inpatient (hospital-based) or outpatient care, or a combination. In addition to treating diseases, doctors practice "preventive health care" that may include Pap smears (to detect early cervical cancer) or testing cholesterol levels to decrease arteriosclerosis.

State medical boards grant licenses to physicians to practice. They also ensure that physicians complete required continuing medical education (CME) programs to keep their medical knowledge up to date. Additionally, medical boards keep records on physicians and may be involved in disciplinary action against physicians when needed. State medical boards can be contacted for information about physicians and some have information about physicians available online.

Though increasing numbers of women are entering the profession, medicine is still a male-dominated field. In particular, women are underrepresented in positions of leadership in medicine, including only a small minority of departmental "chairmen" and medical school deans. Due to the more recent entry of women into medicine, younger women entering the profession may experience a lack of more senior women to serve as mentors or role models. Women's medical societies, such as the American Medical Women's Association and the Association of Women Psychiatrists, have been founded to address issues faced by women in the profession. At a personal level, the length of training required to be a physician implies that women physicians may spend many of their childbearing years in training. In recent years, increasing numbers of women have surpassed obstacles to become successful physicians, and are paving the way for future generations of women to thrive in the field.

SEE ALSO: History of Women's Health (pp. 3–13); Women in the Health Professions (pp. 20–32); Blackwell, Elizabeth

Suggested Reading

Chin, E. L. (Ed.). (2002). *This side of doctoring: Reflections from women in medicine.* Thousand Oaks, CA: Sage.

Ehrenreich, B., & English, D. (1973). *Witches, midwives, and nurses.* Old Westbury, NY: Feminist Press.

Friedman, E. (Ed.). (1994). *An unfinished revolution: Women and health care in America.* New York: United Hospital Fund of New York.

Levin, B. (1988). *Women and medicine: Pioneers meeting the challenge* (2nd ed.). Lincoln, NE: Media.

SUSAN HATTERS FRIEDMAN

Piercing Body piercing has been practiced in many cultures for many centuries. Depending upon the era, the place, and the culture, body piercing has been variously associated with royalty, spirituality, sexuality, and beauty.

Body piercings can be done on almost any part of the body, including ears (lobes and cartilage), eyebrows, nostrils, nasal septums and bridges, tongues, lips, nipples, navels, and male and female genitalia. A piercing is done by passing a hollow needle through the body part, followed by the insertion of body jewelry. The piercing may cause a small amount of bleeding and the area that is pierced may be somewhat swollen and/or sore for several days afterward. A piercing gun should not be used for piercing because it crushes the tissues that are being pierced and the gun cannot be resterilized for the next person, increasing the risk that an infection can be spread from one individual to the next. These infections can range from a bacterial infection to hepatitis or even HIV. The healing time will vary depending upon which part of the body is pierced and how quickly an individual heals in general. Proper care of the piercing will hasten the healing process and reduce the risk of infection or other problems. It could take, for instance, from 4 weeks for the tongue to heal to 1 year for the navel or ear cartilage to heal.

Women may have particular concerns associated with piercing. Some piercers have suggested that women remove nipple piercings if they are going to breast-feed. The pierced area may close once the jewelry is removed and will have to be repierced. Women are also advised to wait to have a navel piercing done if they are pregnant or planning to become pregnant soon and to remove an already existing navel piercing if they are pregnant because the pierced area will stretch.

If you are considering getting a body piercing, it is important to consider the following.

1. It is best to have the piercing done by a professional piercer rather than a friend. A professional piercer will know how to do it safely.

2. Make sure that the parlor where you will have the piercing done is clean and maintains clean equipment. A fresh needle should be used for each client, and you should be able to see the piercer remove the needle from the unopened package. The piercer should be wearing new gloves for each client.

3. Make sure that the area to be pierced is first cleaned. The jewelry that is to be inserted into the freshly pierced site should be sterilized before it is inserted.

4. To avoid infecting the newly pierced site, make sure you wash your hands before touching the site.

5. Clean the pierced area with an antibacterial soap once a day. Softsoap, Provon, and Satin are recommended by many piercers.

6. There may be some discharge and crusting around the site. Remove this with warm water using a cotton swab (Q-tip).

7. Cleaning is usually easiest in the shower. Place a small amount of the antibacterial soap on your fingertips, lather the area, and work the jewelry back and forth several times gently in order to get the soap into the area. Wait 30–60 s and then rinse with warm water, working the jewelry back and forth in order to get all of the soap off.

8. Always support the area that has been pierced when you are washing it.

9. Soaking the pierced site in warm water with sea salts for 10 min a day will hasten healing and help to remove any crusting or discharge.

10. Some piercers recommend taking multivitamins and especially vitamin C and zinc to help the healing process.

11. Avoid overcleaning the area or changing the jewelry too soon because this can lead to other problems and/or infection.

12. If your jewelry is internally threaded, like barbells, be sure to check the ends twice a day to make sure that they are tight.

13. If you have a new piercing on your face or ear, avoid using makeup or hairspray/other hair products near that area until it is healed.

14. Do not wear tight clothes over the pierced area. If you have a navel piercing, do not sleep on your stomach. If you have an ear piercing, try to avoid sleeping on that side.

15. Signs of an infection include swelling or hardness in the area of the piercing, pain, a yellow or green discharge, and a feeling of heat in the pierced area. If any of these symptoms are present, it is wise to consult a physician.

Polyamory

See Also: Acquired immunodeficiency syndrome, Fetish, Hepatitis

Suggested Resources

Association of Professional Piercers: http://www.bodypiercinginfo.biz/index.html

Virtual Hospital: http://www.vh.org/pediatric/patient/dermatology/tattoo/index.html

DAVID VIDRA

SANA LOUE

Plastic Surgery *see* Cosmetic Surgery

PMS *see* Premenstrual Dysphoric Disorder

Polyamory In American culture monogamy, or the lifelong sexual and emotional commitment of two individuals to each other, is the norm. Unspoken and less frequently practiced is polyamory. Polyamory, from the Greek and Latin roots meaning "many loves," describes a diverse range of nonmonogamous relationship styles that heterosexuals, lesbians, gay men, and bisexuals practice. To be successful, individuals in polyamorous relationships typically negotiate a set of rules or agreements around issues such as safer sexual practices, social proximity to other lovers, frequency of contact between lovers, and level of emotional and/or sexual involvement between partners. These agreements make polyamory distinctly different than infidelity or promiscuity as all partners are fully aware of the arrangements. Although infidelity and cheating can occur within the context of polyamory, polyamorous individuals strive to be up-front and open about their desires and practices, which is why polyamory is sometimes referred to as "responsible nonmonogamy."

Although there is some disagreement over the terminology used to describe various multipartner relationships, they can be broadly categorized as primary, secondary, and tertiary. Primary partners are committed to a long-term, supportive sexual and emotional relationship and typically have a high level of involvement in each other's daily lives (e.g., share housing and finances). Secondary partners may also have a long-term, committed sexual and/or emotional relationship, but typically live separately and do not share finances. Tertiary partners may be involved in a relationship for a brief period of time or have a long-term, but infrequent relationship. Although tertiary relationships may be characterized as highly intimate, individuals' lives are typically not as intertwined. It is possible to have any number and combination of primary, secondary, and tertiary partners.

No matter the arrangement, polyamorous relationships are typically characterized by mutual respect and caring for all partners. Because of this, many polyamorous individuals claim that the lifestyle, or "lovestyle," is different from swinging, which involves more casual sex and typically does not allow for emotionally based relationships to develop. This distinction is tenuous, however, because some polyamorous individuals resist such hierarchical classification of relationships and reject such differences. These individuals may refer to their lifestyle as an "open relationship," instead of a "polyamorous relationship."

Multipartner relationships may be open or closed to outside sexual partners. For example, a triad of lovers may decide to be closed and thus only have sexual relations with members of that intimate network. Such closed polyamorous relationships are also called polyfidelity and are often considered a safer sex strategy. An open relationship among a small group of lovers does not have such rules on sexual relationships; however, there is usually an agreement between partners to disclose new sexual relationships and/or to consistently practice safer sex.

Although there has been little research on polyamorous relationships, practitioners often claim that with communication and support these relationships can be just as healthy as traditional monogamy and perhaps healthier than serial monogamy. Polyamory advocates claim that multipartner relationships may be an excellent solution for couples with different sex drives or different emotional or sexual needs. Furthermore, some believe polyfidelity or intimate networks are conducive for childrearing because they mirror the support provided by extended family.

Just as with monogamous relationships, feelings of jealousy are commonly experienced by those who practice polyamory. Unless agreements and commitments between partners have been violated, feelings of jealousy typically indicate an individual's insecurity, inability to trust, or lack of self-esteem. Polyamorous individuals are encouraged to process through feelings of jealousy and grow emotionally from the experience. The ability to do so, however, is a learned, ongoing skill and is usually more successful with the support of a skilled therapist or friends.

Because the Western world is couple-centric and values monogamy, polyamorous individuals often remain closeted or go through a "coming out" process as they accept their own desires and communicate those to others. Polyamorous individuals are often stigmatized as promiscuous, self-centered, irresponsible, and unable to commit, thus experiencing an emotional toll. It is important for polyamorous individuals to find a supportive therapist and community to help deal with and minimize the stigma of multipartner relations.

SEE ALSO: Safer sex

Suggested Reading

Anapol, D. M. (1997). *Polyamory: The new love without limits.* San Rafael, CA: IntiNet Resource Center.

Easton, D., & Catherine, L. (1997). *The ethical slut.* San Francisco: Greenery Press.

Matik, W. O. (2002). *Redefining our relationships: Guidelines for responsible open relationships.* Oakland, CA: Defiant Times Press.

West, C. (1996). *Lesbian polyfidelity.* San Francisco: Booklegger.

SARAH A. SMITH
JULIANNE M. SEROVICH

Polymyalgia Rheumatica

Polymyalgia Rheumatica Polymyalgia rheumatica (PMR) is an inflammatory condition that typically causes pain and stiffness in the neck, shoulders, and pelvic/hip muscles. It occurs almost exclusively in those over the age of 50 and occurs more often with age. PMR usually begins with stiffness in the morning that lasts greater than 1 hr. The stiffness is usually mild in the beginning, but increases with time and may become so severe as to cause difficulty getting out of bed. Occasionally symptoms begin quite abruptly and become incapacitating almost overnight. While the neck, hips, and shoulders have the most pain and stiffness, these areas rarely have swelling. The hands, wrists, and knees are involved less often, but when they are affected, significant swelling may occur in these areas. Symptoms such as fatigue, weight loss, and less commonly fever may occur in about one third of

patients. A severe headache, jaw pain, or new visual symptoms suggest the possibility of temporal arteritis, which can occur along with PMR. This requires immediate medical evaluation, as temporal arteritis can cause sudden irreversible blindness.

The most commonly used test in the diagnosis of PMR is the erythrocyte sedimentation rate (ESR), which indicates inflammation somewhere in the body. In PMR, the ESR level is usually greater than 40 mm/hr. A normal ESR does not rule out the diagnosis, however, and a highly elevated ESR does not necessarily mean more severe disease. The ESR is also elevated in many conditions other than PMR. Other laboratory abnormalities that may occur include mild anemia and occasionally abnormal tests of liver function.

Treatment with moderate doses of corticosteroids, such as prednisone 15–20 mg daily, usually leads to a prompt response with most symptoms resolving in 2–3 days. If adequate doses of corticosteroids do not improve symptoms, the diagnosis of PMR should be reconsidered. The average length of treatment is between 1 and 4 years, with some patients requiring treatment for longer. Corticosteroids can cause multiple side effects and the minimum effective dose should be used. When the corticosteroid dose cannot be lowered to an acceptable level, addition of the drug methotrexate may help. Due to the long duration of corticosteroid therapy, treatment to prevent corticosteroid-induced osteoporosis is often given along with the corticosteroids. This may include measurement of bone density, calcium and vitamin D supplementation, and medications to treat or prevent osteoporosis.

Other inflammatory conditions such as rheumatoid arthritis, infections, and malignancy may rarely mimic PMR. Usually, however, the diagnosis of PMR is clear because of its characteristic symptoms, elevated ESR, and prompt response to treatment. In 10–15% of patients, however, PMR may coexist with another condition called temporal arteritis, or giant cell arteritis. Treatment of temporal arteritis usually requires higher corticosteroid doses than PMR. Since temporal arteritis may develop during the treatment of PMR, symptoms of headache, jaw pain with chewing, or visual symptoms should be evaluated without delay, even in people who have responded well to treatment for PMR.

Most people affected by PMR will respond rapidly to treatment. With careful attention, side effects of treatment are manageable. People with PMR are generally able to lead normal lives with minimal effect on their quality of life or functioning.

Postpartum Disorders

SEE ALSO: Giant cell arteritis, Osteoporosis and osteopenia, Rheumatoid arthritis

Suggested Reading

Hunder, G. G. (2001). Giant cell arteritis and polymyalgia rheumatica. In S. Ruddy, E. D. Harris, & C. B. Sledge (Eds.), *Kelley's textbook of rheumatology* (6th ed., pp. 1155–1164). Philadelphia: W.B. Saunders.

Klippel, J. H. (Ed.). (2001). *Primer on the rheumatic diseases* (12th ed.). Atlanta, GA: Arthritis Foundation.

Salvarani, C., Cantini, F., Boiardi, L., & Hunder, G. (2002). Polymyalgia rheumatica and giant cell arteritis. *The New England Journal of Medicine, 347*, 261–271.

DOUGLAS FLAGG

Postpartum Disorders Any psychiatric illness may occur during the postpartum period. However, the most common disorders having an onset, recurrence, or exacerbation in the postpartum period include mood disorders and anxiety disorders. Difficulty with adjustment and problems in the mother–infant relationship may also occur after childbirth. Women who experienced a psychiatric disorder prior to or during the pregnancy are more likely to experience the symptoms in the postpartum period (up to 1 year after childbirth).

The postpartum period is a vulnerable time for emotional disturbances to occur. Physiologically, there is a rapid shift in hormones, fluid levels, and electrolytes. These changes affect neurotransmitter release and the neurological stress system (hypothalamic–pituitary–adrenal axis and peripheral nervous system) functioning. Psychologically and socioculturally, women and their families are adjusting to parenthood and the new roles they need to perform. This may create changes in the family system, particularly in the marital relationship. All these changes influence the development of postpartum psychiatric disorders.

POSTPARTUM MOOD DISORDERS

Mood disorders are the most common psychiatric illnesses to begin or exacerbate in the first few months to a year after childbirth. Major depression with postpartum onset occurs in 10–15% of women and includes identical symptoms to major depression in the general population of women. Major depression is a psychiatric disorder that is different from the more benign postpartum blues experienced by 50–80% of women just after delivery. Postpartum blues is a time-limited (4–10 days) disturbance of mood reactivity that includes unexpected mood changes (from sadness to elation) in response to seemingly minor details, tearfulness, irritability, and general anxiety, and does not usually interfere with daily functioning or overall enjoyment of life. Postpartum blues may result from a natural process of events following the extreme hormonal changes after delivery. Twenty percent of women experiencing "the blues" will develop major depression in the following months. Postpartum depression may begin in the first few weeks after delivery but is more commonly seen at 3–6 months postpartum. This is a serious disorder that requires treatment. Women with a prior history of a mood disorder or those who have had a previous postpartum depression are more likely to develop major depression after childbirth. Psychosocial factors influencing the development of postpartum depression include marital dissatisfaction, inadequate social support, and stressful life events.

Despite the relatively high prevalence of postpartum depression, many women with the disorder are not identified or treated. Women experiencing depression after the birth of a baby often feel the symptoms are evidence that they are bad mothers, influencing their decision not to disclose their symptoms. Some of the most difficult symptoms to disclose are obsessional thoughts of harming the baby or ambivalence and negative feelings toward the baby. However, the incidence of women with postpartum depression actually harming the baby is very low. Other symptoms include emotional lability, guilt, poor concentration and memory, poor sleep, and fatigue. Many of these symptoms are often labeled as expected in the postpartum period and are thus overlooked as an indication of a more serious illness. Although suicidal ideation is very common the actual rate of suicide is fairly low.

Major depression in the postpartum period has major consequences for mother–infant pairs as well as other family members. Depression can impair a woman's interest in her infant. The symptoms of fatigue, negativity, and general low functioning can also affect how the woman interacts with her infant and other family members. These factors often lead to a decrease in the quality of mother–child interactions, altered maternal responsiveness toward the infant, and increased child behavior and mood disorders later on. Early detection and treatment is essential. Treatment involves interpersonal, cognitive, or family therapy in conjunction with antidepressant medication (e.g., fluoxetine or nortriptyline).

Postpartum psychoses are rare, yet severe disorders still affect 1–2 women per 1,000 births. This rate has not changed in the last 150 years and it is consistent throughout other cultures studied, including women in Africa, the Middle East, and Asia. These data suggest that psychoses in the first 4 weeks after delivery are related more strongly to physiological (biological) factors rather than psychosocial factors. Postpartum psychosis is most often a manifestation of bipolar disorder as there is frequently a depressive, manic, or mixed mood episode occurring with hallucinations and delusions. The mood episodes occur within 2–14 days following delivery and come on suddenly. Early symptoms include restlessness, irritability, and insomnia. Within a very short period of time, extreme mood lability, disorientation, erratic behavior, and hallucinations or delusions begin to emerge. The delusions are often paranoid delusions that center on the infant being evil or in some way dangerous. There is a high risk at this time of suicide, homicide, and infanticide. If untreated, the rate of infanticide has been as high as 4%. In some cases, the experience of psychosis is not associated with a mood disturbance and may be associated with schizophrenia.

Psychoses in the postpartum period could also be caused by other medical conditions that are common during this time, such as thyroid disease, vitamin B12 deficiency, and Tay–Sachs disease. Medication such as some antibiotics, medications to stop lactation, or mood-altering drugs can also induce psychosis.

Once potential medical and drug causes are examined, early and aggressive treatment is needed. Treatment typically includes inpatient hospitalization, mood stabilizers (e.g., lithium), antipsychotic medication (e.g., olanzapine or Zyprexa), and occasionally benzodiazepines (e.g., lorazepam or Ativan).

POSTPARTUM ANXIETY DISORDERS

Although not as common as the mood disorders, anxiety disorders also occur in the postpartum period and are frequently comorbid with a mood disorder. The diagnoses include generalized anxiety disorder (GAD), obsessive–compulsive disorder (OCD), and post-traumatic stress disorder (PTSD). These disorders may develop with or without panic attacks.

GAD occurs in 4.3% of all women and as many as 10% of postpartum women. It is highly comorbid with depression and panic disorder. GAD occurs when there is excessive and persistent worry and anxiety that lasts for at least 6 months and causes significant distress or impairment.

OCD occurs in 3–5% of postpartum women and may be a new onset or a recurrence of a previous illness. The disorder is characterized by intrusive, obsessional thoughts. Occasionally the obsessions are associated with rituals or compulsive behaviors to relieve anxiety about the particular obsession. New mothers who develop OCD typically have obsessional thoughts about harming the baby. Unlike the hallucinations and delusions of postpartum psychosis, these thoughts are very frightening and provoke extreme anxiety. Women who suffer from these intrusive thoughts know the thoughts are wrong and do not harm their infants.

PTSD develops in the postpartum period generally after a certain event triggers a stress reaction or a panic attack. The event may be remembrance of a previous trauma, a very traumatic delivery, extreme suffering, a long hard labor, or an emergency cesarean section. The risk of developing PTSD following delivery is higher in women who have experienced difficult births in addition to neonatal death or stillbirth.

Treatment of anxiety disorders after childbirth is usually a combination of psychotherapy and medication. Cognitive-behavioral therapy is very effective in the treatment of anxiety disorders. Selective serotonin reuptake inhibitors (e.g., fluoxetine or Prozac and others), tricyclic antidepressants (e.g., clomipramine or Anafranil and others), and benzodiazepines (e.g., lorazepam or Ativan and others) are some of the medications used to alleviate the symptoms of anxiety disorders.

Adjustment to life as a mother or even to being a mother of multiple children can be very stressful, especially if there are additional medical or family concerns. Adjustment disorders may develop under such conditions. These disorders are characterized by marked distress to a known stressor, such as childbirth, changing roles, loss of income, and marital discord, which is in excess of what would be expected. Adjustment disorders in the postpartum period often involve depressed mood and anxiety as the main symptoms without symptoms of a significant mood disorder.

Any of the postpartum disorders can contribute to difficulties in the mother–infant relationship. Mothers experiencing postpartum psychiatric illness may be unable to care for their infant, may be afraid to harm the infant, or may reject the infant. In some instances, delayed attachment results from these conditions and requires additional treatment for the mother and the infant.

SEE ALSO: Anxiety disorders, Bipolar disorder, Depression, Mood disorders

Suggested Reading

Dunnewold, A. L. (1997). *Evaluation and treatment of postpartum emotional disorders.* Sarasota, FL: Professional Resource Press.

Gold, L. H. (2002). Postpartum disorders in primary care: Diagnosis and treatment. *Primary Care: Clinics in Office Practice, 29*(1), 27–41, vi.

Miller, L. J. (Ed.). (1999). *Postpartum mood disorders.* Washington, DC: American Psychiatric Press.

Sadock, B. J., & Sadock, V. A. (2003). *Kaplan & Sadock's synopsis of psychiatry: Behavioral sciences/clinical psychiatry* (9th ed.). Philadelphia: Lippincott, Williams & Wilkins.

Stotland, N. L., & Stewart, D. E. (Eds.). (2001). *Psychological aspects of women's health care: The interface between psychiatry and obstetrics and gynecology* (2nd ed.). Washington, DC: American Psychiatric Press.

Wisner, K. L., & Stowe, Z. N. (1997). Psychobiology of postpartum mood disorders. *Seminars in Reproductive Endocrinology, 15*(1), 77–89.

AMY L. SALISBURY

Postpartum Period The postpartum period, also known as the puerperium, lasts from the delivery of the infant until about 8 weeks after the delivery. Most of the anatomic and physiologic changes a woman experiences in pregnancy will have returned to the normal state by this 8-week time. The new mother will experience many changes during this postpartum period. The most important changes will be discussed.

The uterus rapidly returns to the normal, nonpregnant size over the first few weeks after delivery. Following delivery, there is a heavy, bloody vaginal flow, known as lochia, for several hours, which transitions into a reddish brown discharge by the fourth day postpartum. This discharge then transitions to a yellow-brown mucous discharge, lochia serosa, which lasts until approximately 25 days after delivery. However, 10–15% of women will still have some lochia serosa at the time of their 6-week postpartum visit with their obstetric provider.

Many women have an episiotomy or spontaneous laceration at the time of their delivery, which will be initially uncomfortable. Such women should delay intercourse for at least 3 weeks to allow healing of the wound and reabsorption of any suture used in the repair. Iced sitz baths appear to assist women by reducing pain and swelling. A woman should initially fill a sitz basin with tepid water, then add the ice cubes, with the episiotomy area remaining submerged in the bath for 20–30 minutes. Topical anesthetic sprays are often started in the hospital or birthing center after delivery. Pain from hemorrhoids, either from swelling or prolapse from the anus, may be managed with topical creams and witch hazel compresses (Tucks pad), and extra dietary fiber to ensure soft bowel movements.

Many couples do not resume sexual activity until after the 6- to 8-week postpartum examination by the obstetric provider. Though unnecessary to wait before resuming sexual relations at this time, for some women with minimal birth trauma, the sex drive (libido) is generally diminished for weeks to months due to fatigue and other family adjustments to the newborn infant. The couple interested in spacing pregnancies will want to consider a contraceptive choice before resuming sexual activity. Women who are breast-feeding "on demand," with the breast milk as the exclusive source of the infant's nutrition, will generally have several months of suppressed ovulation. The addition of another method of contraception, either hormonal (like the progestin-only contraceptive pill) or a barrier method (like a diaphragm or condom), will provide additional pregnancy protection. When women first become sexually active after a delivery, it is common to experience some vaginal dryness and discomfort. Use of additional lubrication (like Astroglide) and open communication with the partner regarding discomfort is essential.

Women are strongly encouraged to breast-feed their newborn infant. Breast milk provides the optimal nutrition for babies and is convenient and affordable. Breast-fed babies have less infectious illness and future problems with obesity. Maintenance of breast-feeding for at least the infant's first year of life is encouraged. Women returning to work after recovering from delivery can continue to provide breast milk, either by pumping and storing breast milk, or if available and close to the workplace, breast-feeding during work breaks.

The new mother will experience a full range of emotions during the first few weeks after delivery, including joy and contentment as well as sadness and a sense of being overwhelmed. A very common condition, affecting as many as 85% of new mothers, is a condition known as "postpartum blues" or "baby blues." The condition typically begins 3 or 4 days after birth and may last several days. Symptoms include mood swings (happy one minute, crying the next), feelings of depression, a hard time concentrating, a poor appetite, and sleeping difficulty. These symptoms will generally resolve by 10 days after the delivery. Some women have worse symptoms of depression, which lasts longer. This condition, known as "postpartum depression," is much more serious and requires evaluation by a health care professional. Women with postpartum depression will have symptoms that include loss of interest in activities, loss of appetite, low energy, a hard time falling asleep and staying asleep, frequent crying, and feelings of sadness, worthlessness, and hopelessness. A woman may also experience thoughts of harming herself. It is essential that women experiencing these symptoms be promptly evaluated and treated. Fortunately, the newer antidepressant medications, along with counseling, can result in significant improvements. Several of these medications can also be used safely in women who wish to continue breast-feeding.

SEE ALSO: Libido and desire, Postpartum disorders

Suggested Reading

Epperson, C. N. (1999). Postpartum major depression: Detection and treatment. *American Family Physician, 59*(8), 2259–2260.

Johnson, R. V. (Ed.). (1994). *Mayo Clinic complete book of pregnancy and baby's first year.* New York: William Morrow.

Gabbe, S. G. (Ed.). (2002). *Obstetrics: Normal and problem pregnancies* (4th ed.). New York: Churchill Livingstone.

Morrow, M. H. (2000). Postpartum depression. In R. Rakel (Ed.), *Saunders manual of medical practice* (pp. 636–639). Philadelphia: W.B. Saunders.

Suggested Resources

Postpartum Support International: http://www.postpartum.net/

KEITH A. FREY

Posttraumatic Stress Disorder Posttraumatic stress disorder (PTSD) is an anxiety disorder

that follows exposure to a traumatic event. Research shows that 10.4% of women and 5.0% of men develop PTSD at some point in their lives. The precise reason for the twice greater prevalence of PTSD in women is not known, though a combination of biological causes (e.g., hormones) and environmental causes (e.g., gender socialization) are most likely responsible.

A traumatic event is the experiencing or witnessing of actual or threatened death or serious injury. In women the most frequent traumas are childhood sexual abuse, rape, domestic violence, and traumatic labor and delivery.

The symptoms of PTSD are divided into three categories. The first is the persistent reexperiencing of the traumatic event. This reexperiencing can take the form of intrusive recollections, recurrent dreams, reliving of the experience, hallucinations, flashbacks, and intense psychological distress and/or anxiety on exposure to cues that symbolize the traumatic event.

The second category of symptoms is avoidance of stimuli associated with the trauma and numbing of responsiveness. The avoidance can take the form of efforts to avoid thoughts, feelings, activities, places, or people associated with the trauma. The avoidance can also be manifested by the inability to recall important aspects of the trauma. The numbing can take the form of diminished interest in significant activities, a feeling of detachment or estrangement from other people, restricted range of feelings and emotions (e.g., love or intimacy), and a sense of a foreshortened future.

The third category of symptoms are those of increased arousal. Profound difficulty falling or staying asleep is a hallmark of PTSD. Other symptoms of increased arousal are irritability or outbursts of anger, hypervigilance, exaggerated startle response, and difficulty concentrating.

The majority of individuals who experience a trauma manifest some of the above symptoms, but in approximately 50–66% of cases the symptoms begin to improve within 4 weeks. If the significant symptoms persist after 1 month, then a diagnosis of PTSD can be made.

Individuals with chronic PTSD commonly develop additional psychiatric illnesses. Depression and alcohol and/or substance abuse are the most common comorbid illnesses, but there is also an increased prevalence of panic disorder, generalized anxiety disorder, obsessive–compulsive disorder, and mania. The occurrence of the aforementioned comorbid illnesses can complicate the course and treatment of PTSD.

Preconception Care

Psychotherapy and medication are the two major forms of treatment of PTSD. The most commonly used psychotherapeutic treatments are known as cognitive–behavioral interventions. The goals of these techniques include: (a) helping patients to confront traumatic memories rather than avoid them; (b) decreasing avoidance of normal activities; (c) reducing anxiety associated with traumatic memories; and (d) correcting beliefs that have decreased self-esteem or the ability to function (e.g., inordinate guilt or feelings of helplessness).

The second major form of treatment of PTSD is medication. The group of medications that is known as antidepressants actually improves PTSD whether depression is present or not. The most effective medications in this category are the selective serotonin reuptake inhibitors, that is, medications that increase the availability of the neurotransmitter serotonin in the brain.

Future research on PTSD is focused on understanding how trauma adversely effects the biological functioning of the brain as a means of refining the treatment of the disorder. Recent research on an area of the brain known as the amygdala promises to enhance the understanding of how traumatic memories are recorded and reexperienced. Such research could lead to improved treatment of PTSD and could perhaps lead to prevention of the disorder in those exposed to traumatic events.

See Also: Anxiety disorders, Depression, Mood disorders, Panic attack

Suggested Reading

Foa, E. B., Keane, T. M., & Friedman, M. J. (Eds.). (2000). *Effective treatments for PTSD.* New York: Guilford Press.

Miller, L. J., & Wiegartz, P. (2002). Posttraumatic stress disorder: How to meet women's specific needs. *Current Psychiatry, 2*(2), 25–26, 35–38.

Yehuda, R. (Ed.). (1998). *Psychological trauma.* Washington, DC: American Psychiatric Press.

David S. Liebling

Preconception Care Preconception care is the promotion of the health and well-being of a woman and her partner before pregnancy. The optimal time to identify, manage, and treat many potential pregnancy conditions and complications is before pregnancy occurs. The goal of a preconception office visit with a primary care doctor is to identify and assess those medical and social conditions that may put the mother and her baby at risk. The benefits of intentionally preparing for a pregnancy relate to the important and critical period of fetal organ development that occurs in the first 10 weeks after fertilization. The traditional first prenatal visit is too late to impact on pregnancy complications impacted by prescription and nonprescription drugs, alcohol, and poor diet.

THE PRECONCEPTION HISTORY

The primary care physician will want to approach the preconception evaluation systematically. A woman should come to a preconception office visit prepared to discuss the following aspects of their health history:

- Medications
- Exposure to possible toxins
- Age, family history, and genetic disorders
- Infections and immunizations
- Social habits
- Diet and exercise
- Any chronic illnesses

Medications

A key challenge is to identify those medications and chemicals that are potentially harmful to the fetus before conception and discourage their use during the preconception and early pregnancy periods. All current prescription and nonprescription medications as well as herbal supplements must be reviewed.

Work, Home, and Hobby—Exposure to Toxins

Many toxic exposures are teratogenic (damaging to the fetus), including occupational exposure to organic solvents, anesthetic gases, and antineoplastic agents. Women planning a pregnancy should minimize use of common household products such as paint and paint removal products, bleaches, lye, and oven cleaners. There is no convincing evidence of adverse pregnancy outcomes for women exposed to common sources of electromagnetic field radiation, such as office and home computer use, electric blankets, and heated waterbeds.

Age, Family History, and Genetic Disorders

Many women are postponing pregnancy because of educational and career goals, therefore advanced maternal age is becoming more common. The older woman is more likely to have concerns about chromosomal abnormalities and infertility as well as an increased likelihood of chronic medical illness. Advanced maternal age contributes to the risk of chromosomal abnormalities, as does advanced paternal age over 60. The preconception period is the perfect opportunity to educate parents about a woman's fertility "biologic time clock" (particularly after the age of 35 years), and the purposes and techniques of prenatal diagnosis. A detailed review of the woman's family history and ethnicity for genetic disorders (for such disorders as cystic fibrosis, sickle-cell anemia, and Tay–Sachs disease) and malformations (such as neural tube defects) is important during a preconception office visit. A genetic counselor or maternal–fetal specialist may need to be seen if there is a personal or family history of a child with a potential genetic disorder, or advanced maternal age.

Infections and Immunizations

Hepatitis B is the most common type of hepatitis in the United States. Risk factors for hepatitis B include multiple sexual partners, sexually transmitted diseases, blood transfusions, and intravenous drug abuse in both the patient and her sexual partner. All women should be screened for hepatitis B, and those patients at high risk should have more detailed testing. Most women who might transmit the HIV infection to their fetus are asymptomatic. Vertical transmission (from mother to baby) results in approximately a 25% chance of fetal infection from an untreated HIV-positive mother, a risk that can be significantly reduced with preconception or early pregnancy treatment. During the preconception period, women should be educated about high-risk behavior as well as given advice on contraception. All sexually active women should be offered HIV testing.

Toxoplasma gondii is a parasite that can cause fetal growth retardation and congenital anomalies. Approximately 30% of adults in the United States have serologic evidence of prior exposure. Screening is controversial because evidence that treatment prevents congenital disease is lacking. Patients can reduce their risk by avoiding the high-risk practices of eating raw or uncooked meat, changing cat litter, and failing to wash kitchen knives after preparing raw meat products.

Congenital cytomegalovirus (CMV) infection occurs in 1% of all live births in United States, and causes major neonatal illness in 5–10% of these cases. Most congenital CMV is a result of a primary (first time) infection during pregnancy. No specific recommendations for health care and day care workers have emerged, other than universal precautions—thorough hand washing and use of protective gloves and garments. However, day care workers caring for children in the 12- to 36-month age group have the highest risk of occupational CMV infection and, if seronegative (no blood evidence of antibodies as protection), may want to consider shifting their job to care for either infants or older children to reduce their exposure.

The preconception visit should include an evaluation and update of standard adult immunizations. These would include tetanus, rubella, hepatitis, and varicella (chicken pox). Finally, pregnancy is considered a high-risk condition for influenza. Women expected to be at least 3 months pregnant during the influenza season (November to April) should be vaccinated.

Social Habits

A woman's psychosocial and mental health can have a significant impact on a pregnancy. Ongoing use of alcohol, tobacco, and illicit drugs should end due to the risks to the woman and her future baby. Unfortunately, approximately a third of women in the United States drink alcohol during their pregnancy. However, even modest amounts of alcohol consumption during pregnancy can cause persistent neurobehavioral deficits in children. Approximately 18% of pregnant women report smoking tobacco and will be at risk for such complications as abruptio placentae (placental abruption and bleeding), preeclampsia (toxemia), and preterm labor.

Diet and Exercise

A balanced diet, along with the achievement or maintenance of an ideal body weight improves pregnancy outcomes. Women with eating disorders should be evaluated and treated prior to pregnancy. Most general diets, including vegetarianism, will be safe during pregnancy. More restrictive diets, such as lactovegetarians (who eat no eggs) and vegans (who eat only plants), will require supplementary calcium, zinc, iron, and vitamins B and D. High-dose vitamin supplements should be avoided. Daily folic acid intake of 0.4 mg should begin at least 1 month prior to pregnancy and continued through the first trimester. For women who have had a child with a neural tube defect, a higher dose of folic acid (4.0 mg) is recommended and has been shown to decrease the recurrence rate of neural tube defects. The Food and Drug Administration has recently warned that women who may become pregnant, and those pregnant and lactating, should avoid certain fish (such as shark, swordfish, and king mackerel) because of methyl mercury. This form of mercury can cause harm to the developing fetal nervous system.

The current evidence continues to demonstrate marked benefit to both the mother and fetus for women who exercise during pregnancy. The current recommendation is for women to continue their prepregnancy activity level when they become pregnant. Specific guidelines for maximum heart rate ranges during pregnancy should be discussed.

Chronic Illnesses

The woman contemplating a pregnancy who has a chronic illness should seek the advice of her physician. Examples of such illnesses include asthma, high blood pressure, and heart and kidney disease. The physician's goal will be to optimize the health status for the existing illness prior to pregnancy, and alert the woman to any additional risks.

SEE ALSO: Diet, Exercise, Immunization, Pregnancy, Prenatal care, Toxoplasmosis

Suggested Reading

Frey, K. A. (2002). Preconception care by the nonobstetrical provider. *Mayo Clinic Proceedings, 77*(5), 469–473.

Frey, K. A. (2002). Preconception care. *Primary Care Reports, 8*(25), 222–227.

KEITH A. FREY

Preeclampsia Preeclampsia, otherwise known as "toxemia," is a disease unique to pregnancy that affects approximately 5–8% of all pregnant women. Preeclampsia is part of the spectrum of hypertensive disorders of pregnancy, which accounts for approximately 18% of all maternal deaths in the United States.

By definition, preeclampsia is unique to pregnancy and usually occurs after 20 weeks' gestation. Preeclampsia has traditionally been diagnosed clinically with a triad of signs including two of the following three: edema (swelling), hypertension (high blood pressure), and proteinuria (protein in the urine). The edema is significant if it occurs in the face and hands (as opposed to legs and feet), but this has recently become the least important symptom in the diagnosis. Preeclampsia can be associated with a dramatic weight gain over a short period of time. Hypertension is defined as two blood pressure readings of greater than 140/90 taken in the seated position greater than 6 hr apart. Prior to 20 weeks' gestation, an elevation in blood pressure is usually unrelated to the woman being pregnant, and preeclampsia is a disease that typically occurs later than 20 weeks' gestation. Proteinuria is defined as ≥300 mg protein in a 24-hr collection of urine or greater than or equal to 1+ protein dipped on a clean catch urine.

Risks factors for developing preeclampsia include: first pregnancy; more than one fetus (twins, triplets, etc.); having had preeclampsia in a prior pregnancy; diabetes; molar pregnancies; chronic hypertension; systemic lupus erythematosus (SLE); kidney disease; obesity; older age; thrombophilias (blood clotting disorders); and family history. The exact etiology of preeclampsia is unclear, but we have some clues. For example, preeclampsia is not only unique to pregnancy, but it is also unique to the placenta versus the fetus. This is demonstrated by the fact that molar pregnancies (without fetal tissue) are at high risk for preeclampsia as well as pregnancies complicated by abnormal placentas. There is evidence that changes of preeclampsia start as early as the first trimester of pregnancy with abnormal blood vessels in the early placental tissue. This may predispose a patient to release of "toxins," hence the older term toxemia. The only cure for preeclampsia is delivery or evacuation of the uterus. However, preeclampsia may be temporized depending on the severity of the disease and the health of the mother and fetus.

Preeclampsia is stratified into mild and severe. Severe preeclampsia is also subdivided into severe preeclampsia based on blood pressure (≥160/110 mm Hg as measured with a blood pressure cuff) or proteinuria (≥5 g in 24 hr), HELLP syndrome (hemolysis [the breakdown of red blood cells], elevated liver enzymes, and low platelets), and eclampsia. Other indicators of severe preeclampsia are maternal symptoms and fetal symptoms. Maternal signs and symptoms are headache, blurry vision or flashing lights, mid or right upper quadrant abdominal pain, oliguria (low urine output), pulmonary edema (water on the lungs), heart failure, and kidney failure. Fetal signs are oligohydramnios (low amniotic fluid) and intrauterine growth restriction (failure to grow appropriately in the uterus).

Eclampsia is perhaps the most severe form of preeclampsia and is defined by the presence of seizures with no other known seizure etiology. Prophylaxis against seizures is typically administered for the severe preeclamptic patient and often the mild preeclamptic patient. The most common and most effective seizure prophylaxis (preventive) is intravenous magnesium sulfate. The standard dose is 4 g IV (intravenous) over 20 min and then 2 g IV per hour. Seizures are most likely to occur during labor and in the first 24 hr after delivery. The most commonly associated prodromal (warning) symptoms of an eclamptic seizure are a headache and visual changes. Seizures have also been reported up to 2 weeks postpartum but if they occur more than 48 hr postpartum, other reasons for the seizure must be considered.

Management of preeclampsia and eclampsia depends on the severity as stated above. Eclampsia and HELLP syndrome necessitate delivery regardless of gestational age. Mild preeclampsia can be monitored closely until either the fetus' lungs are mature or a gestational age of 36 weeks is reached. Severe preeclampsia should also be delivered expeditiously unless the diagnosis is based on elevated blood pressure that can be controlled with medication or based solely on proteinuria. Patients who have severe preeclampsia but are delaying delivery due to fetal immaturity should be managed at a tertiary care center as an inpatient with daily maternal and fetal testing.

SEE ALSO: Diabetes, Hypertension, Preconception care, Pregnancy, Renal disease, Seizures, Systemic lupus erythematosus

Suggested Resources

http://www.acog.com

JANET M. BURLINGAME

Pregnancy
Pregnancy is a time of great anticipation and immense physiologic change for a woman. A woman's body goes through significant anatomic and hormonal changes during pregnancy in order to support the development of her growing baby. The estimated date of delivery or "due date" is generally 40 weeks after the first day of the last menstrual period. Ultrasound can also be used to establish the dating of the pregnancy if the last menstrual period is uncertain. Pregnancy is divided into trimesters for the purposes of discussing common milestones and problems at each period of development. Maternity care providers often refer to the "gestational age" in weeks during ongoing care; gestational age includes the 2 weeks prior to conception.

The first trimester includes the weeks between the last menstrual period and 12 weeks of pregnancy. Conception occurs in the fallopian tube 1–5 days after an ovum (egg) is released from the ovary and is fertilized by a sperm. The first division of cells occurs 12 hr later and the fertilized egg continues to divide every 12–15 hr thereafter. When the fertilized egg drops out of the fallopian tube into the uterus it contains hundreds of cells. Implantation of the fertilized ovum (now called a blastocyst) occurs 4–8 days after ovulation. The corpus luteum, a structure on the ovary that is a remnant from the ovarian follicle that released the egg, secretes the female hormone, progesterone. This hormone prevents the endometrial (uterine) lining from shedding, thus allowing the blastocyst to remain implanted in the uterus. Occasionally, a fertilized ovum will not be able to exit the fallopian tube. This results in a condition called ectopic pregnancy. Ectopic pregnancies put the mother at significant risk for intra-abdominal bleeding as the fallopian tube is not designed to support a developing embryo.

Within 12 days after conception, the placenta, a collection of both embryonic and maternal cells, begins to form. This organ exchanges nutrients from the maternal blood supply for waste products from the fetus. The developing embryo attaches to the placenta via the umbilical cord. The placenta and ovaries all contribute to increased levels of progesterone, estrogen, and beta-human chorionic gonadotropin (beta-hCG, the "pregnancy hormone") that are necessary to maintain a normal pregnancy.

At 5 weeks' gestation (3 weeks after conception) the embryo is $\frac{1}{7}$ in. long and has developed three separate cell layers. One layer develops into the neural tube (brain, spinal cord, nerves, and backbone). A second layer becomes the heart and blood vessels, bones, muscles, and genitourinary system. The heart begins to beat 21–22 days after conception. The third (inner) layer develops into the urinary bladder and esophagus, stomach, and bowel.

Pregnancy

Three weeks later the embryo is $\frac{1}{2}$ in. long and the arms and legs have begun to develop. Transvaginal ultrasound can easily detect an embryo with a heartbeat at this time.

At 8 weeks' gestation (5 weeks after conception) the embryo is $1\frac{1}{4}$ in. long. The beginnings of all major organs are formed and the skeleton and ears are beginning to develop.

At the end of the first trimester, or 11–14 weeks' gestation (9–12 weeks since conception), the embryo is 3 in. long and weighs $1\frac{1}{2}$ oz. All organ systems are in place and the brain, nerves, and muscles start to function. The embryo has begun to make small movements although the woman is not able to feel them due to its small size. The genitalia now have recognizable male or female characteristics.

The first trimester is a period of critical organ development. Infections and environmental toxins (tobacco products, illicit drugs, alcohol, medications, and chemical exposures) can cause abnormalities in development, particularly 3–8 weeks after conception (5–10 weeks' gestation). Examples of problems that can occur include abnormal development of the brain and spinal cord (neural tube defects) and miscarriage. The risk of neural tube defects can be decreased by ensuring maternal intake of at least 400 mg of folic acid daily prior to conception. Over 80% of miscarriages occur in the first 12 weeks of pregnancy. They are most commonly caused by abnormal division of the embryonic cells or abnormalities of the fetal chromosomes that lead to abnormal organ development. Common symptoms of miscarriage include cramping and bleeding.

Many women experience nausea and vomiting, increased fatigue, frequent urination, breast tenderness, and dizziness during the first trimester. Nausea and vomiting are due to the hormonal changes, primarily increased progesterone and beta-hCG, that occur with early pregnancy. Up to 70% of women experience these symptoms, which typically begin at 6–8 weeks' gestation and diminish after 13–16 weeks. Fatigue is due to increased metabolic demands on the female body. A pregnant woman begins to produce more blood cells and her heart rate increases to accommodate the need to pump blood to the placenta and developing embryo. The increasing size of the uterus and increased efficiency of the maternal kidneys both contribute to urinary frequency, a condition which eases during the second trimester. Increased maternal estrogen and progesterone both cause breast tenderness, enlargement, and tingling. These hormones also promote further breast development throughout the pregnancy to support lactation. Dizziness due to hormonal changes as well as changes in heart rate and blood volume may also be worsened by fatigue and nausea. Concerning symptoms that should be reported to the maternity care provider during the first trimester of pregnancy include vaginal bleeding and cramping, abdominal pain, and painful urination.

The second trimester includes 13–27 weeks of gestation (11–25 weeks after conception). At 15–18 weeks' gestation (13–16 weeks after conception) the fetus is $3\frac{1}{2}$ in. long and weighs 7 oz. The eyebrows and scalp hair are beginning to develop. By 19–22 weeks' gestation (17–20 weeks after conception) the fetus is $7\frac{1}{2}$ in. long and weighs 1 lb. At this time, vernix, a white creamy substance, forms on the skin in order to protect it from the amniotic fluid. The fetal kidneys have begun to make urine and all internal organs are formed. The fetus is able to hear and react to sound. At the end of the second trimester (21–25 weeks after conception or 23–27 weeks' gestation) the fetus has little body fat. It is 11–15 in. long and weighs $1\frac{1}{2}$–2 lb. The lungs have begun to secrete surfactant, a chemical which will prepare the fetal lungs to breathe air after birth.

From a maternal standpoint, the second trimester is often referred to as the "golden period." Fatigue and nausea have improved and the body has not yet changed enough to feel awkward. Most women begin to experience fetal movement, described as "fluttering" or "tapping" between 18 and 20 weeks' gestation. The uterus is rapidly increasing in size and will be measured at each prenatal visit. It typically reaches the level of the maternal umbilicus by 20 weeks' gestation and increases by 1 cm per week thereafter. Lower blood pressure and increased heart rate may predispose the mother to light-headedness with rapid changes in position. There may be an increase in vaginal discharge due to increased hormonal levels. Common physical complaints at this time include leg cramps and low back pain. Slowing of bowel motility due to progesterone can cause increased heartburn and constipation. Anticipated maternal weight gain during this portion of pregnancy is 1 lb per week.

The third trimester encompasses 28–40 weeks' gestation (26–38 weeks after conception). A fetus between 28 and 31 weeks' pregnancy is able to open its eyes. The lungs are more developed but often require support for breathing if born prematurely. At this stage, the fetus weighs 2–3 lb and is 12–16 in. long.

Between 32 and 36 weeks' gestation, the fetal lungs continue to mature and the sucking reflex, required for feeding, is improving. Premature infants at this stage of development vary in their need for support of temperature, feeding, and breathing. These fetuses range from 3 to 6 lb and are 16–19 in. long.

Typical maternal symptoms during the third trimester include shortness of breath due to increased pressure of the growing fetus and uterus on the diaphragm. Some pregnant women experience sciatic nerve pain (sharp pain or numbness in the buttock radiating into the leg) due to pressure of the uterus on this nerve. Sharp or stabbing pain in the vaginal area is not uncommon as the cervix begins to change in preparation for childbirth. This is generally not concerning unless accompanied by abdominal pain or bleeding. Increased urination and difficulty finding a comfortable sleeping position result in maternal sleep disturbances.

At 37–40 weeks' gestation the fetus is considered full term. Less than 3% of women will deliver on their due date at 40 weeks' gestation. Average weight at the time of delivery is 6–9 lb with a length of 18–21 in. Many pregnancies may continue for 1–2 weeks after the due date. Labor may commence at any time. The baby is fully developed, and if healthy, is ready for delivery and life outside the mother. A pregnancy is not considered abnormally prolonged until it has exceeded 42 weeks.

SEE ALSO: Labor and delivery, Miscarriage, Neural tube defects, Pregnancy testing, Prenatal care

Suggested Reading

Baxley, E. G. (2001). Physiologic changes and common discomforts of pregnancy. In S. D. Ratcliffe (Ed.), *Family practice obstetrics* (2nd ed.). Philadelphia: Hanley & Belfus.

Johnson, R. V. (Ed.). (1994). *Mayo Clinic complete book of pregnancy and baby's first year.* New York: William Morrow.

Nilsson, L., & Hamberger, L. (1990). *A child is born.* New York: Bantam Doubleday Dell.

Suggested Resources

The Visible Embryo: http://www.visembryo.com/baby/

ANDREA DARBY-STEWART

Pregnancy Testing
Early and accurate diagnosis of pregnancy is important in order to determine the estimated date of delivery and to allow the pregnant woman to make decisions regarding her reproductive care. There are several different ways to diagnose intrauterine pregnancy including increased blood or urine levels of the pregnancy hormone beta-human chorionic gonadotropin (beta-hCG), ultrasound visualization of an embryo in the uterus, and the presence of audible fetal heart tones.

Within 12 days after conception, the placenta, a collection of fetal and maternal cells, begins to form and secrete the hormone beta-hCG. The levels of beta-hCG double every 2–3 days and are detectable in both blood and urine. Concentrations of this hormone vary depending on the individual and the stage of pregnancy.

Home pregnancy tests use monoclonal antibodies to detect the presence of beta-hCG in the urine. Some tests are able to detect very low levels of this hormone (approximately ten millionths of an International Unit) several days before a missed menstrual period. However, due to the very low levels of hormone in the urine and inherent inaccuracies of the test, up to 50% of early pregnancies may be missed if a woman depends only on this early urine testing. Home urine pregnancy tests are most accurate if taken 1 week after the missed menstrual period. A positive home pregnancy test should be followed up by an appointment with a maternity care provider (family physician, midwife, or obstetrician) to confirm the diagnosis of pregnancy and discuss ongoing care.

While urine tests are designed to detect either the presence or absence of beta-hCG, serum pregnancy tests can be used to quantify the amount of this hormone in the blood. The absolute amount of beta-hCG may be used by a woman's health care provider to follow the progress of the early pregnancy. A level that does not double every 2–3 days may be suggestive of a nonviable pregnancy.

Ultrasound of the uterus can provide confirmation of an intrauterine pregnancy as well as an accurate estimate of the due date. Typically, by 6 weeks' gestation (4 weeks after conception), a transvaginal ultrasound can detect an embryonic pole and heartbeat. It is possible to hear the fetal heartbeat through the abdominal wall using a Doppler device at 10–12 weeks' gestational age (8–10 weeks after conception).

SEE ALSO: Pregnancy, Prenatal care, Ultrasound

Premenstrual Dysphoric Disorder

Suggested Reading

Johnson, R. V. (Ed.). (1994). *Mayo Clinic complete book of pregnancy and baby's first year.* New York: William Morrow.
When the test really counts. Part one: Earliest pregnancy detection. (2003, February). *Consumer Reports,* 45–47.

KEITH A. FREY

Premarital Agreement *see* Prenuptial Agreement

Premenstrual Dysphoric Disorder

Hippocrates first documented mood and bodily symptoms related to the menstrual cycle. In 1931 the term "premenstrual tension" was introduced. This related to a set of symptoms that appeared a week before menses and resolved with the start of menses. In the 1950s, Greene and Dalton coined the term "the premenstrual syndrome" (PMS), but PMS has not been in the forefront of medical science until more recently. In contrast, popular culture has long discussed PMS. It is both a well-known term to the layperson and now the subject of examination by the American Psychiatric Association. PMS is the diagnosis frequently given by primary care physicians and obstetrician–gynecologists. Mental health practitioners favor the term "premenstrual dysphoric disorder" (PMDD).

The continuum of PMS complaints varies with each individual. Physical symptoms include headaches, breast pain, fatigue, weight gain, appetite changes, and bloating. Emotional symptoms are irritability, depressed mood, and mood swings. Both the physical and emotional symptoms must occur in the latter half of the menstrual cycle usually ending when menstrual flow begins. Approximately 70% of menstruating American women have some type of premenstrual complaints. Only 3–5% of these women have problems severe enough to interfere with life activities, meriting a diagnosis of PMS or PMDD. For these women, the physical and emotional symptoms can significantly interfere with relationships at work and home, leading to potential economic problems and divorce.

Obtaining the correct diagnosis is crucial for the patient. Many common psychiatric disorders produce similar symptoms. Environmental factors such as the presence of active domestic violence and past sexual abuse play into the reporting of premenstrual problems. Some women may be more comfortable seeing their gynecologist as opposed to seeing a psychiatrist due to how they view psychiatric care. Ethnic and racial groups around the globe have symptoms but describe different severity levels and different manifestations of their PMS.

Risk factors include age in the late 20s to mid-30s, and for some women, a history of mental health difficulty as well as a family history of PMS. Patient evaluation for PMS/PMDD requires careful screening to rule out various disorders that may present to the physician as related to premenstrual difficulties. The key feature of both PMS and PMDD is the timing of symptoms to the latter half of the menstrual cycle (the luteal phase). After eliciting a listing of medical problems, a careful psychiatric history is crucial. Depression, anxiety/panic, eating disorders, or even substance abuse belie the true cause of their symptoms. Making the diagnosis even more challenging is the fact that the luteal phase of the menstrual cycle can exacerbate all of the above psychiatric illnesses. Asking about domestic violence or sexual abuse completes the necessary history.

In order to assess the relationship of the symptoms to the luteal phase of the menstrual cycle, a prospective recording of changes in mood, irritability, carbohydrate cravings, weight gain, and the like must be obtained. The diagnosis of PMDD requires prospective recording of two menstrual cycles. Using a graph-like system, the patient should code symptom type and severity underneath the sequential days of the cycle.

The underlying causes of PMS have not been completely elucidated. Endocrine studies show that PMS is not related to a simple excess or deficiency in hormone status. Genetic factors exist as well. Identical twins have similar scoring of their PMS symptoms in comparison to fraternal twins.

The interaction of ovarian steroid hormones with the central nervous system neurotransmitters may be the true basis for PMS. The role of the neurotransmitter compound serotonin appears to be significant. This substance is also believed to be involved in a host of psychiatric disorders. Animal data indicate that ovarian hormones influence serotonergic brain activity. Lower levels of serotonin are believed to cause symptoms of depressed mood, irritability, impulsiveness, as well as the increased desire for carbohydrates. The natural central nervous system opiate compounds along with gamma-aminobutyric acid (GABA) and adrenaline-related neurotransmitters may also be involved.

Treatment approaches for PMS/PMDD vary widely, but only a few have undergone rigorous evaluations. Some pharmacological treatments have been studied thoroughly, whereas healthy lifestyle changes have not been evaluated under controlled studies. Antidepressants called selective serotonin reuptake inhibitors (SSRIs), such as fluoxetine (Prozac), can be administered daily or during the luteal phase of the cycle. Related compounds sertraline (Zoloft) and paroxetine (Paxil) also may be effective. These medications show efficacy both on emotional symptoms as well as some of the physical symptoms especially bloating, breast tenderness, and appetite. Adverse effects include low libido that complicates continuous dosing of these medications. The tricyclic antidepressant clomipramine showed positive results. Medication for anxiety such as alprazolam (Xanax), as well as the novel anxiolytic agent buspirone may be reasonable alternatives. Gonadotropin-releasing hormone (GnRH) analogs provide relief by stopping ovarian function. However, GnRH analogs may not relieve the severe emotional problems of PMS/PMDD and will potentially cause osteoporosis and symptoms of menopause. There have been mixed results using standard oral contraceptives, because they may improve only a few of the physical symptoms and do not always lead to improvement of the emotional symptoms. Using oral contraceptives in a continuous fashion (eliminating placebo pills, that is, the pills that do not contain hormones) may be more successful. Danazol, an androgenic synthetic hormone, may help in treating mood and physical symptoms of PMS along with relief of premenstrual migraine headache. Unfortunately, danazol and other medications also have some unwanted side effects.

Nonpharmacological approaches, though not as well researched, appear to help many women. The elimination of caffeine, alcohol, chocolate, and sugar may provide some relief. Calcium supplementation of 1,200 mg a day showed better-than-placebo (pills that do not contain any drug) rates of improvement in mood and emotional difficulties. Pyridoxine (vitamin B6) in doses under 100 mg a day may provide some efficacy, though adverse effects such as insomnia and neuropathy may complicate therapy. Aerobic exercise can be very helpful. Psychotherapy and patient education offer help to many women as well.

SEE ALSO: Anxiety disorders, Bipolar disorder, Menstrual cycle disorders, Mood disorders, Oral contraception, Psychologists, Psychotherapy

Suggested Reading

Group Health Cooperative. (1992). *Premenstrual syndrome.* Seattle, WA: Group Health Cooperative.

Harrison, M. (1999). *Self-help for premenstrual syndrome.* New York: Random House.

Htay, T. T., et al. (2002). *Premenstrual dysphoric disorder.* http://www.emedicine.com/med/topic3357.htm

Lark, S. (1993). *Premenstrual syndrome self-help book: A woman's guide to feeling good all month.* New Providence, Bahamas: Celestial Arts.

Ling, F. W., et al. (Eds.). (1998). *Premenstrual syndrome and premenstrual dysphoric disorder: Scope, diagnosis, and treatment.* Washington, DC: Association of Professors of Gynecology and Obstetrics.

Yonkers, K. A., & Davis, L. L. (2000). Premenstrual dysphoric disorder. In *Kaplan and Sadock's comprehensive textbooks of psychiatry* (pp. 1952–1958). Philadelphia: Lippincott, Williams & Wilkins.

SHARON ABEGG

Premenstrual Syndrome *see*
Premenstrual Dysphoric Disorder

Prenatal Care
A pregnancy is an exciting and wonderful event in a woman's life, one which incorporates remarkable physical changes, intense emotions, and growth in important relationships. About 50% of pregnancies are unplanned, which may have consequences to the physical health of the mother and fetus, as well as emotional turmoil. Planning and preparing for a pregnancy will often improve the outcome and is the subject of the entry Preconception care.

PREGNANCY CARE

One of the most important steps a woman can take when she either suspects a pregnancy or notes a positive home pregnancy test is to establish an early appointment with the obstetric provider. In the United States, there are both physician and nonphysician health care professionals who provide pregnancy care through the delivery of the infant. The physician specialties include obstetricians and some family physicians. Nonphysician professionals include two kinds of midwives: the certified nurse midwife and the lay midwife. The availability of each of these four types of pregnancy care providers varies by region in the United States.

An early prenatal appointment is essential to establish an accurate "due date," or what the physician calls an "EDC" (estimated date of confinement). A woman should try to make her first prenatal appointment within 2–3 weeks of missing her period or noting a positive home pregnancy test. Any bleeding, cramping, or severe abdominal pain warrants an urgent physician appointment, either with the primary care physician or seeking emergency department services if needed.

Perhaps the most accurate way to settle on the EDC is by a woman's first day of her last menstrual period (called the "LMP"). A woman should try to keep an accurate record of the first day of the onset of her monthly period for several months prior to a pregnancy. She should also note any additional spotting or abnormalities of her menstrual flow. If a woman has irregular menstrual cycles, or had recently ended the use of oral contraceptive pills to get pregnant, then the obstetric provider will generally order an early (first trimester) ultrasound to establish an accurate EDC.

The first prenatal visit will include a comprehensive review of the medical and family history, a physical examination, and routine laboratory work. The newly pregnant woman should come to this appointment with a well-organized list of her past medical problems, medication allergies, prior surgeries, and family medical history. Additionally, any family history of genetic disorders or mental retardation should be known. The woman should clarify if she has either had chicken pox or received the chicken pox (varicella) vaccine. The woman should have a list of all her current prescription, nonprescription, and herbal medications. The physical examination will include a pelvic exam with updating, the Pap smear, and the obtaining of cultures to exclude infections that may affect the pregnancy. Routine blood and urine testing will establish the woman's blood type and Rh status, complete blood count (indirectly assessing iron levels), and tests for prior evidence of immunity to rubella (German measles), hepatitis B, and HIV. This first prenatal visit is an excellent time to ask any questions about the pregnancy, upcoming tests, and to clarify any "advice" received from well-meaning friends and relatives.

Common issues that pregnant women face include work concerns, travel advice, exercise, nutrition, and sexual intimacy:

1. *Work concerns.* Most occupational activities are safe to continue during a pregnant. The obstetric provider should be aware of the nature of the pregnant woman's work, and offer advice if the workplace includes exposure to potentially toxic chemicals and extremes in temperature and physical activity.

2. *Travel advice.* Automobile and air travel are safe for the majority of the pregnancy. Most major airlines restrict air travel during the last few weeks of pregnancy, and generally the pregnant woman will want to be close to her home and obstetric provider anyway. Whether by car or air, the pregnant woman should stretch every 1–2 hr to minimize any risks to lower leg swelling and potential blood clots. Seat belts should be worn throughout the pregnancy, with the shoulder belt worn as usual and the lap belt fastened low over the hips.

3. *Exercise.* In general, overall physical conditioning provides benefits for both the mother and baby. In addition to the sense of well-being, mothers-to-be who are physically fit, benefit from improved sleep patterns and bowel habits. Women are encouraged to maintain their prepregnancy level of fitness, and not try to significantly increase their workouts once pregnant. The obstetric provider will provide advice on which forms of exercise are safest and most effective, as well as maximum heart rate limitations for the pregnant state.

4. *Nutrition.* A diet that is adequate in calories and balanced in nutrients is an important component of healthy pregnancy. There are many accurate resources to access complete pregnancy-related nutritional information (some listed under Suggested Reading at the end of this entry). Several points to know include the importance of folic acid (at least 0.4 mg daily) and adequate intake of iron and calcium. Additionally, certain fish are to be avoided during pregnancy and lactation (breastfeeding) due to possible high levels of methylmercury. The list of fish to avoid includes: shark, swordfish, king mackerel, and tilefish.

5. *Sexual intimacy.* Generally, a pregnant woman may continue to enjoy sexual intimacy throughout her pregnancy, unless the obstetric provider instructs otherwise. Often sexual desire is diminished in the first trimester due to nausea and fatigue. In the third trimester, finding a comfortable position for intercourse will require open communication between the couple. Achieving orgasm, or a climax, is also safe throughout

pregnancy, again unless restricted due to pregnancy complications by your obstetric provider.

ROUTINE PRENATAL VISITS

After the initial prenatal visit, the obstetric provider will see most women monthly until the last months of the pregnancy. These shorter visits focus on any new concerns the woman has, checking for certain symptoms (such as headaches, leg swelling, uterine contractions, vaginal bleeding), and physical findings. The weight and blood pressure are measured at each visit, the urine is checked for sugar (diabetes) and protein (kidney problems), the baby is checked for adequate growth (by measuring the mother's abdomen), and the baby's heart tones are noted. Women are encouraged to bring along a list of any questions or concerns. In the last 8 weeks of the pregnancy, the visits become more frequent—often every 1–2 weeks.

Several additional tests are offered at certain times in the pregnancy:

1. *Serum alpha-feto protein test.* This test of the pregnant woman's blood provides a screen for congenital anomalies in the baby called neural tube defects (like spina bifida, where there is an incomplete formation of the spinal cord and its coverings) and the chromosomal anomaly called Down's syndrome. The test actually involves evaluating the levels of four chemicals in the blood (so now known as a "Quad" screen) and must be accurately timed between 15 and 19 weeks of the pregnancy. Though only a screening test, any abnormality may or may not represent a true anomaly in the fetus, and may necessitate further testing by ultrasound or amniocentesis.

2. *Genetic counseling and amniocentesis.* These services are offered to women with a personal or family history of genetic abnormalities, or if the woman will be 35 years or older when she delivers. An amniocentesis is a procedure in which a sample of the fluid surrounding the fetus (amniotic fluid) is withdrawn through a needle. The needle is guided by an ultrasound through the woman's abdomen in such a way as to minimize any risks to the baby. The fluid is analyzed for the specific chromosomes.

3. *Ultrasound.* The majority of pregnant women are offered at least one ultrasound, and the optimal timing for a single ultrasound is midway through the pregnancy (18–20 weeks). This study provides images of the fetus without the use of the radiation needed in standard x-rays (and therefore felt to be safe). The ultrasound will assess the baby for adequate growth, organ development, and placental location.

4. *Gestational diabetes screening.* Some women are at risk to develop a form of diabetes in pregnancy known as gestational diabetes. In this condition, the mother-to-be's blood sugars are higher than normal, and can lead to pregnancy complications, such as a very large baby at delivery and placental abnormalities. Most women are screened between 26 and 28 weeks of the pregnancy for this condition by a simple blood sugar test 1 hr after drinking a sugar solution. When identified, the condition is usually well controlled with a specific diet alone. In rare circumstances, treatment with insulin may be required.

5. *Blood antibody testing and RhoGam administration.* Human beings have one of several "types" of blood, depending on the genetic profile acquired from their parents. Blood is typed by two systems: ABO (types A, B, O, AB) and Rh (types positive and negative), and each individual will have a blood type with both designations (such as "O positive" or "AB negative"). Women with an Rh-negative blood type (about 15% of the population) may become "sensitized" by their baby's blood during a pregnancy, which can affect future pregnancies. To prevent this potential complication, women with an Rh-negative blood type are given an injection of a medication called "RhoGam" at approximately 28 weeks and again after their delivery.

6. *Cultures for group B streptococcus.* Approximately 30% of women will have a common bacterium, the group B streptococcus, present in the vagina at the time of their delivery. This bacterium often is present without any signs of an active infection like a vaginitis or bladder infection, but can infect the baby during the passage through the birth canal. To identify pregnant women at risk of this infection and offer antibiotics during labor and delivery, a simple vaginal culture is done about 1 month prior to the delivery date.

CHILDBIRTH EDUCATION

To fully understand and plan for the birth experience, the pregnant woman and her partner should attend childbirth education classes. These programs are often taught by experienced childbirth educators or nurses, and provide an understanding of the labor and birth process. These education classes include information on pain management, labor signs, help in designing a personal birth plan, and a tour of the hospital birthing center. Additionally, many programs offer classes on the care of the infant and breast-feeding. Most couples find these childbirth programs help in allaying fears, guiding toward more informed choices about the delivery, and building a sense of "team" between the woman and her partner.

LABOR

The culmination of the pregnancy process is the delivery of a healthy baby. A pregnancy is at full term at 40 weeks of gestation, when measured from the first day of the last menstrual period. A woman will generally enter the beginning of labor between 37 and 41 weeks of gestation. Labors that begin before 37 weeks, or beyond 41 weeks, require special attention by the obstetric provider and the pediatric staff. The onset of labor is signaled by rhythmic uterine contractions that gradually increase in frequency, intensity, and duration. Occasionally the "bag of water" (amniotic fluid) will rupture before the onset of labor contractions. The woman may note a blood-tinged mucus discharge from the vagina 1–2 days prior to the onset of labor, often called the "mucus plug." The obstetric provider will give instructions on when and how to contact the birthing center during the early labor stages.

The labor process is divided into three stages: The first stage is the longest and begins with the onset of contractions that dilate the cervix (birth canal). This first stage varies in length, with first-time mothers having the longest stage. The second stage begins with the full dilation of the cervix and is completed with the birth of the baby. This second stage generally lasts from 1 to 3 hr and includes a time when the mother actively assists the delivery of the baby by "pushing" or bearing down. The third and final stage of the birthing process includes the passage of the placenta or "afterbirth," and is generally completed within 30 min of the birth of the baby.

SEE ALSO: Diabetes, Diet, Exercise, Labor and delivery, Nutrition, Pelvic examination, Physical examination

Suggested Reading

Johnson, R. V. (Ed.). (1994). *Mayo Clinic complete book of pregnancy and baby's first year.* New York: William Morrow.

Gabbe, S. G. (Ed.). (2002). *Obstetrics: Normal and problem pregnancies* (4th ed.) New York: Churchill Livingstone.

Homan, D. D. (2000). *Pregnancy.* In R. Rakel (Ed.), *Saunders manual of medical practice* (pp. 636–639). Philadelphia: W.B. Saunders.

KEITH A. FREY

Prenuptial Agreement

A prenuptial agreement is an agreement made before a marriage that concerns arrangements for when the marriage ends by divorce or death of one of the parties. These agreements are also known as premarital agreements or antenuptial agreements. These agreements usually describe how the parties' money and possessions will be divided, although some agreements cover additional topics, such as arrangements for children from prior marriages or children that the marriage may produce.

Premarital agreements are often used when one or both of the people to be married have children from a previous relationship and there is a desire to keep assets available for those children rather than having those assets awarded to a new spouse. These agreements are also used when there is a great disparity between the incomes or assets of the people who are to marry and the person with greater resources wants to keep those resources in the event of a divorce. For example, the person who is wealthy may seek to limit the amount of property or support that the new spouse could claim upon divorce, and may seek an agreement that a certain sum would be awarded if the marriage lasts for a year and greater amounts would be awarded if the marriage lasts longer.

These agreements are contracts, and courts usually enforce contracts, which means that courts can make people live up to their agreements. But historically courts did not enforce premarital agreements because the agreements were thought to promote divorce. With the increasing frequency of divorce, courts are increasingly enforcing prenuptial contracts.

These agreements are not typical contracts, like for the sale or purchase of products. Prenuptial agreements are made between people who love and trust each other and will be promising to spend the rest of their lives together. Because of this relationship between the parties, courts look at these agreements much more carefully before enforcing them.

Courts often find out whether each person had a lawyer to represent them in making the agreement. This is not required for most other contracts, but may be required before a prenuptial agreement can be enforced. The wealthier person will almost surely have a lawyer prepare the contract and the court may require a separate lawyer for the person with less resources.

Courts may also require that each party tell the other what income and assets she or he has. This is done to make sure that the person with fewer resources knows what kind of income or assets she or he is agreeing to do without in the event of divorce.

Sometimes prenuptial agreements are not enforced because they were made under duress. This means that someone was forced to sign the agreement or given little choice. Agreements that are proposed immediately prior to the wedding may be examined for duress.

SEE ALSO: Divorce

Suggested Reading

Haman, E. (1998). *How to write your own premarital agreement.* Naperville, IL: Sphinx.

Lindey, A., & Parley, L. (1999). *Lindey and Parley on separation agreements and antenuptial contracts.* New York: Matthew Bender.

SHEILA SIMON

Preventive Care
Prevention of disease and injury is a major part of routine health care. It is important to identify risk factors that predispose patients to a myriad of different illnesses. By identifying risky behaviors or abnormalities, such as high blood pressure, these problems can be modified or eliminated entirely, thus reducing the woman's risk of future illnesses. In order for a population to be screened or counseled for any given illness, it must be a common illness that causes a significant burden of suffering in people. It must be proven that the early detection of these problems in persons before they develop symptoms actually helps them to live better and longer. Screening for cancers is a major part of preventive care and these are addressed in other sections. Screening for high blood pressure, a key component of preventive care, is covered in the entry Hypertension.

EVALUATION OF CHOLESTEROL

There is clear evidence that high cholesterol is a cause of coronary artery disease (heart disease) and that lowering the level of cholesterol can reduce the risk of heart disease. The American College of Physicians and the U.S. Preventive Services Task Force recommend that screening for high cholesterol begin at the age of 45 for women. Screening women younger than 45 years of age is not recommended by these two groups unless the patient has known heart disease, a family history of heart disease, or unless she has multiple other risk factors for coronary artery disease. The National Cholesterol Education Program (NCEP) suggests that screening begin at the age of 20 and that blood tests be checked every 5 years. The NCEP delineates between high-risk and low-risk persons. The NCEP defines risk factors for coronary artery disease as age, family history of early coronary artery disease, current smoker, hypertension, diabetes, and a low level of high-density lipoprotein (HDL), the protective form of cholesterol. Screening is usually done with a serum total cholesterol. High is considered over 200 mg/dl. If there are two of the above risk factors, it is appropriate to measure a fasting lipid panel to determine the levels of low-density lipoprotein (LDL), triglycerides (TGs), and HDL. Unless the LDL level is very high, coupled with multiple risk factors for heart disease, treatment usually begins with dietary restriction of fat. However, based on the NCEP guidelines, immediate initiation of drug therapy may also be indicated based on risk factors, along with the absolute level of cholesterol, specifically the LDL.

IMMUNIZATIONS

Vaccination Status

At the age of 50 years, vaccination status should be reviewed for all patients. The tetanus–diphtheria boosters should be given every 10 years throughout a person's life. Unfortunately, compliance with this regimen has been poor. Therefore, tetanus cases continue to occur.

Influenza Vaccine

Immunizations for influenza are recommended for normal-risk adults between the ages of 65 and 75 years. Younger persons who qualify for an influenza vaccination include those with chronic diseases of the heart, lungs, and kidneys or other diseases causing immunosuppression (decrease ability to fight infection). Diabetics and persons who live with diabetics are also high-priority patients for this vaccination. Public health authorities are increasingly recommending offering influenza vaccination to all healthy adults.

The pneumonia vaccine should be given once between the ages of 65 and 75 years in normal-risk adults. If a patient received the pneumococcal vaccine before the age of 65, she should receive a second dose 5 years after that vaccination was given. Patients younger than 65 who are at high risk for pneumococcal disease include the following: Those with chronic diseases of the heart, lungs, and kidneys, diabetics, alcoholics, persons with serious liver disease, patients with immunosuppression, patients with no spleen (either through illness, surgery, or a nonfunctioning spleen), and patients with lymphoma or a history of multiple myeloma would qualify at a younger age. The pneumococcal vaccination is a 23-valent vaccine and it contains capsular materials from 88% of the strains responsible for serious illness from pneumonia in the United States. It does decrease the rate of pneumonia.

Hepatitis A Vaccine

Hepatitis A vaccine is a vaccine prepared from virus and is very effective in the populations of healthy volunteers in whom it has been studied. Hepatitis is a viral infection of the liver that is usually self-limited but causes a great deal of suffering for the patient. Hepatitis A vaccine should be considered for international travelers going to developing countries, persons relocating to areas of poor sanitation, military personnel, intravenous (IV) drug users, and persons with occupational risks (such as sanitation workers).

Hepatitis B Vaccine

Hepatitis B vaccine is now routinely given to children and adolescents not previously vaccinated, and should be considered in persons at increased risk including women with multiple sexual partners, injection drug users, and health care workers. The effect lasts at least 7 years and does decline over time.

Varicella Vaccine

The varicella vaccine should be considered for women without a history of chicken pox or antibodies

to the varicella-zoster virus who work in high-risk environments, including day-care centers or health care settings. It is important that women of childbearing age not become pregnant for 3 months after having received this vaccine. (Pregnant women in the third trimester who do not have history of chicken pox or antibody evidence of previous infection should be considered for varicella immunoglobulin if they are exposed to an individual with chicken pox.)

SUBSTANCE ABUSE

Alcohol Abuse

The use of alcohol causes many serious health problems in adults. Women are affected to a greater extent because it takes less alcohol in women to cause the adverse effects than in men. It is felt that they have a decreased level of a liver enzyme that detoxifies alcohol, and being smaller, they have a lower volume of distribution of the alcohol. Seventeen to nineteen percent of persons, men and women, in the primary care setting have evidence of risky drinking behaviors. Thirteen to thirty-five percent of persons, at some point in their lifetime, will have some problem with alcohol abuse and dependence. As this is such a common disorder, it is important that patients share honestly with regard to the amount and the frequency that they use alcohol. Lack of being forthcoming with this information leads to underrecognition of alcohol use, and misses an important opportunity to get help for the drinking problem. For patients who are dependent on alcohol, their physician can refer them to the appropriate groups or specialist to help them. Alcohol treatment programs are also available and can improve abstinence from alcohol and increase the intervals between relapse.

Drug Abuse

Part of preventive care is to assess a person's use of illicit drugs. For many reasons, especially out of concern for legal and social implications, many patients will understate the use of illicit drugs. Marijuana is the most commonly used drug, followed by cocaine. Women over the age of 18 are half as likely to use illicit drugs, as are men. Drug use carries serious risks including the risk of HIV infection due to injection drug use and the fact that drug use is commonly involved in motor vehicle injuries. While the U.S. Preventive Services Task Force does not recommend routine screening for drug abuse with either questionnaires or serum or urine testing, the task force does acknowledge that a careful drug history is important on other grounds. It is very important for your future to share this information openly with your physician.

Tobacco Dependence

Tobacco smoke causes much disease and a great deal of suffering in men and women. It is definitely a positive factor in many cancers, as well as in heart disease and emphysema. It is the most preventable cause of premature death. In 1994, nearly one fourth of women smoked. Lung cancer is now more common in women than breast cancer.

One year after stopping smoking, there is a 50% reduction in the risk of heart disease death or heart attack. The stroke risk reduces 2 years after, and after 10–15 years, approaches that of a nonsmoker. The cancer risk drops more slowly with lung cancer being 50% at 10 years, and esophagus and oral cavity cancers are reduced by 50% at 5 years.

It is important for the smoker to involve her physician in her smoking cessation plan. Advice from the physician can help to motivate the patient and provide information that may help when there is a temptation to smoke. There are methods to stop smoking, including working with the physician to set a quit date, identification of barriers to stopping smoking, and dealing with the temptation that might lead one back to smoking. Drug therapy is available to help a person wean from the effects of nicotine. The withdrawal symptoms can begin 24 hr after the last cigarette and last for several weeks. These symptoms can be extremely bothersome and often intolerable. Most smokers gain approximately 10 lb after they stop smoking. The Agency for Healthcare Research and Quality (AHRQ) recommends a nicotine patch initially. Another drug used for treatment of nicotine dependence is bupropion, which is an antidepressant. It has shown good success in increasing the number of persons who quit smoking. It does carry some adverse effects and the physician and patient must weigh these.

EXERCISE

It is extremely important that physical activity be a part of one's life. Hypertension, diabetes, obesity, osteoporosis, anxiety, and depression are all less common in those who participate in regular exercise. The majority of Americans tend to lead a very sedentary lifestyle. It is not necessary to be involved in an organized exercise program, although it is desirable. However, many patients do not have the time or the access to the facilities to get into a regular program. What is important in an exercise program is to make it easily achievable and easily adopted into the person's life. The goal is that adults do a total of 30 min or more of continuous or intermittent moderate to intense physical activity on most days of the week. Walking, hiking, stair climbing, aerobics, rowing, swimming, and other sports such as tennis and racquetball are excellent ways to achieve this 30 min of exercise. Gardening, housework, and other active tasks apply to the 30 min recommended physical activity per day. It need not be an organized activity on a court or in a gym! For those who are accustomed to an inactive lifestyle, starting a walking program is an excellent way to achieve success in the area of exercise. It is important to understand that there will be muscle aches at the beginning of any program and to not be discouraged when this occurs.

INJURY PREVENTION

Injuries are the fifth leading cause of death overall and the most common cause of death in persons under the age of 40. Smoke detectors, air bags, and seat belt use are paramount in injury prevention. It is important that firearms in the home are in a secure and safe place at all times. It is important to keep the water temperature at a safe level to avoid burns and secure all rugs to avoid falls in the home.

NUTRITION IN THE PRIMARY CARE SETTING

A healthy diet is paramount to reducing one's risk for chronic diseases. Four of the ten causes of death, heart disease, cancer, stroke, and diabetes, are all associated with unhealthy diets. An optimal diet is low in fat, especially saturated fat, trans-fats, and cholesterol. The other characteristics of a good diet include one that is high in fruits, vegetables, and whole-grain products containing fiber. The Dietary Guidelines for Americans recommend 3–5 daily servings of vegetables and vegetable juices, 2–4 daily servings of fruits and fruit juices, and 6–11 daily servings of grain products. Saturated fat should make up less than 10% of the calories and no more than 30% of calories should come from fat.

OSTEOPOROSIS PREVENTION

Healthy women should ingest between 1,000 and 1,500 mg of elemental calcium per day, either through diet or oral supplements. Vitamin D deficiency, which can reduce the absorption of calcium through the intestines, is common, thus a supplement of 400–800 IUs per day is recommended. It is important that one engage in daily physical activity, especially weight-bearing exercise, including walking, jogging, and climbing stairs.

FOLIC ACID

There is evidence that folic acid is instrumental in the prevention of neural tube defects in babies (spina bifida) and is recommended for women considering pregnancy and definitely during pregnancy.

SEE ALSO: Cancer screening, Cardiovascular disease, Coronary risk factors, Diet, Exercise, Immunization, Nutrition, Physical examination, Smoking, Substance use, Tobacco

Suggested Reading

Barker, L. R., Burton, J. R., & Zieve, P. D. (Eds.). (2003). *Principles of ambulatory medicine* (6th ed.). Philadelphia: J.B. Lippincott.

Carlson, K. J., Eisenstat, S. A., Frigoletto, F. D., Jr., & Shift, I. (1995). *Primary care of women*. St. Louis, MO: C.V. Mosby.

Suggested Resources

The American College of Physicians, American Society of Internal Medicine, Ambulatory Medicine and Oncology sections, The Medical Knowledge Self Assessment Program 12.

KATHLEEN WOLNER

Prison Health In 1998 more than 950,000 women were under correctional supervision, comprising about 7% of the overall imprisoned population in the United States. Women represent the fastest growing incarcerated population. The highest percentage has been convicted of property crimes such as check forgery and illegal credit card use. The next largest percentage has been convicted of nonviolent drug offenses, followed by violent felonies. The majority of violent felonies are associated with women's attempts to defend themselves or their children from abuse. Ninety percent of women in prison are single mothers, 40% having children under the age of 18; 58% have not finished high school; 54% are women of color; 80% have incomes of less than $2,000 per year; and 92% have incomes under $10,000 per year.

The imprisonment of women impacts both the family and the community. When women go to prison, their children often end up in foster care; in many cases the women lose their parental rights altogether. Alternatively, other family members may care for the children but often they are older and may need additional care themselves.

In general, the health status of women prisoners is poor. This is a result of many factors. The majority of people in prison are poor and/or minorities who have lacked access to health care throughout their lives and often have not received prior medical treatment. Consequently, many female prisoners suffer from late-stage disease complications such as cirrhosis and diabetes; communicable diseases such as HIV, hepatitis B, and tuberculosis; and diseases of addiction, such as end-stage alcoholism and drug addiction. Many incarcerated women are survivors of physical and sexual abuse, which puts them at a greater risk for developing life-threatening illnesses such as HIV/AIDS, hepatitis C, and human papillomavirus/cervical cancer. Women in correctional institutions are often victims of sexual abuse by prison staff or by predatory prisoners. Women who give birth while incarcerated often remain restrained during delivery, are denied labor support from family members, and are not permitted to breast-feed. In addition, they are often required to relinquish their infant within 72 hr of delivery. There are some model programs in existence where the mother is allowed to be with her child during her prison sentence, but these programs are few and far between.

An estimated 25% of all women in prison suffer from mental health illnesses such as major depression, bipolar disease, schizophrenia, posttraumatic stress disorder, and addiction disorder. Death from suicide is common in prison. Some believe this is a result not only of a mental illness but also because of the isolative and disempowering nature of imprisonment, solitary confinement, overcrowding, longer prison sentences, and an often hostile prison environment. Mental health care providers are in short supply within correctional institutions. Correctional officers often lack an understanding about appropriate management of mental illnesses and treat mentally ill prisoners as if they are or will become violent, restraining or placing them in isolation, which often serves to aggravate the psychiatric condition. Many prisons have reduced funding for rehabilitation programs for prisoners with addictions, even though tougher laws are resulting in more people being imprisoned for nonviolent drug crimes.

Access to care and the quality of care received vary between federal prison and state and county correctional institutions. In many states, a request for care is first reviewed by a medical technical assistant (MTA) who often has minimal medical training. The MTA decides whether or not the prisoner will see a physician. Even if the prisoner is granted permission to see the prison doctor, it does not mean they will get timely care. Many prisoners must wait all day to see a physician. If the clinic closes before they are seen, they have to come back the next day. Many prisoners work within the institution and they forego their pay for the days spent waiting to obtain care. In some prisons, a missed day of work results in another day added to their prison sentence. Additionally, some states require a prisoner to contribute a co-pay for care. Such policies act as a disincentive for a prisoner to seek medical attention when they need it, often resulting in a medical condition that is more advanced, threatening, and difficult to manage.

Prisoners face a confidentiality problem when receiving their medication. They must wait in line to receive their medication. In some states, medications like those for HIV are dispensed in a unique packet that signifies to others in line the confidential medical condition of a prisoner. This can result in prisoners' avoidance of testing or treatment for some conditions. The dispensing of medication is also interrupted during security situations, which can result in the development of drug resistance or the exacerbation of a medical condition. Many prisons require patients to take the medication in the "med line," which can interfere with the patient's ability to take the medication properly, for instance, with food.

Preventive care such as regular Pap smears and breast exams are nearly nonexistent in prison systems, as are health education programs and materials. If a prisoner is referred to an outside physician there is often difficulty with continuity of care and refusal or inability of prison medical staff to follow the outside physician's order.

Many health care workers see prisoners as unlawful, dangerous, and irreparable. A belief that prisons should "lock prisoners up and throw away the key"

and that prisoners should "lose their rights" makes it easier for the prison systems to continue with a system of less than adequate health care for inmates. These biases also exist among health care workers treating former prisoners.

The relative inaccessibility of care and the lack of preventive measures while incarcerated can lead to worsening medical conditions which, when eventually treated, are more costly. The price is paid either by the prison system, by the public health system when a prisoner eventually returns to the community, by the community itself in potential transmission of disease, and/or by the prisoner or former prisoner in terms of pain, suffering, and deteriorated health.

SEE ALSO: Domestic violence, Prostitution, Violence

Suggested Resources

Prison Activist Resource Center, women and prison, eleven things you should know about women in the United States. Retrieved March 10, 2003, from http://prisonactivist.org/women
Understanding prison health care. (2002, June 13). Retrieved March 10, 2003, from http://movementbuilding.org
United States Department of Justice, Office of Justice Programs, Bureau of Justice Statistics. (2003, January 8). Retrieved March 24, 2003, www.ojp.usdoj.gov/bjs/crimoff.htm#findings

JUDITH TRENTMAN

Probate Probate stems from the Latin word *probare* meaning "to prove" and derives its usage from the practice in medieval England of heirs having to prove their right of inheritance of land to the king's court. At that time in history, land conferred wealth and power upon its owner and its transfer was carefully controlled. The early Americans continued the practice of judicial oversight of property transfer but expanded it to include both real and personal property. Today, the term probate generally refers to the laws regarding the process of settling a decedent's estate under the supervision of the court, and in a broader sense of the word refers to the administration of estates, guardianship, adoptions, and/or trusts with court oversight.

Today, courts charged with oversight of the probate process may be called Probate Court, Surrogates Court, Orphans Court, Chancery Court, Circuit Court, or Court of the Ordinary and may be presided over by a judge, surrogate, or magistrate. These are courts of local jurisdiction, such as a county, parish, or other designated district and are governed by the laws of the state or commonwealth and their own local rules.

The contemporary process of "proving" a will begins with the submission of the will itself to the Probate Court. The will is accompanied by an application or petition to probate the will, which details the name of the decedent and his or her date and place of death. The petition must also include the names and addresses of all interested parties, which may include next of kin, beneficiaries named under the will, and persons otherwise named or mentioned in the will. Those interested parties have a set period of time after the submission of the will in which to object to its validity. If no objections are made, a will is considered to be "self-proved," if it was executed according to governing law. If objections are made, the Court must then decide the validity of the will.

The Court must approve the appointment of a person to administer the estate. This person is referred to as an executor if named in the decedent's will to administer the estate, or may be called an administrator or personal representative, if the decedent left no will or the person designated such in the will was unable to serve in that capacity. The Court generally looks to the next of kin to fulfill this administrative role.

The process of estate administration, greatly simplified, includes: the gathering of the decedent's assets, appraisal and inventory of those assets, payment of the debts of the decedent and costs associated with administering the estate, calculation and payment of estate or inheritance taxes and income taxes, distribution of specific bequests or remaining assets under the terms of the will or as directed by law, and accounting to the Court of the disposition of the assets.

Requirements as to how the administration of an estate is conducted and the time frame in which it must be completed may be dependent on the size and complexity of the estate and vary from state to state, but most states have enacted laws to streamline and simplify this process. Many states have also adopted all or part of the Uniform Probate Code to give some consistency to this process across the country.

"Small" estates, estates with assets whose value is under an amount prescribed by law, may be distributed to the heirs without a formal administration of the estate but must still have the will submitted to Court and have the distribution approved by the Court. This process may be referred to as "relief from administration" or "small estate administration," or other names. This

process is less time consuming and generally less costly than a full estate administration.

Even with the current push to make the probate process easier, many people still seek to avoid probate and its negative associations. These negatives include the Court having authority superior to the family in the probate process, fees paid to the executor or administrator, attorney fees, and court costs. In addition, documents filed in the Probate Court are open to public review. Assets that avoid the probate process are those held jointly with survivorship rights with another person, property titled as "payable on death" (POD) or "transfer on death" (TOD), assets payable to a designated beneficiary, and possessions gifted to others before death. Real and personal property may also be transferred to or titled in the name of a trust, a document designed to specifically direct the use and disposition of the assets it holds. Avoidance of probate by any of the means above may have its own costs and its own negative consequences depending on the individual's circumstance. Simple wills are still often recommended to "catch" any property not titled or transferred correctly.

Although probate has changed in meaning and scope through the years, it still stands as a means to "prove" and supervise the transfer of a decedent's estate with judicial oversight and public openness, accessible by persons of all ranges of wealth.

SEE ALSO: Inheritance, Marital status

Suggested Reading

Jasper, M. C. (1997). *Probate law.* New York: Oceana.
Ostberg, K. (1990). *Probate: Settling an estate: A step-by-step guide.* New York: Random House.

Suggested Resources

American Bar Association website: http://www.abanet.org and your local Bar Association.

JANET L. LOWDER
MARIAN J. STER

Promotoras Promotoras (or peer health educators) are individuals from a specific community who serve as a link between the members of their community and the health care system. These individuals are trained to provide education on health issues of importance to the community as well as referrals to a variety of services, such as disease screening and treatment, primary care services, and social services. There are many terms used for peer health educators (e.g., lay health advisor, community health worker, lay community educator, natural helper, outreach worker), with "promotora" specifically referring to women who are native Spanish speakers conducting outreach to other Spanish-speaking women they know or may associate with. Although the peer education model is used for both men and women, most peer health education programs target women, regardless of what term is used to describe the outreach activities, given the traditional roles of women as guardians of the health of their family and healers in the community.

The use of promotoras/peer health educators is not restricted to just Spanish-speaking populations. Most programs that target communities considered, by the health care system, to be "hard to reach" use the promotora model as a means to deliver health-related messages and/or services through community-based outreach programs. The women are individuals who are trusted by the community or who will be able to gain that trust. There are many examples of programs that target women of different ethnicities (e.g., lay health advisors to increase breast cancer screening among African American women), different age groups (e.g., peer educators to reduce smoking on high school, college, and university campuses), and individuals with a specific health need (e.g., diabetic health promoters to educate other diabetics about nutrition and special health care needs) or a risk behavior (e.g., drug users in recovery employed as outreach workers to reduce disease transmission among active drug users). Some programs use community health advisors to increase screening for diseases such as breast and cervical cancers among women living in rural settings, where access to health care services may not be convenient or easy.

While promotora or peer educator models for community-based health promotion activities may have started out as a means to reach populations not seen in the health care system, they have evolved into models that incorporate theories of community empowerment, adult learning, and leadership development. Some promotora programs view the training of a cadre of health promoters as a means to increase community involvement with the local health system and to help individuals develop leadership skills so they can advocate on behalf of the community they represent. The promotora serves as a "bridge" between the formal health system and the community by providing services to residents in a culturally appropriate manner, while increasing the ability of the health system to provide health care in ways that respect the culture and health beliefs of the population.

The key to the success of promotora models for providing health education and health promotion services is that the promotoras are recruited from the neighborhoods where services are needed; the women generally have extensive social networks, are often already turned to for health advice, and may serve a leadership role within the community (e.g., the owner of a local business, the spouse of a local religious leader, a community organizer). Research has shown that promotoras have certain characteristics that contribute to their success, including compassion, a sense of connectedness to the community, and a commitment to community service.

SEE ALSO: Gender, Healers

Suggested Reading

Eng, E., Parker, E., & Harlan, C. (1997). Lay health advisor intervention strategies: A continuum from natural helping to paraprofessional helping. *Health Education & Behavior, 24*(4), 413–417.

Ramos, I. N., May, M., & Ramos, K. S. (2001). Environmental health training of *promotoras* in *colonias* along the Texas–Mexico border. *American Journal of Public Health, 91*(4), 568–570.

Schulz, A. J., Israel, B. A., Becker, A. B., & Hollis, R. M. (1997). "It's a 24-hour thing...a living-for-each-other concept": Identity, networks, and community in an urban village health worker project. *Health Education & Behavior, 24*(2), 465–480.

Scott, B. S. (2003). Latina promotoras educate farmworkers. *Closing the gap*, January/February. Washington, DC: Department of Health and Human Services, Office of Minority Health Resource Center.

LINDA S. LLOYD

Prostitution Though estimates vary significantly due to the illicit nature and social stigma of prostitution, research suggests that more than one million people, or 1% of the population, currently "work the streets and parlors" of the United States as prostitutes. Prostitution, often referred to as the oldest "trade" or profession, reportedly dates back to the historic times of ancient Greece, but one may assume that prostitution infected the earliest civilization and every society since then at varying rates. Research on prostitution in 19th-century New York City documents that as many as 10–15% of its young women prostituted themselves on a temporary or long-term basis, outpacing the income of many major developing economic industries of the time.

Street prostitution varies by city type, ranging from 10–20% in larger cities to 50% in smaller cities. Gender estimates for prostitutes similarly vary city by city, with larger cities believed to have a higher concentration of male prostitutes, upward of 20–30%, while in certain cities (e.g., San Francisco), it is estimated that up to 25% of female prostitutes are transgender. Although the overwhelming majority of prostitutes are adult women, statistics indicate that in the United States, girls as young as 14 years are induced into prostitution. Most prostitutes arrested and sentenced are "street-working" prostitutes and disproportionately women of color, although women of color constitute a minority of prostitutes. While estimates ignore prostitutes working indoor venues, such as sauna, massage parlors, and escort services, it is believed that up to 50% of prostitutes work such venues.

Clients of prostitutes, or "johns," are primarily male. Prostitution-related arrests indicate that the johns, unlike the prostitutes, are rarely arrested and infrequently jailed. Though the demographics of clients differ, the rates of johns frequenting prostitutes have significantly decreased over the years. A 1948 study reflected 69% of American men reporting having had sex with a prostitute, versus a 1997 study reporting a rate of 18%. Many clients are married (50–70%), inclusive of clients of male prostitutes who often identify themselves as heterosexual. Men in the military and between the ages of 53 and 60 years are more likely to frequent prostitutes.

Health implications of prostitution center on the transmission of sexual diseases. While prostitution reportedly accounts for 3–5% of sexually transmitted infections (STIs) in the United States (compared to 30–35% attributable to teenagers), research conducted by the Centers for Disease Control cites no known proven cases of HIV transmission from prostitutes to their clients. Prevention efforts focus on reducing STIs and the spread of HIV infection through condom promotion. Ironically, in some circles, prostitutes have been called "sexual ambassadors" playing a significant role in educating clients about measures to ensure safe sex through condom use. However, health access of prostitutes differs drastically according to whether they work the street or indoor venues. Street prostitutes seek health access from community-based organizations and community clinics, while those working indoor venues tend to have access to more comprehensive health care. Major mental health problems tied to prostitution are violence and drug use. The majority of violence is perpetuated by the clients and the domestic partners of prostitutes, with up to 80% reporting having been physically assaulted. Moreover, prostitutes report being raped between 8 and 10 times on average per year. Rates of substance use and addiction are high, reaching up to 84% for street prostitutes. However, it is not clear if prostitution causes drug use or drug use results in prostitution, given that roughly 50% used drugs prior to becoming a prostitute.

Reasons for becoming a prostitute vary depending on the perspective of the study. While some psychological perspectives argue that prostitution is a defense mechanism against lesbian desires, most argue that it is due to a history of either severe maternal deprivation or physical or sexual childhood abuse resulting in a lack of self-esteem or an abnormal desire to please others. Sociological explanations for prostitution point to the economic factors involved in prostitution, positing that prostitution enables the financially dependent or suffering women to be economically independent from, or equal to, men. The feminist perspective is both radical and liberal. Radical feminists believe that prostitution is a wholly degrading experience: The prostitute is reduced to merchandise with the customer focused only on the service and not the personality. The liberal feminist views prostitution as a contract between parties that was entered into freely, arguing that victimization espoused by radicals is overstated. Where these two views converge is on the criticism of involuntary prostitution whereby, through cultural, economic, familial need, and governmental arrangements, women are sold or forced into prostitution. The majority of prostitutes, especially those who have experienced abuse, tend to adopt the radical feminist perspective. Studies indicate that poor living conditions, unhealthy neighborhoods, neglected homes, inadequate education, and early coercive sexual experiences are common social denominators among prostitutes.

Internationally, one must examine closely the role of the military and sexual tourism. During wartime, the military has significantly impacted prostitution globally due to large concentrations of males with limited females. American folklore reports that the word "hooker" was derived from General James Hooker who provided women for his military troops during the Civil War. The military presence in parts of Southeast Asia (especially during the Vietnam War) created the current flourishing prostitution tourism industry fondly referred to as "sun, sea, sand, and sex." Though reinforced by the ideology of cultural male supremacy and subordination of women, the economic contribution of prostitution in Thailand continues to hold great significance. A 1991 study reported that the trafficking of women and children generated greater profits than the trafficking of drugs or illicit arms, resulting in Thailand being labeled the "prostitution capital of the world." However, HIV disease has significantly impacted the international tourism racketeering and drug trade with sex trading focusing primarily away from older and possibly infected women to younger girls and even children.

SEE ALSO: Drugs, Feminism, Gender, Violence

Suggested Reading

Cleves-Mosse, J. (1993). *Half the world, half a chance. An introduction to gender and development.* UK and Ireland: Oxfam.

Elias, J. E., Bullough, V. L., Elias, V., & Brewer, G. (Eds.). (1998). *Prostitution, whores, hustlers, and johns.* New York: Prometheus Books.

Sanger, W. W. (2002). *The history of prostitution. Its extents, causes and effects throughout the world.* Amsterdam: Fredonia Books.

SUSANNE MONTGOMERY
HEATHER DIAZ

Psychoanalysis

Psychoanalysis is an intensive treatment method based on the observation that people are usually unaware of the factors responsible for their symptoms, difficulties at work, relationships, moods, irrational fears, and a general inability to enjoy life and live up to their potential. Psychoanalysis is also a basic psychological theory of normal as well as pathological human development and personality formation. Psychoanalysis emphasizes relationships, awareness of defensive processes, understanding of basic needs and wishes, and recognition of transference in all human relationships. Transference is the influence of past relationships and feelings on present relationships. Psychoanalytic understanding of how the mind functions is the basis of psychoanalytic treatment and psychodynamic "talking therapy." It originated in Sigmund Freud's discovery of the unconscious and how it reveals itself in dreams, slips of the tongue, and unintended actions.

Freud (1856–1939) learned that the most effective way to help patients is to urge them to say whatever comes to mind without censor ("free associating"—free from conscious control) while lying on a couch, not influenced by visual feedback from the doctor. In this way a patient could become aware of the impulses he or she is repressing from consciousness because they are in conflict with his or her moral standards or the requirements of reality and the society in which we live. This awareness, as well as learning how the past created some of the conflicts hidden in the unconscious, may relieve painful emotional symptoms and maladaptive behaviors interfering with relationships, work, and play. Insight is made possible by reliving the intense feelings of the past in the present relationship with the analyst in the confidential, respectful atmosphere established in this long-term exclusive treatment relationship. It allows a patient to correct the misfit of past experience and a child's perception with the present experience and understanding of the adult.

Freud published his basic theory in 1900 in his book *The Interpretation of Dreams.* Freud's theory evolved through several phases as he continued learning from listening to his patients. He first concentrated on making the unconscious conscious. The unconscious was considered to be mainly the repository of the biologically based sexual and aggressive drives. Freud focused on the sexual drives; he named the energy fuelling them "libido." Freud described the following overlapping stages of psychosexual development: oral (age 0–2 years) where the infant's life-preserving and sensual drives center in the mouth and its functions, anal (2–3 years) with its pleasure in retaining and expelling feces, phallic (age 3–5) with its focus on the intense penile and clitoral sensations, leading to the genital–oedipal phase (5–6 years) involving love and a wish for exclusive possession of the parent of the opposite sex and hostile competition with the parent of the same sex. Because of fear of retaliation from the perceived competitor, the child eventually displaces these desires to outside persons while identifying with the competitor, taking in real and imagined prohibitions as building blocks for his or her conscience. These various phases have the potential for conflicts if not managed well by the environment. Unmanageable conflict leads to anxiety, inhibitions, and symptoms. Freud next focused on the agencies regulating psychic forces: the Id—repository of the drives, the Ego—the mediating, executive function of the personality, and the Superego—repository of moral injunctions and ideals we want to live up to. Anxiety is a signal of unmanageable conflict between these agencies. The three greatest fears of childhood are the fear of loss of love, the fear of losing the object of one's love, and ultimately the fear of loss of oneself. Any one of these can be symbolized by castration anxiety, the fear of injury to his genitals in the male's case, and the fantasy of having been injured in the female's case because of the absence of a penis, leading to "penis envy."

Freud was the product of a patriarchal repressive society. He had a masculine-centric attitude, with a misogynist's view of women. Freud confessed his inability to understand women, comparing them to a dark continent. In spite of this he encouraged and trained some brilliant women analysts whose contributions clarified female development and enriched psychoanalytic knowledge in general.

Psychoanalytic knowledge has evolved over the past 100 years beyond Freud's original formulations. Anna Freud contributed to ego psychology with her description of the necessary and adaptive function of defenses. She also developed child analysis. She demonstrated the importance of mother–child attachment and the traumatic effects of early separations from mother. It was her work that influenced such innovations in hospital procedures as allowing parents to stay with their hospitalized children.

Helena Deutsch (1944) described the importance of a woman being in control of her childbirth experience. This influenced some of the changes in maternity ward procedures and support for natural childbirth. She also clarified that relationships are more important to women than to men, leading to inhibition of aggression and, at times, striving to be peacemakers at any price.

Greta Bibring studied the psychological processes during pregnancy showing the need of the pregnant woman for a supportive close relationship with another woman if her mother is not available. This developmental phase in a woman's life is also a chance to rework the often intensely ambivalent, early mother–daughter tie.

Melanie Klein established the equivalence of a child's play with free associations, thus enabling work with very young children, and made a major contribution to object relations theory. She elucidated the centrality of the early mother–child relationship and clarified the distortions created by the child's projection of its own impulses and fantasies on to the mother/other

and reaction to that distorted perception of the mother/other as actuality. She also established the importance of aggression in a person's life. Melanie Klein was a pioneer in alerting us to how helpful it is to be aware of the countertransference of the therapist as a clue to how the patient affects others in their way of relating, as well as to the underlying fantasies in their interactions.

Infant and child observations established the fact that genital identity is set by age 18–24 months dependent on the perception and labeling by the environment as well as the child's identification with the adults in its life, independent of its genetic sex. The genital identity does not in itself influence the sexual object choice of the individual. The latter is probably multidetermined. Freud was aware of the bisexual tendencies in one's mental life, in view of an individual's attachment and potential for identification with both parents as well as possible innate, biological factors. Penis envy is now seen as also secondary to cultural discriminations, or defensive against a fear of injury in intercourse. It has its counterpart in the boy's womb envy—the ability to have babies. Little girls are aware of their inner and outer genitals and experience pleasurable sensations from them; if inhibited in this, sexual as well as a general learning disability may result. Menarche is normally an organizing, positive experience, consolidating a girl's identity. Menopause can thus be experienced as a loss on many levels. Women have other psychological issues besides sexuality, such as a need to be appreciated as individuals capable of intellectual achievements, feeling comfortable with self-assertion and competitive striving, and finding a way to integrate this with their sexual and maternal needs.

Current psychoanalytic research, based on observation of infant–mother interaction, formulated an attachment theory that has demonstrated an ability to predict personality development based on the quality of the infant's attachment to mother. The importance of the earliest experience for attachment led to the "rooming-in" of newborn and mother at the hospital; it was found that besides making for better child development it also protects the child from parental abuse. The importance of a secure attachment of mother and child in the first 3 years of life has also highlighted the current conflict women have between ambitious careers and motherhood, as well as the problem of day care for the working mother and her child.

Fathers are important, representing the outside world and its reality, thus helping in the eventual separation from mother and autonomy of the child. A father's appreciation of his daughter also helps in her valuing her femininity and being a person in her own right. A father's encouragement facilitates a woman's success in pursuing a career.

Psychoanalysis is an effective treatment for many people who have not been helped in briefer therapies. Low-cost treatment for psychoanalysis or psychotherapy is usually available through local psychoanalytic institutes.

SEE ALSO: Cognitive-behavioral therapy, Psychotherapy

Suggested Reading

Richards, A. D., & Tyson, P. (Eds.). (1996). The psychology of women: Psychoanalytic perspectives. *Journal of the American Psychoanalytic Association, 44*(Suppl.).

Suggested Resources

American Psychoanalytic Association website: http://www.apsa.org

RACHEL M. BAKER

Psychologists

Clinical psychologists perform multiple roles in the mental health care system. They work in hospitals, private offices, schools, and large outpatient mental health facilities. Psychologists receive advanced training in the assessment, diagnosis, and psychosocial treatment of mental health difficulties. To be a clinical psychologist, one must earn a PhD in clinical psychology or a related field. Typically, earning a PhD in clinical psychology takes 5–7 years of post-undergraduate education. To practice as a psychologist, one must also document a certain number of hours of clinical work with patients, pass a nationally administered test, and subsequently be licensed by a state board. To maintain this license, psychologists in most states must continue to be educated about issues in the field, and must submit documentation of certain number of hours of such education on a regular basis.

Often psychologists are sought out for their expertise in talk therapy. Psychologists cannot generally prescribe medications, but can deliver evidence-based talk therapies like cognitive–behavioral therapy (CBT). CBT in particular has been shown to be very helpful in treating a variety of disorders relevant to women, for example, posttraumatic stress disorder and depression, two mental health difficulties that are diagnosed more often in women than in men. Knowledge of assessment and diagnostic procedures is another area of strength for clinical psychologists. They are trained in the use of assessment tools and use assessment results to guide appropriate treatment. In regard to women's health care, it is interesting that many psychologists are women.

SEE ALSO: Cognitive-behavioral therapy, Couples therapy, Psychoanalysis, Psychotherapy

NORAH C. FEENY

Psychosomatic Disorder

The term psychosomatic disorder generally refers to a medical disorder that is caused by psychological factors. Although the term continues to be used extensively in the medical community, "psychosomatic disorders" largely has been replaced by the term "somatoform disorders," and is referred to as such in the most recent version of *Diagnostic and Statistical Manual of Mental Disorders*. There are several types of somatoform disorders including conversion disorder, somatization disorder, and hypochondriasis. The fundamental commonality of all somatoform disorders is the experience of physical symptoms that are not fully explained by a medical condition or by another mental disorder and cause significant functional impairment in life realms such as family, career, and social activity. The physical symptoms are not voluntarily or consciously produced. In fact, the individual who experiences these symptoms truly believes there to be an underlying physical condition in spite of the medical evidence demonstrating otherwise. The combined prevalence rate for somatoform disorders varies greatly by sample, although findings of 10% or more are not uncommon in medical settings.

Conversion disorder is one type of somatoform disorder in which there are motor symptoms (paralysis, difficulty swallowing) and/or sensory symptoms (blindness, deafness) that suggest a neurological condition but do not have medical basis and often appear or worsen during or after stressful life events. For a diagnosis of somatization disorder, there must be an established history of somatic complaints prior to the age of 30 that include multiple pain sites, gastrointestinal problems (diarrhea, nausea), sexual problems (sexual dysfunction, irregular menses), and one pseudoneurological symptom such as those experienced with conversion disorder. With hypochondriasis, the ability of individuals to function in their lives becomes impaired due to a preoccupation with having a serious illness related to the misinterpretation of bodily experiences (rapid heartbeat, sweating). This preoccupation continues to exist despite thorough medical workup and continual reassurance. Individuals with somatoform disorders are often seen with great frequency in medical clinics and are considered costly to the health care system due to the number of medical tests and specialist consultations they often receive before a psychiatric diagnosis can be reached. Somatoform disorders as a whole seem to occur more frequently in women although the gender makeup does vary from culture to culture.

The etiology of somatoform disorders is often unclear and the complex interaction of biological, environmental, social, and psychological factors produces a symptom presentation unique to the individual. However, theories on somatoform disorders continue to remain grounded in the belief that individuals who involuntarily block psychological distress and/or traumatic experiences from the conscious mental state will experience the distress on a physiological level. It has been theorized that women may experience somatoform disorders in greater numbers related to the higher rates of lifetime sexual and physical abuse (traumas) that they experience. Subsequently, when trauma is combined with female gender role expectations like internalizing (vs. expressing) negative emotions and a caretaking focus on others (vs. themselves), the result is limited outlets for the body to express distress. Additionally, physical illness is generally considered a more "legitimate" and less stigmatized malady than psychological illness in American society; hence, there is even greater reason to keep psychological distress buried and continue to manifest it physically. This reality often makes the treatment of these individuals difficult and lengthy for medical and mental health providers. Alternatively, some feminist theorists have speculated that the higher rates of somatoform disorders in women may be grounded in the inherent power differential in the male-dominated medical profession such that a woman's somatic complaints are often minimized and hastily attributed to a psychiatric origin, particularly when the medical diagnosis is challenging to ascertain.

Recent medical interest in mind–body relationships and research advances in fields like psychoneuro-immunology have increased awareness about the meaningful reciprocal relationship between emotional and physical states in psychological disorders (depression, posttraumatic stress disorder) and in physical disorders (HIV, autoimmune disorders, cancer). Consequently, a wide array of research-based treatments such as biofeedback, relaxation, and cognitive–behavioral therapy are now available to treat individuals with the more commonplace psychosomatic symptoms of everyday stress as well as the more disabling somatoform disorders.

SEE ALSO: Anxiety disorders, Cognitive-behavioral therapy, Mood disorders

Suggested Reading

Asaad, G. (1996). *Psychosomatic disorders: Theoretical and clinical aspects.* New York: Brunner/Mazel.

Schumacher Finell, J. (Ed.). (1997). *Mind body problems: Psychotherapy with psychosomatic disorders.* Northvale, NJ: Jason Aronson.

Shorter, E. (1993). *From paralysis to fatigue: A history of psychosomatic illness in the modern era.* New York: The Free Press.

LARA M. STEPLEMAN

Psychotherapy

Psychotherapy can be defined as "the treatment of mental or emotional disorders, or of related bodily ills by psychological means." Another source defines it as "the art of alleviating personal difficulties through the agency of words and a personal, professional relationship." There are many different types of psychotherapy, each of which has its own premise for success, utility, and sometimes inherent limitations. Following are the most widely used and accepted psychotherapeutic modalities, with an overview of each.

PSYCHOANALYSIS

Psychoanalysis is typically reserved for patients whose emotional difficulties arise solely from the *past.* The therapeutic relationship focuses on bringing forth repressed material that has encumbered a patient's ability to optimally manage life's provocations. Repression is a defense mechanism characterized by withholding a feeling or idea from conscious awareness.

The process of psychoanalysis utilizes the concepts of transference, countertransference, interpretation, therapeutic alliance, and resistance. *Transference* refers to unconscious feelings the patient has toward the analyst (positive or negative), typically founded upon the patient's relationships/conflicts with parental figures. *Countertransference* refers to the analyst's responses to the patient, also typically based in the unconscious. *Interpretation* is the analyst's understanding and explanation of psychologically based events. *Therapeutic alliance* refers to the relationship between analyst and patient, based upon trust and cooperation. *Resistance* implies a patient's withholding of information from the analyst, either conscious (lengthy silences) or unconscious (repressed feelings, desires).

Psychoanalysis is a longstanding process, usually comprising 3–6 years, or longer; individual sessions occur four or more times a week, the patient typically assuming the recumbent position on a couch, with the analyst seated out of view. This is said to foster the therapeutic process of regression and obtaining necessary repressed material. Disorders most effectively treated with psychoanalysis are usually limited to anxiety disorders (phobias, obsessive–compulsive disorders), dysthymia (mild depression), and some sexual, personality, and impulse control disorders.

PSYCHOANALYTIC PSYCHOTHERAPY

Although based on psychoanalytic concepts, this modality focuses on a patient's current conflicts and behaviors, and how this affects one's self-perception and relationships with others. There are two basic types of psychoanalytic psychotherapy: (a) supportive or relationship-oriented and (b) expressive or insight-oriented.

Supportive therapy is typically used when a patient has encountered a time-limited crisis situation, or decompensation, and lacks the ego strength to manage the challenge entirely independently. Expressive therapy, on the other hand, is *not* problem focused, but instead allows the patient to acquire new insights into one's behaviors and interactions with others, assuming rather intact ego strength.

The therapy is also one-on-one, but a couch is not used in the process, treatment can be short lived (a few sessions for a particular problem) or comprise

several years (1–3 sessions/week), and there is much less emphasis, if any, on the concepts of regression and transference. Unlike psychoanalysis, psychoanalytic psychotherapy is used to treat most psychiatric disorders.

BRIEF PSYCHOTHERAPY

Also utilizing psychodynamic concepts, this type of therapy is appealing because of its shorter duration. Conflict resolution, transference, interpretation, and resistance are all central elements of the brief psychotherapies, of which there are several. Examples include brief focal psychotherapy, time-limited psychotherapy, short-term dynamic psychotherapy, and short-term anxiety-provoking psychotherapy. The duration of therapy may be up to 1 year, but typically averages a few months.

CRISIS INTERVENTION

Seemingly obvious, this therapy is very time-limited, brief, and serves to resolve a crisis situation that has caused a person to manifest psychiatric symptoms. It is typically used for individuals who have developed maladaptive coping mechanisms to crisis-oriented situations, which when repeated over time produce greater and more intense difficulties in managing such experiences. The patient eventually develops psychiatric symptoms that further interfere with optimal functioning.

The goal of therapy is to facilitate learning new and adaptive coping skills by using reassurance, environmental manipulation, and suggestion, ultimately reducing the patient's anxiety. Duration of treatment is anywhere from 1–2 sessions to 1–2 months, with the hope that what is learned in therapy is used in future crises to prevent regression back to unhealthy or maladaptive responses.

GROUP PSYCHOTHERAPY

There are a variety of group therapy approaches, all of which utilize the "group experience" to render individual personality change.

Supportive group therapy, for example, encourages reality testing by group members and focuses on present environmental change and adaptation. *Psycho-analytic* group therapy, conversely, emphasizes the role of past life experiences and restructuring personality dynamics. *Transactional* group therapy iterates the importance of "here-and-now" patterns of behavior, while *behavioral* group therapy uses conditioning methods to effect change for persons with phobias and other dysfunctional learned behaviors. *Self-help groups* are a type of group therapy characterized by their homogeneity and "sameness" of individual members. The goal for each person is typically to relinquish very similar unwanted behaviors.

Those appropriate for group therapy would be motivated to create/accept change and would be capable of performing the group task. Those who cannot tolerate a group setting or who have markedly unacceptable behaviors for the group milieu would obviously be inappropriate candidates for this type of therapy.

FAMILY THERAPY

Used typically to treat families in conflict, this therapy modality can be very complex and versatile. The family is viewed as a unit, which is determined by the behaviors of its individual related members. One's symptoms are not so much the focus of treatment as are family dynamics and interactions. Directive control of the sessions by the therapist is imperative, so as to limit further deterioration (during the session) of already dysfunctional relationships.

Frequency of treatment is typically once a week, and duration can be weeks to years. Main goals are improved interpersonal and generational relationships, and overall conflict reduction/resolution.

MARITAL THERAPY

This type of psychotherapy addresses issues of conflict in the context of a couple's relationship. Reasons for seeking treatment can be emotional, economic, sexual, social, parental, interpersonal, etc. The goal is to facilitate change within the relationship, by modifying unhealthy behaviors, and working toward improving interpersonal development.

Marital therapy can be an option when individual therapy has failed to improve marital conflict, or when marital issues are the source of conflict. It should be noted that for a chance at successful outcomes, both partners must be involved and motivated for treatment.

BIOFEEDBACK

This is a rather unique type of psychotherapy in which a person changes maladaptive, involuntary, physiologic responses oneself, by means of conscious mental control. Feedback instruments relay personal data to the patient (e.g., heart rate, muscle tension), which can then be modified by that person using conscious mental regulation.

Equipment most often used are the electromyogram (EMG—measures muscle movement), electroencephalogram (EEG—measures brain waves), galvanic skin response (GSR—measures skin temperature), and thermistor (measures skin temperature). Conditions that may respond to biofeedback are migraine and tension headaches, cardiac arrhythmias, asthma, enuresis, fecal incontinence, Raynaud's syndrome, temporomandibular joint (TMJ) pain, blood pressure irregularities, and hyperactivity.

BEHAVIOR THERAPY

Behavior therapy focuses on specific problems, using learning theory and emphasizing standard conditioning techniques. There are various types of therapies used to target identified behaviors (rather than entire areas of dysfunction), and unlike other psychotherapies they do not require one to have insight into the source of the distress. Also, it is usually shorter in duration than the other psychotherapies.

Systematic desensitization, one type of behavior therapy, exposes the patient to increasing levels of anxiety while visualizing feared situations. Steps involved are relaxation training (imagery and muscle relaxation), hierarchy construction (a list of anxiety-provoking scenes increasing in severity), and desensitization of the stimulus (scenes are imagined while in a relaxed state, from least to most anxiety producing).

Graded exposure, another behavioral therapy, uses the same premise as systematic desensitization, but without relaxation training and the patient is exposed to real-life anxiety-provoking situations.

Flooding, often used for specific phobias, requires the patient to repeatedly confront the feared event, without escape, which over time, reduces anxiety and allows the patient to gain a sense of control. No relaxation training is used.

Participant modeling emphasizes patient observation, and eventual mimicking of others who confront the feared or anxiety-provoking event. An example of this would be the therapist who gradually leads the person with agoraphobia into a dreaded situation.

Aversion therapy, another less often utilized behavioral therapy, is used for impulse control problems such as paraphilias and addictions. This is facilitated by presenting the patient with a noxious stimulus after engaging in the undesirable behavior. Examples of such include social disapproval, medications that induce vomiting, and electrical stimuli, to name a few.

HYPNOSIS

The hypnotic state is one which resembles sleep, but is characterized by heightened focal concentration and receptivity to the suggestion of another person (Kaplan & Sadock, 1991). It is a type of therapy often used to uncover repressed memories, to change unwanted behaviors/habits (smoking, overeating, etc.), to treat chronic pain, and to induce anesthesia.

Persons undergoing hypnosis are put into a "trance" state that has varied levels: light, medium, or heavy. Posthypnotic suggestions are typically made during deep trance states. Because hypnotic induction is based upon trust, paranoid patients and those with very rigid, controlling personality structure are not appropriate candidates for this type of therapy.

COGNITIVE THERAPY

This type of psychotherapy is often used to treat depressive conditions. It is based on the premise that cognitive distortions (negative thought patterns) are the basis for causing depressive symptoms (anhedonia, apathy, low motivation, etc.). The goal of treatment is to change one's thinking, by first identifying cognitive distortions, then finding alternatives to the thought patterns, and finally putting them into practice (mentally and behaviorally). It is believed that this in turn can alleviate depressive symptoms.

Cognitive therapy is of short duration (4–6 months of weekly sessions) and requires commitment and motivation of the patient given there is an established agenda at the outset, interspersed with homework assignments between sessions. In addition to depression, cognitive therapy has been applied to panic and somatoform disorders, paranoid syndromes, impulsive behaviors, and obsessive–compulsive disorders.

SEE ALSO: Cognitive-behavioral therapy, Psychoanalysis, Psychologists

Suggested Reading

Beck, J. S. (1995). *Cognitive therapy: Basics and beyond*. New York: Guilford Press.

Kaplan, H. I., & Sadock, B. J. (1991). *Synopsis of psychiatry* (6th ed.). Baltimore: Williams & Williams.

Manning, D. W., & Frances, A. J. (1990). *Combined pharmacotherapy and psychotherapy for depression*. Washington, DC: American Psychiatric Press.

Storr, A. (1990). *The art of psychotherapy* (2nd ed.). New York: Routledge.

Weinberg, G. (1984). *The heart of psychotherapy*. New York: St. Martin's Press.

GRETCHEN K. GARDNER

PTSD   *see* Posttraumatic Stress Disorder

Puberty   Puberty is a dynamic period of development characterized by maturation of the genital organs, rapid changes in body size, shape, and composition, and the emergence of secondary sex characteristics. It marks the first time that adolescents are capable of sexual reproduction. Pubertal development is influenced by a wide array of biological and environmental variables and marked by substantial alterations in mood and behavior. Variations may be associated with several factors, including but not limited to ethnic background, nutrition, exercise, and body weight. Physiological changes that occur during puberty may have important long-term implications for women's health. We close with a set of recommendations for future research and strategies to foster healthy adolescent development among health care providers.

BIOLOGICAL PROCESSES

The age of onset of puberty is earlier for girls than for boys and varies anywhere from 9 to 13 years. One of the hallmarks of puberty is the growth spurt

Puberty

accompanied by significant weight gain. The sequence of biological events that occur during puberty encompass a broad spectrum of cellular and somatic changes initiated by the hypothalamus and affecting the pituitary gland, both structures in the brain. The hypothalamus stimulates the pituitary gland to produce the gonadotropin-releasing hormone (GnRH). GnRH causes the hormones estrogen and testosterone to be released followed by the release of the growth hormone (GH) by the pituitary gland. This process begins a cascade of events where the internal sex organs (e.g., ovaries) increase in size, followed by the development of the breast buds. Next there is an increase in body hair on the legs, under the arms, and in the pubic region. As the levels of estrogen and testosterone steadily increase, there is an increase in body weight and height, followed by a widening of the hips. The last event of pubertal development for girls is usually the onset of menstruation, or menarche (see Menarche). Once menarche is achieved, changes in height and weight begin to slow down and within a short period of time, the young girl has reached her adult height and achieved reproductive maturity. Although there is some variation in the timing of specific stages, most adolescents follow the same sequence of events except under unusual circumstances such as malnutrition or excessive exercise.

The onset of puberty can begin at any time between age 9 and 13 to be considered within the normal range, but several studies have examined the effects of early and late puberty on girls. In general, girls who mature at the same time as their peers or later than their peers fare much better than those who mature before their peers. Girls who reach puberty before age 11 are defined as early maturers, although this classification may vary according to context and ethnicity. The definition of early maturation is generally relative to one's peers; if the girl reaches puberty before her peers, she is considered an early maturer. Early maturation in girls has been associated with higher rates of mental health problems such as anxiety, depression, and eating disorders. Early maturation is also related to elevated rates of high-risk behaviors such as smoking, drug use, delinquent behaviors, and early sexual intercourse. The mechanism by which early maturation leads to these negative outcomes is unclear. Some research implicates increased testosterone levels whereas other data suggest that girls who mature early face a host of expectations associated with adulthood for which they are unprepared. The lack of congruity between girls' physically mature appearance and

psychological immaturity has been postulated as one explanation for these girls' poor adjustment. Moreover, early maturing girls' first boyfriends are usually 2–3 years older than them, thereby increasing their exposure to higher risk activities.

ENVIRONMENTAL INFLUENCES

Recent trends in adolescent development (e.g., height, timing of puberty) provide evidence that environmental factors influence pubertal processes. For example, girls are maturing earlier today than ever before, with the onset of public hair and breast development reported at 8.9 years for African Americans and 10.5 among Caucasians, respectively. Research documents the important role of nutrition and exercise in pubertal development. Specifically, undernutrition is related to later age at menarche and delayed pubertal maturation, whereas obesity is associated with early sexual maturation. Similarly, moderate physical activity or exercise has been linked to cardiovascular benefits and favorable body changes, but excessive physical activity such as the kind often required by some sports (e.g., gymnastics, wrestling) negatively affects adolescent development by slowing growth and maturation.

IMPLICATIONS FOR WOMEN'S HEALTH IN ADULTHOOD

Several studies indicate that certain physiological processes during puberty may have implications for women's health in adulthood, including the timing of puberty, the development of bone density, and the strength of immune functioning. The timing of puberty has consequences for estrogen exposure; earlier pubertal onset is associated with greater estrogen exposure and increased exposure to estrogen is linked to a higher incidence of adult reproductive cancers (i.e., breast and uterine). Similarly, bone density is affected by the interrelationships among endocrine changes, diet, and exercise during adolescence, and the absence of bone accretion increases the likelihood of osteopenia in adulthood. Finally, important immune functions develop during adolescence that may predispose women to infections and autoimmune diseases.

FUTURE RECOMMENDATIONS

The *Journal of Adolescent Health* recently published a series of papers outlining several priorities for future research on adolescent health and fostering healthy adolescent development. The work group on physical health made several recommendations for future research on pubertal processes, including but not limited to: (a) understanding the neurobiological mechanisms that regulate the onset of puberty; (b) identifying the complex factors that influence the pubertal endocrine process (e.g., diet, stress); (c) clarifying the role of estrogen in controlling bone growth, maturation, and mineral accretion; (d) differentiating the relative influences of nutritional excess, fat metabolism, and genetic risk factors on later cardiovascular risk; (e) examining how sleep during adolescence affects self-control, emotion regulation, and school performance; and (f) investigating how nutrition, adolescent obesity, calcium, and bone accretion have long-term effects on osteoperosis and cardiovascular risk.

A second set of recommendations may be directed at adolescent health care providers. These providers can help girls adjust to pubertal changes in positive ways by providing accurate information, encouraging open communication and questions, and facilitating effective coping in response to alterations in mood, behavior, and biology. Adolescent health care providers have a unique opportunity to educate adolescents and families about the normal developmental processes associated with puberty and to help them identify and solve problems that occur.

SEE ALSO: Birth control, Body image, Menarche

Suggested Reading

Archibald, A. B., Graber, J. A., & Brooks-Gunn, J. (in press). Pubertal processes and physiological growth in adolescence. In G. R. Adams & M. Berzonsky (Eds.), *Handbook of adolescence*. Malden, MA: Blackwell Publishers.

Brooks-Gunn, J. & Reiter, E. O. (1990). The role of pubertal processes. In S. S. Feldman & G. R. Elliott (Eds.), *The Developing Adolescent*. Cambridge: Harvard University Press.

Paikoff, R. L., & Brooks-Gunn, J. (1991). Do parent-child relationships change during puberty? *Psychological Bulletin, 110*, 47–66.

Suggested Resources

http://www.plannedparenthood.org/TEENISSUES/TEENMAINHTM/ Girls and Puberty/html (a Planned Parenthood website)

GERI R. DONENBERG

Puerperium   *see* Postpartum Period

Quality of Life

Quality of life, as a concept, has various meanings and definitions. The World Health Organization has defined quality of life as "an individual's perception of their position in life in the context of the culture and value system in which they live and in relation to their goals, expectations, standards, and concerns. It is a broad ranging concept affected in a complex way by the person's physical health, psychological state, level of independence, social relationships and their relationships to salient features of the environment."

Quality of life research can be applied to various disciplines, such as politics and economics, but is primarily used in medical contexts. In a medical context, quality of life is referred to as "health-related quality of life." Health-related quality of life research measures the way illness, disease, and treatment affects a patient's welfare. The idea is that the information gained directly from patients can help health care professionals assess the patient's condition. The results of such data assist health professionals in determining, among other things, whether a particular course of treatment should be continued, or if a different course of treatment would be more beneficial. Quality of life data enable health professionals to compare treatments, monitor the overall progress of individual patients, and receive a better understanding of an individual patient's beliefs regarding his or her treatment and well-being.

Quality of life research can be done in various ways. A health professional, for example, can conduct an open-ended interview with the patient. Most quality of life research, however, is done through questionnaires. While questionnaires can be administered through an interview, most are self-administered.

Quality of life questionnaires measure, usually by assigning a numeric value to each answer, the patient's perceptions, beliefs, feelings, and expectations regarding different domains. Common domains include physical health, psychological health, social relations, level of independence, environment, and spirituality, religion, or personal beliefs. For each domain, various questions are asked to give the health professional an idea of the patient's appraisal of his or her well-being in that area. For example, when attempting to gage a patient's physical health, the questionnaire may include questions concerning energy, fatigue, pain or discomfort, sleep or rest, health habits, sensory functions, mobility, nutrition, and illness symptoms. Similarly questions used to assess psychological health may include inquiries regarding body image, appearance, negative and positive feelings, self-esteem, education, learning and the opportunity for continued learning, concentration, memory, emotional functioning and fulfillment, anxiety, stress, depression, and the ability to cope.

There are over 800 questionnaires that measure health-related quality of life. These questionnaires, however, can generally be labeled as either generic or specific.

Generic questionnaires are designed to assess many domains of health-related issues, and are based on a broad and global concept of quality of life. There are two types of generic questionnaires: health profiles and health indices. Health profiles include inquiries concerning a large range of health-related domains and uses questions related to various aspects of subjective health status. As the patient answers each question, a numerical score based upon the patient's answer is figured for each domain. Health indices questionnaires also ask various health-related questions. However, unlike the health profile questionnaires, health indices questionnaires combine the scores each answer generates into a single number. The number is then placed in a range, with, for example, 0 being death and 1.0 being perfect health.

The numerical score, or scores, arrived at using generic questionnaires contribute to a health care professional's understanding of a patient's needs, as it reflects the patient's perception of his or her life. This perception is important because a patient has a unique perspective on his or her quality of life that cannot necessarily be arrived at by others. A paraplegic, for example, might perceive his or her quality of life as not differing much from that of able-bodied individuals. However, an evaluation of the paraplegic's quality of life that is performed by an able-bodied individual may result in a lower score than the paraplegic himself or herself would have arrived at. Such a result could be partially explained by the fact that, for example, an able-bodied individual may place a higher value on the ability to stand and walk than the paraplegic does. Bringing the patient's perceptions to the attention of the health professional promotes the development of a comprehensive treatment plan. The health care professional can learn what aspects of the patient's life the patient is satisfied with or believes need improvement. This information permits the health care professional to put more or less weight on various treatment goals. If a patient's primary objective, for example, is pain management, awareness of this objective will help a health care professional develop a treatment plan that places more emphasis on this goal. Knowing the patient's perception of his or her overall condition could also assist the health care physician in making decisions concerning the effectiveness or continuation of various treatments.

Specific health-related quality of life questionnaires are designed to measure the quality of life of patients with a specific condition. There are four basic types of specific questionnaires:

1. *Domain specific.* This type of questionnaire only inquires as to one domain. For example, the questionnaire could be designed to solely assess the patient's psychological health.

2. *Disease specific.* This form of questionnaire is concerned with the quality of life of individuals with specific conditions. Thus, a questionnaire that measures the health-related quality of life for individuals with spinal cord injuries would be disease specific.

3. *Population specific.* This type of questionnaire is used to determine the health-related quality of life in the population being studied. This type of questionnaire is often used to gain information about subgroups like adolescents and nonsmokers.

4. *Symptom specific.* These questionnaires are used to gain information about one symptom. By concentrating on one symptom, like insomnia, the results of this type of questionnaire can provide physicians with valuable information about the disease, various forms of treatment, and any changes that may result from treatment.

Once an individual's health-related quality of life has been determined, the health professional and patient can take steps to improve the patient's quality of life. The steps taken to improve the individual's health-related quality of life could vary from stress relief to pain management. Improving one's health-related quality of life is extremely individualized and will vary with each patient's state of health.

Every individual could improve his or her health-related quality of life. For the average individual, their health-related quality of life could generally be improved by taking steps to, among other things, reduce stress, improve nutrition, increase relaxation and exercise levels, increase energy level, strengthen social bonds, improve self-image and self-esteem, and reduce fatigue.

Improving the health-related quality of life for individuals who suffer from an injury, illness, or disease is more complicated because these individuals often deal with additional symptoms, such as chronic pain and fatigue, which the average person does not face. The injured, ill, or diseased may also face mobility and independence issues. Improving the health-related quality of life for these individuals might include: finding a successful treatment regime, decrease illness symptoms, and discovering methods that will increase both mobility and independence, create strong channels of support, strengthen coping mechanisms and spirituality, decrease depression, and increase emotional functioning.

Individuals nearing the end of their life, including the elderly and terminally ill, often face a hard decision: quantity of life or quality of life. Rather than taking measures to extend their lives, many individuals choose to improve the quality of the life they have remaining. Individuals who are nearing death are often concerned with issues including pain control, fatigue, symptom management, autonomy, maintaining a sense of control over decision-making, avoiding a prolonged death, strengthening the relationships with loved ones, the burden of physical care, spirituality, burial arrangements, and the burden placed on loved ones who may have to make decisions concerning life-sustaining treatment.

An individual who is facing death can improve his or her quality of life, at least to a degree, by addressing some of the above-mentioned concerns. For example, the individual can work with physicians to find a regime that could help manage symptoms and pain.

Legal documents, such as advance directives, could also be utilized to relieve the individual of decision-making concerns. For instance, the individual could execute a living will, thereby making his or her wishes concerning life-sustaining treatment known. The individual could also execute a document known as a durable power of attorney. A durable power of attorney would permit the individual to retain decision-making power as long as he or she remains legally competent. The document also allows the individual to elect a person to act as a decision-maker if the individual were to become incompetent. By discussing the dying individual's wishes with the elected decision-maker, the individual can ensure both his or her health care wishes are known and the elected decision-maker is willing to accept the responsibility of respecting those wishes. A second form of durable power of attorney could also help improve the quality of life of the dying. By executing a durable power of attorney over property, an individual, who may become unable to manage financial affairs, can ensure his or her property and bills will be managed by a person of his choice.

Further, the execution of a will and the prearrangement of burial planning could also be utilized to make the dying individual's intentions known. Such measures relieve the dying individual's reluctance to leave loved ones with the burden of making such decisions.

Whether an individual is in perfect health or is dying from a terminal disease, measures can be taken to improve his or her health-related quality of life. Moreover, the data collected in quality of life research, which reveals valuable information about diseases, treatments, and health care in general, can be utilized to improve the quality of life of future patients.

SEE ALSO: Disability, Durable power of attorney for health care, Hospice, Living wills

Suggested Reading

Andrews, F. (Ed.). (1986). *Research on the quality of life.* Ann Arbor: University of Michigan, Institute for Social Research.

Camilleri-Brennan, J., & Steele, R. J. C. (1999). Measurement of quality of life in surgery. *Journal of the Royal College of Surgeons of Edinburgh, 44,* 252–260.

Crammer, J. (1999). Quality of life assessment in clinical practice. *Neurology, 54*(Suppl. 2), S49–S52.

Larson, D., & Tobin, D. (2000). End of life conversations: Evolving practice and theory. *Journal of the American Medical Association, 28,* 1573–1578.

Singer, P., Martin, D., & Kelner, M. (1999). Quality of life care: Patients' perspective. *Journal of the American Medical Association, 281,* 163–168.

Suggested Resources

The American Geriatrics Society. (1996, January 1). New York. http://www.americangeriatrics.org/products/positionpapers/quality.shtml

University of Bergen, Department of Public Health and Primary Health Care, The Center for Quality of Life Research in Nursing Science Section for Nursing Science. (2000, September 5). Bergen, Norway. http://www.uib.no/isf/people/doc/qol/comp0002.htm

BRANDY GLASSER

Queer The term *queer* evolved through different historical contexts during the 20th century. Prior to the Stonewall rebellion in 1969, which marked the beginning of the gay liberation movement, queer, in the context of describing a person, was used almost exclusively as a derogatory term against homosexuals. As the gay liberation movement gained momentum, a new meaning surfaced that signified a radical act of gay pride in defiance of *heteronormativity* and was evidenced in slogans such as "We're here; We're queer; Get used to it!" Heteronormativity describes a binary gender system, in which only two sexes are recognized, where sex is equated with gender and gender with a heterosexual orientation.

At the same time, lesbian feminists were concerned with legitimizing lesbian as an identity within the general context of women's oppression, which necessitated defining parameters. Out of this emerged separatist movements, proscriptions against butch and femme gender roles, anti-sadomasochism and/or anti-dominance/

submission stances, and exclusionary taxonomies such as "women-born, women-identified women." This process led to an identity politic that alienated and marginalized increasing numbers of women. Additionally, *homonormative* strategies (we're just like you except for one thing) employed by lesbian and gay organizations to gain civil rights served to further marginalize individuals. Among those ostracized were transgendered persons, bisexuals, intersexed persons, and butch and femme lesbians. Others were also ostracized, irrespective of sexual orientation. These individuals, who do not fit the prevailing cultural norms of gender, include drag queens and drag kings, transsexual persons, leather fetishists, transvestites, and others who do not adhere to cultural standards of monogamous partnerships.

Similar to the gay liberation movement, these groups adopted queer as an umbrella term in a radical act of defiance and pride. However, in this case it was in defiance of lesbian and gay homonormativity *in addition to* heteronormativity. This meaning of queer exposes the hypocritical stance of gay liberation, in that queers can be visible only so long as they fit within the prevailing parameters of acceptability. Thus, these marginalized groups are queer even within lesbian and gay circles. In effect, they are *queer* queers.

All three usages of queer remain prevalent today. However, against this backdrop, queer studies emerged as an academic discipline sustained by a well-articulated theoretical framework. Queer theory proposes that sexual identities are a function of representations. It assumes that representations preexist and define, as well as complicate and disrupt, sexual identities. Whereas the gay liberation movement fought to legitimize an acceptable homosexual identity and in the process free from oppression marginalized sexual minorities, queer theorists seek to destabilize cultural ideals of normality and foster the freedom people need to create their own sexualities.

Although same-sex dynamics have been a focal point of queer theorists, the benchmark of the coming out narrative that commonly solidifies contemporary gay and lesbian identities is not used to evaluate these dynamics. Queer theory rejects teleological views of sexuality and identity, tending more toward coalition politics. It is skeptical of viewing some identities as authentic and others as lacking, inauthentic, or deviant. Instead, queer theory concentrates on what individuals want and do.

See Also: Femininity, Gender, Gender role, Hermaphroditism, Homosexuality, Intersexuality, Lesbian, Masculinity, Transgenderism, Transsexuality

Suggested Reading

Jagose, A. (1997). *Queer theory: An introduction.* New York: New York University Press.

Spargo, T. (1999). *Foucault and queer theory.* Kallista, Australia: Totem Books.

Turner, W. B. (2000). *A genealogy of queer theory* (American Subjects Series). Philadelphia: Temple University Press.

ANGELA PATTATUCCI ARAGON

Rape The Latin word "to steal or carry off" is *rapere* and described the behavior of ancient Romans who stole their wives from other tribes. Laws delivered by Moses in Deuteronomy 22:22–28 categorized rape and what occurred to victims and perpetrators. The tragedy of rape continues today of children, adolescents, and adults, including the very elderly. The frequency rises so dramatically during wartime that even collecting firewood or bringing water to one's family carries incredible risk.

Female victims are more frequent than males by a ratio of 13.5:1 in the United States with the highest prevalence (5/1,000) in male and female adolescents between 16 and 19 years old. It is estimated in this country that more than 25% of women at some point in their lives will experience nonconsensual sexual penetration of their anus, vagina, or mouth.

Sexual assault includes multiple types of inappropriate or forced sexual behaviors. Under this heading, there is molestation or noncoital activity between an adult and a child as well as various types of rape, forced sexual intercourse. Statutory rape exists when an adult (over 18 years of age) sexually penetrates a child or adolescent. Gang rape involves one victim with multiple perpetrators. Date or acquaintance rape exists when the perpetrator is known. Two thirds to three quarters of adolescent rapes are perpetrated by an acquaintance or family member.

Adolescent victims are more likely than adults to have used alcohol or drugs, but less likely to have been physically injured. Adolescents and young adults are at higher risk for receiving the date rape drug flunitrazepam (Rohypnol), which is profoundly sedating for up to 12 hr.

The risk of developing a sexually transmitted disease (STD) varies with region of the country, age, and sex among other factors. Syphilis, gonorrhea, HIV, herpes, papillomavirus, chlamydia, candida, and gardnerella are reported. The Centers for Disease Control and Prevention updates guidelines regularly for prophylaxis of STDs within the first 72 hr and recommendations to monitor the development of STD-related symptoms—initially for all STDs and again at 6 months for HIV.

A needed history and physical examination is frequently quite difficult. The victim, who has already been terrorized, often does not want to relive the account in her mind and can feel violated by a physical examination. Ideally a police officer, physician, nurse, and rape crisis volunteer who are well trained in rape intervention will be on hand. Emotional support is provided with careful explanation of why particular questions are asked, why an intimate detailed physical examination is necessary, or why photos are taken and specimens properly collected. This is not easy under any circumstances, but especially when the victim is a younger child, is disabled and suffering from contractures, or elderly with dementia.

There are multiple reasons for rape, but sexual tension is not high on the list. Most rapists live with a sexual partner and prostitution is also available. Power through violence is misidentified as healthy male aggression or animal instinct gone awry. Although society's desire to reestablish the family is sound, promoting an individual's "license to abuse" is not. When some males perceive their patriarchal rule threatened, they rationalize violence to assure female subordination.

These men may have difficulty communicating to women in any other manner. Poor interpersonal skills and a sense of insecurity lead to attacks that humiliate and degrade women. Some are merely angry while others are sadistic. Up to 40% of rapes are meant as punishment and 5% are only satisfied by torture or murder.

A psychological interpretation is that many rapists were abused as children and grow up with low self-esteem, resentment, and hostility. Impulsive behavior and poor ego structure lead some to acknowledge a likelihood to commit rape if they can escape punishment.

The motivation to rape during times of war includes revenge, genocide, and ethnic cleansing. Women and girls living in refugee camps or left in their homes when husbands and sons are off to war are at great risk for rape, STDs, and pregnancy. Women may also be forced into sexual acts to gain passage for themselves and their families at a border crossing. Not only do they experience posttraumatic stress disorder and depression, but also they may be rejected by their clan and sent away if they become pregnant after the rape. These acts are directed at humiliation of the males who are off fighting and are unable to protect their women. A woman and her family may feel tremendous disgrace if she becomes pregnant after this act of violence. The babies are at high risk for neglect, abandonment, or infanticide. It is no wonder that women who have been molested are frequently afraid to let anyone know what has occurred. Feeling powerless and fearful of retaliation, they may not seek medical help for prophylaxis of infection or reconstructive surgery for injuries.

The tragedy of rape is clearly not often punished during war despite efforts of some humanitarians to address these wrongs. However, even in this country where there is relative peace, only 9.5% report nonmarital attempted rapes or 6% of those who survive rape. Many drop the charges before committal if interrogators imply by questioning that the woman may have encouraged it in some way. Many perpetrators negotiate for a lesser offense. Only 10% of the 6–9.5% who report (0.6–0.95% of all cases) will actually see conviction of the perpetrator. There is much to be done to improve the compassion and care for victims of abuse, as well as provision of education about prevention and procurement of treatment and legal protection.

SEE ALSO: Domestic violence, Gangs, Incest, Pedophilia, Sexual abuse, Sexually transmitted diseases, Violence

Suggested Reading

Bamberger, J. D., Waldo, C. R., Gerberding, J. L., & Katz, M. H. (1999). Postexposure prophylaxis for human immunodeficiency virus (HIV) infection following sexual assault. *American Journal of Medicine, 106*(3), 323–326.

Burgess, A. W., Dowdell, E. B., & Brown, K. (2000). The elderly rape victim: Stereotypes, perpetrators, and implications for practice. *Journal of Emergency Nursing, 26*(5), 516–518; quiz 529.

Kaplan, D. W., Feinstein, R. A., Fisher, M. M., Klein, J. D., Olmedo, L. F., Rome, E. S., et al., & Committee on Adolescence. (2001). *Pediatrics, 107*(6), 1476–1479.

Moore, L. (1998). *Nursing Standard, 12*(48), 49–54; quiz 55–56.

The Revised English Bible (pp. 167–168). (1989). Deuteronomy. Cambridge: Oxford University Press.

Reynolds, M. W., Peipert, J. F., & Collins, B. (2000). Epidemiologic issues of sexually transmitted diseases in sexual assault victims. *Obstetrical and Gynecological Survey, 55*(1), 51–57.

Schafran, L. H. (1996). Rape is a major public health issue. *American Journal of Public Health, 86*(1), 15–17.

Shanks, L., & Schull, M. J. (2000). Rape in war: The humanitarian response. *Canadian Medical Association Journal, 163*(9), 1152–1156.

KATHLEEN N. FRANCO
DAVID L. BRONSON
MOHAMMED ALISHAHIE

Raynaud's Phenomenon Raynaud's phenomenon is a condition in which exposure to cold or emotional stress causes skin discoloration and pain. This occurs most often in the fingers, but can also affect the toes, the tip of the nose, and tips of the ears. Raynaud's phenomenon can occur itself or may be a symptom of an underlying disease.

During an attack, the skin color changes to white, blue, or red. The color changes are caused by spasm of blood vessels. On exposure to a stress, such as cold or an emotional situation, blood vessels narrow (vasospasm) causing the skin to appear pale. Because blood flow is reduced, the skin then turns blue. When the causative condition (cold or stress) is removed, after a period of about 10–15 minutes, rewarming occurs, turning the skin red. The diagnosis of Raynaud's phenomenon is based on a description or observation of these color changes in the setting of a typical exposure.

Approximately 4–15% of the population describe symptoms of Raynaud's. Most of these people have no other symptoms or signs of an underlying disease, toxin exposure, or occupational risk. This is defined as primary Raynaud's phenomenon. Nearly 80% of patients diagnosed with primary Raynaud's are female. Attacks generally begin between the ages of 15 and 25 in otherwise healthy individuals. Symptoms are mild and no damage to blood vessels or destructive skin damage occurs. Treatment includes using protective clothing and avoiding excessive exposure to conditions that cause symptoms. Medications that cause narrowing of blood vessels should be discontinued or changed if medically advisable. Any tobacco use should be avoided.

Attacks that begin at a later age are usually more severe and more likely to result from an underlying disease. Systemic sclerosis (also known as scleroderma), a rheumatological disease, is the most common underlying disease. Secondary Raynaud's can also be caused by other rheumatological diseases (lupus, vasculitis), drugs and toxins (amphetamines), structural diseases of the blood vessels (atherosclerosis), occupational disorders (hand–arm vibration syndrome), and certain blood conditions (cryoglobulinemia).

In systemic sclerosis, nearly 90% of the patients also have Raynaud's. In these people, Raynaud's is more severe and can involve skin ulcerations on the fingers or toes. In the worst case, gangrene can occur and surgical amputation is necessary. This kind of Raynaud's is caused by more than the simple vasospasm of primary Raynaud's. Changes in the normal lining of the blood vessels lead to scarring, clot formation, and chronic damage. Because the vessels are damaged to start with, vasospasm can lead to blockage of the blood vessels. One distinguishing feature of secondary Raynaud's that occurs with systemic sclerosis is the abnormal appearance of the small blood vessels of the finger nailbeds when viewed on close inspection.

Treatment for both primary and secondary Raynaud's includes topical nitrate creams and a class of medications known as calcium channel blockers. Traditionally, these medications are used to treat heart disease and high blood pressure. Here, their role is to decrease vasospasm and stabilize blood vessel membranes. Unfortunately, in cases where gangrene develops, amputation may be the only treatment option.

SEE ALSO: Autoimmune disorders, Scleroderma

Suggested Reading

Klippel, J. H. (Ed.) (2001). *Primer on the rheumatic diseases* (12th ed.). Atlanta, GA: Arthritis Foundation.
Ruddy, S., Harris, E. D., & Sledge, C. B. (Eds.) (2001). *Kelley's textbook of rheumatology* (6th ed.). Philadelphia, PA: W. B. Saunders.

Suggested Resources

Arthritis Foundation at www.arthritis.org National phone number 1-800-283-7800.
National Organization for Rare Disorders Inc. (NORD) at www.rarediseases.org

JULIANNE S. ORLOWSKI

Reduction Mammoplasty *see* Breast Reduction

Regional Rheumatic Pain

Regional rheumatic pain is a family of syndromes including tendonitis, tenosynovitis, and bursitis. These conditions, although commonly seen in medical practice, are challenging to diagnose. They are usually diagnosed without laboratory testing or x-rays.

These conditions of the musculoskeletal system are the result of repetitive overuse along with abnormal body position or mechanics. Tendons, which attach muscle to bone, may be more vulnerable to injury if a person does not stretch before strenuous exercise. Bursae, which act as cushion around joints and in between muscles, can be subjected to extensive periods of pressure or force, causing inflammation. Less common causes for these conditions include aging, disuse, muscle atrophy or weakening, poor circulation, calcium deposits, or diseases such as arthritis. The health care provider should obtain a thorough history of patient activities, recent illnesses or trauma, and changes in habits or daily lifestyle. A detailed musculoskeletal exam should include pressing on painful areas, moving joints through their full range of motion both voluntarily and with manipulation, and resistance testing of the muscles. Knowing the anatomy of the affected area is important in making a diagnosis (Table 1).

Shoulder pain is one of the most common complaints among older people as well as in young athletes. Overuse and calcium deposition are the most common causes of inflammation in this area. The shoulder has many parts, making it difficult to determine the source of the pain. Three components of the shoulder are

Table 1. Common overuse syndromes by region

Location	Syndrome
Shoulder: Rotator cuff tendons and bursa	Rotator cuff tears, subacromial or subdeltoid bursitis
Elbow: Flexor and extensor carpi radialis tendons and sheaths	Medial epicondylitis (golfer's elbow) and lateral epicondylitis (tennis elbow)
Wrist: Abductor and extensor pollicus longus tendon and sheath	DeQuervain's tenosynovitis
Wrist: Flexor and extensor tendons and sheaths	Tenosynovitis of the wrist
Knee: Prepatellar bursa	Prepatellar bursitis (housemaid's knee)
Heel: Retrocalcaneal bursa	Retrocalcaneal bursitis (pump bump)

often affected by overuse syndromes: (a) the rotator cuff muscles and their tendons, (b) the subacromial bursa, and (c) the subdeltoid bursa. Acute rotator cuff tendonitis usually causes pain on voluntary movement of the arm away from the body, while chronic tendonitis causes a dull ache and difficulty performing daily tasks. Rotator cuff tendonitis is confirmed if the impingement test causes pain. If injection of lidocaine into specific shoulder bursa causes relief of pain with motion, then bursitis is the likely cause.

Elbow pain is also most commonly caused by overuse, although chronic elbow pain may be associated with bony abnormalities, calcifications, or nerve problems. Lateral epicondylitis, or tennis elbow, causes tenderness directly over or just in front of the lateral epicondyle, which is the bony prominence on the outer side of the elbow. Pain occurs with everyday activities such as shaking hands, opening a can, or lifting objects. This tenderness is due to inflammation or a tear of the tendon at that location. Medial epicondylitis, or golfer's elbow, demonstrates pain with resistance to wrist movement downward as well as point tenderness over the medial epicondyle, the bony prominence on the inner side of the elbow.

DeQuervain's tenosynovitis involves the tendons that pull the thumb up into the hitchhiker position. This condition is usually a result of overuse of the thumb from gripping pens or pencils too tightly or in mothers diapering their children using safety pins. Pain is elicited with pressure on the wrist at the base of the thumb. Swelling can develop in the area. The Finkelstein test confirms the diagnosis. First, fold the thumb over the palm and close the fingers over the thumb. Bending the wrist sideways away from the thumb will cause pain in a positive test. Tenosynovitis of the wrist is caused by excessive writing, typing, or other repetitive movements of the area.

Prepatellar bursitis, or housemaid's knee, is often caused by frequent kneeling. History of such activity as well as visible swelling usually makes the diagnosis clear. In contrast to problems within the knee joint, the knee has full range of motion without pain. Pressure directly over the bursa on the lower half of the kneecap may reproduce the pain. Increased pain and tenderness with warmth and redness may mean the bursa is infected. The clinician should note a history of any recent trauma and obtain fluid from the bursa to see if it is infected. Infection is treated with antibiotics, and antibiotics are often given until infection is ruled out.

People with trochanteric bursitis will complain of hip pain, but the patient is able to point directly to the outside of the upper thigh. This pain is worse when the patient lies on the affected side or wears a purse or tool belt over the area. Heel bursitis, also known as "pump bump," causes pain in the area around the Achilles tendon and the back of the heel bone. Pain is usually increased by having the patient move the foot downward. Swelling and a hard bump may be present. Improper footwear can cause pressure and irritation in this area, hence the name "pump bump."

TREATMENT

Treatment aims at reducing symptoms and preventing reoccurrence. Avoiding the activity that causes overuse is extremely important. If the patient cannot do this, then the activity (e.g., typing) should be performed with proper alignment and posture. Rest and immobilization with possible splinting will relieve current inflammation. Once the inflammation decreases, physical therapy may be helpful in increasing muscle flexibility, strength, and endurance. Heat compresses are useful for tendonitis while cold compresses provide relief for bursitis, although some patients prefer the opposite.

Nonsteroidal anti-inflammatory medication is a mainstay for these disorders, sometimes along with other pain relievers. Injection of a mixture of corticosteroids and anesthetics into the affected area provides short-term relief, reduces inflammation, and helps confirm the diagnosis.

SEE ALSO: Arthritis

Suggested Reading

Klippel, J. H., Crofford, L. J., Stone, J. H., & Weyand, C. M. (Eds.). (2001). *Primer on the rheumatic diseases* (12th ed.). Atlanta, GA: Arthritis Foundation.
Snider, R. K. (Ed.). (2001). *Essentials of musculoskeletal care* (2nd ed.). Rosemont, IL: American Academy of Orthopaedic Surgeons.

Suggested Resources

American Academy of Orthopaedic Surgeons patient information website: orthoinfo.aaos.org

AMITA SAPRA
LORI B. SIEGEL

Renal Disease Renal (kidney) disease is a significant health care problem. As of 2000 (the most recent data available from the U.S. Renal Data Service report), the federal government's cost of providing renal replacement therapy to patients with end-stage renal disease (ESRD) was over 12 billion dollars. Over the past decade, the increase in ESRD program costs has outpaced that of the general Medicare program by approximately 50% and presently accounts for 5.8% of the Medicare program. This is up from 4.5% over the past decade. Most of the increase is due to an increase in the patient population that has nearly doubled to 260,000 people. It is estimated that 20 million people have some form of renal disease in the United States, many of whom will progress to ESRD. Within the ESRD program, women are disproportionately represented in the Medicaid and Medicare populations.

MANIFESTATIONS OF RENAL DISEASE

As with hypertension, most people with renal disease are initially asymptomatic (without symptoms). Screening urinalysis or blood work are the most common ways with which renal disease is initially detected. Screening urinalysis in children or young adults as part of camp or school health examination may reveal hematuria (blood in urine) or proteinuria (protein in urine). Adults, as part of an insurance examination or routine annual examination, may show, in addition to hematuria or proteinuria, evidence of renal insufficiency by an elevation of the serum blood urea nitrogen (BUN) or creatinine (both BUN and creatinine are naturally occurring substances in the blood). An abnormal urinalysis is noted when there are more than 3–5 red blood cells (rbc) per high-powered field (hpf) on a microscope-viewed slide, or the detection of protein on the dipstick dipped in a urine sample. In order to measure the amount of protein, a 24-hour urine collection or spot urine (one-time urine collection sample) for protein and creatinine will need to be obtained. To screen for abnormal proteins, a urine protein electrophoresis and immunoelectrophoresis (specialized procedures that stratify/categorize urine proteins) may need to be performed.

Renal involvement can reflect prerenal causes, postrenal causes, or intrinsic (renal tissue) disease. *Prerenal* causes most commonly reflect abnormalities in renal blood flow (from congestive heart failure, volume depletion, or cirrhosis of the liver) that become manifest (or more pronounced) if someone is also ingesting certain medications such as anti-inflammatory drugs. Generally speaking, there is a disproportionate rise in the BUN compared to the creatinine (>15–20:1 ratio). The urinalysis (both dipstick and microscopic) is typically normal. Hypertension may also be a reflection of renal hypoperfusion (low blood flow) even in the absence of abnormalities in renal function studies. The presence of hypertension in a woman in her late teens and early 20s, or the presence of marked hypertension in a woman without a family history of hypertension raises the possibility of fibromuscular dysplasia (narrowing of arteries due to thickening of artery wall lining).

Postrenal causes typically manifest as hydronephrosis (dilated kidney) or hydroureter (dilated ureter—tube from the kidney to the urinary bladder). Acquired causes of urinary tract obstruction (UTO) include intrinsic and extrinsic processes. Intrinsic causes include direct disease of the kidney and/or related disorders such as kidney stones, blood clots, impaired bladder function (neurogenic bladder) in diabetes mellitus, ureteral or urethral strictures, and tumors of the renal pelvis, ureter, or bladder. Extrinsic processes include reproductive tract causes such as pregnancy, fibroids, endometriosis, cancer of the cervix or ovaries, kidneys, or ureter or bladder. Depending on the etiology, the urinalysis may be abnormal, for example, hematuria with stones or tumors.

PATIENTS WITH HEMATURIA AND PROTEINURIA

In order to understand the patient's condition, the physician will need an appropriate medical history and must conduct a physical examination. If there is isolated hematuria, the physician must evaluate whether it is renal (in the kidney) or nonrenal (related structures such as the bladder or ureter). Renal causes may manifest with abnormal changes in rbcs when the red cells are viewed under a microscope. These abnormalities include rbc casts (abnormal clumping of blood cells), rbcs that have "buds" or "nipples," or rbcs that are fragmented. If these changes are not present or predominant, then the physician must conduct a urologic evaluation. In cases where it is suspected that the patient has intrinsic disease, the patient is generally evaluated initially with an ultrasound. However, radiologic imaging of patients with suspected postrenal causes is generally performed with a CT scan of the abdomen and pelvis. If the evaluation points to a renal cause, then additional laboratory testing may be in order (e.g., blood testing for autoimmune disease such as lupus, or for inflammation of the blood vessel walls known as vasculitis) along with a consideration of a renal biopsy (removal of a small piece of kidney tissue for microscopic inspection).

The detection of isolated proteinuria almost invariably reflects a renal cause. Protein excretion is measured and based upon the clinical setting, a protein electrophoresis and immunoelectrophoresis may be performed. Additional blood testing may be obtained. After the initial evaluation, a renal biopsy may be in order. The detection of hematuria and proteinuria most often reflects a renal cause and would be evaluated as described above.

If renal insufficiency is present, then it is necessary to determine whether it reflects an acute (short term) or chronic (long term) process. A renal ultrasound is usually more accurate than a CT scan to determine size. Small kidneys reflect chronicity. If the clinical picture is suggestive of an acute process, then a renal biopsy is generally in order. Abnormal laboratory values for BUN and creatinine only first appear after the loss of at least 50% of renal function. Therefore, early in the course of renal failure, the BUN and creatinine are not sensitive markers. In addition, since creatinine is a reflection of muscle mass, small-framed individuals and women will have normal creatinine values at the lower limits of the normal range.

RENAL DISEASE IN WOMEN

Although most renal disorders occur with nearly equal frequency in males and females, there are certain diseases more likely to occur in women. The two most common are lupus nephropathy (LN) and analgesic nephropathy (AN).

Systemic lupus erythematosus (SLE) occurs 13 times more frequently in females than males and is more common and severe in blacks. It afflicts young individuals especially in the third and fourth decades. Lupus nephropathy is typically more severe in children and in blacks. Although the cause is unknown, there is a role for genetic and hormonal factors. At the time of diagnosis of SLE, an abnormal urinalysis or renal insufficiency is already present in approximately 50% of patients. Over time approximately 75% of patients will manifest renal involvement with renal insufficiency present in about 30%. Generally speaking, specific therapy using immunosuppressants (medications to treat abnormal autoimmune system functioning) is considered when severe proteinuria and/or severe renal insufficiency are present. Given the complexities of the decision-making process, therapy is coordinated by a nephrologist (a doctor who specializes in the kidneys) and/or a rheumatologist. The renal prognosis has improved significantly over the past few decades.

Analgesic nephropathy occurs 5–7 times more frequently in women. It is more commonly diagnosed in the southeastern United States. Chronic headaches, joint pain, and other chronic pain syndromes are the most common reasons for consuming analgesics. The development of AN requires long-term ingestion of combination analgesics (e.g., aspirin, acetaminophen, caffeine). Epidemiologic studies have noted the regular ingestion of at least six tablets daily for more than 3 years. At the time of diagnosis, patients usually have nocturia (need to urinate during times the individual should be sleeping at night), sterile pyuria (white blood cells in the urine), anemia, and hypertension. Stopping consumption of combination analgesics is necessary.

PREGNANCY AND THE KIDNEY

Normal pregnancy results in changes in renal function. These changes are important to appreciate in the evaluation of women who are being seen for possible renal disease. By the end of the first trimester, the glomerular filtration rate (amount of urine processed/filtered by the kidney) increases by approximately 50%. The blood pressure decreases substantially over the first 28 weeks of pregnancy and increases slightly thereafter till delivery.

PREGNANCY AND RENAL DISEASE

Pregnancy in women with renal disease can affect the natural history of the underlying disorder, and renal disease can affect the maternal and fetal outcomes. *Effect of pregnancy on renal disease* generally depends upon the severity of the underlying renal disease and the presence of hypertension at the time of conception. Overall, proteinuria increases in nearly 50% of women and hypertension worsens in nearly 25% of women. With normal renal function or mild renal insufficiency, less than 10% of women will manifest a permanent decline in renal function. When the creatinine is more than mildly elevated, the risk of worsening renal insufficiency has been shown to increase by approximately 40%. Due to amenorrhea (lack of menstruation) or anovulatory menstrual cycles (menstruation without ovulation), the ability to conceive when the creatinine is very elevated (more than 3 mg/dl) and carry the fetus to term is generally very low.

Pregnancy in women with diabetes and SLE is not uncommon. In the diabetic patient without underlying nephropathy, pregnancy does not appear to increase the subsequent development of diabetic nephropathy (kidney damage due to diabetes). As with other forms of renal disease, renal insufficiency (creatinine $\geq$ 1.5 mg/dl) at the time of conception has been associated with irreversible deterioration of renal function. In one study, about 45% of patients were affected.

Effect of renal disease on pregnancy is a reflection of the severity of renal insufficiency. Mild renal insufficiency is associated with an increase in preterm labor

(approximately 20%), stillbirth (approximately 5%), and small for gestational age (SGA) infants (approximately 24%). Superimposed preeclampsia (pregnancy-associated disorder with abnormal blood pressure) occurs in about 10% of patients. In moderate and severe renal insufficiency, preterm labor, perinatal mortality, and other complications are more common. Uncontrolled hypertension (mean arterial pressure > 105 mm Hg at conception) has been estimated to be associated with a 10-fold increase in relative risk of fetal death.

In women with diabetic nephropathy, both perinatal morbidity and mortality have improved markedly in association with excellent blood sugar control. As in the nondiabetic patient with renal disease, the risk of complications of pregnancy, including preeclampsia, is increased with worsening renal insufficiency.

In women with SLE and preexisting LN, predictors of adverse fetal outcome include proteinuria (approximately 60% fetal loss), presence of abnormal blood (antiphospholipid), antibodies (approximately 75% fetal loss), and hypertension (approximately 30% fetal loss). Due to the small number of patients studied with renal insufficiency at the outset of pregnancy, the role of renal insufficiency on fetal outcome is presently unclear. In patients with SLE and LN (irrespective as to whether LN preceded pregnancy or first occurred during pregnancy), overall fetal loss has improved over the past three decades. Between 1990 and 2000, fetal loss occurred in 30% of pregnancies.

GENERAL APPROACH TO THERAPY

Specific treatment strategies for the multiple etiologies (causes) of renal disorders are beyond the scope of this text. There is a common therapeutic approach to patients with renal disease. This approach involves: (a) excellent blood pressure control (blood pressures ~120/80 mm Hg); (b) the use of specific medications such as angiotensin-converting enzyme inhibitors (ACEI) and angiotensin receptor blockers (ARB); (c) control of elevated blood fats/lipid (hyperlipidemia) with diet, exercise, and statin drugs; (d) restriction of dietary salt intake; (e) avoidance of excess protein intake; (f) control of elevated blood phosphorus concentrations with diet and use of medications that serve as phosphate binders; (g) control of metabolic acidosis (excessive accumulation of blood acid) with sodium bicarbonate.

Since an elevation in the serum creatinine to values just above the upper limits of normal generally reflects a loss of at least 50% of renal function, a referral to a nephrologist at this time is recommended.

SEE ALSO: Autoimmune disorders, Cardiovascular disease, Diabetes, Hypertension, Pregnancy, Systemic lupus erythematosus

Suggested Reading

Appel, G. B., Radhakrishnan, J., & D'Agat, V. (2000). Secondary glomerular disease. In B. M. Brenner (Ed.), *Brenner and Rector's the kidney* (pp. 1350–1448). Philadelphia, PA: W. B. Saunders.

Berger, B. E. (2003). Interstitial renal disease. In D. E. Hricik, R. T. Miller, & J. R. Sedor (Eds.), *Nephrology secrets* (pp. 136–139). Philadelphia: Hanley & Belfus.

Falk, R. J., Jennette, J. C., & Nachman, P. H. (2000). Primary glomerular disease. In B. M. Brenner (Ed.), *Brenner and Rector's the kidney* (pp. 1263–1349). Philadelphia: W. B. Saunders.

Hou, S. (1999). Pregnancy in chronic renal insufficiency and end-stage renal disease. *American Journal of Kidney Disease, 33,* 235–252.

Jungers, P., & Chauveau, D. (1997). Pregnancy in renal disease. *Kidney International, 52,* 871–885.

Mackie, A. D. R., Doddridge, M. C., Gamsu, H. R., et al. (1996). Outcome of pregnancy in patients with insulin-dependent diabetes mellitus and nephropathy with moderate renal impairment. *Diabetic Medicine, 13,* 90–96.

Moroni, G., Quaglini, S., Banfi, G., et al. (2002). Pregnancy in lupus nephritis. *American Journal of Kidney Disease, 40,* 713–720.

Sanders, C. L., & Lucas, M. J. (2001). Medical complications of pregnancy. *Obstetrics and Gynecology Clinics, 28,* 593–600.

United States Renal Data System (USRDS). (2002). *Annual data report: Atlas of end-stage renal disease in the United States* (National Institutes of Health, National Institute of Diabetes and Digestive and Kidney Diseases). Bethesda, MD.

BRUCE E. BERGER

Reproductive Technologies

Robert Edwards and Patrick Steptoe made a significant contribution to the treatment of infertility in 1978, with the successful birth of Louise Brown after in vitro fertilization (IVF). Twenty-two years later, the Centers for Disease Control and Prevention (CDC) reported that IVF resulted in 25,228 live births in the United States. The success of IVF has been estimated to be one live birth in every five IVF cycles. While the use of sperm donation and intrauterine insemination (IUI) with either partner or donated sperm has been available for many years, it is advances in assisted reproductive technologies (ART) that have revolutionized the care and management of couples dealing with infertility.

There are a number of different technologies available including IVF, intracytoplasmic sperm injection (ICSI), preimplantation genetic diagnosis (PGD), and third party reproduction (donor egg, donor sperm, surrogacy).

Invitro fertilization is a procedure that involves removing eggs from a woman's ovaries and fertilizing them outside her body in a glass dish. The embryos that are produced are then transferred into the woman's uterus through the cervix. The first step is to treat the woman with hormones to produce multiple eggs. Most women produce at least 4–6 eggs capable of being fertilized, but some may produce as many as 20–30 eggs. The eggs are removed and placed in a sterile dish along with sperm. Fertilization and early cell division takes place in the dish and can be seen under the microscope. Once the fertilized eggs have divided into 6- to 8-cell-stage embryos, they are returned to the uterus and are expected to implant in the uterus and continue with a normal pregnancy. The success of IVF has been estimated to be one live birth in every five IVF cycles. Two variations of IVF are gamete intrafallopian transfer (GIFT) and zygote intrafallopian transfer (ZIFT). GIFT uses the same initial procedure, but instead of waiting for fertilization to take place in the dish, the eggs and sperm are placed directly into the fallopian tubes using a laparoscope through small incisions in the abdomen. ZIFT involves placing the egg that was fertilized (zygote) in the dish directly into the fallopian tubes instead of the uterus.

Intracytoplamic sperm injection was developed by researchers in Brussels in 1992 and involves the direct microinjection of a single sperm into the cytoplasm of a single egg (oocyte). This technique was developed to help males who are infertile due to very low sperm count or very limited numbers of healthy sperm. This procedure has been reported to dramatically increase fertilization rate by 50–80%, with a successful pregnancy rate of about 20–30% for couples with male infertility. Since the first reports of successful pregnancies after ICSI, there has been an effort to assess the genetic risks that may be associated with this technique as ICSI bypasses the natural mechanisms of sperm selection during reproduction. While there have been some reports of the occurrence of birth defects in children conceived after ICSI, the incidence of a congenital malformation is estimated to be 2.5–3%, which is similar to that of the general population. Also, some causes of male infertility can be genetic and passed on, so male offsprings might have reproductive problems as adults.

Preimplantation genetic diagnosis is a relatively new technique developed 10 years ago that combines advances in molecular genetics and ART. Preimplantation genetic diagnosis is a technology that can be used during IVF to test for genetic disorders in the embryo, prior to being transferred back into the uterus. Once the embryos are obtained, they are placed under a microscope and a single cell is removed from each embryo with a glass needle (pipette). That cell can then be tested for the presence of the genetic disorder the couple was at risk for. Embryos that are unaffected—do not have the genetic disorder—can then be transferred into the uterus. For example, Tay–Sachs disease, Duchenne muscular dystrophy, Down syndrome, and cystic fibrosis are a few of the genetic disorders that have been successfully bypassed by using PGD. Preimplantation genetic diagnosis was developed for couples for whom pregnancy termination after conventional prenatal diagnosis was not an option. The risks of PGD are similar to those of IVF, namely, multiple fetal pregnancies. Preliminary studies show no risk for spontaneous abortions or birth defects; however, the data from long-term follow-up of children conceived after PGD have yet to be collected.

Third-party reproduction refers to using donated gametes (eggs or sperm), donated embryos, or a donated uterus (surrogacy or a gestational carrier) by a third person (the donor) to an infertile couple (the recipient). There are genetic issues involved with donated eggs, sperm, and embryos in particular. Gamete donors undergo genetic screening according to guidelines established by the American Society for Reproductive Medicine (ASRM) in 1997. In addition, some programs offer donated embryos from couples who have gotten pregnant following IVF and no longer need the other remaining fertilized eggs. Donor eggs are often recommended when a woman has a uterus but her ovaries do not produce healthy eggs, or ovaries were previously removed due to cancer or infection. Using IVF techniques, the egg donor is given hormone medication to stimulate ovulation and then the eggs are retrieved. These are then mixed with the infertile woman's partner's sperm or donated sperm and the resulting embryo is transferred back into the recipient. Donor sperm is used when the male is infertile. The sperm can be injected directly into the uterus (IUI) and conception occurs naturally or can be mixed in the laboratory with eggs to create embryos. When using donated sperm, it is recommended that it be frozen for several months to rule out the presence of infectious diseases such as HIV. Surrogacy (having another woman carry the pregnancy) is considered when a woman does not have a uterus because of a previous hysterectomy or was born without a uterus. In this case, either the couple's eggs and sperm or donor eggs and

sperm can be used. Using the same IVF techniques, the embryo is transferred into the surrogate mother.

While all of these ART have provided many new options for infertile couples, the achievement of a pregnancy using ART can have physical, emotional, and social consequences. One adverse consequence of IVF is an increased rate in multiple fetal pregnancies. These can be potentially harmful for both mother and fetus due to higher rates of cesarean sections, prematurity, low birthweight, infant death, and disability. According to the CDC, the multiple-infant birth rate after ART was 38% in 1998, compared to only 3% in the general population. Moreover, despite advances in ART, IVF still remains relatively unsuccessful. Only about 22% of ART cycles performed in the United States in 2000 in all aged women resulted in a live birth. Women who are under the age of 35 have the highest success rates and women over the age of 40 have lower success rates. Finally, ART is expensive. Costs vary depending on the center and what is done. Costs can range from a few thousand dollars per cycle to $10,000 per cycle.

See Also: Menstrual cycle disorders, Miscarriage, Pregnancy

Suggested Resources

American Society for Reproductive Medicine (ASRM). (2002, April 27). Frequently asked questions about infertility (online). Available: http://asrm.org/Patients/faqs.html

American Society for Reproductive Medicine (ASRM). Patients Home page (online). Available: http://www.asrm.org/Patients/mainpati.html

CDC's Reproductive Health Information Source (online). Available: http://www.cdc.gov/nccdphp/drh/art.htm

http://www.asrm.org/

http://www.sart.org/patients.htm

Anne L. Matthews

Restraining Orders One of the most important things a victim can do to save his or her life is to file an order for protection, also known as a restraining order. In response to domestic violence and other abuse, the law developed the restraining order, which is a legal order created to protect a person from harm. Since a legal order carries the weight of the law, an abuser must abide by it or face legal penalties. All restraining orders are defined at the state level rather than at the federal level. However, there is only slight variation among the states as to the types of available restraining orders, who can obtain it, and under what circumstances it can be issued. Although domestic violence is one of the most common reasons for a restraining order, other instances include but are not limited to stalking, harassment, and sexual abuse.

There are various types of restraining orders such as the traditional restraining order, harassment orders, temporary restraining orders, and civil protection orders. Deciding what type of restraining order to petition for depends on your specific situation, but ultimately the judge or commissioner decides what type of restraining order can be issued. *Traditional restraining orders* are issued if the abuser is your spouse, boyfriend, related to you by blood, or is someone you have had a significant sexual relationship with. A second type of order of protection is a *harassment restraining order*, which only takes an hour to complete, but unlike a traditional restraining order, it cannot be amended. Typically, a harassment restraining order is obtained only if the victim does not qualify for a traditional restraining order. Alternatively, *temporary restraining orders* are often used in divorce proceedings to prevent a party from disposing of any marital assets or to protect one party from the vindictive actions of the other party. Also, issued under divorce or annulment court proceedings are *civil restraining orders*, which can only be enforced by the court. Furthermore, if one party violates a civil restraining order, it does not excuse the other party from abiding by the court orders, even if an attorney or an advocate advises otherwise.

The fundamental function of most restraining orders is to prevent harm and the manner in which this is done depends on provisions in the restraining order. Several different types of provisions are: stay away, no contact, cease abuse, support, exclusive use, restitution, relinquish firearms, custody visitation, and child support provisions. *Stay away provisions* order the abuser to not be at or near your work, school, home, or other places. *No contact provisions* order the abuser to stop all calls, faxes, gifts, mail, emails, or other communication. *Cease abuse provisions* order the abuser to not threaten or harm you. *Support provisions* order the abuser to provide financial support, by continuing to pay the mortgage or other temporary financial support. *Exclusive use provisions* order the abuser to cease all use of the home and/or car. *Restitution provisions* order the abuser to reimburse you for medical costs, property damages, or other damages resulting from the abuse. *Relinquish firearms provisions* order the abuser to surrender all weapons and ammunition. *Custody visitation provisions* order the abuser to only visit the child under supervised visitation and can order that the transfer of the child only occur under safe supervision.

An abuser is guilty of violating an order if he or she fails to do what the order required or does something that the order prohibits. Violation of a restraining order subjects the abuser to fines, prison, or both. Restraining orders can be enforced against the abuser by the court or police, depending on the provision violated. Generally, the police can enforce the following provisions: no contact, stay away, cease abuse, exclusive use, and child custody. Therefore, it is critical to contact local law enforcement immediately when such an order is violated; if that is not possible, then a police report should be filed as soon as possible. In most states, witnesses or proof of the violation are not required. Reporting every violation to the police will strengthen the case against the abuser because police reports are heavily relied upon by the court to determine the penalty and other courses of action. On the other hand, violation of child support provisions can only be addressed by filing a motion for contempt in court, which leads to a court hearing to determine how the abuser violated the order and the applicable penalty.

To obtain a restraining order, contact either a domestic violence advocate at a crisis center, an attorney, or your local police department. Given that restraining orders are legal documents and take a few hours to fill out, professional assistance in filling out the forms is recommended. Advocates are particularly specialized in filing restraining orders and know how to help you qualify for available fee waivers, and are a great source of other relevant aid. For example, advocates can advise you on which important documents should be included with the restraining order application, make sure you are safe when the order is delivered to the abuser, and can assist you in finding safe housing if necessary.

An alarming number of people do not obtain restraining orders because of a common misconception that it will make an abusive situation worse. Although this perception is ill-founded, of the 1.5 million women in the United States who report physical and/or sexual abuse, only 20% seek restraining orders. However, it has been proven in recent studies that women who obtained a 12-month restraining order were fives times *less likely* to experience abuse than women who refused restraining orders. In contrast, studies show that temporary restraining orders, as opposed to long-term restraining orders, are not as effective since they are only valid for a short period of time.

Rh Disease

In conclusion, the restraining order has altered the power equation between an abuser and the victim. No longer is a victim alone to defend herself. The power of the law will rise up to protect her through the restraining order, ordering no harm be done to her. Although each state dictates its own law on the scope and power of a restraining order, each state offers this basic protection. Should you consider obtaining a restraining order, contact a local crisis center or the police to find out what the process and law is in your state. Remember you are not alone; there is a legal system in place to enforce your protection.

SEE ALSO: Child custody, Divorce, Domestic violence, Homicide, Rape, Sexual harassment, Stalking

Suggested Resources

Cooper & Forbes. (1999). Cooper, Linda D. *Restraining orders, civil protection orders, temporary protection order.* (2003, May 14). http://library.lp.findlaw.com/articles/file/

Discovery Health Channel. (2002, August 6). *Court orders can protect battered women.* (2003, May 14). http://health.discovery.com/news/afp/20020805/battered_print.html

Larsen, D. *All about restraining orders; Part 1: The differences between OFPs and HROs.* (2003, May 14). http://incestabuse.about.com/library/weekly/aa100902b.htm

Law Info.com. (2000). *Temporary restraining orders.* (2003, May 14). http://www.lawinfo.com/legal-audio/real/4257.htm

Women's Law Initiative. *More information on domestic violence.* (2003, May 14); http://www.womenslaw.org/more_info.htm

ELIZABETH M. VALENCIA

Rh Disease Rh disease is known as hemolytic (having to do with the blood) disease of the newborn (erythroblastosis fetalis). Rh refers to the Rh system (antigen groups include C, D, E) on blood cells and specifically the D-antigen. Rh disease develops when antibodies form in an individual with Rh-negative (lack of D-antigen) blood after exposure to red blood cells that have a D-antigen (Rh-positive) within the blood. Antibodies are cells of the immune system that identify other cells or compounds in the body or blood that the immune system perceives as dangerous. Among racial groups, the Rh-negative blood group is more common among whites (15%) than African Americans (5–8%) or Asians/Native Americans (1–2%).

Rh disease has a wide variety of presentations from mild hemolysis (anemia caused by the breakdown of red blood cells) to hydrops fetalis (a severe, life-threatening problem of severe edema [swelling] in the fetus and newborn). An Rh-negative woman during her first pregnancy will probably have some exposure to fetal blood; if the fetus is Rh-positive, the woman may develop antibodies (IgG) to the D-antigen on the fetal red blood cells. The infant from the first pregnancy may exhibit few or no signs of hemolysis (red blood cell breakdown) and only have mild signs of jaundice after birth. During subsequent pregnancies, a fetus, if Rh-positive, may be at increased risk for complications due to mother's Rh-negative blood group.

LABORATORY EVALUATION

In the case of suspected Rh incompatibility (the mother being Rh-positive and the fetus Rh-negative), laboratory data of infant and maternal blood groups should be identified. The infant will need a variety of specialized blood tests (a Coomb's test, hemoglobin, reticulocyte count, total and direct bilirubin level, and a blood smear). In the presence of hemolytic disease, some of these blood tests will be abnormal (the Coomb's test will be positive, there will be evidence of anemia on the hemoglobin, the reticulocyte count will be increased, there will be abnormal cells on the blood smear, and the total [unconjugated] bilirubin will be elevated).

INFANT PRESENTATION OF Rh DISEASE

The characteristic presentation of an infant (Rh-positive) born to a mother (Rh-negative) will be yellowing of skin and whites of the eyes (jaundice) within the first day of life. While the infant was in utero, the bilirubin was cleared by the placenta. The infant will not be able to handle the red cell waste products (bilirubin by-products) being produced by the breakdown (hemolysis) of red blood cells occurring due to the maternal antibodies that have crossed into the infant's blood prior to delivery via the placenta. Jaundice due to hemolysis of red blood cells puts infants at greater risk for kernicterus (a buildup of bilirubin in the brain), which may include symptoms of flaccidity (weakness), opisthotonus (a spasm of the spine and extremities), seizures, apnea, and even death.

Treatment of Rh disease includes a specialized form of light exposure therapy (phototherapy) and possibly blood exchange transfusion (remove damaged blood and replace with healthy blood).

Infants with a more severe presentation of Rh disease, hydrops fetalis, require immediate diagnosis and supportive therapy. Signs of more severe disease include pallor (anemia), edema (hypoalbuminemia), pleural and cardiac effusions (fluid around the lungs and heart), hepatosplenomegaly (enlarged liver and spleen), petechiae (a rash of tiny red bumps from a low platelet count that does not blanch when pressed on), or ascites (fluid in the abdomen). These infants will often need the care of a neonatal intensive care unit for monitoring, temperature stabilization, respiratory support, correction of abnormal blood acid balance (metabolic acidosis), and exchange transfusion. An exchange transfusion involves exchanging two blood volumes of the infant's blood with the donor's blood. The exchange transfusion should help to remove bilirubin and hemolyzing red blood cells (about 85%).

PREVENTION OF Rh DISEASE

Prevention of Rh disease is done by screening maternal blood type. If the woman is Rh-negative, she should have a specific blood product, anti-D gamma globulin or RhoGAM, given between 20 and 28 weeks gestation, at the end of pregnancy (delivery, miscarriage, or abortion) or in the case of blood transfusion, amniocentesis or vaginal bleeding during the pregnancy. An Rh-negative woman should be monitored during pregnancies for increasing levels of antibody. If the Rh-antibody levels are increasing or there is previous history of an infant with Rh disease, then close fetal monitoring is required with ultrasound and specific procedures that sample small pieces of the placenta, or tissues and fluids that surround the fetus (chorionic villus sampling, amniocentesis, or percutaneous umbilical blood sampling). The overall incidence of Rh-negative mothers with multiple pregnancies having an infant with hemolytic disease is around 5%.

RhoGAM has revolutionized Rh disease for most mothers and babies. What was once a commonly devastating and deadly disease is now one seen much more rarely and less severely.

SEE ALSO: Labor and delivery, Neonatal care ethics, Pregnancy, Prenatal care, Reproductive technologies

Suggested Reading

Behrman, R. E., Kliegman, R. M., & Jenson, H. B. (Eds.). (2000). Hemolytic disease of the newborn. *Nelson's textbook of pediatrics* (pp. 521–525). Philadelphia: W.B. Saunders.

Gabbe, S. G., Niebyl, J. R., & Simpson, J. L. (Eds.). (2002). Rh disease. *Obstetrics, normal and problem pregnancies* (pp. 893–915). New York: Churchill Livingstone.

Stockman, J. A. (2001). Overview of the state of the art in Rh disease: History, current clinical management, and recent progress. *Journal of Pediatric Hematology/Oncology, 23*(8), 554–562.

DEANNA DAHL-GROVE

Rheumatoid Arthritis Rheumatoid arthritis (RA) is an autoimmune disease in which the joints are the primary target of progressive inflammation and destruction. This disease affects about 1% of the U.S. population and is nearly three times more common in women than men. It can occur at any age and tends to increase in frequency with age. However, it most commonly begins between ages 30 and 60. There is not one particular test that can easily establish the diagnosis of RA. Rather, the diagnosis is based on a constellation of clinical, laboratory, and x-ray findings.

Despite extensive research, the cause of RA is still not well understood. Autoimmune diseases occur when the immune system, the body's natural defense mechanism against infection, mistakenly identifies "self" as a target to attack. Over the years, a number of bacteria and viruses have been suspected as possible triggers for the development of RA, but none has been consistently identified. Familial studies and studies of twins suggest that genetic factors are important in developing RA. Certain genetic markers, if present, not only suggest susceptibility, but may also indicate how severe the disease is likely to be. However, clustering in families is not common and genetic influences alone do not explain why a particular patient develops RA. Cigarette smoking is the only environmental factor that has been shown to be associated with the development of RA. In summary, RA is a process which occurs in a genetically predisposed individual as a result of a yet unidentified trigger.

The primary target of inflammation in RA is the joint. The interior of the joint is lined by a membrane called the synovium which secretes a lubricating fluid called synovial fluid. When the synovium becomes inflamed, as occurs in RA, certain molecules and enzymes that can damage tissue are released. These mediators of inflammation can attack cartilage, ligaments, tendons, and bones. Unchecked, the damage from this inflammation can become permanent.

Most commonly, RA develops over a period of several weeks as a gradually progressive joint inflammation. Most often, the same joints are affected on both sides of the body. Typically, the joints involved include, the small joints of the hands and feet, wrists, elbows, shoulders, knees, and ankles. In addition, the spine in the neck may be affected. Over time, this can lead to instability of the neck with potentially serious neurologic complications. Early in the disease, the disease may initially appear asymmetric, making the diagnosis less clear. Other possible diagnoses should always be considered, such as other types of arthritis, infection, or other rheumatic diseases such as lupus.

Early on, the joint symptoms are reversible and related to ongoing inflammation. Later in the course of the disease, irreversible joint damage may occur. Patients describe morning stiffness which is due to synovial inflammation. Unlike degenerative arthritis (osteoarthritis) in which this stiffness is brief (minutes) in duration, the morning stiffness associated with RA generally lasts 1 hour or more. Upon physical examination, joints which are more superficial and easily examined, such as the small joints of the hand or the knee, may show active signs of inflammation such as warmth, swelling, or redness. Over time, if this chronic inflammation continues untreated, the lining of the joints become scarred, cartilage is destroyed, and the bony surfaces of the joints become eroded, resulting in irreversible destructive damage. At this point, joint deformities become obvious and joint function is limited. Therefore, the goal of therapy is early identification of disease and aggressive treatment of the inflammatory process in order to prevent permanent joint damage.

RA causes problems in other organ systems as well. Initially, some individuals experience fevers, weight loss, and fatigue. Up to 50% of patients with RA may develop rheumatoid nodules, which are firm, soft accumulations of connective tissue typically located over pressure points such as the outer surface of the forearm or the Achilles tendon. Other patients develop a diffuse skin rash as part of their RA. RA can also involve the heart, lungs, and neurologic system. Inflammation of the lining of the lungs (pleurisy) or the heart (pericarditis) may occur. Fluid accumulation (effusions) may affect these organs as well. These findings vary from asymptomatic to severe, and may require increased immunosuppressive therapy or drainage of the fluid.

Neurologic manifestations in RA may occur in several ways. First, arthritis which affects the cervical spine may lead to instability, pinched nerves, and problems with movement or sensation. These symptoms gradually get worse. Because of the possibility of cervical spine instability, care should be taken to avoid any unnecessary manipulation of the neck in a patient with RA. Prior to elective surgery, an anesthesiologist should consult with a rheumatologist regarding intubation of a patient with possible cervical instability. RA can also affect peripheral nerves. Nerves pass through compartments, which are also occupied by synovium and tendon sheaths. If these structures become inflamed, the nerves can be compressed. This causes symptoms which change with joint position or according to the degree of inflammation. Finally, the blood vessels supplying peripheral nerves may become inflamed. This causes neurologic symptoms that occur more abruptly and are not altered with a change in position.

The American College of Rheumatology has established criteria for the diagnosis of RA based on clinical, laboratory, and x-ray changes. Clinical criteria include prolonged morning stiffness, arthritis of multiple joints in a symmetric pattern, and rheumatoid nodules. Laboratory tests and x-rays also help confirm the diagnosis of RA. One particular blood test, the rheumatoid factor (RF), can be found in nearly 85% of patients with RA. If present in high titers, it may predict more severe and unremitting disease as well as an increased risk for nonjoint manifestations of the disease. This lab test alone does not make the diagnosis of RA and in fact may be negative early on in RA. It is also important to realize that this test may be positive in healthy individuals or in those with other autoimmune, infectious, or cancerous conditions. Blood tests which can be followed as markers of inflammation include the erythrocyte sedimentation rate (ESR), C-reactive protein (CRP), and platelet count. Many individuals will also have anemia (low blood count) or low albumin (protein), which are frequently seen in patients with chronic diseases. Drainage of joint fluid may be performed to assess the degree of inflammation and to rule out infections. Rarely, a biopsy of joint synovium is performed to look for pathologic features that would support (or rule out) a diagnosis of RA.

X-rays are performed periodically throughout the course of the disease. Early changes may reveal soft tissue swelling and thinning of the bones near the joints. As the disease advances, x-rays show bony erosions, joint space narrowing, and progressive joint destruction. One of the primary goals of therapy is to delay and prevent such destructive changes. Repeated x-rays are often done to monitor response to treatment. Checking hand or foot x-rays over the course of the disease helps the rheumatologist to judge whether the current therapy is working.

Treatment of RA addresses a number of important goals. From the patient's perspective, perhaps the most important goals are improvement of joint pain and swelling and preservation of joint function. These goals are important to the physician as well, but the physician is also trying to prevent further joint damage, reduce long-term disease-related illness and death, and carefully monitor for harmful side effects of medication. In general, there are two main classes of drugs for the treatment of RA. One group of medications focuses on controlling symptoms by decreasing pain and inflammation. The other type of medication focuses on preventing further disease progression and improving long-term outcomes.

The first category of medications includes non-steroidal anti-inflammatory drugs (NSAIDs), cyclooxygenase-2 (Cox-2) inhibitors, and corticosteroids. These medications are effective in the treatment of inflammation and pain but do not prevent further disease progression. It is not recommended that any of these medications be used as the only therapy for the long-term treatment of RA.

The mainstay of therapy for long-term treatment of RA are the disease-modifying antirheumatic drugs (DMARDs). These medications vary in their mechanisms of action but in general alter the immune system by reducing its abnormal response as well as blocking pathways involved in the inflammatory process. The choice of a DMARD depends on a number of considerations. Clearly, the degree of disease activity and severity is important. Whether the patient has other diseases or certain lifestyle behaviors (such as alcohol consumption and increased risk of liver toxicty with certain drugs) is important as well. Finally, the patient's willingness to comply with drug monitoring and drug dosing plays a role. In general, all of the DMARD class of medications increase the risk of developing infections because they suppress the immune system. A careful evaluation of the risks and benefits of each medication should be discussed and weighed against the risks of untreated disease.

In conclusion, RA is a disease process primarily affecting the joints but potentially involving other organ systems as well. It is diagnosed by a combination of clinical, laboratory, and radiographic findings. Treatment is individualized to each patient with the primary objectives of reducing of inflammation and preserving joint function.

See Also: Arthritis, Autoimmune disorders

Suggested Reading

Klippel, J. H. (Ed.). (2001). *Primer on the rheumatic diseases* (12th ed.). Atlanta, GA: Arthritis Foundation.
Ruddy, S., Harris, E. D., & Sledge, C. B. (Eds.). (2001). *Kelley's textbook of rheumatology* (6th ed.). Philadelphia: W.B. Saunders.

Suggested Resources

Arthritis Foundation at www.arthritis.org National phone number 1–800–283–7800.
National Organization for Rare Disorders, Inc. (NORD) at www.rarediseases.org

JULIANNE S. ORLOWSKI

Rhythm Method *see* Natural Family Planning

Rosacea Rosacea is a common facial skin condition that most frequently affects fair-skinned Caucasian women and men of northern European ancestry. While the precise etiology (cause) of rosacea is unknown, it is probably due to some combination of factors in predisposed individuals resulting in an abnormality of the blood supply to the skin (cutaneous vasculature). The earliest sign of rosacea is recurrent episodes of flushing that may be triggered by a variety of exacerbating factors including hot beverages, spicy foods, alcohol, sunlight, or emotional stress. Over time, the redness of the skin (erythema) may become permanent rather than episodic and more inflammatory changes ensue including swelling (edema), bumps (papules), and blisters (pustules). Phymas, disfiguring fibrotic changes in the skin, are a late stage of rosacea and are seen more commonly in men. An index of suspicion should be maintained for rosacea that affects the eye area (ocular rosacea), which is common and often unrecognized, but has the potential to cause discomfort as well as possible corneal ulceration.

Avoidance of irritating stimuli that cause flushing is an essential first step of treating rosacea. A frequent complaint of rosacea patients is hyperirritability of the skin characterized by stinging and burning with application of topical preparations. Avoidance of products that produce this symptom and employing gentle skin care can also improve the condition. Daily use of a gentle moisturizer with a broad-spectrum, nonchemical sunscreen is essential. Skin atrophy as a result of chronic sun damage can further accentuate the prominent blood vessels. Cosmetics can be used if they are mild and do not irritate the skin; the use of cosmetics to camouflage the redness and blemishes goes a long way toward benefiting self-esteem in this highly visible condition.

Therapy of rosacea has included both topical and systemic agents, with treatment regimens based primarily on disease severity. Antibiotics are the most common prescription drugs for rosacea, and most dermatologists employ a tiered approach based on the severity of the condition. Topical metronidazole products are the most common first-line therapies. Combination therapy with systemic antibiotics, particularly those in the tetracycline class, is prescribed for inflammatory lesions as well as ocular involvement. Rosacea fulminans, a severe inflammatory variant of rosacea seen most commonly in young women, may require oral corticosteroids or the retin medication, isotretinoin. Swelling of the nose with fibrosis resulting in a bulbous appearance, known as rhinophyma, is much more commonly seen in men. Rosacea tends to be cyclic in nature and systemic medications can often be tapered while maintaining a regimen of gentle skin care, daily sunscreen, and avoidance of known factors that trigger flares. Recognition and treatment of rosacea early in its onset provides the most favorable long-term prognosis.

SEE ALSO: Edema, Skin disorders

Suggested Reading

Quarterman, M. J., Johnson, D. W., Abele, D. C., et al. (1997). Ocular rosacea: Signs, symptoms, and tear studies before and after treatment with doxycycline. *Archives of Dermatology, 133*, 49–54.

Torok, H. M. (2000). Rosacea skin care. *Cutis, 66*, 14–16.

Wilkin, J. K. (1994). Rosacea: Pathophysiology and treatment. *Archives of Dermatology, 130*, 359–362.

MARY GAIL MERCURIO

Rubella Rubella is commonly referred to as German measles or 3-day measles. This disease is a common and relatively mild disease of childhood. The disease is caused by an RNA virus (genus: Rubivirus, family: Togaviridae) and humans are the only known host. Rubella is passed by secretions; nasopharyngeal, blood, stool, or urine. The virus can be recovered from secretions 7 days before symptoms start and up to 7 days after the rash disappears. The incubation period is 14–21 days and usually 16–18 days. Rubella outbreaks often occur in late winter and early spring. Outbreaks, which have occurred since the vaccine development, are usually in environments where close contact with other individuals occurs such as dormitories or health care environments.

CLINICAL COURSE

Rubella, in postnatal infection, begins with swollen lymph nodes in the head and neck regions, in particular, the occipital lymph nodes. Within 5 days, a mild enanthem of rose-colored spots may be noted on the soft palate. Sore throat, conjunctivitis, and enlarged spleen are the next symptoms, followed by fever, usually low grade ($< 38.5°C$; 101°F), and rash. The rash begins in the face and then proceeds to the trunk and extremities. The rash has discrete maculopapular (raised but flat) and slightly erythematous (red) lesions that last about 3 days. Other symptoms that may occur are anorexia, headache, and malaise. Less common symptoms include polyarthritis, usually of small joints of hands and feet among women, and paresthesias (abnormal sensations in the extremities), tendonitis, purpura (small, raised purple skin lesions), testicular pain, and encephalitis (inflammation of the brain), which is a rare complication. Some individuals may be asymptomatic during infection (25–50%). Generally, laboratory evaluation during the disease course is not indicated, but, if performed, a white blood cell (WBC) count may be low or normal, and a platelet count may be low. Other diseases that can resemble the rash of rubella are scarlet fever, rubeola (measles), roseola, mononucleosis, enteroviral infections, drug rashes, and secondary syphilis. The treatment of rubella is mainly supportive care.

PREVENTION

The vaccine was developed in 1969. The vaccine that is currently used is a live virus (RA 27/3) developed from human diploid cells and confers nasopharyngeal immunity. The vaccine is routinely given to children between 12 and 15 months and revaccination occurs between 4 and 6 years old, in combination with measles and mumps (MMR). The number of rubella outbreaks has been dramatically reduced since the introduction of the vaccine. Vaccination given by single subcutaneous injection causes protective antibodies in approximately 98% of individuals and the immunity is lifelong. Reinfection among individuals who have had the immunization is 14–18% and among individuals who had natural immunity, 3–10%. Postpubertal women need to avoid pregnancy within 3 months of vaccination. Contraindications to vaccination include sensitivity to vaccine components, immunodeficiency, and persons taking antimetabolic drugs or prolonged steroids (greater than 14 days). Reactions to the vaccine include fever, lymphadenopathy (swollen glands), rash, arthritis/arthralgia (joint pains), and a more unusual reaction which may occur in young women is paresthesia in hands and knees.

Rubella virus may be isolated from the throat, blood, urine, or spinal fluid of affected infants and detected by cell culture or by several different tests based on detecting viral proteins or genetic material. Infants with congenital rubella may shed virus up to 1 year after birth. Pregnant women should avoid contact with infants known to have congenital rubella.

SEE ALSO: Birth control, Immunization, Neonatal care ethics, Pregnancy

Suggested Reading

American Academy of Pediatrics. (2000). Rubella. In L. K. Pickering (Ed.), *2000 red book: Report of the Committee on Infectious Diseases* (25th ed., pp. 495–500). Elk Grove Village, IL: Author.

Behrman, R. E., Kliegman, R. M., & Jenson, H. B. (Eds.) (2000). Rubella. *Nelson's textbook of pediatrics* (pp. 951–953). Philadelphia: W. B. Saunders.

DEANNA DAHL-GROVE

CONGENITAL RUBELLA

Congenital rubella occurs when the mother has an active rubella infection and the fetus is exposed in utero. Risk of congenital malformations to the fetus is highest during the first 14 weeks of gestation. If a pregnant woman is exposed to rubella, an antibody test for rubella should be performed to determine immunity. If the mother is not immune, then therapeutic abortion is recommended or if unavailable or unacceptable, then passive immunization (immunoglobulin) may be given. Despite the use of passive immunity shortly after exposure to rubella in pregnant women, infants have been born with congenital rubella.

Infants with congenital rubella have many complications. Ophthalmologic complications include cataracts and retinopathy. Cardiac problems include patent ductus arteriosus and pulmonary artery stenosis. An auditory complication is sensorineural deafness. Neurologic complications are behavioral disorders, meningoencephalitis, and mental retardation. Other complications may include growth retardation, bone disease, hepatosplenomegaly (enlarged liver and spleen), thrombocytopenia (low platelets), purple skin lesions (blueberry muffin rash). The care of infants with congenital rubella is primarily supportive but complex and usually occurs in neonatal intensive care units.

Rural Health Women represent over half (52%) of the 60 million people who live in rural and frontier areas in the United States. In recent years, the image of rural life as simple, healthy, and natural has been replaced with a more complex understanding in which distinct physiological stresses, physical hardships, and community patterns of rural life are also recognized. For example, age-adjusted death rates of rural women are a fourth (24%) higher than for their urban counterparts, and rural women make fewer doctor visits, are more likely to be seriously ill, and are more likely to be admitted to the hospital when they do seek medical attention. In addition, chronic physical illnesses (e.g., diabetes and arthritis), addiction, mental illness, and long-term sequelae of serious conditions associated with urban populations such as HIV and hepatitis are increasingly recognized for their burden among rural women. Rural women may not be able to overcome the additional barriers to optimal health services that exist in nonmetropolitan settings compared to urban areas, including limited access to care, fewer facilities, increased travel time, lack of specialized caregivers, and fewer patients having adequate insurance. Rural health care also poses special ethical problems surrounding health care that are related to overlapping personal and professional relationships, confidentiality, and stigma.

For these reasons, the health care of women who reside in rural areas deserves special attention.

Rural women experience diverse health concerns, encompassing accidents and injuries, addictions, mental illnesses, and reproductive health. About one third of all U.S. births take place in rural areas, and rural women have their first pregnancy earlier in life and have more children than their urban counterparts. However, appropriate, affordable obstetric care is unavailable in many rural counties. Rural women with high-risk pregnancies are more likely to receive care that does not meet national practice standards and to develop complications such as pregnancy loss, preterm labor, premature birth, and poor infant outcome. The infant mortality rate is one fifth (20%) higher in rural areas than in metro areas (7.6 vs. 6.1 deaths per 1,000 live births), and sudden infant death syndrome (SIDS) rates are also much higher in rural areas (90 vs. 57 deaths per 100,000).

Addiction and mental illnesses affect the lives of rural women, indirectly and directly. Although fewer rural residents admit to consuming alcohol (44% rural vs. 54% urban residents), the prevalence of heavy and binge drinking among active drinkers is similar in rural and urban areas. Among heavy drinkers, two thirds (65%) of rural respondents described negative social consequences compared to only two fifths (40%) of urban people. In recent years, the use of illicit substances has increased in rural areas to the levels in urban communities, and rural states and counties have higher arrest rates for substance abuse violations (e.g., driving under the influence, liquor law violations, possession of illegal substances) than nonrural areas. Approximately one quarter of rural women have a diagnosable mental illness, and nearly one half will experience some significant mental health problem sometime during their lives. The consequences of coexisting addiction and mental disorders on physical and mental health can be especially severe among women in remote areas, where few resources and supports exist for them.

Rural women, like urban women, also face issues of domestic violence. Very few empirical studies of rural battered women exist, but it appears that living in rural environments may exacerbate issues contributing to domestic violence, perhaps because of social and physical isolation. In one study, twice as many rural women (25%) as urban women (12%) were likely to be involved in an ongoing violent relationship. Poverty, lack of public transportation, shortages of health care providers, lack of health insurance or underinsurance, and decreased access to any resources may make it more difficult for rural women to escape abusive relationships. Furthermore, the closeness of rural communities may make it difficult for rural women to disclose abuse for fear of breaching their confidentiality. Geographical isolation and the increased availability of firearms and knives common in rural households also increase the potential lethality of domestic attacks upon rural women.

Accidents and trauma are a major concern for rural women. For example, farming has inherent risks for women, and as more women have participated in farming, their rate of machinery-related injuries has increased. Women and children suffer almost twice as many farm-related injuries as men, most (75%) of which are severe, permanent, or fatal. High rates of automobile accidents occur in remote areas, often secondary to alcohol intoxication, and contribute to the high rates of morbidity among rural women. Beyond a heavier burden of physical disability associated with accident and trauma, rural people are nearly twice as likely as city dwellers to die of injuries they sustain, partly due to the limited emergency services and time of travel to services.

Women and men in rural areas experience *infections* that are uncommon or rare in more urban locales. They are more likely to have jobs (e.g., farming) or avocations (e.g., hunting) that expose them to many disease-inducing organisms that are carried by animals and insects (e.g., anthrax, hantavirus, plague, tularemia, Lyme disease, brucella). Rural dwellers are more likely than urban people to be exposed to contaminated water and to improper sanitation systems, which increase risk for a number of illnesses (e.g., giardiasis, hepatitis A). Finally, migrant workers in rural areas present with infections acquired in their country of origin that are uncommon in the United States (e.g., malaria). Because physicians and other clinicians are typically trained in urban environments, when they come to practice in rural communities, they, at least initially, are often less familiar with many of the health risks that are more common in rural than urban areas.

Rural residents also show higher rates of a number of chronic conditions, many of which may relate to conditions specific to rural life. Greater heart disease rates were detected in rural areas beginning in the 1970s and continued into the 1980s and 1990s. A number of studies have revealed greater rates of certain kinds of cancer in rural than urban areas, particularly those associated with exposure to herbicides, pesticides, insecticides, and other carcinogenic substances. Greater respiratory disease (e.g., asthma, organic dust syndrome, chronic bronchitis, lung function changes) rates have been found among farm than nonfarm populations. Residents of rural communities also have higher rates of activity limitations due to chronic conditions, and fewer rural residents perceive their health to be excellent. Some studies have reported that arthritis and related disability are greater in rural areas, but that rural residents are more mobile than their similarly ill counterparts. Some neurologic diseases (e.g., Parkinson's disease, Alzheimer's disease, amyotrophic lateral sclerosis, chronic encephalopathy) associated with exposures to toxic chemicals used by farmers and miners have been found to have greater prevalence in rural than nonrural areas. Obesity and nutritional problems are also higher in rural communities with self-reported levels of obesity for rural residents (23%) being nearly one third higher than urban residents (16%), and rates of diabetes and hypertension may be higher in rural areas due to greater rates of obesity. Finally, for psychiatric illnesses, higher prevalence rates tend to be reported by numerous studies in urban compared to rural areas. However, some believe that psychiatric illness rates may actually be equivalent across geographic areas, and that the difference in regional rates merely reflects the much lower access to psychiatric services in rural areas.

A variety of these rural versus urban differences have been reported in studies that are confined to certain geographic areas of the United States. Some reports have questioned whether the rural–urban disease differences may be attributable largely to differences in education level or socioeconomic differences. Others have suggested that some rural–urban illness rates may be due in part to different reporting probabilities in different locales. Other research suggests that rural people may have some advantages in lifestyle over crowded urban dwellers. Some have suggested that rural populations may be slower to adopt prevention behaviors, suggested in part by the fact that rural areas use preventive health services less frequently. Thus, it may be that intervention strategies to reduce chronic disease may need to be tailored to fit the culture and demands of rural communities. It is clear, however, that sufficient research to examine rural versus urban health differences is lacking, and research to examine such differences as a function of gender is even more sparse.

Certain conditions may be highly stigmatized in small, interdependent communities and often require ongoing medical monitoring and lifestyle changes which can be harder to accomplish due to constraints in rural settings. Health care resources in rural areas and their utilization are limited. For example, more than 95% of the most urbanized counties had psychiatric inpatient services, in contrast to only 13% of rural counties. Although rural areas are home to over one fifth of the population, they contain well less than 1% of the psychiatric beds. Similarly, less than one fifth (17%) of rural general hospitals provide psychiatric emergency services compared to one third (32%) of urban hospitals. Some data suggest that the attitudes and values (e.g., self-reliance, stoicism, shame) of rural women may interfere with their willingness to seek formal, needed health care. Alternatively, care seeking may be sought informally through social networks of rural women. This tendency may change in the coming decades if differences in urban and rural communities diminish, especially if rural women continue to experience the decline in social networks, which have served as a source of support and a buffer to the stresses of rural life.

Special ethical dilemmas can be encountered in rural communities, which are often derived from overlapping relationships wherein caregivers, patients, and families must operate in conflicting roles in smaller communities. Challenges in preserving patient confidentiality are greater in rural areas where people know most if not all members of the community. For example, in rural towns, the doctor, nurse, or clinic staff may attend the same church as the patient, their kids may go to the same school, they may shop at the same store, they may serve in the same community organization, and they may even be related to each other. In one study, physicians reported that more than 5% of their patients interacted with their physician in a nonmedical context, and nearly half reported that over 5% of their patients were friends or family members. Overlapping relationships have the potential to enrich the clinical experience by enmeshing the clinician in the overall activities of the community, but they also have the potential for being exploitative due to problems related to treatment boundaries. Respect for patient privacy is a fundamental element of the doctor–patient relationship, but maintaining confidentiality is especially difficult in small communities often due to this issue of overlapping relations. In fact, rural physicians, especially mental health providers, have been known to create "shadow charts" and use other adaptations in an effort to keep information confidential about a patient.

Despite the considerable stresses of rural life, rural women have strengths and resources, which are often overlooked. Rural women have a history of "hardiness"—of being resilient and self-reliant in meeting their own and their family's needs. Networks of family members, neighbors and friends, healers, and local wise-persons have been diagnosing and treating health problems in rural communities for generations. Rural women have also used self-care and alternative healing practices, at times due to preference and at other times out of necessity. Rural women have thus adapted by being creative in solving health care problems for themselves and their rural families, who represent an important but neglected underserved population in this country.

SEE ALSO: Agricultural work, Alcohol use, Domestic violence, Maternal mortality, Midwifery, Reproductive technologies, Substance use

Suggested Reading

Armitage, K. B., & Sinclair, G. I. (2001). Infectious diseases. In S. Loue & B. E. Quill (Eds.), *Handbook of rural health* (pp. 173–187). New York: Kluwer Academic/Plenum.

Bushy, A. (1998). Health issues of women in rural environments: An overview. *Journal of the American Medical Women's Association, 53*(2), 53–56.

Dennis, L. K., & Pallotta, S. L. (2001). Chronic disease in rural health. In S. Loue & B. E. Quill (Eds.), *Handbook of rural health* (pp. 189–207). New York: Kluwer Academic/Plenum.

Geyman, J. P., Norris, T. E., & Hart, L. G. (2000). *Textbook of rural medicine.* New York: McGraw-Hill.

Hemard, J. B., Monroe, P. A., Atkinson, E. S., & Blalock, L. B. (1998). Rural women's satisfaction and stress as family health care gatekeepers. *Women and Health, 28*(2), 55–77.

Pearson, T. A., & Lewis, C. (1998). Rural epidemiology: Insights from a rural population laboratory. *American Journal of Epidemiology, 148*(10), 949–957.

Roberts, L. W., Battaglia, J., Smithpeter, M., & Epstein, R. S. (1999). An office on Main Street: Health care dilemmas in small communities. *Hastings Center Report, 29*(4), 28–37.

Walker, L. O., Walker, M. L., & Walker, M. E. (1994). Health and well-being of childbearing women in rural and urban contexts. *Journal of Rural Health, 10*(3), 168–172.

Winstead-Fry, P., & Wheeler, E. (2001). Rural women's health. In S. Loue & B. E. Quill (Eds.), *Handbook of rural health* (pp. 135–156). New York: Kluwer Academic/Plenum.

PAMELA MONAGHAN-GEERNAERT
TEDDY WARNER
LAURA WEISS ROBERTS

S

Safer Sex Sexual contact is the most common route of transmission of HIV in women. According to the Centers for Disease Control and Prevention, approximately 50%, or 19.2 million, of the 38.6 million adults living with HIV or AIDS worldwide are women. Furthermore, the majority of women who were reported with AIDS were infected through heterosexual exposure to HIV. Given the importance of sexual transmission in the HIV epidemic, many HIV prevention strategies have focused on identifying and promoting safer sex practices.

Safer sex barriers include male and female condoms and oral barriers such as dental dams. The Surgeon General of the United States and the Centers for Disease Control and Prevention recommend the consistent and proper use of male condoms for personal protection from infection. The clinical and public health importance of consistent condom use was demonstrated in findings from the European Study Group on Heterosexual Transmission of HIV. This study observed that among couples who were serodiscordant for HIV (one partner was HIV negative and the other partner was HIV positive), no seroconversions (becoming HIV positive) were observed among couples who used condoms consistently while among inconsistent condom users, the seroconversion rate was significantly higher, 4.8 per 100 person-years. Thus, consistent condom use can substantially reduce the risk of sexually transmitted HIV infection relative to never or half-time condom use. Although there is substantial evidence that condoms are effective in preventing HIV transmission, the degree of protection afforded by condoms against other sexually transmitted infections (STIs) has not yet been adequately documented. In vitro studies suggest that the latex condom provides excellent protection against a variety of STIs if it does not break or slip off during use. However, condoms are not likely to be effective if they fail during intercourse. Thus, measures of the rates of breakage and slippage are important indicators of condom effectiveness. To reduce the risk of infection associated with vaginal and anal sex, researchers recommend consistent use of latex condoms in conjunction with water-based lubricants only, while fellatio should be performed with nonlubricated latex condoms.

The female condom, made of two flexible polyurethane rings and a loose-fitting polyurethane sheath, has also been approved for contraception and HIV prevention. Research studies have revealed that the female condom has demonstrated efficacy in preventing leakage of HIV in laboratory testing. Other laboratory studies have shown that the female condom serves as an effective barrier to organisms smaller than hepatitis B, the smallest virus known to cause an STI. Another clinical study incorporating women from the United States has demonstrated the female condom to be at least equivalent to the male condom in preventing gonorrhea, trichomoniasis, and chlamydia. Additionally, calculations within this study, based on correct and consistent use, estimate 97.1% reduction in the risk of HIV infection for each act of intercourse.

The most appropriate barriers that can be employed to reduce the risk of transmission of viruses during oral–vaginal sex and oral–anal sex are dental dams. These square sheaths of latex can be placed over the labia and genitalia, or over the anal area, to facilitate safer sex. Currently, Glyde Dams (Glyde USA Inc.) are the only latex dams cleared by the U.S. Food and Drug Administration for protection against STDs for oral–vaginal and oral–anal (rimming) sex. Yet, very little has been documented regarding the efficacy rates of this barrier method.

Precautions can be taken to greatly reduce the risk of contracting HIV and other STIs; however, safer sex practices do not completely eradicate risk. For example, using a condom correctly and every time for vaginal, oral, and anal sex greatly reduces, but does not eliminate, the risk for transmission. The most reliable method that can be employed to avoid sexually contracting HIV is abstinence. While abstinence until establishing a monogamous relationship provides the most certain protection against HIV, it is not a pattern that represents the behavior of most young adults. As a result of this reality, consistent condom use and mastery of safer sex practices is greatly encouraged among individuals who are sexually active outside of monogamous relationships.

SEE ALSO: Acquired immunodeficiency syndrome, Birth control, Condoms, Hepatitis, Lubricants, Reproductive technologies, Sexually transmitted diseases

Suggested Reading

McIlvenna, T. (1999). *The complete guide to safer sex* (2nd ed.). New York: Dembner Books.

Roth, N., & Fuller, L. (Eds.). (1998). *Women and AIDS: Negotiating safer practices, care, and representation.* New York: Harrington Park Press.

Wingood, G. M., & DiClemente, R. J. (2002). *Women's sexual and reproductive health.* New York: Kluwer/Plenum.

CHRISTINA M. CAMP
GINA M. WINGOOD

Sanger, Margaret

Margaret Sanger, America's birth control pioneer, was instrumental in the defeat of "Comstock" laws that made it a crime to distribute information about contraceptive techniques. Sanger and her sister, Ethel Byrne, were both imprisoned several times for violations of Comstock laws. She coined the phrase "birth control" after noticing that in countries with lower birth rates, the percentage of infants who survived increased. Sanger opened the United States' first birth control clinic in 1916. In 1921, she founded the American Birth Control League—the organization now known as Planned Parenthood Federation of America.

Born Margaret Higgins in 1879, Sanger, the sixth of 11 children, grew up in an industrial neighborhood in Corning, New York. Her mother, Anne, suffered from tuberculosis, which was aggravated by 18 pregnancies and 7 miscarriages. The family grew more impoverished with each of the 11 children. Sanger's father, Michael, was a tombstone engraver. He was a well-read, politically outspoken man. He was a socialist and invited one of his heroes, an agnostic, to speak in the neighborhood. The family's poverty increased as a result: the local priest told the parish to "shun him like the devil himself" and to take their business elsewhere.

At 16, Margaret left Corning and began attending Claverack College on a scholarship in 1896. Her older sisters helped finance the school expenses and Margaret waited tables for her room and board. Margaret loved the academic environment at Claverack, but soon had to return to Corning to care for her ailing mother. Anne Higgins died of tuberculosis while Margaret was still a teenager.

After her mother's death, Sanger and her sister looked after their father. When she turned 20, a friend advised her to enter nursing school. In 1900, she entered the three-year nursing program at White Plains Hospital. A doctor introduced Margaret to William Sanger, a draftsman/architect, at a dance. Bill and Margaret were married in 1902. Shortly thereafter, Margaret was diagnosed with tuberculosis. Like her mother, Margaret's disease was aggravated by pregnancy. After giving birth to her son, Stuart, Sanger was so ill that doctors did not believe she would survive. However, Margaret recovered and had a second son, Grant, and a daughter, Peggy.

Bill's mother lived with the couple and cared for the children while Margaret worked as a nurse. Margaret and Bill were active in the Socialist Party, and Margaret was asked to speak at a Socialist meeting. Since she was not familiar with the labor movement, she discussed women's health and hygiene. The audience showed great interest in the topic, and the editor of the Socialist weekly magazine, *The Call*, asked her to write a series of articles. Her articles were entitled "What Every Mother Should Know" and "What Every Girl Should Know." Margaret often accompanied doctors into the crowded slums to deliver children. Time after time, women would ask Margaret how they could keep from having more children. One woman who asked was Sadie Sachs. Sadie was 28 years old and had three children. When she asked her doctor how she could prevent another pregnancy, she was told to have her husband sleep on the roof. When Sadie got pregnant again, she went to an abortionist. Margaret was called to care for her, but Sadie died of complications.

After Sadie's death, Margaret became determined to find out how to teach women to prevent pregnancy. With the 1873 Comstock laws in place, she could not find the information in the United States. When she and Bill moved to France, Sanger discovered that French women had been limiting their families for decades. She spent her days learning the secrets of contraception. Then, she and the children returned to the United States. In 1914, Margaret started a magazine called *The Woman Rebel* "for the advancement of women's freedom." The magazine spoke out in favor of birth control, but did not outline specific contraceptive methods. After Sanger received over 10,000 letters from women asking for the information, she wrote a pamphlet, called *Family Limitation*, which outlined the methods she had learned in France. Before she could distribute the pamphlets, she was indicted for publishing "obscenity" through her magazine. Her husband was also arrested and imprisoned. Although the charges against Sanger were dismissed, she would soon challenge the law again.

Margaret's "birth control movement" had many supporters. She began traveling the country, speaking out in favor of birth control and raising money to open a birth control clinic. Through donations, she raised enough money to open a clinic in Brownsville, Brooklyn. While a growing number of doctors supported birth control, none were willing to be associated with a clinic for fear of reprisals. Margaret and her sister, both nurses, decided to open the clinic anyway and in October 1916, Margaret Sanger and Ethel Byrne opened the first birth control clinic in the United States. Ten days later, she and Ethel were arrested and each received 30 days in jail. As soon as she was released, Margaret resumed her travels and speaking engagements. In 1917, she established a new monthly magazine, the *Birth Control Review*, and in 1921, she started the American Birth Control League as part of a campaign to win mainstream support for birth control.

Margaret would be imprisoned a total of eight times for her activities. But the birth control movement she founded could not be stifled. Support steadily increased, and in 1936, the U.S. Court of Appeals ruled that physicians were exempt from the Comstock law's ban on the importation of birth control materials, thereby giving doctors the right to prescribe or distribute contraceptives. In 1965, the U.S. Supreme Court struck down state statutes that outlawed contraception among married couples in *Griswold v. Connecticut.* Today, the Planned Parenthood Federation of America has 875 health centers in the United States and serves 5 million people a year. Margaret Sanger died at the age of 86 on September 6, 1966.

SEE ALSO: Access to health care; Birth control; Byrne, Ethel; Comstock Laws; Nursing; Pregnancy

Suggested Reading

Gray, M. (1979). *Margaret Sanger, A biography of the champion of birth control.* New York: Richard Marek.
Werner, V. (1970). *Margaret Sanger: Woman rebel.* New York: Hawthorne Books.

Suggested Resources

New York University. (2003). The Margaret Sanger papers project. Retrieved July 9, 2003 from http://www.nyu.edu/projects/sanger
Planned Parenthood Federation of America. (2003). Retrieved March 31, 2003 from http://www.plannedparenthood.org

POLLY HAMPTON

Schizophrenia Schizophrenia is a severe mental illness that affects 1% of the world's population. Contrary to popular opinion, schizophrenia is not a "split personality." Schizophrenia is a chronic disorder in which individuals experience disturbances in thinking and behavior. People with schizophrenia have a higher risk of suicide, and approximately 10% of all people with schizophrenia commit suicide. They also have a higher risk of substance abuse.

Schizophrenia includes psychotic symptoms such as delusions, hallucinations, and thought disorganization. Delusions are beliefs involving a misunderstanding of experiences. The beliefs are held with conviction even when confronted with clear evidence to the contrary. Examples include romantic delusions of jealousy, delusions of being persecuted, or somatic delusions (that something is wrong with their body despite clear evidence that it is not). Delusions may be bizarre; for example, individuals may believe that they receive personal messages from the radio or television, or that their body is under the control of an outside force.

Hallucinations, which are false sensory perceptions, often occur in schizophrenia. Hallucinations may be auditory, visual, tactile, or olfactory. Individuals may hear voices, or see visions, which seem real. These voices may become threatening, or may comment on what they do.

Thinking may become severely disorganized, and individuals may even have problems speaking coherently. Their behavior can also become severely disorganized, including difficulties caring for themselves, showering, or preparing meals, or acting inappropriately in public. Alternatively, individuals with schizophrenia may exhibit "catatonic" behavior, in which they do not react to what is going on around them. For example, patients with catatonic behaviors could appear to be in a stupor, be rigid, resist instruction or movement, or even show excessive purposeless activity.

Associated symptoms that may occur early include social isolation and withdrawal, self-neglect, lack of motivation, and decreased emotional expression. These are known as "negative symptoms," reflecting loss of normal functioning, and can persist even with treatment.

Symptoms should be present for 6 months to merit a diagnosis of schizophrenia. Symptoms cannot be due to substance abuse, but frequently patients with schizophrenia have substance abuse problems as well, perhaps in attempts to deal with their psychotic symptoms. Symptoms in an individual with schizophrenia are variable, and there are several types of schizophrenia. These types include: paranoid type, disorganized type, catatonic type, undifferentiated type, or residual type. Diagnosis of the specific type of schizophrenia is dependent on the category into which the predominant symptoms fall.

Disorders other than schizophrenia may also cause psychotic symptoms. Clinicians need to consider other possibilities when they are diagnosing schizophrenia. Other considerations include a mood disorder with psychotic features (e.g., severe bipolar disorder), delusional disorder (with nonbizarre delusions), schizoaffective disorder (with both significant mood and psychotic symptoms), and schizophreniform or brief psychotic disorder (which have shorter time courses).

Physicians will perform a physical examination and may check various laboratory tests to ensure that psychotic symptoms are not due to a medical problem.

For example, use of steroids can cause psychotic-type symptoms. Minor structural brain abnormalities have been noted in individuals with schizophrenia; however, there is not currently a diagnostic test for schizophrenia. Relatives of people with schizophrenia have an increased risk of developing the disorder themselves.

Schizophrenia is a chronic illness that often interferes with work, family, and school. Currently, there is no cure for schizophrenia, but medications can treat symptoms and decrease the risk of relapse. In the past decade, many better medications have been developed. Antipsychotic medications include haloperidol (Haldol), fluphenazine (Prolixin), risperidone (Risperdal), olanzapine (Zyprexa), quetiapine (Seroquel), ziprasidone (Geodon), and aripiprazole (Abilify). These long-term medications are helpful in treating delusions and hallucinations and may help with social functioning as well. Each medication has its own possible side effects. For example, side effects could include weight gain (with some of the medications), menstrual irregularities, and, in rare instances, a neurologic problem known as tardive dyskinesia (which involves abnormal movements and may develop over the course of many years). Some medications are available as injectables for individuals who have difficulties with adherence. Medications should not be discontinued without discussion with the physician, because of the significant risk of relapse of symptoms of schizophrenia.

Medication management is critical in schizophrenia. Other important treatments include individual psychotherapy, group therapy, and family counseling. Regular follow-up is critical. Individuals with schizophrenia may require hospitalization when their symptoms become dangerous to themselves or others, but in general, they can live at home. Additionally, some individuals with schizophrenia can live in group homes or halfway houses.

ISSUES SPECIFIC TO WOMEN WITH SCHIZOPHRENIA

Men and women have the same lifetime risk of schizophrenia, but in women, schizophrenia develops several years later, often from ages 25 to 35. Women may be diagnosed with schizophrenia through menopause as well. Women with schizophrenia tend to have fewer hospital stays and better social functioning than men with schizophrenia. In women, the focus of therapy may be preservation of roles, such as mother or worker. Sometimes women may delay seeking help because of fear that their children may be removed from their care. However, the sooner that a woman seeks help, the more likely help is to be effective.

Women with schizophrenia should discuss pregnancy with their physicians, and try to plan pregnancy if possible. Risks and benefits of medications during pregnancy to mother and baby should be considered, rather than just discontinuing medications. Different doses of medication may be needed during pregnancy and delivery. Breast-feeding also requires special consideration. Throughout the perinatal period, it is important that psychiatrists are in contact with obstetricians and family doctors so that the patient can get the best care possible.

Postpartum psychosis occurs in approximately 1 out of 1,000 women soon after delivery, and occurs in a significant number of women with schizophrenia. There is a strong risk of recurrence with future pregnancies. Surprisingly, there is more risk of postpartum psychosis in bipolar disorder than in schizophrenia. Physicians and the treatment team may suggest which resources in the community services can be most helpful to mothers with schizophrenia.

The course of schizophrenia in women is believed to be related to their estrogen level, which explains increased symptoms of schizophrenia after delivery and at menopause. Schizophrenia can be a debilitating psychotic illness. Increased knowledge about schizophrenia may lead women with symptoms to see their physicians earlier to begin appropriate treatment, so that their lives may be improved.

SEE ALSO: Bipolar disorder, Mood disorders, Postpartum disorders, Suicide

Suggested Reading

American Psychiatric Association. (1994). *Diagnostic and statistical manual of mental disorders* (4th ed.). Washington, DC: American Psychiatric Association.

Canuso, C. M., Goldstein, J. M., & Green, A. I. (1998). The evaluation of women with schizophrenia. *Psychopharmacology Bulletin, 34*(3), 271–277.

Riecher-Rossler, A., & Hafner, H. (2000). Gender aspects in schizophrenia: Bridging the border between social and biological psychiatry. *Acta Psychiatrica Scandinavia, 102*(Suppl. 407), 58–62.

Seeman, M. V. (2002). The role of sex hormones in psychopathology: Focus on schizophrenia. *Primary Care Clinics in Office Practice, 29*(1), 171–182.

SUSAN HATTERS-FRIEDMAN

Scleroderma

Scleroderma is a group of diseases that involve abnormal growth of connective tissue, which is the "glue" made of proteins and cells that holds the cells of the body together and gives the skin and organs their shape. In some people, scleroderma affects the skin, causing it to become tight and hard. In others, it can affect the blood vessels and internal organs such as the lungs and kidneys. Scleroderma is not contagious and is not considered malignant. It is a common disease, with approximately 40,000–165,000 Americans having the disease. Women suffer from scleroderma three times more often than men.

Scleroderma can be divided into two classes: localized scleroderma and systemic sclerosis. Localized scleroderma is limited to the skin and does not affect internal organs. Localized scleroderma is more common in children. Two common types of localized scleroderma are morphea and linear scleroderma. Morphea usually leads to patches of skin that are thick and firm, and usually fade away in 3–5 years. Linear scleroderma produces a band of thick skin that usually runs down an arm or leg. Localized scleroderma does not develop into the systemic form of the disease.

Systemic scleroderma or systemic sclerosis involves the skin and other organ systems. Typically this develops rapidly with skin thickening over much of the body usually in a symmetrical fashion. Internal organs such as the lungs and kidneys are often involved. People with skin thickening commonly complain of joint pain, fatigue, dryness of the eyes or mouth, swelling of the hands and feet, and weight loss. Patients may also complain of Raynaud's phenomenon, which is a condition in which the small blood vessels of the hands contract when they become cold, which causes the fingertips to turn blue, red, or white. Fortunately, less than one third of patients with systemic scleroderma develop severe internal organ problems.

The cause of scleroderma is unknown. Many believe scleroderma to be an autoimmune disease in which one's own immune system attacks the body. Scleroderma is diagnosed mainly by a medical history and physical exam. The physician may perform lab tests to help to confirm the diagnosis of scleroderma. The lab tests may include looking for two antibodies that are commonly found in the blood of patients with scleroderma (anti-Scl-70 and anticentromere antibodies). These tests may not be positive in all individuals with scleroderma and a skin biopsy may be required to make the diagnosis.

At the present time, there is no treatment that reverses or halts the development of abnormal connective tissue in scleroderma. Treatment of scleroderma consists mainly of relieving symptoms of the disease. Because of the wide variety of symptoms, patients may have many different health professionals involved in their treatment including a dermatologist, a rheumatologist, physical therapists, a nephrologist, and many others.

SEE ALSO: Autoimmune disorders, Raynaud's phenomenon, Skin care, Skin disorders

Suggested Reading

Freedberg, I., Eisen, A., Wolff, K., Austen, K. F., Goldsmith, L., Katz, S., et al. (1999). *Fitzpatrick's dermatology in general medicine* (6th ed.). New York: McGraw-Hill.
Odom, R. B., James, W. D., & Berger, T. G. (Eds.). (2000). *Andrews' diseases of the skin* (9th ed.). Philadelphia: W.B. Saunders.

Suggested Resources

National Institute of Arthritis and Musculoskeletal and Skin Diseases. (2001, July). www.niams.nih.gov

MICHELLE ENDICOTT
PARADI MIRMIRANI

Sclerotherapy

Sclerotherapy Sclerotherapy is a form of treatment for spider veins and varicose veins. Spider veins, or telangiectasias, are small red to blue veins which may appear in up to 50% of women. Varicose veins are larger, blue or purple in color, and may cause pain, throbbing, or burning. The incidence of varicose veins increases as people age. About 41% of women in their 40s have varicose veins, and about 72% of women in their 60s have varicose veins.

Sclerotherapy involves the use of a very fine needle to inject a solution of sclerosing agent directly into the veins to cause damage to the vessel wall. Once the vessel wall is damaged, it will begin to swell and stick together, and the blood in that area will thicken. Over a period of weeks, the damaged vessel and thickened blood are absorbed by the body. Eventually the vein becomes unnoticeable. Repeat treatments may be necessary at 6- to 12-week intervals. There are three kinds of sclerosing agents used: hypertonic (concentrated salt solution), detergent, and chemical irritants. Each class of sclerosing agent destroys the vessel wall in a different way. Selection of a particular sclerosing agent depends on the type and size of vessels being treated. The solution that is injected must make good contact with the vein in order to cause damage. To assist with this process, physicians will encourage the use of support hose or compression bandages for up to two weeks after treatment. Walking is also important because it increases blood flow through the untreated veins. For larger varicose veins, surgical therapy may be required in addition to sclerotherapy.

Sclerotherapy should not be done in someone who is bedridden, since walking following the procedure is necessary. A history of blood clots or previous trauma in the leg should lead to further workup with Doppler ultrasound prior to treatment. A history of suspected allergy to any of the sclerosing agents is a reason to avoid treatment. Treatment of varicose veins during pregnancy should not be done during the first two trimesters and may be considered during the third trimester only if varicose veins are extremely tender or bleeding.

SEE ALSO: Pregnancy

Suggested Reading

Freedberg, I., Eisen, A., Wolff, K., Austen, K., Goldsmith, L., Katz, S., et al. (1998). *Fitzpatrick's dermatology in general medicine* (5th ed., Vol. 2, pp. 2959–2967). New York: McGraw-Hill.
Wheeland, R. G. (1994). *Cutaneous surgery* (pp. 951–979). Philadelphia: W.B. Saunders.

Suggested Resources

www.phlebology.org

MARY G. VEREMIS-LEY
PARADI MIRMIRANI

Seasonal Affective Disorder Seasonal affective disorder (SAD) is a cycling and atypical mood disorder in which the symptoms get worse in winter when there are shortened days with lessened sunlight in temperate climates. It affects women more than men (about 80% are women) and is more common than one might expect with a prevalence of 1–3% of adults. The symptoms include mood changes, increased sleepiness, increased appetite with weight gain, a decreased interest in sex, lethargy and fatigue, all of which begin to increase as the daylight decreases in length. As many as 70% of women who have SAD also have depressive symptoms associated with their menstrual cycle.

Comparing seasonal with nonseasonal depressions, researchers have found less employment and thinking impairment, less hopelessness, and weight loss with SAD. Often anxiety symptoms accompany the depression. Researchers are also beginning to note some differences in biological and psychosocial aspects of SAD such as gender, race, marital status, and employment. Individuals with bipolar I or II disease may also show some seasonality to their illnesses (i.e., worsening of symptoms with less light), although those with major depressive disorders usually do not. Men with SAD have more obsessive/compulsive and suicidal symptoms than women. Those with dark-colored eyes with more pigment may suffer more than those with lighter colored eyes, which allow in more light.

Most of those with SAD will respond to high-intensity light treatments (2,500 lux). This has given support to theories about the cause of seasonality to mood disorders being due to circadian rhythm disturbances, where the rhythms are delayed relative to the sleep/wake and rest/activity cycle. If the circadian rhythm can be phase advanced by light, the individual with SAD may show improvement in the troublesome symptoms. The latter are thought to be involved in the etiology as are theories about melatonin. Melatonin is a hormone that is produced by the pineal gland (in the brain), which may act as a coordinator between light exposure and circadian rhythms, which are related. Melatonin is a hormone which is involved in seasonal reproductive cycles in animals. While the causes are still elusive, treatments do include use of light therapy and aerobic exercise.

SEE ALSO: Bipolar disorder, Depression, Light therapy

Suggested Reading

Sadock, J. B., & Sadock, V. S. (2000). *Comprehensive textbook of psychiatry* (7th ed.). Philadelphia: Lippincott, Williams & Wilkins.

MIRIAM B. ROSENTHAL

Seizures

Epileptic seizures are episodic and sudden attacks that impair some aspect of a person's function. These attacks consist of an alteration of one or more spheres of the brain functions such as sensory perception, motor activity, autonomic control, and level of consciousness. Epileptic seizures are caused by abnormal electrical discharges occurring in the brain. There are a variety of different manifestations of seizures. Although there are specific names given to characterize these various seizures, such as generalized tonic-clonic seizures, complex partial seizures, absence seizures, the manifestation of seizures between individuals can be quite varied, even of seizures in the same category. Within the same individual, however, the seizures are very consistent. Indeed this stereotypic nature of epileptic seizures is one characteristic sought out by physicians to help differentiate epileptic seizures from other paroxysmal events that are not caused by epileptic discharges in the brain.

SEIZURE TYPES

There are some commonly used terms that have been given to various types of seizures. These terms are derived from the International League Against Epilepsy's (ILAE) classification of epileptic seizures. While this is an imperfect classification system and the particulars are clinically insignificant, the terms are widely used and its usage has become generalized. Therefore, we will briefly review some of the more common seizure types in this classification system. Generalized tonic-clonic seizures, previously known as "grand mal seizures," are seizures in which there is a sudden and complete loss of consciousness by the individual, quickly followed by a tensing up of the entire body shortly followed by rhythmic jerking of the extremities. These seizures typically last less than 2 min in duration. These seizures are often associated with a loud groan in the beginning of the seizure called the "epileptic cry" as well as other associated symptoms such as tongue biting and urinary incontinence.

Complex partial seizures are seizures in which there is a loss of awareness that is associated with a blank stare. In contrast to generalized tonic-clonic seizures, the involuntary motor activities during these seizures are less dramatic and often very subtle. These movements may include minor mouth chewing movements, and picking movements of the hands, which are termed "automatisms." During the seizure, the patient is typically unable to respond to questions or interact with persons or their environment usually for a period of 1–2 min. Following these seizures, there is usually a period of confusion that can last seconds to 1–2 hr.

Absence seizures, previously called "petit mal seizures," on the other hand are similar to complex partial seizures in which again there is a loss of awareness with a stare but usually there is a paucity of any other movements expect perhaps some minor eye fluttering. Absence seizures are usually shorter in duration than complex partial seizures and usually are not associated with a period of confusion following the seizure. There are a number of other types of seizures that also occur but are less widely recognized by the general population. (Please refer to the Suggested Reading material at the end of this entry for more information about other seizure types.)

SEIZURE PRECAUTIONS

The most important thing to do if you witness a person having a seizure is to try to minimize the circumstances in which physical injury could result from the seizure. These precautions include clearing the area around the person and rolling the person onto their side if they have fallen, which allows any saliva or vomitus to escape their mouth easily without falling back into their lungs. Do not put your fingers or other objects in a seizing person's mouth as this can result in accidental laceration or amputation of your fingers and damage to the person's dentition or oral cavity. Once the person has stopped seizing, they may often be confused and even agitated. It is useful not to provide too much stimulation to the person in this setting as they may become combative in some circumstances. If a seizure has lasted for longer than 2 min and it does not appear that the person is coming out of the seizure, then it should be considered a medical emergency and a call to 911 should be made. Otherwise, following a typical seizure, the patient's physician may be contacted for further management.

General precautions that the seizure patient can follow include surrendering driving privileges, avoiding tub baths (as seizures even in small pools of water can result in drowning), avoiding sharp moving objects, avoiding hot surfaces, avoid being at heights, swimming only in groups and with individuals who are aware of

the patient's medical history of seizures and can rescue the patient from the water if they have a seizure while swimming. General health precautions that apply not only to seizure patients but to all people include wearing seat belts as a passenger in a car and using helmets while bicycling or skating.

PSEUDOSEIZURE AND OTHER PAROXYSMAL EVENTS

There are many paroxysmal events that individuals can exhibit that may be confused as seizures. During these events, a person has what appears to be a seizure but there is no associated electrical abnormality originating from the brain. These types of events may occur in the setting of other disorders such as migraine headaches, strokes, cardiac disorders, fainting, or pseudoseizures. Pseudoseizures are episodes that may masquerade as seizures but result from a psychiatric disturbance such as a conversion disorder, mood disorder, somatization disorder, or malingering. In these cases, treatment with drugs made to control true seizures (anticonvulsants) is not helpful.

EPILEPSY

Epilepsy is a common disorder affecting approximately 1% of the U.S. population. The diagnosis of epilepsy simply means that the person has a tendency for recurrent seizures. The possibility of having one seizure in a person's lifetime is not unusual. Indeed up to 10% of the U.S. population will have a seizure in their lifetime; however, only 10% of those persons who have had their first seizure will go on to have another seizure. This distinction is important when a physician is considering when to start a medication. In fact, many physicians may not start a seizure medication after a single seizure. The indication to start treating seizures is usually reserved for a person who has had his or her second seizure or history of several seizures in the past. This places them at a higher risk for future seizures. Epilepsy occurs in both women and men in equal percentages. There are some particular issues that affect women who have epilepsy that are unique. These include issues relating to pregnancy, breast-feeding, fertility, birth control, hormonal influences, anticonvulsant effect on female health, and propensity to pass on the disease to their offspring. These are some of the issues that will be discussed in the remainder of this section.

EPILEPSY AND PREGNANCY

There are many unwarranted social stigmas that have been attached to epilepsy. One of the most disturbing is the fallacy that women with epilepsy cannot bear healthy children. Nothing could be further from the truth. Indeed, the vast majority of women with epilepsy who take anticonvulsants bear completely normal children who grow up to be healthy and lead fulfilling lives. Another misconception is the notion that all anticonvulsants should be stopped during pregnancy. The discontinuation of anticonvulsants during pregnancy could lead to increased number of seizures and potential injury to the fetus, which could result in birth defects or miscarriage. Women with epilepsy taking anticonvulsant medications are considered to have high-risk pregnancies but it does not mean that pregnancy itself or anticonvulsants are contraindicated. The high-risk status is to underscore the necessity and importance of frequent, regular doctor visits early in the pregnancy. Ideally each pregnancy should be planned and medical care coordinated with a team of medical specialists, including an obstetrician, a seizure specialist, and a primary care physician. This is to ensure that women with epilepsy's anticonvulsant medications can be optimized and the appropriate prenatal vitamin regimen initiated.

In general, the goal for the medical treatment of epilepsy during pregnancy is to achieve optimal seizure control, defined as no seizures, with the fewest medications, preferably one anticonvulsant, at the lowest dose possible. During pregnancy, anticonvulsant levels are often closely monitored because anticonvulsant levels of both the older anticonvulsants such as phenytoin, carbamazepine, or valproic acid and some of the newer anticonvulsants such as lamotrigine can fall during pregnancy. Among all the established anticonvulsant medications, valproic acid carries the highest risk of fetal malformation, almost a 1–2% risk of neural tube defects. In spite of this, however, valproic acid is considered the drug of choice for particular types of epilepsy, such as Juvenile Myoclonic Epilepsy. Some physicians may suggest that this medication be continued if the highest degree of seizure control for these individuals was seen with valproic acid rather than other medications. In general it appears that the new-generation anticonvulsant

medications carry a lower rate of fetal malformation than the older anticonvulsant medications although the data are still incomplete. The preliminary data from lamotrigine appear to carry no more increased risk than the general population.

Most anticonvulsant medications are minimally secreted in breast milk and should not affect the infant. Therefore, breast-feeding is not generally contraindicated (advised against).

HORMONAL INFLUENCES IN EPILEPSY

Catamenial epilepsy is the cyclic increase in seizure frequency near the time of the menstrual cycle. This pattern was first documented over 100 years ago and is ascribed to normal fluctuation of the female hormones, estrogen and progesterone, during the menstrual cycle. In general, estrogens decrease seizure threshold by inhibiting a neurotransmitter substance in the brain called γ-aminobutyric acid (GABA) and potentiating glutamate, which results in increased excitability. On the other hand, progesterone (a hormone) appears to have the opposite effect. The by-products of progesterone appear to increase GABA's function, which in turn results in increased inhibition and thereby decreasing the propensity for seizures. This "protection" that progesterone may provide is the basis for its use in some people with catamenial epilepsy.

For women with ovulatory cycles, estrogen rises midcycle with ovulation and again during the luteal phase. Progesterone is low throughout the first half of the menstrual cycle, peaks during the luteal phase then rapidly declines, which trigger the menses. Therefore, women may notice increased seizures midcycle during ovulation due to high estrogen levels and perimenstrually due to dropping progesterone levels.

For women with anovulatory cycles, progesterone remains low during the luteal phase so these women may have an irregular pattern of increased seizures throughout the second half of the menstrual cycle due to the unopposed high levels of estrogen.

Furthermore, women taking the antiseizure medication phenytoin may have fluctuations in their medication levels around the time of menstruation (perimenstrual fluctuations) since both phenytoin and the hormone estrogen are metabolized by the same enzyme in the liver (hepatic cytochrome P-450 enzyme system). Increased liver clearance of the anticonvulsant plus the high estrogen levels may precipitate increased seizure activity.

ANOVULATION AND INFERTILITY

Whereas 10% of menstrual cycles are anovulatory (without ovulation) in normal women, up to 35% are anovulatory in women with complex partial seizures. In other studies of women with both complex partial seizures and generalized tonic-clonic seizures, some of the women had endocrine dysfunction consistent with primary ovarian failure (gonadal insufficiency), ovarian failure secondary to other medical causes (hypogonadotropic hypogonadism), or disorders of the ovaries (polycystic ovarian syndrome). While most of these endocrine disorders appear to be a product of seizure-induced hormonal changes, anticonvulsants can also affect hormonal function. For example, valproate has been associated with polycystic ovaries and abnormalities in hormone levels (hyperandrogenism).

Fertility rates for women with epilepsy are reduced by 15% in comparison to the general population. Women whose first seizure was before the age of 10 years are more likely to never have children. The reasons for these observations are not entirely clear but are certainly multifactorial. Major depression may be more common in epileptics and tends to be associated with infertility. One study reported that 33% of women with epilepsy in an outpatient clinic had sexual dysfunction including dyspareunia, vaginismus, and arousal insufficiency.

HORMONAL CONTRACEPTIVES

Despite estrogens being thought of as proconvulsant, hormonal contraceptives have not been reported to increase seizure frequency. However, there is a higher rate of hormonal contraceptive failure in women taking hepatic enzyme-inducing anticonvulsant drugs. Women taking such medication, which includes barbiturates, phenytoin, and carbamazapine, need oral contraceptives with higher levels of the hormone estradiol (at least 50 μg of estradiol rather than the typical 20–35 μg). Contraception failure has also been reported with fixed subdermal levonorgestrel implants (Norplant) due to the increased hepatic metabolism of the medication. Medroxyprogesterone acetate (Depo-Provera) may be a better long-acting option but the injections should be given every 10 weeks, instead of every 12 weeks.

SEE ALSO: Breast-feeding, Headache, Migraine, Mood disorders, Oral contraception, Pregnancy

Suggested Reading

Liporace, J., & D'Abreau, A. (2003). Epilepsy and women's health: Family planning, bone health, menopause, and menstrual-related seizures. *Mayo Clinic Proceedings, 78*, 497–506.

Lüders, H., & Lesser, R. P. (1987). *Clinical medicine and the nervous system: Epilepsy, electroclinical syndromes.* London: Springer-Verlag.

Morrel, M. J. (1997). Sexuality in epilepsy. In J. Engle & T. A. Pedley (Eds.), *Epilepsy* (pp. 2021–2026). Philadelphia: Lippincott-Raven.

Rush, A., & Plum, F. (1998). Neurologic health and disorders. In L. A. Wallis et al. (Eds.), *Textbook of women's health* (pp. 573–575). Philadelphia: Lippincott-Raven.

Woolley, C. S., & Schwartzkroin, P. A. (1998). Hormonal effects on the brain. *Epilepsia, 39*(Suppl. 8), S2–S8.

Wyllie, E. (1993). *The treatment of epilepsy: Principles and practice.* Philadelphia: Lea & Febiger.

Yerby, M. S. (2000). Quality of life, epilepsy advances, and the evolving role of anticonvulsants in women with epilepsy. *Neurology, 55*(Suppl. 1), S21–S31.

ANITA B. VARKEY
DILEEP R. NAIR

Self-Injurious Behavior Although mental health professionals have yet to establish a universally accepted definition of self-injurious behavior (SIB), the term generally encompasses any intentional, nonsuicidal act upon one's own body that results in organ or tissue damage. Notably, acts embodied in cultural practices or rituals that are shared by many members of a given society and may have symbolic significance (e.g., ear piercing in our own culture, the Sun Dance of the Plains Indians) are commonly excluded from this definition. Specific behaviors covered by the umbrella term of SIB vary greatly with respect to severity, with those associated with the least damage (e.g., hair pulling, self-hitting, and skin picking) and those associated with the most damage (e.g., castration, eye gouging, and limb amputation) lying on opposite ends of a continuum. To add to the complexity of the phenomenon, SIB crosses the boundaries of diagnostic categories and similar behaviors may be exhibited by individuals with different psychiatric conditions, such as developmental disabilities, eating disorders, personality disorders, and schizophrenia. Given the heterogeneous nature of SIB, it is useful to classify the behavior into categories. The most widely used system for classifying SIB identifies four major categories: stereotypic, major, compulsive, and impulsive.

Stereotypic SIB is behavior that is fixed, highly repetitive, monotonous, and often rhythmic. It occurs in individuals with mental retardation, autism, and various congenital disorders. It can sometimes result in severe injury and usually includes head banging, self-hitting, skin picking, self-biting, and hair pulling. In individuals with mental retardation, prevalence estimates of SIB range from 3% to 46%. Interestingly, within the female members of this population, rates of SIB appear to fluctuate with the menstrual cycle. Some medications may be helpful in the treatment of stereotypic SIB. However, behavioral interventions utilizing applied behavior analysis have shown the most promise in eliminating these behaviors.

Major SIB includes isolated incidents of severe or life-threatening SIB such as castration, eye gouging, and limb amputation. Frequently, these behaviors have symbolic meaning to the individual. Major SIB is most commonly associated with psychosis due to schizophrenia or a severe mood disorder. Genital mutilation is the most common form of major SIB and appears to be 10 times more common in men than in women. The recommended treatment for major SIB is antipsychotic medication.

Compulsive SIB is classified as compulsive, repetitive, and high-frequency behaviors of mild to moderate severity, such as hair pulling (trichotillomania), skin picking, and nail biting. Individuals with compulsive SIB usually experience the urge to engage in SIB as difficult to resist, as the behavior results in a decrease in tension or anxiety. Some experts have hypothesized that compulsive SIB is related to obsessive–compulsive disorder. While compulsive nail biting is most common in the general population, it is usually benign and decreases in frequency over the life span. Trichotillomania is the most studied of these behaviors, and can cause marked distress. Women and girls more frequently present for treatment of trichotillomania than do boys and men. However, this finding may be confounded by women's greater likelihood of seeking mental health services in general. Effective treatments of compulsive SIB are behavioral treatments including self-monitoring, response prevention, and contingency management strategies (e.g., rewarding the absence of the behavior). Medications are also sometimes used in addition to behavior therapy.

Impulsive SIB includes behavior such as skin cutting, skin burning, and self-hitting. This behavior generally functions to temporarily relieve distress that is perceived as intolerable. Impulsive SIB is commonly associated with borderline personality disorder, with estimates that 70–75% of these individuals have engaged in at least one act of SIB. It is also seen in individuals with antisocial personality disorder, eating disorders, dissociative disorders, and posttraumatic stress disorder. It is associated with having had traumatic experiences, particularly childhood sexual abuse experiences. Available data suggest that women are more likely than men to engage in impulsive SIB. Treatment of impulsive SIB frequently focuses on helping individuals replace the SIB with more adaptive strategies for tolerating and expressing painful emotions. Dialectical behavior therapy for borderline personality disorder is an effective treatment approach for SIB as it occurs in that population. This treatment emphasizes behavioral analysis of the SIB and intensive skills training in alternative behaviors. Little data are available on pharmacological treatments for impulsive SIB, but certain antidepressant medications may be helpful in alleviating painful emotional states and reducing impulsive SIB.

SEE ALSO: Mental illness, Personality disorders, Schizophrenia, Trichotillomania

Suggested Reading

Conterio, K., & Lader, W. (1998). *Bodily harm: The breakthrough healing program for self-injurers.* New York: Hyperion.

Linehan, M. M. (1993). *Cognitive-behavioral treatment of borderline personality disorder.* New York: Guilford Press.

Simeon, D., & Hollander, E. (Eds.). (2001). *Self-injurious behaviors: Assessment and treatment.* Washington, DC: American Psychiatric Press.

Spradlin, S. E. (2003). *Don't let your emotions run your life: How dialectical behavior therapy can put you in control.* New York: New Harbinger.

AMY S. HOUSE
JENNIFER CERCONE-KEENEY

Sexual Abuse One out of four women will be sexually assaulted in her lifetime. Since the 1970s, the general public has been exposed to information and education regarding the prevalence of sexual violence against women and children, the lasting effects of sexual trauma, and the development of rape crisis programs. In the 1980s, the United States saw the emergence of the "Self Help" and "Recovery" movement, and the shift in perspective from "victim" to "survivor." More recent issues regarding sexual assault since the 1990s include the short- and long-term effects of sexual trauma on the survivor, the impact of sexual assault on the friends and family members of the survivor, the "date rape drugs," the delayed/false memory debate, and the impact of and changes in public policy.

Sexual abuse can be defined as any activity where an individual is used to meet the physical or emotional sexual needs of another person, with disregard to the needs of the victim. Children and adult women of all ages have the potential to be sexually abused or assaulted. Examples of covert sexual abuse, or using an individual to satisfy emotional sexual needs of another, include voyeurism, exhibitionism, witnessing someone else's sexual violation, exposure to pornography, romanticized relationship with parent or adult, exposure to inappropriate nudity, or exposure to masturbation. Overt sexual abuse involves being forced to meet the physical needs of another person. Examples include being touched or massaged in a sexual manner, sexualized back rubs or hand holding, genital or breast fondling or rubbing, oral sex, anal sex, intercourse, mutual masturbation or being used for masturbation, penetration with finger or objects, sexual torture, and rape. Other experiences that include violations of physical and emotional sexual boundaries can also have negative affects. These include a lack of accurate information about puberty or sexuality, lack of right to privacy, too much information too early in a child's development, sexualization by exposure to inappropriate adult sexual behavior, enmeshment in a parent's adult sexual relationships or problems, living with parents who either repress or overdo affection and sexuality or parents who are involved in affairs, uncomfortable hugs that last too long, wet or lingering kisses, or seductive dancing.

Sexual abuse of children includes sexual stimulation or contact that is inappropriate for the age and emotional development of the child. Statistics indicate that between 100,000 and 500,000 children are sexually abused each year. It is estimated that 500,000–1,000,000 children in this country are involved in prostitution and pornography. Most children are sexually abused by someone they know; family members, family friends, neighbors, or other adults involved in their lives.

The impact of sexual abuse goes beyond physical injury and often results in significant emotional difficulties.

Research has shown that children who have been sexually abused often show behavior problems such as opposition to authority, aggression, school problems, and poor social skills. These children also may show symptoms such as depressed mood, anxiety, fear, sleep problems, and physical complaints. They often have low self-esteem, poor social skills, and mistrust others. Some children develop posttraumatic stress disorder (PTSD), which is characterized by a traumatizing event (in this case, sexual abuse), intrusive reexperiencing of the event (such as flashbacks, intrusive thoughts, nightmares), persistent avoidance of stimuli that are associated with the event, and physiological reactivity (paying close attention to cues and emotions, increased levels of adrenaline, increased startle response).

Adult survivors of childhood sexual abuse often experience effects lasting into adulthood that are difficult to overcome without treatment. This may include PTSD symptoms, as well as other body, sexual, mood, anxiety, and self-perception issues. These women may have difficulty with eating disorders, drug and alcohol abuse, self-mutilation, self-destructiveness, failure to be aware of body signals, or poor body image. They may have sexual problems such as believing that sex is dirty, aversion to being touched, difficulty integrating sex and emotions, feeling betrayed by their bodies, "promiscuous" sexual experiences, or avoidance of sex. They may also experience depression, fear of being alone or in the dark, feeling crazy, anger or intense hostility toward the gender of the perpetrator, or limited tolerance for happiness. Self-destructiveness, perfectionism, poor body image, and low self-esteem are common. Relationship problems are also common, including trust issues, pattern of being a victim, power and control issues, and choosing ambivalent relationships.

In our culture, adult women continue to struggle with power and authority in relation to men. Rape is sex without consent and represents the total surrender of power, control, and autonomy over one's body. There are different types of rape including stranger rape, date rape, acquaintance rape, marital rape, gang rape, ritualistic abuse, office rape, and many women are also subjected to sexual harassment.

Women who are sexually abused or assaulted as adults have similar reactions to those of children who are sexually abused, and adults who were sexually abused as children. It is estimated that 4 million women in the United States have suffered from long-term psychological distress related to being raped, often including a diagnosis of PTSD. Due to cognitive maturity that most children have not yet developed, adult women who have been raped may feel that they were partially responsible for the assault. Many women are told, or believe themselves, that if they dressed or behaved in a particular manner, or made certain decisions, they hold some of the blame for the attack. One important part of treatment involves the survivor acknowledging that the assault was in no way her fault.

Treatment in the form of individual and group therapy, recovery groups, and psychoeducational tools can be successful. Treatment for sexual abuse generally include goals such as committing to treatment and forming a therapeutic alliance, acknowledging and accepting the abuse, recounting or "telling the story" of the abuse, breaking down and then expressing feelings, resolving responsibility and survival issues, grieving, restructuring cognitive distortions, self-determination, education and skill building, and forgiveness (of self and possibly the perpetrator).

Not only must sexual abuse survivors cope with the emotional and physical trauma of the events that occurred, they also often must face the police reports, medical assessment and treatment, and the legal system. Although more than 100,000 women report being raped in this country, approximately 60–90% of women who are raped do not report the assault. In part because of unreported rapes, less than 10% of rapists go to jail. There are various reasons why a woman would not report a rape, such as fear due to the rapist's threats, fear of blame or insensitivity from the police, wanting to forget that it happened, not wanting others to find out, and planning not to go to court. Reporting the rape right away is important because the police can provide for the survivor's safety needs, direct her to the appropriate community resources, take her for treatment and for a physical examination that will include collection of evidence. Reporting is also important for the safety of other women; many rapists are serial rapists and will act again.

Obtaining medical attention after sexual assault is important to avoid potential problems, even if the rape occurred weeks prior. A pregnancy test and tests for and treatment of sexually transmitted diseases (STDs) are generally part of the medical examination and treatment process. It is also important for the survivor to consult counseling and psychological support after an assault as well as treatment for any physical injuries. An evidentiary exam includes collecting evidence to show that recent sexual intercourse occurred, documenting signs of force or coercion, and to identify the perpetrator.

Prosecuting and convicting a rapist is generally a long process that is extremely difficult, and often frustrating, for the survivor. Many prosecuting attorneys screen rape cases before making an arrest, making a decision regarding how "good" a case is and the likelihood of a conviction. Survivor attributes, offender attributes, circumstances of the assault, rape laws, and the police investigation all affect the legal case.

Public policy (and the media's coverage) related to sexual assault and abuse reflects changes in our society during the last 30 years and although these changes are positive, there is a long way to go. For example, the pornography industry continues to grow, particularly with the widespread use of the Internet. The male fantasies played out in pornography often portray a woman as a submissive, compliant sexual object. They often depict forms of sexuality that are aggressive and sometimes represent torture. Many forms of pornography act out sexual assaults and rapes, with the women smiling and accepting the man's domination and control. Another example includes recent changes in laws concerning marital rape. Until the late 1970s, wives were widely considered property of their husbands. This perspective led to the belief that forced sex between a husband and wife was not considered rape and therefore also not considered a crime. Most of the states in our country have changed laws regarding marital rape, though there are some states that still exclude marital rape from their laws.

The media has brought the prevalence of "date rape drugs" to the awareness of the general public. The drug Rohypnol is a medication that is prescribed in countries other than the United States for treating insomnia or to be used as a sedative. Although this drug is illegally and recreationally used in this country, it has been associated with date rape as it can induce blackouts, memory loss, and decrease in resistance. Many women have involuntarily and unknowingly ingested this drug, sometimes slipped into a drink by an unknown attacker. Gamma-hydroxybutyrate (GHB) has been abused for its sedative effects as well when used by an offender.

In the past 10 years, the repressed memory/false memory of sexual abuse debate has been discussed at length with varying opinions. The debate centers on the question of existence of an individual repressing (the mind subconsciously "chooses to forget") childhood sexual experiences that are later uncovered as an adult. There are many reports of uncovered memories that individuals believe are true and accurate. Because these individuals had no conscious memory of the abuse until many years later, others speculate that these are in fact false memories that have no basis in truth. Some believe that the false memories were suggested by therapists and psychologists, and accepted by individuals while in treatment for other problems. The False Memory Syndrome Foundation was founded by the parents of a cognitive psychologist who believed that she uncovered repressed memories of childhood sexual abuse by her father. Some parents accused of childhood sexual abuse have (often successfully) sued the therapists of individuals who claim to have uncovered repressed memories of abuse.

The prevention of childhood sexual abuse and the sexual assault of adult women consistently remains a significant priority. It is imperative that parents teach their children body safety (appropriate boundaries regarding private body parts and what to do when another child or adult attempts to violate those boundaries) and dispel myths related to sexual abuse (occurs across all socioeconomic levels and racial lines, children can be offenders, etc.). Parents need to be emotionally and physically available to their children, protect and guide them, keep open communication, and not be afraid to ask direct questions. Parents with a history of sexual abuse should do their own personal work on remaining related issues.

Adult women can also take steps to protect themselves from rape and other sexual assault. Active measures such as making smart choices, carrying protection (i.e., Mace), looking confident when walking alone, locking car doors when driving alone, being familiar with your surroundings, and taking a self-defense course are all positive ways to protect oneself from sexual assault.

See Also: Domestic violence, Incest, Posttraumatic stress disorder, Psychotherapy, Rape, Sexual harassment, Sexually transmitted diseases, Stalking

Suggested Reading

Bass, E., & Davis, L. (1988). *The courage to heal.* New York: Harper & Row.

Ledray, L. E. (1994). *Recovering from rape.* New York: Henry Holt.

Lees, A. B. (1998 workshop Raleigh, NC). *Sexual abuse: Helping adult and child survivors.* Tucson, AZ: Carondelet Management Institute.

Suggested Resources

Incest Survivors Anonymous
P.O. Box 5613
Long Beach, CA 90805
562-428-5599

The National Women's Health Information Center. (2000). Retrieved December 1, 2000, from www.4woman.gov/faq/rohypnol.htm

The National Resource Center on Child Sexual Abuse (NRCCSA)
2204 Whitesburg Dr., Suite 200
Huntsville, AL 35801
1-800-543-7006

USA Rape Hotlines by state: www.nemasys.com/ghostwolf/Resources/Hotlines/USA-rape/index.shtml (updated 3/8/03)

Tira B. Stebbins

Sexual Dysfunction

SEXUAL FUNCTION

The study of sexual function in women, while still in its infancy, has evolved beyond early conceptualizations that focused on mystery and possible associations with witchcraft to psychological explanations that developed in the 19th and 20th centuries. The psychiatric evolution came to fruition in the 20th century with Freudian theories where treatment centered on psychoanalysis. Scientific investigations into sexual function were carried out by Masters and Johnson in the 1960s and furthered by research by Kaplan into psychotherapy and behavioral exercises. In the 20th century, the ability to treat men with erectile dysfunction has increased interest in women's sexual function, particularly in postmenopausal women. This has led to alternative theories of sexual function other than the traditional model as well as a reclassification of female sexual dysfunction.

The traditional model of sexual function for men and women, as proposed by Masters and Johnson, is linear and includes four phases: desire, arousal, climax, and resolution. Newer models describe a more circular relationship between satisfaction and intimacy (Figure 1). Norms for sexual function are difficult to characterize, as dysfunction should imply individual distress, not something that causes distress only in the partner. Although prevalence and incidence data are scarce for rates of sexual activity, the data available support the conclusion that women are sexually active throughout their life span. Data from the National Survey of Family Growth indicate that approximately 40% of women 15–19 years of age have had sexual intercourse within the last 3 months. Although rates of sexual activity decline with age, population-based

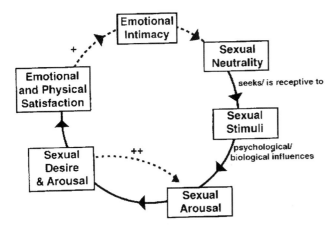

Figure 1. The interrelatedness of intimacy, sexual arousal, desire, and satisfaction.

Source: Copyright 2001 from "Complexities of woman's sexual function" by R. Basson Reproduced by permission of Taylor & Francis, Inc., http://www.routledge-ny.com

studies indicate continued sexual activity in 47% of married women aged 66–71 and a third of women over 78.

Norms of sexual activity are not well characterized for women. Although heterosexual practices are commonly reported among American women, up to 1.2% of women report having sex exclusively with women. Reported frequencies of sexual activity vary with one survey of women reporting sexual activity an average of six times per month. Even though vaginal intercourse is the most commonly reported sexual practice among American women, many women report inability to achieve orgasm with vaginal intercourse, and require direct clitoral stimulation. Additionally, unlike men, desire in women does not always precede arousal. Some women participate in intimacy out of affection for a partner, become aroused, and then experience desire. This response pattern underlines the importance to most women of the relationship that they are in as well as the interdependent nature of the sexual response cycle.

The physical manifestations of the normal female sexual response cycle are described in the four classical phases: excitement, plateau, orgasm, and resolution. The physical effects are all the result of changes in blood flow patterns (engorgement) and increased muscle tension. During the excitement phase, muscle fibers contract in the nipples and increased blood flow causes swelling of the breasts, clitoris, and results in increased vaginal lubrication. The plateau phase is relatively short and involves further engorgement of the breasts and

tissue around the vagina as well as vasodilatation of the skin, which may appear as a temporary flush. Further muscle tension around the vagina creates an anatomic basin at the base of the cervix that helps retain any seminal fluid and the uterus begins rhythmic involuntary contractions. During the orgasmic phase, the uterine contractions continue and there may be involuntary contractions of the lower vagina before the release of the previously building muscle tension and blood engorgement. Resolution is quite variable in length and results in the return of muscle tension and blood flow to the unstimulated state.

FEMALE SEXUAL DYSFUNCTION

Prevalence of sexual dysfunction is difficult to characterize, but from the few studies available appears to be common, with American women reporting rates ranging from 25% to 63%. Common sexual complaints include low sexual desire (22% prevalence), arousal disorders (14% prevalence), and sexual pain disorders (7% prevalence).

In 1998, an international multidisciplinary group met to define areas of sexual dysfunction. To be called a sexual dysfunction or disorder, currently, the symptoms must be recurring (persistent), of significance (pervasive), and cause distress to the woman in question. Symptoms that bother the woman's partner but not the woman herself are not defined as *her* sexual dysfunction. Likewise, if a woman has no interest in sex and it is not distressing to her to have no interest, it is not classified as a sexual dysfunction.

Sexual dysfunctions are further described as being primary (the problem has always been there) or secondary (there was no sexual problem initially but now there is), situational (it only occurs in predictable circumstances) or generalized (the problem occurs in all variations of a situation). Dysfunctions can be psychogenic, having an emotional cause, organic, having a physical cause, or result from a mixture of the two. The current classification system (Figure 2) includes four general areas: (a) sexual desire disorders, (b) sexual arousal disorders, (c) orgasmic disorders, and (d) sexual pain disorders.

Although the types of sexual dysfunction are defined in order to differentiate one from the other, in actuality, women often have symptoms that fall into more than one dysfunction category. The causes of dysfunction are often a combination of physical, emotional,

Sexual Dysfunction

Sexual Desire Disorders	
Hypoactive sexual desire disorder	Deficiency of sexual thought/ fantasies and/or desire for or receptivity to sexual activity
Sexual aversion disorder	Phobic aversion to and avoidance of sexual contact with a sexual partner
Sexual Arousal Disorder	Inability to attain or maintain sufficient sexual excitement, which may be expressed as a lack of subjective excitement, or genital or other somatic responses
Orgasmic Disorder	Difficulty, delay in, or absence of attaining orgasm following sufficient sexual stimulation and arousal
Sexual Pain Disorders	
Dyspareunia	Genital pain associated with sexual intercourse
Vaginismus	Involuntary spasm of the musculature of the outer third of the vagina that interferes with vaginal penetration
Noncoital sexual pain disorder	Genital pain induced by noncoital sexual stimulation

Figure 2. Classification of female sexual dysfunction.

and interpersonal issues, which results in multifactorial etiologies for many of the dysfunctions.

Sexual Desire Disorders

These are further divided into two subcategories, hypoactive sexual desire disorders and sexual aversion disorders. A *hypoactive sexual desire disorder* is defined as a lack of desire for sexual activity, and/or a deficiency or absence of sexual thoughts and fantasies. This manifests by the absence of sexual thoughts, fantasies, or interest in sexual activity. Debilitating physical or emotional conditions and medical treatments or medications may cause hypoactive sexual desire disorder.

A *sexual aversion disorder* refers to fear and avoidance of sexual thoughts and situations. In aversion disorder there may be fear and phobic avoidance in response to any sexually suggestive situation. Aversion disorders may result from traumatic life events such as sexual assault or serious anxiety illnesses such as obsessive–compulsive disorders or phobias.

Example A 32-year-old woman developed a major depression. She tells her physician that the most distressing depression symptom is her utter lack of sexual desire. Molested as a child, she overcame an active fear of sexual intimacy in the context of her supportive relationship. Recovery from her initial sexual aversion makes this recent loss of sexual desire secondary to depression doubly distressing.

Sexual Arousal Disorders

These are defined as the persistent or recurrent inability to attain or maintain sexual excitement. Arousal disorders may be reported as an emotional lessening of excitement or sensation, and can be evident in the physical manifestations of lack of excitement, vaginal lubrication, decreased nipple sensitivity, and decreased clitoral engorgement and swelling. Decreased arousal can be caused by injury or illness that affects pelvic innervation and blood flow and by emotional illnesses that impair interest and enjoyment.

586

Example A 42-year-old woman recently started a new medication for her chronic medical illness. Since starting the medication, she reports that her genitals feel numb. She wants to have sex, but it is as if the physical responses have been disconnected from her desire. Stopping the medication is likely to reverse these sexual arousal disorder symptoms.

Orgasmic Disorder

This is defined as the difficulty or inability to reach orgasm after sufficient sexual stimulation and arousal. The dysfunction may be primary, never having the ability to achieve orgasm, or secondary, having lost the ability to achieve orgasm. Orgasmic disorders may be evident as a diminished intensity of orgasm, or the inability to achieve orgasm. Emotional or physical abuse can cause inability to achieve orgasm, but it can also be caused by medical illnesses or surgery that damages the nerves or blood flow to the pelvis.

Example A 55-year-old woman complains of difficulty achieving orgasm since undergoing total abdominal hysterectomy with bilateral salpingo-oophorectomy for leiomyomata. Her cause of anorgasmia is multifactorial including abrupt disruption of pelvic blood flow, coupled with castration. Both contributed to her inability to achieve orgasm.

Sexual Pain Disorders

Sexual pain disorders are further divided into three subcategories: dyspareunia, vaginismus, and noncoital sexual pain disorders. *Dyspareunia* refers to genital pain that occurs with sexual intercourse. Dyspareunia commonly manifests as pain with penile penetration or deep thrusting.

Vaginismus is the involuntary spasm of the lower third of the vagina making sexual intercourse impossible. These women are incapable of vaginal intercourse, pelvic exams, or wearing tampons.

Noncoital sexual pain disorders refer to pain that occurs with any type of sexual stimulation other than intercourse. Noncoital sexual pain disorders include genital pain that is initiated by sexual stimulation that does not involve intercourse. Pain disorders are usually multifactorial in etiology. Causes include atrophic vaginitis, or thinning of the vaginal wall that occurs during menopause, vaginal infections or inflammatory processes, or emotional or relationship problems.

Example A 65-year-old woman presents with pain with vaginal intercourse since discontinuing hormone replacement therapy. The cessation of hormonal therapy caused vaginal atrophy that in turn caused dyspareunia.

TREATMENT

Just as the causes of dysfunction are often a combination of physical, emotional, and interpersonal issues, treatments are also multifactorial. For this reason, treatments for all the sexual dysfunctions are discussed in general.

Treatment recommendations are best tailored to an individual after a careful diagnostic evaluation. The evaluation begins by taking a history to determine if sexual symptoms are new or longstanding, and if they developed acutely, perhaps in relation to a surgery or starting a medication, or if the onset was insidious over time. A careful health maintenance history, including tobacco, alcohol, and drug use, as well as recreation practices like bicycling, which has been associated with increased risk of sexual dysfunction, is also gathered. A thorough health, surgical, and medication history is in order.

Once the diagnostic possibilities have been gathered and sorted, several treatment approaches are often indicated. The first treatment intervention is often to provide accurate information and education. Medications causing sexual side effects are common and if an equivalent medication that does not cause sexual side effects is available, the solution may be simple. Sometimes sexual activity can be scheduled right before or after taking the offending medication so that sex occurs when the least medication is in the bloodstream. Some medications and devices can be prescribed and used to specifically increase sexual responsiveness. Use of vibrators to increase clitoral stimulation, as well as medications or devices that can increase genital blood flow can also be helpful. Hormonal therapy, including estrogen to increase vaginal lubrication and blood flow, as well as testosterone, which increases desire, can also be used in women to address sexual dysfunction disorders.

Psychotherapy of various types and medication for emotional disorders such as anxiety and depression are frequently recommended. Central to treatment of sexual dysfunction is the need to address partner-related issues, as often the dysfunction is shared between a couple and is causing both distress.

Sexual Harassment

In conclusion, interest in the diagnosis and treatment of female sexual dysfunction has increased in importance to care providers and their patients. As research in this area expands, newer therapies and treatments will become available for women who suffer from these disorders.

SEE ALSO: Dyspareunia

Suggested Reading

Anonymous. (1995). ACOG technical bulletin. Sexual dysfunction. Number 211—September 1995. American College of Obstetricians and Gynecologists [Educational Review]. *International Journal of Gynecology and Obstetrics, 51*, 265–277.

Basson, R. (2001). Are the complexities of women's sexual function reflected in the new consensus definitions of dysfunction? *Journal of Sex and Marital Therapy, 27*, 105–112.

Basson, R., Berman, J., Burnett, A., Derogatis, L., Ferguson, D., et al. (2001). Report of the international consensus development conference on female sexual dysfunction: Definitions and classifications. *Journal of Sex and Marital Therapy, 27*, 83–94.

Kaplan, H. S. (1979). *Disorders of sexual desire.* New York: Brunner/Mazel.

Laumann, E. O., Paik, A., & Rosen, R. C. (1999). Sexual dysfunction in the United States. *Journal of the American Medical Association, 281*, 537–544.

Masters, W. H., & Johnson, V. E. (1966). *Human sexual response.* Boston: Little, Brown.

REBECCA G. ROGERS
TERESITA MCCARTY

Sexual Harassment

The 20th century has seen a drastic increase in the number of women in the workforce. This influx of women into the workforce helps explain an increase of sexual harassment in the workplace. In 2002, there were 14,396 charges of sexual harassment filed with the appropriate state and federal authorities. This is a 37% increase in the amount of complaints filed 10 years ago.

Congress took a major step toward ending sexual harassment in the workplace when it passed the Title VII to the Civil Rights Act of 1964. Under Title VII, it is illegal for an employer to discriminate, on the basis of sex, with respect to compensation, terms, conditions, or privileges of employment. Every state also has promulgated laws prohibiting employers from discriminating on the basis of sex.

There are two basic forms of workplace sexual harassment. The first is known as either quid pro quo or tangible job action harassment. This form of harassment occurs when an employer makes an employment decision based on the employee's refusal to submit to sexual demands. Such employment decisions include, but are not limited to, denial of a promotion, a demotion, denial of a raise, and dismissal. An employer can be held liable for a tangible job action executed by a supervisor who retains authority over the employee.

The second form of sexual harassment involves the creation of a hostile work environment. Hostile work environment harassment occurs when a workplace is permeated with such severe and pervasive discriminatory intimidation, ridicule, and insult that the conditions of the employee's working conditions are altered so as to create an abusive working environment. Conduct that has been found to create a hostile work environment includes: sexual teasing, sexual looks or gestures, deliberate touching, pressure for dates or sexual favors, letters, telephone calls, and exposure to materials of a sexual nature. However, for the conduct to be deemed "harassing" in a legal context, the conduct must have been of such a nature that both the employee and a reasonable person would find it unwelcome. Further, the law requires the conduct be so severe and pervasive as to alter the terms, conditions, or privileges of employment. Whether the harassing conduct is severe and pervasive is determined by looking at the severity of the conduct, the frequency of the encounters, the length of time over which the conduct occurs, the context in which the conduct occurs, the interference with the employee's work performance, and whether the conduct is physically threatening or humiliating.

The law draws a distinction between when a hostile work environment is created by a co-worker rather than a supervisor. When the harassment involves a co-worker, the law requires that the employer knew, or should have known, of the harassment and failed to take corrective action. However, when a supervisor creates the hostile work environment, the law only requires proof that the behavior that occurred was unwelcome, severe, and pervasive. The employer, however, can avoid liability for the supervisor's creation of a hostile work environment if it can show it exercised reasonable care to prevent, and correct promptly, any sexually harassing behavior, and the employee unreasonably failed to take advantage of the preventive or corrective measures.

Sexual harassment can have various effects on those employees subjected to it. Employees who have been exposed to sexual harassment frequently develop, and suffer from, a lack of self-esteem, irritability, headaches, sleep deprivation, nightmares, gastrointestinal disturbances, isolation, loss of appetite, anger, frustration, guilt, and fear. Those who have been sexually harassed may feel helpless, depressed, fluctuate their weight, or increase their alcohol consumption. The employee's work performance is often affected by increased absenteeism, poor work performance evaluations, and deficient work performance. Employees who have been forced to endure sexual harassment commonly suffer from diagnoses including: adjustment disorder, major depression, posttraumatic stress syndrome, somatoform disorders, generalized anxiety disorder, and panic anxiety disorder.

Employees who believe they are being sexually harassed have various options available to them. The employee could file a charge with the Equal Employment Opportunity Commission (EEOC). How the EEOC will proceed with the charge depends on whether the state involved is considered a deferral state or a nondeferral state. If the state is a deferral state, the charge must first be examined by the appropriate state agency. The filing process has been made easier by the EEOC, which will forward the charge to a deferral state if the employee selects the appropriate option on the charge form. The matter will be reexamined by the EEOC after the matter has been with the state agency for a specified amount of time. However, if the state is a nondeferral state, the employee can choose whether to apply with the EEOC or with the state agency.

An employee may, without involving the EEOC, also file a charge with the appropriate state agency, bringing the claim solely under the state's sexual harassment law. This option may be vital to some claims. For example, Illinois' Human Rights Act, unlike Title VII, allows the employee to sue the individual harasser. This would make it easier for the employee to bring a charge against a co-worker harasser. Further, unlike Title VII, some states allow an individual to bring a claim against an employer who retains under 15 employees.

Finally, the employee, after receiving a right to sue letter from the EEOC, can sue the employer in a court of law. If the employee sues under Title VII, the remedies available to the employee include money to compensate for emotional distress and intangible losses, punitive damages to monetarily punish the employers, attorney fees, payment for loss of wages, and injunctive relief ordering the employer to take a certain action (i.e., grant the denied promotion).

SEE ALSO: Discrimination

Suggested Reading

Friedman, S. (1990). *Sex law: A legal sourcebook on critical sexual issues for the non-lawyer.* Jefferson, NC: McFarland.
Jorgenson, L., & Wahl, K. (2000). Workplace sexual harassment: Incidence, legal analysis, and the role of the psychiatrist. *Harvard Review of Psychiatry, 8,* 94–98.
Pepper, W., & Kennedy, F. (1981). *Sexual harassment in employment.* Charlottesville, VA: Michie.
Stein, L. (1999). *Sexual harassment in America: A documentary history.* Westport, CT: Greenwood Press.

BRANDY GLASSER

Sexual Organs

Sexual Organs The female sexual or reproductive organs may be categorized into the internal pelvic organs, the external genitalia, and the outside organs. Changes in the size and function of these organs occur throughout a woman's reproductive life. The most dramatic changes in the size and function of the female reproductive organs occur at puberty and during pregnancy.

The internal female reproductive structures are well protected by the bony pelvis. These structures include the ovaries, fallopian tubes, uterus, and cervix. The vagina connects the uterus to the external genitalia.

OVARIES

The ovaries are responsible for hormone production and ovulation. They are normally about 3–5 cm in length, and shrink to the size of an almond after menopause. One ovary is usually adequate for normal hormonal production. Surgical removal of both ovaries results in the vasomotor symptoms, or "hot flashes," that are common in menopausal women. Menopause occurs when the ovaries cease producing estrogen.

FALLOPIAN TUBES

The fallopian tubes arise from the uterus and reach toward the ovaries. After ovulation, the egg is picked up into the tube. Sperm are transported through the uterus into the fallopian tubes. Fertilization of the egg occurs in the tube. The tube moves the fertilized egg to the uterus for implantation. If a pregnancy implants in the fallopian tube, an ectopic pregnancy results. If this pregnancy grows, the tube may rupture, which can be life threatening.

UTERUS

The uterus, or womb, is normally the size of a small pear, and expands up to 20 times its size during pregnancy. The uterus is composed of several layers of tissue. The innermost layer is called the endometrium. The surface layer of the endometrium sloughs during normal menstruation. Much of the body of the uterus is composed of the myometrium. The myometrium is composed of smooth muscle tissue, which contracts during "menstrual cramps," and is also responsible for contractions during labor. The uterus is covered with a thin layer of tissue called the serosa. Benign conditions, such as fibroids, can dramatically alter the size of the uterus.

CERVIX

The cervix is the opening to the uterus and is the structure that is sampled during a Pap test. The opening of the cervix is referred to as the cervical os. In a woman who has never had children, this often looks like a pin point. Once a woman has given birth, however, the os actually resembles a "smile" or fish mouth. A normal cervix has a consistency of your nose, and is about 3–4 cm in length. During pregnancy, it softens and shortens and eventually dilates until it is 10 cm open during labor. After menopause, the opening to the cervix may become small, narrow, and even stenotic.

VAGINA

The vagina is a tubular, muscular structure, which is sometimes referred to as the "birth canal." It expands up to four times its size during childbirth. After menopause, the tissue of the vagina usually becomes very thin, and may cause dryness and discomfort with sexual intercourse.

The external female genitalia include the mons pubis, clitoris, introitus, labia majora and minora, and the urethra.

MONS

The mons pubis, which overlies the pubic bone, is an area of fatty tissue which is covered with skin and pubic hair.

CLITORIS

The clitoris is an extremely sensitive mound of tissue that is responsible for orgasm. The homolog, or similar structure in the male, is the penis.

LABIA MAJORA AND MINORA

The labia majora and minora surround the vaginal introitus, or opening of the vagina. They are often referred to as the "lips." There is a great variety of size and shape of the labia majora and minora, and this variation among women is normal.

URETHRA

The urethra is the opening to the bladder, located below the clitoris and above the vaginal opening. Its shorter length and close proximity to the vagina is thought to be one of the reasons that cystitis, or urinary tract infections, are so common among young sexually active women.

SKENE'S AND BARTHOLIN'S GLANDS

The Skene's and Bartholin's glands produce mucus and secretions, and are located around the vaginal opening. The Bartholin's gland can form a cyst, which may be asymptomatic, or may become infected. Infection results in a Bartholin's abscess, which is very painful and may require surgical drainage.

SEE ALSO: Ectopic pregnancy, Menopause, Menstruation, Pelvic examination, Puberty, Urinary tract infections, Uterine fibroids

Suggested Resources

http://www.acog.org

KAREN L. ASHBY

Sexually Transmitted Diseases Sexually transmitted diseases, or STDs, refer to a variety of bacterial, viral, and other infections acquired through sexual contact. STDs are common reasons for visits to clinics and physicians' offices. STDs produce significant morbidity and are estimated to cost the health care system billions of dollars each year.

STDs affect women of all social and economic backgrounds. Most STDs, however, occur in men and women between the ages of 19 and 25 years of age. Any sexually active person may be at risk for infection, particularly if he or she has multiple partners. Especially in women, many STDs are asymptomatic, which can increase their transmission and complications, as they are often passed on without knowledge. Screening tests are available for HIV, hepatitis B, syphilis, gonorrhea, and chlamydia.

STD SCREENING

Health care providers can help patients identify their risk factors and assess which screening tests, if any, should be done. The annual gynecological examination is a particular time to ask questions about STDs, and obtain appropriate testing. Screening is also particularly important during pregnancy, or for women planning to become pregnant. Several STDs may result in pregnancy complications, or transmission to the fetus, either during delivery or breast-feeding. Hepatitis B, syphilis, gonorrhea, and chlamydia are all part of routine prenatal screening. All pregnant women should also undergo HIV testing, because the transmission to the unborn fetus can be significantly reduced with appropriate treatment.

STD DIAGNOSIS

Patients and providers must work together to diagnose STDs. Patients may help by learning to identify symptoms and seeking medical treatment early, which may prevent the consequences of many STDs. Barrier methods of contraception, such as male or female condoms, can dramatically reduce transmission of STDs, but are not 100% effective.

The majority of STDs may be diagnosed either by simple office tests or by blood testing. Once a person is diagnosed with an STD, sexual partners should be notified promptly. Which STDs require that the doctor submit a report to local health authorities will vary from state to state.

STD TREATMENT

In most instances, diagnosing and treating an infection promptly will decrease potential long-term complications. In general, most infections that are caused by bacteria can usually be cured with antibiotic therapy (Table 1). However, there are several viral STDs, such as herpes simplex virus (HSV) or human papillomavirus (HPV), that may not be curable by treatment. For

Table 1. Common sexually transmitted diseases

Infection	Cause	Symptoms	Treatment or cure
Trichomonas	*Trichomonas vaginalis* (protozoan)	Foul-smelling vaginal discharge; irritation	Antibiotics—vaginal or oral
Chlamydia	*Chlamydia trachomatis* (bacteria)	None; vaginal discharge, pelvic pain	Antibiotics—oral
Gonorrhea	*Neisseria gonorrhoeae* (bacteria)	None; vaginal discharge, pelvic pain	Antibiotics—oral or IM
Human papillomavirus (HPV)	Human papillomavirus	Mild vaginal itching or burning	Topical medications or surgical removal
Herpes simplex virus (HSV)	Herpes simplex virus	Vaginal burning or painful sores	Antivirals do not cure, but can shorten symptoms
Human immunodeficiency virus (HIV)	HIV	None in early stages	Antiretrovirals can provide long-term control of disease

591

these infections, symptoms can be treated and the infection can be controlled.

STD PREVENTION

Education, particularly for young sexually active men and women, is one of the best ways to prevent the spread of STDs. While research is being done on vaccines for some STDs, prevention is still the best defense.

SEE ALSO: Acquired immunodeficiency syndrome, Chlamydia, Gonorrhea, Herpes simplex virus, Human papillomavirus, Syphilis

Suggested Reading

Gripshover, B., & Valdez, H. (2002). Common sexually transmitted diseases. In J. S. Tan (Ed.), *Experts guide to the management of common infectious diseases* (pp. 271–303). Philadelphia: American College of Physicians.

Suggested Resources

Centers for Disease Control and Prevention website: http://www.cdc.gov/health/ std.htm

KAREN L. ASHBY

Shamans Since early civilization, shamans have been integral in the healing process. The term shaman is derived from "saman," a Russian term which refers to one that uses ecstasy techniques. Shamankas, which are female shamans, and shamans use ecstasy techniques to act as a channel between the spiritual and physical worlds. During a connection with the spirit world, the shaman investigates why a patient suffers from physical, spiritual, or emotional discomforts, meanwhile deciphering a way to heal that patient.

Since shamankas and shamans were the only source of healing and connection to the spirit world, they were widely respected and revered within their community. Adding to their status was the common belief that only a select few possessed the gift of healing and the key to the spirit world. For instance, a child who recovered from an illness on her own strength proved that she was destined to be a shamanka.

Although shaman powers are bestowed on a select few, the gift is not gender biased. Gender, unlike other cultural healing practices, does not alter the healing power of a shamanka or shaman. Nonetheless, shamankas are often sought after more because of certain female characteristics such as a nurturing spirit, warmth, concern, firmness, and assertiveness. However, these characteristics reflect a patient's preference but not the effectiveness of healing.

Patients will seek a shaman's healing for ailments ranging from common colds, broken bones, depression, or evil spirits. Regardless of their sickness, the shaman will take an account of the patient's daily activities, diet, and any unusual occurrences. After gathering this information, the shaman will begin to search for a cure, by using bones, teeth, animal claws, shellfish, snail shells, dried roots, herbs, pieces of wood, stones, and glass as ingredients for remedies.

Generally, a shaman will communicate with the spirit world to bring about healing. Shamans communicate with spirits through trances, which are sometimes induced by alcohol or narcotics. While entranced, the shaman will begin to dance, sing, groan, their spirit will fly to distant lands, ascend into the heavens, and descend into the underworld. The shaman's entrancement and behavior initiates the conversation with the spirits, thus allowing the shaman to find the cause of illness, cures, and fight off evil spirits. Upon returning to the physical world, the shamanka will construct a remedy based on the information that she gathered while entranced.

Although shamans are not licensed medical doctors, they continue to have a significant role in healing, especially in rural communities around the world. As long as sickness and evil plague the world, shamankas and shamans will maintain their role in society as a source of healing and connection with the spirit world.

SEE ALSO: Charismatic healers, Healers

Suggested Reading

Kalweit, H. (1987). *Shamans, healers, and medicine men*. Boston: Shambhala.

Suggested Resources

Branigan, C. Shamanism. Retrieved December 4, 2000, from http://indigo.ie/~imago/cate/overview.html

Dale, C. The history of shamanism. Retrieved 2002 from http://www.mbspirit.net/topics/topi_page.aspx?topicID=18&pageType=38

STEPHANIE CABRERA

Shingles

The pathogenesis (cause) of shingles sounds like science fiction—a virus that causes a common childhood illness lies dormant for 50 or 60 years and then produces a different illness that can lead to severe, lifelong pain. Shingles, or herpes zoster, is caused by a relapse of the varicella-zoster virus (VZV); acute infection with this virus causes chicken pox. VZV is a member of the herpesvirus family, which also includes herpes simplex I and II, and Epstein–Barr virus, which causes mononucleosis. Infection due to this family of viruses is characterized by an acute illness followed by lifelong infection, which is usually clinically silent, although chronic infection, mild relapses, and severe relapse due to immunosuppression can occur. In the case of VZV, following acute infection (chicken pox), the virus remains dormant in the dorsal root ganglia in the spinal cord. Immune system surveillance keeps the virus dormant but the virus "hides" in the genome of the host cell and the immune system cannot eliminate it. Triggered by stress, immunosuppression (decreased functioning of the immune system), or decreased immune surveillance due to the prolonged elapsed time from the primary infection, the virus escapes the immune system and produces a local skin infection. The infection occurs in the area of the sensory nerve (the "dermatome") from which it emanated (i.e., "hiding in the ganglia"). As a result, the skin lesions occur unilaterally (on one side of the body) in patterns predicted by the known distribution of sensory nerves.

The clinical presentation is distinct and a clinical diagnosis can be reliably made when the characteristic vesicular (bubble-like) rash is present. Pain and paraesthesias (altered sensory perception) can precede the rash, and on occasion the pain can be confused with other pathology depending on the location (e.g., pain in abdominal dermatomes may mimic an acute abdomen). The skin lesions may appear initially as small areas of erythema (localized redness of the skin), but evolve into small vesicular lesions developing along the dermatome (nerve distribution area on the skin). The most commonly affected areas are the thoracic (chest) and lumbar (back) dermatomes. The skin lesions are infectious, and nonimmune individuals can contract chicken pox from exposure to the skin lesions of an individual with shingles.

The acute illness lasts 1–2 weeks. The most common complications are pain and superinfection due to bacterial infection (staphylococcus and group A streptococcus). Other complications depend on the location of the infection. Cranial nerve shingles can lead to eye involvement and cranial neuropathies. Ramsay–Hunt syndrome results from shingles of the sensory branch of the trigeminal nerve and is characterized by skin lesions around the ear, hypersensitive hearing (hyperacusis), and paralysis of facial nerves (Bell's palsy). Therapy with acyclovir or other antivirals has been shown in clinical trials to shorten the duration and severity of the acute illness when the therapy is begun within 48 hours of the appearance of the skin lesions. The role of antiviral medications in preventing chronic pain from shingles is discussed below. Management otherwise consists of pain control and monitoring for complications.

Shingles has a lifetime prevalence of 30% and is strongly associated with aging. Less than 5% of individuals 65 and under have a history of shingles; 10% of 75-year-olds and 30% of 85-year-olds have had shingles. About 30% of patients will experience a second episode of shingles in their lifetime, and about 5–10% will have a third episode. Shingles can occur in younger individuals in the absence of immunosuppression, but also may be associated with steroid therapy and immunosuppressing illnesses. Shingles in young adults may be associated with immunosuppression from HIV, and should prompt consideration for HIV testing. With the notable exception of HIV, younger patients with shingles rarely have a related immunosuppressing illness, and the presence of shingles should not generally lead to a search for an underlying problem that is not evident on a routine history and physical examination.

While the acute illness may lead to some morbidity (illness) and may rarely lead to complications, acute shingles is largely self-limited. The most dreaded complication is severe, chronic nerve pain at the site of the infection. Pain due to shingles that persists for more than 30 days is termed postherpetic neuralgia (PHN). Pain due to PHN can be disabling and may require complicated pain management in order for the patient to have sustained symptomatic relief. Therapy with antiviral medications during the acute infection can decrease the severity of PHN. This benefit from antiviral therapy provides a strong indication for their use. There is ongoing research as to whether the use of vaccine to boost immunity in older individuals can prevent shingles.

SEE ALSO: Acquired immunodeficiency syndrome, Herpes simplex virus

Suggested Reading

Gnann, J. W., Jr., & Whitley, R. J. (2002). Herpes zoster. *New England Journal of Medicine, 347*, 340–346.

Whitley, R. J. (2000). Varicella-zoster virus. In G. L. Mandell, J. E. Bennett, & R. Dolin (Eds.), *Principles and practices of infectious diseases* (5th ed., pp. 1580–1585). New York: Churchill Livingstone.

Suggested Resources

http://www.cdc.gov/nip/diseases/varicella/

KEITH B. ARMITAGE

Sigmoidoscopy *see* Colorectal Cancer

Sjögren's Syndrome

Sjögren's syndrome (SS) is a chronic autoimmune disorder of unknown cause that mostly involves the tear glands of the eye and salivary glands of the mouth. It can also cause problems in the lining of the genital, urinary, gastrointestinal, and respiratory tracts. SS occurs alone or as part of many other autoimmune disorders. The severity varies considerably. Most SS patients should be treated by specialists in rheumatology, ophthalmology, dentistry, and other necessary specialties. It is estimated that more than 1 million people in the United States suffer from SS, and 90% are women in their 30s and 40s. Connective tissue diseases associated with SS include rheumatoid arthritis, systemic lupus erythematosus, scleroderma, fibromyalgia, and others. Much is still unknown about the cause of SS, but it is clear that infectious, genetic, and hormonal factors are involved.

SYMPTOMS, SIGNS, AND DIAGNOSIS

A health professional examining an individual for symptoms of SS should ask questions about the patient's eyes and mouth (see Tables 1 and 2).

It also is helpful to note that individuals with SS generally have salivary gland enlargement on both sides although this may not be symmetric. Other diseases that cause salivary gland swelling typically affect only one side.

Table 1. Questions to ask when checking for *eye* symptoms[a]

Have you had daily, persistent, troublesome dry eyes for more than 3 months?
Do you have a recurrent sensation of gravel or sand in the eyes?
Do you use tear substitutes more than three times a day?

[a] Only one positive response is required to consider the patient symptomatic.

Table 2. Questions to ask when checking for *oral* symptoms[a]

Have you had a daily feeling of dry mouth for more than 3 months?
Have you had recurrently or persistently swollen salivary glands as an adult?
Do you frequently drink liquids to aid in swallowing dry food?

[a] Only one positive response is required to consider the patient symptomatic.

If eye symptoms are present, certain tests should be performed to evaluate tear production (Schirmer's test) and quality of tear fluid using microscopic techniques (rose bengal staining). If mouth symptoms are present, objective evidence of salivary gland function is needed. Biopsy examination of the minor salivary glands as well as blood tests must be performed.

To diagnose a patient with SS, it is *required* that either the biopsy or the blood test results be positive, but even positive results on both tests are not enough to definitely diagnose SS. Mouth and/or eye symptoms must be present as well.

Clinical features of SS are similar to those of several other diseases such as hepatitis C infection, AIDS, preexisting lymphoma, certain autoimmune disorders such as sarcoidosis, and medical complications in transplant patients (graft-versus-host disease). A patient with a past history of head and neck radiation therapy could have symptoms similar to SS as well. Lastly, effects of certain medications (anticholinergic drugs) may mimic SS.

TREATMENT

To treat eye symptoms (keratoconjunctivitis sicca), the patient should be instructed to use artificial tears. Some individuals can benefit from more concentrated viscous solutions or hydroxypropylcellulose pellet insertion under the lower eyelids. Ointments can be helpful as well but should only be used at night because they can interfere with vision. Pilocarpine taken internally has been approved for the treatment of mouth symptoms and can help eye symptoms as well.

Mouth symptoms (xerostomia) require frequent dental care, daily use of antimicrobial mouth rinse, and application of topical fluoride. Artificial saliva and lubricants may relieve oral dryness and help with swallowing difficulty. Some people will find that chewing gum or candies (sugar-free to prevent tooth decay) will stimulate secretion in the mouth. Dietary modifications may aid in swallowing as well. As discussed above, drugs like pilocarpine may increase oral salivary secretion, as long as sufficient gland tissue is present. Oral candidiasis, a fungal infection, which commonly results from dry mouth, should be treated by having the patient suck oral lozenges or use vaginal suppositories of antifungal agents like nystatin or clotrimazole. Systemic manifestations can be treated by various immune-altering drugs.

PROGNOSIS AND EDUCATION

The prognosis for individuals with SS is usually good. There is, however, an increased risk of progression to non-Hodgkin's lymphoma. All individuals should be provided with information that will help them cope with the difficulties associated with SS.

SEE ALSO: Autoimmune disorders

Suggested Reading

Klippel, J. H., et al., (Eds.). (2001). *Primer on the rheumatic diseases* (12th ed.). Atlanta, GA: Arthritis Foundation.

Klippel, J. H., & Dieppe, P. A. (1998). *Rheumatology* (2nd ed.). St. Louis, MO: C. V. Mosby.

Klippel, J. H., Dieppe, P. A., & Ferri, F. F. (2000). *Primary care rheumatology*. London: Harcourt.

DANIEL GREENE
LORI B. SIEGEL

Skin Care
The skin is the largest and most exposed organ of the body. Its functions are complex and include serving as a physical and immunologic barrier to external substances, retaining water, regulating body temperature, and acting as a sensory organ. The skin is also an integral part of our self-image and is often a focus of cosmetic and beautifying agents.

The skin consists of three layers. The upper layer, or *epidermis*, is about as thick as a sheet of paper. It is composed of layered skin cells called *keratinocytes*. The outermost part of the epidermis, called the *stratum corneum*, is composed of dead keratinocytes that are shed continuously. The living layer of keratinocytes underneath is called *squamous cells*. The innermost part of the epidermis consists of *basal cells* that are constantly dividing to form new keratinocytes. The bottom skin layer is called the *dermis*, which contains tiny blood and lymph vessels that increase in number deeper in the skin. Cells called *melanocytes* form the transitional layer between the epidermis and dermis. These skin cells produce a brown-black skin pigment called *melanin*, which helps to protect against the damaging rays of the sun and also determines skin coloring. As a person ages, melanocytes often proliferate, forming concentrated clusters that appear on the surface as small, dark, flat, or dome-shaped spots, which are usually harmless moles or liver spots.

Because the skin is exposed to the environment, it is susceptible to damage over time. Ultraviolet rays from sunlight and smoking are the most common causes of environmental skin damage. Sunlight consists of ultraviolet (referred to as UVA or UVB) radiation that penetrates the layers of the skin. UVB radiation primarily affects the outer skin layers and is the primary cause of sunburn. It affects skin cells by damaging the genetic material, the DNA, inside the skin cells. UVA radiation penetrates into the inner skin layers and is responsible for tanning and allergic reactions to sunlight (such as from medication). UVA causes the release of *oxidants*, or oxygen free radicals, that can damage cell membranes and interact with genetic material. Cigarette smoke also produces oxygen free radicals and is known to accelerate wrinkles and aging skin disorders.

Sun protection is one of the most important parts of a skin care regimen. Research has shown that exposure to UV light can cause various skin cancers, the most common being basal cell carcinoma and squamous cell carcinoma. A less common but much more dangerous form of skin cancer, malignant melanoma, may be linked to sunburns in childhood.

UVA and UVB radiations cause dramatically accelerated skin aging, including wrinkling, dryness, visible blood vessels, and changes in pigmentation. Sunlight damages *collagen* fibers (the major structural protein in the skin) and causes accumulation of abnormal *elastin* (the protein that causes tissue to stretch). Large amounts of enzymes called *metalloproteinases* are produced in response to the abnormal elastin that function to remodel the damaged tissue by manufacturing and reforming collagen. In addition to sun damage, smokers have considerably higher levels of these metalloproteinases, which may contribute to the skin-aging effects of smoking. Unfortunately, the reformation process is imperfect and some metalloproteinases actually degrade collagen. The result is an uneven formation of disorganized collagen fibers called *solar scars.* Repetition of this imperfect skin rebuilding over time causes wrinkles.

Healthy skin care and habits can decrease this cumulative injury. Recommendations include:

1. Minimizing sun exposure during peak hours (10 AM to 2 PM).
2. Wearing sun-protective clothing, hats, and sunglasses.
3. Using a broad-spectrum sunscreen (UVA and UVB protection) with a sun-protection factor (SPF) of greater than or equal to 15.
4. Avoiding sunlamps and tanning beds.
5. Avoid cigarette smoke; if you smoke, quit.

Protective sun exposure habits are most beneficial when started in childhood since statistics show that more than one half of a person's lifetime UV exposure occurs during childhood and adolescence. However, it is never too late to incorporate sun protection into a skin care regimen. Medical treatments for reversing some of the effects of sun damage are available and include topical creams, chemical peels, and laser therapy.

Other components of a skin care regimen need not be complicated. Mild, nonperfumed soaps are usually recommended for cleansing the skin, with a moisturizer applied as needed (consider products that have a built-in sunscreen). As we get older, our skin has fewer sweat and oil glands and is less efficient in retaining water, which can lead to dryness and itching. Dry skin can be worsened by frequent bathing or showering, and may be more sensitive to soaps, cosmetics, and certain fabrics. Frequent use of emollients and avoiding aggravating factors are basic measures for dry skin care. For those with oily or acne-prone skin, facial moisturizers are usually not needed and care should be taken to choose cosmetics that are oil-free and noncomedogenic (acne-producing).

SEE ALSO: Acne, Cancer, Dermatitis, Liver spots, Melanoma, Skin disorders, Smoking, Wrinkles

Suggested Reading

Habif (Ed.). (1996). *Clinical dermatology* (3rd ed., pp. 603–604). St. Louis, MO: Mosby-Year Book.
Tourles, S. (1999). *Naturally healthy skin: Tips and techniques for a lifetime of radiant skin.* North Adams, MA: Storey Books.
Glanz, K. (2002). Guidelines for school programs to prevent skin cancer. *MMWR Recommendation Report, 51*(4), 1–18.

Suggested Resources

American Academy of Dermatology: www.aad.org

PARADI MIRMIRANI

Skin Disorders

Skin disorders can be broadly categorized as either rashes or as growths. Rashes are often a result of skin inflammation and can be precipitated by a wide variety of causes. Two common inflammatory diagnoses in women are acne and atopic dermatitis, commonly called eczema. Growths or tumors may be further classified into benign, premalignant, or malignant lesions. The most common tumors are outlined in the following table.

Benign	Premalignant	Malignant
Seborrheic keratoses	Actinic keratoses	Basal cell carcinoma
Skin tags		Squamous cell carcinoma
		Malignant melanoma

Acne is a skin condition that is primarily a disease of adolescence but may persist through the third decade or beyond, particularly in women. Although the precise etiology of acne remains unknown, it is likely multifactorial. The almost universal presence of *Propionobacterium acnes* bacteria in the skin of patients with acne suggests it has a causative role. In addition, certain sex hormones (androgens) are known to regulate sebum or oil from the sebaceous glands and therefore play a role in the development of acne. The lesions of acne include pustules, red papules, and inflammatory nodules, which most commonly affect the face and to a lesser degree the back, chest, and shoulders. The physical appearance of acne can result in significant emotional distress to patients and is ample justification to treat this disorder. In addition, treatment may prevent the major sequelae of acne, namely, permanent and potentially disfiguring scars. Common treatment measures are aimed at decreasing the bacterial load, reducing the level of androgens, and decreasing sebum production.

Atopic dermatitis or eczema is an inflammatory condition of the skin that is typically a chronic and relapsing disorder, which usually starts in infancy and childhood, but may persist into adulthood. Persons with atopic dermatitis are often predisposed to other allergic diseases including hay fever and asthma. The cardinal features of atopic dermatitis are itchy, dry skin which when scratched or irritated can lead to a rash. Common locations for atopic dermatitis are around the eyes and in the creases of the elbows and knees. Many adults with atopic dermatitis may have chronic hand eczema as the only manifestation of their disease. The mainstays of treatment for atopic dermatitis include avoiding common skin irritants, keeping the skin well hydrated with emollients, topical steroid treatments, and control of itching with antihistamines.

Seborrheic keratoses are extremely common skin tumors, usually affecting people older than 50 years but also seen in young adults. These lesions usually arise on the trunk, face, and upper extremities and can range in color from tan to red or even black. Such skin changes can occur as an isolated lesion or hundreds may be present in the same person. Their diagnosis is often made based on a clinically "stuck-on" appearance. Seborrheic keratoses represent a benign proliferation of immature keratinocytes. The tendency for seborrheic keratoses may be inherited in an autosomal dominant fashion. No treatment is necessary for most lesions.

Skin tags are outgrowths of normal skin. Twenty-five percent of adults have skin tags, and there is a familial tendency for these lesions. They usually occur at sites of friction such as the axillae, neck, underneath the breasts, and in the groin area. Treatment is indicated only if lesions are irritating or the individual desires removal for cosmetic reasons.

Actinic keratoses are common premalignant lesions of the skin, resulting from chronic, cumulative sun exposure, and occurring most commonly in fair-skinned people on sun-exposed skin sites including the face and the dorsal hands. Actinic keratoses are characterized by an irregular shape, and scaly or "sandpaper" texture. If left untreated, some actinic keratoses may progress to become cancerous. Treatment options include liquid nitrogen or prescription medications aimed at destroying the premalignant cells.

Basal cell carcinoma is a malignancy of the basal cells in the epidermis. It is the most common human malignancy with approximately 750,000 new cases in the United States each year. Basal cell carcinoma occurs more commonly in men, almost exclusively in whites, and most frequently between the ages of 40 and 80. Predisposing factors include chronic UV sunlight exposure, arsenic, and ionizing radiation. Basal cell cancers are usually noticed as a new growth in sun-damaged skin that is skin colored, sometimes pearly, and has a tendency to bleed. Most basal cell tumors spread locally and do not metastasize. Treatment usually involves surgical excision but is influenced by size and location of the tumor.

Squamous cell carcinomas are malignant tumors of keratinocytes, the main cell type that comprises the skin. Although squamous cell cancer is the second most frequent skin carcinoma, its incidence is increasing greatly. Although squamous cell cancer occurs most commonly in white men older than 55, women with extensive sun exposure or other predisposing factors are affected. Predisposing factors include: UV sunlight exposure, old burn scars, sites of chronic inflammation, radiation therapy, arsenic, immunosuppression, and smoking (lip lesions). A squamous cell carcinoma commonly appears as a new growth that may be scaly and has a tendency to bleed. These tumors can in some cases metastasize depending on the location of the tumor or the predisposing cause. Treatment typically involves excision of the lesion.

Melanoma, which exactly means black tumor, is the malignant proliferation of pigment-producing cells, called melanocytes. Malignant melanoma deserves all the attention given it because of its potentially fatal nature, rapidly increasing incidence, and excellent prognosis if treated early. Malignant melanoma represents 3% of all cancers, with tens of thousands of new cases in the United States annually. Representing 1–2% of all cancer-related deaths, the increase in the melanoma mortality rates is second only to lung cancer. Risk factors for developing malignant melanoma include fair hair and light eyes, extensive sun exposure, history of sunburns in childhood, multiple irregular moles, or a family history of melanoma. However, any patient with a history of change in a longstanding pigmented lesion or a new lesion with suspect features should alert the clinician to the possible diagnosis of melanoma. A mnemonic to remember suspect features of melanoma is:

A = asymmetry
B = borders irregular and blurred

C = color change or variable pigmentation
D = diameter greater than 6 mm
E = elevation of previously flat lesion

Diagnosis is based on excisional biopsy and characteristic histologic findings. The depth of the tumor is of crucial importance in determining prognosis. With a thick melanoma, additional tests are required to evaluate possible metastasis to lymph nodes and other organs. Treatment of melanoma depends on the stage of the tumor: excisions are performed for thin lesion whereas thicker tumors may require adjuvant therapy.

SEE ALSO: Cancer, Dermatitis, Skin cancer, Skin care, Smoking

Suggested Reading

Freedberg, I., Eisen, A., Wolff, K., Austen, K. F., Goldsmith, L., Katz, S., et al. (Eds.). (1999). *Fitzpatrick's dermatology in general medicine* (5th ed., pp. 769, 1464). New York: McGraw-Hill.

Goldstein, B. G., & Goldstein, A. O. (1997). *Practical dermatology* (2nd ed., pp. 128–157). St. Louis, MO: C. V. Mosby.

Suggested Resources

American Academy of Dermatology www.AAD.org

SAROLTA SZABO
RADHA MIKKILLINENI
PARADI MIRMIRANI

Slavery

Slavery was one of the most brutal events in American history, yet in most history courses, little or no information is offered about the health and health care issues of slaves. Furthermore, the existing literature varies greatly in its description of the type of health care given to African/black African American slaves.

In the early 1800s, the United States Congress passed legislation to decrease and subsequently stop the African slave trade. Nonetheless, that same legislation permitted slavery to continue within the borders of the Americas. Each ship's captain had to prepare and keep records of his human cargo. The "records" consisted of the slave's name, age, gender, color, and height. This information was kept with the ship and a handwritten copy was given to the individual who was responsible for the slaves at their point of arrival.

Due to the passage of this legislation and the economic need of the slave owners for a constant stream of laborers, the slave owners began to allow the slaves to mate (the proper term at the time was breed) for the purpose of reproduction and increasing the manpower on the plantation as well as to open up a new economic avenue for the slave owner. During slavery, the men and the women were given work responsibilities according to their age and physical condition. Gender did not play a significant role in the assignment of work. Plantation owners and overseers expected equal amounts of labor from both genders based on their size and age. Female slaves were given cotton-picking equipment consisting of bags, baskets, and sheets that had to be filled to capacity in order to be heavy enough to bring a good fair market value when weighed. The strenuous and heavy labor associated with this work along with inadequate nutrition and exposure to European diseases played important roles in fetal malformation and fetal demise. The age of a pregnant slave also played a crucial role in the high incidence of miscarriages and infant mortality.

The plantation owners depended upon the slave overseer to let them know when a female was pregnant. The overseer depended upon the slave women to tell him when they were pregnant. The women looked for symptoms such as increased urination, ceasing of the menses, enlarged breasts, vomiting, and movement of the child. Once these occurred, the women then reported them to the overseer and the overseer made the decision to allow the women to shift to lighter workloads. However, on many plantations the overseer would not take the word of a slave and would wait until there were visible outward signs of pregnancy. Many times the visible signs did not occur until the female was in the middle of her second trimester.

Female slaves were allowed less than 1 month of downtime during their pregnancies. Those who had infants who survived birth and lived for 1 year received more days out of the field than those who had stillbirths or an infant who died within the first year. There is a significant correlation between the strenuous, heavy labor of the female field hand, the time frame between when the pregnancy was reported and when the female field hand was allowed by the overseer to reduce her workload, and the high incidence of miscarriages, infant malformation, and infant mortality.

In today's world, there is still a higher incidence of miscarriages, infant malformation, and infant mortality rate for black African Americans than their white

European American equivalents. Slavery is no longer an issue, but the poverty, including the low salaries of the working class poor, malnutrition, and lack of immediate medical attention continue to contribute to this problem in the United States.

SEE ALSO: African American, Discrimination, Pregnancy

Suggested Reading

Bankole, K. (1998). *Slavery and medicine: Enslavement and medical practices in antebellum Louisiana.* New York: Garland.

Campbell, J. (1984). Work, pregnancy, and infant mortality among Southern slaves. *Journal of Interdisciplinary History, 14*(4).

Logan, S. L., & Freeman, E. M. (2000). *Health care in the black community, empowerment, knowledge, skills and collectivism.* Binghamton, NY: Haworth Press.

McMillen, S. G. (1991). "No uncommon disease": Neonatal tetanus, slave infants, and the Southern medical profession. *Journal of the History of Medicine and Allied Sciences, 46,* 291–315.

PATRICIA M. HENRY

Sleep Disorders
Poor sleep is one of the most common presenting symptoms heard by modern doctors. Many sleep disturbances are caused by ineffective sleep hygiene, which refers to the sum total of the waking behaviors that affect the quality and quantity of our sleep.

The first step for the physician in the assessment and treatment of a complaint of impaired sleep is to review optimal sleep hygiene practices with a patient. A key component is establishing the bed as a sanctuary for sleep and sex only. Reliable daily sleep and wake times are important as well. The ideal amount of sleep likely varies from person to person, although a recent study revealed that women who reported typically sleeping less than 5 or more than 9 hr per night had a significantly higher risk of coronary heart disease than those who typically slept 6–7 hr nightly, at 10-year follow-up.

Abstaining from rigorous exercise or hot baths or showers too close to bedtime is a practical rule. If unable to fall asleep after 30–45 min in bed, individuals are advised to spend 20–30 min occupied in some activity outside the bedroom and then try to retire again. Caffeine and tobacco should be avoided within 3 hr of bedtime, as should meals and significant fluid intake. Alcohol may promote the initiation of sleep but will reliably decrease the quality and continuity of ensuing sleep.

The comprehensive assessment of a potential sleep disorder includes a thorough history of sleep dysfunction and sleep hygiene, a complete medical and mental health history, a review of current medications, an assessment of drug and alcohol use, a physical examination with guided use of laboratory testing, and an overnight "sleep study," or polysomnogram. Polysomnography is the systematic evaluation of brainwave, ocular, muscular, and respiratory function during sleep. Recorded over the course of a typical night's sleep, this exam may reveal apneas or hypopneas (the absence or slowing of spontaneous respiration, respectively) or abnormal body movements. The latency (duration from bedtime to sleep onset), continuity, efficiency, and architecture of sleep are each assessed. Sleep architecture refers to the duration of and transitions between the unique physiologic phases of sleep.

Five specific stages of sleep are identified: one stage of rapid eye movement (REM) sleep and four stages of non-rapid eye movement (NREM) sleep, identified as stages 1 through 4. Stage 1 NREM is relatively brief and signifies the transition from a waking state to sleep. Stage 2 NREM, significant for "sleep spindles" and "K complexes" on the EEG portion of the polysomnogram, comprises up to 50% of total sleep time. Progressively deeper stages of sleep, stages 3 and 4 ("slow-wave" sleep) occupy up to 20% of sleep time, while REM sleep, in which dream activity and loss of muscle tone occur, occupies up to 25% of sleep time. REM sleep occurs typically every 80–90 min, and periods of REM become longer in duration across the night. NREM stages 3 and 4 are more prominent during the first half of the night, and tend to deteriorate in duration and frequency as we age. Perhaps as a result, up to 50% of American seniors may have a sleep disorder.

There are multiple specific sleep disorders. These can be divided into four main groups: sleep disorders caused by: (a) an independent mental disorder, (b) the use or discontinuation of a substance, or (c) a general medical condition (all are "secondary" sleep disorders), and the "primary" sleep disorders, which include the *dyssomnias*, or disorders of the onset or maintenance of sleep; and the *parasomnias*, or disorders of abnormal behaviors associated with sleep. Parasomnias include conditions such as sleepwalking (somnambulism), sleeptalking (somniloquy), sleep terrors, nightmares, REM sleep behavior disorder, bruxism, and enuresis ("bedwetting").

Mood and anxiety disorders commonly perturb sleep. Sleep disorders secondary to other mental disorders are more common in women than in men.

Sleep Disorders

Up to 50% of individuals with chronic insomnia may have a separate mental disorder responsible for the sleep disturbance. Major depression, bipolar disorder, schizophrenia, adjustment disorders, and anxiety disorders such as panic disorder, generalized anxiety disorder, and posttraumatic stress disorder typically involve an alteration in the amount and timing of sleep. In major depression, for example, sleep latency is prolonged, REM latency decreased, and REM sleep becomes denser. Slow-wave sleep is reduced. The medications used to treat these disorders may also cause disturbances in sleep, such as insomnia, hypersomnia, vivid dreams or nightmares, or bruxism.

Intoxication or withdrawal from drugs and alcohol may cause significant sleep disruption. Alcohol intoxication increases slow-wave sleep and suppresses REM sleep, and causes restless, fitful sleep with increased dreaming. Its use may also worsen sleep apneas. Withdrawal from chronic alcohol use tends to reveal a drop in slow-wave sleep and increase in REM. Caffeine use increases wakefulness and contributes to insomnia, but hypersomnia or fatigue may ensue after an individual dose has worn off. Amphetamines and cocaine tend to cause insomnia with intoxication and hypersomnia with withdrawal. Opioids, sedatives, and many antianxiety medications are acutely sedating, but provoke insomnia when used chronically, as tolerance develops. As with alcohol, a rebound in REM sleep amount may be seen after discontinuation of these agents.

Scores of medical conditions carry with them the risk of sleep impairment. Common culprits include acute infection, dementia, rheumatologic disorders characterized by acute or chronic pain, neurodegenerative disorders, endocrine disorders, cardiopulmonary disease, epilepsy, headaches, and other neurologic disorders. Women are at greater risk for disrupted sleep in pregnancy, postmenopause, and with polycystic ovary syndrome (secondary to a higher risk of sleep-disordered breathing). In hospitals and nursing homes, delirium is a very common cause of sleep disruption. A delirium is an acute confusional state secondary to an acute medical condition or substance that is characterized by impairments in attention, concentration, cognition, and perception. Sleep is often fitful, nonrestorative, and exhibits a day–night reversal pattern.

More common dyssomnias include primary insomnia or hypersomnia, narcolepsy, sleep apnea, restless legs syndrome, and circadian rhythm sleep disorders. Narcolepsy involves daytime sleep attacks, cataplexy (brief episodes of loss of muscle tone, often associated with intense emotion), sleep–wake hallucinations, and sleep paralysis. Onset is typically during adolescence and genetics is believed to have a strong role. The disorder is rare, perhaps affecting 1 in 1,000 persons, and the male:female ratio is roughly 1:1. Treatment goals include ensuring wakefulness by day and the consolidation of sleep at night. Amphetamine stimulants and a newer nonamphetamine medication, modafinil, may promote daytime wakefulness, and sedative-hypnotics may help nighttime sleep.

Sleep apnea may be either central or obstructive in type. Central sleep apnea is rare and involves diminished respiratory drive at the level of the brainstem. Obstructive sleep apnea (OSA) is much more common, affecting from 1% to 10% of the population. The male-to-female ratio is around 3 to 1. OSA is caused by the mechanical obstruction of ventilation by increased palatal and pharyngeal tissues. Obese persons are at greater risk. Excessive daytime sleepiness, morning headaches, loud snoring, and apneas observed by sleeping partners can aid in diagnosis, which is confirmed by polysomnography. Many are first diagnosed between 40 and 60 years of age. Treatment involves weight loss, smoking cessation, reduction of cardiac risk factors (as OSA carries with it an increased risk of high blood pressure), and ventilation through the night with continuous positive airway pressure (CPAP) machines. Surgeries to reduce posterior palatopharyngeal tissues have not been routinely helpful.

Restless leg syndrome involves random, repetitive irregular movements of the feet and legs, and unpleasant aches and pains sensed deeply in the lower extremities. The discomfort often mandates walking or rubbing of the legs by the sufferer for temporary relief. The symptoms occur in the evening and earlier phases of sleep, and respond on a limited basis to dopamine agonists, tricyclic antidepressants, or opiate analgesics. Common causes include peripheral nerve disorders related to diabetes or kidney dysfunction, pregnancy, iron deficiency, and medication side effects. Periodic limb movement disorder is a similar disorder that involves repetitive involuntary movements, which intrude upon normal sleep maintenance and cause nonrestorative sleep and excessive daytime sleepiness. Restless leg syndrome and OSA are the two most common primary sleep disorders in the elderly.

Circadian rhythm sleep disorders include jet lag, shift work, and delayed sleep phase disorders. Jet lag syndrome is seen when people travel two or more time zones, typically west to east, and subsequently have difficulty advancing their sleep schedules. Exposure to light may help delay, and sedative-hypnotic medicines may help advance, sleep onset. Shift work disorders are born of changes from first or second to third shift schedules. Delayed sleep phase disorders result when the onset of sleep is intentionally delayed because of lifestyle concerns and the ensuing normal sleep duration causes social or occupational dysfunction the following day.

Treatment strategies are diverse, as one can see from the multiple causes of sleep impairment found in clinical practice. Optimizing and accentuating the importance of sleep hygiene is vitally important. Other psychiatric and medical conditions should be treated, and offending medications or drugs discontinued. Sedative medications should only be used whenever absolutely necessary and for the shortest possible duration. Benzodiazepine sedative-hypnotics such as lorazepam, diazepam, and alprazolam carry with them a very real risk of acute adverse effects such as slowed respiration, confusion, unsteady gait and falls, and the risk of dependence with chronic use.

SEE ALSO: Alcohol use, Anxiety disorders, Bipolar disorder, Insomnia, Posttraumatic stress disorder, Sleep hygiene, Substance use

Suggested Reading

American Psychiatric Association. (2000). *Diagnostic and statistical manual of mental disorders* (4th ed., text revision). Washington, DC: Author.

Ayas, N. T., White, D. P., Manson, J. E., et al. (2003). A prospective study of sleep duration and coronary heart disease in women. *Archives of Internal Medicine, 163,* 205–209.

Barthlen, G. M. (2002). Sleep disorders [Review]. *Geriatrics, 57,* 34–39.

Coffey, C. E., & Cummings, J. L. (2000). *Textbook of geriatric neuropsychiatry* (2nd ed.). Washington, DC: American Psychiatric Press.

Dancey, D. R., Hanly, P. J., Soong, C., et al. (2001). Impact of menopause on the prevalence and severity of sleep apnea. *Chest, 120,* 151–155.

Kaplan, H. I., & Sadock, B. J. (1998). *Synopsis of psychiatry* (8th ed.). Baltimore: Williams & Wilkins.

Malhotra, A., & White, D. P. (2002). Obstructive sleep apnoea [Review]. *Lancet, 360,* 237–245.

JOHN SANITATO

Sleep Hygiene
Sleep hygiene is an important consideration after underlying causes of sleep disturbance have been addressed from neurological, psychiatric, and medical causes, and acute stressors are not immediate by apparent. Sleep hygiene refers to patterns of behavior and attitudes about sleep for a given person. Probably one of the most significant factors is the misunderstanding that surrounds sleep. There are often significant maladaptive behaviors that can arise when a person develops sleep disturbances. This leads to a negative spiral that tends to exacerbate the symptoms of insomnia. It is imperative at the outset of addressing sleep issues to educate individuals about the natural process of sleep. When pathology has been ruled out, then individuals can be reassured that sleep will occur and this is important to provide relief to the suffering person. Insomnia may undermine an individual's own sleep. This occurs by factors that are under a given person's immediate control and issues which require adaptation to external factors or modification of those factors.

Factors under a person's direct control involve making a choice about what times a person chooses to sleep. It is advisable under most circumstances not to take naps greater than one half hour during the day if one expects to sleep at traditional times at night. Vigorous activities or eating substantially should be avoided close to anticipated times of sleep to alleviate insomnia. Avoidance of stimulants such as caffeine is also important. Forcing yourself to sleep is a common misconception. Going to bed when sleepy and not at arbitrary times needs to be appreciated. The tendency to overcontrol sleep instead of learning to work with an individual's sleep patterns needs flexibility to avoid anxiety or self-induced stress regarding sleep habits. Treatment needs to be directed toward the development of behaviors and adaptations to sleep patterns that are flexible.

It is important that the effect of external factors on sleep needs to be appreciated and again assist individuals in their ability to negotiate these issues. More challenging issues may indicate a need for psychotherapy. Anticipation of a job or endeavor the next day can contribute to anxiety and may compromise sleep. Recognition of the influence of thoughts on sleep patterns may be enough of an influence to change cognitive behaviors, yet, at other times, psychotherapy may be necessary to be able to adapt to changes required.

Chronic sedative use in the absence of applications of these principles is not only not helpful but is in fact counter productive. In fact, chronic sedative use is usually a sign of underlying issues, as previously mentioned, that have not been addressed.

Smoking

To summarize, sleep hygiene involves education and techniques of adaptation that reflect appropriate management of factors direct and indirect that affect sleep function. It is critical to understand the multidimensional nature of sleep hygiene to implement it efficaciously.

SEE ALSO: Anxiety disorders, Insomnia, Mood disorders, Sleep disorders

Suggested Reading

Cartwright, R. D. (1995). Sleep disorders: Diagnosis and treatment. *American Journal of Psychiatry, 152*, 1659–1663.

Cohen, G. D. (1998). Aging to sleep, perchance to dream. *American Journal of Geriatric Psychiatry, 6*, 93–96.

Dupont, R. L. (1999). The secret strength of angels—7 virtues to live by. *American Journal of Psychiatry, 156*, 2011.

Hartmann, E., Baekeland, F., Zwilling, G., & Hoy, P. (1971). Sleep need: How much sleep and what kind? *American Journal of Psychiatry, 127*, 1001–1008.

Hartmann, L. (2001). Sleep in America: National survey results. *Psychiatric News, 36*, 13-a.

Kavanau, J. L. (2000). Sleep, memory maintenance, and mental disorders. *Journal of Neuropsychiatry and Clinical Neuroscience, 12*, 199–208.

Kayumov, L., Rotengerg, V., Buttoo, K., Auch, C., Pandi-Perumal, S. R., & Shapiro, C. M. (2000). Interrelationships between nocturnal sleep, daytime alertness, and sleepiness: Two types of alertness proposed. *Journal of Neuropsychiatry and Clinical Neuroscience, 12*, 86–90.

Morin, C. M., Culbert, J. P., & Schwartz, S. M. (1994). Nonpharmacological interventions for insomnia: A meta-analysis of treatment efficacy. *American Journal of Psychiatry, 151*, 1172–1180.

Noffsinger, S. (1998). Psychiatric aspects of sleep. *Psychiatric Service, 49*, 1099.

Regesteinm, Q. R., & Monk, T. H. (1991). Is the poor sleep of shift workers a disorder? *American Journal of Psychiatry, 148*, 1487–1493.

Schnierow, B. J. (2000). The enchanted world of sleep. *American Journal of Psychiatry, 157*, 1191.

PHILIP L. DINES

Smoking   Approximately 28% of all men and 22% of all women are current cigarette smokers. Factors that influence smoking initiation, addiction, and smoking cessation as well as the health consequences of smoking are generally similar in men and women.

SMOKING INITIATION

Many women start to smoke as teenagers. Current figures indicate that, in 2000, about 30% of high school senior girls have smoked in the past month. Reasons for starting to smoke include smoking for a calming and relaxing effect, smoking to lose weight, smoking as a social activity at parties or dinners, and smoking to increase alertness. According to the Centers for Disease Control, the prevalence of current smoking in women is associated with their educational level, poverty level, and racial/ethnic group. Women with 9–11 years of education smoke more cigarettes than women with 16 or more years of education (33% vs. 11%). Women living below the poverty level smoke more cigarettes than those living at or about the poverty level (30% vs. 22%). Lastly, in 1997–1998, the rates of smoking in the major racial/ethnic groups were as follows:

- American Indian or Alaskan Native—34.5%
- White—23.5%
- African American—21.9%
- Hispanic—13.8%
- Asian/Pacific Islander—11.2%

Two reasons that are often cited for the high rate of smoking in women include: (a) extensive, targeted marketing by the tobacco industry and (b) the addictive quality of nicotine. Since the 1920s, women have been extensively targeted in cigarette advertisements. Marketing efforts on television and in magazines generally presented the woman smoker as an independent, successful, stylish, and intelligent person. Also, regardless of the quantity of cigarettes smoked, smoking is addictive for many women. Nicotine appears to be the primary addictive agent in cigarette smoking. According to the American Lung Association, nicotine reaches the brain just 7 seconds after inhalation, causing a "high," pleasurable or calming effect. However, nicotine is metabolized quickly; smokers soon need more and more nicotine in their system to get similar effects. Shortly after, average smokers are smoking $1-1\frac{1}{2}$ packs of cigarettes a day; they soon become addicted to nicotine and experience withdrawal symptoms when they try to stop smoking. (See Nicotine entry for more details about its addictive properties.)

HEALTH CONSEQUENCES

Thirty years ago, the Surgeon General's Office first reported on the bad health consequences of cigarette smoking. Since then, cigarette smoking has been associated with disease, disability, and death. According to recent estimates, one of every five deaths in the United

States is smoking related. The leading causes of the approximately 430,000 smoking-related deaths each year are lung cancer, chronic obstructive pulmonary disease, and ischemic heart disease.

In his 2001 report, the Surgeon General writes "Clearly, smoking-related disease among women is a full-blown epidemic." Complications of smoking include increased risk for stroke, other cardiovascular and respiratory diseases, and cancer of the mouth, pharynx, larynx, and esophagus. Women smokers also seem to have an increased risk for conception delay, infertility, ectopic pregnancy, spontaneous abortion, and preterm delivery. Clinical studies in both men and women have examined nicotine's effect on the endocrine system. Several disorders that may be associated with cigarette smoking in women include menstrual dysfunction, early menopause, estrogen deficiency disorders, and osteoporosis.

Economically, an estimated $80 billion of total U.S. health care costs each year is attributable to smoking. This figure increases to $138 billion when additional costs from smoking-related fires, medical care costs from secondhand smoke, and care of babies born to smoking mothers are considered.

SMOKING DURING PREGNANCY

According to the 2001 Surgeon General's Report on Women and Smoking, estimates of women smoking during pregnancy range from 12% to 22%. Smoking during pregnancy is associated with increased risk for preterm delivery and lower than average infant birth weight. Therefore, recommendations for pregnant smokers include: stop smoking throughout the pregnancy, obtain self-help materials from your physician/obstetrician, and participate in a stop-smoking program.

SMOKING CESSATION

According to the National Institute on Drug Abuse, nearly 35 million people make a serious attempt to quit smoking each year. About 7% of those who try to quit on their own succeed, defined as being able to stop smoking for more than 1 year. Many smokers try to quit about 7–8 times before they are successful; these numbers mean that most persons return to smoking after a few days of attempting to quit. These high relapse rates reflect nicotine addiction and the resultant difficulty in quitting smoking. Ex-smokers quickly experience mood changes, irritability, and cravings as they withdraw from nicotine. Also, withdrawal symptoms are usually worst during the first few days of abstinence.

Because of the physiological discomforts of nicotine withdrawal, there are numerous methods available that can assist smokers with their cessation efforts. The methods include: self-help materials (many of these can be obtained free from the National Cancer Institute or the American Lung Association), counseling (individual, group, and telephone), and pharmacotherapy. Unfortunately, many insurance companies do not provide coverage for these efforts to quit.

Most persons who try to quit smoking under the care of a physician are encouraged to use one or more of the available pharmacotherapies (although special medical circumstances such as pregnancy/breast-feeding may limit the physician's recommendations). Firstline pharmacotherapy methods include nicotine replacement (gum, patch, inhaler, and nasal spray) and Bupropion SR (Zyban/Wellbutrin), which needs a prescription. These pharmacotherapies have been approved by the U.S. Food and Drug Administration (FDA) for their use for smoking cessation. Studies of Nicotine Replacement Therapy (NRT) and Bupropion SR indicate that these pharmacotherapies are also prescribed to alleviate depressive symptoms or to delay weight gain following smoking cessation.

In women, factors that are associated with success at smoking cessation include pregnancy, weight gain, and social support. Many women stop smoking during pregnancy. However, at least two thirds of women who stop smoking during pregnancy are smoking again by 12 months after delivery. Also, many women worry that they will gain weight if they quit smoking. Studies indicate that the majority of people who quit smoking do gain weight, but the health consequences of continuing to smoke far outweigh the consequences from the weight gain. Lastly, family and friends who support the smoker's cessation effort help improve cessation rates.

SOCIAL ATTITUDES

Social attitudes toward cigarette smoking have changed dramatically over the last 30 years. According to the American Lung Association, smoking used to be thought of as "cool"; now it has become less socially acceptable. In fact, most states restrict smoking by law in public places, while many workplaces have no-smoking policies.

The 2001 Surgeon General's Report on Women and Smoking concludes that what is needed to reduce smoking among women include the following:

- Increased awareness of the impact of smoking on women's health
- Expose and counter the tobacco industry's targeting of women
- Conduct further studies of the relationship between smoking and health outcomes
- Support efforts to reduce exposure to environmental tobacco smoke among women (see entry on Tobacco)

SEE ALSO: Nicotine, Tobacco

Suggested Reading

Froom, P., Melamed, S., & Benbassat, J. (1998). Smoking cessation and weight gain. *Journal of Family Practice, 46,* 460–464.

United States Department of Health and Human Services. (2000, June). *Clinical practice guidelines for treating tobacco use and dependence.* Washington, D.C.: author.

United States Department of Health and Human Services. (2001). *Women and smoking: A report of the surgeon general.* Rockville, MD: Author. [Copies of this report can be obtained through the Office on Smoking and Health of the Centers for Disease Control and Prevention at (770) 488-5705 or www.cdc.gov/tobacco]

Suggested Resources

American Lung Association national website: http://www.lungusa.org

MARILYN DAVIES

Social Security Disability Benefits

Hubert Humphrey observed that "The moral test of government is how it treats those who are in the dawn of life, the children; those who are in the twilight of life, the aged; and those who are in the shadows of life, the sick, the needy and the handicapped." According to the Social Security Administration, the Social Security Act aims to provide for the material needs of individuals and families, protect aged and disabled persons against the expenses of illnesses that may otherwise use up their savings, keep families together, and give children the chance to grow up healthy and secure. These programs, designed to make all of us feel and be more socially secure, include both federal and state benefits commonly known as Social Security retirement or disability benefits, and Supplemental Security Income (SSI), as well as Medicare, Medicaid, and all the public assistance or human services programs sometimes known as Welfare.

Some of the programs are need-based or means-tested, meaning that you must have low income and assets to qualify. Entitlement to other programs, notably Social Security retirement and disability benefits, is earned through Federal Insurance Contributions Act (FICA) paycheck contributions. The worker may think of it as paying an insurance premium on a policy that will entitle her to future benefits, even though today's workers are paying for today's beneficiaries.

The eligibility criteria for the means-tested programs vary; sometimes income guidelines are tied to the Federal Poverty Level. To be eligible for SSI disability benefits, for example, you are allowed to have no more than $2,000 in assets, not counting your home and car, and any income (over a minimal, specified amount) will reduce the benefit, depending on whether the income is earned or unearned. To give people receiving public benefits the incentive to return to work, earned income is often treated more kindly than unearned income when it comes to calculating benefits, and various trial work periods allow disabled people to venture back into the workforce as soon as they can.

To attain insured status or become vested in the Social Security system, a worker must generally have worked 20 out of the last 40 quarters, or 5 of the last 10 years. Quarters of coverage are now known as credits, but whatever the updated term may be, you may want to know, at any given point in your life, whether you are insured or not. As you plan your future (or reflect on your past) as a stay-at-home parent or homemaker, keep in mind that over time, a number of zero years can reduce the amount of retirement benefits available on your own work record (as opposed to that of your wage-earning spouse, or divorced spouse).

While the means-tested SSI benefit for noninsured disabled and elderly people is in the neighborhood of $552/month, the Social Security retirement or disability benefit may be higher, as high as $1,700/month or so, plus auxiliary benefits for dependent children, depending on how much the worker earned and contributed to the system during her working years. Various offsets may apply (workers' compensation, veterans' benefits), to preserve the notion that working should always be more financially attractive than drawing disability benefits. If the Social Security amount is less than the SSI amount, the individual may be eligible for both concurrent benefits.

Perhaps two of the most unsettling aspects of the Social Security benefits system are that disability coverage does not last forever, and that not every disabled person is entitled to government benefits. First, women and others who work in the home should be aware that Social Security Disability Insurance coverage does not typically last more than 5 years after a period of steady work, called your date last insured or DLI. So the mother of the 6-year-old who seriously injures herself in a household or car accident is not likely to be eligible for Social Security disability benefits, no matter how much she contributed to the Social Security system before trading her career in the paid workforce for her unpaid position raising a family. And we all know how much it costs to try to pay someone to do everything a mom does. She is irreplaceable and her work invaluable.

Second, not every disabled person is entitled to government benefits. A claimant may be entitled to disability benefits under one, both, or *neither* of two different programs: Social Security Disability Insurance and Supplemental Security Income (SSI). What this means is that some very disabled people, often women who have not worked much outside the home over the years, will not be entitled to *any* government benefit because they have neither earned the right to draw Social Security benefits on their own work record nor are they impoverished enough to be eligible for SSI.

The Social Security Administration's assessment of disability, considered by many to incorporate quite a rigorous standard, is the same for both programs and turns on a five-step sequential evaluation. The only people who get Social Security Disability or SSI are those found to be totally and permanently disabled. Claimants do not get more money the more disabled they are. To be disabled, a claimant must (a) not be working at an income level known as substantial gainful activity (self-employment is a special case with rules that look at how much time the claimant puts in and how much money the claimant takes out, and how other unimpaired people in that business fare); (b) suffer from a severe medically determinable impairment that lasts at least 12 months; (c) either meet a listed impairment or suffer from an impairment so severe that it (d) prevents return to past relevant work performed in the last 15 years and (e) prevents entry into other jobs existing in significant numbers in the national economy. For this final criterion,

Social Security needs only to prove that the jobs exist somewhere in the United States—it is not a matter of whether there are openings, whether you can get hired, pass the physical exam, or whether you can reach any such jobs by car or bus from where you live.

Social Security's Listing of Impairments covers Musculoskeletal, Respiratory, Cardiovascular, Neurological, Digestive, Genito-Urinary, Hemic and Lymphatic, Endocrine, Multiple Body, and Immune Systems, as well as Special Senses and Speech, Skin, Mental Disorders, and Neoplastic Malignant Diseases. A person who meets a listing—for example, a person who has not just one but *two* amputated limbs, or a 5 ft. 4 in. woman whose gastrointestinal disorder has shrunk her to less than 91 pounds—should qualify instantly for benefits.

The combination of a person's physical and mental impairments may not be listing-level, but may nevertheless be severe enough to reduce the claimant's capacity so much that she cannot sustain full-time employment. The Social Security rules do reflect the basic idea that the older a worker gets, the less we demand, both physically and mentally, of her. Age is key, particularly the 50th and 55th birthdays, unless someone has skills that can be used at a sedentary, desk-type job. Some people are chagrined to learn that Social Security does not cover skilled workers with professional or technical expertise just because they can no longer perform their job as doctor or plumber. A 44-year-old brain surgeon who loses only one hand or one eye may have to prove not only that she can no longer perform surgery, but also that she cannot do a stint as the minimum-wage worker at the circular desk in the middle of the shopping mall who points people in the direction of the shoe store.

Certain other Social Security benefits are part of the safety net woven by the workers. For example, Surviving Spouse benefits are available to widows over 60, or 50 and disabled. In certain limited circumstances, a remarried woman can keep receiving widow's benefits on her deceased husband's earnings record. Older women receiving benefits should always explore the financial implications of remarriage, no matter which time around it is. Disabled Adult Child (DAC) benefits are available to developmentally disabled adult children whose parents retire, become disabled, or die. An interesting sidelight: a DAC may not marry and maintain benefits, unless she marries another DAC. Child's SSI is available to help support severely disabled children, but only if their parents have very little in the way of income and assets. Social Security provides no automatic family benefit to full-time wage-earners with some savings who happen to have a disabled minor child or spouse.

Nationally, about 50% of claimants who apply for Social Security disability benefits are eventually granted benefits. In some regions, it can take over a year, sometimes two, to obtain benefits under this system. If a claimant chooses to hire a lawyer, consider that legal fees are highly regulated to protect vulnerable and often desperate claimants from unscrupulous lawyers. If the case goes all the way to federal court, sometimes the U.S. government will be required to pay the claimant's legal bill under the Equal Access to Justice Act (EAJA), a law intended to help individual citizens fight city hall. If you are receiving private long-term disability (LTD) benefits, do not lightly abandon your SSD claim even if you see no immediate dollar benefit, because Medicare eligibility (after 2 years on SSD) and your retirement benefits can be affected by the decisions you make now.

SEE ALSO: Disability, Medicaid, Medicare

Suggested Reading

House Ways and Means Committee. *The 2000 green book: Background material and data on programs within the jurisdiction of the Committee on Ways and Means* (17th ed.).
Social Security Administration. (2001). *Social Security handbook* (14th ed.).
Social Security Administration (2003). *Social Security: What every Woman should know* (SSA Publ. No. 05-10127, ICN 480667).
Treanor, J. R. (2002). *2002 Mercer guide to Social Security and Medicare* (30th ed.). New York: William Mercer.

JANET L. LOWDER
MARY B. MCKEE

Social Stress Social stress plays a major role in a person's well-being. While many researchers do not differentiate between the terms social stress and stress, social stress is differentiated from physical stress in that physical stress is due to stressors that are directly taxing the physical condition of the body such as excessive physical labor or physical restraint. Social stress has been found to be deleterious to health across a variety of outcomes (see entry on Stress). In a study of mice, socially stressed mice were more likely to die after exposure to infection relative to physically stressed mice. In this study, socially stressed mice were defined as those that were put in a cage for a portion of the day with an aggressive mouse whereas physical stress was defined as being physically restrained in a cylindrical tube for 16 hours a day with no food or water.

Human studies are complicated by the fact that responses to stressors are dependent on the individual experiencing the stressor. The coping mechanisms that follow a stressful event have been described in the Transactional Model of Stress and Coping. In this model, the impact of a stressor is mediated by the person's appraisal of the stressor. Two appraisals are made including a primary assessment and a secondary assessment. The primary assessment allows an individual to decide whether the stressor is good or bad and important or irrelevant. The secondary appraisal ascertains whether the individual believes that they can alter or manage the situation and/or deal with the emotions that come along with the stressor.

These assessments are mediated by different coping mechanisms. Generally, two different coping mechanisms are described. The first is problem management coping (problem-focused), in which efforts are focused on changing the stressor or the stressful situation. This may include problem solving or information seeking. The second coping strategy is emotional regulation coping (emotion-focused), in which efforts are focused on changing one's feelings about the stressor or stressful situation. This may include denial, venting of feelings, avoidance, and seeking social support.

Other lines of research have investigated the degree to which a person engages (i.e., active coping, information seeking, social support) or disengages (i.e., cognitive or behavioral avoidance, denial) from the stressor. When the stressor is very threatening or not perceived to be under one's control, disengaging coping strategies are often used. On the contrary, when the stressor is perceived to be controllable, engaging coping strategies may be more likely. In general, research shows there are psychological benefits to using active coping styles over disengaging coping styles, at least in the long term. Furthermore, avoidant coping styles have been associated with negative health behaviors. These coping mechanisms may be moderated by psychological traits including optimism, locus of control, information-seeking styles along with social support and stress management interventions. While coping efforts may vary over different stressors, coping styles or psychological traits are inherent characteristics of the individual and remain constant over situations.

Women often face different stressful situations than men. Women are more likely to perform multiple roles such as childcare provider and housekeeper as well as working for pay. In addition, women who work for pay are often in occupations where they experience or perceive to experience high psychological demands/high strain coupled with low control. This combination of high strain and low control has been associated with a higher risk of coronary heart disease and worse self-reported health.

Due to the deleterious effects of stress, various recommendations have been made for reducing general stress. These recommendations include making time in your life for leisure activities, setting reasonable goals, getting help with regular chores, not agreeing to do too many things (i.e., learn to say no), engaging in more demanding or enjoyable activities during your body's peak hours, and identifying sources of stress. In addition, several specific physical recommendations have been suggested including breathing deeply, engaging in relaxation techniques, and exercising one's shoulders and neck muscles.

Stress can have a major effect on one's health. It is important to recognize stress as a normal part of life, but also realize that chronic stress can have ill-effects on the body. Understanding the stress process, coping styles, and ways to combat stress is the first step for better well-being.

SEE ALSO: Parenting, Social support

Suggested Reading

Bosma, H., Marmot, M. G., Hemingway, H., Nicholson, A. C., Brunner, E., & Stansfeld, S. A. (1997). Low job control and risk of coronary heart disease in Whitehall II (prospective cohort) study. *British Medical Journal, 314*(7080), 558–565.

Cassel, J. (1976). The contribution of the social environment to host resistance. *American Journal of Epidemiology, 104*, 107–123.

Ibrahim, S. A., Scott, F. E., Cole, D. C., Shannon, H. S., & Eyles, J. (2001). Job strain and self-reported health among working women and men: An analysis of the 1994/5 Canadian National Population Health Survey. *Women and Health, 33*(1–2), 105–124.

Lazarus, R. S. (1993). Coping theory and research: Past, present, and future. *Psychosomatic Medicine, 55*(3), 234–247.

Lerman, C., & Glanz, K. (1997). Stress, coping, and health behavior. In K. Glanz, F. M. Lewis, & B. Rimer (Eds.), *Health behavior and health education: Theory, research and practice* (2nd ed.). San Francisco: Jossey-Bass.

Quan, N., Avitsur, R., Stark, J. L., He, L., Shah, M., Caligiuri, M., et al. (2001, April 2). Social stress increases the susceptibility to endotoxic shock. *Journal of Neuroimmunology, 115*, 36–45.

NATALIE COLABIANCHI

Social Support

Social support is the help and assistance or exchange of resources that is given by others within a person's social network (i.e., a person's web of social relationships) with the intent to enhance the recipient's well-being. Social support was first identified as a protective factor against deleterious effects of stress on health by Cassel in 1976. He suggested furthermore that social support was important in the etiology of many diseases. Since this time, many studies have confirmed the association between the lack of social ties or social networks and mortality for almost every cause of death. It is thought that social support provides a basic human need, namely, the need for companionship, intimacy, and reassurance of self-worth. Furthermore, social support is thought to increase one's sense of personal control by providing information, new contacts, and new ways to solve problems.

While many types of social support have been identified, social support is generally divided into four categories: instrumental support, emotional support, informational support, and appraisal support. Instrumental support includes tangible actions that directly aid the person in need, such as getting groceries, helping someone to an appointment, cooking, cleaning, etc. Emotional support is often the support given by an intimate partner or confidant, although it can be given by others. It includes support that provides love, understanding, trust, sympathy, and/or caring. Informational support is the provision of advice or aid that a person can use to address their problem(s). One segment of this support has been to referred to as "weak ties," which have shown to be quite powerful for activities such as finding a job or health care provider. Finally, appraisal support is communications related to the provision of advice or dialogue useful for self-evaluation.

In general, the association between social support and health does not follow a dose–response effect, but rather low levels of social support are most harmful with a leveling-off of the effect at some threshold level. Furthermore, the type of social support that is most helpful may vary by age or stage of development. For example, after the passing of a spouse, close dense networks have been found to be important (i.e., emotional support), but later in the process, more diffuse networks with access to new social ties and information are more helpful (i.e., informational support). In addition, not all support given is equally effective. In general, those who have experienced the same stressor and are at the same social position are thought to provide the most effective social support because they would likely be more empathic and more likely to provide relevant support regardless of type (i.e., emotional, information, appraisal, or instrumental).

Social support can influence health in at least three ways. First, it may facilitate health-promoting behaviors. Second, it may give an individual a sense of meaning in their lives, and third, it may produce feelings and thoughts that promote health (i.e., reduction in stress). Several specific research studies on social support are worth noting. First, several animal studies have shown the negative effect of isolation on health. Specifically, female monkeys housed alone developed more atherosclerosis than female monkeys housed in small groups. Furthermore, monkeys caged alone had higher heart rates under average conditions compared to those that lived in groups.

In an interesting human study, participants were asked to give a public talk. Half of the participants (randomly assigned) were told that there would be someone available to them before they presented in case they needed any help (although in reality no help was provided nor asked for). The other half of the participants were not offered this avenue of support. The researchers found that systolic and diastolic pressure were higher both before the public talk and during the talk in the group that was not offered any support when compared to the group that was told there would be someone there to help them if they needed it.

Social isolation has been shown to be related to all-cause mortality across 13 cohort studies in many countries. Specifically, in Alameda County, those who did not have many social ties to others were 2–3 times more likely to die during the follow-up period (9 years) compared to those with many social ties. The risk for dying was not associated with any one disease but rather a multitude of different diseases including: ischemic heart disease, cancer, and circulatory disease. Other conflicting studies have shown this risk for men but not for women.

The role of social support and specific diseases has not shown a consistent effect across studies. However, over the last several years there have been several studies that have shown social ties have a protective effect on survival after myocardial infarction and for those with serious cardiovascular disease. Similarly, social support has been shown to be important for those recovering from stroke. Finally, having social contact may provide resistance against the development of infection including the common cold. In a study where participants were given nasal drops with rhinovirus, those with more social ties were less likely to develop a cold, had less mucus associated with the cold, and shed less virus even after controlling for virus-specific antibody, virus type, age, gender, season, BMI, education, and race. Furthermore, there was a dose–response of decreased colds to increased diversity of social network.

The earliest literature for social support focused on the association between social relations and health for men. As the research expanded to include women, many studies found that the same associations were not found for women or the associations were weaker, although some studies have shown similar effects for men and women. The health benefits of marriage, a potential form of social support, have been the subject of many research studies. Studies have consistently shown that married persons have better health outcomes than divorced or separated persons and that single men have poorer health outcomes than married persons, although single women do not have poorer health outcomes than married persons. While several theories have been advanced to explain why married women could have poorer health relative to single women, it has been hypothesized that as women gain increasing opportunities in the workforce and with changes in marital roles, these differences will disappear.

Men and women may also differ in the types and quantity of social support received and given. Women tend to have both larger and more varied social networks. Furthermore, they are more likely to report having a close confidant who is not their spouse. They generally spend more time than men giving and receiving support and are said to have a wider range of opportunities for emotional support. On the other hand, women are more likely to have negative interactions with those members of their network and have more negative effects from marital conflict relative to men. It is important to consider these gender differences when trying to examine the association between support and health, as different ways of quantifying support may lead to different conclusions. For example, researchers found that when information from up to four close people was used to describe support, gender differences was attenuated, and in some cases eliminated when examining physical and psychological health.

When conceptualizing social support, it is important to view social support within the broader spectrum of the social relationships in which social support exists. Social support is provided by one's social network, which is one's web of personal social relationships. Social networks can vary by size, density, boundedness, and homogeneity. They have also been described by intensity and complexity. Size in a social network represents the number of members in one's network; density is the extent to which members know and interact with one another; boundedness is the degree to which the relationships are based on traditional group structures; homogeneity is the extent to which they are similar. Intensity in a social network is the extent to which the relationship offers emotional closeness, and complexity is the extent to which the relationship serves different functions. Social relationships also vary in the extent of frequency of contact, duration, and reciprocity.

While one's social network provides the opportunity for social support, it also provides opportunities for social influence or norms, social engagement, person-to-person contact, and access to resources and material goods. Within a network, the existence of normative behavior has an important influence on the behaviors of others. In particular for adolescents, peer behavior is one of the best predictors for behavior. So, for example, if a large percentage of people within a network smoke, the nonsmokers may be more likely to take up the habit. Norms can affect various health behaviors such as smoking, alcohol use, and eating patterns as well as health utilization patterns.

In addition to social support and social norms, social networks also provide opportunities for social engagement or social participation, including such activities as social functions, church-going, getting together with friends, and the like. These activities help define and reinforce one's social role in both the family and community, which provides a sense of belonging and attachment. It is believed that this sense of belongingness can give meaning to one's life, which results in longevity. Person-to-person contact can influence disease directly via contact with others who are infectious. Finally, social networks can influence access to material goods and resources, such as job opportunities and quality health care.

These five mechanisms through which social networks can influence disease in turn can affect health behavior, psychological pathways, and physiologic pathways. Health behaviors do not appear to explain a large amount of the relationship between social networks and mortality, although methodological difficulties may be in part to blame. Psychological mechanisms including self-efficacy, self-esteem, depression, and coping styles are influenced by social networks generally and social support specifically. Social support has been shown to influence smoking cessation and depression through enhanced self-efficacy. Furthermore, it is thought that self-efficacy mediates the relationship between social networks and engaging in health-promoting behaviors such as exercise. In addition to self-efficacy, social support is associated with emotional states including depression, and has been shown to moderate the effect of stress on depression. Finally, the pathway between social networks and disease can also be physiological, via immune system functioning, allostatic load, transmission of infectious disease, and cardiovascular reactivity to name a few. Unfortunately, this is the least researched aspect of social networks and social support and much of the work that has been done in this area is in animal studies only.

The pathway from social networks to the subsequent five psychosocial mechanisms (social support, social influence, social participation, person-to-person contact, and access to resources) as well as the specific pathways to illness (i.e., health behaviors, psychological pathways, and physiological pathways) are all preceded by larger social forces including culture, socioeconomic factors, historic social change, politics, and policies. This results in a complex framework of pathways and mechanisms through which social networks and social support influences health. The challenge is to develop better measures and utilize causal modeling to elucidate these pathways and mechanisms in order to better understand these important relationships.

SEE ALSO: Marital status, Stress

Suggested Reading

Arber, S., & Khlat, M. (2002). Introduction to "social and economic patterning of women's health in a changing world." *Social Science and Medicine, 54*, 643–647.

Berkman, L. F. (1995). The role of social relations in health promotion. *Psychosomatic Medicine, 57*(3), 245–254.

Berkman, L. F., & Glass, T. (2000). Social integration, social networks, social support, and health. In L. F. Berkman & I. Kawachi (Eds.), *Social epidemiology.* New York: Oxford University Press.

Callaghan, P., & Morrissey, J. (1993). Social support and health: A review. *Journal of Advanced Nursing, 18*, 203–210.

Fuhrer, R., & Stansfeld, S. A. (2002). How gender affects patterns of social relations and their impact on health: A comparison of one or multiple sources of support from "close persons." *Social Science and Medicine, 54*, 811–825.

Heaney, C. A., & Israel, B. A. (1997). Social networks and social support. In K. Glanz, F. M. Lewis, & B. K. Rimer (Eds.), *Health behavior and health education: Theory, research and practice* (2nd ed.). San Francisco: Jossey-Bass.

House, J. S. (1981). *Work stress and social support.* Reading, MA: Addison-Wesley.

House, J. S., Landis, K. R., & Umberson, D. (1988). Social relationships and health. *Science, 241*(4865), 540–545.

Israel, B. A. (1982). Social networks and health status: Linking theory, research and practice. *Patient Counselling and Health Education, 4,* 65–79.

Turner, H. A. (1994). Gender and social support—taking the bad with the good. *Sex Roles, 30*(7–8), 521–541.

NATALIE COLABIANCHI

Socioeconomic Status Socioeconomic status (SES) is a concept intended to describe one's position in society. While SES is one of the terms most often used to describe this concept in the literature, SES has also been called social class, social status, socioeconomic position, and social inequality (although some of these terms are also used to represent distinct concepts). SES was originally described by Karl Marx as a group's relation to the means of production, but has been more recently described by Weber to include three dimensions: class, status, and party or power. Since these factors describe one's relationship to their work and others, these factors are not an inherent property of an individual, but rather are created by society. Consequently these social relationships exist prior to the factors by which SES is operationally measured (i.e., income, education, and occupation).

SES is a strong and consistent predictor of morbidity and premature mortality. This relationship has been observed for centuries. Even with the relatively recent improvements in standards of living and medical care across the globe, this relationship still holds. Furthermore, this relationship between SES and health is seen across the span of SES levels. This is often referred to as the SES gradient. For example, the upper class has better health outcomes than the upper-middle class, the upper-middle class has better health outcomes than the middle class, and so on.

Often the relationship between SES and disease is so strong that it does not matter which measure of SES is used. However, for some diseases, the effect of SES and disease differs depending on the measure of social class.

The mixed results may be a result of methodological differences across studies or may signify that the different measures of SES are distinct but related components. Furthermore, as will be described, each measure of SES has its own limitations.

Education is the most popular single indicator of SES, likely due to the simplicity of measurement, its ability to categorize the nonactive labor force, and because of its association with many lifestyle characteristics. For most adults, this measure is more stable than either occupation or income. However, one limitation is that education levels vary by the age cohort of the individual. Many more people have graduated from high school and college in the past 20 years compared to the years prior. Furthermore, the earning potential of someone who was a high school graduate in the 1950s is different than a person graduating with a high school degree in the 1990s. Mandatory minimum age requirements for leaving school and increased opportunities for greater education are resulting in homogeneity of the population's years of education. A further complication with using education is deciding how to categorize education. Often "years of schooling" is used, however, some have argued that academic degrees are more relevant. Furthermore, types of degrees earned and area of education may also be relevant.

The income measure of SES can be used as a quantitative measure but is often grouped into categories due to people's reluctance and/or inability to report their exact income. The sensitivity of this information is often problematic since many are unwilling to give out their income level, even in broad categories. Further complications with this measure include that it is relatively unstable over time and is age-dependent since income tends to rise throughout one's career and then drop after retirement. Furthermore, income does not necessarily equate to purchasing power or available money and household size, and regional differences in costs of living can also affect income.

Occupation is the most complex of the three single SES measures. There are several standard scales by which SES occupational status can be measured. However, many of these scales are based on data that were collected over 20 years ago and the categories were based on the judgments of persons with various degrees of familiarity with each occupation.

In addition to measurement problems with single indicators of SES, there are also problems with defining SES for special groups. For example, woman's social class is often determined on the basis of her husband (if married) and sometimes by her father if unmarried. Furthermore, many of the scales developed for measuring occupation were created based exclusively on the male workforce. Occupational scales have been deemed less useful for assessing occupation status for African Americans, since it has been suggested that African Americans assign social class on a different scale than whites. Furthermore, the financial rewards for the same level of education are greater for white males compared to African American males. Finally, measuring the occupation and income for the elderly can be difficult, since many are in retirement. One must decide whether they will use their last job, the job they held for the longest period of time, or some other measure.

The strong relationship between SES and health has prompted many to consider how SES affects health. Research has shown that no one factor can be shown to account exclusively or entirely for the effects between SES and health, although several factors have been described repeatedly. Many have attributed the health gradient that exists among levels of SES to differential access to medical care. Research has shown that those with lower SES are more likely to have less access to care. However, lack of access to care is not sufficient to explain the entire relationship between SES and health since countries that have universal access to health care, such as England, still experience the SES gradient. Furthermore, since there are differences in health all along the SES spectrum, and those at the medium and high levels of SES are all likely to have access to care, it is unlikely that access to health care explains the difference entirely. Of course, access to care means more than just insurance coverage and those with lower SES may have more difficulty finding available doctors and may have more problems getting to the doctor (due to transportation or job conflicts). In addition, some have proposed that the quality of doctors may be different in areas of low-SES residents.

Poor health behaviors, such as smoking, poor diet, and lack of exercise, have an inverse linear relationship with SES. For example, smoking rate for those with less than a high school education is 45%, compared to 19% for those with advanced degrees. Similarly, the risk factors that go along with these behaviors, such as high cholesterol levels, obesity, and high blood pressure, are associated with lower SES. Recently, researchers have investigated the reasons why those with lower SES engage in unhealthy risk behavior more often than those with higher SES. Some proposed reasons include increased advertising and access to cigarettes and alcohol in the neighborhood in which they live as well as decreased availability of healthy foods.

Physical environment has also been proposed as a factor related to the relationship between SES and health. The lower an individual is in the SES hierarchy, the more likely that that they will be exposed to adverse environmental conditions at work or at home, such as exposures to carcinogens or pathogens, and sanitation problems.

There is increasing evidence that stress plays an important role in the development of disease, in particular, heart disease and susceptibility to infection. Studies have shown that those with lower SES status are more likely to report being exposed to stressful events. Furthermore, the perception of the stressfulness of these events may be directly related to SES since those with higher education levels or more income may have more resources to resolve or reduce the impact of these events.

Many adolescents who grow up poor are thought to discount the future, perhaps because they do not feel that they will live into adulthood. This theory, called Fuch's time preference theory, can explain both lower educational attainment and poor health behaviors, since both would require an investment in the future.

Many studies have reported health disparities across different racial and ethnic groups. Many have attributed these differences to SES since, in general, minorities are disproportionately represented in lower SES groups. To substantiate this, many studies have found no racial or ethnic differences after controlling for SES. However, other studies have found that controlling for SES does reduce the racial and ethnic differences but does not eliminate it completely. Many have attributed these residual differences in part to racial discrimination.

Some researchers have argued that even if you would consider all these factors that are related to SES and would control for them, studies would still find an association of SES and health because SES is a fundamental cause of disease. In general, studies focus on a single disease and a single cause at a single point in time. However, risk factors and the potential social factors that affect health are dynamic and change over time. As new risk factors emerge, those with higher SES are in a more favorable position to know about the risks and have the means to protect themselves against these new risks.

SES is clearly an important factor in health outcomes. Given the various ways to measure SES along with the multitude of factors that are associated with SES, researchers have argued for further research into SES, specifically its theoretical conception as well as standardized or at least consistent measurement of SES in all public health databases. Other suggestions include considering various time periods to measure one's SES, for example, childhood SES versus adult SES. Another important avenue of investigation is determining the relevant level of SES, meaning individual, household, and/or neighborhood, since it has been found that an individual's SES and their neighborhood's SES can have independent effects on their health.

Additional research is also needed to examine whether and how the effects of SES may be different for women compared to men. Most of the research up until the late 1980s focused exclusively on men and how their occupation affected health. However, there are many economic issues that are specific to women. Single mothers and women who live alone are vulnerable to living in poverty. There are a growing number of single-parent households, of which the majority are headed by females. Female-headed households have median incomes below those of male-headed households or married households. Consequently, these women face the same stressors from assuming various roles (i.e., childcare, household management, paid work), but have less monetary resources to combat these stressors. The increase in single-parent households is a function of increased childbearing outside of marriage and, more often, because of divorce. Further research is needed to examine how changes in SES after a divorce affect women's health relative to men, particularly, since a decline in the standards of living is often seen in the first year after a divorce for women.

There are still inequalities in pay for women in the same positions as men and women are more likely to carry out unpaid work. Presently, it is not clear the degree to which the dual role of paid and unpaid (i.e., household duties) work affects women's health. Finally, there are important cohort effects in the SES of women. Women across generations have experienced very different social and economic environments and it is important to incorporate a life course perspective when examining the association between women and SES.

Given the increasing disparity in health outcomes and increasing income inequality, understanding SES is an important goal for public health practitioners. It is only through understanding the mechanism through which SES exerts its effects that we will be able to address these growing health disparities.

SEE ALSO: Disparities in Women's Health and Health Care (pp. 13–20)

Suggested Reading

Adler, N. E., Boyce, T., Chesney, M. A., Cohen, S., Folkman, S., Kahn, R. L., et al. (1994). Socioeconomic status and health. The challenge of the gradient. *American Psychologist, 49*(1), 15–24.

Adler, N. E., Boyce, W. T., Chesney, M. A., Folkman, S., & Syme, S. L. (1993). Socioeconomic inequalities in health. No easy solution. *Journal of the American Medical Association, 269*(24), 3140–3145.

Arber, S., & Khlat, M. (2002). Introduction to "social and economic patterning of women's health in a changing world." *Social Science and Medicine, 54*, 643–647.

Feinstein, J. S. (1993). The relationship between socioeconomic status and health: A review of the literature. *Milbank Quarterly, 71*(2), 279–322.

Krieger, N., Williams, D. R., & Moss, N. E. (1997). Measuring social class in US public health research: Concepts, methodologies, and guidelines. *Annual Review of Public Health, 18*, 341–378.

Liberatos, P., Link, B. G., & Kelsey, J. L. (1988). The measurement of social class in epidemiology. *Epidemiologic Reviews, 10*, 87–121.

Link, B. G., & Phelan, J. (1995). Social conditions as fundamental causes of disease. *Journal of Health and Social Behavior,* Spec. No, 80–94.

Lynch, J., & Kaplan, G. (2000). Socioeconomic position. In L. F. Berkman & I. Kawachi (Eds.), *Social epidemiology.* New York: Oxford University Press.

Marmot, M. G., Fuhrer, R., Ettner, S. L., Marks, N. F., Bumpass, L. L., & Ryff, C. D. (1998). Contribution of psychosocial factors to socioeconomic differences in health. *Milbank Quarterly, 76*(3), 403–448.

Strobino, D. M., Grason, H., & Minkovitz, C. (2002). Charting a course for the future of women's health in the United States: Concepts, findings and recommendations. *Social Science and Medicine, 54*, 839–848.

NATALIE COLABIANCHI

Spirituality Spirituality is not easily defined. By its very nature it is personal and private. Spirituality concerns our human awareness of and relationship to those aspects of life that are intangible. Spirituality involves our awareness of being a part of something greater and more powerful than ourselves, yet something we cannot touch or see. Unlike science, spirituality seeks to know the intangible. It involves a belief in a power outside of our own existence. One definition of spirituality is "my relationship with that which exceeds me utterly." This definition suggests the relationship of spirituality to the human experience of awe and wonder. It generates our sense of unity with and a reverence for all existence.

Spirituality differs from religion although the two are closely connected. Religion refers to a codified or organized system of beliefs, values, codes of conduct, and rituals. Religious practice is often taken as one indication of the strength of belief or commitment that an individual has to their spiritual life. However, this is found to be an inadequate measure. Spirituality is broader than religious practice and religious practice may sometimes interfere with spiritual awareness.

Current studies suggest that the medical benefits derived from spirituality are directly related to the strength of belief and the intrinsic involvement of the individual in their spiritual commitment. Religious practice in and of itself does not necessarily relate to the depth or strength of one's faith. Health benefits are derived from the sincerity and importance that the individual attaches to his or her spiritual involvement whatever form this may take.

Spirituality is also concerned with establishing one's sense of life's meaning. Meaning derived from spirituality should be differentiated from the philosophical approach to meaning. A philosophical belief finds an existential meaning for a particular life experience. It does not reference any external power or being and is an intellectual understanding. While important, it does not include a spiritual dimension. For many people, spirituality is vital in establishing life's meaning. More than 70% surveyed reported that religious faith was the most important influence in their lives.

SCIENCE, MEDICINE, AND SPIRITUALITY

The separation of spirituality from health and healing is unique to Western medicine. Throughout time and cultures, spiritual belief and practices were inherently linked with healing practices. The age of enlightenment began the move toward empirical study, which began to dominate much of Western thinking. In the 18th and 19th centuries, science struggled to replace religion as the most appropriate way to understand nature. The scientific method produced discoveries that dramatically changed our lives including our approach to health and illness. While we enjoy the fruits of scientific progress, we are confronted with the negative outcomes from eliminating spirituality from our relationship to nature. This disjuncture is vitally important in the area of health and healing.

In recent years, medical researchers have turned their attention to the role of spirituality in medicine and health care. This burgeoning interest stemmed largely from a small number of studies suggesting that spiritual beliefs and practices improve health, well-being, and responses to medical care. Prior to the 1990s, medical science and religion had become so separate in Western culture that David Larson referred to spirituality as the "forgotten factor" in modern medicine. Medical studies ignored the role of religious or spiritual practices assuming they had no role in health outcome.

It has been suggested that the increasing use of alternative, nontraditional approaches to health care is the public's response to mainstream medicine's neglect of spirituality. In two recent national surveys, 70% of patients reported a belief that spiritual faith and prayer could aid in recovery from illness. Another 64% believe that physicians should talk to patients about spiritual issues as a part of their health care and indeed that physicians should pray with patients if the patients requested this.

Although scientific research ignored spirituality and religion, the general U.S. population placed a high value on spiritual and religious beliefs and practices. The Gallup organization conducted scientific polling regarding religious beliefs and practices among Americans over the last four decades. These studies showed that the proportion of Americans who believe in God remained remarkably constant. Ninety-six percent of Americans reported they believed in God in 1944 and ninety-four in 1986. In the general public, 66% considered religion to be the most important or a very important aspect of their lives and 40% reported that they attended services on a weekly basis.

A review of 212 studies examining the effects of religious commitment on health care outcomes found that 75% demonstrated a positive benefit of religious commitment. Of these studies, only 7% demonstrated a negative effect. This is not to suggest, however, that spirituality is a replacement for modern medical care. Rather, it is a potentially important addition. Ralph Snyderman, MD, Chancellor of Health Affairs at Duke University Medical Center, put this very well: "In the health care setting, science without spirituality is incomplete and spirituality without science is ineffective."

SPIRITUALITY AND PHYSICAL HEALTH

Studies are now available that suggest an active spiritual practice, most often in the form of religious practice, is beneficial to physical health. Other studies further suggest that spiritual practice helps in healing if one does become ill. A study published in 1999 included 21,000 U.S. adults followed over an extended period of time. The researchers found that attending religious services more than once a week correlated with an extended life span of at least 7 years. The impact was even greater for African Americans for whom weekly church attendance correlated with an additional 14 years. Regular, weekly attendance of religious services was the strongest predictor for living longer of all the relevant factors that they could identify. Another large study followed a group for 28 years and found that frequent church attenders were 25% less likely to die than the infrequent attenders.

Cardiovascular disease and hypertension are illnesses most extensively studied in relationship to spirituality and religious practices. Among the studies all but one suggested that religious commitment is associated with lower blood pressure and lower rates of hypertension. One study found that men who placed high importance on religion and had high attendance rates at religious services had mean blood pressure readings (diastolic pressures 5 mm) lower than those who did not place high importance on religious issues. It has been shown that a reduction of a mean blood pressure by as little as 2–4 mm could reduce cardiovascular disease by 10–20%. This reduction could also influence whether or not antihypertension medication is prescribed. Another study reported that people who attended religious study once a week and prayed or studied the Bible at least once a day were 40% less likely to have high blood pressure than those who do so less frequently or not at all.

Older adults were found to be less likely to be hospitalized if they regularly attended religious services. Further, older adults with religious affiliations who are hospitalized had stays that were two and a half times shorter than those without religious affiliations. Another study of 1,718 older adults found that those who attended church regularly had healthier immune systems. A study done at Dartmouth Medical School found that a constant predictor of who survived heart surgery was the strength of a patient's religious commitment. Elderly heart patients who were socially active and found strength in their religious faith were 14 times less likely to die following surgery. A study of heart transplant patients at the University of Pittsburgh found that those with strong beliefs and who participated in religious activities complied better with their medical regime and had better psychical functioning and

emotional well-being at their 12-month follow-ups. Even among smokers, regular church attendance provided some protection from hypertension. Smokers who regularly attended church were four times less likely to have high blood pressure than smokers who did not attend.

A study published in 1984 suggested that spirituality measured as church attendance was important for lowering mortality rates among women. In this study, 2,700 persons were followed for 8–10 years. Only one social factor effectively lowered mortality rates for women and this was increased church attendance. In this study, church attendance was not found to be protective for men. In another study, the risk of dying of atherosclerotic heart disease among women was about twice as high among infrequent church attenders compared to those who attended church weekly or more. This study also found that death rates from pulmonary emphysema and suicide were more than twice as high and death from cirrhosis of the liver was nearly four times as high among women who were infrequent church attenders. It is likely that cirrhosis was the result of higher alcoholism among women who chose not to attend church regularly.

Hip fractures are a serious cause of morbidity among elderly women. A study showed that elderly women recovering from hip fractures revealed that those with the best surgical outcome were those to whom God was a source of strength and comfort, and among those who frequently attended religious services.

In the 1990s, the Templeton Foundation began awarding grants to medical schools to support the addition of spiritual considerations in their curriculum. This has expanded to support teaching about spirituality in residencies in psychiatry, family practice, internal medicine, and obstetrics and gynecology. Some medical schools are developing programs in alternative medicine following the lead of Andrew Weil at the University of Arizona.

MENTAL HEALTH

The relationship of spirituality to mental health is an interesting one. Studies of the last several years have suggested that spiritual and religious practices support mental health in different ways. Some suggest that spiritual practice helps to improve self-esteem and especially that meditative practice will improve an overall state of greater calm and optimism. Involvement in a spiritual or religious community may also provide a supportive community and the consequent benefits of this.

Traditionally, psychiatry has taken a skeptical, if not a sometimes hostile, attitude toward spirituality or religion. This may relate to the fact that such problems as psychosis, depression, and hysteria were the last areas to be won over from the church as areas more relevant to medical concern. Freud, who dominated psychiatric thinking for the first half of the 20th century, proclaimed his own atheistic orientation and understood religious belief as illusions and generated by deep unacknowledged wishes. Albert Ellis, a psychologist, stated that "religiosity in many respects is equivalent to irrational thinking and emotional disturbance." Psychiatric clinicians tend to be less religious than the general population. While only 6% of the U.S. population claim to be agnostics or atheists, 21% of psychiatrists and 28% of clinical psychologists claim to be agnostic or atheists.

Despite this history and general difference in attitudes between psychiatric practitioners and the general public, there is an increasing interest in the role of spirituality and religion in mental health and in psychiatric treatment. Four major journals in psychiatry were reviewed between the years of 1978 and 1982. During those 5 years, a religious measure was used in less than 3% of all the quantitative studies. With the increased interest in spirituality and religion, however, this trend is changing. Research involving an assessment of spiritual and religious practice is becoming more sophisticated. Measures of spiritual and religious practice now include an assessment of practices, such as ceremonies, prayer and social support, beliefs involving relations to God or a higher power, attitudes, especially those regarding meaning pertaining to personal purpose, values, and ethics, and others. Assessment tools are now developed in terms of their reliability and validity in measuring different dimensions of spiritual and religious practice. Of these dimensions, a relationship with God or higher power and social support reveal a positive valance correlating with mental health.

Several studies have documented a positive impact of spiritual and religious practice on the overall state of mental well-being. These studies include reactions to life stress as well as a stable sense of well-being. Two large-scale epidemiological studies which examined the overall rate of psychological distress in a general population both found that the religiously committed had less psychological distress than those with less commitment. Studies that assessed religious status and psychological status at different points in time demonstrate improvement in psychological functioning following religious participation. A study published in 1991 of 720 randomly sampled adults found that persons who attended religious services reported lower levels of psychiatric distress than infrequent attenders or non-attenders. This was true regardless of age, education, gender, marital status, or race. In addition to general well-being, they found that as the level of religious attendance increased, the adverse consequences of stress were reduced. Some studies have also indicated that spiritual and religious practices may be important and play a positive role in reducing depression and the rate of suicide. For example, a study published in the *American Journal of Psychiatry* in 1990 looked at the rate of depression among elderly women recovering from hip fractures. Among the patients with stronger belief and practices, there was less depression and it increased a positive impact on recovery time.

Several studies indicate that spiritual and religious involvement reduces the risk of suicide. One large-scale study found that persons who did not attend church were four times more likely to kill themselves. Another study found that the rate of church attendance predicted suicide rates more effectively than any other factor including unemployment. Other studies have found that religious persons report experiencing fewer suicidal impulses. It has been proposed that religion might help prevent suicide because religious commitment and community provide a unique source of self-esteem, social support, and a moral accountability to a higher power. Groups with higher religious commitment have been found to have a more negative attitude toward suicidal behavior.

Many studies indicate that spirituality and religious practice play an important role in substance abuse. This has been most studied in the area of alcohol abuse where studies reveal that alcohol abusers rarely had strong religious commitment. One study found that 89% of alcoholics had lost interest in religion in their teenage years whereas of the community controlled subjects, 48% had an increased interest in religion and 32% said their interest had remained unchanged. Whether or not the religious tradition specifically teaches against alcohol use, those who are active in a religious group consume substantially less alcohol than those who are not active. Alcoholics Anonymous (AA) has proven to be one of the most effective treatments for alcohol addiction. It is of interest that AA uses religion in the form of invoking a higher power to help alcoholics recover from addiction.

Studies have confirmed that other forms of drug abuse show similar correlations to spiritual and religious commitments. The religious commitment measure of frequency of church attendance was more strongly associated with drug abstinence than other religious variables, such as religious feelings or parental religious commitment. A study of 14,000 young people found that the measure of "importance of religion" to the person was the best predictor in indicating lack of substance abuse. This implies that the controls operating here are deeply internalized values and norms rather than fear or peer pressure. Drug abuse appears to be related to the absence of religion in a person's life.

Family stability and illogical activities are indirect measures of emotional well-being. Studies have shown that religious and spiritual commitments are important in these areas as well. Persons in long-lasting marriages, in some studies, ranked religion as one of the most important prescriptions for a happy marriage. Another study found that the most important predictor of marital stability was church attendance. These studies raise the concern that divorce rates may be lower among religious people because of constraints against divorce. Studies that look specifically at self-reported marital satisfaction do find that a happy marriage does correlate with religious and spiritual commitment. Indeed, another study reported that very religious women report greater happiness and satisfaction with marital sex than either moderately religious or nonreligious women. Divorce has further implications for mental health; for example, divorced or separated men had four times the risk for outpatient or inpatient psychiatric care, and separated or divorced women had a fivefold increased risk. Personal church attendance has also been found to correlate in a negative way with juvenile delinquency.

Scientists have become interested in the psychological changes brought about by spiritual practices. Early studies looked at changes in cortisol, the stress hormone, and the autonomic nervous system. Advances in neuroscience allow researchers to observe actual changes in the brain from meditation and prayer. In a recent book *Why God Won't Go Away*, the authors suggest that the human experience of spirituality is deeply rooted in the brain itself. The work of Jon Kabat-Zinn suggests that spiritual practice may provide treatment. He studied the effect of mindfulness meditation on individuals diagnosed with anxiety disorders. Those who participated in intensive meditation showed marked improvement in their symptoms.

Spirituality is an important aspect of human life. Traditionally all cultures have incorporated spirituality in religious practices. Healing was often incorporated in these practices. Western medicine developed with the scientific method and largely in opposition to religious institutions. Now public consensus and scientific evidence are requiring a reconsideration of this separation. While modern medicine has much to offer to our health and healing, it will be enriched by attending to the spiritual needs of patients.

SEE ALSO: Anxiety disorders, Cardiovascular disease, Depression, Hypertension, Meditation, Yoga

Suggested Reading

Benson, H. (1975). *The relaxation responses.* New York: William Morrow.

Dossey, L. (1993). *Healing words: The power of prayer & the practice of medicine.* New York: HarperCollins.

Kabat-Zinn, J. (1990). *Full catastrophe of living: Using the wisdom of your body and mind to face stress, pain and illness.* New York: Delacorte.

Newberg, A., D'Aquli, E., & Rause, V. (2002). *Why God won't go away.* New York: Ballantine Books.

NANCY K. MORRISON

Sports Injuries Women have become increasingly involved in sporting activity over the past 30 years. In 1972, Title IX—a federal antidiscrimination law—led to a significant increase in female sports participation. The Title IX amendment prohibits gender discrimination in secondary and postsecondary educational institutions receiving federal funds. This has led to more women competing at the high school, college, and professional levels. Women also participate in a greater variety of sports, including traditionally male-dominated sports. For example, women not only compete in gymnastics, figure skating, and softball, but also in soccer, lacrosse, hockey, and American football.

As a result of increased female sports participation, orthopedic injuries are emerging that are more common and unique to female athletes. Anatomic differences and poor training regimens have contributed to the increase in sports injuries for women.

Anatomic and physiologic differences between men and women play a role in the incidence and type of sports injury. The three most common injuries are the knee, shoulder, and foot.

Patellofemoral disorders and *anterior cruciate ligament* (ACL) injuries of the knee have a higher incidence in female athletes than in males. Patellofemoral disorder refers to a group of syndromes that arise from the knee extensor mechanism and the surrounding soft tissue attachments. The knee extensor mechanism consists of the quadriceps muscle (commonly known as the anterior thigh), patella (or kneecap), and patellar tendon. Several anatomic differences contribute to the increased incidence of patellofemoral disorders in female athletes. These anatomic differences include underdeveloped quadriceps and hamstring muscles, knee recurvatum (hyperextension), and patellar misalignment. Patellofemoral injuries cause an irritation and inflammation of the undersurface of the patella. Women often report pain behind the patella, buckling knees, and stiffness after prolonged sitting. Treatment for these conditions ranges from conservative therapy and exercise to surgical procedures.

Anterior cruciate ligament injuries are more common in females participating in sports that involve jumping and pivoting, such as basketball, soccer, and volleyball. The ACL provides knee stability and prevents forward movement of the femur (thigh bone). Theories suggest that ligament laxity, intercondylar notch dimensions and limb alignment, and low ratios of hamstring-to-quadriceps strength contribute to the higher incidence of ACL injuries in women. Ligament laxity refers to decreased tensor strength of the ACL and may be hormone dependent. For example, the hormone relaxin, secreted during the luteal phase of the menstrual cycle (the time between ovulation and the onset of the next menses), is postulated to cause greater ACL laxity in women, leading to more frequent ACL injury. Additionally, women generally have wider pelvises than men, which increase the angle that the femur connects to the knee joint and may result in increased force transmission to the ACL. A related biomechanical factor is the narrower intercondylar notch dimensions in women. The ACL passes through the intercondylar notch of the femur before fanning out and connecting to the tibia (shin bone). It is postulated that cutting and jumping movements in athletes with narrow femoral notches may weaken and fray the ACL. Finally, women generally

have a lower ratio of hamstring-to-quadriceps strength, indicating a relative deficit in hamstring strength. Jumping and pivoting motions require that the quadriceps and hamstring muscles oppose and act in concert with each other. For example, landing from a jump and bending the knees involves eccentric contraction of the quadriceps (lengthening of muscle fibers) and concentric contraction of the hamstrings (shortening), whereas recovery requires the opposite action. Female athletes with low ratios of hamstring-to-quadriceps strength, rely on quadriceps activation for both landing and recovery, creating a high probability for ACL injury.

ACL injuries most often involve a partial or full-thickness tear of the ligament. Women who sustain these injuries develop pain, swelling, and instability of their knee. Most often surgical intervention is necessary to repair the damaged ligament.

The shoulder joint is another common area of injury in female athletes. Sports that involve overhead movements such as swimming, racquet sports, and throwing sports frequently cause shoulder pain. Rotator cuff impingement syndrome commonly occurs in overhead sporting activity. Impingement syndrome occurs when the shoulder rotator cuff tendons become impinged underneath the acromion (the flat bone covering the rear of the shoulder) with overhead arm movement. This condition occurs because of less developed shoulder girdle musculature. As a result, the rotator cuff muscles and tendons must work harder to perform the demands placed on them. With rotator cuff impingement syndrome, the tendons become irritated and inflamed leading to bursitis, tendonitis, and potential tearing. Treatment primarily involves therapy to alleviate the inflammation and build strength in the shoulder and upper extremity muscles.

Increased shoulder capsular laxity is an anatomic difference between females and males that also causes shoulder pain. Capsular laxity refers to the movement, or translation, of the head of the humerus (upper arm bone) with respect to the socket, or glenoid. With capsular laxity, the shoulder joint is unstable causing pain in the shoulder and upper arm. Thus, laxity in the shoulder capsule may become a problem in repetitive overhead arm movements. Similar to rotator cuff impingement syndrome, a progressive strengthening program improves stability, thereby alleviating pain.

Anatomic foot differences are also a common problem area in female athletes. Studies suggest that women's foot problems, particularly bunions and other toe deformities, may be inherited but often arise from poor footwear. Athletic footwear has traditionally been designed for the male population with smaller versions available for females. However, the female foot is not simply a smaller version of the male foot. A female's wider forefoot and narrow hindfoot need a shoe design to properly accommodate these differences. Improperly fitted athletic shoes can cause hallux valgus (bunion) deformity, hammertoe, and plantar calluses. These problems typically cause foot discomfort and hinder athletic performance.

A major contributor to sports injury in female athletes is a lack of proper training. Coaching has focused on winning the game rather than training and proper conditioning for a particular sport. Sport-specific conditioning strengthens muscles that prevent fatigue and overuse-type injuries such as patellofemoral and shoulder impingement syndromes. Teaching proper jumping and landing techniques reduces the risk of twisting injuries that cause ligament damage. Studies show that a decreased injury rate is directly correlated with proper training and conditioning. In fact, the primary treatment for many nonsurgical athletic injuries starts with a rehabilitation program that focuses on conditioning the injured joint to meet the demands of sports activity.

The significant increase in women's sports participation the past 30 years has led to female injury patterns not previously recognized or studied. Recognizing female anatomic differences and the necessity of proper training will provide a better understanding for treating and preventing injuries.

SEE ALSO: Arthritis, Exercise, Foot care, Menstruation, Osteoarthritis, Tendonitis, Women's Health Initiative

Suggested Reading

Allred, A. P. (2003). *Atta girl: A celebration of women in sports*. Terre Haute, IN: Wish.

Beim, G., & Winter, R. (2003). *The female athlete's body book: How to prevent and treat sports injuries in women and girls*. New York: McGraw-Hill/Contemporary Books.

Levy, A. M., & Fuerst, M. L. (1993). *Sports injury handbook: Professional advice for amateur athletes*. New York: John Wiley & Sons.

O'Connor, B., Fasting, K., Dahm, D., Wells, C., et al. (2001). *Complete conditioning for the female athlete*. Terre Haute, IN: Wish.

Shamus, E., & Shamus, J. (2001). *Sports injury prevention and rehabilitation*. New York: McGraw-Hill/Appleton & Lange.

Sibley, C., & Smith, S. (2001). *Games girls play: Understanding and guiding young female athletes*. New York: St. Martin's Press.

MARY ANTHONY

Stalking

Stalking is a pattern of behaviors which includes repeated annoyance and harassment through unwanted contact with another person. Stalking is a form of violence and occurs in a wide variety of ways, including threatening or unwanted phone calls, following the victim home or to public places, damaging property, or constantly surveilling activities and whereabouts. Some stalkers may seek out members of the victim's family and attempt to either intimidate or use the family to gain information about their victim. Stalking is not limited to threats or anger. A stalker may also profess great love and affection for his/her victim, and may even appear desperate and vulnerable. All 50 states currently have antistalking laws, and there is a federal antistalking law as well. Women are frequently stalking victims: A 1998 study by the National Institute of Justice found that 78% of stalking victims are women.

There are three basic types of stalkers: delusional or "obsession" stalkers, intimate partner stalkers, and vengeful stalkers. Delusional stalkers are those who have not had any substantial relationship with the victim. The stalker incorrectly believes he/she has a relationship with the victim, or can form a relationship through the stalking activities. Celebrity stalking is a form of delusional stalking. Two particularly well-known stalking cases involved actresses. Jodie Foster was stalked by John Hinckley, Jr. Mr. Hinckley shot President Ronald Reagan in an effort to impress the actress. Rebecca Schaeffer, a teen actress, was shot and killed by her stalker in 1989. Noncelebrities can also be the victim of delusional stalkers. A stalker may become obsessed with someone he/she sees in a public setting, such as on the bus or in a restaurant. As in the case of celebrities, this type of stalking can escalate from adoration to violence against the victim or others.

Intimate partner stalkers are those who have had a romantic relationship with their victim. Intimate partner stalking accounts for more than 60% of the stalking cases in the United States and Canada. Forty-two percent of intimate partner stalking is committed by a spouse or partner. In many cases, the stalker was abusive during the relationship. When the victim leaves the abuser, he/she uses stalking to continue to control the former partner. Intimate partner stalking may take the form of repeated, unwanted requests for a reconciliation attempt. The stalker may interpret any interaction with the victim as an indication that the relationship will continue. Interfering with the victim's social life is a common tactic of intimate partner stalkers. The stalker may confront the victim in a public place, hoping she/he will talk with him/her in order to avoid "making a scene." Intimate partner stalking is the most dangerous form of stalking: there is a 75% greater chance of being killed by this type of stalker than any other type.

Vengeful stalkers are those seeking to "get even" with their victim for some real or imagined misdeed. The stalker may be a former co-worker, student, or even, as in the cases involving abortion providers, a protester. Unlike other stalkers, the vengeful stalker does not have any positive feelings toward his/her victim. They are very likely to be psychopathic and physically violent.

Regardless of the particular category they fall into, most stalkers share some common characteristics: low self-esteem, refusal to take no for an answer, obsessive personality, "moody," above-average intelligence, manipulative, and violent tendencies. While many stalkers have similar personality traits, stalkers do not come from any one socioeconomic group. Stalking can (and does) occur in all segments of society.

Regardless of the stalker or the victim, stalking creates apprehension and fear. Stalkers may or may not physically harm their victims. However, any type of stalking is dangerous and must be handled seriously because there is no reliable way to predict a stalker's future violent behavior. The first step in dealing with a stalker (or potential stalker) is to clearly communicate that ANY contact is unwanted and if there is any more contact, you will call the police. This is sometimes referred to as a "no-contact statement." A no-contact statement can be done in person, on the phone, or in a letter or email. As soon as a victim begins to feel uncomfortable with the stalker's behavior, she/he should issue a no-contact statement. A "wait and see" approach can be dangerous when it comes to stalking.

If the harassment continues after the no-contact statement, the victim will need to contact the police in order to file a report of stalking. Victims should keep a log of the stalker's behavior that includes dates, times, places, and witnesses to stalking behavior. The log will facilitate building a case against the stalker. After reporting a stalking, the victim should obtain a copy of the police report. In addition to reporting all instances of harassment, the victim should keep all evidence: threats, cards, notes, emails, gifts, and the like.

Stalking victims may want to obtain a restraining order against their stalker. Restraining orders provide no protection in and of themselves, but give the police the ability to arrest stalkers in situations where they otherwise could not. There are community resources available to help the victims of stalkers. These resources may provide help with restraining orders and a variety of information on prosecuting stalkers.

SEE ALSO: Divorce mediation, Domestic violence, Homicide, Restraining orders

Suggested Reading

Dunn, J. (2002). *Courting disaster: Intimate stalking, culture, and criminal justice.* New York: Aldine de Gruyter.

Gedatus, G. (2000). *Perspectives on violence—Stalking.* Mankato, MN: Capstone Press.

Snow, R. (1998). *Stopping a stalker: A cop's guide to making the system work for you.* New York: Plenum Press.

Spence-Diel, E. (1999). *Stalking: A handbook for victims.* Holmes Beach, FL: Learning.

POLLY HAMPTON

Stomachache   *see* Abdominal Pain

Stomach Pain   *see* Abdominal Pain

Stress   The association between stress and health has been documented for decades. Stress can affect health both directly through its physiological effects and indirectly from maladaptive behaviors such as overeating or smoking. While great advances have been made in our understanding the role of stress and its deleterious effects on health, much still remains to be elucidated.

The term "stress" is used to represent a variety of concepts including: (a) an environmental situation; (b) appraisal of this situation; (c) the response to the situation or appraisal; and (d) a person's capacity to respond to environmental situations in general. The latter three are described here while the first is referred to as a stressor.

Much of the early work on stress focused on the "fight-or-flight" reaction to stress originally described by Cannon in 1932. This work was extended by Hans Selye as a three-step process called the general adaptation syndrome (GAS). Selye speculated that people exhibited changes in response to stressors including an alarm reaction, resistance, and exhaustion. Each stage would produce both physiological and behavioral changes, so if curative measures were not taken, then both physical and psychological deterioration would occur.

Stress was speculated to help species survive under a variety of conditions. The early response to acute stress enables the organism to face the stressor by enhancing immune function and increasing blood pressure and heart rate to prepare them to meet the physical demands from the stressor, and in the longer run, make more fuel available for sustained activity. However, as seen from observations of animals in their natural habitat, the stressors are most often for a limited duration. The stress system was not designed to adequately face stressors of lingering duration, such as unemployment or unreasonable job demands. When the system is overburdened by constant or consistent stressors, there is a chronic "wear and tear" that can render the organism more vulnerable to disability and disease.

While the "fight-or-flight" response has been studies for many years, recent research has suggested that women may respond differently to stressors than men. Some researchers argue that while women do experience the "fight-or-flight" phenomena when under acute stress, another stress response that women utilize is the "tend and befriend." "Tend and befriend" means that women under stress will nurture themselves and their children (i.e., tend) and will form alliances with others (i.e., befriend). This stress response also is associated with the survival of species in that females would need to protect their young in stressful situations.

Stress is described as one of several factors (e.g., lifestyle, sleep) that contribute to allostatic load, which was described by McEwen and Stellar in 1993. When the body is subjected to consistent and repeated strain, the body is predisposed to disease. This state is called allostatic load. Allostatic load can affect health states via three mechanisms. First it can affect the primary mediators, meaning the chemical mediators such as cortisol, norepinephrine, and the like. Alternatively, it can affect the systems that are mediated by the primary mediators, such as cellular events. Finally, allostatic load can affect health states by secondary mediators, meaning via more integrated processes such as blood pressure or metabolic profiles.

Stress has been shown to be involved in a variety of illnesses including hypertension, atherosclerosis, osteoporosis, irritable colon, and peptic ulcers. Stress has also been related to exacerbation of multiple sclerosis and hampering control of both types of diabetes. Fibromyalgia, chronic fatigue syndrome, and rheumatoid arthritis are related to processes resulting from chronic stress. Finally, it has been estimated that approximately two thirds of all visits to the family doctor are for stress-related disorders.

While stress has been associated with a number of illnesses, it is difficult to identify the precise mechanism that is responsible for disease. Animal studies of mice and primates allow for controlled studies, which have shown that inducing psychological stress results in distinct illness including atherosclerosis and hypertension. However, studies in humans are complicated by the fact that responses to stressors are variable and characteristics of the individual experiencing the stressor become important. In addition, the duration, frequency, and severity of stressors are also difficult to measure. Over the past 30 years, social scientists have grappled with these measurement and conceptual difficulties and have tried to refine measurements and theoretical frameworks to better elucidate the complicated role between stress and subsequent illness or disease.

In the 1960s and 1970s, social scientists expanded the lines of research on stress and developed ways to identify and measure potential stressors. Life event scales were developed to measure both positive and negative life events that might be considered stressful. Researchers found that those who reported high scores on the scales (meaning more stressful life events) were also more likely to experience illness compared to those with low scores. This research was extended to measuring the participant's subjective rating of the impact of the event, rather than just whether the event happened. This meant that a given event could be perceived differently depending on the person experiencing the event. Researchers believed it was the subjective perception that was important in determining deleterious effects of stress.

Subsequent research has shown that some personality types and/or psychological states are related to stress and disease. Early research focused on "type A" personalities, which are characterized by aggressiveness, haste, hurriedness, competitiveness, and the like. This personality trait is considered a risk factor for cardiovascular disease and angina, although conflicted research exists that finds no effect or effects only for certain groups of individuals (i.e., men in white-collar jobs).

Psychological states also include dispositional coping styles, which are enduring traits of an individual thought to influence coping efforts. These coping styles can moderate the association between stress and coping efforts. Optimism is the most widely researched dispositional coping style. Optimism is defined as having positive rather than negative expectations for the future. These positive expectations are consistent over time and across situations. Optimistic individuals have been found to recover faster after myocardial infarction and experience fewer physical symptoms during life stressors. Furthermore, optimists have been shown to have better psychological adjustment during and after major illnesses such as cancer and HIV.

Another dispositional trait that has received a lot of attention is locus of control. Locus of control is defined as a person's belief in his or her ability to control events through their own efforts. Persons with an internal locus of control believe that they can control events through their efforts (i.e., the environment is controllable) while those who have an external locus of control feel that outside influences control events in their lives. Those with an internal locus of control have been found to have different coping mechanisms for stress. Specifically, people with an internal locus of control are more likely to use acting coping styles and increase their efforts to control the outcome.

Two different information-seeking styles, monitoring and blunting, have been shown to be related to various health-related outcomes. Monitoring is the seeking of relevant information and is related to a perceived heightened risk and excessive worry. This excessive worry has been related to negative outcomes, such as increased nausea and vomiting in cancer patients undergoing chemotherapy. Blunting, on the other hand, is the avoidance of such information. While monitoring has been shown to have negative effects from excessive worrying, it can also have beneficial effects. Monitors may be more likely to actively seek important health information when they are ill or suspect that they are ill and may also be more likely to adhere to recommended health practices.

Several factors have been shown to buffer or moderate the effects of stress, in particular, social support and stress management interventions. A buffering or moderating effect means that stress would not be deleterious under certain situations where there was a protective element. Social support has beneficial direct effects on well-being but has also been shown to have "stress-buffering" effects on well-being. In addition, stress management interventions such as biofeedback have shown promise in reducing the harmful effects of stress.

Women, in particular, can face stress from a variety of different areas including love relationships, personal success, job stress, physical health, parent–child relationships, personal time, and social relationships. The stress from each of these areas has been shown to vary across age groups. Furthermore, many women today face challenges from trying to balance stress from multiple areas simultaneously, such as stress from work, children, and love relationships. While men often face more immediate occupational hazards, women are more prone to stress-related illnesses. In addition to dealing with the multiple roles previously described, women as a group are less likely to be in positions of power and therefore less likely to be able to control their environment, a situation which has been shown to be related to increased stress. Researchers have speculated that women today may be disadvantaged in that they are expected to achieve a (previously deemed) "male" standard of achievement at work and at the same time achieve an old-fashioned female standard for perfection at home as well.

SEE ALSO: Parenting, Social support

Suggested Reading

Cannon, W. B. (1932). *The wisdom of the body.* New York: Norton.

Cohen, S., Kessler, R. C., & Gordon, L. U. (1997). *Measuring stress: A guide for health and social scientists.* New York: Oxford University Press.

Cohen, S., & Wills, T. A. (1985). Stress, social support, and the buffering hypothesis. *Psychological Bulletin, 98*(2), 310–357.

Lazarus, R. S. (1993). Coping theory and research: Past, present, and future. *Psychosomatic Medicine, 55*(3), 234–247.

Lerman, C., & Glanz, K. (1997). Stress, coping, and health behavior. In K. Glanz, F. M. Lewis, & B. Rimer (Eds.), *Health behavior and health education: Theory, research and practice* (2nd ed.). San Francisco: Jossey-Bass.

Lovallo, W. R. (1996). *Stress and health.* Thousand Oaks, CA: Sage.

McEwen, B. S. & Stellar, E. (1993). Stress and the individual's mechanisms leading to disease. *Archives of Intestinal Medicine, 153*, 2093–2101.

Taylor, S. E., Cousino-Klein, L., Lewis, B. P., Gruenewald, T. L., Gurung, R. A., & Updegraff, J. A. (2000). Biobehavioral responses to stress in females: Tend-and-befriend, not fight-or-flight. *Psychological Review, 107*(3), 411–429.

Vanltallie, T. B. (2002). Stress: A risk factor for serious illness. *Metabolism, 51*(6), 40–45.

NATALIE COLABIANCHI

Stretch Marks
Striae gravidarum, also known as "stretch marks," arise during pregnancy in the majority of women. Common locations include the abdomen,

Stroke

breasts, buttocks, and thighs. Although the exact etiology is unknown, mechanical stress on connective tissue due to increased size of the various portions of the body is thought to be important. There are no significant differences between skin markings due to skin stretching (striae distensae) of different etiologies, and they can also occur in the settings of disorders of the endocrine system (Cushing's syndrome), steroid therapy, and rapid weight fluctuations (adolescents undergoing a growth spurt or bodybuilders).

Clinically striae gravidarum appear as wavy linear bands in the skin with their long axis parallel to the lines of skin tension. They are often characterized by their stage of evolution and are classified as recent or old. Striae are initially raised with a red or purple coloration. Early lesions may be associated with mild burning or itching. Over time they become flat or indented and flesh-colored to white with a fine wrinkled texture. Gradually, some striae may resolve over time and become inconspicuous, particularly in the case of adolescent striae occurring in the setting of growth spurts.

Histopathologic findings (those seen under a microscope) demonstrate that stretch marks are a form of scar. In early lesions, the dermal layer of skin reveals inflammatory cells with fragmentation of the collagen and elastic fibers, critical skin components to maintain structure and resiliency. In later lesions, the epidermis, which is the outermost layer of the skin, shows significant atrophy (thinning of the skin).

Striae distensae are primarily a cosmetic problem; however, if extensive, the disfigurement can be quite distressing. Early therapeutic interventions afford the most superior results, but there is no highly effective treatment for this condition. Medications that are applied directly to the skin (topical retinoids) have been shown to improve the appearance; however, they are contraindicated during pregnancy and lactation. Serial chemical peels and laser therapies have also been shown to improve the clinical appearance of striae distensae.

SEE ALSO: Pregnancy, Skin care

Suggested Reading

Fox, J. L. (1997). Pulse dye laser eliminates stretch marks. *Cosmetic Dermatology, 10,* 51–52.

Kang, S., Kim, K. J., & Griffiths, C. E. M. (1996). Topical tretinoin improves early stretch marks. *Archives of Dermatology, 132,* 519–526.

Zheng, P., Lavker, R. M., & Kligman, A. M. (1985). Anatomy of striae. *British Journal of Dermatology, 112,* 185–193.

MARY GAIL MERCURIO

Stroke   Strokes are the third leading cause of death in the United States, following coronary heart disease and cancer. The Centers for Disease Control estimates that every 45 seconds, someone in the United States suffers a new or recurrent stroke; every 3.1 minutes, someone in the United States dies of a stroke. Overall, men are 1.6 times more likely than women to have a stroke. However, this statistic can be misleading. While men are more likely to have a stroke than women when they are younger, by age 55, the risk is equal among women and men. Furthermore, women are nearly twice as likely as men to die of a stroke, making strokes the second leading cause of death in women after coronary heart disease.

The two most important things to know about strokes are that many are preventable, and that prompt diagnosis and treatment can save lives. Everyone should learn about the risk factors and the warning signs of stroke.

DEFINITION AND CAUSES

A stroke, or cerebrovascular accident (CVA), is a type of injury to the brain that occurs in one of two ways. The most common type of stroke is a nonhemorrhagic or ischemic stroke which occurs when a vessel that supplies blood to an area of the brain is blocked, leading to the death of brain cells that are normally supplied by the oxygen carried in the blood. A hemorrhagic stroke occurs when a damaged blood vessel bleeds directly into the brain, also leading to the death of brain cells in that area. The area of cell death that results in either type of stroke is called an infarct.

Ischemic strokes are most often caused by atherosclerotic thrombosis or cerebral embolism, each account for one third of all strokes. Atherosclerotic thrombosis is the development of stenosis (narrowing) or complete blockage of a blood vessel by a lipid-containing plaque. Because this is a slow process, there may be warning signs such as transient stroke symptoms before an actual stroke occurs. Cerebral embolism occurs when a fragment of a blood clot (thrombus) or atherosclerotic plaque breaks off and then lodges in a smaller blood vessel thus blocking blood flow. People with strokes caused by emboli have often had no warning signs beforehand. Some rarer causes of ischemic strokes are infectious or connective tissue diseases or a sudden increase in blood's tendency to form a clot caused by other medical conditions.

Hemorrhagic strokes may be caused by a ruptured aneurysm (a bulging or outpouching of an arterial wall, usually the result of an artery with developmental defects from birth) or a ruptured arteriovenous (AV) malformation (an abnormal connection between the arterial and venous systems, also the result of developmental defects). They can also be caused by a hypertensive crisis, in which someone's blood pressure increases so severely that even normal blood vessels will rupture and bleed. In any of these cases, bleeding may occur either very gradually or happen abruptly without warning.

SYMPTOMS

The initial symptoms of stroke are varied such as: sudden numbness or weakness of the face, arm, or leg, particularly on one side of the body; sudden confusion, or trouble speaking or understanding; sudden trouble with walking, dizziness, or loss of balance or coordination; or a sudden, severe headache with no known cause. The variety of presenting symptoms reflects the many different specialized areas of the brain in which a stroke can occur. A small stroke that occurs in the motor cortex of the brain, for example, may produce only a physical symptom such as weakness in one leg. On the other hand, a stroke in the language centers of the brain can produce sudden problems with communication such as slurred or incomprehensible speech. It is not uncommon for people to ignore the initial warning signs of a stroke if it is mild, or for other people to mistake the initial signs of a stroke for alcohol intoxication.

Sometimes, a person develops symptoms of a stroke that last less than a day, often lasting just a few minutes or hours. When this happens, it is called a transient ischemic attack (TIA). Transient ischemic attack may be caused by a partly occluded blood vessel, a small embolus that resolves, or intermittent small amounts of blood leakage from an aneurysm. TIAs should always prompt a rapid medical evaluation because the data show that approximately one third of people who have TIAs will eventually have a stroke. One recent study showed that of people evaluated in a hospital for TIAs, there was an 11% incidence of stroke just in the next 90 days.

TREATMENT AND PREVENTION

The treatment for acute strokes is still quite limited. If someone is having an ischemic stroke, and arrives at a hospital quickly enough, in some instances medication can be given that will break apart any clots that may be blocking the blood supply to that area of the brain. However, this type of medication is quite powerful and is not without its own risks. Also, if someone does not immediately come to the hospital when the first signs of a stroke arise, it is usually too late to give the medication. Once a stroke has occurred, treatment is generally limited to physical or speech therapy to improve functioning in the areas that have been affected by the stroke. Some people have complete or almost complete recoveries from strokes, while others are left with speech or motor problems that are permanent.

However, it is vital to remember that many strokes are preventable. The modifiable risk factors that are linked to having strokes include hypertension, cholesterol level of greater than 240 mg/dl, smoking, physical inactivity, obesity, carotid stenosis, alcohol consumption of more than five drinks per day, and atrial fibrillation. Smoking, for example, raises the chance of having a stroke to 1.5 times that of someone in the general population; hypertension raises the chance 3–5 times greater than normal. Not surprisingly, these risk factors are also generally associated with atherosclerosis, so that modifying these risk factors can also reduce the risk of having heart attacks and other health problems.

Of course, some risk factors are not themselves modifiable, such as being older or of non-Caucasian descent, having coronary heart disease or congestive heart failure, or a family history of stroke or TIAs. Also, there are physical disorders that increase the risk of having a stroke, such as sickle-cell anemia, certain bleeding disorders, or vasculitis caused by systemic lupus erythematosus, polyarteritis nodosa, or other conditions. However, the presence of these risk factors should lead individuals to pay even closer attention to prevention efforts aimed at the modifiable risk factors.

The evidence suggests that the most effective ways to reduce the chance of having a first stroke are good blood pressure control, using antithrombotic medicine (such as warfarin or aspirin) if an individual has a history of atrial fibrillation, and using aspirin or other antiplatelet therapy if an individual has had a myocardial infarction. Other things that are likely to help include lifestyle changes or the use of lipid-lowering medications to keep low-density lipoprotein (LDL) cholesterol below 130 mg/dl and smoking cessation. If an individual has already had a stroke, treatment of hypertension and hyperlipidemia, antithrombotic therapy (for atrial fibrillation), antiplatelet therapy (for myocardial infarction), and carotid endarterectomy (if an individual has carotid stenosis of 70% or greater and is not a high surgery risk) are all well-proven risk reduction methods.

Several risk factors for stroke are specific to women, including pregnancy, the use of oral contraceptives (OCs), or the use of hormone replacement therapy (HRT). A number of studies have shown an increased risk of strokes during pregnancy or childbirth, but this risk has been decreasing steadily over time. A 1996 study showed no increased risk for ischemic stroke during pregnancy itself, but did show a risk that was 8.7 times greater than normal during the first 6 weeks postpartum. The pregnancy-related causes of strokes are mainly preeclampsia or eclampsia (characterized by severe hypertension, protein in the urine, and edema developing during the pregnancy or within 48 hr postpartum); postpartum cerebral angiopathy (characterized by severe hypertension, headache, nausea and vomiting, and seizures or other neurologic signs developing minutes to weeks after delivery); and cerebral venous thrombosis (characterized by headaches and focal neurologic symptoms that develop during pregnancy or within a month of delivery). Immediate medical attention should be sought if these symptoms occur related to a pregnancy.

Oral contraceptive use and the risk of stroke are often overstated. While the early studies did show a link between OC use and strokes, most women now take newer OCs that have lower estrogen doses or contain desogestrel and most studies have shown these do not appear to elevate the risk of stroke, though not all studies agree. However, women who already have higher risk of strokes, such as those who smoke, have hyperlipidemia or hypertension, or are over 35, should talk carefully with their doctors before initiating or continuing use of OCs. Also, since OCs are known to increase clotting factors in the blood, women with certain clotting disorders should not take OCs.

The use of HRT has been extensively scrutinized in recent years. Initially, HRT was hoped to be something that would decrease women's risk of stroke or coronary heart disease, and certainly the early studies generally seemed to support this belief, showing either a modest benefit or no difference in risk, with a couple of notable exceptions. However, in 2002, several researchers published a meta-analysis of previous research data on HRT. The data showed that HRT increased the risk of thromboembolic strokes, though not subarachnoid or intracerebral strokes, to 1.2 times that of other women. In addition, the risk of having any venous thromboembolism was shown to be increased by HRT to 2.1 times normal, and in the first year of use was 3.5 times normal. Another study published in 2002 showed no overall association of ischemic or hemorrhagic stroke with HRT, but did show a twofold increase in risk of those types of strokes during the first 6 months of hormone use. Because of the new data on HRT risks including stroke and breast cancer, HRT is no longer routinely recommended. However, in certain circumstances, the benefits of HRT may outweigh the potential risks, and some women will still choose to take hormones.

SEE ALSO: Acute myocardial infarction, Coronary artery disease, Giant cell arteritis, Hormone replacement therapy, Oral contraception, Pregnancy, Smoking, Systemic lupus erythematosus, Venous thromboembolism

Suggested Reading

Bushnell, C., & Goldstein, L., (1999). Ischemic stroke: Recognizing risks unique to women. *Women's Health in Primary Care, 2,* 788–804.

Letmaitre, R., Heckbert, S., Pstay, B., Smith, N., Kaplan, R., & Longstreth, W., Jr. (2002). Hormone replacement therapy and associated risk of stroke in postmenopausal women. *Archives of Internal Medicine, 162,* 1954–1960.

Nelson, H., Humphrey, L., Nygren, P., Teutsch, S., & Allen, J. (2002). Postmenopausal hormone replacement therapy. *Journal of the American Medical Association, 288,* 872–881.

Straus, S., Majumdar, S., & McAlister, F. (2002). New evidence for stroke prevention: Scientific review. *Journal of the American Medical Association, 288,* 1388–1395.

United States Department of Health and Human Services. (2003). *A public action plan to prevent heart disease and stroke: Executive summary and overview.* Atlanta, GA: Centers for Disease Control and Prevention.

JULIE SCHULMAN

Student Health

Student Health College students are a sizeable and diverse group of people. In 1995, one quarter of people in the United States between 18 and 24 years of age were either full- or part-time college students, making colleges and universities an important setting for addressing common health issues for young adults. In 2004, nearly 14 million students will enroll in the 3,600+ undergraduate colleges and universities in the United States; just over half (57%) of those will be women. According to the National Center for Education Statistics (NCES), approximately one third of undergraduates are nonwhite and only half are of traditional college age (18–24 years). The NCES recently noted that "more than a quarter (27%) of undergraduates had dependents, 13% were single parents, and 80% were employed, including 39% who were employed full time." According to self-reports, about 1 in 10 college students have some kind of disability. Approximately 3.5 million college students in the United States do not have health insurance. These individuals may face substantial barriers in seeking access to health care. It is for these reasons that college students represent a little discussed but important and distinct health population in our country.

To better understand the prevalence of health-risk behaviors among college students, the Centers for Disease Control (CDC) sponsored the 1995 National College Health Risk Behavior Survey (NCHRBS), which was conducted with 4,609 U.S. undergraduates (age 18 and older) at 2- and 4-year institutions across the nation. The purpose of the NCHRBS was to monitor six areas identified as priority health risk factors: behaviors that contribute to unintentional and intentional injury; tobacco use; alcohol and other drug use; sexual behaviors that contribute to unintended pregnancy and sexually transmitted diseases (STDs), including HIV; unhealthy dietary behaviors; and physical inactivity. The results of the NCHRBS are summarized below, followed by some discussion of health resources available to students.

Alcohol consumption is a significant public health problem among college students. Episodic heavy drinking is more prevalent among college students than among their peers of the same age who do not attend college. Alcohol use in this manner is strongly linked with serious injury and injury-related deaths, particularly involving motor vehicle accidents. Alcohol use among college students is also related to unsafe sexual behavior, violence, and academic problems. One third (34.5%) of students reported episodic heavy drinking during the 30 days preceding the survey and 27.4% reported drinking and driving during the month prior to the survey.

Tobacco use. The health effects of tobacco use are the single most preventable cause of death in the United States. Nevertheless, more than one quarter (29%) of college students reported currently smoking cigarettes. Although fewer college students (16.5%) are frequent cigarette smokers, it is clear that even modest levels of tobacco use may place students at risk for long-term addiction and associated health problems.

Illicit drug use. Nationwide, 48.7% of college students reported using marijuana at some point during their lifetime (i.e., "lifetime use"), while only 11.6% of women college students reported current marijuana use. While 14.4% of college students had used some form of cocaine during their lifetime, fewer than 1 in 100 students reported cocaine use during the 30 days prior to the NCHRBS. Lifetime inhalant abuse (e.g., sniffing glue, breathing the contents of aerosol spray cans, or inhaling any paints or sprays to get high) was reported by 7% of undergraduate women. Nationwide, 20.5% of college students reported lifetime use of "other illegal drugs," such as LSD, PCP, "ecstasy," mushrooms (i.e., hallucinogens), speed, ice, or heroin. Among women, white students (22.2%) were significantly more likely than black (4.5%) and Hispanic (14.1%) students to have ever used other illegal drugs. However, only 1.6% of women reported current "other illegal drug" use. White (1.8%) and Hispanic (2.1%) women were significantly more likely than black women (0.1%) to report current use of "other illegal drugs." Current combination of illegal drugs and alcohol was reported by 6.8% of female college students, with white female students (8.3%) being significantly more likely than black female students (1.9%) to report current combined illegal drug and alcohol use.

STDs and unintended pregnancies pose a significant risk for many college students. STDs of particular importance for college students include HIV/AIDS, chlamydia, genital warts/HPV/condyloma, hepatitis B and C, herpes, gonorrhea, trichomoniasis, pubic lice, syphilis, urinary tract infections (UTIs), and yeast infections. Nationwide, only 38.8% of college students had ever had a blood test for HIV. Rates of unintended pregnancy among persons aged 15–24 years are higher than for any other age group. In 1988, almost two thirds of births to females aged 15–24 years were unintended. The NCHRBS indicates that of students who had had sexual intercourse during the 3 months preceding the survey, only 29.6% had used a condom at the last sexual intercourse and 34.5% had used birth control pills. Increased use of both condoms and effective methods

625

of contraception among college students is necessary to decrease rates of STD and unintended pregnancy. Many STDs have no or minimal symptoms or might be mistaken for other common ailments (e.g., a yeast infection), but can lead to serious health problems, such as infertility or a compromised immune system, or even death if untreated. Consistent condom use is very important in preventing most STDs, but does not guarantee protection. Routine testing to facilitate early diagnosis and treatment of STDs is critical, not only for the infected person, but to avoid transmission to others.

Mental health issues, many of which were not directly assessed by the NCHRBS, are common problems on college campuses, including depression, anxiety, gender identity issues, and eating disorders. For instance, 10.3% of college students nationwide had seriously considered attempting suicide during the 12 months preceding the NCHRBS. Some psychiatric disorders appear for the first time during the college years, such as schizophrenia, which is characterized by auditory and/or visual hallucinations, unusual beliefs, disordered thoughts, social withdrawal, and diminished relatedness.

Unhealthy diet and physical inactivity. Approximately one in five (20.5%) college students was overweight based on their body mass index (BMI). Survey results indicated that 73.7% of students had failed to eat five or more servings of fruits and vegetables during the day preceding the survey, 21.8% had eaten three or more high-fat foods during the day preceding the survey, and few students had engaged in vigorous (37.6%) or moderate (19.5%) physical activity at recommended levels. Men (26.6%) were significantly more likely than women (10.3%) to have participated on a college or university sports teams (intramural or extramural).

Gender-specific health risks. The NCHRBS found there were several health risks that were significantly different for college men and women. For example, men were more likely than women to report the following negative health behaviors: rarely or never wearing safety belts when riding in or driving a car; drinking alcohol and driving a car or other vehicle; drinking alcohol while boating or swimming; carrying a weapon or gun; physical fighting; current smokeless tobacco use; current tobacco use; current alcohol use; current, frequent alcohol use; current episodic heavy drinking; current marijuana use; lifetime inhalant use; lifetime illegal steroid use; current other illegal drug use; current combined illegal drug and alcohol use; initiating alcohol use, marijuana use, and sexual intercourse at age less than 13 years; having six or more sex partners during their lifetime; alcohol and drug use at last sexual intercourse; and eating more than two servings of foods typically high in fat content.

Sexual assault is another serious concern among college students, particularly among young women. The Sexual Experiences Survey conducted during 1984–1985 indicated that 15% of females reported having been raped and an additional 12% reported that someone had attempted to rape them since age 14. According to self-reports, one in five female college students had been forced to have sexual intercourse during her lifetime. This finding was confirmed by the NCHRBS, with women students more likely than male students to report ever being forced to have sexual intercourse against their will.

In terms of other risk behaviors and negative health issues, women more commonly indicated not using a condom at last sexual intercourse or using condoms inconsistently. They had a more pronounced pattern of thinking they were overweight, attempting weight loss through dieting, excessive exercise, vomiting, taking laxatives, or taking diet pills. The majority of women students indicated that they had not participated in vigorous physical activity or strengthening exercises on a consistent basis, and fewer women than men proportionately participate on a college sports team.

Student health resources are available to help college students protect and maintain their mental, physical, and emotional well-being. College students face major developmental challenges in each of these domains, often while under considerable pressure from a variety of sources: academic, economic, self-imposed, peer, familial, or social stress. Student Health Centers, available on most campuses, are an excellent resource to help students successfully navigate these obstacles while usually providing clear privacy protections for student-patients. While resource issues appear to be common on college campuses, many have special programs to address specialized mental, physical, and emotional health care needs of college students.

Medical services offered by student health centers commonly include contraceptive information, prescription, and follow-up; pregnancy testing, counseling and referrals; annual gynecological exams; STD testing, diagnosis, and treatment; primary care services and referrals; preventive health checkups; and mental health counseling. Many provide some services for free and offer low-cost insurance plans that enable students to gain access to their full range of services. While many programs currently exist that are aimed at helping colleges and universities address health-risk behaviors among their students by increasing access to health-related information, education, and services, there is still room for improvement. Many cities and towns in which colleges are located also offer Rape Crisis Centers and hotlines available to those who have experienced sexual assault. Some of these centers are run in collaboration with local universities to facilitate student access, and the contact information for counselors and hotline volunteers is often listed in school directories.

Many student health centers take a "wellness" approach which looks beyond an absence of sickness to emphasize optimal physical, mental, and emotional well-being. These centers have programs to educate students about a preventive way of living that focuses on personal responsibility for making the lifestyle choices and self-care decisions that will improve quality of life. This includes educating and improving college students' choices about nutrition, physical activity, stress management, responsible sexual behavior, and leading a balanced lifestyle. Wellness is a positive, day-to-day approach to a long, healthful, active life.

SEE ALSO: Acquired immunodeficiency syndrome, Alcohol use, Cannabis, Chlamydia, Condoms, Health insurance, Rape, Reproductive technologies, Safer sex, Sexually transmitted diseases, Smoking, Substance use, Teen pregnancy, Tobacco

Suggested Reading

Division of Adolescent and School Health National Center for Chronic Disease Prevention and Health Promotion. (1997). Youth risk behavior surveillance: National College Health Risk Behavior Survey—United States, 1995. *CDC MMWR Surveillance Summary, 46*(SS-6), 1–54. Also available at http://www.cdc.gov/mmwr/preview/mmwrhtml/00049859.htm

Roberts, L. W., Warner, T., Lyketsos, C., Frank, E., Ganzini, L., Carter, D. D., et al. (2000). Caring for medical students as patients: Access to services and care-seeking practices of 1027 students at nine medical schools. *Academic Medicine, 75*(3), 272–277.

Roberts, L. W., Warner, T., Lyketsos, C., Frank, E., Ganzini, L., Carter, D. D., et al. (2001). Perceptions of academic vulnerability associated with personal illness: A study of 1027 students at nine medical schools. *Comprehensive Psychiatry, 42*(1), 1–15.

Suggested Resources

Amherst College, Student Services, Health Education Library Project: Book suggestions, http://www.amherst.edu/~healthed/libraryprojecttopics.html

Go Ask Alice: Columbia University's Health Question and Answer Internet Service. http://www.goaskalice.columbia.edu/

United States Department of Health and Human Services. Healthfinder—Your guide to reliable health information. http://www.healthfinder.gov/library/

MEGAN V. SMITHPETER
MELINDA K. ROGERS
LAURA WEISS ROBERTS

Substance Use

Substance Use Human beings have used mood-altering drugs—or drugs of potential abuse—for hundreds of thousands of years. Their use is due to the fact that all these drugs directly or indirectly produce quick surges of a neurotransmitter or brain chemical called dopamine. Dopamine is a substance which when released in the brain results in a feeling of pleasure or euphoria, in other words a "high." Each drug of use, abuse, and addiction that has been carefully studied has been shown to result in this increase in dopamine and pleasurable euphoria.

CLASSES OF MOOD-ALTERING DRUGS

Although this effect of dopamine is the characteristic that results in the use of these drugs, they also have many other brain effects. It is these other brain effects that dictate the type or *class* of the drug. There are four main classes of mood-altering drugs: stimulants, opioids, sedative hypnotics, and hallucinogens. Table 1 lists the drugs that fall into each of these classes.

Stimulants are drugs that result in the release of varying amounts of norepinephrine or adrenaline in addition to dopamine. This release of adrenaline results in dilated or widening of the pupils, increased attention, increased reflexes, increased blood pressure and heart rate, increased alertness, decrease need for sleep, and decreased appetite. Therefore, stimulants produce euphoria from the release of dopamine, and stimulation from the release of adrenaline.

Opioids are drugs, natural or synthetic compounds related to opium, that affect the mu or morphine receptor in the brain. As a consequence they produce constriction of the pupils, dry eyes, dry mouth, constipation, sedation or sleepiness, slowing of the heart rate and breathing rate, decrease in blood pressure, and pronounced pain relief.

The sedative hypnotic class of drugs is made up of substances that work on the gamma-aminobutyrate (GABA) receptor system of the brain. Gamma-aminobutyrate neurons are cells that excite and activate the brain, leading to wakefulness and at times even anxiety. Sedative hypnotic substances tend to depress or quiet down GABA nerve cells, causing a relief of anxiety, sleepiness, and when used at too high a dose result in coma or even death. Sedative hypnotic substances, like the more potent amphetamines and cocaine, tend to produce a high degree of judgment impairment as a consequence of overuse and intoxication. Thus, bizarre behavior contrary to the patient's upbringing is commonplace with intoxication. These sedative hypnotics range from relatively weak substances like alcohol to very potent ones like the "date rape" drug Rohypnol. An additional danger of sedative hypnotics is that they clearly increase in potency of effect when used in combination, markedly increasing the chances of serious overdose.

Hallucinogens are a diverse group of substances that alter perception as part of their central nervous system or brain effect. This group includes LSD, phencyclidine (PCP), marijuana, and many naturally occurring hallucinogens from a variety of plants. Hallucinogens as a group, like the opioids, tend to produce a low degree of judgment impairment as a consequence of overuse and intoxication. The altering of perception seems to include many different effects such as visual distortions, spatial distortions, and loss of time perception.

Mood-altering drugs are primarily used for their ability to trigger a quick rise in dopamine, and thus an elevation in mood or euphoria. These same drugs have additional actions and effects that can generally be categorized into one of the above four classes. Virtually all of the drugs listed in Table 1 can be used, or abused, or trigger the development of an addiction.

THE CONTINUUM OF MOOD-ALTERING DRUG USE

Alcohol use, and to some extent other drug use, has been characterized as existing in our society as a gradual continuum. The levels of use are *abstinence, low-risk or casual use, risky use or "substance abuse,"* and *chemical dependence or addiction*. Definitions of each of these use levels follow.

Abstinence

These people are nonusers of mood-altering drugs, do not use even in low-risk amounts, and are more often older women or members of a relatively more fundamentalist sect of the major religions. Another smaller yet critically important group of abstainers are those people with a history of chemical dependence or addiction who are currently abstinent in an effort to deal with the addiction.

Table 1. Four main classes of mood-altering drugs

Stimulants	Opioids	Sedative-hypnotics	Hallucinogens
Caffeine	Opium	Alcohol	Phencyclidine
Nicotine	Heroin	Benzodiazepines	LSD
Cocaine	Prescription opioids	Diazepam	Marijuana
"Crack"	Codeine	Lorazepam	Kat
Methamphetamine	Morphine	Clonazepam	Mescaline
"Crank"	Hydromorphone	Aprazolam	Mushrooms
"Speed"	Oxycodone	Rohypnol etc.	Jimsonweed
Psychostimulants	Methadone	Barbiturates	
Amphetamine	Buprenorphine		
Methylphenidate			
Cylert			
Dexadrine			
Diet pills			

628

Abstinence is prevalent among three groups in society, those with a strong, relatively conservative or fundamentalist religious belief, those with a strong family history of addiction who do not want to take the risk of activating the disease in themselves, and those individuals with the disease of addiction who are in recovery and thus not using.

The most important issue in abstinence, for those who are in recovery from addiction, is to maintain complete abstinence from mood-altering drugs. Although there are very rare instances when medications that are mood-altering drugs must be prescribed, the long-term intake of these medications is generally very dangerous for persons in recovery and should be avoided. Common reasons for relapsing back to addiction are (a) trying to go back and control one's use of the previously addicting drug, (b) trying to use mood-altering drugs other than the one that was the previous addicting drug, and (c) being prescribed mood-altering drugs on a long-term basis by a physician and reactivating addiction.

Low-Risk Use

These people are low-level intermittent users of mood-altering drugs who do not binge, use only in socially acceptable situations, and have little if any evidence of health risk from their use. The federal government has published "Sensible Drinking Guidelines" for adult men and women that provide clear information about what drinking levels are associated with no detectable health risks. Interestingly, these guidelines stipulate at least a 30% lower level of alcohol use for women than for their male counterparts.

This is generally a very stable pattern of use, only in social situations, and always keeping to within the "sensible use guidelines" referenced above. True social users never have to try to limit their use, consciously construct rules around their use, cut back on their use because of an embarrassing situation, and the like. Persons with addiction problems constantly try to become low-risk "social" users, by cutting back and trying to control their use. In reality, low-risk users never have to think about controlling their use, it just happens unconsciously.

It is difficult to discuss low-risk use of drugs other than alcohol in American society where possession of other drugs is illegal and thus carries serious potential consequences. The limited data that are available from other countries seem to indicate that some nonalcohol mood-altering drugs might be available to a community for low-risk or "social" use purposes. However, for the foreseeable future, possession will remain illegal in this country, and thus low-risk use is not a term that can be applied to nonalcohol mood-altering drug use.

Substance Abuse

Substance abusers are individuals who use more alcohol than is considered "healthy," or who use any amounts of nonalcohol mood-altering drugs. Although the use patterns tend to fall within their general peer group norm, and there are rare adverse consequences from the use, they tend to binge at levels that have clearly been shown to be a risk to health, and use to levels of intoxication that significantly impair their judgment and moral values. They are also individuals who do not meet the criteria for chemical dependence or addiction. It is generally thought that substance abuse is a *behavior* that many people participate in during late adolescence and early adulthood, which evolves either into low-risk use or addiction, and that is under a good deal of voluntary control.

Although not a disease or illness, substance abuse is responsible for a tremendous amount of pain and suffering in our society, including the majority of "date rapes," and much young adult nonsexual interpersonal violence as well as destruction of property. In effect, although substance abuse is a behavior and not an illness, and it rarely involves problems for any person who might be an abuser, it is very common with an estimated 70–85% of the population in their teens and 20s passing through some period of substance abuse. As a result, there is a large amount of societal morbidity (pain and suffering) that occurs as a result of substance abuse.

Substance abusers tend to be intermittent binge users, using to risky levels of intoxication. This use tends to be self-limited in time with a gradual decrease over time and "maturity." Some individuals labeled as "abusers" are probably addicted, and over time their use escalated (while that of many of their general peer group abates). This accounts for the phenomena of some substance abusers seeming to progress to addiction. The most appropriate intervention or treatment of substance abuse is to counsel the individual (a) against use of illegal and illicit drugs, (b) against the underage use of legal drugs, (c) away from binging behavior, and (d) toward staying within the "sensible drinking guidelines."

Chemical Dependence or Addiction

Chemical dependence or addiction is clearly a chronic disease of the brain that bears no relationship with morality, education, social class, or ethnicity. It is a primarily genetic illness that clusters fairly heavily in families. Addiction is characterized by the *repetitive, intermittent, loss of control over the use of a mood-altering drug that causes problems in a person's life.* As a consequence, addiction is not defined in terms of quantity and frequency of use, but rather in terms of patterns (loss of control) and consequences (repeated problems) of use.

The essential problem in addiction is this loss of control, and the resulting bizarre/uncharacteristic/erratic/irresponsible behaviors. Thus, the domains in a person's life where problems from addiction arise tend to be the following: self-respect/close love relationships/social relationships/financial problems/legal problems/work problems/and finally medical or psychiatric problems. Individuals with addiction or chemical dependence have developed one or more alcohol-related or drug-related problems such as a Driving Under the Influence of Alcohol (DUI), medical complications, family problems, or other behavioral consequences. The types of problems range from minimal—such as one or two blackouts in young adulthood, followed by family concern about the person's drinking—to severe, including loss of work, or loss of family.

The societal costs of addictions are overwhelming. Tobacco dependence is the leading preventable cause of death in America, with 470,000 premature deaths per year. Fetal alcohol syndrome is the leading cause of preventable birth defects in our country. Over 70% of domestic violence is addiction related, 70% of child abuse and 90% of childhood sexual abuse are thought to be addiction related. The economic costs of addiction are estimated at 80–110 billion dollars per year, and addictions are considered the nation's number one health problem!

SCREENING, INTERVENTION, AND TREATMENT

Screening

It can be difficult to figure out if a person's use of mood-altering drugs is low risk, abuse, or dependence. Most of our societal belief systems regarding these issues are flawed, and therefore many of our "community screening criteria" are relatively weak. In general, the community misses the presence of substance abuse and dependence far more often than they are identified. Up to 90% of people with drinking problems are not noticed by their family, friends, faith communities, educational institutions, or health care providers. Clearly we as a society need better screening tools. One useful questionnaire is the f-CAGE or "family CAGE." This stands for the first letter in key words from four screening questions: Cut down, Annoyed, Guilty and Eye-opener as shown in Table 2. Each positive response to a question on the f-CAGE, especially when it represents a repetition of behavior, has a 40% chance of addictive disease. The reason for this is the fact that the f-CAGE assesses for abnormal patterns and consequences of substance use and identifies repetitive loss of control and adverse consequences.

Intervention

Intervention with persons who have substance abuse or dependence problems is a difficult but potentially very useful task. The most important part of intervening by one's self with a friend who has a substance use problem is to be sure to actually do it. The most basic approach is to share one's concern with the affected person about the substance use. It is helpful not

Table 2. The f-CAGE questionnaire

C	Does anyone in your family ever periodically feel a need to *cut down* on their use of alcohol or other drugs?
A	Does anyone in your family ever get *annoyed* by comments made by friends or family about his/her use of alcohol or other drugs?
G	Does anyone in your family ever feel *guilty*, embarrassed, or even bashful about things they say or do while using alcohol or other drugs?
E	Does anyone in your family ever need *eye-openers* or to drink or drug in the morning to "get started" or "settle their nerves"?

to be judgmental, to focus on the use and the consequences and not on the person. The strategy is to separate the person from the addictive disease and behaviors associated with the disease when sharing concerns. This minimizes arguments and helps keep communication open. Phrases such as "I know it is not you, it is the drinking…" are very helpful. Other more specific suggestions are available through the references.

The Crisis Family Intervention is worth mentioning for several reasons, even though it is beyond the expertise of family member or loved one. First, over the past decade or two it has become the most successful approach to involve patients in treatment for chemical dependence. Second, family members are periodically asked to participate in the interventions. The crisis intervention is basically a group confrontation with the chemically dependent person, carefully organized, rehearsed, and choreographed by a trained "intervention counselor." Each member of the group is a "significant other" of the patient, and is prepared to state several experiences where the drinking/drugging of the patient adversely affected that group member. With the weight of all of this objective evidence, presented by friends and family members, the "wall of denial" for most patients breaks down enough to help get that patient into a treatment program. Phrases and techniques that are coached by the intervention counselor include the following: "It's not you, it is the drinking." "It hurts me too much to see you continue in this painful disease." "You did not develop this on purpose, but you've got it." "We care about you, but hate your drinking." "I will not argue; this is what you did, this is when you did it, and this is how it made me feel." Obviously, there are a few common threads in these phrases:

1. Exhibiting positive regard toward the individual and negative regard toward the drinking at all times.

2. Obtaining specific data about specific events in order to adequately confront such patients.

3. Validating the disease via statements about the obvious pain of this progressive illness—which ruins family, job, financial, legal, spiritual, and physical health—gives the patient permission to become less defensive.

4. Acknowledging that patients with chemical dependence do not try to catch it, but need treatment anyway, can relieve some degree of guilt, and make patients even less defensive. When organized and supervised by a well-trained intervention counselor, a crisis intervention can motivate up to 80% of patients who are resisting treatment to change their minds and enter a treatment program.

Treatment

Treatment of substance abuse primarily entails education about dangers of overuse and binging, efforts to eliminate illegal drug use altogether, and support in limiting use of alcohol to within the sensible drinking guidelines. Treatment for substance abuse is primarily education and advice, coupled with the reprimand of and intolerance for future intoxicated and disinhibited behavior.

Treatment of addiction requires a focus on eliminating mood-altering drug use. Therefore, abstinence is the treatment goal and most treatment efforts are aimed at achieving abstinence and maintaining abstinence long term. There are several levels of addiction treatment available, and each will be briefly described:

Detoxification

This is a short, 1- to 7-day inpatient or outpatient stay during which patients are detoxified from one or more mood-altering substances. A "detox" is indicated if a patient gives a history of not being able to "get sober or straight" at all on her/his own.

Inpatient Treatment (Rehabilitation)

This refers to an inpatient stay on a residential unit for a variable period of time ranging from 7 days to 6 weeks. Admission criteria as well as programs tend to vary, but generally accept insured patients who have finished the worst of their withdrawal. Some programs accept uninsured patients. While enrolled, patients spend their time being educated about addiction, recovery, and Alcoholics Anonymous (AA) in group therapy, individual counseling, family counseling sessions, and doing reading and writing homework assignments.

Advantages of these programs include protected environments, intensive education and therapy, and new friends and associates who are drug- and alcohol-free. Disadvantages include cost and thus limited access to this treatment as well as separation from the realities

631

of life during treatment. For some patients, separation from their environment via residential treatment will be essential for establishing a period of drug-free time to allow treatment and recovery to begin.

Outpatient Treatment (Rehabilitation)

With limited insurance resources but a commitment to treat the illness of chemical dependence, more and more emphasis is being placed on flexible outpatient programs. These programs offer most of what the inpatient programs do, except that it is "day treatment" or "evening treatment" and, thus, less expensive.

Advantages are a longer period of treatment for the same or less cost, a chance for patients to continue to work or care for their home while participating, and the opportunity to interact with the environment (home, work, etc.) while exploring, through treatment, the strategies to use in that environment to stay sober and develop a recovery plan. Disadvantages include the cost not being covered by insurance, large co-pay percentages, limited number of programs available, and a less structured environment and greater tendency for relapse during treatment.

Self-Help Programs (AA, NA, CA, etc.)

The self-help programs, notably AA, were developed in the 1930s and 1940s, and were the first successful approaches to recovery from chemical dependence. Though difficult to describe and nearly impossible to explain, AA works as a fellowship of individuals, all of whom have alcoholism or drug dependence and all of whom meet regularly to act as support for each other's efforts to live without drinking or drugging. Daily meetings, which take place in all communities, are free and are open to all people in need. They follow a general outline of opening with a recitation of the Twelve Steps and Twelve Traditions of AA, followed by a member telling his/her story of life with and without alcohol, and closing with a discussion and then the Lord's Prayer. Though clearly spiritual in orientation, AA is not religious and mainly concentrates on how to live sober. Advantages include cost (free), accessibility, convenience, and success. Disadvantages include preconceived notions/prejudices on the part of patients so they refuse to attend, and the fact that what is good treatment for many is not sufficient for everyone.

When using 12-step meetings, it is important for women in early recovery to try to attend at least some "women-only closed" meetings. A women-only meeting should be the person's "home group" and utilizing a person from the home group for a "sponsor" is very important. These recommendations are made to counteract the strong tendency toward male–female socializing at times in formal and self-help treatment programs. It is clearly not in the best interests of a woman's recovery to develop a relationship in treatment. In fact, unstable romantic relationships are such a strong predictor for relapsing back to addiction that it is recommended not to begin any new relationships for the first 12–18 months of sobriety.

Family Treatment Resources

There are several resources available to help family and friends educate themselves about chemical dependence in the references. After family members have read these materials, they will be more likely to agree to referral for individual counseling or family therapy. There are self-help organizations also available for family members of people with chemical dependence problems, including AlAnon, Alateen, Tough Love, and Families Anonymous. In addition, family members can benefit from individual counseling or family therapy when dealing with a loved one who has addiction problems.

SEE ALSO: Addiction, Addiction ethics, Club drugs, Cocaine, Heroin, Inhalant abuse, Injection drug use, Marijuana

Suggested Reading

American Psychiatric Association. (1994). *Diagnostic and statistical manual of mental disorders* (4th ed.) Washington, DC: American Psychiatric Association.

Alcoholics Anonymous. (1976). Third edition. New York: Alcoholics Anonymous World Services.

Barker, L. R., & Whitfield, C. L. (2002). Alcoholism. In L. Barker, J. R. Burton, & P. D. Zieve (Eds.), *Principles of ambulatory medicine* (pp. 258–259). Baltimore: Williams & Wilkins.

Institute of Medicine, Division of Mental Health and Behavioral Medicine. (1990). *Broadening the base of treatment for alcohol problems.* Washington, DC: National Academy Press.

Mooney, A. (1992). *The recovery book.* New York: Workman.

National Institute on Alcohol Abuse and Alcoholism. (1995). NIAAA sensible guide to drinking *The physicians guide to helping patients with alcohol problems* (NIH Publication No. 95-3769). Washington, DC: U.S. Department of Health and Human Services, Public Health Service, National Institutes of Health.

Principles of Addiction Medicine. (2003). Vol. 3. Washington, DC: American Society of Addiction Medicine.

Rogers, R. L., & McMillin, C. S. (1992). *Freeing someone you love from alcohol and other drugs.* New York: The Body Press.

Valliant, G. E. (1983). *The natural history of alcoholism: Causes, patterns, and paths to recovery.* Cambridge, MA: Harvard University Press.

TED PARRAN, JR.

Suicide Suicide is when a person intentionally ends his or her life. Over the ages society has had differing views regarding this act—from acceptance, in that this is a choice, to considering it as a sin. Currently it is felt that suicide is rather complex resulting from social stressors, psychology, and biological factors. In the United States, approximately 30,000 people kill themselves every year, while it is believed that a much larger number of people attempt suicide. Suicide is the ninth overall cause of death in this country.

There are many factors that are felt to be associated with risk to attempt and complete suicide. These include gender, age, marital status, psychiatric illness, substance abuse, occupation, physical health, and history of suicide attempts. Men kill themselves three times as often as women, whereas women attempt four times as often as men. It is felt that the reason for this may be related to the methods employed. Men attempting suicide commonly use more lethal methods, such as guns and hanging. Women tend to overdose more frequently in their attempts. However, new studies indicate that women are using firearms more often than they had previously.

Age is another associated factor and suicide rates increase with age. Suicides peak for men after the age of 45, while that of women is at 55 years. Younger people tend to attempt suicide more often and are less likely to succeed than older people as a trend. Currently, the suicide rate is rising most rapidly in younger people and is specific to men 18–24 years old. People who are married have a lower risk of suicide and this is reinforced if they are parents. Occupation plays a role as well in the risk for suicide. Unemployment is a risk factor for suicide as are high-stress professions, such as medicine.

Medical illness can be a large factor in suicide. When people have chronic medical problems that impact their quality of life, the risk for killing themselves increases. In the treatment of some medical illnesses, the medications used can result in a mood disorder such as depression, which again can place people at higher risk. Psychiatric illnesses are another risk factor for suicide. It is estimated that almost 95% of people who kill themselves have a mental illness. The predominant ones are the depressive disorders with 80% of suicides having this class of illness. People with these types of disorders who kill themselves are usually in a depressive episode. It is noted that they will kill themselves either at the beginning or the end of a depressive period. Along with mental illness is comorbid substance abuse, which is seen commonly. People with schizophrenia are also at risk for suicide and account for 10% of the people with mental illness who kill themselves. This group of people has the onset of their illness during early adulthood, and those who commit suicide usually do so within the first few years after diagnosis. People with alcohol dependence are at risk and it is estimated that 15% will kill themselves. Approximately 80% of those alcohol-dependent people who commit suicide are males. Many of the people with mental illness have other factors in common—significant social isolation, feeling hopeless, and unemployment—that in and of themselves are risk factors for suicide.

It is felt that perhaps the best predictor for suicide is a past suicide attempt. Some data show that up to 40% of people with depression who kill themselves have attempted suicide in the past. Further studies have been examining the intent to die associated with prior attempts. It is believed that this will show that people who attempt suicide with a high intent to die will be at higher risk of completed suicide.

Warning signs of suicide are felt to be seen in approximately 80% of people who succeed at this. These signs can be the person telling others about their thoughts, preoccupation with death, or discussing feeling hopeless. Much attention has also been drawn to the evaluation of art—paintings, songs, and poetry that revolve around the topic of death. Another common warning sign is when people give away their valued personal belongings. While it is frequently thought that asking about suicide will plant this idea onto an otherwise nonsuicidal person, research suggests that this is not the case. On the other hand, asking about suicidal thoughts many times can aid in finding treatment for an underlying depression and thus prevent a suicide. It is felt that most suicides are preventable as suicidal thoughts are usually temporary and secondary to a depressed mood.

Syphilis

CAUSES

Over the years many different theories have been proposed to explain why people commit suicide. As mentioned previously, depression plays a large role, but there are various possible causes for depression. The French sociologist Emile Durkheim hypothesized that both social and cultural influences play a role in depression. He described multiple types of suicide where integration in a social group, or lack thereof, can result in one killing himself or herself. Psychological factors have been examined as possible explanations to suicide. For example, Sigmund Freud felt that suicide was a result of an earlier repressed wish to kill someone else. Recent media coverage of famous people who commit suicide has brought speculation that this can cause others, specifically adolescents, to kill themselves. Currently there are no data to support this thought.

Biological factors have also been investigated. Genetics is a known risk factor and suicide runs in families. One study in an Amish population in Pennsylvania found 26 suicides in just 4 families. However, in this study, the family members all had psychiatric illnesses. Because of this, it is felt that suicide itself may not be genetically inherited, but rather the psychiatric illness is hereditary and this is what puts a person at higher risk. Neurobiochemistry also appears to play a role in suicide. In a study of people who killed themselves by violent means, it was found that there was a lower serotonin level in their brains compared to depressed people who did not commit suicide. Serotonin is a neurochemical believed to be one of the main chemicals involved in depression.

PREVENTION

It is felt that suicide is many times preventable as it is usually secondary to fleeting thoughts while in a depressive episode. In the 1950s, most communities in the United States started suicide hotlines; however, these are only helpful to those who call. People in the community, such as teachers and police, are educated in how to recognize the risk factors for suicide. Many times when someone is suicidal and intent on killing themselves, psychiatric hospitalization is appropriate. Suicide has a large impact on the people who were close to the person who ended his/her life. These people, left behind, can blame themselves and may not want to talk about the event secondary to the social stigma attached to suicide. There are many support groups for families who have lived through a suicide, which can be useful in coping with this tragedy.

SEE ALSO: Depression, Mental illness, Mood disorders, Schizophrenia, Self-injurious behavior, Substance use, Violence

Suggested Reading

American Psychiatric Association. (1994). *Diagnostic and statistical manual of mental disorders* (4th ed.). Washington, DC: American Psychiatric Association.

ISABEL SCHUERMEYER

Sun Spots   *see* Liver Spots

Syphilis   Syphilis is a sexually transmitted disease caused by the bacterium *Treponema pallidum.* Syphilis is a potentially progressive disease that if untreated may cause debilitating disease of the entire body. Syphilis currently is of particular concern because it is believed to increase the transmission of HIV.

Syphilis is transmitted during sexual or nonsexual contact with a person who is infected. The bacterium initially spreads from the infected person to the skin or genital area of the uninfected person. Syphilis can also be transmitted in utero. Syphilis cannot be spread by toilet seats, doorknobs, swimming pools, hot tubs, shared clothing, or eating utensils.

The symptoms of syphilis vary according to the stage of disease. The stages of syphilis are divided into primary, secondary, latent, and tertiary disease. The initial lesion of primary syphilis is a genital ulcer called a "chancre." It may appear between 10 and 90 days after a person comes in contact with the bacteria. Newly infected people are often unaware of the ulcer, since it is painless and usually disappears within 3–6 weeks with or without treatment. Secondary syphilis is usually characterized by a skin rash. The rash can appear anywhere on the body, but is almost always on the palms of the hands and soles of the feet. It does not itch, and may be very faint and not noticeable. The rash usually disappears within several weeks. Other symptoms during this stage may include fever, fatigue, headache, and swollen lymph glands. If syphilis remains untreated, the disease may go into the latent stage. People at this point usually have no further signs or symptoms of disease. Tertiary syphilis is characterized by systemic disease, but not all patients who develop secondary syphilis will develop tertiary syphilis. At this point, the bacteria can damage almost any part of the body, particularly the nervous system, bones, and joints. This stage can last for years or even decades. Untreated syphilis can be responsible for blindness and neurological problems, mental illness, heart disease, and potentially death.

Clinical symptoms of syphilis, especially the early symptoms, can be confusing, mimicking other diseases. The diagnosis of syphilis is made by a blood test. Because the blood test can have "false positives," another blood test is always used to confirm the diagnosis. Identifying the syphilis bacteria under the microscope is another way of diagnosing the disease, but requires specialized equipment not available to most physicians.

Syphilis usually responds well to injectable penicillin. There are other antibiotics available for patients who have penicillin allergies. Unfortunately, during the first stages of syphilis, many people do not realize that they are infected, and usually do not seek treatment. Once a person is treated, the blood test can be followed to make sure that the infection is gone. People with more advanced stages of syphilis usually require longer courses of treatment. Patients who present with syphilis should always be tested for HIV. Ulcers due to syphilis increase the risk of acquisition of HIV, and advanced HIV infection alters the clinical presentation of syphilis and makes central nervous system complications more likely.

Women who have syphilis early in their pregnancy have a higher rate of miscarriage. Pregnant women who do not miscarry have a 40–70% chance of passing syphilis on to their unborn child, depending on the stage of their disease. Congenital syphilis can cause serious fetal and neonatal complications, including stillbirth, neonatal jaundice (yellow skin), swollen limbs and spleens, and skin ulcers and rashes. All women should be tested at their first prenatal visit for syphilis, and women who are at higher risk for acquiring syphilis should be tested again later in their pregnancy.

Syphilis, like many sexually transmitted diseases, can be prevented by practicing safe sex and using latex condoms properly and consistently. While initial syphilis infection may not always be preventable, getting screened if you are at high risk, and being treated early, reduces the likelihood that complications of late-stage disease will develop.

SEE ALSO: Acquired immunodeficiency syndrome, Chlamydia, Gonorrhea, Herpes simplex virus, Human papillomavirus, Sexually transmitted diseases

Suggested Reading

Gripshover, B., & Valdez, H. (2002). Common sexually transmitted diseases. In J. S. Tan (Ed.), *Experts guide to the management of common infectious diseases* (pp. 271–303). Philadelphia: American College of Physicians.

Suggested Resources

Center for Disease Control website: http://www.cdc.gov/health/std.htm

KAREN L. ASHBY

Systemic Lupus Erythematosus

Systemic lupus erythematosus (SLE) is an autoimmune, multisystem disease with a wide variety of symptoms. The primary immunological defect is the production of antibodies against one's own self. These molecules cause tissue injury principally in the skin, joints, kidneys, nervous system, heart, and the lungs and surrounding linings. SLE affects 1 in 2,000 individuals in the general outpatient population. Women of childbearing age are most commonly affected. A genetic predisposition to SLE is likely since first-degree relatives have a much higher frequency of disease. Environmental factors, including ultraviolet light, emotional stress, and certain drugs, may also play a role by bringing on the disease or worsening it. Thus, SLE is a complex disease of many potential causes, including genetic and environmental factors, which results in an immune system that fights against normal tissues.

The symptoms of SLE vary, but usually include nonspecific features such as fatigue, fever, and weight loss. SLE potentially can affect almost every body part. Because of this variability and the fact that other diseases may resemble SLE, diagnostic criteria have been developed. Although the list of criteria is a handy checklist, it is only a guide and is used primarily for research studies. In a research study, a patient must have 4 of the 11 criteria to meet the diagnosis of SLE. However, in practice, patients are often treated as symptoms arise and may not have 4 criteria even though treatment is warranted.

The skin is most commonly involved. The characteristic malar or "butterfly rash" is a red and swollen rash extending over the bony part of the nose and across the cheeks, often associated with sun exposure and getting sick from the sun. Painful joints are the most common initial symptoms of SLE. Arthritis may involve the hands, wrists, and knees on both sides of the body. This pattern also occurs in rheumatoid arthritis (RA), but unlike RA, permanent deformity does not develop. The kidney is one of the most important organs affected by SLE, and kidney failure is the most common cause of death. Inflammatory reactions within the kidney lead to deposition of proteins that can cause a variety of problems including leakage of blood and protein into the urine. Nervous system involvement is also common and may involve the brain, nerves, and automatic functions such as blood pressure and pulse rate. SLE affects the heart by causing swelling and irritation of the heart. This may produce a scratching sound when listening with a stethoscope. More than one third of SLE patients have some form of lung disease during their lifetime, mostly involving the lining around the lung. The eye, the gastrointestinal tract, and liver may also be involved.

LABORATORY FEATURES

Since SLE causes various changes in the blood itself, the complete blood count (CBC) is important in evaluating the disease. Up to 80% of patients will have anemia, due to many potential causes such as iron deficiency or destruction of blood cells by the immune system. This may result in not only decreased red blood cells but also decreased white blood cells and platelets. A low platelet count can cause nosebleeds and bleeding in the skin and gums. At times, this may be the only manifestation of SLE.

Blood tests look for proteins and cells directed against otherwise normal proteins in the blood. Some of these tests include a positive antinuclear antibodies (ANA), antibodies to double-stranded DNA, and anti-Sm (Smith) antigen. A positive ANA may be found with autoimmunity but does not automatically diagnose SLE, since there are many conditions that may cause a false-positive ANA. Complement proteins, which are involved in inflammation, can also be measured and are often greatly decreased, especially if there is active

kidney involvement. Overall, these tests or measurements of antibodies are important for baseline evaluation, but treatment of SLE should not be based on serological test results alone. More importantly, treatment should be based on the history and physical exam of each individual.

TREATMENT

Due to the various drug treatments available, treatment should be based on the patient's symptoms and their severity. Education is extremely important. The patient, along with his or her support network, should be provided information about SLE, support groups and organizations, and strategies to maintain his or her quality of life.

Drugs commonly used in the treatment of SLE include nonsteroidal anti-inflammatory drugs (NSAIDs), corticosteroids, antimalarials, and several immunosuppressants.

NSAIDs are frequently used for musculoskeletal pain, inflammation, and headaches. Patients should be monitored for common side effects including gastrointestinal bleeding, liver or kidney damage, and high blood pressure.

Corticosteroids are often used for the immediate relief of life-threatening symptoms. Topical creams and joint injections should be used sparingly. Long-term use of corticosteroids should be avoided due to many potential side effects.

Antimalarial medications are commonly used for fatigue, skin, and musculoskeletal symptoms. Antimalarials are generally well tolerated and help avoid the need for corticosteroids. The most significant risk involves eye toxicity and a thorough eye examination by an ophthalmologist is required every 6 months.

Cyclophosphamide, a strong immunosuppressant, is used for severe organ-system disease, particularly for kidney damage due to SLE (lupus nephritis). Side effects include bone marrow suppression, bleeding from the bladder, and severe hair loss (alopecia). Regular laboratory monitoring is required. Other immunosuppressive medications, such as azathioprine and methotrexate, are often used as an alternative agent for the treatment of nephritis or to avoid corticosteroids for nonkidney symptoms.

Alternative therapies and experimental drugs under investigation include stem cell research and biologic therapies. However, more studies of long-term effects and effectiveness will be needed before these treatments can be used in the management of SLE.

SEE ALSO: Autoimmune disorders

Suggested Reading

Klippel, J. H., et al. (Eds.). (2001). *Primer on the rheumatic diseases* (12th ed.). Atlanta, GA: Arthritis Foundation.

Klippel, J. H., & Dieppe, P. A. (1998). *Rheumatology* (2nd ed.). St. Louis, MO: Mosby.

Klippel, J. H., Dieppe, P. A., & Ferri, F. F. (2000). *Primary care rheumatology*. London: Harcourt.

KATHERINE WREN
SHIRLEY LEE
LORI B. SIEGEL

Tampon Tampons are used to collect menstrual fluid. They are made of either synthetic fibers such as rayon or natural fibers such as cotton. These fibers are manufactured into a compact tubular shape that allows for easy insertion into the vagina. Tampons come in different levels of absorbency. This allows the woman to select the tampon to meet the demands of her menstrual flow. Women should select the lightest absorbency needed to provide effective coverage. If the tampon is difficult to remove or does not need to be changed in 4 hours, it may be too absorbent. If any signs of irritation appear in the vaginal area, consider changing brands or switching to sanitary pads.

Tampon users should be aware of the signs of toxic shock syndrome such as high fever, low blood pressure, and sunburn—like rash, vomiting, and diarrhea. One brand of tampon, Rely tampons, was removed from the market after studies demonstrated that there was an increased risk of toxic shock syndrome associated with their use. This increased risk has not been associated with the use of any other brand of tampon.

SEE ALSO: Menstruation, Toxic shock syndrome

Suggested Reading

Chin, H. (1997). *On call: Obstetrics and gynecology* (p. 283). Philadelphia: W.B. Saunders.
Scott, J., et al. (1999). *Danforth's obstetrics and gynecology* (8th ed., p. 287). Philadelphia: W.B. Saunders

SUSAN WIEDASECK

Tattoos Tattoos have been used in many cultures to identify beauty, position or status, and worth. They mark rites of passage, such as a life cycle event (marriage, pregnancy, childbirth, death), change in an individual's social position, the progression from childhood to puberty, and the initiation into social and different family groups. For instance, both men and women of the Maori tribe of New Zealand are tattooed beginning at puberty. Individuals may also choose to have tattoos done for artistic, spiritual, or other personal reasons. There are similarities between the tattoos of men and women but the tattoos of the female Moko were generally confined to the chin and lips and were designed to attract a mate. It was thought that having a full set of very blue lips was the ultimate in beauty.

A tattoo is a permanent coloration of the second layer of skin (dermis) that is produced by puncturing the skin and inserting indelible inks of a chosen color in a selected pattern or design. The designs that are favored have changed over time and may differ depending upon the particular social context. For instance, some individuals who are members of the armed services prefer patriotic or military tattoos. Other individuals may wish to have the names of their loved ones tattooed on their bodies, while still others use tattoos to memorialize specific events or experiences. Still others wish to use tattoos to have permanent makeup and have their eyebrows and their eyeliner done permanently.

In deciding whether or not to have a tattoo done, it is important to remember that a tattoo remains with you permanently. Decide ahead of time how public you wish to be about your tattoo; some people want the world to see their tattoos, while others prefer to have them done in a more private area of their bodies so that they choose who can see it and when. Although it is possible to have a tattoo removed, this procedure is timely and can be costly. The following guidelines may be helpful in selecting a tattooist.

1. Make sure that the establishment is licensed if the state in which it is located requires that tattooists be licensed.

2. Check the cleanliness of the tattoo parlor.

3. Make sure that the tattooist is using a technique for tattooing that minimizes the possibility of any type of infection. It is important that he or she uses new needles and new ink for each client; all equipment should be "single use." Used ink from one client should not be poured back into a larger container. Ink should not be poured into a cap that has been used to hold the ink for someone else's tattoo. New ink should be used in a new disposable container for each client. The tattoo artist should be wearing gloves while tattooing and should change his or her gloves for each client. A failure to follow proper procedures could result in the transmission of HIV/AIDS, hepatitis, bacterial infections, and other blood-borne diseases.

4. Make sure that the tattooist is willing to make accommodations for your ability to tolerate the pain associated with the tattoo procedure. For instance, some individuals find it difficult to sit for a tattoo for more than 20 minutes due to their pain threshold. The tattoo artist should be willing to schedule more sessions of smaller length to accommodate this.

5. You should feel comfortable with the tattoo artist. Make sure that he or she understands what you want. Feel free to ask to see photographs of his or her work to make sure that the artist's style matches yours.

6. Many tattoo artists charge from $125 to $250 an hour, depending upon their skill and experience and the complexity of the design that you are requesting. Do not choose a tattooist on the basis of price. A "bargain" may be no bargain if the tattoo artist does not follow appropriate infection control procedures or does not have the requisite skill and experience to provide the design requested.

After receiving a tattoo, it is important that it receive the requisite care. These guidelines are often used to care for a tattoo.

1. After receiving the tattoo, the tattooist will often apply an ointment and bandage. Leave the bandage on for the instructed period of time, which may range from 2 or 3 hours to up to 12 hours.

2. Remove the bandage carefully. If it sticks to the skin, use warm water to gently remove it.

3. Carefully rinse off any dried blood from the tattoo. (Some, but not all, individuals may have some bleeding when they first get the tattoo.)

4. Do not put a new bandage on the tattoo.

5. For up to a few days, the tattooed area will feel as if you have a bad sunburn. Do not use sunburn products on your skin.

6. Wear loose clothing in the area of the tattoo for at least a few days in order to avoid irritating the area. Women who are tattooed near the breast area may choose not to wear a bra for a few days or may use a bra that does not have an underwire and is made from a stretchy fabric.

7. Do not use alcohol, Vaseline, or petroleum jelly on the tattoo.

8. For 1 week, apply Neosporin or a similar cream to the tattoo two or three times a day.

9. Avoid strenuous exercise for at least 2 weeks in order to allow the skin to heal.

10. Do not expose the tattooed area to chlorine (as in swimming pools) or the sun for 2 weeks.

11. Do not soak in a sauna, steambath, or bathtub for at least 1 week to reduce the risk of any type of infection.

12. After the first week, use a good body lotion on the tattoo to keep it moist.

13. In a period of 1–2 weeks, the skin on the tattoo will become dry and somewhat harder and will fall off. This is normal. During this time, it is likely that your tattoo will itch a great deal. Do not scratch or pick at the tattoo or pull off the drying/flaking skin. Use the lotion to ameliorate the itching.

SEE ALSO: Acquired immunodeficiency syndrome, Hepatitis

Suggested Reading

Krakow, A. (1994). *The total tattoo book*. New York: Warner Books.

Schiffmacher, H., & Riemschneider, B. (1996). *1000 tattoos*. Cologne: Taschen.

Suggested Resources

Alliance of Professional Tattooists: http://www.safe-tattoos.com

DAVID VIDRA
SANA LOUE

Tay–Sachs Disease

Tay–Sachs disease (TSD) is a fatal genetic disorder named after Warren Tay (1843–1927) and Bernard Sachs (1858–1944). Tay was a British ophthalmologist who, in 1881, described the occurrence of cherry-red spots ("Tay's spots") on the retinas of three siblings. Sachs was an American neurologist who, in 1887, described cellular changes occurring in the disorder. Sachs also recognized the disorder's familial nature and later, after seeing more cases, noted that most cases occurred in infants of eastern European Jewish descent.

CLINICAL PRESENTATION

Infants with TSD typically seem to be normal until age 3–6 months. Often, infants will have a porcelain-like complexion and long eyelashes. The onset of the illness is usually insidious, but the disease progresses rapidly. Normal development slows, and the baby may show an increased startle response. Infants will start to lose already-developed skills, such as sitting up unsupported and crawling. By age 2 years, most children exhibit slowed mental functioning and recurrent seizures. Children eventually become blind, deaf, mentally retarded, and paralyzed. Swallowing difficulties may lead to the placement of feeding tubes. Twenty-four-hour care, either in a care facility or in the home, is typically required due to the multitude of medical complications. They usually have chronic respiratory difficulties from the age of 2 years on, and death is often due to pneumonia. Children with TSD die early, generally by age 5.

CAUSE OF TAY–SACHS DISEASE

Children with TSD lack an important enzyme, hexosaminidase A (hex-A), which breaks down lipids in the brain and central nervous system. The absence of hex-A causes a lipid called GM2 ganglioside to accumulate in brain cells, damaging them irreversibly. Other disorders of hex-A production may be included under the name TSD, such as juvenile-, chronic-, and adult-onset hex-A deficiency. These other disorders tend to have slower courses, but life span is shortened.

Tay-Sachs disease has been linked to alterations in chromosome 15—more than 50 mutations have been identified in the gene. The disorder appears to have originated in a population of eastern European (Ashkenazi) Jewish families in the early 1800s. The disease is by no means an exclusively Jewish genetic disease, although approximately 85% of patients with TSD are Jewish. While 1 in 30 people of central or eastern Jewish descent carry the gene for TSD, approximately 1 in 300 people in the general population carry the gene as well. Clusters of cases have also been described in populations of French Canadians and Louisiana Cajuns. It is an autosomal recessive genetic condition, meaning that both parents must be carriers of the recessive TSD gene (each has the TSD in their genetic makeup), and pass the recessive gene on to their child for the child to develop the disease. For two carriers, the chance of having an unaffected (healthy), noncarrier offspring (no TSD gene) is 25%. For these same two carriers, the chance of having a nondiseased but carrier offspring (has TSD gene) is 50%. For these same two carriers, the chance of having a child with TSD is 25%. If only one parent is a carrier, no children will inherit two copies of the recessive gene, so none will have TSD. However, each child of such a union has a 50% chance of inheriting the recessive gene, and thus being a carrier himself or herself.

DETECTION AND TREATMENT

There is no known cure for TSD; medical therapy is supportive. Attempts to treat the disorder using a specific type of enzyme replacement (hex-A enzyme replacement) have been unsuccessful because this protein cannot cross the blood–brain barrier and get to the affected brain cells. Tay-Sachs disease can, however, be detected both before birth (prenatally), by procedures that sample the fluid or tissue around the fetus (amniocentesis or chorionic villus sampling), and after birth, via a simple blood test. Since 1971, screening programs have been in effect and have greatly reduced the incidence of TSD in the United States through genetic counseling, use of alternative reproductive options, and therapeutic abortion. Blood testing reveals how much hex-A is present, and by inference how many working genes the person has. An infant with TSD has no circulating hex-A. Carriers, individuals who have one normal gene and one recessive gene, have approximately half the normal amount of hex-A. When carriers are identified, relatives should be tested to detect other potential carriers. It is very important for carrier couples to participate in genetic counseling to assess risks and potential alternative reproductive options such as adoption or artificial insemination with noncarrier sperm.

SEE ALSO: Adoption, Genetic counseling, Neonatal care ethics, Reproductive technologies

Suggested Reading

Ford, L., & Nissenbaum, M. (1998). Tay–Sachs Disease. In L. Phelps (Ed.), *Health-related disorders in children and adolescents: A guidebook for understanding and educating* (pp. 636–640). Washington, DC: American Psychological Association.

Bellenir, K. (Ed.). (1996). Tay–Sachs disease. *Genetic disorders sourcebook*. Detroit, MI: Omnigraphics.

PAULA L. HENSLEY

Teen Pregnancy
Currently, approximately 15 million girls under the age of 20 in the world have a child each year. Estimates are that 20–60% of these pregnancies in developing countries are mistimed or unwanted. In the United States, the percent of teenage pregnancies that are unintended is estimated at 78%. The rates of teen pregnancy are not equivalent across societies. Rates of adolescent pregnancy vary by a factor of almost 10 from as low as 12 pregnancies per year per 1,000 adolescents in the Netherlands to rates of more than 100 adolescents per year per 1,000 in the Russian Federation. The rates of women having a child before age 20 are higher in the United States compared to similar countries. For example, 22% of women report having a child before age 20 in the United States, compared to 15% in Great Britain and 11% in Canada. These differences are even greater when comparing birth rates among younger teenagers. When one controls for poverty and ethnicity, some, but not all, of this difference disappears.

In the early 1990s, over 1 million teenagers aged 15–19 became pregnant each year in the United States. This figure represents a peak of increasing rates of teen pregnancy through the 1980s and early 1990s. In the latter part of the 1990s through the first part of the new century, rates have begun to decline. Now it is estimated that just below 900,000 teenagers become pregnant each year. Reasons cited for the decline over the past decade include increased formal sex education programs, stabilization in the proportion of teenagers having sex at an early age, improved communication between child and parent, and improved contraceptive use. Similar trends are found in other Western countries, suggesting that similar social forces may play a role.

Older teenagers (i.e., 18- to 19-year-olds) have higher rates of birth than do younger teens aged 15–17 years old. Eighteen- to nineteen-year-olds make up over 60% of the births. Furthermore, rates of pregnancy across racial groups are not equal. In 1996, the rates among 15- to 19-year-olds for white non-Hispanic girls were 66 per 1,000, 179 per 1,000 for African American girls, and 165 per 1,000 for Hispanic girls.

Teenage pregnancy was not recognized as a national problem until the 1970s. Reasons include that the number of adolescent mothers increased dramatically when the baby boomers reached their teenage years. In addition, while birth rates were relatively high prior to this time, it was during the 1970s when the traditional trajectory for a pregnant adolescent changed, meaning that a pregnant adolescent did not necessarily get married and form a traditional family unit. For example, during the 1950s, almost 70% of first births were to married adolescents. In contrast, in 1997, 78% of adolescent mothers were unmarried. In addition, the majority of adolescents who give birth are of low socioeconomic status.

These changes have resulted in large economic consequences. In 1990, the government spent over 25 billion dollars for health and social services for adolescent mothers and their children. It has been estimated that the cost for adolescent childbearing to taxpayers in 1996 exceeded that of delayed childbearing by 7 billion dollars. In addition to the economic disadvantages, adolescent pregnancy can also result in negative social consequences. When teens give birth, they are less likely to finish school and are more likely to have large families and be single parents. Moreover, children born to mothers aged 15–17 have poorer health including lower cognitive development and higher rates of behavior problems, as well as worse educational outcomes. Children born to adolescent mothers are also more likely to become teen parents themselves when compared to children born to older mothers. Furthermore, they are less likely to grow up in a home with fathers. Boys of adolescent mothers are almost three times more likely to engage in criminal behavior and be sent to prison compared to sons of older moms. Of course, it is difficult to disentangle the effects of poverty from those of teen childbearing. Poverty has for a long time been thought of as the consequence of teenage childbearing, however, these effects may be overstated in that poverty is also a catalyst for teenage childbearing.

In part because of these consequences, several different movements or activities have been implemented to combat teen pregnancy. First and foremost, there has been an increase in education programs. Along with individual instruction, efforts have been made to involve parents and families in educational programming as well as to have multicomponent prevention programs (i.e., schoolwide activities, media campaigns). In addition, there has been an increased effort to provide contraception to adolescents via family planning services and school-based health, such as HIV prevention education. While the focus of such programs is to prevent HIV infection, the methods through which to achieve this (i.e., condom use, abstinence) also result in decreased teenage pregnancy. Furthermore, Section 510 was added to Title V of the Social Security Act in 1996 which allocated $50 million a year in programming for abstinence education over several years. Finally, programs that focus on youth development generally, and education and life opportunities specifically have been implemented to encourage adolescents to delay childbearing.

See Also: Acquired immunodeficiency syndrome, Adolescence, Birth control, Condoms, Pregnancy, Sexually transmitted diseases

Suggested Reading

Darroch, J. E., Singh, S., & Frost, J. J. (2001). Differences in teenage pregnancy rates among five developed countries: The roles of sexual activity and contraceptive use. *Family Planning Perspectives, 33*(6), 244–250.

Kirby, D. (1999). Reflections on two decades of research on teen sexual behavior and pregnancy. *Journal of School Health, 69*(3), 89–94.

Kirby, D. (2001). *Emerging answers: Research findings on programs to reduce teen pregnancy.* Washington, DC: National Campaign to Prevent Teen Pregnancy.

Miller, F. C. (2000). Impact of adolescent pregnancy as we approach the new millennium. *Journal of Pediatric and Adolescent Gynecology, 13*(1), 5–8.

Singh, S., & Darroch, J. E. (2000). Adolescent pregnancy and childbearing: Levels and trends in developed countries. *Family Planning Perspectives, 32*(1), 14–23.

Natalie Colabianchi

Temporal Arteritis *see* Giant Cell Arteritis

Temporomandibular Joint Disorders The National Institute of Dental and Craniofacial Research of the National Institutes of Health indicates that 10.8 million people in the United States suffer from temporomandibular joint (TMJ) problems at any given time. While both men and women experience TMJ problems, 90% of those seeking treatment are women in their childbearing years.

Temporomandibular joint disorders (TMD) are one of the many causes of headache, facial pain, neck pain, and related symptoms. The TMJ differs from any other joints in the body in that it has a hinge action similar to the movements of the knees, and a sliding action similar to movements of the wrists.

To locate the TMJ, place your fingers on each side of your face, just in front of your ears and gently open and close your mouth. Upon opening the mouth, the rounded end of bone at the top of the lower jaw, known as the condyle, will glide along a groove in the bone on the temple area (known as the temporal bone). Upon closing the mouth, the condyle will slide back to its original position. This can be felt by holding the fingers over the TMJ. A very thin soft disk lies between the condyle and the temporal bone. This disk acts as a shock absorber for the TMJ during daily functions such as chewing, talking, and yawning. It is during these actions that the TMJ and its surrounding muscles may be affected, resulting in any one of a number of uncomfortable conditions including TMD.

TMD generally falls into three main categories:

1. Extracapsular (outside of the TMJ) or myofascial (surrounding muscle) pain. This is the most common form of TMD, which involves discomfort or pain in the muscles that control jaw function, as well as the neck and shoulder muscles. The pain involved stems from abnormalities in the tissues or muscles around the TMJ.

2. Intracapsular disorders or internal derangement of the TMJ refer to disorders within the joint itself. There is an abnormal joint structure interfering with or restricting normal joint function during movement of the jaw (mandibular movement). This involves a dislocated jaw, displaced disk, or injury to the condyle.

3. Degenerative joint disease. This includes disease of the bone in the jaw such as osteoarthritis or rheumatoid arthritis in the TMJ.

SIGNS AND SYMPTOMS

1. Pain or discomfort in front of the ears, in the ears, in or behind the eyes, at the base of the skull, in the temple areas, at the top of the head, or in the cheekbone area.
2. Inability to chew hard or sticky foods, to talk for long periods of time, or to open the mouth very wide.
3. Clicking, popping, or grating noises in the joint during movement.
4. Inability to put the teeth together without pain, dislocation of the jaw, or locking of the jaw.
5. Other symptoms that do not seem related such as dizziness, fatigue, or visual problems.

A physical examination will include taking a proper history of mouth-related problems. Palpation (hands-on physical examination of the joint by the practitioner) properly done is a very effective tool in detecting tender, uncomfortable, and painful areas. Further clinical investigation may include specialized diagnostic procedures such as making a model of the joint and x-ray (radiographic) analysis.

The clinician may find one or more of the following during physical examination:

1. Facial asymmetry, such as different eye levels, deviation of the nose or chin to one side, too much or too little height in the lower third of the face.
2. Limited or excessive range of mouth opening.
3. Abnormal pattern of movement of the lower jaw on opening or closing.
4. Malocclusion (bad bite), such as missing, shifted, rotated, or tipped teeth.
5. Abnormal joint sounds such as clicking or cracking (crepitation).
6. Muscle rigidity.
7. Radiographic (x-ray) findings such as displaced or poorly shaped condyles.
8. Soft tissue findings such as disk displacement.

A significant percentage of patients will respond to conservative noninvasive (nonsurgical) treatment that includes thorough patient education. Nonsurgical treatment options include physical therapy; biofeedback with an occupational therapist; nonsteroidal anti-inflammatory medications; or a night guard, splint, or other mouth (orthotic) device that helps patients stop clenching or grinding their teeth while they sleep.

Dentists and specialists in the field of dentistry such as orthodontists, oral surgeons, and prosthodontists can be of great assistance in identifying and treating TMDs.

SEE ALSO: Arthritis, Headache, Sleep disorders

Suggested Reading

Abdel-Fatteh, R. (1992). *Evaluating TMJ injuries.* New York: Wiley.
Fricton, J. R., Koening, R. J., & Hathaway, K. M. (1998). *TMJ and craniofacial pain: Diagnosis and management.* Philadelphia: W.B. Saunders.
Okeson, J. P. (1992). *Management of temporomandibular disorders and occlusion* (3rd ed.). St. Louis, MO: Mosby-Year Book.

NORMAN DELOACH, JR.
JOY A. JORDAN

Tendonitis *see* Regional Rheumatic Pain

Thalidomide Thalidomide, now recognized as the cause of an epidemic of infant malformations, was originally a tranquilizer developed by Ciba, a Swiss pharmaceutical company in 1953. It was one of many chemical compounds discovered in the post-World War II decade. After briefly testing thalidomide, Ciba abandoned the product because the company observed no marketable pharmacological effects.

In 1954, the German company Chemie Gruenthal acquired thalidomide and marketed it as an anticonvulsant for epileptics. Again, it had no efficacy. They began trials for its use as an antihistamine, which also failed. The trials, however, demonstrated that the drug was well tolerated and was effective as a sedative and sleep aid. Gruenthal also found that it was particularly effective for pregnant women suffering from morning sickness.

In 1957, Gruenthal began marketing thalidomide in Germany for nausea and morning sickness. The drug quickly became the "drug of choice" to help pregnant

Thalidomide

women with severe morning sickness. It was advertised as a nontoxic medication, with no side effects, and completely safe for pregnant women. All of these claims were untrue. A major side effect associated with long-term use is peripheral neurosis, an often irreversible numbing of the hands and feet. Most insidious were the teratogenic effects (ability to cause birth defects), which were undiscovered because the drug was not tested on pregnant animals.

The first baby suffering from complications due to thalidomide was born on Christmas Day, 1956, a few months prior to the marketing release in Germany. It would be roughly $4\frac{1}{2}$ years until Dr. McBride, an obstetrician in Sydney, Australia, would first publicly report a connection between thalidomide and birth defects. No action was taken to remove the product from shelves in Germany until 1961, when these results were confirmed by Dr. Lenz in Germany. Prior to that time, as many as 20,000 children were born from mothers who took thalidomide. Thousands more were stillborn or miscarried.

Thalidomide actually has a limited window of teratogenic activity (activity causing malformations), which consists of a 15-day period during the first trimester of pregnancy. Common malformations that may result from its use during this period include deafness, blindness, cleft palate, malformed organs, no arms, no legs, no fingers, and even flippers growing from the shoulders.

Sadly, thalidomide babies are still being born in Third World countries due to the availability of the drug on the black market. Today, there are approximately 5,000 thalidomide survivors worldwide.

Thalidomide was never approved in the United States for morning sickness, mostly due to the efforts of a young physician, Frances Kelsey, who was then serving as an investigator for the U.S. Food and Drug Administration (FDA). Dr. Kelsey was given the thalidomide approval as an "easy start" for her career. The agency thought that since the drug was already approved in almost every European country, it would be an uncomplicated process. Fortunately for many would-be U.S. thalidomide consumers, Kelsey was a physician-pharmacologist with a profound interest in fetal development. She refused to approve the drug until the fetal interactions of the drug were shown to be safe. She fought a several-year battle against drug approval with the Richardson–Merrell corporation (the U.S. Gruenthal licensee) until it was shown in the global community that the drug was dangerous to fetal development, and the application was terminated.

The thalidomide crisis and subsequent infant malformation epidemic provided the motivation to establish more stringent drug testing and approval procedures worldwide. In the United States, the Food, Drug and Cosmetic Act (FDCA) has required FDA approval for new drugs since 1938, but it was not until 1962, after the thalidomide crisis, that the FDCA was amended to require new drug sponsors to demonstrate the safety and effectiveness of their products prior to receiving FDA approval.

In recent years, thalidomide has experienced a comeback. In addition to being an effective sedative, thalidomide gas been found to be helpful in modulating the immune system (an immunomodulatory drug). The FDA first approved its use in 1998 for the treatment of lesions associated with leprosy. Researchers are also examining its usefulness for the treatment of breast, prostate, and brain cancer, macular degeneration (an overgrowth of new blood vessels in the eye covering the retina), and HIV.

The FDA still recognizes thalidomide as a very dangerous drug and has imposed unprecedented regulatory controls on its distribution. The regulations promote a zero tolerance policy for thalidomide exposure during pregnancy. The System for Thalidomide Education and Prescribing Safety (S.T.E.P.S.) program is a comprehensive information package for prescribers and patients. It requires a 100% patient registry and requires that heterosexual women who have sex while taking the medication must use *at least* two forms of birth control. Additionally, heterosexual men must use condoms because thalidomide is present and can be transmitted in semen.

Despite its tainted history and potentially dangerous consequences, thalidomide is a true story of a pharmaceutical comeback. While in the past it caused harm and heartache, scientists are now using the once-negative aspects of the drug as the basis of possible cures for some of our most dangerous and elusive diseases.

SEE ALSO: Pregnancy

Suggested Resources

Burkholz, H. *Giving thalidomide a second chance.* US FDA, September–October 1997. Retrieved April 17, 2003, from http://www.fda.gov/fdac/features/1997/697_thal.html

Extraordinary People. *History of thalidomide.* Canadian Broadcasting Corporation. Retrieved April 17, 2003, from http://www.tv.cbc.ca/witness/thalidomide/extrahis.htm

Lenz, W. *The history of thalidomide.* Thalidomide Victims Association of Canada. Retrieved April 17, 2003, from http://www.thalidomide.ca/english/history.html

Physician's desk reference electronic library. Thalomid Capsules (Celgene) (ref: thalidomide). Thompson Medical Economics, 2002.

JOHN FRISBEE

The Pill   *see* Birth Control, Oral Contraception

Thyroid Diseases

PHYSIOLOGY

The thyroid gland secretes the hormones T_4 (thyroxine) and T_3 (triiodothyronine) which then control metabolism. These hormones act on a wide variety of tissues and in each organ may have slightly different effects. Thyroid hormone secretion is under the control of thyrotropin (a thryoid-stimulating hormone, TSH) which is secreted by the pituitary gland. The normal serum T_4/T_3 levels and the activation of thyroid hormone receptors inversely regulate TSH secretion; the higher the level of thyroid hormones in the blood, the lower the TSH level and vice versa. The hallmark of underactive thyroid (primary hypothyroidism), therefore, is an elevated TSH level. Occasionally, thyroid hormone levels are within the normal range and the TSH is elevated, yet these patients are still appropriately considered to have hypothyroidism. Similarly, hyperthyroidism is characterized by a decreased (usually undetectable) TSH level.

The thyroid gland traps the important chemical iodine and through a series of biochemical reactions synthesizes T_4 and T_3. If there is inadequate iodine available (e.g., iodine deficiency), then lack of thyroid hormone synthesis and secretion may result in increased TSH secretion and possibly thyroidal enlargement.

Tissues contain specific nuclear receptors that bind T_4/T_3. These receptors cause a variety of proteins to be formulated which enhance metabolism. Each organ or tissue may have varying amounts of T_4/T_3 receptors and different specific proteins and actions may result from receptor activation.

THYROID FUNCTION TESTS

Thyrotropin (TSH)

Serum TSH is the best indicator of thyroid hormone levels at the tissue level. All abnormal TSH concentrations must be investigated even if the serum T_4 and T_3 levels are within the normal range.

Thyroxine

In the past, total T_4 measurements and indirect assessment of binding proteins had been used as had Free T_4 estimates. These tests, however, were imperfect and now have been replaced by a direct "free T_4" measurement. Free T_4 measurements are more accurate and reliable. Free T_4 measurements, nonetheless, are still imperfect and their use during pregnancy, for example, has been somewhat problematic.

Triiodothyronine

Free T_3 assays have not become widely available as a routine test. Serum T_3 concentrations need not be performed routinely but may be especially helpful in the evaluation and treatment of hyperthyroid patients.

Thyroid Antibodies

Substances produced in the blood which activate the immune system (antibodies) against specific types of thyroid components (thyroglobulin and thyroid peroxidase) develop in patients with autoimmune thyroid disease. These antibody levels (titers) are typically elevated in patients with some types of autoimmune diseases which affect the thyroid gland such as Hashimoto's thyroiditis, and may be elevated in patients with Graves' disease (autoimmune thyroid disease), but usually at a lower titer.

OTHER TESTS

A radioactive iodine uptake (RAIU) test (normal range about 8–30%) is useful to help diagnose hyperthyroidism, as the test should be elevated. A very low RAIU test (less than 5%) is also useful when seen in a patient with hyperthyroidism as this suggests the presence of (less severe) subacute, silent, or postpartum thyroiditis. An RAIU test cannot be used in a pregnant or breast-feeding woman.

Thyroid scans are not used often now and the older practice of using them to determine if a thyroid lump (nodule) was "cold" or nonfunctional (suggesting a higher risk of being cancerous) has fallen into disfavor because of the advent of fine needle aspirations (FNA; using a fine needle to remove a small amount of thyroid tissue for testing). On the other hand, it is relevant to perform an isotope (specialized imaging technique) scan to assess whether a thyroid nodule is "hot" or autonomous. A "hot" nodule concentrates most of the isotope and the remaining extranodular tissue (tissue outside of the nodule) concentrates little, if any, isotope. Isotope scans are recommended in patients with solitary nodules (and in some patients with multinodular goiters) with a low TSH.

Thyroid sonograms, another specialized imaging technique to evaluate the consistency of the thyroid gland, are important to help diagnose the presence and size of thyroid nodules and are used to follow changes in the nodule(s) over time.

HYPERTHYROIDISM

Graves' Disease

Hyperthyroidism clinically is typically associated with signs or symptoms of anxiety, nervousness, weight loss, palpitations, tachycardia, warm, moist skin, hand tremor, sweating, and heat intolerance. The most common cause in young women is Graves' disease. Graves' disease is caused by the formation of specific TSH receptor antibodies that stimulate thyroid hormone synthesis and secretion resulting in increased serum free T_4, T_3, and, as a result, an undetectable TSH. One unusual aspect of Graves' disease is that some of its manifestations may be a result of the antibodies, rather than a direct consequence of thyroid hormone excess. Eye findings and pretibial myxedema (swelling seen in thyroid disease) are two such disorders. Possible ophthalmic manifestations include lid lag, proptosis (protruding eyes), conjunctivitis, diplopia (double vision), and rarely impaired visual acuity.

Treatment of Graves' disease hyperthyroidism can be either long-term antithyroid agents in an effort to induce a remission, surgery, or radioactive iodine. Specific antithyroid medications (e.g., propylthiouracil [PTU] or methimazole) can be used in an effort to induce a permanent remission. This treatment is very effective in normalizing thyroid function tests but only infrequently produces a long-lived remission when they are discontinued. Patients must be carefully monitored for potential adverse effects of PTU or methimazole including skin rash, hepatotoxicity (liver toxicity), arthralgias (joint pains), and bone marrow suppression. Pregnant women who are definitively diagnosed as having Graves' hyperthyroidism can be treated with low-dose PTU. The goal is to maintain the free T_4 in the upper normal range for pregnancy with the T_3 within the normal range. Because of the potential side effects of antithyroid agents and the low likelihood that they will induce a long-lived remission when discontinued, most clinicians use antithyroid agents to cause normal thyroid function in the short term, but then utilize a more permanent definitive therapy such as radioactive iodine.

The most commonly utilized treatment for Graves' hyperthyroidism is radioactive iodine (RAI) therapy. RAI therapy is safe and effective. Rarely, it may worsen ophthalmopathy (eye problems). The goal of RAI therapy is to render the patient hypothyroid (lowered thyroid functioning) so that lifelong thyroid supplement therapy is then prescribed with periodic monitoring. Efforts to administer a dose of RAI sufficient to render the patient euthyroid (normal thyroid functioning), rather than hypothyroid, are difficult to achieve routinely due to differing thyroid gland sensitivity, and unless the patient is rendered hypothyroid, the persistent presence of detectable TSH receptor antibodies may result in recurrent hyperthyroidism. RAI must not be used in pregnant or lactating women. Women of childbearing potential should delay becoming pregnant until at least 6 months after receiving RAI therapy.

Surgery is rarely used as the primary treatment modality for Graves' hyperthyroidism except in patients with suspicious thyroid nodules and in patients who desire surgery, after discussion of the therapeutic options. The decision as to which treatment modality to employ should be jointly reached with the health care team and the patient and family.

Other Causes of Hyperthyroid

Patients with multinodular goiters (multiple nodules) and solitary autonomous nodules (single nodules) also may be hyperthyroid. Definitive treatment for these patients generally is surgery or RAI therapy but antithyroid agents may restore euthyroidism (normal thyroid functioning). Patients with inflammation of the thyroid gland or thyroiditis, typically evolve through phases of hyperthyroidism and hypothyroidism. Occasionally, permanent thyroid function abnormalities may persist. Taking L-thyroxine (thyroid supplementation) may be associated with abnormal thyroid function (either too high or too low) and these patients should have frequent thyroid hormone evaluations. Elderly patients may present with very subtle findings suggestive of hyperthyroidism, and the sole manifestation could be a cardiac arrhythmia, such as atrial fibrillation (a type of irregular heart rate). Other manifestations could be congestive heart failure, muscle weakness, or a flat affect. Taken together, this presentation is referred to as "apathetic hyperthyroidism."

Subclinical hyperthyroidism is defined as a TSH that is decreased below the normal range in conjunction with a normal serum free T_4 and T_3. Subclinical hyperthyroidism is part of a continuum of hyperthyroidism and usually, but not always, the signs and symptoms are less severe than in patients with overt hyperthyroidism (suppressed TSH, elevated free T_4/T_3). Subclinical hyperthyroidism has been found to be associated with an increased risk of atrial fibrillation (a type of irregular heart rate) and with enhanced bone loss, especially in patients over about age 50 years.

HYPOTHYROIDISM

Hypothyroidism may manifest as signs or symptoms of lethargy, cold intolerance, difficulty concentrating, slowed thinking (mentation) and reflexes, dry skin, slowed heart rate (bradycardia), hair loss, and constipation. Primary hypothyroidism is characterized by an elevated TSH in conjunction with a low free T_4 and T_3. The most common causes of primary hypothyroidism include types of autoimmune disorders that affect the thyroid gland such as Hashimoto's thyroiditis, deliberate destruction of the thyroid gland (e.g., RAI, surgery), and congenital abnormalities. The thyroid gland itself may or may not be enlarged depending upon the etiology. Hypothyroidism may be associated with reproductive abnormalities and blood lipid (cholesterol/fat) elevations. Symptoms of hypothyroidism may be nonspecific and frequently patients will attribute subjective symptoms of tiredness, for example, to hypothyroidism, when, in fact, thyroid hormone is not playing a role. Other autoimmune disorders such as

diabetes mellitus, Addison's disease (adrenal insufficiency), premature ovarian failure, and pernicious anemia (anemia due to reduced red blood cell production) may also occur in increased frequency in patients who have autoimmune thyroid disease (Hashimoto's thyroiditis).

Chronic or severe hypothyroidism may present as severe lowered body temperature (hypothermia), mental confusion, and perhaps even coma (usually in conjunction with several of the more routine signs and symptoms noted above).

Patients being evaluated for thyroid disease should also have a thorough physical examination and a routine laboratory testing to include complete blood count (CBC) and comprehensive metabolic profile. Patients with primary hypothyroidism may require a thyroid sonogram to assess thyroid structure. Thyroid antibody measurements may help to diagnose autoimmune thyroid disease as the etiology.

In routine patients, L-thyroxine therapy is used for the treatment of most patients with primary hypothyroidism with an equilibrium period of 4–6 weeks. A slower initiation schedule may be used in elderly patients or those with cardiac disease in order to avoid an increase in cardiac arrhythmias or worsen angina pectoris.

Subclinical hypothyroidism is defined by an elevated TSH level with a normal Free T_4 concentration. This condition is part of a continuum of mild hypothyroidism to overt hypothyroidism (elevated TSH with decreased Free T_4). The signs and symptoms of subclinical hypothyroidism vary, but, in general, are subtle in comparison to patients with more overt disease. Patients with subclinical hypothyroidism should have a thorough history and physical examination and laboratory studies to include CBC, comprehensive metabolic profile, and probably a lipid profile.

THYROID NODULES AND GOITER

Thyroid Nodules

The critical issue with regard to thyroid nodules is to try to discern nodules that harbor malignancy from those that are benign. About 80–90% of all thyroid nodules are benign. The approach to thyroid nodules is controversial and varies between physicians. Thyroid nodules larger than approximately 1 cm usually require evaluation and monitoring. An FNA interpreted by an experienced specialist in cell disorders (cytologist) should be performed. Clinical findings such as family or personal history of thyroid cancer, radiation exposure to the neck area, identifiable or palpable cervical lymph nodes, a nodule that is very firm or adherent to surrounding tissue, hoarse voice, male gender and age greater than 40, nodule growth and probably nodule size greater than 3–4 cm increase concern that the nodule harbors thyroid cancer. These comments are guidelines and clinical findings are important and may, for example, suggest a thyroidectomy (thyroid removal) be performed even in the context of a benign aspiration. Thyroid function tests, CBC, and comprehensive metabolic profile should be obtained routinely in a patient being evaluated for a thyroid nodule.

A thyroid aspiration interpretation can be read as either benign, suspicious, malignant, or indeterminate. A patient with a benign aspiration can be followed with baseline and periodic examination and repeated sonograms to assess nodule changes. The false-negative rate of a benign aspiration is about 2–5% so a repeat aspiration is recommended in 3–12 months helping confirm the original diagnosis. Nodules larger than 3–4 cm have a higher false-negative rate. A suspicious aspiration usually requires surgery. The chance of a nodule harboring thyroid cancer when the aspiration is suspicious is probably about 20%, although this depends on the individual cellular (cytologic) characteristics as well as the experience of the cytologist. Sometimes the clinical findings are sufficiently worrisome that surgery should be recommended even if the aspiration is benign. If the nodule is relatively small and the patient has few worrisome clinical features, then the patient may be followed with periodic neck exams and sonograms until it is clear that the nodule is benign. If a nodule grows while a patient is being followed, a repeat thyroid aspiration is usually indicated. If the FNA shows malignancy, then a near-total or total thyroidectomy should usually be performed. An indeterminate cytology should be repeated, perhaps with sonographic guidance.

Goiters

The term "goiter" refers to diffuse enlargement of the thyroid gland usually noted on physical examination and confirmed by specialized imaging studies, such as sonogram. Occasionally, thyroid function tests are abnormal in patients with goiter, but usually they are normal. Functional abnormalities, of course, must be addressed.

Although still controversial, it is believed that each nodule in a patient with a multinodular (multiple nodules) goiter has the same chance of harboring malignancy as does a solitary thyroid nodule. Practically speaking, every nodule larger than 1 cm may not be able to be aspirated, even if sonographic guidance is used. One approach is to perform sonograms on most patients with goiters and to try to aspirate (usually under sonographic guidance) nodules larger than 1 cm. However, judgment must be utilized. Interpretation of the FNA and the clinical approach is similar to that noted for patients with thyroid nodules. It is important to monitor patients with goiters (and benign aspirates) with periodic examinations and sonograms. If a nodule is enlarging, repeat aspiration should be performed, when possible. Possible indications for surgery in patients with a goiter include: suspicious or malignant aspiration, enlarging nodules or goiter, tracheal (windpipe) compression, impingement on the nerves in the neck (recurrent laryngeal nerve), or additional worrisome features. In large goiters, it may be helpful to obtain additional tests such as pulmonary function tests, swallowing studies, and/or chest computerized tomogram (CT). These tests help to define size, location of nodules, and compression of other organs and may be used to monitor the individual over time.

There are some reports of using RAI therapy to treat euthyroid goiter patients. This treatment is still undergoing investigation. Most euthyroid patients with goiters do not have indications for treatment (e.g., abnormal thyroid function tests, compression) so they can be followed with periodic examination and radiologic studies with FNAs as appropriate.

SEE ALSO: Anxiety disorders, Cancer, Constipation, Hair loss, Insomnia, Pregnancy

Suggested Reading

American College of Obstetricians and Gynecologists, Committee on Primary Care. (1997, October). *Primary and preventive care, primary care review for the obstetrician–gynecologist.* Washington, DC: Author.

American College of Physicians. (1998). Clinical guideline, part 1: Screening for thyroid disease. *Annals of Internal Medicine, 129,* 141–143.

Cooper, D. S. (1998). Subclinical thyroid disease: A clinician's perspective. Editorial. *Annals of Internal Medicine, 129,* 135–138.

Franklyn, J. A. (1994). The management of hyperthyroidism. *New England Journal of Medicine, 330,* 1731–1738 [erratum *New England Journal of Medicine* 1994, *331,* 559].

Griffin, J. E. (1990). Hypothyroidism in the elderly. *American Journal of Medical Science, 299*, 334–345.

Helfand, M., & Redfern, C. C. (1998). Clinical guideline, part 2: Screening for thyroid disease: An update. American College of Physicians. *Annals of Internal Medicine, 129*, 144–158.

Lazarus, J. H., Hall, R., Othman, S., Parkes, A. B., Richards, C. J., McCulloch, B., et al. (1996). The clinical spectrum of postpartum thyroid disease. *QJM, 89*, 429–435.

Shrier, D. K., & Burman, K. D. (2002). Subclinical hyperthyroidism: Controversies in management. *American Family Physician, 65*, 431–438.

Stathatos, N., Levetan, C., Burman, K. D., & Wartofsky, L. (2001). The controversy of the treatment of critically ill patients with thyroid hormone. *Best Practice and Research Clinical Endocrinology and Metabolism, 15*(4), 465–478.

Uzzan, B., Campos, J., Cucherat, M., et al. (1996). Effects on bone mass of long term treatment with thyroid hormones: A meta-analysis. *Journal of Clinical Endocrinology and Metabolism, 81*, 4278–4279.

KENNETH D. BURMAN

TMJ *see* Temporomandibular Joint Disorders

Tobacco According to the National Institute on Drug Abuse, there are many species of tobacco plants; the tabacum species is the major source of tobacco products today. Tobacco products include cigarettes, cigars, pipes, and smokeless tobacco. According to the 1999 National Household Survey on Drug Abuse, 57 million Americans are current smokers and 7.6 million use smokeless tobacco. The use of cigars, pipes, and smokeless tobacco among women is low, but cigar smoking may be increasing. In 1999, almost 10% of high school girls under age 18 had past-month cigar use. Forms of smokeless tobacco include chewing tobacco and snuff. Chewing tobacco is leaf tobacco that is chewed and sucked in after it is placed between the cheek and the teeth. Snuff is finely ground tobacco that is placed between the cheek and gum or between the lower lip and gum.

HEALTH CONSEQUENCES OF TOBACCO USE

All tobacco products cause lung diseases (lung cancer, emphysema, and chronic bronchitis) and cancers of the mouth, throat, and larynx. In the United States, deaths from tobacco-related cancers contribute to over 30% of cancer mortality. Globally, lung cancer is one of the most deadly of the tobacco-related diseases; these rates are expected to increase because of increased cases in developing countries. Data from a 1998 study indicate that U.S. women have the highest death rate from lung cancer in the world.

Women smokers also seem to have an increased risk for conception delay, infertility, ectopic pregnancy, spontaneous abortion, and preterm delivery. Other disorders that may be associated with cigarette smoking in women include menstrual dysfunction, early menopause, estrogen deficiency disorders, and osteoporosis.

ENVIRONMENTAL TOBACCO SMOKE (ETS)

ETS is classified as a Group A carcinogen (known to cause cancer in humans). According to the National Center for Chronic Disease Prevention and Health Promotion, ETS causes about 3,000 lung cancer deaths per year among adult nonsmokers and causes serious respiratory problems in children (such as asthma and upper respiratory infections). A major problem with ETS is that most persons affected by it have no control over ETS. Many schools, work sites, and public gathering places are now enforcing smoke-free environments to protect nonsmokers from ETS.

TOBACCO CONTROL

In 1996, the Agency for Health Care Policy Research (AHCPR) produced guidelines for smoking cessation, which supported the involvement of all health professionals in tobacco control efforts. Societal efforts to reduce tobacco use and to reduce exposure to ETS have increased over the last 10 years. Societal strategies include counteradvertising, increasing tobacco taxes, laws that prohibit minors' access to tobacco products, and banning smoking in workplaces and in public places.

INTERVENTIONS FOR TOBACCO USE

In 2000, the U.S. Department of Health and Human Services published clinical practice guidelines for treating tobacco use and dependence. Many states have demonstrated programs called "best-evidence"-based programs, which show a successful reduction of smoking rates among women and girls. Also, the American Lung Association (ALA) supports research and other programs to help people to quit using tobacco. Because it is so difficult to stop smoking, many public health efforts are now focusing on prevention of tobacco use, particularly in young people. Most adult smokers start their tobacco use as teenagers.

SEE ALSO: Cancer, Lung cancer, Nicotine, Smoking, Substance use

Suggested Reading

Landis, S. H., Murray, T., Boldlen, S., & Wingo, P. A. (1998). Cancer statistics, 1998. *Cancer Journal for Clinicians, 48,* 6–29.

Sarna, L. (1999). Hope and vision prevention: Tobacco control and cancer nursing. *Cancer Nursing, 22*(1), 21–28.

United States Department of Health and Human Services. (1996). Smoking cessation. Clinical Practice Guideline No. 18. Rockville, MD. (AHCPR Publication No. 96-0692, April). Available at http://www.os.dhhs.gov. Last accessed January 12, 2004.

United States Department of Health and Human Services. (2000, June). Clinical practice guidelines: Treating tobacco use and dependence. Available at http://surgeongeneral.gov/tobacco/clinpack.html. Last accessed January 12, 2004.

Suggested Resources

American Lung Association National website: http://www.lungusa.org

National Center for Chronic Disease Prevention and Health Promotion, Tobacco Information and Prevention Source (TIPS)

MARILYN DAVIES

Torsion   *see* Pelvic Pain

Toxemia   *see* Preeclampsia

Toxic Shock Syndrome   Toxic shock syndrome is a serious illness that occurs in response to the absorption of a bacterium called *Staphylococcus aureus* (*S. aureus*) into the general circulation. Most cases occur in women who are menstruating. In order for toxic shock syndrome to develop, the person must be colonized with the bacterium *Staph aureus* and there must be a port of entry for the bacteria.

Common sites of entry can be abrasions in the vaginal area or on the skin. Women who use tampons that are too absorbent are at risk for developing this syndrome because insertion and removal of the tampon can cause microabrasions that can allow the *Staph aureus* to enter the general circulation. After this occurs, the bacteria produce a powerful toxin that causes an acute illness. Symptoms include fever of over 102°F, low blood pressure, shock, sunburn-like rash, vomiting, and diarrhea. Toxic shock can be fatal.

All women who are tampon users should be aware of the signs of toxic shock. Tampons should not be worn in a greater absorbency than needed. Tampons should not be left in for longer than 3–4 hours. If toxic shock syndrome is suspected, a health care provider should be notified immediately.

SEE ALSO: Menstruation, Tampon

Suggested Reading

Chin, H. (1997). *On call: Obstetrics and gynecology* (p. 283). Philadelphia: W.B. Saunders.

Scott, J., et al. (1999). *Danforth's obstetrics and gynecology* (8th ed., p. 287). Philadelphia: W.B. Saunders.

SUSAN WIEDASECK

Toxoplasmosis   Toxoplasmosis, caused by a one-celled parasite called *Toxoplasma gondii* (*T. gondii*), is one of the most widespread infections in the world, affecting roughly 50% of the world's population, regardless of gender. Generally a mild, harmless infection, toxoplasmosis is of grave concern to two groups of patients: pregnant women and those with suppressed immune systems, due to HIV infection or chemotherapy treatments.

LIFE CYCLE

The parasite *T. gondii* is capable of infecting all warm-blooded mammals and birds. It is found in cats, sheep, rodents, swine, cattle, and humans. Cats hold the unique distinction of being the only definitive host for this organism, for it is only in the cat that the organism can progress through all of the stages of its life cycle. Up to 60% of all domestic cats harbor toxoplasma in their body.

The organism enters the cat through the digestive tract, typically when the cat eats an infected rodent or bird. The cat's immune response attacks the organism, but rather than being killed, the organism enters a new phase where it is protected from the immune system and continues to survive. The cat (and only the cat) then excretes in its feces a form of the organism that is highly contagious if ingested. But this phase of the infection only lasts about 20 days in the cat's life, after which the cat (while still harboring the parasite) is no longer capable of transmitting infection.

All other animals infected with toxoplasma continue to harbor the organism in their body for the rest of their lives but they are not contagious and the organism is not excreted in their feces, which is why all other hosts are referred to as intermediate hosts.

HUMAN INFECTION

About 30% of Americans and Britains have had toxoplasmosis, but in France as many as 65% (in some regions as high as 95%) have had it. The symptoms are generally so mild that people testing positive for toxoplasmosis rarely know when they became infected.

Studies on risk factors for infection have shown that the main cause of infection is from eating undercooked meat, particularly sheep or lamb. The French tend to eat more dishes using uncooked or undercooked meat, thus their higher rate of toxoplasmosis exposure. Unwashed vegetables can transmit the organism as it can survive in soil. Cat ownership, in some studies, has not been shown to be a risk factor for toxoplasmosis infection, presumably because there are so few days in the cat's life where their feces actually contain infectious organisms.

If someone has had toxoplasmosis once, they are forever immune afterwards, but if later in life they develop an immunodeficiency condition (such as HIV or cancer chemotherapy), then they can become reinfected (called recrudescence) and can develop a life-threatening infection in the brain called encephalitis.

TOXOPLASMOSIS AND PREGNANCY

Toxoplasmosis, while harmless to the mother, can have disastrous consequences for the fetus. In early pregnancy, infection is less common but has more severe consequences. These include miscarriage or severe birth defects such as blindness, mental retardation, or cerebral palsy which occur in 10% of cases of congenital toxoplasmosis. Fetal infection more commonly occurs in the latter half of pregnancy but fetal manifestations are not typically evident. In fact, 90% of babies born with late-onset congenital toxoplasmosis look normal at birth, with only some of them developing serious vision or hearing problems, or seizures many years later.

Documented infection can and should be treated during pregnancy. This has been shown to help reduce fetal harm and prevent some cases of congenital toxoplasmosis. It is estimated that from 1 to 10 out of 10,000 babies born in the United States have congenital toxoplasmosis, about 400–4,000 cases per year.

TOXOPLASMOSIS TESTING

The most common method of detecting toxoplasma infection is through antibody testing. Blood tests detect the presence of IgG or IgM antibodies to the toxoplasma parasite. Positive IgG indicates past exposure and is evidence of immunity. Positive IgM usually indicates current infection, but there have been problems with commercial testing for IgM resulting in a high level of false positives. Universal screening is not practiced in the United States.

Therefore, it is recommended that all pregnant women testing positive for IgM have repeat tests run at a toxoplasma reference laboratory. The Toxoplasma Serology Laboratory in Palo Alto, California (www.pamf. org, 1-650-853-4828) is a U.S. Centers for Disease Control (CDC) reference laboratory. Testing done by these highly specialized laboratories can determine whether a previous positive blood test was actually a false positive. By having such data available for counseling, health care providers have been able to reduce anxiety and possible consideration of pregnancy terminations for perceived toxoplasmosis by 50%.

PREVENTION

1. Avoid contact with cat litter or wear gloves. Wear gloves while gardening because the organisms can live in the soil. Cats also like to defecate in children's sandboxes.

2. Cook all meat, particularly sheep, beef, and pork, to a minimum of 150°F (66°C). Cook poultry to 180°F.
3. Thoroughly wash all fruits and vegetables, or peel them. Using soap and hot water, wash all surfaces that have come into contact with raw meat or poultry.
4. Do not drink unpasteurized milk or milk products, especially goat's milk products.

SEE ALSO: Acquired immunodeficiency syndrome, Miscarriage, Pregnancy

Suggested Reading

Howard, B., Chow, G., & Fairchok, M. (2002). Congenital toxoplasmosis. In S. Ransom, M. Dombrowski, M. Evans, & K. Ginsburg (Eds.), *Contemporary therapy in obstetrics and gynecology* (pp. 328–329). Philadelphia: W.B. Saunders.

Lopez, A., Dietz, V., Wilson, T., & Jones, J. (2000). Preventing congenital toxoplasmosis. *Morbidity and Mortality Weekly Report, 49,* 57–75. Also available at http://www.cdc.gov/mmwr/preview/mmwrhtml/rr4902a5.htm

Suggested Resources

Toxoplasmosis Fact Sheet, March of Dimes from http://www.marchofdimes.com/aboutus/681_1228.asp

BRYAN S. JICK

Transgenderism A simple definition of transgenderism is any form of dress and/or behavior interpreted as contravening traditional gender roles. Transgenderism comprises a diverse collection of individuals expressing one of three basic facets. First, there are those who transform to the opposite gender within the *heteronormative* dichotomy. (Heteronormativity describes a binary gender system, in which only two sexes are recognized, where sex is equated with gender and gender with a heterosexual orientation.) These individuals are referred to as transsexuals in the medical literature and typically seek surgical solutions to confirm their transidentity. Those who move across or blend genders represent the second group. Crossing involves moving to the other side of the gender binary system (either partially or completely) but rejecting the need for surgery to confirm identity. Thus, the emphasis is on crossing and not on surgical transformation. Those who blend genders combine or harmonize aspects to create a unique presentation. However, blending and crossing still give reflexive credibility to the heteronormative categories. There are still two genders. In the third facet, a transgendered person is one who has transcended the boundaries of the heteronormative gender binary system. An unequivocal gender attribution can neither be made nor in most cases does the individual permit a category to be assigned. Gender ceases to exist for these individuals.

Transgenderism is often represented as a challenge to the social construction of gender. However, this may be an oversimplification. Although the existence of transpeople exposes the dubiousness and fragility of the conventional female/male dichotomy, transpeople still live in a social context that acknowledges only females and males. The true challenge may rest with the ability of transgendered persons to earn and maintain a transgender attribution in the face of a socially sanctioned process that constrains others to assign them to heteronormative female and male categories.

In theory, transgenderism may appear to be an innovative subversion of traditional gender categories and roles. However, in practice, it may actually serve to reinforce the heteronormativity it seeks to destabilize. For example, establishing transgender as an official identity creates a boundary between gendered persons and transgendered persons. The unfortunate consequence is that this separation enables the remainder of the population to locate transpeople into a category of *other* and helps them to be even more secure about dividing themselves along established gender lines.

Numerous other societies have accommodated transgenderism as a legitimate third gender category. Examples include the Hijiras of India, Native American Berdaches, Eunuchs of the Byzantine Empire, the Mahu of Tahiti, Philippine Baklas, the Kathoey of Thailand, Indonesian Warias, and the Fafafines of Samoa, among others. Many societies throughout history have also accommodated transgenderism in the performing arts. Because women were forbidden to appear on stage in past centuries, men were required to take the roles of women. The ongoing Japanese Kabuki Theater, where the tradition of performing a female role on stage is passed from father to son, and the long-abandoned tradition of castrato sopranos in the Italian Opera, where young boys were castrated to preserve their soprano singing voices, are two examples.

Societies with strong Christian traditions tend to be less tolerant of transgenderism. However, even in societies where it is accommodated, tolerance does not necessarily translate to acceptance. Persecution of transpeople can be found everywhere. Moreover, the focus on describing the diversity under the transgendered umbrella tends to divert attention away from the social and political consequences of forming a transgender identity and the historical progression that made it possible.

See Also: Femininity, Gender, Gender role, Homosexuality, Intersexuality, Lesbian, Masculinity, Queer, Transsexuality

Suggested Reading

Bornstein, K. (1995). *Gender outlaw: On men, women, and the rest of us.* New York: Vintage Books.

Kessler, S. J., & McKenna, W. (1985). *Gender: An ethnomethodological approach.* Chicago: University of Chicago Press.

Nanda, S. (1999). *Gender diversity: Crosscultural variations.* Prospect Heights, IL: Waveland Press.

Wilchins, R. (1997). *Read my lips: Sexual subversion and the end of gender.* Ann Arbor, MI: Firebrand Books.

ANGELA PATTATUCCI ARAGON

Transsexuality

Transsexuality Transsexuality is a clinical diagnosis representing the most extreme manifestation of gender dysphoria—a psychological condition in which a person's gender identity is opposite that of their assigned sex at birth. Simply stated, the individual believes that they were born into the wrong body, a situation that occurs in approximately equal frequency for individuals originally assigned female or male at birth. Although the medical establishment and popular media have freely used the term *transsexual* as a descriptive term for these individuals, a growing activist movement has rejected this designation in lieu of using *transpeople* or *transwoman* or *transman*.

Transsexuality as a distinct and treatable medical condition is a relatively recent phenomenon. However, incidences of women who lived their lives as men and men who lived their lives as women have been recorded throughout history in many societies. Several theorists have proposed that transsexuality is a variation in the gestational sex development pathway. However, unlike intersex conditions in which the variation rests in sexual differentiation of the gonads (see entries on Intersexuality and Hermaphroditism), for transsexuality the proposed variation is instead located in sexual differentiation of the brain. This hypothesis is conceptually appealing and is in fact supported by a number of studies on animals, but the definitive link for humans has remained elusive.

Because transsexuality cannot be detected visually or by any simple medical test, the transmale or transfemale appears to be a typical female or male with primary and secondary sexual characteristics congruent with their assigned sex at birth. Consequently, people often erroneously conclude that transsexuality is an emotional or psychological problem, that with a little self-discipline, or with counseling, transpeople can act normally and accept their original sex assignment. However, decades of psychiatric interventions, some bordering on barbarism, failed to effect even a single instance of a positive and permanent outcome—in this case, defined as adjustment to a gender identity and associated gender role congruent with the transperson's assigned sex at birth. In response to this resounding failure, psychiatrist and endocrinologist Dr. Harry Benjamin emerged in the 1950s with a new and radical treatment for transsexuality. He reasoned that if the mind could not be changed to correspond to the body, then the body should be changed to match the mind.

Benjamin's efforts ushered in the era of gender reassignment surgery, and with it a shift in focus from altering minds to reshaping bodies. The procedure is a combination of hormone treatment and major surgery to transform the appearance of genitalia and secondary sex characteristics. Methods have evolved over the years to become progressively more sophisticated and in some cases have driven advances in other areas of reconstructive surgery. However, a third, but unexplored, option to deal with transsexuality was to educate people about the ways in which gender is socially constructed in societies—in effect, to give societies an *attitude reassignment* (see entries on Queer and Transgenderism). This option is admittedly oriented toward a long-term solution, but it neither requires changing the minds of individuals nor their bodies. It also correctly locates transsexuality as a symptom of a greater problem—the strict adherence by societies to rigidly defined binary gender categories that are presumed to be mutually exclusive extensions of biology. In fact, some theorists argue that gender dysphoria would all but disappear as a psychological condition if societies simply embraced diversity and treated people with greater compassion and respect.

Although the issues and challenges that intersex and transpeople face are for the most part different, they have one common thread. The medical establishment manages both conditions with a surgical solution that is designed to erase evidence of human diversity. In both situations, bodies are surgically altered to "normalize" their appearance. For the intersexed, this is done without individual consent, whereas for transpeople, this is done with individual consent.

In addition to facing an array of personal, social, and financial challenges before surgical intervention, transpeople often encounter legal obstacles after the procedure has been completed. In the United States, policies surrounding legal recognition of gender reassignment, along with requirements for divorce (if the individual was married prior to surgery), child custody and visitation rights, future marriage, and adoption are in the hands of state legislatures and vary considerably. Additionally, a majority of states in the United States makes it legal to openly discriminate against transpersons, as well as homosexuals, in employment and housing. Policies vary internationally as well.

An unfortunate byproduct of the medicalization of transsexuality is that the gender reassignment procedure has grown to become inappropriately viewed as a cure rather than a treatment. Although gender reassignment surgery may the best short-term solution at the present time when all things are considered, a cure for transsexuality should render the treatment obsolete. When viewed from this perspective, it is clear that the cure does not rest at the individual level (changing bodies), but rather at the societal level through changing the normative values that societies hold about gender.

SEE ALSO: Femininity, Gender, Gender role, Homosexuality, Intersexuality, Lesbian, Masculinity, Queer, Transgenderism

Suggested Reading

Bloom, A. (2002). *Normal: Transsexual CEO's, crossdressing cops, and hermaphrodites with attitude.* New York: Random House.

Bornstein, K. (1995). *Gender outlaw: On men, women, and the rest of us.* New York: Vintage Books.

Brown, M. L., & Rounsley, C. A. (2003). *True selves: Understanding transsexualism—For families, friends, co-workers, and helping professionals.* San Francisco: Jossey-Bass.

ANGELA PATTATUCCI ARAGON

Trichomoniasis Trichomonads are motile, flagellate, protozoan organisms known to cause a diverse spectrum of diseases in humans. Most of these diseases are rare. The single exception is *Trichomonas vaginalis*, the most significant of these parasites, which infects between 3 and 5 million American women each year. The organism causes an inflammation of the vaginal wall, or vaginitis, in women who contract this disease. The disease is usually sexually transmitted and the incidence is high particularly in populations at risk for other venereal diseases, such as those attending clinics for sexually transmitted diseases, those with multiple sexual partners, and those infected with HIV. *T. vaginalis* also causes genital infections in men; because these tend to be asymptomatic, the true incidence of infection in this population is unknown.

The clinical presentation of trichomoniasis is variable. It is estimated that between one fourth and one half of infected women are asymptomatic; in symptomatic women, the most common complaints are usually of malodorous vaginal discharge, discomfort with urination, and vulvovaginal irritation, pain, or burning. A history of unprotected sexual intercourse is usually present. On pelvic examination, a yellow-green discharge, usually described as "frothy," may be present in the vagina. Other signs may include vulvovaginal erythema (redness) and a "strawberry" appearance of the cervix. The latter finding is caused by microscopic hemorrhages in the surface tissue in the cervix (exocervical mucosa). In men, *T. vaginalis* infection is usually asymptomatic. Symptomatic men may experience urethral burning, pain with urination, or rarely a penile discharge.

Diagnosis of infection with *T. vaginalis* in women is usually made by examination of vaginal secretions. Characteristics that are suggestive of trichomoniasis include a yellow-green, frothy discharge, with pH level (acid level) of greater than 4.5. Conclusive proof of disease includes the microscopic identification of the organisms on a wet-mount slide of vaginal secretions. The diagnosis can also be made if the organism is identified in samples recovered from the exocervix (such as those obtained via Pap smear); however, this method is less sensitive and is therefore not currently recommended. In men, a diagnosis of trichomoniasis may be more difficult to establish and microscopic examination of both a urethral sample and a urine sample may be necessary. In both sexes, the ability to detect the disease may be increased by combining direct microscopic evaluation with cultures of infected material. Most importantly, women with trichomoniasis should also be screened for other coexistent sexually transmitted diseases.

Treatment of trichomoniasis is fairly straightforward and, in most cases, exceedingly successful. The mainstay of therapy is the antibiotic metronidazole, which is highly active against most strains of *T. vaginalis*. The drug can be administered as a single, oral dose (usual dose 2 g) to cure the majority of cases of trichomoniasis. This single-dose regimen tends to be easier for most individuals to take. For individuals unable to tolerate this dose or for those with recurrent disease after the single-dose regimen, a 7-day course of therapy, consisting of a gram of metronidazole daily, administered in two divided doses, is recommended. In rare cases of true antibiotic resistance in the organism, higher dose metronidazole, topical paromomycin, and tinidazole have all been shown to be efficacious in eradicating the disease. All infected women should be counseled regarding the necessity of having their sexual partners seek treatment, as reinfection from an asymptomatic sexual partner (partner with no symptoms) remains a common cause of relapsing disease after treatment. Reinforcement of safe sex practices remains critical.

It is generally recommended that all individuals diagnosed with *T. vaginalis* infection undergo antibiotic treatment. Although many men and some women are diagnosed while asymptomatic, they may become symptomatic at a later date or may unknowingly transmit the organism to others through unprotected sexual contact. Additionally, some studies have suggested that women with untreated trichomoniasis may be more susceptible to HIV disease, due to the damage of surface tissue (disruption of native mucosal barriers) by inflammation. Pregnant women who contract *T. vaginalis* may be more likely to deliver premature or low-birthweight infants. Although it has not been established conclusively that cure of infection in expectant mothers will prevent these negative events, current guidelines also support treatment of women with trichomoniasis during pregnancy (gestational trichomoniasis).

SEE ALSO: Condoms, Safer sex, Sexually transmitted diseases

Suggested Reading

Centers for Disease Control and Prevention, Division of Parasitic Diseases. (1999). Parasitic disease information, *Trichomonas infection*. Atlanta. Retrieved October 15 from http://www.cdc.gov

Paavonen, J., & Stamm, W. E. (1987). Lower genital tract infections in women. *Infectious Diseases Clinics of North America, 1*(1), 179–198.

Schwebke, J. R. (2002). Update of trichomoniasis. *Sexually Transmitted Infections, 78*, 378–379.

USHA STIEFEL

Trichotillomania

Trichotillomania, a disorder of chronic hair pulling, is classified in the *Diagnostic Statistical Manual of Mental Disorders,* fourth edition (DSM-IV) as an impulse control disorder. The individual experiences a recurrent and generally irresistible urge to engage in hair pulling, resulting in significant hair loss. This may occur at multiple sites, most often on the scalp, but also on the eyebrows, eyelashes, pubic area, underarm (axillary area), and beard. A sense of tension is experienced just before the hair pulling or if the individual resists pulling. As the hair is pulled, the patient experiences a sense of pleasure, gratification, or relief. To be considered as trichotillomania in the DSM-IV, hair pulling must not be caused by any medical, dermatological, or psychiatric disorder and should cause clinically significant distress and impairment in social, occupational, or other important areas of functioning.

Trichotillomania was previously considered a rare condition. Recent studies suggest a lifetime prevalence of 2–3%, children more often than adults and female:male ratio of 7:1 or higher, perhaps because females are more likely to seek medical care. It predominantly develops in the first two decades of life with a mean age of onset at 13 years. As with obsessive–compulsive disorder (OCD), patients with trichotillomania are secretive about their symptoms and tend to disguise hair loss with hair styles and hair prosthetics. They may be embarrassed by the hair loss or reluctant to seek treatment, thus delaying recognition of the disorder. The course of the disease varies, from chronic to episodic to permanent remission. Two styles of hair pulling have been proposed. Patients with a "focused style" center their complete attention on the pulling activity. The majority of patients have an "automatic style" and practice hair pulling parallel to other situations like reading or watching television. Hair pullers often describe a combination of both styles.

Hair pulling results in alopecia (hairless areas on the scalp), which occurs in irregular patches and is identifiable by its distinctive pathology on scalp biopsy. On skin surface (histopathologic) examination, there is no scarring, inflammation, or abnormalities of the scalp or skin. Short broken strands are mixed with a few longer, normal hairs. Hair pulling of trichotillomania is not reported to be painful. The diagnostic evaluation of trichotillomania includes a number of different medical conditions and psychiatric pathology like OCD. Patchy hair loss can be seen in patients with syphilis, tinea capitis (head lice), and systemic lupus erythematosus (a disorder of the immune system), but is usually accompanied by inflammation. Alopecia can cause either generalized or patchy hair loss. When patches occur, they are sharply bounded and lack any normal hair. Unlike patients with trichotillomania, medical conditions like hypothyroidism and lithium toxicity cause generalized hair loss. Hair pulling of OCD is performed consciously to avoid anxiety and may be associated with other rituals. Hair pulling of trichotillomania, on the other hand, is pleasurable, performed in response to anxiety, and is associated with denial and minimum awareness.

Medical complications of trichotillomania can include infection and scarring at the site, change in color or texture of the hair, slowed or stopped hair growth, and indirect complications leading to fear of embarrassment such as avoiding physical examinations, and the like. Trichophagy or hair ingestion may accompany hair pulling, sometimes leading to development of a trichobezoar (hairball). Anorexia (lack of appetite), stomach pain, obstruction, anemia (low blood count), and malnutrition may develop secondary to trichobezoar formation. Repetitive arm and hand movements involved in hair pulling can cause carpal tunnel syndrome and other neuromuscular disorders. Psychiatric comorbidities (conditions occurring at the same time) include major depression, generalized anxiety disorder, eating disorder, Tourette's syndrome (a syndrome of involuntary tics), body dysmorphic disorder (abnormal perception of body form), alcohol or other substance dependence and abuse, simple or social phobia. Prevalence of OCD in these patients is extremely high (13%), as compared to the general population (2–3%).

Although trichotillomania may be multidetermined (caused by multiple factors), its onset has been linked to stressful situations in more than 25% of all cases. Disturbances in mother–child relationships, fear of being left alone, and recent object loss are often cited as important contributing factors. Neurobiological investigations show evidence of abnormal patterns of brain neurotransmitters (serotonin) and involvement of the parts of the brain called the basal ganglia and frontal lobes, similar to that seen in people with OCD and Tourette's syndrome. Baseline levels of amino acids in spinal fluid (cerebrol spinal fluid 5-hydroxyindoleacetic acid levels) in individuals with trichotillomania seem to correlate with response to serotonin reuptake inhibitors (some types of antidepressant medications). Severity of assessment of trichotillomania can be assessed by different questionnaires: Trichotillomania Questionnaire, Massachusetts General Hospital Hairpulling Scale, Trichotillomania Symptom Severity Scale, Trichotillomania Impairment Scale, and Physician's Rating of Clinical Progress Scale.

Treatment options include medication, behavioral techniques, and hypnosis. Selective serotonin reuptake inhibitors (SSRI) remain the most popular pharmacological intervention and have the most evidence-based support. Very scientifically rigorous research studies (double-blind placebo-controlled studies) have documented positive treatment responses to the antidepressant medications clomipramine, fluvoxamine, and fluoxetine. Lithium may lead to decreased hair pulling and mild to moderate hair growth but relapse often occurs. Lithium can cause hair loss by itself, especially if there is a coexistent zinc deficiency. Treatment with naltrexone has shown mixed results and there are case reports documenting efficacy of buspirone, levonorgestrel, and fenfluramine. Neuroleptics have been successfully used in cases of hair pulling associated with severe mental disorders such as autism and with conditions in which individuals have conditions of abnormal perception, such as psychosis.

The most widely studied, preferred, and popular treatment is the behavioral technique of habit reversal. It includes the principle of awareness training, which consists of monitoring all urges to pull, actual occurrences of pulling, and feelings immediately before and after the pulling. Habit reversal also includes competing response training which requires substituting an incompatible behavior like clenching an object when experiencing the urge to pull out hair. Relaxation training, overcorrection like extensive hair brushing, and prevention training are other components of behavioral therapy. Hypnosis may be used independently or as complementing other techniques. The focus is on helping the individual become more aware of what he or she is doing and reinforcing behavioral control over hair pulling. In addition, cognitive-behavioral therapy can assist the patient in counteracting maladaptive thought patterns. Ongoing research is hopeful with up-to-date information available online through the Trichotillomania Learning Center (http://www.trich.org).

SEE ALSO: Anxiety disorders, Body image, Depression, Obsessive–compulsive disorder

Suggested Reading

American Psychiatric Association. (1994). *Diagnostic and statistical manual of mental disorders* (4th ed., pp. 618–621). Washington, DC: American Psychiatric Association.

Christenson, G. A., & Crow, S. J. (1996). The characterization and treatment of trichotillomania. *Journal of Clinical Psychiatry, 57*(Suppl. 8), 42–49.

Hautmann, G., Hercogova, J., & Lotti, T. (2002). Trichotillomania. *Journal of the American Academy of Dermatology, 46,* 807–821.

Hyman, B. M., & Pedrick, C. (1999). *The OCD workbook.* Oakland, CA: New Harbinger.

Kaplan, H. I., & Sadock, B. J. (1998). *Synopsis of psychiatry.* Baltimore: Lippincott, Williams & Wilkins.

KATHLEEN N. FRANCO
RASHMI S. DESHMUKH

Trigeminal Neuralgia

Trigeminal neuralgia is a descriptive term applied to cases of brief, excruciating, electric-shock-like pains affecting one side or the other of the face. The term derives from combining *neuralgia*, meaning pain originating aberrantly in a nerve, with *trigeminal*, the name of the nerve responsible for carrying sensation from the face. It has also been referred to as *tic douloureux*, a misnomer applied to the facial wincing (mistakenly labeled tics) that often results from the episodic pains. The pains of trigeminal neuralgia typically last only seconds at a time. They are often described by patients as seeming electrical (such as "like a bolt of lightning"), and can be among the most excruciating the person has ever experienced in his or her lifetime. Pains typically occur only in the lower half of the face, in the distribution of the second and third divisions of the nerve. Most people with this condition experience periods of frequent pains, interspersed with other periods of relative quietude. Many people find that they have a "trigger zone," an area of facial skin or oral mucous membrane in which light touch or other normal sensation can induce paroxysms of pain.

The disorder typically begins when someone is in their 50s or 60s, and affects women slightly more frequently than men. In the overwhelming majority of cases, trigeminal neuralgia arises for unknown reasons; it does not mean that there is an underlying neurological disorder. However, in a very small minority of sufferers, the condition is caused by a small tumor, vascular malformation, or area of inflammation. It is therefore very important that a physician evaluate any sufferer of pain potentially consistent with this disorder, and make note of any symptoms other than the pains. Symptoms that may be particularly important are facial numbness between pains, and current or past episodes of (a) numbness or tingling in the face or elsewhere in the body, (b) loss of vision, blurry vision, or double vision, (c) ringing or rushing noises in the ears, or hearing loss, (d) balance disturbances, (e) weakness or clumsiness of any part of the body, especially of the face or mouth, (f) difficulty speaking or swallowing, or (g) fainting or lightheadedness. Presence of any of these signs is worrisome for the presence of abnormal vein patterns (vascular malformation), tumor, or the inflammation of multiple sclerosis, and should prompt the clinician to proceed with contrasted magnetic resonance imaging (MRI) of the brain, which is far more sensitive than standard CT (computerized assisted tomography—CAT scan) for brainstem disease. Presentation of the disorder before the age of 50 should likewise prompt specialized imaging of the nervous system (neuroimaging). It is also important to be aware of any other symptoms that accompany the pain, such as tearing, excessive salivation, facial flushing, or altered sensation elsewhere besides the face; these signs may suggest that the underlying diagnosis (real problem) is cluster headache.

The first choice (preferred) treatment of trigeminal neuralgia is the antiseizure medication carbamazepine. Many people obtain complete relief from this agent. The drawbacks of carbamazepine are potential damage to the blood-producing apparatus of the bone marrow (bone marrow suppression), potential liver toxicity, and many possible interactions with other medications, particularly oral contraceptive pills. Any woman starting carbamazepine who is taking birth control pills should discuss the issue both with the physician starting the carbamazepine, and with her gynecologist. Carbamazepine may be associated with a higher rate of birth defects among infants of mothers who took carbamazepine during pregnancy. This increase in risk is moderate and a woman of childbearing age taking carbamazepine must take extra precautions to avoid pregnancy, and discuss the risks and potential alternative treatments with her physician if she wishes to become pregnant.

Other medications for trigeminal neuralgia have been tried, and reported to be beneficial to some individuals. In particular, a modified form of carbamazepine, oxcarbazepine, has now been on the market for a few years, and appears to have fewer adverse effects. Other medications that have been tried and found effective in a few individuals include phenytoin, lamotrigine, gabapentin, baclofen, and clonazepam.

In many people for whom medications fail, there is an option of progressing to surgical treatment. In many cases, the abnormal sensory transmission underlying the pains is due to compression of the trigeminal nerve by an abnormal brain artery; surgery to relieve this compression, in those with this cause, can be 80% effective or better. This option must, however, be utilized only after a reasonable trial of medication, and only in individuals who are otherwise without medical illness. This is because the surgery involved, while generally safe in the hands of an experienced neurosurgeon, is nonetheless fairly risky. An alternative procedure does exist, for those in whom medications have been fruitless but are poor candidates for the more risky arterial surgery, but has risks of its own.

Trigeminal neuralgia rarely spontaneously resolves, and treatments are generally not completely curative. In this sense, trigeminal neuralgia is essentially a lifelong, incurable disorder. In most individuals, however, symptoms can be adequately controlled, by medicine or surgery, to permit carrying on in life with minimal disruption from pain.

SEE ALSO: Chronic pain, Neuropathy, Pain, Seizures

Suggested Reading

Goodman, J. M. (2002). Approach to the patient with facial pain. In J. Biller (Ed.), *Practical neurology* (2nd ed.). Philadelphia: Lippincott, Williams & Wilkins.

Rozen, T. D., Capobianco, D. J., & Dalessio, D. J. (2001). Cranial neuralgias and atypical facial pain. In S. D. Silberstein, R. B. Lipton, & D. J. Dalessio (Eds.), *Wolff's headache and other head pain* (7th ed.). New York: Oxford University Press.

MATTHEW A. ECCHER

involves ligating, or surgically interrupting the fallopian tubes. This prevents the egg (ovum) from being transported to the uterus, and also blocks the passage of sperm through the tubes.

There are several methods of tubal ligation. It is generally performed laparoscopically as an outpatient procedure under general anesthesia. A laparoscope is a narrow telescope which is inserted through the belly button after the abdomen is filled with gas. Another small incision is usually made above the pubic bone, and the tubes can be ligated with rings or bands, or cauterized (burned). Alternatively, at the time of cesarean section, the tubes may be ligated. After a vaginal delivery, a surgical procedure called a "mini-laparotomy" can be performed under epidural, spinal, or general anesthesia. This involves making a small incision below the umbilicus and locating and ligating the tubes through the incision. This does not normally increase a woman's hospital stay.

There are some risks to this surgical procedure. A very small percentage of women will have serious complications related to general anesthesia. Another potentially serious complication is injury to the bladder, bowel, or blood vessels during the operation.

Occasionally, tubal ligation fails, and the woman becomes pregnant. The pregnancy rate after tubal ligation is about 1 in 200, and is higher for younger women.

Another serious problem after tubal ligation is regret, which is more common in younger women, and in women who remarry. Tubal ligation may be reversed, but this requires a major surgical procedure. Following a tubal ligation reversal, approximately 50–80% of women will become pregnant, depending upon the type of tubal ligation that was performed.

Most providers will also counsel women about other alternatives prior to performing a tubal ligation. Tubal ligation is often a good choice for women who are positive in not desiring future pregnancy.

SEE ALSO: Birth control, Pregnancy

KAREN L. ASHBY

Tubal Ligation Tubal ligation, often referred to as "tying the tubes," is one of the most popular methods of fertility control in the United States. This is the most commonly used method of contraception among married or previously married women. The procedure

Turner Syndrome Turner syndrome (TS), alternately referred to as Turner's syndrome, monosomy X, and gonadal dysgenesis, was first described in 1938 by Dr. Henry Turner in a case report of several girls with short stature, no secondary sexual characteristics, arms that bent outwards at the elbows (called *cubitus valgus*), neck webbing, and a low posterior hairline. These characteristics are now recognized as cardinal signs of TS, which occurs in approximately 1/2,000 live female births. There are approximately 60,000 girls and women with TS in the United States; approximately 800 infants are born with TS in the United States every year. All TS children are girls and of short stature, on average 4 ft, 7 in. tall, if not treated with growth hormone. Other signs and symptoms are lymphedema (swelling, often in the hands and feet), a broad chest, a short fourth or fifth metacarpal, low-set ears, a small mandible, strabismus (tendency for eyes to wander or cross), and numerous pigmented nevi (moles). We now understand that there are additional associated abnormalities, including lack of development of the ovaries (ovarian dysgenesis) leading to infertility in the majority of women, curvature of the spine (scoliosis), abnormal bone development (bone dysplasia), inner ear defects, a highly arched palate, kidney malformations, and cardiovascular anomalies (such as a malformed heart [tricuspid] valve, narrowing of the major blood vessel in the chest [aorta], and weakening of the wall of the aorta, which can lead to devastating splitting/tissue breakdown [dissection and rupture]). Other medical complications may include high blood pressure, diabetes, arthritis, obesity, hearing loss, exaggerated scar formation, cataracts, and hypothyroidism. Obtaining health insurance can be difficult for patients with TS; some plans may also refuse to pay for treatments such as growth hormone, as discussed below. Little information about life expectancy exists; current studies are examining this question.

CAUSES OF TURNER SYNDROME

In TS, all or part of one of the X chromosomes is lost near the time of conception. The "pure" form of TS, which was the first form identified and represents approximately 50% of cases, is designated 45X or 45XO, meaning that one of the X chromosomes did not get passed to the child by a parent. "Mosaicism" (approximately 30% of cases) occurs in the developing cell, when cell division fails to properly duplicate the genetic material. In these situations the girl has some cells with the usual number of chromosomes, 46XX, and others that are missing an X. In approximately 20% of girls with TS, both X chromosomes are present, but there are structural abnormalities of one X chromosome. The

chromosomal abnormality is not caused by anything either parent has done, and there is no known way to prevent the disorder. Older maternal age is not a factor.

DIAGNOSIS

Only about 1% of pregnancies of TS fetuses result in live births, with spontaneous abortion being the usual consequence of this chromosomal abnormality. Early diagnosis is critical for possible prevention and treatment of the signs and symptoms of TS. The diagnosis is made by chromosomal testing (karyotype), which may be done before birth (prenatally) as part of a specialized procedure to examine the fluid or tissue surrounding the fetus (amniocentesis or chorionic villus sampling procedure). TS may be suspected during ultrasound if the test reveals a heart defect or a specific type of fluid accumulation around the neck (lymphatic fluid). Approximately half of TS girls are diagnosed during infancy due to physical features consistent with the disorder, although many escape detection. Later on, short stature and failure to develop secondary sexual characteristics such as breasts or public hair often indicate a problem. On rare occasions, diagnosis is delayed until adulthood when a woman seeks care for loss of the menstrual period and/or infertility.

TREATMENT

Current recommendations for treatment include use of growth hormone (with or without androgens) to ameliorate short stature, estrogen to initiate the development of secondary sexual characteristics, attention to learning and possible learning disabilities, consideration of social and emotional development, and close medical screening and follow-up of associated medical problems. A specialist in childhood endocrine disorders (pediatric endocrinologist) typically prescribes and directs the hormonal treatment. Growth charting is used to track growth; when the girl's height drops below the 5th percentile (growth category) on a standard growth chart, growth hormone is usually started. This may be done as early as age 2 years. Treatment with growth hormone may be combined with low-dose hormone treatment (androgens) after the girl has reached the age of 9 years to further aid growth. Estrogen accelerates skeletal maturation, so treatment with this hormone is often delayed until the age of 12–15 years to allow for

Turner Syndrome

more growth. Only 1% of girls with TS menstruate without estrogen treatment. Estrogen therapy initiates puberty changes—breast development, uterus growth, and body contour changes. After 1–3 years, the hormone progesterone is added to begin the menstrual cycle. Female hormone therapy is typically continued until around the age of 50 years, when menopause would usually occur.

Girls with TS have a high rate of nonverbal learning disabilities, such as visual-spatial difficulties and trouble with math. Early detection and work with specialists can help the child learn strategies to deal with the deficits, which if left unaddressed can contribute to social difficulties. Attention to the girl's emotional growth and development is extremely important as she may feel different from other girls due to her slower growth and sexual development. Support groups fill a critical need in this area as girls with TS meet others with the syndrome, and parents receive practical advice and support.

SEE ALSO: Access to health care, Health insurance, Hormone replacement therapy

Suggested Reading

Ginther, D. W., & Fullwood, H. (1998). Turner syndrome. In L. Phelps (Ed.). *Health-related disorders in children and adolescents: A guidebook for understanding and educating* (pp. 691–695). Washington, DC: American Psychological Association.

Powell, M. P., & Shulte T. (1999). In S. Goldstein & C. R. Reynolds (Eds.), *Handbook of neurodevelopmental and genetic disorders in children*. New York: Guilford Press.

Rosenfeld, R. G. (1992). *Turner syndrome: A guide for physicians*, Second Edition. Houston, TX: The Turner Syndrome Society.

Suggested Resources

The Turner Syndrome Society of the United States (TSS-US) website: www.turnersyndrome.org

PAULA L. HENSLEY

Ultrasound Ultrasound is a specialized diagnostic procedure which allows clinicians to visualize internal body parts or structures. What is the science behind this fascinating tool? Just as a violin string vibrates to produce sound, a solid ceramic "crystal" inside a protected casing (the probe) is set to vibrate by an electrical signal. The frequency, or pitch, is higher than humans can recognize. These sound waves travel outward and are reflected back as echoes, then being "heard" by the same probe which released them. Computer-based processing allows the sending and receiving of signals from multiple sites on the crystal to occur so rapidly that use of the entire array to form a picture makes it almost instantaneous. Thus, "real-time" movement is observed as the image is updated at a rate of many times per second. The two-dimensional image is created because, just like in fish-finding sonar, the length of time it takes for the sound to travel to and from the surface reflecting the echo indicates the depth. The returned echo is translated electronically into digital information, which can be processed further. What one sees is that a very dense structure will create a strong echo which appears white. Full transmission of the sound waves (no echo) will leave the image black. A spectrum of gray indicates the range of densities and the whole result is like an artist's canvas and shows a "slice" of whatever the target tissue is.

The quality of ultrasound has improved dramatically since the first two-dimensional images in the mid-1970s. The electronics, computerized processing, speed, fine detail, and the display of motion using graphs and color have made it not only easier to perform but also widened the applications. Not content to settle for only one two-dimensional picture at a time, the acquisition of the same type of sound echo information from multiple adjacent "slices" forms a volume of digital data. These data can be selectively processed to reveal any chosen slice or the surface of a solid structure inside water, such as the fetal face inside amniotic fluid.

Contrast between water (fluid), which transmits sound waves, and dense tissue, which reflects sound waves, provides the clearest images. Ultrasound is thus most useful in examining structures where that difference is present, such as unborn babies in amniotic fluid, heart and vessels containing blood, joints with fluid, gallbladders with bile, kidneys and the collecting system containing urine, and the like. Where such contrast does not naturally exist, it has been specially introduced, such as the infusion of saline into the nonpregnant uterine cavity to perform sonohysterography.

A variety of probe sizes, shapes, and sound wave frequencies are available to "see" at shallow and deep levels or inside body cavities. One example is the intravaginal probe, which provides good views of early pregnancy and the nonpregnant uterus. Due to probe technology, a full bladder is rarely needed anymore for obstetrical or gynecologic exams and in fact may hinder or mislead the examiner.

In obstetrics, the number of babies, their sizes, their organ structures including brain, the shape of their limbs and bones, the appearance of the face and other features are eagerly sought by prospective parents. From such things, we postulate due date, adequacy of growth, and probability of being "normal." Also important to the medical caregivers is information about the baby's environment: placenta, amniotic fluid, uterus, and cervix.

Such things may imply an increased risk later on in the pregnancy. Sometimes we can be virtually certain about what these observations mean; at other times we must consider a range of possibilities with no answer expected during the pregnancy. To accomplish further testing or even treat a few conditions, ultrasound can be used to guide placement into the uterus of a needle, catheter, or fiber-optic scope. As pregnancy advances, observations of fetal movement, blood flowing to the placenta through the umbilical cord, and blood distribution to fetal brain or other organs may reassure or conversely reveal a problem indicating whether delivery or some other action on behalf of the baby is needed. One big caution bears repeating: Fetal weight estimated from ultrasound measurements in late pregnancy should be taken with a big grain of salt.

Although obstetrics was the first use to rapidly grow, ultrasound has become essential to gynecology as well as cardiology and almost all areas of medicine. Abnormal vaginal bleeding, pelvic pain, a mass or large lump felt on physical examination, possible cancer, fibroids, and many other gynecologic concerns can be clarified by looking with ultrasound.

Ultrasound examinations are rarely uncomfortable. Patients are often examined while on their backs, and a change of position is used either to see better in a specific way or to assist in patient comfort. No harmful effects have been observed in the many years of ultrasound use, even heavy use during a complicated pregnancy. Based on research, for example, effects on tissue culture, the possibility of biological effects has not been completely ruled out, however, particularly with extensive use in early pregnancy. Thus, casually looking at an unborn baby just for fun is not recommended.

SEE ALSO: Abdominal pain, Cancer screening, Pelvic examination, Pregnancy testing, Prenatal care, Uterine fibroids

Suggested Resources

http://www.acog.org

SUSAN E. RUTHERFORD

United States Civil Rights Act of 1964

Congress passed the most significant legislation affecting equal rights in 1964. The Civil Rights Act made it illegal to discriminate against a person because of his or her race, color, religion, national origin, or sex. This law essentially gave minorities equal access to education, employment, and other opportunities. In addition, the Civil Rights Act made discrimination and segregation illegal in public places, state programs, and community programs. The Equal Employment Opportunity Commission, which was created by the Civil Rights Act, was formed to monitor and enforce the mandate of this law.

Support for the Civil Rights Act began with marches and demonstrations by the Southern Christian Leadership Conference and the Student Nonviolent Coordinating Committee. The brutality unleashed on these peaceful protesters led to President Kennedy's support to pass a federal civil rights law in 1963. In support of the law, Dr. Martin Luther King held a public demonstration called "Jobs and Freedom" in Washington, DC. Over 250,000 people attended and heard Dr. King's "I Have a Dream" speech.

Although the viability of the civil rights legislation was threatened by the assassination of President Kennedy, the push for civil rights law continued when Vice President Lyndon B. Johnson became President. However, several strong Southern senators led a campaign against the civil rights legislation by initiating and sustaining the longest filibuster in history, which lasted for a total of 8 weeks. Despite the Southern senators' strong opposition, they were unsuccessful in preventing the legislation from becoming law. The filibuster was finally defeated by cloture, which allowed 60 senators to vote and end the filibuster. As a result, the Civil Rights Act of 1964 became law.

Even though the Civil Rights Act of 1964 made discrimination against women illegal, the Equal Employment Opportunity Commission did not enforce the ban on gender discrimination. More work was needed to ensure equality for women. The momentum of the Civil Rights Act of 1964 encouraged women's rights organizations such as the National Organization for Women to continue their campaign for equality. These organizations pushed for either a constitutional amendment or a Supreme Court ruling that would further the prohibition of gender discrimination. Although the constitutional amendment known as the Equal Rights Amendment failed, the Supreme Court ruled that gender discrimination violated the 14th amendment's Equal Protection Clause. Other enacted laws that prohibited gender discrimination such as the Pregnancy Discrimination Act of 1978, were passed due to the groundwork established by the Civil Rights Act of 1964.

The abolition of gender discrimination in the workplace was a major goal of the Civil Rights Act of 1964. This Act continues to make it illegal for an employer to treat an employee differently because of his or her sex. Company policies that discriminate against women and job advertisements that discourage women from applying are violations of the Civil Rights Act. The provisions apply regardless of the physically demanding nature of the job or high turnover rates. The Civil Rights Act prohibits virtually all unilateral discrimination against women.

Over time, the Civil Rights Act of 1964 has been amended to expand the law against discrimination. In 1972, the Civil Rights Act was amended to prohibit discrimination by private employers. In addition, the Act was amended in 1980 to prohibit discrimination against persons with disabilities, which includes those with physical, mental, and health disabilities such as AIDS. The 1991 amendment expanded employment discrimination protection for women and minorities.

Today, the effect of the Civil Rights Act of 1964 is visible in the workplace and educational systems. The number of women employed since 1950 has risen over 70%. In education, the number of female students becoming doctors and lawyers has risen dramatically in the last 40 years. Equal access to education has enabled women to study engineering and become astronauts for NASA. Business ownership among women has skyrocketed because of the equal opportunity provided by the Civil Rights Act of 1964.

The 1964 Civil Rights Act was a landmark legislation that furthered and expanded civil rights and equality under the law. It was the first step toward giving every man or woman, regardless of race, an opportunity to pursue any educational career he or she wishes, to own businesses, and to receive equal treatment in the workplace. It allowed U.S. citizens to fully exercise their rights, regardless of sex, color, national origin, or religion.

SEE ALSO: Affirmative action, Discrimination, Sexual harassment

Suggested Reading

O'Connor, K., & Sabato, L. J. (2000). *The essentials of American government, continuity and change.* Boston: Addison Wesley Longman.
Patterson, T. E. (1994). *The American democracy* (2nd ed., pp. 176, 188, 193, 197, 255). New York: McGraw-Hill.
Sack, S. M. (1998). *The working woman's legal survival guide.* Paramus, NJ: Prentice-Hall.

ELIZABETH M. VALENCIA

Urinary Incontinence and Voiding Dysfunction

The function of the bladder is to store urine that is produced in the kidneys and transported to the bladder via the ureters (tubes leading from the kidneys to the bladder). The bladder should store urine effortlessly and painlessly until a socially appropriate situation arises for its evacuation. Voiding (urinating) should be voluntary, painless, and result in the near-complete emptying of the bladder. Urinary incontinence is defined as the involuntary loss of urine that is objectively demonstrable. There are various reasons why a woman develops urinary incontinence. It is important to determine the mechanism responsible for leakage since treatment strategies will vary accordingly. Difficulty in emptying the bladder is termed voiding dysfunction and has various causes and manifestations.

Incontinence affects an estimated 13 million Americans. The prevalence increases with age and varies widely among various studies from 2% to 27% depending upon the population studied and the definitions given for incontinence as well as the method of data collection. An increasing number of vaginal deliveries seems to correlate with the presence of incontinence.

TYPES OF URINARY INCONTINENCE

The most common type of incontinence in women is stress incontinence, which is defined as involuntary loss of urine that occurs coincident with increased intra-abdominal pressures. These can occur during coughing, sneezing, laughing, exercising, or even while getting up from a seated position.

Urge incontinence is the involuntary leakage of urine coincident with a strong urge to urinate. This is often accompanied by urinary frequency (going more than eight times during the day), urgency ("when I gotta go, I gotta go!!!"), and nocturia (awakening frequently at night to urinate). This condition has been recently termed overactive bladder. Mixed incontinence refers to having features of both conditions of stress and urge incontinence.

Overflow incontinence is less common in women, and is associated with incomplete emptying of the bladder and maintaining excessive urine in the bladder (a high residual volume) even after voiding. Such voiding dysfunction can be the result of neurological disease, medications, acute inflammatory conditions of the tube

663

leading out from the bladder (urethra) and/or genital structures (vulva), obstruction from surgery, prolapse (inversion) of the bladder, or a variety of other pelvic, endocrinologic, or psychogenic conditions. In addition to overflow incontinence, other consequences may occur such as frequent urinary tract infections, symptoms of overactive bladder, and in rare instances damage to the kidneys.

Other rare conditions that result in urinary incontinence include fistulas, which are abnormal communications between the urinary tract and other organs. The most common urinary fistula is one between the bladder and vagina, termed a vesicovaginal fistula, which leads to constant leakage of urine from the vagina. In the United States, this occurs most commonly following hysterectomy, whereas in the Third World, the most common reason is childbirth. Other causes of incontinence are congenital due to abnormal development of the urinary tract, and remain very rare.

EVALUATION

Keeping in mind the definition of incontinence ("...loss of urine that is objectively demonstrable"), a primary goal of medical evaluation is to demonstrate the leakage experienced. This may require multiple attempts of coughing or other maneuvers in an attempt to replicate in the office, what occurs in daily life. An equally important goal of initial evaluation is ensuring that there is no reversible cause of incontinence, which if found, should be addressed. Reversible causes of incontinence include disorders of consciousness/alertness (delirium), urinary tract infection, disorders of the vaginal walls (vaginal atrophy), medications, psychological, endocrine (hormonal) disorders, restricted mobility making it difficult to get to the bathroom on time, and severe constipation with stool buildup (impaction). A pelvic exam is needed to look for any pelvic organ invasion (prolapse), signs of atrophy (lack of the effects of estrogen on the vagina), and other gynecologic abnormalities that may affect the urinary tract system. The exam should also include a targeted neurological evaluation focusing on the lower spinal nerves in the area of the lower pelvis (sacrum).

When evaluating abnormal bladder function, evaluation of the "postvoid residual volume" is very important, that is, urine still in the bladder after voiding has taken place. This can be done by specialized visualization techniques (ultrasound) or catheterization (using a

small tube) of the bladder. Urine is obtained for urinalysis and culture to rule out urinary tract infection and the presence of microscopic amounts of blood in the urine. After the first visit, many centers require the patient to keep a bladder diary for several days in which she measures and records all urine volumes of each void for the period of time the diary is being kept.

More specialized testing called urodynamics (measuring how well the bladder functions) may be necessary to increase diagnostic accuracy. Some practitioners prefer urodynamic studies on all patients who are being considered for surgery to improve counseling regarding the risks and benefits and to help determine the type of surgery that would be most appropriate for the particular situation. Urodynamics usually involves pressure measurement of the bladder via a bladder catheter (small tube) and simultaneous intra-abdominal pressure measurement by a catheter in the rectum or vagina. The bladder is filled, and attempts are made to elicit urinary incontinence that mimics the symptoms at home at different bladder volumes. Further tests are done to evaluate how well the tubes leading out from the bladder function (urethral competence), and usually the patient is asked to void with the catheters in place to ascertain the bladder's function during the voiding process. In many cases additional information is obtained by specialized measurements of nerve conduction by the urethral muscle (electromyographic [EMG] recordings) during the entire study, which usually lasts 30–60 minutes overall.

TREATMENT

Initial therapy of urinary tract infections, vaginal atrophy, and/or constipation is instituted, and improvement monitored; if incontinence persists despite adequate therapy, further diagnostic and therapeutic options are explored. The bladder diary is useful in ruling out excessive fluid intake, which should be addressed before instituting specific therapy. Most women will maintain adequate hydration with drinking 50–60 ounces of fluid a day. Dietary restriction of substances considered to be bladder irritants, most notably alcohol and caffeine, is instituted. Early intervention with adequately performed and persistently done Kegel exercises may cure mild cases of incontinence and improve many others. Kegel exercises are specialized and easy-to-learn exercises which strengthen the pelvic muscles. Biofeedback and electrical stimulation may be used to increase the effectiveness of Kegel exercises alone for stress or urge incontinence as well as mixed incontinence.

Specific therapy regarding urge incontinence (overactive bladder) includes bladder retraining, which is designed to gradually increase the bladder's ability to hold urine for increasingly longer periods of time. Biofeedback and electrical stimulation are commonly used methods for the treatment of urge incontinence, and tend to be more effective when done while on medication. Medications used to treat urge incontinence and the overactive bladder work by calming the bladder muscle and reducing its contractility. These include various preparations such as the medications tolterodine, oxybutynin, hyoscyamine, propantheline, and imipramine. The most common side effects include dry mouth and constipation.

In patients who continue to have severe symptoms of urgency, frequency, and/or urge incontinence, and for whom all other options have failed, implantation of a medical devise (sacral neuromodulation) may offer significant benefit. This involves surgically implanting an electrode in the pelvis (sacral region) and connecting it to a small external generator. If it is found during the testing phase that the therapy is effective, an implantable programmable battery is placed (similar to the battery used for cardiac pacemakers). Other, more aggressive surgery is possible, but is rarely used nowadays.

Specific therapy for stress incontinence beyond Kegel exercises and biofeedback may include nonsurgical as well as surgical modalities. For mild degrees of stress incontinence that occurs during specific and well-defined circumstances (such as playing tennis), it may be helpful to take the medication pseudoephedrine just prior to the activity. Another option is using a relatively small anti-incontinence device inserted into the vagina (pessary), which works by supporting the urethra during times of increased intra-abdominal pressure.

Many surgeries have been proposed for the treatment of stress incontinence. Some of these surgeries can be done abdominally (conventional surgery) or laparoscopically (using a small tube inserted into the abdomen), although laparoscopic procedures have been shown to have inferior long-term success rates. Injection of bulking agents into the tube leading out from the bladder (urethra) is also a simple procedure that has some success in treating certain patients with stress incontinence. Various sling procedures have been described where a strap of material, either fascia (covering of muscle) from the patient, from a donor, other biological tissue, or artificially produced, is placed under the urethra to provide a new supportive platform for restoring continence. The ends of the strap must be attached to appropriate tissue to create the support needed. The various sling procedures differ not only in the source of the sling material, but also in the way it is suspended. All surgeries carry risks along with the potential benefits they provide. Unique risks of surgeries for stress incontinence include possible difficulty in bladder emptying, development of overactive bladder symptoms, and erosion of permanent materials used for the repair through the vagina, and rarely through surrounding structures.

For patients with mild mixed incontinence, the medication imipramine is especially useful. Biofeedback and electrical stimulation has also shown benefit. Another strategy is treating the worst component first with type-specific approaches, and then tackling the other component if needed.

Overflow incontinence and voiding dysfunction with incomplete bladder emptying is first addressed by having the women with incontinence use a procedure called clean intermittent catheterization (CIC). This involves the patient catheterizing herself with a special short rigid catheter, usually several times a day. The technique does not need to be done under sterile conditions, rather under clean conditions. The procedure is relatively easy to learn and quick to do at home or in a public restroom. Most patients do very well with this; however, some will continue to have problems with recurrent urinary tract infections or other difficulties. If the cause of the dysfunctional voiding is not due to blockage of the tube leading out from the bladder obstruction, as may occur from prolapse or following surgery for stress incontinence, these patients may be candidates for sacral neuromodulation (see earlier explanation of this procedure), which is effective in restoring normal voiding. Diagnostic procedures that evaluate the functional capability of the bladder (urodynamic studies) are important in the diagnosis of voiding dysfunction to guide therapy.

SEE ALSO: Kegel exercises, Pelvic organ prolapse, Urinary tract infections

Suggested Reading

Adam, R. A., & Preston, M. R. (2002). Urinary incontinence: Diagnosis and treatment. *Women Health, Gynecology Edition, 2*(4), 218–229.

Agency for Healthcare Policy and Research. (1992). *Urinary incontinence in adults* [Publication 93-0552]. Rockville, MD: United States Department of Health and Human Services.

RONY ADAM

Urinary Tract Infections

Urinary tract infections (UTIs) are one of the most common medical problems that cause women to seek medical attention. In most cases UTIs are a nuisance; a medical problem that produces uncomfortable symptoms that appropriate outpatient treatment can quickly alleviate. While usually a benign condition, UTIs do have the potential to become a serious medical problem, requiring hospitalization and aggressive therapy.

UTIs are defined as the presence of bacteria anywhere in the urinary tract. Most commonly, UTIs result from bacteria growing in the bladder, and producing cystitis, a term that is often used interchangeably with UTIs. Cystitis refers to infection limited to the bladder, while the term UTI includes other structures such as the kidneys, ureters, and urethra. UTIs can be defined as complicated and uncomplicated. Complicated UTIs refer to cases in which there are functional or anatomic abnormalities of the urinary tract, underlying host abnormalities, or infection of the kidneys or ureters. Uncomplicated UTIs refer to cases without these factors and account for 80% of cases. Complicated UTIs require more aggressive or prolonged treatment and are associated with increased morbidity. In greater than 99% of cases, bacteria gain access to the urinary tract by ascending via the urethra; in rare cases, infection can result from the spread of bacteria to the kidney via the bloodstream or other routes.

UTIs are very common among sexually active young women, with approximately one third of women having a UTI within 10 years of the onset of sexual activity. Most UTIs in sexually active young women are uncomplicated cystitis. There are about 25 million cases of acute cystitis per year in the United States, with most of these cases treated by physicians. Sexual activity predisposes women to UTIs by inoculation of urinary tract pathogens into the urethra and by acquisition of strains of *Escherichia coli* (see below) that are urinary tract pathogens. Many women are prone to frequent UTIs and contract them commonly after sexual activity. Some women are more susceptible to UTIs due to cell surface markers in the bladder that favor bacterial colonization, and other factors. Women with frequent uncomplicated UTIs sometimes employ a self-treatment strategy without physician intervention for each episode.

Elderly women are more susceptible to bacterial colonization of the bladder. The reasons for this are not fully known but are thought to be related to anatomic changes that lead to incomplete voiding and estrogen deficiency. Elderly women may have significant numbers of bacteria in their bladder without having any symptoms; this is termed "asymptomatic *bacteriuria*." Prospective studies have shown that asymptomatic bacteriuria in elderly women resolves spontaneously and does not require antibiotic therapy. There is no reason to screen for *bacteriuria* and treat asymptomatic elderly women. When symptomatic UTIs do occur in the elderly, they are more often complicated due to factors such as the presence of bladder catheters, anatomic or functional abnormalities, and other comorbidities.

UTIs in pregnancy can cause preterm labor and low birthweight. Physiologic and anatomic changes related to pregnancy make pregnant women more susceptible to UTIs and more likely to have complications. In contrast to elderly women, asymptomatic *bacteriuria* in pregnant women has been shown to lead to complicated UTIs, and should be treated. Screening and treating asymptomatic *bacteriuria* in the first trimester has been shown to decrease the incidence of complicated UTIs later in pregnancy.

Women with uncomplicated UTIs present with pain and burning on urination, difficulty voiding, and frequent urination. There may be visible blood in the urine, which can be quite dramatic. The onset of these symptoms can be very acute. There may be some overlap in symptoms between UTIs and urethritis due to sexually transmitted diseases (STDs) such as herpes, gonorrhea, and chlamydia, which can also produce burning on urination. A urinalysis demonstrating the presence of white blood cells and bacteria in the urine will differentiate between burning on urination from UTI versus urethritis from STDs. Frail elderly women with UTIs may present with more subtle findings such as lethargy and decreased oral intake without specific symptoms related to the urinary tract.

UTIs involving the kidney (termed pyelonephritis) produce additional symptoms compared to simple cystitis. In addition to burning and frequency, patients with pyelonephritis present with flank pain and tenderness, fever chills, nausea, and vomiting. Other conditions that produce symptoms that overlap with those of pyelonephritis include pelvic inflammatory disease, acute appendicitis, kidney stones, and diverticulitis. Acute pyelonephritis can be complicated by sepsis, and patients are often admitted for inpatient therapy.

The bacterium that most often causes UTIs is *E. coli*, which is a normal inhabitant of the gastrointestinal (GI) tract and perineum. There are specific strains of *E. coli* that are pathogenic (disease-causing) for the urinary tract due to their ability to adhere to the lining of the bladder and other factors. Colonization with one of these "uropathogenic" strains of *E. coli* may lead to recurrent bouts of UTIs, which then stop once this strain is eliminated. In addition to *E. coli*, a variety of other bacteria that are normal inhabitants of the GI tract cause UTIs, including *Klebsiella, Enterococcus*, and *Proteus Staphylococcus saprophyticus* is a common pathogen (disease-causing agent) in sexually active young women. Patients residing in long-term care facilities, hospitalized patients, and patients with chronic bladder catheters may become infected with pathogens that are difficult to treat including bacteria that have acquired resistance to commonly used antibiotics.

Treatment of acute uncomplicated cystitis consists of a short course of antibiotics (3 days) and adequate hydration (fluid intake). Complicated UTIs require a longer course of antibiotics, usually 7–10 days. Patients with pyelonephritis are often admitted and treated with intravenous antibiotics. The specific antibiotics used will depend on issues of cost, changing susceptibility patterns of UTI pathogens, and the patient's history of allergies and prior treatment. Cranberry juice has not been shown to be effective in treating an established UTI, but may be beneficial in preventing UTIs by impeding bacteria from adhering to the bladder wall. Adequate fluid intake can also help prevent UTIs as bacteria are flushed out of the bladder by urination before an infection is established. For women who have UTIs frequently after sexual activity, drinking one or two glasses of water resulting in increased urine production has been shown to prevent UTIs.

SEE ALSO: Gonorrhea, Herpes simplex virus, Sexually transmitted diseases

Suggested Reading

Ronald, R. A. (2002). Urinary tract infections in adults. In J. S. Tan (Ed.), *Experts guide to the management of common infectious diseases* (pp. 229–250). Philadelphia: American College of Physicians.

Suggested Resources

National Kidney and Urologic Disease Information Clearinghouse website: http://kidney.niddk.nih.gov/kudiseases/pubs/utiadult/index.htm

KEITH B. ARMITAGE

Uterine Cancer   Among the three most common gynecologic cancers of the female reproductive system, uterine cancer is the most common in the United States. Approximately 37,000 women will be diagnosed with uterine cancer each year. Fortunately, the overall cure rate for uterine cancer is high with greater than 80% of women developing uterine cancer being cured. The uterus, situated in the female pelvis, is comprised of a muscular wall surrounding the uterine cavity, which is also known as the endometrial cavity. Cancers of the uterus can arise from either the lining of the uterine cavity or from the muscular wall of the uterus. Uterine cancers arising from the lining of the cavity, termed the endometrium, are commonly referred to as endometrial cancers. Uterine cancers arising from the muscular wall are referred to as uterine sarcomas. Because over 95% of uterine cancers are endometrial cancers, these terms are often used synonymously. Since the great majority of uterine cancers are endometrial cancers, most of the discussion in this section will focus on endometrial cancers, although in general, uterine sarcomas are managed similarly to endometrial cancers.

RISK FACTORS

Although younger women may develop uterine cancers, as in many other cancers, uterine cancer tends to arise in older women with an average of diagnosis at approximately 60 years of age. One important risk factor in developing uterine cancer is increased estrogen hormone exposure. Estrogens are a class of female hormones that are a potent growth stimulator of the endometrium. Estrogens are sometimes administered as hormone replacement therapy to treat conditions associated with perimenopause and menopause. When administered alone for hormone replacement therapy, estrogen increases a woman's risk of developing endometrial cancer. The progestins, another class of female hormones, counteract the proliferative effects of estrogen on the endometrium and are therefore often given along with estrogens in women on hormone replacement therapy for the main purpose of reducing the increased risk of developing endometrial cancer due to estrogen.

Several other risk factors for developing endometrial cancer are related to the principle of increased estrogen exposure. One such risk factor is obesity. This is because one area of production of estrogens other than the ovary is in adipose tissue or fat cells. Women who are obese, therefore, have higher endogenous production of estrogens. Women who have had a history of using oral contraceptives (birth control pills) have a reduced lifetime risk of developing uterine cancers.

DIAGNOSIS

Most women who have uterine cancers will have symptoms of some type of abnormal vaginal bleeding. This can range from minimal vaginal spotting or a bloody vaginal discharge to heavy bleeding in between periods or during periods. Any woman with irregular vaginal bleeding, and especially menopausal women who have any type of vaginal bleeding should see a physician for further evaluation. A physician will then decide, based on history and examination, whether such symptoms need to be further evaluated for cancer. As part of the evaluation, additional tests may include an endometrial biopsy, uterine dilation and curettage, hysteroscopy, or a pelvic ultrasound.

An endometrial biopsy is commonly done in the office in which a small narrow tube (thinner than a pencil) made of either plastic or metal is inserted through the entrance of the cervix (the lower portion of the uterus that extends into the vagina) into the uterine cavity followed by aspiration of a small amount of tissue from the uterine cavity. This procedure can cause cramping and pain very briefly. Most women are able to tolerate this office procedure very well. Potential problems associated with this procedure include an inability to successfully insert the biopsy tube into the uterine cavity due to a cervical stenosis (excessive narrowing of the opening of the cervix). Other problems that may occur from endometrial biopsies but are rare may include infection or uterine perforation (creating a hole in the uterus).

A dilation and curettage (commonly referred to as D&C) is another method a physician may select to evaluate for the possibility of uterine cancer. This is a procedure usually performed in the operating room under anesthesia in which the entrance to the cervix is opened (dilated) followed by a scraping (curettage) of the

uterine cavity. Both the endometrial biopsy and D&C provide tissue from the endometrial cavity for submission to the pathologist (a physician who examines the tissue under a microscope to determine whether there is cancer). Risks of a D&C include the same as for an endometrial biopsy; however, because the D&C is a more invasive procedure, there are additional risks including the risk of anesthesia. Despite being a more invasive procedure, a physician may select a D&C over an endometrial biopsy for several reasons including the following:

1. Women may not be able to tolerate an endometrial biopsy in the office.
2. A significant narrowing of the entrance of the cervix may prevent successful sampling of the endometrial cavity.
3. Women who have heavy uterine bleeding may require a D&C as not only a diagnostic procedure, but also as a therapeutic procedure to stop the heavy bleeding.
4. There may be situations in which a physician may need a greater sampling of tissue and a D&C may be able to provide this better than an endometrial biopsy.

At the time of the endometrial biopsy or D&C, a hysteroscopy may also be performed as part of the evaluation. Hysteroscopy is a procedure in which a "telescope" is inserted into the uterine cavity allowing direct visualization of the cavity. In addition to these tests that are available, a physician may also select pelvic ultrasound to evaluate uterine bleeding. Pelvic ultrasonography is a radiologic evaluation in which sound waves are used to visualize the pelvic organs including the uterus. Current technology allows visualization of the thickness of the endometrial cavity, which is almost always thickened in endometrial cancers. However, many other noncancerous conditions may cause an increased thickness in the endometrial cavity.

TREATMENT AND PROGNOSIS

The primary treatment of uterine cancer is surgery. The surgery that is performed includes a hysterectomy (removal of the uterus) and bilateral salpingo-oophorectomy (removal of the attached ovaries and fallopian tubes). In addition, other biopsies including removal of lymph nodes in the pelvis and in the abdomen may be performed during surgery to determine if there is spread of the cancer. Radiation therapy may be offered as an alternative to surgery in women who are unable or unwilling to have surgery. Nevertheless, surgery is the preferred method of treatment as it results in a higher cure rate when compared with radiation therapy. Cure rates for surgery have been reported to be between 80% and 94% compared with 60% and 80% for radiation therapy.

After surgery, the woman may, however, be offered radiation therapy as adjuvant therapy. This is sometimes done for women with spread of uterine cancer to the lymph nodes or who have other high-risk features portending a higher risk for cancer recurrence. Rarely, for young women who wish to maintain the ability to get pregnant, hormonal therapy with progestins may be a consideration, but only if the cancer is considered a very early cancer.

During the consultation regarding endometrial cancer, a physician may use terms such as stage and grade to characterize the cancer. The stage of a cancer ranging from Stage I to Stage IV refers to the extent of spread of the cancer with Stage I being a cancer confined to the uterus and Stage IV indicating spread beyond lymph nodes and uterus, usually advanced spread. The grade of the cancer refers to the degree of differentiation of the cancer cells or how aggressive the cancer cells appear under the microscope. Pathologists currently grade endometrial cancers from 1 to 3 with grade 1 indicating a well-differentiated or not so aggressive appearing cancer, a grade 3 indicating a poorly differentiated or aggressive-appearing cancer, and a grade 2 in between. Important prognostic factors of endometrial cancer, meaning factors that indicate how well the cancer will respond to treatment, include the stage, grade, and status of lymph node involvement. Fortunately, uterine cancer has a high cure rate because most women with uterine cancer are diagnosed at an early stage, confined to the uterus. The overall cure rate of uterine cancer is greater than 80%. For the majority of women who are diagnosed with cancer confined to the uterus, the cure rate is greater than 90%.

SEE ALSO: Cancer, Cancer screening, Dilation and curettage, Endometriosis, Hysterectomy, Pap test, Ultrasound, Vaginal bleeding

Suggested Resources

http://www.acog.org

PAUL S. LIN

Uterine Fibroids Uterine fibroids are the most common of the noncancerous (benign) tumors of the uterus. The medical term that is synonymous with uterine fibroids is leiomyoma. The cause of fibroids is unknown. However, the hormone estrogen plays a dominant role, since fibroids and associated symptoms are prevalent during the reproductive years and decline during menopause. Fibroid-related symptoms resolve during the menopause and rarely occur during puberty or adolescence. The mean age group for symptoms related to fibroid tumors is between 30 and 50 years old. The incidence of uterine fibroids ranges from 10% to 50%. Factors affecting the incidence include age, race, genetics, and family history. Luckily, most women with uterine fibroids are asymptomatic. Some fibroids may undergo cancerous (malignant) transformation, but fortunately, this is rare. In fact, leiomyosarcoma (the cancerous change of fibroids) is detected in only 0.1% of women with fibroids.

The uterus is normally about the size of a small lemon. There are three regions within the uterus: the inner wall (endometrium), the middle wall (myometrium), and the outer wall (serosal layers). Fibroids even though originating in the myometrium can extend to any or all of these regions. Fibroids are defined as an increase in the smooth muscle component of the uterus. Generally, those originating in the endometrium (called submucosal fibroids) or myometrium (called intramural fibroids) will result in changes within the menstrual cycle. Fibroids originating in the serosa and myometrium tend to be associated with symptoms of pressure on the bladder or the bowels. The size of fibroids can range from the size of a lentil pea to the size of a watermelon. Likewise, the weight may range from a few ounces to several pounds.

Symptoms from uterine fibroids include changes in menstruation, pain, infertility, urinary pressure or urinary retention, constipation, backache, leg pain or swelling, dyspareunia (painful sexual intercourse), pregnancy-related complications, infertility, and increased abdominal girth. In the past, patients were often advised to undergo removal of all or part of the affected uterine tissue (myomectomy or hysterectomy) if the size of the uterus was greater than the size of a normal uterus at 12 weeks in pregnancy. This is no longer true. Today, the caveat is "if your fibroids don't bother you, we don't bother them."

Some patients can experience a range of menstrual complaints associated with fibroids. These include heavier cycles, blood clots, longer duration of menses, and irregular menstruation, constant vaginal discharge, or episodic bloody/fluid (serosanguineous) discharge. Severely affected patients may decrease physical activities and miss work, due to incessant need to change sanitary pads and tampons. Patients who chronically suffer from heavier menstrual cycles may develop anemia (low blood counts) and fatigue.

Other patients have symptoms related to pressure on the bladder. These include complaints of urinary frequency and urgency. Nocturia (having to urinate several times during the night) is also common. Less frequent complaints are stress urinary incontinence, acute urinary retention, urinary tract infections, and pain or difficulty urinating (dysuria). When fibroids enlarge to 16–20 cm, they may put pressure on the ureters, leading to hydronephrosis (swelling of the tube connecting the kidney to the bladder). This may lead to kidney damage on rare occasions.

The least common structure associated with the presence of fibroids is the bowel. Common bowel-related complaints include severe constipation and painful bowel movements.

Collectively, "bulk" symptoms include pelvic heaviness, feeling full, abdominal pressure, and backache. Some patients will also complain of heaviness or a sense that "something is falling out" of the vagina. Some may experience discomfort with intercourse. These symptoms may increase in intensity 1–2 weeks before the menstrual cycle and resolve after menstruation.

Finally, patients with fibroids may note increasing menstrual cramps and pain (dysmenorrhea). Menstrual cramps may escalate 1–2 weeks before menses and be further exacerbated with the menses.

The impact of fibroids on pregnancy and infertility is debatable. Luckily, most women with fibroids do not have reproductive problems. However, fibroids have been associated with premature labor and delivery, persistent breech presentation, postpartum uterine bleeding, more complicated cesarean sections, and early pregnancy-related bleeding. The location of uterine fibroids plays an important role in patients with infertility. Large submucosal fibroids obstructing the endometrial cavity can be associated with difficulty for the egg to implant in the wall of the uterus as is necessary for normal pregnancy (poor placentation), poor sperm migration, and blockage of the fallopian tubes. Likewise, intramural fibroids may impinge on the fallopian tubes or distort the interior of the uterus (endometrial cavity) making pregnancy more difficult. It is important that women experiencing recurrent miscarriages or infertility undergo a thorough evaluation.

The diagnosis of uterine fibroids is often suspected by clinical history and the pelvic examination. Confirmation can be made with pelvic or transvaginal ultrasound. Patients with a normal uterine size but heavy menses may undergo specialized diagnostic procedures that help visualize the uterus better (hysteroscopy is an imaging procedure that can be done in the doctor's office) to determine the presence of uterine fibroids, which line the endometrial cavity.

Many factors must be considered when advising a patient with fibroids. Choice of therapy depends upon reproductive desires of the patient, age, size and number of fibroids, and desire for maintaining the uterus. Sometimes, expectant management is indicated in women who are perimenopausal. Patients with minimal complaints nearing menopause may be reassured about resolution of fibroid symptoms once menopause occurs. Some fibroid-related complaints might be simply treated with nonsteroidal medication, low-dose oral contraceptive pills, or hormone (GnRH) therapy. Luckily there are many conventional surgical procedures as well as minimally invasive techniques to treat uterine fibroids. Hysterectomy always solves fibroid-related bleeding and bulk symptoms. However, hysterectomy should rarely be advised in women wanting children. Myomectomy, which involves just the removal of uterine fibroids, should be considered in women who wish to preserve their fertility or in women opposing hysterectomy.

Currently there are several methods available to perform myomectomy including procedures that take place via a small tube (hysteroscopic, laparoscopic procedures), vaginal, or by conventional exploratory laparotomy (conventional surgery). The surgical choice depends upon the size, number, and location of the fibroids. Finally, a newer form of nonsurgical therapy called uterine fibroid embolization (UFE) is a minimally invasive technique performed by a specially trained radiologist (interventional radiologist) who selectively blocks the flow of blood to the fibroid. The blocked blood flow essentially causes the fibroid to break down and resolve.

Patients now have a vast array of options to treat uterine fibroids. Fortunately, most fibroids are benign. For this reason, patients should never feel rushed into making a clinical or surgical decision. Patients with symptomatic uterine fibroids should seek a compassionate and well-trained gynecologist who is knowledgeable about all fibroid options. The decision to proceed with surgery or other minimally invasive options should be made rationally.

SEE ALSO: Dysmenorrhea, Infertility, Menstrual cycle disorders

Suggested Reading

Bradley, L. D., Falcone, T., & Magen, A. B. (2000). Radiographic imaging techniques for the diagnosis of abnormal uterine bleeding. *Obstetrics and Gynecology Clinics of North America, 27*(2), 245–276.

Clark, A., Black, N., Rowe, P., et al. (1995). Indications for and outcome of total abdominal hysterectomy for benign disease: A prospective cohort study. *British Journal of Obstetrics and Gynaecology, 102*(8), 611–620.

LINDA D. BRADLEY

Vaginal Bleeding Normal menstruation begins between the ages of 10 and 17 years. Once ovulatory cycles ensue, women will have regular and predictable bleeding every 24–35 days, lasting 3–7 days with a predictable amount of flow. Most women lose 2–4 tablespoons of blood with each menses (30–40 ml). The majority of blood loss occurs over 1–2 days, and scantier amounts of bleeding will occur during the remainder of the cycle. Some women may have 1–2 days during the course of menstruation, when bleeding stops and then spontaneously resumes. Subjectively, each woman will serve as her own control, experiencing menstruation individually and uniquely. Slight variations in pattern, duration, and amount will be alarming and lead a patient to seek an evaluation.

Abnormal uterine bleeding is a common and significant problem during puberty, adolescence, reproductive, and postmenopausal years. Approximately 10 million women annually suffer from abnormal bleeding; many suffer in silence. Menstrual cycle-related complaints account for almost one third of all visits to gynecologists. Depending on the time during the reproductive life cycle, complaints and presentations among women vary widely. In addition, the causes for bleeding vary with the time during the life cycle. In the adolescent, heavy and prolonged bleeding can be severe enough and lead to an emergency room visit but tend to be for benign reasons. During the reproductive years, pregnancy-related concerns and uterine pathology must be addressed. Among postmenopausal women, the new onset of bleeding will require an urgent visit to the gynecologist to exclude malignancy.

The impact of abnormal uterine bleeding and subsequent treatment can be profound. At one extreme, heavy bleeding can be associated with hypotension (low blood pressure), anemia, and subsequent blood transfusions. At the other, it may be associated with the inability to enjoy work, hobbies, or coitus. Women who experience unpredictable and heavy menses often complain of a poor quality of life, with restrictions of work, travel, or sports. They may feel confined and afraid to leave their homes because of their fear of social embarrassment from soiling through clothing and furniture due to unpredictable and uncontrolled bleeding.

Recently the American College of Obstetrics and Gynecology (ACOG) recommended the more descriptive terminology of anovulatory uterine bleeding (AUB) to refer to bleeding not caused by anatomic, organic, or systemic pathological conditions. The spectrum of menstrual abnormalities associated with AUB is generally related to the hormonal abnormalities in the menstrual cycle. These are associated with the loss of regulatory control of the hypothalamic–pituitary–ovarian axis. Symptomatically, the menstrual changes can include changes in the duration and amount of the blood flow.

Many factors can be associated with bleeding from the genital tract. These include pregnancy-related complications, vaginal, cervical, and uterine disease, cancer, systemic diseases, infection, trauma, drugs, and iatrogenic causes. The most common pregnancy-related complications include: miscarriage, incomplete abortion, implantation bleeding, and ectopic pregnancy. Vaginal bleeding can also be caused by anatomic abnormalities within the reproductive tract. These include vaginal polyps, vaginal infections and lacerations, foreign bodies, vaginal cancer, or cervical bleeding. Causes of cervical bleeding include cervical polyps, ectropion (unhealed sore), eversion, cervical cancer, and infections. Uterine abnormalities can include: endometrial atrophy or polyps, fibroids, adenomyosis, endometrial hyperplasia, endometrial cancer, and infections. Rarely does fallopian tube cancer or ovarian cancer present as abnormal vaginal bleeding, but these diagnoses must be considered during evaluation of the patient.

A detailed history and physical examination must be obtained in any woman presenting with abnormal bleeding. Systemic diseases must be excluded by a detailed history. Physical inspection of the vulva, vagina, and cervix must be performed on all patients. Thorough bimanual and rectal examinations are important.

Once a thorough physical examination has been performed, laboratory testing and imaging become imperative adjuncts to the evaluation process. Generally, initial laboratory studies will include a complete blood count with platelets and a thyroid-stimulating hormone test. Other laboratory testing including coagulation studies, liver function tests, and hormonal panels may be selected based on the findings during the history or physical examination.

Several diagnostic techniques are available including endometrial biopsy, transvaginal ultrasound, hysteroscopy, saline infusion sonography (SIS), and magnetic resonance imaging (MRI). Findings obtained from the history and physical examination will dictate which modalities are chosen. The therapy chosen for patients with abnormal uterine bleeding may include a medical or surgical approach or a combination of both. For women with anovulatory menstrual cycles, many effective medical therapies are available. These include oral contraceptive pills, progestin therapy, hormone-impregnated intrauterine devices, nonsteroidal anti-inflammatory drugs, or GnRH analogues. Sometimes correction of other hormones may be needed when their imbalance is determined to be a contributing cause of the bleeding. The choice of medical therapies will be determined by the desire for future childbearing, lack of contraindications for therapy, cost, compliance issues, and the absence of other organic, anatomic, or systemic disease.

Surgical therapies may utilize minimally invasive therapy with removal of polyps or fibroids via operative hysteroscopy (a procedure done with a small tube placed in the uterus). In cases where no anatomic pathology is found and patients desire preservation of the uterus (but not childbearing), patients may be offered a procedure called an endometrial ablation. Hysterectomy may be the ultimate procedure when other therapies have failed or when women expect 100% relief from abnormal bleeding.

Finally, abnormal uterine bleeding affects many patients and spans the reproductive life cycle. The causes of abnormal vaginal bleeding span the gamut from reproductive tract abnormalities to systemic disease. In some cases, the bleeding can be debilitating, in others it is just a minor nuisance. However, a thorough history, physical examination, and carefully chosen imaging and laboratory tests will quickly delineate the etiology, pointing the way to appropriate medical or surgical therapy.

SEE ALSO: Ectopic pregnancy, Hysterectomy, Menstrual cycle disorders, Oral contraception, Pelvic examination, Physical examination, Uterine fibroids

Suggested Reading

Jones, K., & Bourne T. (2001). The feasibility of a "one stop" ultrasound-based clinic for the diagnosis and management of abnormal uterine bleeding. *Ultrasound Obstetrics and Gynecology, 17*, 517–521.

Munro, M. G. (2000). Abnormal uterine bleeding in the reproductive years. Part I pathogenesis and clinical investigation. *Journal of the American Association of Gynecologic Laparoscopists, 6*(4), 393–416.

LINDA D. BRADLEY

Vaginismus   Vaginismus is defined as the involuntary spasm of the pelvic muscles surrounding the outer third of the vagina. Such spasm may interfere with or prevent sexual intercourse. In some cases, vaginismus may prevent insertion of almost anything into the vagina, including tampons, fingers, or speculums used in gynecologic examinations.

The psychiatric diagnosis of vaginismus is described in the *Diagnostic and Statistical Manual of Mental Disorders,* fourth edition (DSM-IV). The essential feature of the disorder is the "recurrent or persistent involuntary contraction" of the involved vaginal muscles, which interferes with sexual intercourse. To make the diagnosis of vaginismus, the symptoms must (a) cause marked distress or interpersonal difficulty, (b) cannot be better accounted for by another major

Vaginismus

psychiatric disorder, and (c) cannot be due exclusively to the direct physical effects of a medical condition. Although pain is not part of this definition, most women with vaginismus either experience pain or fear pain with vaginal penetration. That being the case, distinguishing vaginismus from dyspareunia (genital pain with sexual intercourse) can be difficult. The diagnosis should be confirmed by careful pelvic examination, preferably by a thoughtful, sensitive physician well versed in the care of women with sexual dysfunction.

The rate of vaginismus in the general population is estimated at 1% or less. The rate is higher in women referred to sexual dysfunction and medical clinics, ranging between 5% and 42%. The spasm of vaginismus is typically triggered by anticipation of or actual attempts at vaginal penetration. Responses and reactions of women with the disorder vary. Fear of pain or other factors can prevent any attempts at sexual intercourse for some women, while other women and their partners do attempt penetration but report the sensation of "the penis hitting a brick wall" approximately 1 inch into the vagina.

Vaginismus is a significant and very troubling problem for women who experience it and for their partners. It is considered one of the main causes of "unconsummated marriage," and may make conception impossible. It is almost always the source of strong feelings on the part of the woman and her partner. It may also prevent adequate gynecological care. Feelings such as frustration, embarrassment, humiliation, and inadequacy are common among women with this disorder. This is not to say that women with vaginismus are always sexually unresponsive. In fact, the opposite is true: Many women with the disorder are sexually responsive, experience orgasm with clitoral stimulation, and engage in satisfying, nonpenetrative sexual relationships.

A large number of possible causes for vaginismus have been proposed. The most widely accepted view is that vaginismus is a conditioned response to any unpleasant stimulus affecting the pelvic/genital region or sexual functioning of a woman. That is, the spasm that is characteristic of vaginismus may have at one time been a voluntary reaction on the part of a woman when encountering an unpleasant event or stimulus affecting the pelvic area (such as pain, surgery, or forceful intercourse). Later, when faced with stimuli that the woman perceives as similar to the original unpleasant stimulus, the spasm becomes "conditioned" or automatic and occurs involuntarily. This response of spasm is then reinforced by phobic avoidance of vaginal penetration and by beliefs that such penetration is harmful or painful.

Treatment of vaginismus is usually two-pronged, and includes (a) eliminating erroneous beliefs or thoughts which reinforce the response of involuntary muscle spasm and (b) desensitization exercises to eliminate anxiety about vaginal penetration and allow resolution of the fear response (muscle spasm). The first treatment aim is accomplished through education (e.g., about the size of the vagina and likelihood of pain) and by challenging erroneous beliefs and thoughts. The second aim is accomplished through relaxation exercises and gradual exposure to vaginal penetration. The woman is taught to gradually begin exploring her genital region, both visually and manually, and then to begin insertion of her fingers or dilators into the vaginal area, proceeding from smallest to largest. It is of utmost importance that the patient controls this process and how rapidly it proceeds. Many treatment programs also include vaginal muscle exercises to teach voluntary control over such muscles.

Treatment is individualized to a woman's needs and wishes. For example, women who do not consider sexual intercourse important but wish to bear children may consider artificial insemination. When to include partners in treatment is an individualized decision. Problems such as impotence and premature ejaculation are common among male partners of vaginismic women. The partners should be treated at the same time, although many such problems will improve with treatment of the woman's vaginismic response. Physical problems that act to reinforce the vaginismic response should be treated as well.

Originally, sex therapists such as Masters and Johnson reported cure rates of virtually 100% for vaginismus. Currently, reported cure and improvement rates are less dramatic, but most therapists report good success rates. Many factors play into the course of this disorder. The woman's motivation to overcome the condition is the most important. Greater marital/relationship satisfaction, type of vaginismus (e.g., acquired rather than lifelong), and overall sexual comfort and enjoyment may all be associated with better response to treatment. Finally, the outcome of treatment is variable. Some women may be able to tolerate vaginal penetration but never find it truly pleasurable, while others will experience great pleasure and/or orgasm during coitus and will be able to include vaginal intercourse in a rich, satisfying sexual life thereafter.

SEE ALSO: Dyspareunia, Pain, Sexual dysfunction

Suggested Reading

Kaplan, H. S. (1974). *The new sex therapy: Active treatment of sexual dysfunctions.* New York: Brunner/Mazel.
Lamont, J. A. (1978). Vaginismus. *American Journal of Obstetrics and Gynecology, 131*(6), 633–636.
Leiblum, S. R., & Rosen, R. C. (Eds.). (2000). *Principles and practice of sex therapy* (3rd ed.). New York: Guilford Press.

GRAY B. CLARKE

Varicose Veins *see* Sclerotherapy

Veils

A veil is a length of cloth worn by women as a covering for the head and shoulders, and often in Eastern countries for the face. The practice of veiling began in Mesopotamian cultures as early as 4,000–5,000 years ago as an adaptation to desert life, that is, for protection against the sun, wind, and sand. A variety of religions and cultures with roots in the Middle East and Mediterranean regions incorporated the practice of veiling. Veiling was seen as a ritual to purify, and Greeks, Jews, Hindus, and Christians all practiced veiling. Catholics in particular used the ritual of veiling for covering things and persons. In Catholicism, for example, the *paten* veil covers the bread before consecration while the *chalice* veil covers the wine. Nuns, brides, and young girls receiving communion all wear veils. Although the practice of veiling predates Islam, it has been embraced and spread by that religion. Many Muslims view the practice of veiling as a symbol of virtue, modesty, and privacy for women.

DIFFERENT TYPES OF VEILS

In the Middle East there are many terms used to describe a variety of veils. The type of veil used depends on what body part is to be covered and the geographic region in which it is to be used. There are dozens of veils used in the Middle East; below are descriptions of the most commonly used veils. *Hijab* means to cover or screen in classical Arabic. Muslim women use the word to refer to a variety of styles in which one uses scarves and large pieces of cloth to cover their hair, neck, and sometimes shoulders. The hijab often leaves the entire face open. Most Muslim women living in the United States wear the hijab.

The *chador* is a full-body cloak that conservative Muslim women in Iran wear outdoors. Depending on how it is designed, the chador may or may not cover the face. In 1979, the Iranian revolution led by the Ayatollah Khomeini brought about required veiling in its strictest form, the chador. Government officials arrested and sometimes flogged unveiled women. Today Iranian women are required to veil, but in the less strict hijab form rather than chador. A similar full-body cloak is called the *abaya* in Saudi Arabia. Saudi Arabian women are also required to wear the abaya outdoors under penalty of arrest.

The *nikab* is a veil that covers everything below the bridge of the nose and the upper cheeks, and sometimes also covers the forehead. It is most commonly worn by women with roots in Pakistan and Morocco. The nikab is worn with a head scarf and body cloak.

The *burka* comes in many variations but in its most conservative form, it thoroughly covers the full body and face of the person wearing it, leaving only a mesh-like screen to see through. The *burka* is most associated with the Taliban regime, which ruled in Afghanistan from 1996 to 2001. Women were beaten in public if they refused to wear the *burka*.

EXPRESSION OR OPPRESSION

The veiling of Muslim women has fueled and continues to fuel fierce debate. Although there are no laws requiring veiling in most Middle Eastern countries, conservative and traditionalist Muslims justify their pro-veiling stance on a number of grounds:

1. Traditionalist Muslims argue that men's sexuality can be ignited through unregulated social contact with women. Thus, the purpose of a veil is to regulate social contact and to "protect [a woman's] virtue and to safeguard her chastity from lustful eyes and covetous hands."
2. Traditionalist Muslims argue that the veil is a symbol of the Muslim woman's obedience to Islamic principles.
3. Some individuals feel that veiling reflects cultural and ethnic identity.

Muslim feminists, on the other hand, have argued that veiling is a means of oppression:

1. The veil clearly marks Islamic women who wear it and places unveiled Muslim women in the position of justifying why they do not wear it.

2. In some Middle Eastern countries, most notably Afghanistan, Saudi Arabia, and Iran, unveiled women are flogged, arrested, or beaten by government officials and family members.

3. The forced veiling of women can be seen as a tool for exercising political power, control, punishment, and obedience.

HOW VEILS AFFECT WOMEN'S HEALTH

While the beliefs and customs of veiling are a mystery to many Western health care professionals, most acknowledge that they appear to have a substantial influence on the delivery of health care services in the United States. A recent study on breast cancer screening found that Muslim women who practice veiling felt uncomfortable participating in recommended cancer screening programs. Muslim women expressed concern over exposing their bodies to men and non-Muslim women except in circumstances where there were obvious symptoms of disease present, thus making disease prevention activities difficult. The study concluded that failure to accommodate the beliefs, customs, and lifestyle of Muslim women into health care delivery could significantly affect their participation in health care.

SEE ALSO: Cancer screening, Discrimination, Ethnicity, Feminism, Spirituality

Suggested Reading

Bartkowski, J. P., & Ghazal Read, J. (2003). Veiled submission: Gender, power, and identity among evangelical and Muslim women in the United States. *Qualitative Sociology, 26*(1), 71–92.

Merriam-Webster's collegiate dictionary (10th ed.). (1994). Springfield, MA: Merriam-Webster.

Moghadam, V., & Faegheh, S. (2002). The veil unveiled: The hijab in modern culture. *International Journal of Middle East Studies, 34*(3), 597–599.

Sanders, E. (2001, October 5). Interpreting veils. *The Seattle Times.*

Underwood, S. M., Shaikha, L., & Bakr, D. (1999). Veiled yet vulnerable. *Cancer Practice, 7*(6), 285–289.

NANCY MENDEZ

Venous Thromboembolism

Venous thrombosis is the presence of a blood clot within a superficial or deep vein and the resultant inflammation in the blood vessel wall. Thrombosis most commonly occurs in the legs, but can also occur in the arms. Signs of thrombosis include tenderness in the involved veins, presence of a palpable "cord" in the leg, increased tissue swelling and rigidity, and distension of superficial veins. A careful history eliciting risk factors as well as a physical examination guide the clinician to a proper diagnosis, and diagnostic testing such as duplex venous ultrasonography or venography (specialized scans of the veins and venous walls) helps to confirm the diagnosis. Left untreated, patients with deep venous thrombosis (DVT) are at increased risk of pulmonary embolism (PE), a condition in which the blood clot travels through the venous system to arteries in the lungs.

Risk factors for venous thrombosis were summarized by Rudolf Virchow in 1856: (a) local trauma to the vessel wall; (b) hypercoagulability (increased tendency for clotting of blood); and (c) stasis (pooling or nonmovement of the blood). Over a century later, it is still believed that these factors play a critical role in the formation of thrombus, but also that genetic abnormalities predispose individuals to develop thrombosis when exposed to particular environmental stressors. An "inherited" predisposition to hypercoagulable states can result from deficiencies in factors in the blood that prevent clotting, such as anticoagulant proteins C or S, antithrombin III, and plasminogen. The most frequently inherited predisposition to clot formation is due to the presence of a genetic mutation, factor V Leiden, which increases clotting. Genetic mutations are genes that differ in some individuals from those typically seen in the "normal" population. Given the important role of genetic abnormalities, a careful family history should be obtained from anyone who presents with a venous thromboembolism.

Environmental conditions that lead to venous stasis or endothelial (blood vessel wall) damage promote venous thrombosis, especially among individuals who already have clinical or subclinical tendency to form clots. Approximately 50% of thrombotic events, or clots, in patients with inherited hypercoagulable (increasing clotting) states are associated with acquired risk factors. Some of the more common conditions that can precipitate venous thrombosis are surgery, trauma, immobilization, prolonged travel (such as in cramped airplane seats), cancer, systemic arterial hypertension, indwelling venous catheters, morbid obesity, and cigarette smoking.

Moreover, patients with a history of DVT are at significantly increased risk for recurrent thrombotic events.

Conditions that uniquely place women at increased risk are the use of oral contraceptive pills (OCPs) or hormone replacement therapy (HRT), as well as pregnancy and the postpartum state. OCPs are used by over 70 million women worldwide, including 18 million Americans, making OCP use a key contributor to thrombosis in young women. While the risk of thrombosis increases within 4 months of beginning OCPs, it is unaffected by duration of therapy and returns to baseline levels within 3 months of discontinuation. Women who use OCPs suffer from venous thromboembolism about 3–4 times more than nonusers. This amounts to a total of only about one to four cases per 10,000 oral contraceptive users and should not raise alarm. Women with a genetic predisposition to clotting, such as factor V Leiden genetic mutation, are at significantly increased risk for thrombotic events. The risk of OCPs has decreased with the use of lower estrogen pills. On the other hand, third-generation OCPs containing new progestogens (desogestrel and gestodene) increase the thrombotic rate.

In postmenopausal women, HRT carries a small but significant increase in the risk of venous thromboembolism. In the first randomized, large-scale HRT trial, the Heart and Estrogen/Progestin Replacement Study, HRT was associated with a nearly threefold increased risk of venous thromboembolism. Similarly, the Women's Health Initiative (WHI), which randomized over 16,000 women in an estrogen/progestin versus placebo study, found a twofold increased risk of venous thromboembolism in women treated with HRT. In summary, although these large and carefully done studies demonstrated a statistically significant increase in the rate of thrombotic events with HRT, the number of thrombotic events was still relatively small.

Pregnancy and the postpartum period are well-established risk factors for venous thromboembolism, yielding a greater than fivefold increased risk. Older age is associated with even higher risk. DVT during pregnancy occurs in the left leg more frequently than in the right leg and involves the iliofemoral (pelvic/leg vein) system. The cause of pregnancy-related thrombosis involves all three components of Virchow's original triad: (a) stasis due to the compression of large veins by the pregnant uterus, (b) hypercoagulability due to an increase in blood clotting factors and decrease in anticlotting factors, and (c) endothelial (blood vessel lining) injury, which is worsened at the time of delivery. The risk of venous thromboembolism is further increased in women with a history of venous thrombosis or inherited thrombophilia (tendency to form clots). Thus, screening for these disorders should be provided during prenatal visits, and preventive therapy with subcutaneous low-dose heparin during pregnancy followed by warfarin for 4–6 weeks after delivery may be considered for women at increased risk. This may prevent an "at-risk" woman from developing a DVT.

Anticoagulation is the cornerstone of the treatment of venous thromboembolism. Since patients with DVT are at risk for PE, treatment should be instituted promptly with oral warfarin plus intravenous heparin. After about 5 days, the heparin can be stopped. Warfarin is usually continued for 4–6 months for DVT or at least 6 months for PE. In some patients, if the clot is recurrent or due to an irreversible cause, such as cancer, then anticoagulation may be continued indefinitely. Because warfarin is teratogenic (may cause abnormal fetal development), it is contraindicated in pregnancy. Alternative therapies are available to patients who have contraindications to anticoagulation. Awareness of risk factors and treatment options by both clinicians and patients should decrease the morbidity and mortality associated with this disorder.

See Also: Cardiovascular disease, Coronary risk factors, Hypertension, Oral contraception, Pregnancy

Suggested Reading

Blumenthal, R. S., & Bush, T. (1999). Hormone replacement therapy and the prevention of coronary artery disease. In P. Charney (Ed.), *Coronary artery disease in women: What all physicians need to know* (pp. 264–288). Philadelphia: American College of Physicians.

Hulley, S., Furberg, C., Barrett-Connor, E., et al., for the HERS Research Group. (2002). Noncardiovascular disease outcomes during 6.8 years of hormone replacement therapy. Heart and Estrogen/progestin Replacement Study follow-up (HERS II). *Journal of the American Medical Association, 288*, 58–66.

Writing Group for the Women's Health Initiative Investigators. (2002). Risks and thromboembolic disease and combined oral contraceptives: Results of international multicentre case-control study. *Lancet, 346*, 1575–1582.

Writing Group for the World Health Organization Investigators. (1995). Venous benefits of estrogen plus progestin in healthy postmenopausal women: Principal results from the Women's Health Initiative randomized controlled trial. *Journal of the American Medical Association, 288*, 321–333.

Amir R. Haghighat
Nanette K. Wenger

Violence

Violence is a major contributor to premature death, injury, and disability both in the United States and throughout the world. Each day throughout the world, an average of 4,400 people die from violent acts, for a total of 1.6 million deaths each year. Since many violent deaths are unreported, this estimate is an undercount. Many more people survive acts of violence, and they and their families must often deal with long-term consequences such as disabilities and psychological trauma.

Violence is generally classified into four categories: interpersonal violence, self-harm (such as suicide and suicide attempts), legal intervention (such as capital punishment), and war. This section will focus on interpersonal violence.

Homicide is the most severe act of interpersonal violence. Worldwide, homicide is the 17th leading cause of death. In the United States, homicide is the third leading cause of death for those aged 1 through 34. Homicide rates rose dramatically in the United States between the 1970s and 1993, but then decreased to rates similar to those seen in the late 1960s. While increases in homicide rates are attributed in part to increases in related crime, urban poverty, and inner-city strife, as well as more accurate reporting of cause of death, recent decreases in homicide rates are attributed to the growing economy, community-based prevention programs, increased and more effective law enforcement activities, and anticrime legislation. The observed decreases are likely due in part to combinations of all of these as well as other undocumented factors.

In the United States, nonfatal violent victimizations are measured nationally through the National Crime Victimization Survey. This survey includes rape, sexual assault, robbery, aggravated assault, and simple assault victimizations among those over 12 years of age. In 2000, approximately 6.6 million violent victimizations occurred, or about 29.1 per 1,000 persons over age 12. This is the lowest level of violent victimizations since the survey began in 1973.

Men are more likely than women to be victims of violent crime. In 2000, men experienced 42% more violent crimes, 125% more robberies, and 159% more assaults than women. The only exception is for rape and sexual assault victimizations, in which women are the more likely victims.

Violent crimes against women are more likely than those against men to be perpetrated by someone they know. In over 65% of violent victimizations reported by women, they identified a nonstranger as the perpetrator. This compares to only 44% of victimizations reported by men. A higher percentage of women (21%) than men (3%) reported being victimized by an intimate partner. Over 60% of rapes and sexual assaults were committed by someone known to the woman, including intimate partners (18%), friends/acquaintances (42%), or other relatives (2%).

Men are also more likely than women to perpetrate violent crimes. Each year, women commit approximately 2 million violent offenses, or about 14% of all violent crimes. Three out of four violent crimes committed by women were simple assaults, and about 75% of their victims were also women. Women comprise 22% of all arrestees, 16% of convicted felons, and 16% of the correctional facility population.

Over the last decade, there has been a growing concern about violence perpetrated by adolescents. Surveys have identified that between 30% and 40% of adolescent males and 15–30% of adolescent females have perpetrated a violent crime by the age of 17. The Bureau of Justice Statistics reported in 1997 that persons aged 12–24 comprised 22% of the total population, 35% of murder victims, and 49% of serious violent crime victims. Differences in violent crime perpetration and victimization between men and women are most marked among the younger age groups.

Violence is preventable. Although many believe violent acts to be random events, they actually occur in predictable patterns. Identification of these patterns has led to an understanding that violence is predicated by a complicated interplay between individual, community, and societal characteristics. Violence can be prevented or reduced through actions that modify the characteristics that predicate violence.

At the individual level, factors such as poor communication skills, past violent victimization or witnessing violent acts, low levels of education, and unemployment can lead to violent victimization and perpetration. Violence is also consistently linked with a lifestyle that includes alcohol and drug use, guns, precocious sexual activity, and nonviolent criminal behavior. However, individual predictors of violent behavior usually have a weak effect, and the ability to predict whether specific individuals are likely to become violent is extremely poor. Most individuals who exhibit predisposing factors for violence, such as being a victim of child abuse, do not become violent. Knowledge of individual risk factors is, however, crucial to identify populations at high risk and to design effective intervention programs.

Community factors include poverty, high unemployment, lack of development of the built environment (e.g., dilapidated neighborhoods), and lack of community cohesion. Isolation or segregation of some subpopulations and tolerance for violence are examples of societal factors. Interventions that focus on changing these environmental components can be highly effective because they have the potential to reach a larger number of people. These programs, however, should be implemented in conjunction with programs that address high-risk populations of individuals.

Knowledge about the prevention of violence is rich but fragmented across a number of professional disciplines. A sufficient body of research has not yet been developed that can determine which of the many components of violence are most successfully modifiable, and most programs have not been adequately evaluated. However, most programs that have been highly effective combine interventions that address both individual and multiple components of the environment.

Research into perpetration of violent crimes has revealed two primary categories of violent offenders: those who initiate violent behavior after puberty and those who do so before puberty. Early onset of violent behavior is a very strong predictor of repeated or lifelong violent behavior. Developmental research has identified that early childhood experiences strongly influence the trajectory of brain development, further supporting a strong link between early childhood experiences and later behavior. Developmental research has also found that as a whole, aggressive children and children with behavioral disorders are not more likely to become offenders of violent crimes. In combination, this research implies that direct or indirect violence victimization as a child is a stronger predictor of future violent behavior than a child's personality tendencies.

Based on this research, it is not surprising that prevention programs that focus on early childhood development have proven the most effective. One large review of federally funded violence prevention programs found that early childhood home visitation programs that focus on parenting skills and safe environments were the most effective at preventing the onset of violent behavior. Programs that focus on building communication and problem-solving skills have also shown positive effects, both for children and adults. However, investment in such programs is the

most cost-beneficial when implemented among children and adolescents who live in urban, high-poverty neighborhoods, where the murder rate is often 20 times the national rate.

Knowledge about the causal pathway of violent behavior and how to intervene and prevent such behavior is growing and improving. An evidence-based approach to prevention that encourages collaboration between different agencies and professional backgrounds will contribute to ongoing efforts to reduce violence.

SEE ALSO: Disability, Domestic violence, Mortality, Sexual abuse

Suggested Reading

Sherman, L. W., Gottfredson, D., MacKenzie, D., Eck, J., Reuter, P., & Bushway, S. (1997). *Preventing crime: What works, what doesn't, what's promising* [NCJ 165366]. Washington, DC: U.S. Department of Justice, Office of Justice Programs.
United States Department of Health and Human Services. (2001). *Youth violence: A report of the Surgeon General*. Rockville, MD: author.
United States Department of Justice, Bureau of Justice Statistics. (2001). *Criminal victimization 2000: Changes 1999–2000 with trends 1993–2000*. Washington, D.C.: author.
World Health Organization. (2002). *World report on violence and health*. Geneva: author.

CORINNE PEEK-ASA

Vitamins Vitamins are a group of substances found in foods that are essential for growth, health, and preservation of life itself. The relationship between important food components and health and well-being had been known for hundreds of years, but the specific role of these components was discovered in the 20th century. Vitamins are grouped together as either fat soluble or water soluble.

FAT-SOLUBLE VITAMINS

Fat-soluble vitamins will dissolve in fat and oil, and any extra amount more than the body needs is stored in body fat. Because fat-soluble vitamins can build up in the body, excessive intake of these vitamins can cause toxicity.

679

Vitamins

Vitamin A

Vitamin A occurs in nature in two forms: retinol (the active form of vitamin A) and carotenoids (precursors used by the body to make vitamin A). Vitamin A helps to maintain skin and the lining of certain internal organs. It is also important for normal vision in dim light. Night blindness, in which the eyes adapt poorly to the dark, is an early sign of vitamin A deficiency. If the deficiency is not corrected, it can lead to eye damage and blindness. This vitamin is essential for normal bone and tooth development, is used in the synthesis of hydrocortisone (a steroid hormone) from cholesterol, and helps stabilize cell membranes. Some carotenoids may have the ability to protect cells from cancer-causing changes.

Liver, fish, and egg yolk are rich sources of vitamin A. The main source of vitamin A in the diet is from carotenes found in dark yellow, green, and orange fruits and vegetables. Fortified milk has added vitamins A and D. Too much vitamin A is toxic and causes loss of hair, anorexia, pain in the joints, and enlargement of the liver and spleen.

Vitamin D

Vitamin D occurs in two forms known as vitamin D2 (ergocalciferol), the vitamin D precursor found in plants, and vitamin D3, the main form present in animal cells. Vitamin D3 is formed in the skin when exposed to ultraviolet light. Vitamin D is a steroid and works like a steroid hormone.

Vitamin D helps in mineralization of bones by regulating calcium and phosphorus absorption from the intestine, and preventing calcium loss into the urine. Deficiency of vitamin D can cause poor mineralization of bone, resulting in osteomalacia in adults and rickets in children.

The amount of vitamin D formed by the action of sunlight on the skin depends on the intensity of sunlight, length of sun exposure, and skin pigmentation. Weak sunlight due to air pollution or during winter may not provide the amount of light needed to form enough vitamin D in the skin. Food sources of vitamin D include animal foods like eggs, liver, butter, and fatty fish. Milk contains added vitamin D.

Symptoms of vitamin D toxicity include increased urination, frequent urination at night, weight loss, diarrhea, and nausea. Severe toxicity leads to calcification and hardening of the soft tissues in the blood vessels, heart, stomach, and kidneys.

Vitamin E

Vitamin E is an important antioxidant. Some studies show that vitamin E might protect against chronic conditions like heart disease, cancer, and cataracts, but other studies do not bear this out. Researchers are working to find out whether vitamin E is beneficial in the prevention of coronary artery disease or whether it has no effect. More research is needed before the answer becomes clear.

Vitamin E is needed for normal growth and helps in the intestinal absorption of unsaturated fatty acids. Most of the vitamin E in the blood is carried on lipoproteins, and any condition that affects levels of blood fat and cholesterol (lipids) also alters the amount of vitamin E in the blood.

Vitamin E is found in vegetable oils, nuts, seeds, and wheatgerms. The amount of vitamin E in the diet depends on the amount and kind of fat consumed. Vitamin E requirements increase with the intake of polyunsaturated fatty acids. Toxic effects of this vitamin are unknown.

Vitamin K

Vitamin K exists in two forms. Vitamin K1 is produced by green plants and vitamin K2 is produced by animals and also by the intestinal bacteria. Vitamin K is needed to make blood factors needed for normal clotting. Deficiency of vitamin K causes a delay in blood clotting. This vitamin also helps in growth.

Food sources of vitamin K are liver, cauliflower, spinach, and other green leafy vegetables. People who are taking blood thinners such as warfarin (Coumadin) need to be careful to limit their intake of vitamin K because it interferes with the effect of the blood thinners. A deficiency of vitamin K can be produced by the elimination of dietary sources or by prolonged treatment with antibiotic, which kills the intestinal bacteria.

WATER-SOLUBLE VITAMINS

Water-soluble vitamins will dissolve in water and any extra amount more than the body needs is excreted in the urine. These vitamins are obtained from the daily diet and are not stored in the body.

Vitamin C

Vitamin C (ascorbic acid) is involved in the formation of collagen. Collagen helps to maintain body structure. Collagen is found in cartilage, bone, teeth, and the lining of blood vessels. Vitamin C is important in wound healing and helps the body respond to stress, injury, and infection.

Vitamin C helps convert folic acid to the active form folinic acid, is used in the synthesis of steroid hormones from cholesterol, in the release of iron for transport in the body, and in the conversion of ferric iron to ferrous iron in the gastrointestinal tract. Vitamin C is also a powerful antioxidant.

Vitamin C is present in fresh, frozen, or raw fruits and vegetables. Dairy products are poor sources of vitamin C. Prolonged cooking at high temperature destroys vitamin C. To retain vitamin C in cooked foods, cooking should be done with the minimum amount of water for the shortest possible period of time in a covered pot. Steaming of fruits and vegetables helps to retain vitamin C.

Thiamine

Thiamine functions as a coenzyme in the breakdown of carbohydrates. It regulates muscle tone of the gastrointestinal tract and the heart. It is essential for normal functioning of nerves.

Deficiency of thiamine results in a disease called beriberi. Nerve, heart, and brain damage occur in beriberi. The nerve damage causes numbness and tingling of the legs and wasting and weakness of the muscles of the extremities. Mental depression may occur. Chronic alcoholism can lead to thiamine deficiency, which results in a disease called Wernicke's syndrome. The symptoms of Wernicke's syndrome include confusion, abnormalities of muscle movement, and problems moving the eyes.

Some sources of thiamine include lean pork, organ meats, wheatgerm, whole grains, dried beans, nuts, seeds, enriched flour, and brewer's yeast.

Riboflavin

Riboflavin is a yellow pigment with green fluorescence. This vitamin is used in the conversion of vitamin B6 and folate to their active forms. It is involved in several metabolic reactions. A deficiency of riboflavin leads to cracks in the skin at the corners of the mouth (cheilitis or angular stomatitis). The tongue may develop a magenta hue because of inflammation (glossitis). Changes in the eyes include eye inflammation, invasion of the cornea by blood vessels, and eye pain in bright light. Inadequate dietary intake and chronic alcoholism can cause riboflavin deficiency.

Good sources of riboflavin are milk, meat, fish, poultry, and whole-grain or enriched cereal and cereal products. Riboflavin is relatively insoluble and therefore it is not lost by the usual cooking methods.

Niacin

Niacin occurs as nicotinic acid in plants and nicotinamide in animal tissues (this is not the same as nicotine which is found in tobacco). Niacin is an important component of coenzymes I and II, and plays an important role in cellular respiration. It is also involved in the metabolism of proteins, fats, and carbohydrates. The precursor of niacin is tryptophan, which is also one of the essential amino acids found in protein. Therefore, a diet deficient in protein can also cause niacin deficiency.

Deficiency of niacin leads to a condition called pellagra. This is also called the disease of the three Ds: dermatitis (skin inflammation), diarrhea, and dementia. Niacin deficiency may occur in chronic alcoholism and gastrointestinal disorders.

Niacin has the ability to reduce serum lipids (blood fats and cholesterol) and decrease the release of fatty acids from fat tissues. Niacin is sometimes prescribed in large amounts to lower cholesterol levels. At these high doses, niacin can cause side effects in some people such as flushing or liver problems. Proteins from animal foods are the richest sources of niacin. Most vegetables contain about 1% tryptophan and are a moderately good source of niacin.

Folic acid

This is also known as folacin or folate. Folic acid is involved in the synthesis of choline, DNA, RNA, and amino acids. Folic acid along with vitamin B12 is important in the production of red blood cells in the bone marrow. Severe folic acid deficiency causes a type of anemia in which large immature red blood cells are released into the bloodstream.

Intestinal bacteria synthesize folic acid. The richest sources of folic acid are liver, asparagus, spinach, wheat, yeast, and dried beans. Dark green leafy vegetables are also good sources of this vitamin.

Vitamins

Mild folic acid deficiency has been linked to birth defects in the brain and spinal cord (anencephaly and spina bifida). To prevent these birth defects, women who may become pregnant should take at least 0.4 mg (400 μg) of folic acid daily. This amount is contained in most adult multivitamins. Women who previously had an affected child or who have spina bifida themselves should take 4,000 mg (4 g) daily, under the supervision of their doctor.

Vitamin B12 (cobalamin)

Vitamin B12 is used in the synthesis of DNA and RNA. It is necessary for the synthesis of the myelin sheath that encases nerve fibers. It is also involved in the metabolism of carbohydrates and fats and in the development of mature red blood cells. Like folic acid deficiency, deficiency of vitamin B12 results in a type of anemia in which large immature red blood cells are released into the bloodstream. It can also cause nerve damage, impaired cell division, and altered protein synthesis.

Vitamin B6

Vitamin B6 occurs naturally in three forms: pyridoxine, pyridoxal, and pyridoxamine. Vitamin B6 is essential for the conversion of tryptophan to niacin, the breakdown of glycogen to glucose, the metabolism of unsaturated fatty acids, synthesis of antibodies, and formation of neurotransmitters in the brain from amino acids. Vitamin B6 deficiency causes seborrheic dermatitis, glossitis (inflamed magenta-colored tongue), cheilitis (cracks in the corners of the mouth), nerve damage, and blood disorders. Fish, poultry, meats, walnuts, peanuts, wheatgerm, and brown rice are good sources of vitamin B6.

Biotin

Biotin is a sulfur-containing vitamin. As a component of many enzymes, biotin is involved in carbohydrate and fat metabolism. It is also involved in the breakdown of some amino acids. It is vital to growth and maintenance of skin, hair, nerves, and bone marrow. Biotin is widely distributed in foods. Liver and yeast are the richest sources, but nuts, meats, and seafood are also good sources of biotin.

Pantothenic acid

The term pantothenic acid is derived from the Greek word *pantothene* meaning "everywhere." It is widely distributed in plants and animals. Pantothenic acid has a vital role in the metabolism of carbohydrates, proteins, and fats for energy. It is involved in the release of energy and the synthesis of fatty acids, steroids, cholesterol, acetylcholine, and the porphyrin ring of the hemoglobin molecule.

Kidney, liver, eggs, yeast, wheatgerm, and dried peas are the richest sources of this vitamin. Pantothenic acid is widely distributed in many types of foods.

SEE ALSO: Diet, Nutrition, Prenatal care

Suggested Reading

Chan, A. C. (1998). Vitamin E and atherosclerosis. *Journal of Nutrition, 128*(10), 1593–1596.

Combs, G. F. (1998). *The vitamins: Fundamental aspects in nutrition and health* (2nd ed.). San Diego, CA: Academic Press.

DeLuca, H. F. (1982). New developments in the vitamin D endocrine system. *Journal of the American Dietetic Association, 80*(3), 231–237.

Farrington, K., Miller, P., Varghese, Z., Baillod, R. A., & Moorhead, J. F. (1981). Vitamin A toxicity and hypercalcaemia in chronic renal failure. *British Medical Journal Clinical Research Edition, 282*(6281), 1999–2002.

Institute of Medicine, Food and Nutrition Board. (1998). *Dietary reference intakes for thiamin, riboflavin, niacin, vitamin B-6, folate, vitamin B-12, pantothenic acid, biotin, and cholin.* Washington DC: National Academy Press.

Shils, M. E., et al. (Eds.). (1999). *Modern nutrition in health and disease* (9th ed.). Baltimore: Williams & Wilkins.

RAJKUMARI RICHMONDS

Weight Control   Maintaining a healthy weight is just one part of a healthy lifestyle. Being either overweight or underweight can be unhealthy, and many people who are not obese are interested in maintaining a healthy weight. Often, overweight or obese people are also interested in maintaining their weight.

Many people find that they can lose weight to a certain point, and then find it increasingly difficult to lose more weight or keep the weight off. The body seems to have a "set point," below which the body acts as though it were starving: metabolism slows, appetite increases, and weight loss may seem impossible. The set point is not always the same as the ideal body weight. Sometimes the set point is at a weight considered obese. In 1995, researchers discovered the hormone leptin. When leptin was given to leptin-deficient obese mice, they returned to a normal weight. Unfortunately, leptin is not useful in treating human obesity. Very few obese humans are leptin-deficient: Most obese people actually make lots of leptin in their fat cells. There are probably other regulatory hormones that govern the set point which have not been discovered yet.

When diet and exercise do not lead to dramatic weight loss, a better strategy may be to maintain a realistic weight. Continued efforts at dieting may contribute to poor self-image, nutritional deficiencies, or eating disorders. The goal of being "healthy at any weight" involves deciding on a realistic, maintainable weight and choosing healthy diet and exercise habits to maintain that weight. Healthy lifestyle habits can lead to an improved energy level, a more positive emotional outlook, and a positive body image based on staying active and enjoying life.

According to the National Institute of Diabetes and Digestive and Kidney Diseases, adults should adopt the following healthy habits in order to maintain their weight. (a) Eat breakfast every day. People who eat breakfast are less likely to overeat later in the day. (b) Choose whole grains more often. Try whole-wheat breads and pastas, oatmeal, brown rice, or bulgur. (c) Select a mix of colorful vegetables each day. Different colored vegetables provide different nutrients. (d) Have low-fat, low-sugar snacks on hand at home, at work, or on the go, to combat hunger and prevent overeating. (e) Eat three meals every day instead of skipping meals or eating a snack instead of a meal. (f) Drink plenty of water. Aim for about eight 8-ounce glasses each day. (g) At restaurants, eat only half your meal and take the rest home. (h) Visit museums, the zoo, or an aquarium. You and your family will walk for hours and not realize it. (i) Take a walk after dinner instead of watching TV. (j) Get plenty of sleep.

Children should drink water or low-fat milk more often than sugary sodas or juices. Involving children in meal preparation may increase their interest in eating what is served. Pregnant women should eat high-fiber foods and drink plenty of water to avoid constipation. They should also eat foods rich in folate, iron, calcium, and protein, or get these nutrients through a prenatal supplement. Remaining active is important during pregnancy, but certain activities such as contact sports may be dangerous. Pregnant women should discuss their physical activities with their health care provider.

Older adults should emphasize high-fiber foods like whole-grain breads and cereals, beans, vegetables, and fruits, especially if they are prone to constipation. To prevent osteoporosis and maintain an active lifestyle, older adults should consume at least three servings of low-fat milk, yogurt, or cheese a day, or take a calcium and vitamin D supplement. Although older adults often feel less thirsty, adequate water intake is still important. Physical activity should be part of each day's activities. Several short walks throughout the day can be enough to help seniors stay healthy and active. Older people sometimes become socially isolated, and staying connected with family, friends, and community can help maintain physical activities as well as maintaining emotional health.

SEE ALSO: Body mass index, Diet, Exercise, Nutrition, Obesity, Sports

Suggested Reading

Levine, J. A., & Bine, L. (2001). *Helping your child lose weight the healthy way: A family approach to weight control.* New York: Citadel Press.

Jonas, S., & Konner, L. (1997). *Just the weigh you are: how to be fit and healthy, whatever your size.* Shelburne, VT: Chapters Publishing.

Suggested Resources

Centers for Disease Control and Prevention, National Center for Chronic Disease Prevention and Health Promotion: Nutrition and physical activity website: www.cdc.gov/nccdphp/dnpa/recommendations.htm

National Institutes of Health/National Institute of Diabetes and Digestive and Kidney Diseases: Weight loss and control web site: www.niddk.nih.gov/health/nutrit/nutrit.htm

ALICIA M. WEISSMAN

Witchcraft *see* Mental Illness, Shamans

Woman's Medical College of Pennsylvania

Woman's Medical College of Pennsylvania (WMC), widely but erroneously called "Women's," was founded as The Female Medical College of Pennsylvania in Philadelphia in 1850, and renamed in 1867. With the support of Philadelphia-area Quaker physicians and businessman–philanthropist William J. Mullen, the College was incorporated, in the era of reform movements for women's rights, improved health care, and the abolition of slavery, for the purpose of instructing females in the science and art of medicine. Prominent Quaker activist of the time, Lucretia Mott, advocating for educational opportunities to enable women to participate equally in compassionate works of social reform, stated that a mind has no sex. Women were still virtually excluded from medical education, and WMC provided an environment free of male domination in which women could study and practice medicine with other women, while it promoted the health of women and their children through education and clinical care.

As at other medical schools of the era, 2 years of study with a preceptor and the ability to write literary English were required for admission. The first curriculum included lectures and dissection, with students attending lectures for about 5 months in the fall and winter. Clinical experience was provided initially at the Woman's Hospital of Philadelphia, founded by Quaker women including Ann Preston, a member of the College's first class and later dean of the College. The financial hardship of the early years was to become an enduring problem.

Although the founding board of directors and the first faculty were composed entirely of men, the women of the Medical College were not readily accepted into mainstream (male) Philadelphia medicine. The Philadelphia County Medical Society held that women were unfit for the practice of medicine, and enjoined its members from professional dealings with college professors or graduates. Graduation of the first class of eight students was held with the attendance of fifty police officers to maintain order.

In 1875, the College moved into the first building designed for its own use, and initiated a period of growth, which included its being among the first medical schools in the United States to require a 4-year curriculum. Botanist and chemist Rachel Bodley (dean from 1874 to 1888) promoted the entry of women into medical missionary work, which became a tradition at the College and contributed to its reputation abroad. Anna Broomall (WMC graduate and professor) established an outpatient maternity service for senior students who provided maternity care to poor women of South Philadelphia and emphasized prenatal care. Clara Marshall (WMC graduate and dean from 1888 to 1917) expanded resources for clinical training, overseeing establishment of a hospital adjacent to the College. WMC established its tradition of providing a door of opportunity for women students from diverse backgrounds, including a freed slave, and students from Japan, India, and Syria.

Despite the acceptance, in the early 1900s, of a few women at previously all-male medical schools, WMC continued to provide a professional home for women faculty and students, while it adapted to educational reforms mandated by the 1910 Report for the Advancement of Teaching (the "Flexner Report") to the Carnegie Foundation. By 1921, of the 19 medical schools begun for women, only WMC remained. Despite struggling to maintain its enrollment, in 1930, the College moved to a site in the East Falls section of Philadelphia, which continues to house clinical, research, and hospital space. The College strengthened its research program, providing a receptive environment for women scientists such as WMC graduate Catharine Macfarlane, a gynecologist whose research confirmed the value of periodic examinations in cancer detection, and biochemist-physiologist Phyllis Bott, whose "micropuncture" technique elucidated kidney function. The 1960s brought the ironic necessity of coeducation, required by government mandates for equal educational opportunities. WMC was renamed Medical College of Pennsylvania (MCP), and men were first awarded the MD degree in 1972.

Financial pressure in the era of managed care precipitated the merger in 1993 of MCP with Hahnemann University in Philadelphia, to form "MCP Hahnemann School of Medicine." In 1998, the merged medical school was placed under the management of Drexel University in Philadelphia; Drexel University College of Medicine, in the tradition of WMC of Pennsylvania and Hahnemann Medical College, preserves the goals of the original school at the Institute for Women's Health and Leadership.

The special contribution of the female sensibility to the practice of medicine is described by graduate Rosalie Slaughter-Morton in the inscription on the College's 1916 bas relief "The Woman Physician," by Clara Hill:

> DAUGHTER OF SCIENCE—PIONEER, THY TENDERNESS HATH BANISHED FEAR; WOMAN AND LEADER IN THEE BLEND, PHYSICIAN, SURGEON, STUDENT—FRIEND.

SEE ALSO: Blackwell, Elizabeth; Education; Feminism; Gender role; Healers; Physicians

Suggested Reading

Morantz-Sanchez, R. (1985). *Sympathy and science: Women physicians in American medicine.* Oxford: Oxford University Press.
Peitzman, S. J. (2000). *A new and untried course: Woman's Medical College and Medical College of Pennsylvania 1850–1998.* New Brunswick, NJ: Rutgers University Press.

Suggested Resources

MCP archives and special collections of women in medicine. Drexel University College of Medicine Archives and Special Collections, Drexel University College of Medicine Conference Center, Philadelphia. http://med.library.drexel.edu/archives

LAURENTINE FROMM
STEVEN J. PEITZMAN

Women's Health Initiative

The National Institutes of Health (NIH) in 1990 established the U.S. Office of Research on Women's Health. In 1991, this office launched its first national study on women's health called the Women's Health Initiative. The Women's Health Initiative was initiated because there had been insufficient medical research relating to women's health. Such research is critical because many diseases are unique to women and, therefore, treatments designed specifically for women are needed. Over $625 million was allocated to conduct this 15-year study on health issues affecting postmenopausal women between the ages of 50 and 79 years. The recommended research focus consisted of the study of (a) health disparities between men and women; (b) health issues affecting postmenopausal women for whom few data are available; and (c) health issues affecting women of differing social, economic, and ethnic backgrounds.

The Women's Health Initiative has a tripartite agenda: (a) Clinical Trials, (b) Observational Studies, and (c) the Community Prevention Study. Together, the NIH and the National Heart, Lung, and Blood Institute conduct the Clinical Trials and the Observational Studies. The Community Prevention Study was carried out by the Centers for Disease Control and Prevention (CDC). The Women's Health Initiative was designed to focus on breast cancer, colon cancer, rectal cancer, osteoporosis, and heart disease. These diseases are responsible for most of the deaths, disabilities, and the decreased quality of life among postmenopausal women.

Osteoporosis was selected because one out of every six women suffers from hip fractures, and hip fractures occur four times more often in women than in men. As a result, it is a more frequent risk for women than cancer. Second, heart disease is currently the leading cause of death in women. As many as 240,000 women suffer heart attacks due to heart disease. Third, breast cancer kills more than 46,000 women per year, ranking second in cancer deaths among women.

Furthermore, over 183,000 cases of breast cancer are diagnosed each year. Fourth, colon and/or rectal cancers kill over 28,000 women each year. Each year 51,000 cases of colon cancer and 16,500 cases of rectal cancer are diagnosed in women. Colon cancer ranks third in cancer deaths among women.

The Clinical Trials involve over 68,000 women who will be studied for 9 years. The major studies under way include Dietary Modification, Calcium/Vitamin D Supplementation, and Hormone Replacement Therapy. The Dietary Modification trial focuses on the impact that high fiber, fruit, vegetable, and low-fat intake have on the prevention of cancers and heart disease. The Calcium/Vitamin D Supplement trial focuses on the impact the supplements have on reducing the risk of osteoporosis, hip fractures, and colon and rectal cancer. The Hormone Replacement Therapy trial focuses on the impact estrogen supplements have on reducing the risk of osteoporosis and colon cancer (terminated in 2002). These trials are being conducted across the nation at 40 clinical centers where women were recruited between 1993 and 1998.

The Observational Study tracks the lifestyles and health of over 100,000 women for 8–12 years. The study focuses on the impact exercise and healthy behaviors have on disease prevention. The last recruitment phase for this study was in 1998.

The Community Prevention Study followed 64,500 women from all social, economic, and ethnic backgrounds. For 5 years this Study was carried out at eight university-based prevention centers. The purpose of the Community Prevention Study was to identify the best local programs that lead to healthy lifestyles among women over the age of 40. Healthy programs such as diet, exercise, smoking cessation, vitamin supplements, mammogram checkups, education, and outreach were evaluated to identify the most effective practices.

Today, the Women's Health Initiative is still being conducted. However, while still in Clinical Trials, the Hormone Replacement Therapy trial was abruptly terminated. In 2002, the U.S. Food and Drug Administration (FDA) stopped the trial because the research data indicated that the health risks were beginning to outweigh the benefits. An increased incidence of breast cancer, heart attack, stroke, and blood clots in the legs and arms among healthy women outweighed the benefits gained due to reductions in hip fractures and colon cancers. Since these findings were based on women using hormone replacement therapy for more than 3 years, women considering its use for

shorter periods of time can still gain some benefits. Therefore, the FDA strongly encourages women to consult their physicians for medical advice.

In conclusion, the Women's Health Initiative is the first major step toward increasing the medical data on women available to doctors and researchers. This information will help the development of new treatments for heart disease, breast cancer, osteoporosis, and colon and rectal cancer. Although the Hormone Replacement Therapy trial was stopped, much has been learned about the role of estrogen supplements as a treatment for women. Furthermore, the information from the Observational and Community Prevention studies will help our communities promote healthy practices that are effective in disease prevention and improving the quality of life for women.

SEE ALSO: Cancer, Clinical trials, Coronary risk factors, Hormone replacement therapy, Osteoporosis and osteopenia, Quality of life, Vitamins

Suggested Reading

Bowden, D. J., Hunt, J. R., Kaplan, R. M., Klesges, R. C., Langer, R. D., Mathews, K. A., et al. (1997). Women's Health Initiative. Why now? What is it? What's new? *American Psychologist, 52,* 101–116.

Clifford, C., Finnegan, L. P., Harlan, W. R., McGowan, J. A., Pinn, V. W., & Rossouw, J. E. (1995). The evolution of the Women's Health Initiative: Perspective from the NIH. *Journal of the American Medical Women's Association, 50,* 50–55.

Hamdy, R. C. (2002). Lessons learned from the Women's Health Initiative study. *Southern Medical Journal, 95*(9), 951–965.

Liu, J. (1998). The Women's Health Initiative: Goals, rationale, and current status. *Menopausal Medicine, 6*(2), 1–4.

Suggested Resources

Food and Drug Administration. (2003). FDA statement on the results of the Women's Health Initiative. Retrieved August 13, 2002, from http://www.fda.gov/cder/drug/safety/WHI_statement.html

National Heart, Lung, and Blood Institute. (2003). Women's Health Initiative. Retrieved February 19, 2002, from http://www.nhlbi.nih.gov/whi/references.html

ELIZABETH M. VALENCIA

Wrinkles Human skin, like all other organs of the body, undergoes changes with aging. In addition to intrinsic or chronologic changes, environmental exposure can be a major cause of skin damage and wrinkling.

Over time, the skin's network of elastin and collagen fibers which provide elasticity to the skin is altered. The thickness of the skin (epidermis and dermis) and the underlying layer of fat decreases. There is a decrease in the number of pigment-forming cells, immune cells, and blood vessels. Superficial skin lines form due to repetitive contractions of the small muscles of the face. These universal and presumably inevitable changes in the skin along with the exacerbating factor of gravity lead to wrinkling and sagging of the skin.

Ultraviolet light emanating from sunlight also plays a major role in causing wrinkles in exposed skin. Unlike intrinsic aging, which depends on the passage of time, damage due to ultraviolet light, or photoaging, depends primarily on the degree of lifetime sun exposure and skin pigment. Individuals who have outdoor lifestyles, live in sunny climates, and are lightly pigmented will experience the greatest degree of photoaging. In photodamaged skin there is an abundance of deranged elastic tissue and disorganized collagen, blood vessels are dilated, and immune cells are decreased. Research has shown that the overproduction of oxidants or free radicals is a crucial factor in causing such changes. These unstable molecules are normally produced by chemical metabolism in the body; however, with environmental assaults, they are produced in excessive amounts that can damage cellular and even genetic elements. Cigarette smoke and air pollutants such as ozone are other environmental factors that may promote wrinkles by increasing production of free radicals.

An abundance of antiaging therapies are available to women today. The most widely available of these are antiaging or antiwrinkle creams. The choice of creams depends on many factors, but the consumer is cautioned to consider whether the efficacy of the cream has been proven and documented in scientific, peer-reviewed journals. Many creams are not classified as drugs and are therefore not held to the rigorous standards of documenting efficacy. Currently, retinoic acid, a natural form of vitamin A, is the only cream approved by the FDA as safe and effective for treating some signs of photoaging. Alpha hydroxy acids have also shown considerable evidence in laboratory studies in reversing effects of the sun.

Professional treatments for wrinkles include chemical peels, implants, dermabrasion, laser resurfacing, botulinum toxin injections, and plastic surgery. The choice of treatment is highly individualized and is dependent on the person's age, degree of photoaging, and chronologic aging among other factors. For example, fine wrinkling and textural changes commonly seen with photoaging may be best treated with chemical peels or laser resurfacing. In contrast, lines caused by facial expression and movement of the muscles of the face (frown lines) may be best treated with botulinum toxin injections or implants. In addition to the above treatments, prevention remains the easiest means of decreasing wrinkles. Recommendations include avoidance of excessive sun exposure, sunscreen use, and smoking cessation.

SEE ALSO: Environment, Liver spots, Skin care, Skin disorders, Smoking, Vitamins

Suggested Reading

Pinnell, S. R. (2003). Cutaneous photodamage, oxidative stress, and topical antioxidant protection. *Journal of the American Academy of Dermatology, 48*, 1–19.

Yaar, M., & Gilchrest, B. A. (1999). Aging of skin. In I. M. Freedberg, A. Eisen, K. Wolff, et al. (Eds.), *Dermatology in general medicine* (5th ed., pp. 1697–1706). New York: McGraw-Hill.

Suggested Resources

American Academy of Dermatology. www.aad.org

PARADI MIRMIRANI

Yeast Infection

Yeast vaginitis (candidiasis) is an infection or inflammation of the vagina caused by a fungus, usually the yeast-like fungus *Candida albicans (C. albicans)*. It is the second most common type of vaginal infection. It is estimated that approximately 75% of all women in the United States will have a yeast infection at least once in their lifetime. Therefore, it is important for women to be aware of this condition.

It is believed that the *Candida* may live in small amounts in the healthy vagina. The predominant organism of the vagina is lactobacillus. The presence of lactobacillus helps in the maintenance of the normal vaginal pH of 4.5 or less. Any condition that alters or disturbs the vaginal flora, or this normal pH balance, can promote multiplication of other organisms including *C. albicans*, resulting in infection. Conditions that increase the risk for yeast infection are pregnancy, obesity, diabetes mellitus, the use of some drugs such as corticosteroids, broad-spectrum antibiotics, oral contraceptives, or high-carbohydrate diets. In addition, douching, hot weather along with the use of tight-fitting clothes, or nonabsorbent underwear can contribute as well. Women who are immunocompromised (such as patients with HIV or those receiving chemotherapy) are also at increased risk for yeast infection.

The severity of symptoms varies among women, but patients with vulvovaginal candidiasis usually present with a white, curd-like, cheesy vaginal discharge which adheres to the vaginal wall, intense vulvovaginal pruritus and erythema (swollen, red, itchy, tender labia), a burning sensation following urination, and pain during sexual intercourse (dyspareunia). For most women, the major system is vaginal itching. The discharge of a yeast infection is not malodorous. Diagnosis is usually made by presenting symptoms, physical examination, and by the presence of pseudohyphae with yeast buds on wet mount using potassium hydroxide (KOH).

Treatment may be prescribed as topical or oral antifungals. Topical antifungals are usually in the form of vaginal tablets, creams, or suppositories. An oral antifungal commonly used is fluconazole (Diflucan), which may be given in a single dose. Topical agents include butoconazole (Femstat), clotrimazole (Gyne-Lotrimin), miconazole (Monistat), tiaconazole (Vagistat), and terconazole (Terazol). Clotrimazole and miconazole (Monistat) are over-the-counter agents. Topical antifungal treatment may be used as 1-, 3-, 5-, 7-, or 14-day regimens. Women with recurrent yeast infection, defined as more than four episodes in 1 year, may be put on suppressive therapy with oral ketoconazole 100 mg daily for up to 6 months.

Preventive measures include keeping the genital area clean; avoiding the use of douches, vaginal deodorants, and tight-fitting and nonabsorbent undergarments. Nylon underwear should be replaced by cotton alternatives. Under circumstances where antibiotic use is necessary, the health care provider may offer concurrent antifungal prophylaxis. Discontinuing oral contraceptives or other hormones may be necessary in some patients to control the recurrence of infection. The health care provider may recommend good diabetic control and weight loss in the very overweight patient. Dietary modification, such as the use of acidophilus-based products and limited simple sugars and carbohydrates, may also be recommended.

SEE ALSO: Diabetes, Pregnancy, Sexual organs

Suggested Reading

DeCherney, A. H., & Lauren, N. (2003). Current obstetrics and gynecologic diagnosis and treatment. *Benign disorders of the vulva and vagina* (9th ed., pp. 652–653). New York: McGraw-Hill.

Tierney, L. M., McPhee, S. J., & Papadakis, M. A. (2003). Current medical diagnosis and treatment. *Gynecology* (42nd ed., p. 703). New York: McGraw-Hill.

JOYCE HYATT

Yoga The meaning of the word yoga may be defined as yolking, union, or a bringing together of the mind, body, and soul; the bridging and forming a relationship with oneself and with ultimately how one lives in harmony with the world. The practice of yoga brings with it strength to the body, relaxation to the mind, and renewal to the spirit.

Yoga was developed in India approximately 5,000 years ago. It has been practiced as a way to achieve health and wellness for thousands of years. Some people start to do yoga for its physical benefits. Others are aware of its benefits in assisting in the reduction of stress and tension. With the proper instruction, yoga may be used therapeutically to help heal problems that arise from acute or chronic injuries or genetic predisposition in the structure and function of the body.

Yoga offers a way to slow down and breathe and to be present in the moment and to bring awareness to the body. In the experience of stretching, breathing, and relaxation, the flow of life returns. For many students, yoga enables one to flow through the day as against reacting to it, and feel more present in their daily activities with less stress.

WHAT IS YOGA?

If you ask most Westerners this question, most will reply that yoga is a form of exercise. Yoga actually encompasses many aspects of life. They are postures (*asanas*) for the exercise to strengthen, balance, and increase the flexibility of the body from an anatomical aspect. They have benefit not only to the muscles but also to organ, structural, and hormonal systems. Other practices of yoga include meditation and *pranayama* (breath control), the study of texts, guidelines on how to treat your body, and ways to behave toward others as well as the letting go of attachment to material possessions and suggestions for diet.

HATHA YOGA

Hatha yoga is the most common type of yoga practiced in the United States. It is a physical path of yoga focusing on the use of asanas to receive benefits to the body. The different types of yoga teaching styles taught are generally related to the teacher who developed the type of posture sequence or the place in India from which the particular sequence or practice of yoga originated. There are styles of practice and adaptations to fit almost any fitness level and constitution. "Hatha" literally means sun and moon. It may be thought of as the union of opposites and refers to the powerful balancing aspects of doing asanas. A few of the hatha yoga teaching styles include Viniyoga, Ashtanga yoga, Power yoga, Iyengar yoga, Bikram or Hot yoga, Sivananda yoga, and Kundalini yoga.

ASANAS

Asanas are the postures of yoga. Each posture has benefits to the body. Standing postures are grounding in nature and help to build confidence as well as strength and bring focus to the mind. Most postures in which the body moves forward relax the mind and help to reduce stress. Twists encourage detoxification resetting of the internal organs. Inversions reverse the force of gravity; they help to undo the effects of the downward pull of gravity and aid in digestion as well as decreasing the effects of aging. Postures which lift the heart bring energy to the body and hope to the mind. Consult with your health care provider as to your abilities to begin a practice of yoga. Initial practice of Asanas (postures) should be performed under the supervision of a qualified yoga instructor. A qualified instructor will be able to assist you in choosing Asanas suited to your particular needs. They also will guide you in the safest and best practices for performing each Asana. It is important to keep in mind that yoga is a practice and a process rather than a goal to be achieved.

CHOOSING AN INSTRUCTOR

The following guidelines may prove helpful in choosing a yoga instructor:

1. If you would not choose the person as a friend, chances are you will not enjoy him or her as an instructor.
2. Find someone whose teaching methods complement your learning style.
3. An instructor should work with you as an individual, addressing any issues that arise due to past injuries or particular problems surrounding flexibility or genetic predisposition.
4. The best yoga experiences result from a willingness of the instructor and student to cocreate an environment that is conducive to learning.

SEE ALSO: Complementary and alternative health practices, Meditation, Physical therapy

Suggested Reading

Fraser, T. (2001). *Total yoga: A step-by step guide to yoga at home for everybody.* London: Thorsons.
Iyengar, B. K. S. (2001). *Yoga: The path to holistic health.* New York: Dorling Kindersley.
Kraftsow, G. (1999). *Yoga for wellness, healing with the timeless teachings of viniyoga.* New York: Penguin Putnam.

Suggested Resources

http://www.yogasite.com
http://www.yoga411.com
http://www.yogaalliance.org
http://yogajournal.com

LaGenia Bailey

Youth   Middle childhood is a time of discovery, consolidation, and strengthening of key competencies. During this period of development, ranging between ages 6 and 12 years, physical skills mature, personality traits solidify, and social interactions become more sophisticated. Parents remain at the center of children's social world, but peers become increasingly important. Although biology provides a timetable for development, cultural and contextual factors can slow, nurture, or hinder growth. Thus, developmental shifts during childhood are best understood within a broad social context that includes individual factors as well as family, peers, neighborhoods, and culture.

STATUS OF CHILDREN

In his 2002 State of the Union address, George W. Bush adopted the Children's Defense Fund policy to "Leave No Child Behind." Unfortunately, 2 years later, very little has improved in the lives of American children. Every 11 seconds, an American child is reportedly abused or neglected, and every 2 hours and 40 minutes, an American child is killed by gunfire. One in five U.S. children live in poverty and substandard conditions (e.g., unsanitary housing, poor nutrition) during their first 3 years of life, the most critical time for brain development. Children in poverty are more likely to contract illnesses, have untreated medical and dental problems, and are less likely to receive important immunizations. One in eight American children do not have health insurance, and a majority of our nation's fourth graders cannot read and do math proficiently. Nearly 12 million American children are poor, 1.2 million are homeless on any given night, and 7 million are home alone or without adult supervision after school. Child homelessness is increasing as the rates of adult unemployment surge. These conditions place youth at high risk for serious mental health, behavioral, and physical problems and have important implications for children's intellectual and emotional development.

CHILD DEVELOPMENT IN CONTEXT

Physical Development

Whereas adolescence precipitates enormous changes in physical development (see entry Adolescence in this volume), middle childhood represents slow but regular change. Girls and boys appear similar in weight and height during childhood, although girls begin to mature before boys. There is wide variation in height and weight during this period, but the brain is virtually fully developed. Losing baby teeth is a significant developmental milestone. As their bodies grow in strength and size, children develop better balance and coordination and new motor skills. Research indicates that physical acuity develops at similar rates among boys and girls during middle childhood, but boys begin to excel girls during adolescence.

Cognitive Development

Jean Piaget studied children's mental processes, including their ways of perceiving, remembering, believing, and reasoning. Piaget observed that children progress through a series of stages in their ability to process mental phenomenon. Children between 6 and 12 years of age begin to use symbols (mental images, words, gestures) in sophisticated ways to represent objects and events. For example, they are able to perform mental operations (e.g., simple math), but have difficulty anticipating or considering alternatives. Children at this age can experiment with an idea, observe the results, and then experiment again until they get it right. They can classify objects according to a characteristic like size or color, and they develop skills of conservation or the knowledge that objects or amounts remain the same even if their physical appearance is rearranged. By age 7, children's language becomes less egocentric and more socialized. Children begin to use communication to exchange information and engage in conversation. Their use of communication reflects concern for the listener's needs by considering intentions rather than merely external stimuli.

It is widely recognized that cognitive functioning is influenced by many factors, including individual differences, culture, and the context in which children live. This is perhaps best understood in the study of social cognition, or the ways children understand, interpret, and respond to their social worlds. The social context and life experiences vary among children, and recent research has determined that youth process information differently and respond uniquely to external stimuli. For example, aggressive children have been found to interpret ambiguous social cues in a hostile manner and thereby react aggressively, whereas nonaggressive children tend to have more benign reactions to such situations. Thus, cognitive development is a multidimensional and complex process that depends on social environment, unique predispositions, and life experiences.

Socioemotional Development

Children's socioemotional development has been the subject of considerable discussion and theoretical writing. Individually centered theories propose that a child's personality develops through the resolution of crises or issues at different developmental stages. As the child confronts and masters the crisis, he or she is able to move to the next developmental stage. By all accounts, school is a central influence during middle childhood. Social interactions increasingly revolve around classmates and peers, even though parents continue to be a critical force in children's development. The ability to function in school is one of the major factors that determine youths' quality of life.

Some models of personality development are based on Western values and support increased autonomy and separation from the family as markers of successful personality growth. These may not apply to children from diverse cultural backgrounds. Contextual models, on the other hand, suggest that personality is shaped by individual temperament as well as interactions with parents, peers, schools, communities, culture, and society. The latter theories underscore the importance of interpersonal factors and contextual influences (e.g., exposure to crime and poverty, media messages, cultural beliefs) on personality development. Compared to youth further along the developmental continuum, younger children are in the unique position of discovering their world according to restrictions set by their caregivers. Unlike adolescents, children make few independent decisions. They are unable to function alone in the larger society because their abilities to understand and interpret information are not yet fully developed. In this way, parents serve as "gatekeepers" assuming responsibility for shaping the interactions and experiences of their children according to their own biases, culture, social status, and perceptions. Taken together, these experiences lay the foundation for future development.

Moral Development

Theories of moral development have evolved over the years. Jean Piaget proposed that morality developed through a sequence of invariant stages according to children's cognitive abilities. He argued that earlier stages form the foundation for later ones, and for young children, rules are unalterable, must be obeyed, and are judged solely in terms of their consequences. As children

691

age, however, they are able to view rules more flexibly and understand that they are established and maintained through reciprocal social agreement. Children begin to recognize that intentions are an important factor when judging a behavior as right or wrong. Inspired by Piaget, Lawrence Kohlberg defined morality by an individual's sense of justice. Greater rationality and attention to the "law" was viewed as more advanced moral thinking. In 1982, Carol Gilligan challenged this definition of morality and argued that consideration of others and interpersonal relationships are important factors in moral decision-making. Gilligan observed that girls scored lower than boys on Kohlberg's stage theory, because they focused on maintaining relationships and caring about others when making moral judgments. Gilligan also noted that women's moral choices reflected a concern for the welfare of others, whereas men's moral imperative was to respect rights and protect the rights to life and self-fulfillment. She redefined morality as consisting of two parts, a "morality of care" and a "morality of justice." There has been considerable debate about gender differences in moral thinking, but it is likely that the most advanced moral decision-making combines a concern for others and attention to justice.

Risk and Resilience

Many factors influence children's developmental trajectories. Risk factors increase the possibility of maladjustment while protective factors prevent negative outcomes despite the presence of risk. Children are more vulnerable to certain risk factors at particular periods of development. For instance, peer pressure is more salient during adolescence than early childhood, and exposure to alcohol during the first trimester of pregnancy is more dangerous than exposure during the third trimester. As the number of risk factors increase, the likelihood of negative outcomes is greater (e.g., risky sexual behavior, crime, mental health problems). Despite exposure to risk factors, many children are resilient. Several protective factors predict childhood resilience in the face of risk, including greater intelligence and higher self-esteem; parental warmth, support, and firm control; the presence of a supportive adult; value on achievement; and strong community ties.

CONCLUSIONS AND RECOMMENDATIONS

Despite the Bush administration's assertion that no child should be left behind, the nation's children continue to experience considerable adversity including poverty, abuse and neglect, homelessness, absence of health insurance, exposure to crime and violence, and poor reading and math skills. U.S. children of color are disproportionately affected by poverty, low birthweight, early mortality, and the absence of prenatal care. These experiences strongly influence children's physical, cognitive, emotional, and social development, and determine successful passage into adulthood. Nonetheless, important initiatives have been implemented to improve the lives of young children and families, such as low-cost health clinics, early head start programs, and greater attention to important health issues like nutrition and obesity. Since 1973, the Children's Defense Fund (CDF) has successfully led the charge to educate the nation about the needs of children, identify important directions for prevention, and advocate for improved access to care. Through ongoing advocacy, research, and technological assistance, we will ensure that no child is left behind.

SEE ALSO: Adolescence, Peer relationships

Suggested Reading

Children's Defense Fund. (2003, July). Broken promises: How the Bush administration is failing. *America's Poorest Children*. Retrieved from http://www.childrensdefense.org/pdf/broken_promises.pdf

Erwin, P. (1993). *Friendship and peer relations in children*. New York: John Wiley & Sons.

Gilligan, C. (1982). *In a different voice: Psychological theory and women's development*. Cambridge, MA: Harvard University Press.

Miller, P. A. (1993). *Theories of developmental psychology*. New York: W.H. Freeman.

Singer, D. G., & Revenson, T. A. (1997). *A Piaget primer: How a child thinks*. Madison, WI: International Universities Press.

Sroufe, L. A. (1996). *Emotional development: The organization of emotional life in the early years*. Cambridge: Cambridge University Press.

Suggested Resources

Children's Defense Fund: http://www.childrensdefense.org/pdf/broken_promises.pdf

GERI R. DONENBERG

Contributors

Antonia Abbey, PhD, Department of Community Medicine, School of Medicine, Wayne State University, Detroit, Michigan

Sharon Abegg, MD, Olympia, Washington

Rony Adam, MD, Department of Gynecology and Obstetrics, Emory University, Atlanta, Georgia

Josephine Albritton, MD, Medical College of Georgia, Augusta, Georgia

Mohammed Alishahie, MD, Cleveland Clinic Foundation, Cleveland, Ohio

Teresa Trogdon Anderson, MD, MA, FAAP, Division of General Pediatrics, University of New Mexico Children's Hospital, Albuquerque, New Mexico

Mary Anthony, DO, Parma, Ohio

Pamela Arbuckle, DDS, HPP, Alameda County Medical Center, Department of Ambulatory Health Care Services, Oakland, California

Keith B. Armitage, MD, Department of Medicine, University Hospitals of Cleveland, Case Western Reserve University School of Medicine, Cleveland, Ohio

Karen L. Ashby, MD, University Hospitals of Cleveland, Cleveland, Ohio

Virginia E. Ayres, PhD, Lake City, Pennsylvania

LaGenia Bailey, PharmD, BCPP, RYT, Chicago, Illinois

Rachel M. Baker, MD, Department of Psychiatry, Case Western Reserve University, Cleveland, Ohio

C. Barve, Department of Psychiatry, Institute for Juvenile Research, Chicago, Illinois

Mohamed A. Bedaiwy, MD, Cleveland Clinic Foundation, Department of Obstetrics and Gynecology, Cleveland, Ohio

Gina Bell, MD, Rosalind Franklin University of Medicine and Science, North Chicago, Illinois

Bruce E. Berger, MD, Division of Nephrology, University Hospitals of Cleveland, Cleveland, Ohio

Janet Blanchard, MD, Lake Hospital Systems, Mentor, Ohio

Michael Bogenschutz, MD, Department of Psychiatry, Vice Chair, Addiction and Substance Abuse Program, University of New Mexico School of Medicine, Albuquerque, New Mexico

Denise Bothe, MD, Department of Pediatrics, Rainbow Babies and Children's Hospital, Cleveland, Ohio

Linda D. Bradley, MD, Director of Hysteroscopic Services, The Cleveland Clinic Foundation, Cleveland, Ohio

Contributors

David L. Bronson, MD, Cleveland Clinic Foundation, Cleveland, Ohio

Laurie G. Broutman, MD, Rosalind Franklin University of Medicine and Science, North Chicago, Illinois

Janet M. Burlingame, MD, Cleveland Clinic Foundation, Department of Obstetrics and Gynecology, Cleveland, Ohio

Kenneth D. Burman, MD, Endocrine Section, Washington Hospital Center, Washington, DC; Department of Medicine, Uniformed Services University of the Health Sciences, Bethesda, Maryland; and Department of Medicine, Georgetown and George Washington Universities, Washington, DC

Sandra J. Buzney, JD, MSW, Lowder and Hickman, Cleveland, Ohio.

Stephanie Cabrera, Southern Illinois University at Carbandale, School of Law, Carbondale, Illinois

Tambra K. Cain, Southern Illinois University at Carbondale, School of Law, Carbondale Illinois

Christina M. Camp, PhD, Department of Behavioral Science and Health Education, School of Public Health, Emory University, Atlanta, Georgia

Elaine A. Campbell, NorthEast Ohio Health Sciences, Cleveland, Ohio

Robert G. Carlson, PhD, Center for Interventions, Treatment, and Addictions Research, Wright State University School of Medicine, Dayton, Ohio

James F. Carter, MD, Department of Obstetrics and Gynecology, Medical University of South Carolina, Charleston, South Carolina

Jennifer Cercone-Keeney, MS, Medical College of Georgia, Department of Psychiatry, Augusta, Georgia

Donna T. Chen, MD, Health Evaluation Sciences, Psychiatric Medicine, and Biomedical Ethics, Department of Health Evaluation Sciences, Department of Psychiatric Medicine, and Center for Biomedical Ethics; University of Virginia Health System, Charlottesville, Virginia

Elizabeth Christensen, Department of Geography, San Diego State University, San Diego, California

Gray B. Clarke, MD, Department of Psychiatry, University of New Mexico School of Medicine, Albuquerque, New Mexico

Paula J. Clayton, MD, University of New Mexico, Albuquerque, New Mexico

Natalie Colabianchi, PhD, Case Western Reserve University, School of Medicine, Department of Epidemiology and Biostatistics, Cleveland, Ohio

Jason H. Cole, MD, Emory University School of Medicine, Division of Cardiology, Grady Memorial Hospital, Atlanta, Georgia

Nathan A. Craig, Southern Illinois University at Carbondale, School of Law, Carbondale, Illinois

James Craine, Department of Geography, San Diego State University, San Diego, California

Deanna Dahl-Grove, MD, Rainbow Babies and Children's Hospital, Cleveland, Ohio

Raminta Daniulaityte, PhD, Center for Interventions, Treatment, and Addictions Research, Wright State University School of Medicine, Dayton, Ohio

Andrea Darby-Stewart, MD, Mayo Thunderbird Family Medicine, Scottsdale, Arizona

Marilyn Davies, PhD, Department of Psychiatry, University Hospitals of Cleveland, Cleveland, Ohio

Chad Deal, MD, Shaker Heights, Ohio

Norman DeLoach, Jr., DDS, MS, Cleveland Heights, Ohio

Christina M. Delos Reyes, MD, Department of Psychiatry, Case Western Reserve University School of Medicine, Cleveland, Ohio

Leslie K. Dennis, MS, PhD, Department of Epidemiology, College of Public Health University of Iowa, Iowa City, Iowa

Rashmi S. Deshmukh, MD, General Psychiatry, Cleveland Clinic Foundation, Euclid Cleveland, Ohio

Heather Diaz, Loma Linda University, School of Public Health, Loma Linda, California

Elaine K. Diegmann, CNM, ND, FACNM, UMDNJ/SHRP Nurse Midwifery Education Program, Newark, New Jersey

Philip L. Dines, MD, PhD, Department of Psychiatry, St. Vincent Charity Hospital, Cleveland, Ohio

Geri R. Donenberg, PhD, Department of Psychiatry, Institute for Juvenile Research, Chicago, Illinois

Paul J. Draus, PhD, Center for Interventions, Treatment, and Addictions Research, Wright State University School of Medicine, Dayton, Ohio

Mary M. Duennes, RN, BSN, MA, CHTP/I, Good Samaritan Hospital, Cincinnati, Ohio

Laura B. Dunn, MD, Department of Psychiatry, University of California, San Diego, California

Claire Duvernoy, MD, University of Michigan Health System, Veterans Affairs Medical Center, Cardiology Section, Ann Arbor, Michigan

Matthew A. Eccher, MD, Department of Neurology, University Hospitals of Cleveland, Case Western Reserve University, Cleveland, Ohio

Deborah Rosch Eifert, PhD, Shaker Heights, Ohio

Michelle Endicott, DO, Department of Dermatology, University Hospitals of Cleveland and Case Western Reserve University, Cleveland, Ohio

David Faddis, MD, Huntington Hospital, Pasadena, California

Tommaso Falcone, PhD, Cleveland Clinic Foundation, Department of Obstetrics and Gynecology, Cleveland, Ohio

Ashley Faulx, MD, Division of Gastroentrology, University Hospitals of Cleveland, Euclid Cleveland, Ohio

Norah C. Feeny, PhD, Department of Psychiatry, Case Western Reserve University, Cleveland, Ohio

Barbara Fisher, MPH, Consumer Center for Health Education and Advocacy, San Diego, California

Douglas Flagg, MD, North Royalton, Ohio

Kathleen N. Franco, MD, MS, Director, Psychosomatic Medicine, Cleveland Clinic Foundation, Cleveland, Ohio

S. Franco, MD, University of Miami School of Medicine, Division of Pulmonary and Critical Care, Miami, Florida

Judith M. Frank, MD, The Jewish Home and Hospital Lifecare System, New York, New York

Keith A. Frey, MD, Mayo Thunderbird Family Medicine, Scottsdale, Arizona

John Frisbee, Southern Illinois University at Carbondale, School of Law, Carbondale, Illinois

Laurentine Fromm, MD, MCP, Department of Psychiatry, Drexel University College of Medicine, Philadelphia, Pennsylvania

Matthew A. Fuller, PharmD, BCPS, BCPP, FASHP, Louis Stokes Cleveland Department of Veterans Affairs Medical Center, Pharmacy Service, Brecksville, Ohio

Gretchen K. Gardner, MD, North East Ohio Health Services, Chesterland, Ohio

Cynthia M.A. Geppert, MD, PhD, Albuquerque Veterans Affairs Medical Center, and Assistant Professor and Assistant Director, Institute for Ethics, University of New Mexico Health Sciences Center; Department of Psychiatry, University of New Mexico School of Medicine, Albuquerque, New Mexico

Habibeh Gitiforooz, MD, Department of Obstetrics and Gynecology, Cleveland Clinic Foundation, Cleveland, Ohio

Marilyn Glassberg, MD, University of Miami School of Medicine, Division of Pulmonary and Critical Care, Miami, Florida

Contributors

Brandy L. Glasser, JD, Southern Illinois University at Carbondale, School of Law, Carbondale, Illinois

Valerie Godfrey, DDS, University of California, San Francisco School of Dentistry, Department of Stomatology, San Francisco, California

Carmen Gota, MD, Cleveland Clinic Foundation, Cleveland, Ohio

Debra J. Graham, MD, Case Western Reserve University School of Medicine; Surgical Service, Louis Stokes Cleveland Department of Veterans Affairs Medical Center, Cleveland, Ohio

Daniel Greene, MD, Rosalind Franklin University of Medicine and Science, North Chicago, Illinois

Charles Grover, Lowder and Hickman, Cleveland, Ohio

Victor Groza, PhD, Mandel School of Applied Social Sciences, Case Western Reserve University, Cleveland, Ohio

Amir R. Haghighat, MD, Emory University School of Medicine, Grady Memorial Hospital, Cardiology Division, Atlanta, Georgia

Polly Hampton, Southern Illinois University at Carbondale, School of Law, Carbondale, Illinois

Joseph P. Hanna, MD, Department of Neurology, MetroHealth Medical Center, Cleveland, Ohio

Geoffrey Harris, MD, University of Miami School of Medicine, Division of Pulmonary and Critical Care, Miami, Florida

Bruce Hartsell, Department of Social Work, California State University, Bakersfield, California

Susan Hatters Friedman, MD, University Hospitals of Cleveland, Cleveland, Ohio

Lenwood W. Hayman, Jr., MD, Department of Physiology, School of Medicine, Wayne State University, Detroit, Michigan

Patricia M. Henry, PhD, Department of Social Work, California State University, Bakersfield, California

Paula L. Hensley, MD, University of New Mexico, Albuquerque, New Mexico

Roberto Hernandez, Southern Illinois University at Carbondale, School of Law, Carbondale, Illinois

Lindsey Houlihan, MSSA, Mandel School of Applied Social Sciences, Case Western Reserve University, Cleveland, Ohio

Amy S. House, PhD, Medical College of Georgia, Department of Psychiatry, Augusta, Georgia

Debra Hrouda, MSSA, LISW, Department of Psychiatry, University Hospitals of Cleveland, Cleveland, Ohio

Phyllis D. Hulewat, LISW, Center for Marital and Sexual Health, Beachwood, Ohio

Joyce Hyatt, CNM, MS, UMDNJ/SHRP, Nurse Midwifery Education Program Newark, New Jersey

Margaret Jakubowicz, MSN, RN, NP-C, Francis Bolton School of Nursing, Case Western Reserve University; Louis Stokes Veterans Administration Medical Center, Cleveland, Ohio

Bryan S. Jick, MD, FACOG, Pasadena, California

Joy A. Jordan, DDS, National Dental Association, Washington, D.C.

Kristi Y. Jordan, PhD, Institute for Juvenile Research, Department of Psychiatry, University of Illinois at Chicago, Chicago, Illinois

Evanne Juratovac, RN, MSN, CS, Clinical Nurse Specialist, Geriatric and Consultation/Liaison Psychiatry, University Hospitals of Cleveland, University Hospitals Health System; Clinical Faculty, Case Western Reserve University, School of Medicine and School of Nursing, Cleveland, Ohio

Helen C. Kales, MD, Department of Psychiatry, University of Michigan, and Director, Geriatric Psychiatry Clinic, HSR&D, VA Ann Arbor Healthcare System, Ann Arbor, Michigan

Marshall B. Kapp, JD, Southern Illinois University at Carbondale, School of Law, Carbondale, Illinois

Yasmina Katsulis, MPhil, Yale University, New Haven, Connecticut

Asra Kermani, MB, BS, Dallas Veterans Affairs Medical Center; Assistant Professor, University of Texas Southwestern Medical Center, Department of Internal Medicine, Dallas, Texas

Margaret F. Kinnard, MD, Departments of Medicine and Biostatistics and Epidemiology, Case Western Reserve University School of Medicine, University Hospitals of Cleveland; Louis Stokes Veterans Administration Medical Center, Cleveland, Ohio

Susan Kirsh, MD, University Hospitals of Cleveland, Department of Medicine, Cleveland, Ohio

Siran M. Koroukian, PhD, MSN, MHA, Department of Epidemiology and Biostatistics, School of Medicine, Case Western Reserve University, Cleveland, Ohio

Joan D. Koss-Chioino, PhD, George Washington University, Washington, DC 20006

Jennifer S. Kriegler, MD, Case Western Reserve University, Cleveland, Ohio; Director, American Migraine Center, Lyndhurst, Ohio

Marie Kuchynski, MD, University Primary Care Practices, Brunswick, Ohio

Kathleen Lamping, MD, South Euclid, Ohio

Ginette Lange, CNM, FNP, PhD, Nurse-Midwifery Educational Program, UMDNJ/SHRP, Newark, New Jersey

Rachel Lange, MD, University of Miami School of Medicine, Division of Pulmonary and Critical Care, Miami, Florida

Shirley Lee, MD, Rosalind Franklin University of Medicine and Science, North Chicago, Illinois

Sonya L. Lefever, MD, Emory University School of Medicine, Grady Memorial Hospital, Atlanta, Georgia

Merrill S. Lewen, MD, Huntington Memorial Hospital, Pasadena, California

W. Lance Lewis, MD, Emory University School of Medicine, Division of Cardiology, Grady Memorial Hospital, Atlanta, Georgia

Yuying Li, Department of Geography, San Diego State University, San Diego, California

David S. Liebling, MD, Case Western Reserve University, School of Medicine, Cleveland, Ohio; PTSD Services, Louis Stokes Cleveland Veterans Administration Hospital, Brecksville, Ohio

Paul S. Lin, MD, Women's Hospital, Los Angeles, California

Linda S. Lloyd, DrPH, Vice President, Programs, Alliance Healthcare Foundation, San Diego, California

Sana Loue, JD., PhD, MPH, Case Western Reserve University, School of Medicine, Department of Epidemiology and Biostatistics, Department of Bioethics, Cleveland, Ohio

David J. Lourie, MD, Huntington Memorial Hospital, Pasadena, California

Janet J. Lowder, JD, Lowder and Hickman, Cleveland, Ohio

M. MacDougall, MD, Department of Psychiatry, University Hospitals of Cleveland, Cleveland, Ohio

Susan M. Maixner, MD, Division of Geriatric Psychiatry, Director, Outpatient Geriatric Psychiatry Clinic, University of Michigan, Ann Arbor, Michigan

Melissa Rivera Marano, PsyD, Freehold, New Jersey

MaryAnne E. Markowski, CNM, MS, University of Medicine and Dentistry of New Jersey, Westfield, New Jersey

Lorna A. Marshall, MD, Center for Fertility and Reproductive Endocrinology, Virginia Mason Medical Center, Seattle, Washington

Gary Martz, MD, Beachwood, Ohio

Anne L. Matthews, PhD, Counseling Training Program, Department of Genetics, Case Western Reserve University, Cleveland, Ohio

Contributors

Jan Matz, RNC, NorthEast Ohio Health Services, Beachwood, Ohio

Teresita McCarty, MD, Department of Psychiatry, University of New Mexico School of Medicine, Albuquerque, New Mexico

Jill Adair McCaughan, PhD, Department of Community Health, Center for Interventions, Treatment, and Addictions Research, School of Medicine, Wright State University, Dayton, Ohio

Mary B. McKee, JD, Lowder and Hickman, Cleveland, Ohio

Margaret L. McKenzie, MD, Cleveland Clinic Foundation, Willoughby Hills Family Health, Willoughby Hills, Ohio

Nancy Mendez, Case Western Reserve University School of Medicine, Department of Epidemiology and Biostatistics, Cleveland, Ohio

Mary Gail Mercurio, MD, University of Rochester, Rochester, New York

Dorothy M. Meyer, MSN, APRN, BC, Veterans Aministration Medical Center, Cleveland, Brecksville, Brecksville, Ohio

Mara Meza, San Diego, California

Radha Mikkillineni, MD, Department of Dermatology, University Hospitals of Cleveland and Case Western Reserve University, Clevland, Ohio

Manuel Miranda, Department of Geography, San Diego State University, San Diego, California

Paradi Mirmirani, MD, Department of Dermatology, University Hospitals of Cleveland and Case Western Reserve University, Cleveland, Ohio

Pamela Monaghan-Geernaert, PhD, University of New Mexico Health Sciences Center, Institute for Ethics, Albuquerque, New Mexico

Ruth Monchek, CNM, MSN, Nurse-Midwifery Educational Program, University of Medicine and Dentistry of New Jersey, Newark, New Jersey

Susanne Montgomery, PhD, Loma Linda University, School of Public Health, Loma Linda, California

Tahereh Moradi, PhD, MPH, Ohio State University, James Cancer Hospital and Solove Research Institute, Columbus, Ohio

Rebecca H. Moran, MD, Department of Pediatrics, University of New Mexico School of Medicine; University of New Mexico Health Sciences Center Institute for Ethics, Albuquerque, New Mexico

Nancy K. Morrison, MD, Department of Psychiatry, Albuquerque, New Mexico

Nancy Myers-Bradley, North Coast OB/GYN, Berlin, Ohio

Dileep R Nair, MD, MetroHealth Medical Center; Cleveland Clinic Foundation, Department of Neurology, Cleveland, Ohio

Karen Olness, MD, Department of Pediatrics, Rainbow Babies and Children's Hospital, Cleveland, Ohio

Anne O'Meara, MD, University of Southern California, Keck School of Medicine, Division of Gynecologic Oncology, Women's and Children's Hospital, Los Angeles, California

Daniel P. O'Shea, Office of AIDS Coordination, San Diego, California

Robert S. O'Shea, MD, MSCE, Department of Biostatistics and Epidemiology, Case Western Reserve University School of Medicine, Cleveland, Ohio

Cynthia Olschewsky, OTR/L, Department of Rehabilitation Services, Psychiatric Occupational Therapy Division, University Hospitals of Cleveland, Cleveland, Ohio

Julianne S. Orlowski, DO, Chesapeake, Virginia

Susan Paparella-Pitzel, PT, MS, University of Medicine and Dentistry of New Jersey, Newark, New Jersey

Michele Parkhill, Department of Community Medicine, School of Medicine, Wayne State University, Detroit, Michigan

Ted Parran, Jr., MD, FACP, University Hospitals of Cleveland, Continuing Medical Education, Case Western Reserve School of Medicine, Cleveland, Ohio

Angela Pattatucci Aragon, PhD, Center for Evaluation and Sociomedical Research, Graduate School of Public Health, University of Puerto Rico Medical Sciences Campus, San Juan, Puerto Rico

Corinne Peek-Asa, PhD, Departments of Occupational and Environmental Health and Epidemiology, Injury Prevention Research Center, University of Iowa, Iowa City, Iowa

Steven J. Peitzman, MD, Drexel University College of Medicine, Philadelphia, Pennsylvania

Adam I. Perlman, MD, MPH, Institute for Complementary and Alternative Medicine, UMDNJ School of Health Related Professions, Newark, New Jersey

Stephen G. Post, PhD, Case Western Reserve University, School of Medicine, Department of Bioethics, Cleveland, Ohio

Beth E. Quill, MPH, Management and Policy Sciences, University of Texas at Houston, School of Public Health, Houston, Texas

L.A. Rebhun, PhD, Yale University, Department of Anthropology, New Haven, Connecticut

Rajkumari Richmonds, PhD, Parma, Ohio

Candace B. Risen, LISW, Case Western Reserve University School of Medicine, Cleveland, Ohio; Center for Sexual and Marital Health, Beachwood, Ohio

Laura Weiss Roberts, MD, Department of Psychiatry and Behavioral Medicine, Medical College of Wisconsin, Milwaukee, Wisconsin

Melinda K. Rogers, BS, University of New Mexico, Health Sciences Center Institute, Institute for Ethics, University of New Mexico Health Sciences Center, Albuquerque, New Mexico

Rebecca G. Rogers, MD, Department of Obstetrics and Gynecology, Division of Urogynecology, University of New Mexico, Albuquerque, New Mexico

Lynda D. Roman, MD, Pasadena, California

Miriam B. Rosenthal, MD, Case Western Reserve University, MacDonald Women's Hospital, Cleveland, Ohio

Deborah S. Rossman, Lowder & Hickman, Cleveland, Ohio

Susan E. Rutherford, MD, Obstetrix Medical Group, Tacoma, Washington

Christopher Saenz, Department of Community Medicine, School of Medicine, Wayne State University, Detroit, Michigan

Martha Sajatovic, MD, University Hospitals of Cleveland, Case Western Reserve University, School of Medicine, Cleveland, Ohio

Amy L. Salisbury, PhD, RN, CS, Cranston, Rhode Island

Amita Sapra, MD, Rosalind Franklin University of Medicine and Sciences, North Chicago, Illinois

Robert W. Sanders, EMT-D, Rosalind Franklin University of Medicine and Sciences, North Chicago, Illinois

John Sanitato, MD, University Hospitals of Cleveland, Cleveland, Ohio

Karyn S. Schoem, MSW, School of Social Work, Geriatric Center, University of Michigan, Ann Arbor, Michigan

Isabel Schuermeyer, MD, Department of Psychiatry, University Hospitals of Cleveland, Cleveland, Ohio

Julie Schulman, MD, Consultation-Liaison Psychiatry, Aurora, Colorado

Julianne M. Serovich, PhD, Marriage and Family Therapy, The Ohio State University, Columbus, Ohio

Rakesh Sharma, PhD, Cleveland Clinic Foundation, Department of Obstetrics and Gynecology, Cleveland, Ohio

Mary C. Shemo, MD, FAPA, Psychiatric Alliance of the Blue Ridge, Clinical Research Center, Charlottesville, Virginia

Contributors

Lori B. Siegel, MD, Rosalind Franklin University of Medicine and Science, North Chicago, Illinois

Sheila Simon, JD, Southern Illinois University at Carbondale, School of Law, Carbondale, Illinois

Anne Simpson, MD, Department of Internal Medicine, Division of Geriatrics/Gerontology, University of New Mexico, Albuquerque, New Mexico

Sarah A. Smith, MA, Department of Human Development and Family Science, The Ohio State University, Columbus, Ohio

Megan V. Smithpeter, BA, UNM HSC Institute for Ethics, University of New Mexico Health Sciences Center, Albuquerque, New Mexico

George M. Soliman, MD, Emory University School of Medicine, Division of Cardiology, Grady Memorial Hospital, Atlanta, Georgia

Dan Sorescu, MD, Department of Medicine, Division of Cardiology, Emory University School of Medicine, Grady Memorial Hospital, Atlanta, Georgia

Gail E. Souare, MPH, Souare Consulting, San Diego, California

Linda Agresta Sprinzl, PhD, Mayfield Heights, Ohio

Lorann Stallones, MPH, PhD, Department of Psychology; Director, Colorado Injury Control Research Center, Colorado State University, Fort Collins, Colorado

Tira B. Stebbins, MA, Department of Psychiatry, Case Western Reserve University, leveland, Ohio

Lara M. Stepleman, PhD, Department of Psychiatry Medical College of Georgia, Augusta, Georgia

Marian J. Ster, Lowder & Hickman, Cleveland, Ohio

Usha Stiefel, MD, University Hospitals of Cleveland, Division of Infectious Diseases, Cleveland, Ohio

Marie Haring Sweeney, PhD, Document Development Branch, Education and Information Division, National Institute for Occupational Safety and Health, Cincinnati, Ohio

Sarolta Szabo, MD, Department of Dermatology, University Hospitals of Cleveland and Case Western Reserve University, Cleveland, Ohio

Kamala Tamirisa, MD, University of Michigan Health Systems, Ann Arbor, Michigan

Nimish J. Thakore, MD, Department of Neurology, MetroHealth Medical Center, Cleveland, Ohio

Sapna Thomas, MD, Division of Gastroenterology, University Hospitals of Cleveland; Louis Stokes Veterans Administration Medical Center, Cleveland, Ohio

Judith Trentman, School of Law, Southern Illinois University at Carbondale, Carbondale, Illinois

Wulf H. Utian, MD, PhD, The Cleveland Clinic; Department of Reproductive Biology, Case Western Reserve University, Cleveland, Ohio; The North American Menopause Society, Mayfield Heights, Ohio

Elizabeth M. Valencia, Southern Illinois University at Carbondale, School of Law, Carbondale, Illinois

Anita B. Varkey, MD, Cook County Hospital; Rush Medical College, Department of Medicine, Chicago, Illinois

Carmen M. Verhosek, Lowder & Hickman, Cleveland, Ohio

Mary G. Veremis-Ley, DO, Department of Dermatology, University Hospitals of Cleveland and Case Western Reserve University, Cleveland, Ohio

David Vidra, Body Work Productions, Cleveland, Ohio

Dora L. Wang, MD, University of New Mexico School of Medicine, Albuquerque, New Mexico

Teddy D. Warner, PhD, Department of Psychiatry, School of Medicine; Interim Codirector, HSC Institute for Ethics, University of New Mexico, Albuquerque, New Mexico

John R. Weeks, PhD, International Population Center, Department of Geography, San Diego State University, San Diego, California

Alicia M. Weissman, MD, Crystal Run Healthcare, Middletown, New York

Nanette K. Wenger, MD, Emory University School of Medicine, Division of Cardiology, Grady Memorial Hospital, Atlanta, Georgia

Susan Wiedaseck, CNM, Denville, New Jersey

Andrea Willey, MD, Department of Dermatology, University Hospitals of Cleveland and Case Western Reserve University, Cleveland, Ohio

Gina M. Wingood, PhD, Department of Behavioral Science and Health Education, School of Public Health, Emory University, Atlanta, Georgia

Marc D. Winkelman, Department of Neurology, MetroHealth Medical Center, Cleveland, Ohio

Kathleen Wolner, MD., Centerville, Ohio

Katherine Wren, MD, Rosalind Franklin University of Medicine and Science, North Chicago, Illinois

Karin Small Wurapa, MD, MPH, Perinatal Health Center, Columbus Health Department, Columbus, Ohio

Elina Yamada, M.D., University of Michigan Health Systems, Ann Arbor, Michigan

Natalie K. Yeaney, Division of Neonatology, Rainbow Babies and Children's Hospital; Case Western Reserve University, Department of Pediatrics, Division of Neonatology, Cleveland, Ohio

Diane Young, MD, Department of OB/GYN; The Cleveland Clinic Foundation, Willoughby Hills, Ohio

Ellen Zambo-Anderson, PT, MA, GCS, UNDMJ-SHRP, Newark, New Jersey

Maria Cecilia Zea, PhD, Department of Psychology, George Washington University, Washington, DC

Melissa Zupancic, RN, MSN, CS, APRN, BC, Veterans Administration Medical Center, Brecksville, Ohio

Index

Index

Index

Index